DORLAND'S POCKET

MEDICAL
DICTIONARY

CONSULTANTS

BERNARD D. DAVIS, M.D.

Chairman, Department of Bacteriology and Immunology
Harvard Medical School
Boston, Massachusetts

VICTOR A. McKUSICK, M.D.

Professor of Medicine
Johns Hopkins University School of Medicine
Baltimore, Maryland

RONAN O'RAHILLY, M.D.

Chairman, Department of Anatomy
St. Louis University
St. Louis, Missouri

DORLAND'S POCKET

MEDICAL
DICTIONARY

21st edition

Abridged from
Dorland's Illustrated Medical Dictionary

with a series of 16 color plates:
The Human Body—Highlights of Structure and Function

W. B. SAUNDERS COMPANY
Philadelphia, London, Toronto

Listed here is the latest translated edition of this book together with the language of the translation and the publisher.

Italian (20th Edition)–Editrice Ambrosiana, Milan, Italy

PREFACE

As in the previous edition, this Dictionary, like its younger but larger counterpart (Dorland's Illustrated Medical Dictionary), from which it is largely derived, is officially entitled Dorland's Pocket Medical Dictionary, for Dr. W. A. Newman Dorland, whose name as editor appeared on the title page from the time of its inception in 1898, and whose death, at the age of 92, occurred in September 1956.

The purposes and ideals which motivated its publication for seventy years, however, remain the same: to present the latest in medical terminology and to fulfill, in a compact and convenient format, the three primary functions of a dictionary—the provision of spelling, pronunciation, and meaning. Here, readily available at your fingertips, you will find spelled, pronounced and defined the time-proved terms, as well as newcomers to the vocabulary of medicine and its allied fields.

With the changing emphasis and increasing knowledge in medicine and the related sciences, scores of words have been redefined, some have been omitted as no longer useful, and thousands of new terms have been added. To further increase the usefulness and scope of the book, without increasing its overall size, irregularly formed plurals are presented on the singular forms which constitute the main entries (e.g. **brachium** . . . pl. *brachia*; **lumen** . . . pl. *lumina*). Entries on nouns also include adjectival forms of the specific words (e.g. **allele** . . . adj., **allelic**; **allergen** . . . adj., **allergenic**). Many more abbreviations, in this letter-conscious age, have also been included.

As was true of the first edition, this book is not intended to take the place of the larger dictionary, which is indispensable to a thorough understanding of the language of medicine. The aim has still been to make the "selection of words as complete as possible," in order to "develop the possibilities of a pocket lexicon to a degree not heretofore attained," even by the preceding editions of this work. Although the definitions, of necessity, are brief, "endeavor has been to make them clear, adequate, and to the point." These statements from the Preface to the First Edition, seventy years ago, remain applicable today.

It is hoped that the reader will find this brief lexicon a helpful tool in every respect. The criticisms and suggestions of its users are solicited, to aid in maintaining an increasingly high standard of comprehensiveness, authority and usefulness in future editions.

W. B. SAUNDERS COMPANY

ACKNOWLEDGMENTS

In the past, Dorland's Pocket Medical Dictionary was almost entirely a distillation of and selection from the larger Dorland's Illustrated Medical Dictionary. In this edition an attempt has been made to provide terms and definitions appropriate to the purposes of the Pocket Dictionary and independent of the parent work. Therefore advice and data were solicited from consultants and contributors. These have provided invaluable counsel in making this edition an accurate representation of changes in the vocabulary of science that have occurred since publication of the Twenty-Fourth Edition of Dorland's Illustrated Medical Dictionary. This Twenty-First Edition of the Pocket Dictionary also owes a great debt of gratitude to the Editorial Consultants and Contributors to the larger work.

It is therefore our privilege to acknowledge the able and unstinted help of those listed as Consultants opposite the title page and of those listed here as Contributors:

Harry L. Arnold, Jr., M.D., Straub Clinic, Honolulu, Hawaii

Laura W. Barr, Registered Nurses' Association of Ontario, Canada

Alexander G. Bearn, M.D., Rockefeller University, New York, New York

Christine Brown, Royal College of Nursing and National Council of Nurses of the United Kingdom, London, England

William R. DeLay, American Academy of General Practice, Kansas City, Missouri

L. Joan Cray, Queen's Institute of District Nursing, London, England

Warren G. Guntheroth, M.D., University of Washington, Seattle, Washington

Henry P. Laughlin, M.D., Bethesda, Maryland

Adam G. N. Moore, M.D., Boston, Massachusetts

Margaret L. Parkin, Canadian Nurses Association, Ottawa, Canada

Peyton Rouse, M.D., Rockefeller University, New York, New York

W. B. SAUNDERS COMPANY

CONTENTS

NOTES ON USE OF THIS BOOK

PRONUNCIATION

THE PRONUNCIATION of words is represented by the same simple phonetic respelling which appeared in the previous edition, using a minimum of diacritical markings. Only the macron and breve are used, the macron, where necessary, to indicate the long sound, and the breve, to indicate the short. An unmarked vowel not followed by a consonant has the long sound; an unmarked vowel followed by a consonant has the short sound. A long vowel which syllabication requires to be followed by a consonant is marked with a macron (e.g., ab″āl-yen-a′shun). A short vowel which constitutes or ends a syllable is marked with a breve (e.g., ab-dom′ĭ-nal). The primary accent in a word is indicated by a bold face, single accent. The secondary accent is indicated by a light face, double accent.

When, on successive words, the first syllables are pronounced in the same way, these syllables are included in the phonetic respelling of only the first of the sequence of terms. If the accent varies or other change occurs in the pronunciation of these syllables, even when they involve the same letters, the entire pronunciation of the word is indicated in the phonetic respelling. For example:

> **erythroblast** (ĕ-rith′ro-blast).
> **erythroblastemia** (ĕ-rith″ro-blas-te′me-ah).
> **erythroblastoma** (-blas-to′mah).
> **erythroclasis** (ĕr″ĭ-throk′lah-sis).
> **erythrocyanosis** (ĕ-rith″ro-si″ah-no′sis).

ABBREVIATIONS

Abbreviations used in the text of the definitions are few and fairly obvious. They include

adj. (adjective)	Ger. (German)	L. (Latin)
Fr. (French)	Gr. (Greek)	pl. (plural)

In elaboration of entries which are themselves abbreviations, the words "Abbreviation for . . ." have been omitted, as a further means of reducing size of the book.

COMBINING FORMS IN MEDICAL TERMINOLOGY*

The following is a list of combining forms encountered frequently in the vocabulary of medicine. A dash or dashes are appended to indicate whether the form usually precedes (as *ante-*) or follows (as *-agra*) the other elements of the compound or usually appears between the other elements (as *-em-*). Following each combining form, the first item of information is the Greek or Latin word, or both a Greek and a Latin word, from which it is derived. Those words that are not printed in Greek characters are Latin. Information necessary to an understanding of the form appears next in parentheses. Then the meaning or meanings of the word are given, followed where appropriate by reference to a synonymous combining form. Finally, an example is given to illustrate the use of the combining form in a compound English derivative.

a-	a- (n is added before words beginning with a vowel) negative prefix. Cf. in-³. ametria
ab-	ab away from. Cf. apo-. abducent
abdomin-	abdomen, abdominis. abdominoscopy
ac-	See ad-. accretion
acet-	acetum vinegar. acetometer
acid-	acidus sour. aciduric
acou-	ἀκούω hear. acouesthesia. (Also spelled acu-)
acr-	ἄκρον extremity, peak. acromegaly
act-	ago, actus do, drive, act. reaction
actin-	ἀκτίς, ἀκτῖνος ray, radius. Cf. radi-. actinogenesis
acu-	See acou-. osteoacusis
ad-	ad (d changes to c, f, g, p, s, or t before words beginning with those consonants) to. adrenal
aden-	ἀδήν gland. Cf. gland-. adenoma
adip-	adeps, adipis fat. Cf. lip- and stear-. adipocellular
aer-	ἀήρ air. anaerobiosis
aesthe-	See esthe-. aesthesioneurosis
af-	See ad-. afferent
ag-	See ad-. agglutinant
-agogue	ἀγωγός leading, inducing. galactagogue
-agra	ἄγρα catching, seizure. podagra
alb-	albus white. Cf. leuk-. albocinereous
alg-	ἄλγος pain. neuralgia
all-	ἄλλος other, different. allergy
alve-	alveus trough, channel, cavity. alveolar
amph-	See amphi-. ampheclexis
amphi-	ἀμφί (i is dropped before words beginning with a vowel) both, doubly. amphicelous
amyl-	ἄμυλον starch. amylosynthesis
an-¹	See ana-. anagogic
an-²	See a-. anomalous
ana-	ἀνά (final a is dropped before words beginning with a vowel) up, positive. anaphoresis
ancyl-	See ankyl-. ancylostomiasis
andr-	ἀνήρ, ἀνδρός man. gynandroid
angi-	ἀγγεῖον vessel. Cf. vas-. angiemphraxis
ankyl-	ἀγκύλος crooked, looped. ankylodactylia. (Also spelled ancyl-)
ant-	See anti-. antophthalmic
ante-	ante before. anteflexion
anti-	ἀντί (i is dropped before words beginning with a vowel) against, counter. Cf. contra-. antipyogenic
antr-	ἄντρον cavern. antrodynia
ap-¹	See apo-. apheter
ap-²	See ad-. append
-aph-	ἅπτω, ἀφ- touch. dysaphia. (See also hapt-)
apo-	ἀπό (o is dropped before words beginning with a vowel) away from, detached. Cf. ab-. apophysis
arachn-	ἀράχνη spider. arachnodactyly
arch-	ἀρχή beginning, origin. archenteron
arter(i)-	ἀρτηρία elevator (?), artery. arteriosclerosis, periarteritis
arthr-	ἄρθρον joint. Cf. articul-. synarthrosis
articul-	articulus joint. Cf. arthr-. disarticulation
as-	See ad-. assimilation
at-	See ad-. attrition
aur-	auris ear. Cf. ot-. aurinasal
aux-	αὔξω increase. enterauxe
ax-	ἄξων or axis axis. axofugal
axon-	ἄξων axis. axonometer

*Compiled by Lloyd W. Daly, A. M., Ph.D., Litt. D., Allen Memorial Professor of Greek, University of Pennsylvania.

ba-   βαίνω, βα- go, walk, stand.
           hypno*batia*
bacill-   *bacillus* small staff, rod. Cf.
           bacter-. actino*bacill*osis
bacter-   βακτήριον small staff, rod. Cf.
           bacill-. *bacter*iophage
ball-   βάλλω, βολ- throw. *ball*istics.
           (See also bol-)
bar-   βάρος weight. pedo*bar*ometer
bi-¹   βίος life. Cf. vit-. aero*bic*
bi-²   *bi*- two (see also di-¹). *bi*lobate
bil-   *bilis* bile. Cf. chol-. *bil*iary
blast-   βλαστός bud, child, a growing
           thing in its early stages. Cf.
           germ-. *blast*oma, zygoto*blast.*
blep-   βλέπω look, see. hemia*blep*sia
blephar-   βλέφαρον (from βλέπω; see
           blep-) eyelid. Cf. cili-. *bleph*-
           *ar*oncus
bol-   See ball-. em*bol*ism
brachi-   βραχίων arm. *brachi*ocephalic
brachy-   βραχύς short. *brachy*cephalic
brady-   βραδύς slow. *brady*cardia
brom-   βρῶμος stench. podo*brom*idrosis
bronch-   βρόγχος windpipe. *bronch*os-
           copy
bry-   βρύω be full of life. em*bry*onic
bucc-   *bucca* cheek. disto*bucc*al
cac-   κακός bad, abnormal. Cf. mal-.
           *cac*odontia, arthro*cac*e. (See
           also dys-)
calc-¹   *calx, calcis* stone (cf. lith),
           limestone, lime. *calc*ipexy
calc-²   *calx, calcis* heel. *calc*aneotibial
calor-   *calor* heat. Cf. therm-. *calo*-
           rimeter
cancr-   *cancer, cancri* crab, cancer. Cf.
           carcin-. *cancr*ology. (Also
           spelled chancr-)
capit-   *caput, capitis* head. Cf. cephal-.
           de*capit*ator
caps-   *capsa* (from *capio;* see cept-)
           container. en*caps*ulation
carbo(n)- *carbo, carbonis* coal, charcoal.
           *carbo*hydrate, *carbon*uria
carcin-   καρκίνος crab, cancer. Cf.
           cancr-. *carcin*oma
cardi-   καρδία heart. lipo*cardi*ac
cary-   See kary-. *cary*okinesis
cat-   See cata-. *cat*hode
cata-   κατά (final a is dropped before
           words beginning with a
           vowel) down, negative. *cata*-
           batic
caud-   *cauda* tail. *caud*ad
cav-   *cavus* hollow. Cf. coel-. con*cav*e
cec-   *caecus* blind. Cf. typhl-. *cec*o-
           pexy
cel-¹   See coel-. amphi*cel*ous
cel-²   See -cele. *cel*ectome
-cele   κήλη tumor, hernia. gastro*cele*
cell-   *cella* room, cell. Cf. cyt-.
           *cell*iferous
cen-   κοινός common. *cen*esthesia
cent-   *centum* hundred. Cf. hect-.
           Indicates fraction in metric
           system. [This exemplifies the

custom in the metric system
of identifying fractions of
units by stems from the
Latin, as centimeter, decimeter, millimeter, and mul-
tiples of units by the similar
stems from the Greek, as
hectometer, decameter, and
kilometer.] *centi*meter, *centi*-
pede
cente-   κεντέω puncture. Cf. punct-.
           entero*cente*sis
centr-   κέντρον or *cenrum* point, center.
           neuro*centr*al
cephal-   κεφαλή head. Cf. capit-. en-
           *cephal*itis
cept-   *capio, -cipientis, -ceptus* take,
           receive. re*cept*or
cer-   κηρός or *cera* wax. *cer*oplasty,
           *cer*omel
cerat-   See kerat-. a*cerat*osis
cerebr-   *cerebrum.* *cerebr*ospinal
cervic-   *cervix, cervicis* neck. Cf.
           trachel-. *cervic*itis
chancr-   See cancr-. *chancr*iform
cheil-   χεῖλος lip. Cf. labi-. *chei*-
           *lo*schisis
cheir-   χείρ hand. Cf. man-. macro-
           *cheir*ia. (Also spelled chir-)
chir-   See cheir-. *chir*omegaly
chlor-   χλωρός green. a*chlor*opsia
chol-   χολή bile. Cf. bil-. hepato-
           *chol*angeitis
chondr-   χόνδρος cartilage. *chondro*-
           malacia
chord-   χορδή string, cord. peri*chord*al
chori-   χόριον protective fetal mem-
           brane. endo*chori*on
chro-   χρώς color. poly*chro*matic
chron-   χρόνος time. syn*chron*ous
chy-   χέω, χυ- pour. ec*chy*mosis
-cid(e)   *caedo, -cisus* cut, kill. infanti-
           cide, germi*cid*al
cili-   *cilium* eyelid. Cf. blephar-.
           super*cili*ary
cine-   See kine-. auto*cine*sis
-cipient   See cept . in*cipient*
circum-   *circum* around. Cf. peri-.
           *circum*ferential
-cis   *caedo, -cisus* cut, kill. ex*cis*ion
clas-   κλάω, κλασ- break. cranio*clast*
clin-   κλίνω bend, incline, make lie
           down. *clin*ometer
clus-   *claudo, -clusus* shut. Maloc-
           *clus*ion
co-   See con-. *co*hesion
cocc-   κόκκος seed, pill. gono*cocc*us
coel-   κοῖλος hollow. Cf. cav-. *coel*-
           enteron. (Also spelled cel-)
col-¹   See colon-. *col*ic
col-²   See con-. *col*lapse
colon-   κόλον lower intestine. *colon*ic
colp-   κόλπος hollow, vagina. Cf. sin-.
           endo*colp*itis
com-   See con-. *com*masculation
con-   *con*- (becomes co- before vowels
           or *h;* col- before *l;* com- be-

fore *b*, *m*, or *p*; cor- before *r*) with, together. Cf. syn-. con-traction

contra-   *contra* against, counter. Cf. anti-. *contra*indication

copr-   κόπρος dung.Cf.sterco-.*copro*ma

cor-[1]   κόρη doll, little image, pupil. iso*cor*ia

cor-[2]   See con-. *cor*rugator

corpor-   *corpus*, *corporis* body. Cf. somat-. intra*corpor*al

cortic-   *cortex*, *corticis* bark, rind. *cortic*osterone

cost-   *costa* rib. Cf. pleur-. inter*cost*al

crani-   κρανίον or *cranium* skull. peri-*crani*um

creat-   κρέας, κρεατ- meat, flesh. *cre*-*at*orrhea

-crescent   *cresco*, *crescentis*, *cretus* grow. ex*crescent*

cret-[1]   *cerno*, *cretus* distinguish, separate off. Cf. crin-. dis*crete*

cret-[2]   See -crescent. ac*cret*ion

crin-   κρίνω distinguish, separate off. Cf. cret-[1]. endo*crin*ology

crur-   *crus*, *cruris* shin, leg. brachio-*crur*al

cry-   κρύος cold. *cry*esthesia

crypt-   κρύπτω hide, conceal. *crypt*orchism

cult-   *colo*, *cultus* tend, cultivate. *cult*ure

cune-   *cuneus* wedge. Cf. sphen-. *cune*iform

cut-   *cutis* skin. Cf. derm(at)-. sub-*cut*aneous

cyan-   κύανος blue. antho*cyan*in

cycl-   κύκλος circle, cycle. *cycl*ophoria

cyst-   κύστις bladder. Cf. vesic-. nephro*cyst*itis

cyt-   κύτος cell. Cf. cell-. plasmo-*cyt*oma

dacry-   δάκρυ tear. *dacry*ocyst

dactyl-   δάκτυλος finger, toe. Cf. digit-. hexa*dactyl*ism

de-   *de* down from. *de*composition

dec-[1]   δέκα ten. Indicates multiple in metric system. Cf. dec-[2]. *deca*gram

dec-[2]   *decem* ten. Indicates fraction in metric system. Cf. dec-[1]. *deci*para, *deci*meter

dendr-   δένδρον tree. neuro*dendr*ite

dent-   *dens*, *dentis* tooth. Cf. odont-. inter*dent*al

derm(at)-   δέρμα, δέρματος skin. Cf. cut-. endo*derm*, *dermat*itis

desm-   δεσμός band, ligament. syn-*desm*opexy

dextr-   *dexter*, *dextr*- right-hand. ambi*dextr*ous

di-[1]   *di*- two. *di*morphic. (See also bi-[2])

di-[2]   See dia-. *di*uresis.

di-[3]   See dis-. *di*vergent.

dia-   διά (*a* is dropped before words

beginning with a vowel) through, apart. Cf. per-. *dia*gnosis

didym-   δίδυμος twin. Cf. gemin-. epi-*didym*al

digit-   *digitus* finger, toe. Cf. dactyl-. *digit*igrade

diplo-   διπλόος double. *diplo*myelia

dis-   *dis*- (*s* may be dropped before a word beginning with a consonant) apart, away from. *dis*location

disc-   δίσκος or *discus* disk. *disco*-placenta

dors-   *dorsum* back. ventro*dors*al

drom-   δρόμος course. hemo*drom*ometer

-ducent   See duct-. ad*ducent*

duct-   *duco*, *ducentis*, *ductus* lead, conduct. ovi*duct*

dur-   *durus* hard. Cf. scler-. indura-tion

dynam(i)-   δύναμις power. *dynam*oneure, neuro*dynam*ic

dys-   δυσ- bad, improper. Cf. mal-. *dys*trophic. (See also cac-)

e-   *e* out from. Cf. ec- and ex-. *e*mission

ec-   ἐκ out of. Cf. e- eccentric

-ech-   ἔχω have, hold, be. syn-*ech*otomy

ect-   ἐκτός outside. Cf. extra-. *ecto*-plasm

ede-   οἰδέω swell. *ede*matous

ef-   See ex-. *ef*florescent

-elc-   ἕλκος sore, ulcer. enter*elc*osis. (See also helc-)

electr-   ἤλεκτρον amber. *electr*otherapy

em-   See en-. *em*bolism, *em*pathy, *em*physis

-em-   αἷμα blood. an*em*ia. (See also hem(at)-)

en-   ἐν (*n* changes to *m* before *b*, *p*, or *ph*) in, on. Cf. in-[2]. *en*celitis

end-   ἔνδον inside. Cf. intra-. *end*-angium.

enter-   ἔντερον intestine. dys*enter*y

ep-   See epi-. *ep*axial

epi-   ἐπί (*i* is dropped before words beginning with a vowel) upon, after, in addition. *epi*glottis

erg-   ἔργον work, deed. en*erg*y

erythr-   ἐρυθρός red. Cf. rub(r)-. *eryth*-*r*ochromia

eso-   ἔσω inside. Cf. intra-. *eso*-phylactic

esthe-   αἰσθάνομαι, αἰσθη- perceive, feel. Cf. sens-. an*esthe*sia

eu-   εὖ good, normal. *eu*pepsia

ex-   ἐξ or *ex* out of. Cf. e-. *ex*cretion

exo-   ἔξω outside. Cf. extra-. *exo*-pathic

extra-   *extra* outside of, beyond. Cf. ect- and exo-. *extra*cellular

faci-   *facies* face. Cf. prosop-. brachio-*faci*olingual

-facient   *facio, facientis, factus, -fectus*
            make. Cf. poie-. cale*facient*

-fact-   See facient-. arte*fact*

fasci-   *fascia* band. *fasci*orrhaphy

febr-   *febris* fever. Cf. pyr-. *febr*icide

-fect-   See -facient. de*fect*ive

-ferent   *fero, ferentis, latus* bear, carry.
            Cf. phor-. e*fferent*

ferr-   *ferrum* iron. *ferr*oprotein

fibr-   *fibra* fibre. Cf. in-[1]. chondro-
            *fibr*oma

fil-   *filum* thread. *fil*iform

fiss-   *findo, fissus* split. Cf. schis-.
            *fiss*ion

flagell-   *flagellum* whip. *flagell*ation

flav-   *flavus* yellow. Cf. xanth-. ribo-
            *flav*in

-flect-   *flecto, flexus* bend, divert. de-
            *flect*ion

-flex-   See -flect-. re*flex*ometer

flu-   *fluo, fluxus* flow. Cf. rhe-. *flu*id

flux-   See flu-. af*flux*ion

for-   *foris* door, opening. per*for*ated

-form   *forma* shape. Cf. -oid. ossi-
            form

fract-   *frango, fractus* break. re-
            *fract*ive

front-   *frons, frontis* forehead, front.
            naso*front*al

-fug(e)   *fugio* flee, avoid. vermi*fuge*,
            centri*fug*al

funct-   *fungor, functus* perform, serve,
            function. mal*funct*ion

fund-   *fundo, fusus* pour. in*fund*ib-
            ulum

fus-   See fund-. dif*fus*ible

galact-   γάλα, γάλακτος milk. Cf. lact-.
            dys*galact*ia

gam-   γάμος marriage, reproductive
            union. a*gam*ont

gangli-   γάγγλιον swelling, plexus. neu-
            ro*gangli*itis

gastr-   γαστήρ, γαστρός stomach. cho-
            langiо*gastr*ostomy

gelat-   *gelo, gelatus* freeze, congeal.
            *gelat*in

gemin-   *geminus* twin, double. Cf.
            didym-. quadri*gemin*al

gen-   γίγνομαι, γεν-, γον- become, be
            produced, originate, or
            γεννάω produce, originate.
            cyto*gen*ic

germ-   *germen, germinis* bud, a grow-
            ing thing in its early stages.
            Cf. blast-. *germ*inal, ovi*germ*

gest-   *gero, gerentis, gestus* bear, carry.
            con*gest*ion

gland-   *glans, glandis* acorn. Cf. aden-.
            intra*gland*ular

-glia   γλία glue. neuro*glia*

gloss-   γλῶσσα tongue. Cf. lingu-.
            tricho*gloss*ia

glott-   γλῶττα tongue, language. *glott*ic

gluc-   See glyc(y)-. *gluc*ophenet-
            idin

glutin-   *gluten, glutinis* glue. a*glutina*-
            tion

glyc(y)-   γλυκύς sweet. *glyc*emia, *glycyr*-
            rhizin. (Also spelled gluc-)

gnath-   γνάθος jaw. ortho*gnath*ous

gno-   γιγνώσκω, γνω- know, discern.
            dia*gno*sis

gon-   See gen-. amphi*gon*y

grad-   *gradior* walk, take steps. re-
            tro*grad*e

-gram   γράφω, γραφ- + -μα scratch,
            write, record. cardio*gram*

gran-   *granum* grain, particle. lipo-
            *gran*uloma

graph-   γράφω scratch, write, record.
            histo*graph*y

grav-   *gravis* heavy. multi*grav*ida

gyn(ec)-   γυνή, γυναικός woman, wife.
            andro*gyn*y, *gyn*ecologic

gyr-   γῦρος ring, circle. *gyr*ospasm

haem(at)-   See hem(at)-. *haem*orrhagia,
            *haemat*oxylon

hapt-   ἅπτω touch. *hapt*ometer

hect-   ἑκτ- hundred. Cf. cent-. In-
            dicates multiple in metric
            system. *hect*ometer

helc-   ἕλκος sore, ulcer. *helc*osis

hem(at)-   αἷμα, αἵματος blood. Cf. san-
            guin-. *hem*angioma, *hemat*o-
            cyturia. (See also -em-)

hemi-   ἥμι- half. Cf. semi-. *hemi*ageusia

hen-   εἷς, ἑνός one. Cf. un-. *hen*ogenesis

hepat-   ἧπαρ, ἥπατος liver. *gastro*-
            *hepat*ic

hept(a)-   ἑπτά seven. Cf. sept-[2]. *hept*-
            atomic, *hept*avalent

hered-   *heres, heredis* heir. *hered*oim-
            munity

hex-[1]   ἕξ six. Cf. sex-. *hex*yl-. An *a* is
            added in some combinations.

hex-[2]   ἔχω, ἑχ- (added to σ becomes
            ἕξ-) have, hold, be. cach*exy*

hexa-   See hex-[1]. *hexa*chromic

hidr-   ἱδρώς sweat. hyper*hidr*osis

hist-   ἱστός web, tissue. *hist*odialysis

hod-   ὁδός road, path. *hod*oneuromere.
            (See also od- and -ode[1])

hom-   ὁμός common, same. *homo*-
            morphic

horm-   ὁρμή impetus, impulse. *horm*one

hydat-   ὕδωρ, ὕδατος water. *hydat*ism

hydr-   ὕδωρ, ὑδρ- water. Cf. lymph-.
            achlor*hydr*ia

hyp-   See hypo-. *hyp*axial

hyper-   ὑπέρ above, beyond, extreme.
            Cf. super-. *hyper*trophy

hypn-   ὕπνος sleep. *hypn*otic

hypo-   ὑπό (o is dropped before words
            beginning with a vowel)
            under, below. Cf. sub-. *hypo*-
            metabolism

hyster-   ὑστέρα womb. colpo*hyster*opexy

iatr-   ἰατρός physician. ped*iatr*ics

idi-   ἴδιος peculiar, separate, distinct.
            *idi*osyncrasy

il-   See in-[2,3]. *il*linition (in, on),
            *il*legible (negative prefix)

ile-   See ili-. [ile- is commonly used
            to refer to the portion of the

intestines known as the ileum]. *ileostomy*

ili-   *ilium (ileum)* lower abdomen, intestines [ili- is commonly used to refer to the flaring part of the hip bone known as the ilium]. *iliosacral*

im-   See in-², ³. *immersion* (in, on), *imperforation* (negative prefix)

in-¹   *ís, ινós* fiber. Cf. fibr-. *inosteatoma*

in-²   *in* (*n* changes to *l*, *m*, or *r* before words beginning with those consonants) in, on. Cf. en-. *insertion*

in-³   *in-* (*n* changes to *l*, *m*, or *r* before words beginning with those consonants) negative prefix. Cf. a-. *invalid*

infra-   *infra* beneath. *infraorbital*

insul-   *insula* island. *insulin*

inter-   *inter* among, between. *intercarpal*

intra-   *intra* inside. Cf. end- and eso-. *intravenous*

ir-   See in-², ³. *irradiation* (in, on), *irreducible* (negative prefix)

irid-   *ίρις, ίριδος* rainbow, colored circle. *keratoiridocyclitis*

is-   *ίσος* equal. *isotope*

ischi-   *ίσχιον* hip, haunch. *ischiopubic*

jact-   *iacio, iactus* throw. *jactitation*

ject-   *iacio, -iectus* throw. *injection*

jejun-   *ieiunus* hungry, not partaking of food. *gastrojejunostomy*

jug-   *iugum* yoke. *conjugation*

junct-   *iungo, iunctus* yoke, join. *conjunctiva*

kary-   *κάρυον* nut, kernel, nucleus. Cf. nucle-. *megakaryocyte*. (Also spelled cary-)

kerat-   *κέρας, κέρατος* horn. *keratolysis*. (Also spelled cerat-)

kil-   *χίλιοι* one thousand. Cf. mill-. Indicates multiple in metric system. *kilogram*

kine-   *κινέω* move. *kinematograph*. (Also spelled cine-)

labi-   *labium* lip. Cf. cheil-. *gingivolabial*

lact-   *lac, lactis* milk. Cf. galact-. *glucolactone*

lal-   *λαλέω* talk, babble. *glossolalia*

lapar-   *λαπάρα* flank. *laparotomy*

laryng-   *λάρυγξ, λάρυγγος* windpipe. *laryngendoscope*

lat-   *fero, latus* bear, carry. See -ferent. *translation*

later-   *latus, lateris* side. *ventrolateral*

lent-   *lens, lentis* lentil. Cf. phac-. *lenticonus*

lep-   *λαμβάνω, ληπ-* take, seize. *cataleptic*

leuc-   See leuk-. *leucinuria*

leuk-   *λευκός* white. Cf. alb-. *leukorrhea*. (Also spelled leuc-)

---

lien-   *lien* spleen. Cf. splen-. *lienocele*

lig-   *ligo* tie, bind. *ligate*

lingu-   *lingua* tongue. Cf. gloss-. *sublingual*

lip-   *λίπος* fat. Cf. adip-. *glycolipin*

lith-   *λίθος* stone. Cf. calc-¹. *nephrolithotomy*

loc-   *locus* place. Cf. top-. *locomotion*

log-   *λέγω, λογ-* speak, give an account. *logorrhea*, *embryology*

lumb-   *lumbus* loin. *dorsolumbar*

lute-   *luteus* yellow. Cf. xanth-. *luteoma*

ly-   *λύω* loose, dissolve. Cf. solut-. *keratolysis*

lymph-   *lympha* water. Cf. hydr-. *lymphadenosis*

macr-   *μακρός* long, large. *macromyeloblast*

mal-   *malus* bad, abnormal. Cf. cac- and dys-. *malfunction*

malac-   *μαλακός* soft. *osteomalacia*

mamm-   *mamma* breast. Cf. mast-. *submammary*

man-   *manus* hand. Cf. cheir-. *maniphalanx*

mani-   *μανία* mental aberration. *manigraphy*, *kleptomania*

mast-   *μαστός* breast. Cf. mamm-. *hypermastia*

medi-   *medius* middle. Cf. mes-. *medifrontal*

mega-   *μέγας* great, large. Also indicates multiple (1,000,000) in metric system. *megacolon*, *megadyne*. (See also megal-)

megal-   *μέγας, μεγάλου* great, large. *acromegaly*

mel-   *μέλος* limb, member. *symmelia*

melan-   *μέλας, μέλανος* black. *hippomelanin*

men-   *μήν* month. *dysmenorrhea*

mening-   *μῆνιγξ, μήνιγγος* membrane. *encephalomeningitis*

ment-   *mens, mentis* mind. Cf. phren-, psych- and thym-. *dementia*

mer-   *μέρος* part. *polymeric*

mes-   *μέσος* middle. Cf. medi-. *mesoderm*

met-   See meta-. *metallergy*

meta-   *μετά* (*a* is dropped before words beginning with a vowel) after, beyond, accompanying. *metacarpal*

metr-¹   *μέτρον* measure. *stereometry*

metr-²   *μήτρα* womb. *endometritis*

micr-   *μικρός* small. *photomicrograph*

mill-   *mille* one thousand. Cf. kil-. Indicates fraction in metric system. *milligram*, *millipede*

miss-   See -mittent. *intromission*

-mittent   *mitto, mittentis, missus* send. *intermittent*

mne-   μιμνήσκω, μνη- remember. pseudomnesia

mon-   μόνος only, sole. monoplegia

morph-   μορφή form, shape. polymorphonuclear

mot-   moveo, motus move. vasomotor

my-   μῦς, μυός muscle. inoleiomyoma

-myces   μύκης, μύκητος fungus. myelomyces

myc(et)-   See -myces. ascomycetes, streptomycin

myel-   μυελός marrow. poliomyelitis

myx-   μύξα mucus. myxedema

narc-   νάρκη numbness. toponarcosis

nas-   nasus nose. Cf. rhin-. palatonasal

ne-   νέος new, young. neocyte

necr-   νεκρός corpse. necrocytosis

nephr-   νεφρός kidney. Cf. ren-. paranephric

neur-   νεῦρον nerve. esthesioneure

nod-   nodus knot. nodosity

nom-   νόμος (from νέμω deal out, distribute) law, custom. taxonomy

non-   nona nine. nonacosane

nos-   νόσος disease. nosology

nucle-   nucleus (from nux, nucis nut) kernel. Cf. kary-. nucleide

nutri-   nutrio nourish. malnutrition

ob-   ob (b changes to c before words beginning with that consonant) against, toward, etc. obtuse

oc-   See ob-. occlude.

ocul-   oculus eye. Cf. ophthalm-. oculomotor

-od-   See -ode¹. periodic

-ode¹   ὁδός road, path. cathode. (See also hod-)

-ode²   See -oid. nematode

odont-   ὀδούς, ὀδόντος tooth. Cf. dent-. orthodontia

-odyn-   ὀδύνη pain, distress. gastrodynia

-oid   εἶδος form. Cf. -form. hyoid

-ol   See ole . cholesterol

ole-   oleum oil. oleoresin

olig-   ὀλίγος few, small. oligospermia

omphal-   ὀμφαλός navel. periomphalic

onc-   ὄγκος bulk, mass. hcmatoncometry

onych-   ὄνυξ, ὄνυχος claw, nail. anonychia

oo-   ᾠόν egg. Cf. ov-. perioothecitis

op-   ὁράω, ὀπ- see. erythropsia

ophthalm-   ὀφθαλμός eye. Cf. ocul-. exophthalmic

or-   os, oris mouth. Cf. stom(at)-. intraoral

orb-   orbis circle. suborbital

orchi-   ὄρχις testicle. Cf. test-. orchiopathy

organ-   ὄργανον implement, instrument. organoleptic

orth-   ὀρθός straight, right, normal. orthopedics

oss-   os, ossis bone. Cf. ost(e)-. ossiphone

ost(e)-   ὀστέον bone. Cf. oss-. enostosis, osteanaphysis

ot-   οὖς, ὠτός ear. Cf. aur-. parotid

ov-   ovum egg. Cf. oo-. synovia

oxy-   ὀξύς sharp. oxycephalic

pachy(n)-   παχύνω thicken. pachyderma, myopachynsis

pag-   πήγνυμι, παγ- fix, make fast. thoracopagus

par-¹   pario bear, give birth to. primiparous

par-²   See para-. parepigastric

para-   παρά (final a is dropped before words beginning with a vowel) beside, beyond. paramastoid

part-   pario, partus bear, give birth to. parturition

path-   πάθος that which one undergoes, sickness. psychopathic

pec-   πήγνυμι, πηγ- (πηκ- before τ) fix, make fast. sympectothiene. (See also pex-)

ped-   παῖς, παιδός child. orthopedic

pell-   pellis skin, hide. pellagra

-pellent   pello, pellentis, pulsus drive. repellent

pen-   πένομαι need, lack. erythrocytopenia

pend-   pendeo hang down. appendix

pent⟨a⟩-   πέντε five. Cf. quinque-. pentose, pentaploid

peps-   πέπτω, πεψ- (before σ) digest bradypepsia

pept-   πέπτω digest. dyspeptic

per-   per through. Cf. dia-. pernasal

peri-   περί around. Cf. circum-. periphery

pet-   peto seek, tend toward. centripetal

pex-   πήγνυμι, πηγ- (added to σ becomes πηξ-) fix, make fast. hepatopexy

pha-   φημί, φα- say, speak. dysphasia

phac-   φακός lentil, lens. Cf. lent-. phacosclerosis. (Also spelled phak-)

phag-   φαγεῖν eat. lipophagic

phak-   See phac-. phakitis

phan-   See phen-. diaphanoscopy

pharmac-   φάρμακον drug. pharmacognosy

pharyng-   φάρυγξ, φαρυγγ- throat. glossopharyngeal

phen-   φαίνω, φαν- show, be seen. phosphene

pher-   φέρω, φορ- bear, support. periphery

phil-   φιλέω like, have affinity for. eosinophilia

phleb-   φλέψ, φλεβός vein. periphlebitis

phleg-   φλέγω, φλογ- burn, inflame. adenophlegmon

phlog-   See phleg-. antiphlogistic

phob-   φόβος fear, dread. claustrophobia

phon-   φωνή sound. echophony

phor- See pher-. Cf. -ferent. exo-*phoria*

phos- See phot-. *phos*phorus

phot- φῶς, φωτός light. *phot*erythrous

phrag- φράσσω, φραγ- fence, wall off, stop up. Cf. sept-[1]. dia-*phragm*

phrax- φράσσω, φραγ- (added to σ becomes φραξ-) fence, wall off, stop up. em*phraxis*

phren- φρήν mind, midriff. Cf. ment-. meta*phren*ia, meta*phren*on

phthi- φθίνω decay, waste away. ophthalmo*phthisis*

phy- φύω beget, bring forth, produce, be by nature. noso-*phyte*

phyl- φῦλον tribe, kind. *phyl*ogeny

-phyll φύλλον leaf. xantho*phyll*

phylac- φύλαξ guard. pro*phylac*tic

phys(a)- φυσάω blow, inflate. *phys*ocele, *phys*alis

physe- φυσάω, φυση- blow, inflate. em*physe*ma

pil- *pil*us hair. epi*pil*ation

pituit- *pituit*a phlegm, rheum. *pituit*ous

placent- *placent*a (from πλακοῦς) cake. extra*placent*al

plas- πλάσσω mold, shape. cine*plas*ty

platy- πλατύς broad, flat. *platy*rrhine

pleg- πλήσσω, πληγ- strike. di*pleg*ia

plet- *pleo*, -*pletus* fill. de*plet*ion

pleur- πλευρά rib, side. Cf. cost-. peri*pleur*al

plex- πλήσσω, πληγ- (added to σ becomes πληξ-) strike. apo*plex*y

plic- *plico* fold. com*plic*ation

pne- πνοιά breathing. traumato*pne*a

pneum(at)- πνεῦμα, πνεύματος breath, air. *pneum*odynamics, *pneum*ato-thorax

pneumo(n)- πνεύμων lung. Cf. pulmo(n)-. *pneumo*centesis, *pneumon*ot-omy

pod- πούς, ποδός foot. *pod*iatry

poie- ποιέω make, produce. Cf. -*facient*. sarco*poie*tic

pol- πόλος axis of a sphere. peri-*pol*ar

poly- πολύς much, many. *poly*spermia

pont- *pons*, *pontis* bridge. *pont*o-cerebellar

por-[1] πόρος passage. myelo*por*e

por-[2] πῶρος callus. *por*ocele

posit- *pono*, *positus* put, place. re-*posit*or

post- *post* after, behind in time or place. *post*natal, *post*oral

pre- *prae* before in time or place. *pre*natal, *pre*vesical

press- *premo*, *pressus* press. *press*ore-ceptive

pro- πρό or *pro* before in time or place. *pro*gamous, *pro*cheilon, *pro*lapse

proct- πρωκτός anus. entero*proct*ia

prosop- πρόσωπον face. Cf. faci-. di-*prosop*us

pseud- ψευδής false. *pseud*oparaplegia

psych- ψυχή soul, mind. Cf. ment-. *psych*osomatic

pto- πίπτω, πτω- fall. nephro*pto*sis

pub- *pubes* & *puber*, *puberis* adult. ischio*pub*ic. (See also puber-)

puber- *puber* adult. *puber*ty

pulmo(n)- *pulmo*, *pulmonis* lung. Cf. pneumo(n)-. *pulmo*lith, cardio*pulmo*nary

puls- *pello*, *pellentis*, *pulsus* drive. pro*puls*ion

punct- *pungo*, *punctus* prick, pierce. Cf. cente-. *punct*iform

pur- *pus*, *puris* pus. Cf. py-. sup-*pur*ation

py- πύον pus. Cf. pur-. nephro*py*osis

pyel- πύελος trough, basin, pelvis. nephro*pyel*itis

pyl- πύλη door, orifice. *pyl*ephlebitis

pyr- πῦρ fire. Cf. febr-. galacto*pyr*a

quadr- *quadr*- four. Cf. tetra-. *quadr*i-geminal

quinque- *quinque* five. Cf. pent(a)-. *quinque*cuspid

rachi- ῥαχίς spine. Cf. spin-. enceph-alo*rachi*dian

radi- *radius* ray. Cf. actin-. irradia-tion

re- *re*- back, again. *re*traction

ren- *renes* kidneys. Cf. nephr-. ad-*ren*al

ret- *rete* net. *ret*othelium

retro- *retro* backwards. *retro*deviation

rhag- ῥήγνυμι, ῥαγ- break, burst. hemor*rhag*ic

rhaph- ῥαφή suture. gastror*rhaph*y

rhe- ῥέω flow. Cf. flu-. diar*rhe*al

rhex- ῥήγνυμι, ῥηγ- (added to σ becomes ῥηξ-) break, burst. metror*rhex*is

rhin- ῥίς, ῥινός nose. Cf. nas-. basi-*rhin*al

rot- *rota* wheel. *rot*ator

rub(r)- *ruber*, *rubri* red. Cf. erythr-. bili*rub*in, *rub*rospinal

salping- σάλπιγξ, σάλπιγγος tube, trumpet. *salping*itis

sanguin- *sanguis*, *sanguinis* blood. Cf. hem(at)-. *sanguin*eous

sarc- σάρξ, σαρκός flesh. *sarc*oma

schis- σχίζω, σχιδ- (before τ or added to σ becomes σχισ-) split. Cf. fiss-. *schis*torachis, rachi*schis*is

scler- σκληρός hard. Cf. dur-. *scler*o-sis

scop- σκοπέω look at, observe. endo-*scop*e

sect- *seco*, *sectus* cut. Cf. tom-. *sect*ile

semi- *semi*- half. Cf. hemi-. *semi*-flexion

sens- *sentio*, *sensus* perceive, feel. Cf. esthe-. *sens*ory

sep-
sept-¹ σήπω rot, decay. sepsis
        saepio, saeptus fence, wall off, stop up. Cf. phrag-. nasoseptal
sept-² septem seven. Cf. hept(a)-. septan
ser-   serum whey, watery substance. serosynovitis
sex-   sex six. Cf. hex-¹. sexdigitate
sial-   σίαλον saliva. polysialia
sin-   sinus hollow, fold. Cf. colp-. sinobronchitis
sit-   σῖτος food. parasitic
solut- solvo, solventis, solutus loose, dissolve, set free. Cf. ly-. dissolution
-solvent See solut-. dissolvent
somat- σῶμα, σώματος body. Cf. corpor-. psychosomatic
-some   See somat-. dictyosome
spas-   σπάω, σπασ- draw, pull. spasm, spastic
spectr- spectrum appearance, what is seen. microspectroscope
sperm(at)- σπέρμα, σπέρματος seed. spermacrasia, spermatozoon
spers- spargo, -spersus scatter. dispersion
sphen- σφήν wedge. Cf. cune-. sphenoid
spher- σφαῖρα ball, hemisphere
sphygm- σφυγμός pulsation. sphygmomanometer
spin-   spina spine. Cf. rachi-. cerebrospinal
spirat- spiro, spiratus breathe. inspiratory
splanchn- σπλάγχνα entrails, viscera. neurosplanchnic
splen- σπλήν spleen. Cf. lien-. splenomegaly
spor-   σπόρος seed. sporophyte, zygospore
squam- squama scale. desquamation
sta-   ἵστημι, στα- make stand, stop. genesistasis
stal   στέλλω, σταλ- send. peristalsis. (See also stol-)
staphyl- σταφυλή bunch of grapes, uvula staphylococcus, staphylectomy
stear- στέαρ, στέατος fat. Cf. adip-. stearodermia
steat- See stear-. steatopygous
sten-   στενός narrow, compressed. stenocardia
ster-   στερεός solid. cholesterol
sterc- stercus dung. Cf. copr-. stercoporphyrin
sthen- σθένος strength. asthenia
stol-   στέλλω, στολ- send. diastole
stom(at)- στόμα, στόματος mouth, orifice. Cf. or-. anastomosis, stomatogastric
strep(h)- στρέφω, στρεπ- (before τ) twist. Cf. tors-. strephosymbolia, streptomycin. (See also stroph-)

strict- stringo, stringentis, strictus draw tight, compress, cause pain. constriction
-stringent See strict-. astringent
stroph- στρέφω, στροφ- twist. anastrophic. (See also strep(h)-)
struct- struo, structus pile up (against). obstruction
sub-   sub (b changes to f or p before words beginning with those consonants) under, below. Cf. hypo-. sublumbar
suf-   See sub-. suffusion
sup-   See sub-. suppository
super- super above, beyond, extreme. Cf. hyper-. supermotility
sy-   See syn-. systole
syl-   See syn-. syllepsiology
sym-   See syn-. symbiosis, symmetry, sympathetic, symphysis
syn-   σύν (n disappears before s, changes to l before l, and changes to m before b, m, p, and ph) with, together. Cf. con-. myosynizesis
ta-   See ton-. ectasis
tac-   τάσσω, ταγ- (τακ- before τ) order, arrange. atactic
tact-   tango, tactus touch. contact
tax-   τάσσω, ταγ- (added to o becomes ταξ-), order, arrange. ataxia
tect-   See teg-. protective
teg-   tego, tectus cover. integument
tel-   τέλος end. telosynapsis
tele-   τῆλε at a distance. teleceptor
tempor- tempus, temporis time, timely or fatal spot, temple. temporalar
ten(ont)- τένων, τένοντος (from τείνω stretch) tight stretched band. tenodynia, tenonitis, tenontagra
tens-   tendo, tensus stretch. Cf. ton-. extensor
test-   testis testicle. Cf. orchi-. testitis
tetra- τέτρα- four. Cf. quadr-. tetragenous
the-   τίθημι, θη- put, place. synthesis
thec-   θήκη repository, case. thecostegnosis
thel-   θηλή teat, nipple. thelerethism
therap- θεραπεία treatment. hydrotherapy
therm- θέρμη heat. Cf. calor-. diathermy
thi-   θεῖον sulfur. thiogenic
thorac- θώραξ, θώρακος chest. thoracoplasty
thromb- θρόμβος lump, clot. thrombopenia
thym-   θυμός spirit. Cf. ment-. dysthymia
thyr-   θυρεός shield (shaped like a door θύρα). thyroid

tme-   τέμνω, τμη- cut. axonotmesis
toc-   τόκος childbirth. dystocia
tom-   τέμνω, τομ- cut. Cf. sect-. appendectomy
ton-   τείνω, τον- stretch, put under tension. Cf. tens-. peritoneum
top-   τόπος place. Cf. loc-. topesthesia
tors-   torqueo, torsus twist. Cf. strep-. extorsion
tox-   τοξικόν (from τόξον bow) arrow poison, poison. toxemia
trache-   τραχεῖα windpipe. tracheotomy
trachel- τράχηλος neck. Cf. cervic-. trachelopexy
tract-   traho, tractus draw, drag. protraction
traumat- τραῦμα, τραύματος wound. traumatic
tri-   τρεῖς, τρία or tri- three. trigonid
trich-   θρίξ, τριχός hair. trichoid
trip-   τρίβω rub. entripsis
trop-   τρέπω, τροπ- turn, react. sitotropism

troph-   τρέφω, τροφ- nurture. atrophy
tuber-   tuber swelling, node. tubercle
typ-   τύπος (from τύπτω strike) type. atypical
typh-   τῦφος fog, stupor. adenotyphus
typhl-   τυφλός blind. Cf. cec-. typhlectasis
un-   unus one. Cf. hen-. unioval
ur-   οὖρον urine. polyuria
vacc-   vacca cow. vaccine
vagin-   vagina sheath. invaginated
vas-   vas vessel. Cf. angi-. vascular
vers-   See vert-. inversion
vert-   verto, versus turn. diverticulum
vesic-   vesica bladder. Cf. cyst-. vesicovaginal
vit-   vita life. Cf. bi-[1]. devitalize
vuls-   vello, vulsus pull, twitch. convulsion
xanth-   ξανθός yellow, blond. Cf. flav- and lute-. xanthophyll
-yl-   ὕλη substance. cacodyl
zo-   ζωή life, ζῷον animal. microzoaria
zyg-   ζυγόν yoke, union. zygodactyly
zym-   ζύμη ferment. enzyme

A

A. accommodation; ampere; anode (anodal); anterior; axial; total acidity.

a [L.] *arteria* (artery); atto.

a- word element [L.], *without; not.*

Å Angstrom.

A₂ aortic second sound; both ears.

A.A. achievement age; Alcoholics Anonymous.

aa [L. pl.] *arteriae* (arteries).

āā ana (*of each*).

A.A.A. American Academy of Allergy; American Association of Anatomists.

āāā amalgam.

A.A.A.S. American Association for the Advancement of Science.

A.A.B.B. American Association of Blood Banks.

A.A.C.P. American Academy for Cerebral Palsy.

A.A.D.P. American Academy of Denture Prosthetics.

A.A.D.S. American Academy of Dermatology and Syphilology; American Association of Dental Schools.

A.A.E. American Association of Endodontists.

A.A.G.P. American Academy of General Practice.

A.A.I. American Association of Immunologists.

A.A.I.D. American Academy of Implant Dentures.

A.A.I.N. American Association of Industrial Nurses.

A.A.M.A. American Association of Medical Assistants.

A.A.M.R.L. American Association of Medical Record Librarians.

A.A.O. American Association of Orthodontists.

A.A.O.O. American Academy of Ophthalmology and Otolaryngology.

A.A.O.P. American Academy of Oral Pathology.

A.A.O.S. American Academy of Orthopedic Surgeons.

A.A.P. American Academy of Pediatrics; American Academy of Pedodontics; American Academy of Periodontology; Association for the Advancement of Psychotherapy; Association of American Physicians.

A.A.P.B. American Association of Pathologists and Bacteriologists.

A.A.P.M.R. American Academy of Physical Medicine and Rehabilitation.

A.A.P.S. American Association of Plastic Surgeons.

A.B. [L.] *Ar'tium Baccalau'reus* (Bachelor of Arts); axiobuccal.

ab word element [L.], *from.*

ab- word element [L.], *from; off; away from.*

abacterial (a″bak-te′re-al) free from bacteria.

abalienation (ab′āl-yen-a′shun) derangement of the mental faculties.

abarognosis (ah-bar″og-no′sis) loss of sense of weight.

abarthrosis (ab″ar-thro′sis) abarticulation.

abarticular (ab″ar-tik′u-ler) not affecting a joint; at a distance from a joint.

abarticulation (ab″ar-tik″u-la′shun) 1. diarthrosis. 2. a dislocation.

abasia (ah-ba′ze-ah) inability to walk because of defective coordination. adj., **aba′sic, abat′ic. a.-asta′sia,** loss of power to stand or walk. **a. atac′tica,** abasia with uncertain movements. **choreic a.,** abasia due to paralysis of the limbs. **paralytic a.,** abasia due to paralysis. **paroxysmal trepidant a.,** abasia caused by paralysis of the legs in attempting to stand. **spastic a.,** paroxysmal trepidant abasia. **trembling a., a. trep′idans,** abasia due to trembling of the legs.

abatement (ah-bāt′ment) decrease in severity of a pain or symptom.

abaxial (ab-ak′se-al) not situated in the axis of the body.

abd., abdom. abdomen; abdominal.

abdomen (ab-do′men) that part of the body lying between the thorax and the pelvis. **carinate a., navicular a.,** scaphoid abdomen. **a. obsti′pum,** shortness of the rectus abdominis muscle. **scaphoid a.,** abdomen whose anterior wall is hollowed.

abdomin(o)- word element, *abdomen.*

abdominal (ab-dom′ĭ-nal) pertaining to the abdomen.

abdominoanterior (ab-dom″ĭ-no-an-tēr′e-or) with the abdomen directed toward the anterior surface of the maternal body; said of the fetus in utero.

abdominocentesis (-sen-te′sis) paracentesis of the abdomen.

abdominocystic (-sis′tik) pertaining to abdomen and gallbladder.

abdominohysterectomy (-his″ter-ek′-to-me) hysterectomy through an abdominal incision.

abdominohysterotomy (-his″ter-ot′o-me) hysterotomy through an abdominal incision.

abdominoposterior (-pos-tēr′e-or) with the abdomen directed toward the posterior surface of the maternal body; said of the fetus in utero.

abdominoscopy (ab-dom″ĭ-nos′ko-pe) examination of the abdomen.

abdominous (ab-dom′ĭ-nus) having a prominent abdomen.

abdominovaginal (ab-dom″ĭ-no-vaj′ĭ-nal) pertaining to abdomen and vagina.

abduce (ab-dūs′) to abduct.

abducens (ab-du′senz) [L.] drawing away.

abducent (ab-du′sent) abducting.

abduct (ab-dukt′) to draw away from a center or median line.

abduction (ab-duk′shun) the act of abducting; the state of being abducted.

abductor (ab-duk′tor) that which abducts.

abenteric (ab″en-ter′ik) situated elsewhere than in the intestine.

1

abepithymia (ab″ep-ĭ-thi′me-ah) paralysis of the solar plexus.

aberratio (ab″er-a′she-o) [L.] aberration.

aberration (ab″er-a′shun) 1. deviation from the normal or usual. 2. imperfect refraction or focalization of a lens. **chromatic a.**, unequal refraction of different length rays, producing a blurred image and a display of colors. **chromosomal a.**, loss, gain or exchange of genetic material in the chromosomes of a cell, resulting in a deletion, duplication, inversion or translocation of genes. **dioptric a.**, spherical aberration. **distantial a.**, blurring of vision of distant objects. **emotional a.**, 1. any emotional response other than that which might ordinarily be expected. 2. an emotional illness, especially one in which the manifestations and symptoms are directly emotional. **mental a.**, mental unsoundness not sufficient to constitute insanity. **spherical a.**, inherent inability of a spherical lens to bring all rays of light to a single focus.

aberrometer (ab″er-om′ē-ter) an instrument for determining amount of aberration.

a-beta-lipoproteinemia (a-ba″tah-lip″o-pro″-te-in-e′me-ah) a condition characterized by the lack of beta-lipoproteins in the blood.

abevacuation (ab″e-vak″u-a′shun) incomplete evacuation.

abiatrophy (ab″e-at′ro-fe) 1. premature and endogenous loss of vitality. 2. a condition due to an inborn defect, but not clinically evident until some time after maturity; also used more generally to designate any disorder with late onset.

abiochemistry (ab″e-o-kem′is-tre) inorganic chemistry.

abiogenesis (-jen′ē-sis) production of life from matter not alive. adj., **abiogenet′ic, abiog′-enous.**

abiological (a″bi-o-loj′ĭ-kal) pertaining to nonliving things; having no relation to biology.

abiology (a″bi-ol′o-je) the study of nonliving things.

abionergy (ab″e-on′er-je) abiotrophy.

abiosis (ab″e-o′sis) absence or deficiency of life. adj., **abiot′ic.**

abiotrophy (ab″e-ot′ro-fe) loss of early ability to function normally because of innate constitutional weakness leading to ultimate breakdown.

abirritant (ab-ir′ĭ-tant) diminishing irritation; soothing.

abirritation (ab-ir″ĭ-ta′shun) diminished irritability; atony.

abiuret (ah-bi′u-ret) not giving the biuret reaction.

ablactation (ab″lak-ta′shun) weaning.

ablastemic (a″blas-tem′ik) not concerned with germination.

ablate (ab-lāt′) to remove, especially by cutting.

ablatio (ab-la′she-o) [L.] detachment. **a. ret′-inae**, detachment of the retina.

ablation (ab-la′shun) removal, especially by cutting.

ablepharon (a-blef′ah-ron) total or partial absence of the eyelids. adj., **ableph′arous.**

ablepsia (a-blep′se-ah) blindness.

abluent (ab′lu-ent) detergent; cleansing.

abmortal (ab-mor′tal) passing from a dead or injured part.

abnerval (ab-ner′val) passing from a nerve through a muscle.

abneural (ab-nu′ral) away from the central nervous system.

abnormality (ab″nor-mal′ĭ-te) 1. the state of being abnormal. 2. a malformation.

abocclusion (ab″ŏ-kloo′zhun) occlusion in which the mandibular teeth are not in contact with the maxillary teeth.

abomasitis (ab″o-ma-si′tis) inflammation of the abomasum.

abomasum (ab″o-ma′sum) the fourth stomach of ruminants.

aborad (ab-o′rad) away from the mouth.

aboral (ab-o′ral) opposite to, or remote from, the mouth.

abort (ah-bort′) to arrest prematurely a disease or developmental process.

abortifacient (ah-bor″ti-fa′shent) 1. causing abortion. 2. an agent that induces abortion.

abortion (ah-bor′shun) 1. interruption of pregnancy before the 21st week, usually implying loss from the uterus of the products of conception. 2. premature arrest of a natural or morbid process. **artificial a.**, induced abortion. **contagious a.**, a disease of cattle due to *Brucella abortus*, and causing premature loss of the developing calf. **criminal a.**, induced abortion not nececcssary to save the life of the mother. **early a.**, abortion within the first six weeks of pregnancy. **habitual a.**, abortion occurring in three or more successive pregnancies; classified as *primary* in a woman who had no previous pregnancy, and *secondary* in a woman who had previously produced at least one fetus weighing more than 500 gm. **incomplete a.**, abortion with retention of the placenta. **induced a.**, abortion brought on intentionally by medication or instrumentation. **inevitable a.**, abortion which cannot be averted. **missed a.**, death in the uterus of a conceptus which is not delivered until weeks or months later. **spontaneous a.**, abortion occurring naturally. **therapeutic a.**, interruption of pregnancy by artificial means for medical considerations. **threatened a.**, signs of premature expulsion of the products of conception.

abortive (ah-bor′tiv) 1. incompletely developed. 2. abortifacient.

abortus (ah-bor′tus) a dead or nonviable fetus (weighing less than 17 ounces, or 500 gm., at birth).

abrachia (ah-bra′ke-ah) congenital absence of the arms.

abrachiocephalia (ah-bra″ke-o-se-fa′le-ah) developmental anomaly with absence of the head and arms.

abrachius (ah-bra′ke-us) a fetal monster without arms.

abrasio (ah-bra′se-o) [L.] abrasion. **a. cor′neae**, the scraping off of corneal excrescences. **a. den′tium**, wearing away of tooth substance.

abrasion (ah-bra′zhun) 1. a rubbing or scraping

off. 2. a rubbed or scraped area on skin or mucous membrane.

abrasive (ah-bra'siv) 1. causing abrasion. 2. an agent that produces abrasion.

abreaction (ab"re-ak'shun) the release of tension and anxiety associated with the emotional reliving of past, especially repressed, events (catharsis).

abreuography (ab"roo-og'rah-fe) photofluorography.

abruptio (ah-brup'she-o) [L.] separation. **a. placen'tae,** premature separation of a normally situated placenta.

abscess (ab'ses) a localized collection of pus caused by suppuration in a tissue, organ or confined space. **alveolar a.,** a localized suppurative inflammation of tissues about the apex of the root of a tooth. **anorectal a.,** one involving the anorectum. **appendiceal a., appendicular a.,** one near the vermiform appendix. **arthrifluent a.,** a wandering abscess originating in a diseased joint. **Bezold's a.,** subperiosteal abscess of the temporal bone. **Brodie's a.,** circumscribed abscess in bone, caused by hematogenous infection, that becomes a chronic nidus of infection. **cold a.,** one of slow development and with little inflammation, usually tuberculous. **diffuse a.,** a collection of pus not enclosed by a capsule. **miliary a.,** one composed of numerous small collections of pus. **milk a.,** abscess of the breast occurring during lactation. **perianal a.,** one beneath the skin of the anus and the anal canal. **phlegmonous a.,** one associated with acute inflammation of the subcutaneous connective tissue. **primary a.,** one formed at the seat of the infection. **ring a.,** a ring-shaped purulent infiltration at the periphery of the cornea. **scrofulous a.,** a cold abscess of tuberculous causation. **shirt-stud a.,** one separated into two cavities connected by a narrow channel. **stitch a.,** one developed about a stitch or suture. **strumous a.,** a cold abscess of tuberculous causation. **thecal a.,** one in the sheath of a tendon. **wandering a.,** one that burrows through the tissues, moving from place to place. **web-space a.,** one in the loose connective tissue and fat at the base of the fingers.

abscissa (ab-sis'ah) the horizontal line in a graph along which are plotted the units of one of the factors considered in the study, as time in a time-temperature study.

abscission (ab-sish'un) removal of a part or growth by cutting.

absent-mindedness (ab'sent-mīnd"ed-nes) preoccupation to the extent of being unaware of one's immediate surroundings.

absorbefacient (ab-sor"bĕ-fa'shent) causing absorption.

absorbent (ab-sorb'ent) 1. characterized by absorption. 2. a solid that attracts other material and incorporates it into its substance.

absorptiometer (ab-sorp"she-om'ĕ-ter) 1. an apparatus for determining the amount of gas absorbed by a fluid. 2. a device for measuring the layer of liquid absorbed between two glass plates; used as a hematoscope.

absorption (ab-sorp'shun) the attraction and incorporation of other material, as through a membrane.

absorptive (ab-sorp'tiv) having the power of absorption.

abstergent (ab-ster'jent) 1. cleansing or detergent. 2. a cleansing agent.

abstr. abstract.

abstraction (ab-strak'shun) 1. the mental process of forming abstract ideas. 2. a state synonymous with absent-mindedness.

abtorsion (ab-tor'shun) a turning outward of both eyes.

abulia (ah-bu'le-ah) inability to perform acts voluntarily or to make decisions. adj., **abu'lic.**

abulomania (ah-bu"lo-ma'ne-ah) mental disease with loss of will power.

abutment (ah-but'ment) the anchorage tooth for a bridge.

A.C. air conduction; alternating current; anodal closure; axiocervical.

Ac chemical symbol, *actinium.*

a.c. [L.] *an'te ci'bum* (before meals).

A.C.A. American College of Angiology; American College of Apothecaries.

acacia (ah-ka'shah) the dried gummy exudate from stems and branches of species of Acacia.

acalcerosis (ah-kal"sĕ-ro'sis) acalcicosis.

acalcicosis (ah-kal"sĭ-ko'sis) a condition due to deficiency of calcium in the diet.

acalculia (a-kal-ku'le-ah) inability to do mathematical calculations.

acampsia (a-kamp'se-ah) rigidity of a part or limb.

acanth(o)- word element, *sharp spine*, or *thorn.*

acantha (a-kan'tha) a spinous process of a vertebra.

acanthaceous (ak"an-tha'shus) bearing prickles.

acanthesthesia (a-kan"thes-the'ze-ah) sensation of a sharp point pricking the body.

acanthion (ah-kan'the-on) a point at the base of the anterior nasal spine.

Acanthocephala (ah-kan"tho-sef'ah-lah) a phylum of elongate, mostly cylindrical organisms parasitic in the intestines of all classes of vertebrates.

acanthocephaliasis (-sef"ah-li'ah-sis) infection with worms of the phylum Acanthocephala.

Acanthocephalus (-sef'ah-lus) a genus of parasitic worms (phylum Acanthocephala).

Acanthocheilonema (-ki"lo-ne'mah) a genus of long, threadlike worms. **A. per'stans,** a species often infecting man.

acanthocyte (ah-kan'tho-sīt) a red blood corpuscle with protoplasmic projections giving it a thorny appearance.

acanthocytosis (ah-kan"tho-si-to'sis) presence in the blood of acanthocytes.

acanthokeratodermia (-ker"ah-to-der'me-ah) hyperkeratosis.

acantholysis (ah"kan-thol'ĭ-sis) loss of cohesion between the cells of the prickle cell layer and between it and the layer above. **a. bullo'sa,** epidermolysis bullosa.

acanthoma (ak"an-tho'mah) a tumor in the prickle layer of the skin.

acanthosis (ak″an-tho′sis) hypertrophy or thickening of the prickle cell layer of the skin. adj., **acanthot′ic. a. ni′gricans,** a dermatosis with roughness and increased pigmentation, either generalized or in the axillae or body folds.

acanthrocyte (ah-kan′thro-sīt) acanthocyte.

acanthrocytosis (ah-kan″thro-si-to′sis) acanthocytosis.

acapnia (ah-kap′ne-ah) decrease of carbon dioxide in the blood. adj., **acap′nic.**

acarbia (ah-kar′be-ah) decrease of bicarbonate in the blood.

acardia (ah-kar′de-ah) developmental anomaly with absence of the heart.

acardiacus (ah″kar-di′ah-kus) [L.] having no heart.

acardius (ah-kar′de-us) a fetal monster without a heart.

acariasis (ak″ah-ri′ah-sis) infestation with mites.

acaricide (ah-kar′ĭ-sīd) an agent that destroys mites.

acarid (ak′ah-rid) a tick or mite of the order Acarina.

acaridiasis (ah-kar″ĭ-di′ah-sis) acariasis.

Acarina (ak″ah-ri′nah) an order of arthropods (class Arachnoidea), including mites and ticks.

acarinosis (ah-kar″i-no′sis) any disease caused by mites.

acarodermatitis (ak″ah-ro-der″mah-ti′tis) skin inflammation due to bites of parasitic mites (acarids). **a. urticarioi′des,** grain itch.

acarologist (ak″ah-rol′o-jist) a specialist in acarology.

acarology (ak″ah-rol′o-je) the scientific study of mites and ticks.

acarophobia (ak″ah-ro-fo′be-ah) morbid dread or delusion of infestation by mites.

Acarus (ak′ah-rus) a genus of arthropods (order Acarina), including mites. **A. folliculo′rum,** Demodex folliculorum. **A. scab′iei,** Sarcoptes scabiei.

acaryote (ah-kār′e-ōt) non-nucleated.

acatalasemia (a″kat-ah-la-se′me-ah) deficiency of catalase in the blood.

acatalasia (a″kat-ah-la′ze-ah) congenital absence of catalase from the body cells.

acatalepsy (ah-kat′ah-lep″se) 1. lack of understanding. 2. uncertainty. adj., **acatalep′tic.**

acatamathesia (ah-kat″ah-mah-the′ze-ah) inability to understand situations as perceived, specific objects or language.

acataphasia (ah-kat″ah-fa′ze-ah) speech disorder, with inability to express one's thoughts.

acathexia (ah″ah-thek′se-ah) inability to retain bodily secretions. adj. **acathec′tic.**

acaudal (a-kaw′dal) having no tail.

acaudate (a-kaw′dāt) acaudal.

acauline (ah-kaw′lin) having no stem.

A.C.C. American College of Cardiology; anodal closure contraction.

accelerator (ak-sel″er-a′tor) [L.] an agent or apparatus that increases the rate at which something occurs or progresses. **linear a.,** an apparatus for the acceleration of subatomic particles. **serum prothrombin conversion a.,** factor VII. **serum thrombotic a.,**, a factor in serum which has procoagulant properties and the ability to induce blood coagulation. **thromboplastin generation a.,** a heat-labile component in plasma which appears to influence the rate of formation of thromboplastin.

accelerin (ak-sel′er-in) factor V.

acceptor (ak-sep′tor) a substance which unites with another substance. **hydrogen a.,** the molecule accepting hydrogen in an oxidation-reduction reaction.

accipiter (ak-sip′ĭ-ter) a facial bandage with tails like the claws of a hawk.

acclimation (ak-lĭ-ma′shun) the process of becoming accustomed to a new climate, soil and conditions.

acclimatization (ah-kli″mah-ti-za′shun) acclimation.

accommodation (ah-kom″o-da′shun) adjustment, especially of the eye for seeing objects at various distances. **absolute a.,** the accommodation of either eye separately. **histologic a.,** changes in morphology and function of cells following changed conditions. **negative a.,** adjustment of eye for long distances by relaxation. **positive a.,** adjustment of eye for short distances by contraction.

accommodometer (ah-kom″ŏ-dom′ĕ-ter) an instrument for measuring accommodative capacity of the eye.

accouchement (ah-koōsh-maw′) [Fr.] childbirth; delivery; labor. **a. forcé,** forcible delivery with the hand.

accrementition (ak″re-men-tish′un) growth by addition of similar tissue.

accretion (ah-kre′shun) accumulation of matter to a part.

accumulator (ah-ku′mu-la″tor) an apparatus for accumulating and storing electricity.

acedia (ah-se′de-ah) a morbid state of apathy and mental depression.

acellular (a-sel′u-lar) not cellular in structure.

acelomate (ah-se′lo-māt) having no coelom or body cavity.

acenesthesia (ah-sen″es-the′ze-ah) loss of sense of well-being or physical existence.

acenocoumarol (ah-se″no-koo′mah-rol) an anticoagulant.

acentric (a-sen′tric) having no center; in genetics, designating an apparent pair of sister chromatids without a centromere.

acephalia (ah″sĕ-fa′le-ah) developmental anomaly with absence of the head.

acephalobrachia (ah-sef″ah-lo-bra′ke-ah) developmental anomaly with absence of head and arms.

acephalocardia (-kar′de-ah) developmental anomaly with absence of head and heart.

acephalocardius (-kar′de-us) a fetal monster without head or heart.

acephalochiria (-ki′re-ah) developmental anomaly with absence of head and hands.

acephalocyst (ah-sef′ah-lo-sist″) a sterile echinococcus cyst.

acephalocystis racemosa (ah-sef″ah-lo-sis′tis ra-se-mo′sah) a hydatid mole of the uterus.

acephalogaster (ah-sef″ah-lo-gas′ter) a fetal monster without head or stomach.

acephalogastria (ah-sef″ah-lo-gas′tre-ah) developmental anomaly with absence of head, chest and stomach.

acephalopodia (-po′de-ah) developmental anomaly with absence of head and feet.

acephalopodius (-po′de-us) a fetal monster without head or feet.

acephalorachia (-ra′ke-ah) developmental anomaly with absence of head and spinal column.

acephalostomia (-sto′me-ah) developmental anomaly with absence of head, with mouth aperture on the upper aspect of the fetal body.

acephalothoracia (-tho-ra′se-ah) developmental anomaly with absence of head and thorax.

acephalous (ah-sef′ah-lus) headless.

acephalus (ah-sef′ah-lus) a fetal monster without a head.

aceratosis (ah-ser″ah-to′sis) deficiency in formation of horny tissue.

acervuline (ah-ser′vu-līn) aggregated; heaped up.

acervuloma (ah-ser″vu-lo′mah) a meningioma containing psammoma bodies.

acervulus (ah-ser′vu-lus), pl. *acer′vuli* [L.] a little heap. **a. cer′ebri,** sandy matter about the pineal gland and other parts of the brain.

acescence (ah-ses′ens) sourness.

acescent (ah-ses′ent) sour; slightly acid.

acestoma (ah″ses-to′mah) a mass of granulations.

acetabular (as″ĕ-tab′u-ler) pertaining to the acetabulum.

acetabulectomy (as″ĕ-tab″u lek′to-me) excision of the acetabulum.

acetabuloplasty (as″ĕ-tab′u-lo-plas″te) plastic repair of the acetabulum.

acetabulum (as″ĕ-tab′u-lum) the cup-shaped cavity in the coxa, receiving the head of the femur.

acetaldehyde (as″et-al′de-hīd) a colorless, volatile liquid, CH_3CHO.

acetaminophen (as″et-am′ĭ-no-fen″) an analgesic and antipyretic.

acetanilid (as″ĕ-tan′ĭ-lid) a colorless crystalline powder, C_8H_9NO; analgesic and antipyretic.

acetannin (es″ĕ-tan′in) acetyltannic acid.

acetarsol (as″et-ar′sol) acetarsone.

acetarsone (as″et-ar′sōn) an odorless white powder, $C_8H_{10}AsNO_5$; used in amebic dysentery and trichomonas vaginitis.

acetate (as′ĕ-tāt) a salt of acetic acid.

acetazolamide (as″et-ah-zol′ah-mīd) a diuretic of the carbonic anhydrase inhibitor type, useful in treatment of various conditions. **sodium a.,** a sodium-containing compound, $C_4H_5N_4NaO_3S_2$.

acetic (ah-se′tik, ah-set′ik) pertaining to vinegar or its acid; sour.

aceticoceptor (ah-se″tĭ-ko-sep′tor) a side chain having an affinity for the acetic acid radical.

acetimeter (as″ĕ-tim′ĕ-ter) an instrument for measuring the acetic acid in a fluid.

acetin (as′ĕ-tin) a glyceryl acetate, $C_3H_5(C_2H_3O_2)_3$.

Acetobacter (ah-se″to-bak′ter) a genus of Schizomycetes (order Pseudomonadales, sub-order Pseudomonadineae, family Pseudomonadaceae) important in completion of the carbon cycle and in production of vinegar.

acetomeroctol (as″e-to-mer-ok′tol) an antiseptic for prevention and control of superficial skin infections.

acetometer (as″ĕ-tom′ĕ-ter) an instrument for measuring acetic acid.

acetone (as′ĕ-tōn) a compound, $CH_3.CO.CH_3$, with solvent properties and characteristic odor, obtained by fermentation or produced synthetically; one of the ketone bodies produced in abnormal amounts in diabetes mellitus.

acetonemia (as″ĕ-to-ne′me-ah) ketonemia.

acetonitrile (-ni′trīl) methyl cyanide, CH_3CN, a colorless acid.

acetonuria (-nu′re-ah) ketonuria.

acetophenazine (-fen′ah-zēn) a mildly sedative substance used as a tranquilizer.

acetophenetidin (-fĕ-net′ĭ-din) a fine white crystalline powder, $C_{10}H_{13}NO_2$; analgesic and antipyretic.

acetous (as′ĕ-tus) resembling or pertaining to vinegar.

acetphenarsine (as″et-fen-ar′sēn) acetarsone.

acetphenetidine (-fĕ-net′ĭ-din) acetophenetidin.

acetrozoate sodium (as″ĕ-tro′zo-āt so′de-um) a radiopaque medium for roentgenographic visualization of blood vessels and kidneys.

acetyl (as′ĕ-til) the monovalent radical, CH_3CO, a combining form of acetic acid. **a. peroxide,** a thick liquid, $(C_2H_3O)_2O_2$, powerful oxidizing agent. **a. sulfisoxazole,** a sulfanilamide used as an anti-infective.

acetylaminobenzine (as″ĕ-til-am″ĭ-no-ben′-zēn) acetanilid.

acetylaniline (-an′ĭ-lin) acetanilid.

acetylation (ah-set″ĭ-la′shun) introduction of an acetyl radical into an organic molecule.

acetyl-beta-methylcholine (as″ĕ-til-ba″tah-meth″il-ko′lēn) mecholyl.

acetylcarbromal (-kar-bro′mal) a sedative drug.

acetylcholine (-ko′lēn) an acetyl derivative of choline having blood pressure-lowering properties, given usually in the form of acetylcholine chloride.

acetylcholinesterase (-ko″lin-es′ter-ās) an enzyme having a higher affinity for acetylcholine than for any other ester.

acetyldigitoxin-α (-dij″ĭ-tok′sin al′fah) a digitalis preparation used to improve function of the failing heart.

acetylene (ah-set′ĭ-lēn) a colorless, combustible gas, C_2H_2, with unpleasant odor.

acetylphenylhydrazine (as″ĕ-til-fen″il-hi′drah-zēn) a hemolytic agent for polycythemia.

Ac-G accelerator globulin.

A.C.G. American College of Gastroenterology.

ACH adrenal cortical hormone.

ACh. acetylcholine.

A.C.H.A. American College of Hospital Administrators.

achalasia (ak″ah-la′ze-ah) failure to relax of smooth muscle fibers at any junction of one part of the gastrointestinal tract with another.

AChE acetylcholinesterase.

acheilia (ah-ki'le-ah) developmental anomaly with absence of the lips. adj. **achei'lous.**

acheiria (ah-ki're-ah) 1. developmental anomaly with absence of the hands. 2. sense as of the loss of the hands, seen in hysteria.

acheiropodia (ah-ki″ro-po'de-ah) developmental anomaly characterized by absence of both hands and feet.

achillobursitis (ah-kil″o-ber-si'tis) inflammation of the bursae about the Achilles tendon.

achillodynia (-din'e-ah) pain in the Achilles tendon.

achillorrhaphy (ak″il-lor'ah-fe) suturing of the Achilles tendon.

achillotenotomy (ah-kil″o-ten-ot'o-me) incision of the Achilles tendon.

achlorhydria (a″klōr-hi'dre-ah) absence of hydrochloric acid from gastric juice.

achloride (ah-klo'rīd) a salt that is not a chloride.

achloropsia (ah″klo-rop'se-ah) blindness to green colors.

acholia (a-ko'le-ah) absence of bile secretion. adj., **acho'lic.**

acholuria (ah″ko-lu're-ah) absence of bile pigments from the urine.

achondroplasia (a-kon″dro-pla'ze-ah) a disorder of cartilage formation in the fetus, leading to a type of dwarfism. adj., **achondroplas'tic.**

achoresis (ak″o-re'sis) diminution of the capacity of an organ.

Achorion (ah-ko're-on) trichophyton.

achrestic (a-kres'tik) caused not by absence of a necessary substance, but by inability to utilize such a substance.

achroacyte (ah-kro'ah-sīt) a colorless cell or leukocyte.

achroacytosis (ah-kro″ah-si-to'sis) excessive development of lymph cells (colorless cells).

achroiocythemia (ah-kroi″o-si-the'me-ah) deficiency or lack of hemoglobin in the red blood corpuscles.

achroma (ah-kro'mah) absence of color.

achromacyte (ah-kro'mah-sīt) a decolorized red blood corpuscle.

achromasia (ak″ro-ma'se-ah) lack of normal skin pigmentation.

achromat (a'kro-mat) a person who is color-blind.

achromate (ah-kro'māt) achromat.

Achromatiaceae (ah-kro″mah-ti-a'se-e) a family of Schizomycetes (order Beggiatoales) whose cells lack photosynthetic pigments.

achromatic (ak″ro-mat'ik) 1. producing no discoloration, or staining with difficulty. 2. pertaining to achromatin. 3. refracting light without decomposing it into its component colors.

achromatin (ah-kro'mah-tin) the faintly staining groundwork of a cell nucleus.

achromatism (ah-kro'mah-tizm) absence of chromatic aberration.

Achromatium (ah″kro-ma'te-um) a genus of Schizomycetes (order Beggiatoales, family Achromatiaceae).

achromatocyte (ak″ro-mat'o-sīt) a decolorized red blood corpuscle.

achromatolysis (ak″ro-mah-tol'ĭ-sis) disorganization of cell achromatin.

achromatophil (ak″ro-mat'o-fil, a″kro-mat'o-fil) not easily stainable.

achromatopia (ah″kro-mah-to'pe-ah) defective visual perception of colors. adj., **achromatop'-ic.**

achromatopsia (ah-kro″mah-top'se-ah) achromatopia.

achromatosis (-to'sis) any disease marked by deficiency of pigmentation.

achromatous (a-kro'mah-tus) colorless.

achromaturia (a-kro″mah-tu're-ah) colorless state of the urine.

achromia (a-kro'me-ah) absence of normal color. adj., **achro'mic.**

Achromobacter (a-kro″mo-bak'ter) a genus of Schizomycetes (order Eubacteriales, family Achromobacteraceae) found in soil or in fresh or salt water.

Achromobacteraceae (a-kro″mo-bak″tē-ra'-se-e) a family of Schizomycetes (order Eubacteriales) generally found in soil or in fresh or salt water.

achromocyte (ah-kro'mo-sīt) a red cell artifact which stains more faintly than intact erythrocytes.

achromodermia (-der'me-ah) colorless state of the skin.

achromophil (ah-kro'mo-fil) achromatophil.

achromotrichia (ah-kro″mo-trik'e-ah) loss of color of the hair.

Achromycin (ak″ro-mi'sin) trademark for preparations of tetracycline.

achroodextrin (ah-kro″o-deks'trin) a kind of dextrin not colored by iodine.

achylanemia (ah-ki″lah-ne'me-ah) a condition in which gastric achylia is associated with simple or hypochromic anemia.

achylia (ah-ki'le-ah) absence of chyle. **a. gas'-trica,** absence of hydrochloric acid and enzymes from the gastric secretion. **a. pancreat'ica,** deficiency of enzymes secreted by the pancreas.

achylosis (ak″ĭ-lo'sis) achylia.

achylous (ah-ki'lus) deficient in chyle.

achymia (ah-ki'me-ah) deficiency of chyme.

acicular (ah-sik'u-lar) needle-shaped.

aciculum (ah-sik'u-lum) a bent, finger-like structure observed in certain flagellates.

acid (as'id) 1. sour. 2. a substance which forms hydrogen ions in solution and from which hydrogen may be displaced by a metal when a salt is formed. **abietic a.,** a compound, $C_{20}H_{30}O_2$, prepared by isomerization of rosin. **abric a.,** crystalline acid, $C_{21}H_{24}N_3O$, from jequirity. **acetic a.,** a saturated fatty acid, CH_3COOH, the characteristic component of vinegar; used in solutions of various strengths, as *dilute acetic acid* (6%) and *glacial acetic acid* (99.4%). **acetoacetic a.,** a compound, $CH_3.CO.CH_2.COOH$; one of the ketone bodies formed in the body in metabolism of certain substances and present in increased amounts in various pathologic states. **acetylsalicylic**

a., aspirin. **acetyltannic a.,** a yellowish or grayish white powder; astringent. **adenylic a.,** a component of nucleic acid, consisting of adenine, ribose and phosphoric acid, found in muscle, yeast and other material. **adipic a.,** a compound, $HOOC(CH_2)_4COOH$, found in beet juice. **alginic a.,** a colloidal substance from brown seaweeds, with a formula of $(C_6H_8O_6)_n$ or $(C_6H_8O_6.H_2O)_2$. **amino a.,** one of a class of organic compounds containing the amino (NH_2) and the carboxyl (COOH) group, occurring naturally in plant and animal tissues and forming the chief constituents of protein; many of them are necessary for human and animal growth and nutrition and hence are called essential amino acids. **amino a., essential,** one that is essential for optimal growth or nitrogen equilibrium. **aminoacetic a.,** glycine. **aminobenzoic a.,** a crystalline compound, $C_7H_7NO_2$, used as an antirickettsial agent. **p-aminobenzoic a.,** a member of the B group of vitamins, $NH_2.C_6H_4.COOH$, a growth factor for certain organisms, and used in treatment of scrub typhus; called also PABA. **epsilon-amino-caproic a.,** a synthetic amino acid which is a potent inhibitor of fibrinolysis, plasminogen activator and plasmin. **aminosalicylic a.,** a white or nearly white bulky powder, $NH_2.C_6H_3.OH.COOH$, used in treatment of tuberculosis, called also PAS. **anisic a.,** C_8H_8O, from anise seed; once used as local antiseptic and antirheumatic. **anthranilic a.,** a crystalline acid, $NH_2C_6H_4COOH$, formed in metabolism of tryptophan and excreted in riboflavin deficiency. **arachic a., arachidic a.,** a saturated fatty acid, $C_{19}H_{39}COOH$, occurring in peanut oil. **arachidonic a.,** an unsaturated fatty acid, $C_{19}H_{39}COOH$, occurring in lecithin and cephalin. **argininosuccinic a.,** a compound normally formed in the ornithine cycle of urea formation in the liver, but not normally present in the urine. **arsenous a.,** arsenic trioxide. **ascorbic a.,** $C_6H_8O_6$, a compound found in many vegetables and fruits, and an essential element in the diet of man and many other animals. **aspartic a.,** a dibasic amino acid, derivable from asparagine, produced by pancreatic digestion; actively anticoagulant. **barbituric a.,** a compound, $C_4H_4N_2O_3$, the parent substance of barbiturates. **benzoic a.,** a crystalline acid, $C_6H_5.COOH$, from coal tar and various resins; used as a preservative in pharmaceutical preparations. **beta-hydroxybutyric a.,** a compound, $CH_3.CHOH.CH_2.COOH$, produced in abnormal amounts in diabetes mellitus; considered one of the ketone bodies, although it does not contain the carbonyl group typical of their structure. **beta-ketobutyric a.,** acetoacetic acid. **bile a's,** organic compounds formed in the liver and secreted in the bile. **boric a.,** a crystalline powder, H_3BO_3, used as a bactericide and fungicide for skin and conjunctiva. **butyric a.,** a saturated fatty acid, C_3H_7COOH, found in butter. **cacodylic a.,** a crystalline compound, $(CH_3)_2ASO.OH$, once used in treatment of skin diseases. **caffeic a.,**

crystalline acid, $C_9H_8O_4$, from coffee. **camphoric a.,** crystalline acid, $C_{10}H_{16}O_4$, from camphor. **camphoronic a.,** $C_9H_{14}O_6$, obtained by oxidation of camphoric acid. **capric a.,** a saturated fatty acid, $C_9H_{19}COOH$, in butter, coconut oil, etc. **caproic a.,** a saturated fatty acid, $C_5H_{11}COOH$, in butter, etc. **caprylic a.,** a saturated fatty acid, $C_7H_5.COOH$, in butter, coconut oil, etc. **carbamic a.,** a compound, NH_2COOH, the parent acid of urethan. **carbazotic a.,** trinitrophenol. **carbolic a.,** phenol. **carbonic a.,** aqueous solution of carbon dioxide, H_2CO_3. **carminic a.,** the active principle of carmine, extracted from cochineal. **carnaubic a.,** a saturated fatty acid, $C_{23}H_{47}COOH$, found in carnauba wax. **cerebronic a.,** a saturated monohydroxy acid, $C_{24}H_{48}O$, from phrenosin. **cerotic a.,** a saturated fatty acid, $C_{25}H_{51}COOH$, found in beeswax, wool fat, etc. **cevitamic a.,** ascorbic acid. **chaulmoogric a.,** a cyclic fatty acid, $C_5H_7(CH_2)_{12}COOH$, from chaulmoogra oil. **chenodeoxycholic a.,** an acid formerly believed to occur mainly in the dog, but found also in human bile. **chloroacetic a.,** an acid in which the three hydrogen atoms of acetic acid are wholly or partly replaced by chlorine. **cholalic a., cholic a.,** an acid formed in the liver from cholesterol which plays, with other bile acids, an important role in digestion. **chondroitin sulfuric a.,** a compound of high molecular weight in skin and connective tissue and, combined with collagen, constituting 20–40 per cent of cartilage. **chromic a.,** chromium trioxide. **chrysophanic a.,** a compound, $C_{15}H_{10}O_4$, present in cascara sagrada, senna and rhubarb. **cinnamic a.,** a crystalline acid, $C_6H_5(CH)_2COOH$, from cinnamon, the balsams and other aromatic resins. **citric a.,** crystalline acid, $C_6H_8O_7$, from various fruits; flavoring agent. **cresylic a.,** cresol. **cyanic a.,** a highly irritant compound, HOCN. **cynurenic a.,** one from dog's urine. **cysteic a.,** an intermediate product in the oxidation of cysteine to taurine. **damalic a.,** an acid, C_7H_8O, occurring in urine. **damaluric a.,** $C_7H_{12}O_2$, occurring in urine. **dehydrocholic a.,** a white, fluffy, bitter, odorless powder used to increase output of bile by the liver. **deoxycholic a.,** one of the bile acids, capable of forming soluble, diffusible complexes with fatty acids. **deoxypentosenucleic a.,** deoxyribonucleic acid. **deoxyribonucleic a.,** one of the nucleic acids. **diacetic a.,** acetoacetic acid. **diallylbarbituric a.,** a long-acting barbiturate. **2,4-diaminobutyric a.,** a naturally occurring amino acid discovered in 1948. **2,6-diaminopimelic a.,** a naturally occurring amino acid discovered in 1950. **djenkolic a.,** an amino acid obtained in 1935 by the hydrolysis of djenkol nuts. **ethacrynic a.,** a powerful diuretic used orally or parenterally, and effective in promoting sodium and chloride excretion. **fatty a.,** monobasic acid produced by oxidation of a primary alcohol, and having the general formula $C_nH_{2n}O_2$. **fellic a.,** $C_{23}H_{40}O_4$, a constituent of bile. **filicic a.,** a substance of uncertain composition derived from male fern. **folic a.,** a term loosely applied to several closely related compounds with vitamin B activity. **folinic a.**, a factor in crude liver, yeast extracts and other biological materials, which is necessary to growth of *Leuconostoc citrovorum*. **formic a.**, colorless, pungent liquid, HCOOH, from secretion of ants, nettles, etc. **formiminoglutamic a.**, a product in the metabolism of histidine, the appearance of which in urine is used as a test of folic acid deficiency. **fuchsin a.**, see under *fuchsin*. **gallotannic a.**, tannic acid. **glucoascorbic** COOH, found in certain plant and bacterial polysaccharides. **gallic a.**, crystalline acid, $C_7H_6O_5$, produced by hydrolysis of tannic acid. **gallotannic a.**, tannic acid. **glucoascorbic a.**, an analogue of ascorbic acid that produces scurvy-like symptoms in some animals. **gluconic a.**, an intermediate product, $CH_2OH(CHOH)_4COOH$, formed in biosynthesis of pentoses. **glucuronic a.**, $CHO(CHOH)_4$-COOH, found in various animal and plant tissues. **glutamic a.**, a crystalline dibasic compound, $COOH.(CH_2)_2.CH(NH_2).COOH$, an important amino acid, but not essential to growth. **glutaric a.**, $C_5H_8O_4$, occurring in various natural products. **glyceric a.**, $CH_2OH.CHOH.COOH$, an intermediate product in the transformation in the body of carbohydrate to lactic acid formed by oxidation of glycerol. **glycocholic a.**, a combination of glycine and cholic acid present in bile. **glycolic a.**, a compound, $CH_2OH.COOH$, an intermediate product in the transformation in the body of serine to glycine. **glyoxylic a.**, a compound, $CHO.COOH$, formed in the oxidative deamination of glycine. **guanidoacetic a.**, an intermediate product in the synthesis of creatine. **helvolic a.**, fumigacin. **hexuronic a.**, ascorbic acid. **hippuric a.**, a compound, $C_6H_5.CO.NH.CH_2.COOH$, formed by conjugation of benzoic acid and glycine. **homogentisic a.**, 2,5-dihydroxyphenyl acetic acid, an intermediate product in the metabolism of tyrosine and phenylalanine, excreted in urine in an inborn error of metabolism. **hyaluronic a.**, a sulfate-free polysaccharide in the vitreous humor, synovial fluid, skin, umbilical cord, tumors and hemolytic streptococci. **hydnocarpic a.**, a cyclic fatty acid, $C_5H_7(CH_2)_{10}$-COOH, from chaulmoogra oil. **hydriodic a.**, an aqueous solution of hydrogen iodide (HI) once used as an alterative. **hydrobromic a.**, an aqueous solution of hydrobromide gas (HBr) once used as a sedative. **hydrochloric a.**, HCl, a normal constituent of gastric juice in man and other animals. **hydrocyanic a.**, a volatile poisonous liquid, HCN, from bitter almonds, peach leaves, cherry leaves, etc. **hydrofluoric a.**, an aqueous solution of hydrogen fluoride gas (HF). **hydrosulfuric a.**, hydrogen sulfide. **hydroxybutyric a.**, an acid, $CH_3CHOHCH_2COOH$, found in the urine and the blood in diabetes. **hypochlorous a.**, unstable compound, HClO; used as disinfectant and bleaching agent. **hypophosphoric a.**, an acid, H_2PO_3, whose salts are hypophosphates. **hypophosphorous a.**, a compound, $PH(OH)_2$, once used as a central nervous sys-

tem tonic. **inorganic a.**, an acid containing no carbon atoms. **inosinic a.**, the parent compound of all purines. **iodic a.**, monobasic acid, HIO_3. **iodoalphionic a.**, a white or yellowish powder, $C_{15}H_{12}I_2O_3$, used as a contrast medium in cholecystography. **iodogorgoic a.**, 3,5-diiodotyrosine. **iopanoic a.**, a cream-colored powder, $C_{11}H_{12}I_3NO_3$, used as an opaque medium in cholecystography. **iophenoxic a.**, triiodohydrocinnamic acid; used as a radiopaque medium for cholecystography. **isolysergic a.**, $C_{16}H_{16}N_2O_2$, one of the main cleavage products of hydrolysis of the alkaloids characteristic of ergot, and the parent compound of the ergotinine group of alkaloids. **keto a's**, compounds containing the groups CO and COOH. **kynurenic a.**, a crystalline acid, $C_9H_5N(OH)COOH$, metabolite of tryptophan found in microorganisms and in the urine of normal mammals. **lactic a.**, $CH_3CHOHCOOH$, a compound formed in the body in anaerobic metabolism of carbohydrate; also produced by bacterial action in milk. **lauric a.**, a saturated fatty acid, $C_{11}H_{23}COOH$, found in spermaceti and coconut oil. **levulinic a.**, an acid, $CH_3CO(CH_2)_2COOH$, from decomposition of pentose sugars of nucleic acid and from the thymus gland. **lignoceric a.**, a saturated fatty acid, $C_{23}H_{47}COOH$, found in arachis oil and various cerebrosides. **linoleic a.**, an unsaturated fatty acid, $C_{17}H_{31}COOH$, found in linseed and cottonseed oils. **lithic a.**, uric acid. **lysergic a. diethylamide**, see *LSD*. **malic a.**, crystalline acid, $C_4H_6O_5$, from juices of many fruits and plants, and an intermediary product of carbohydrate metabolism in the body. **mandelic a.**, white crystalline powder, $C_8H_8O_3$; used in infections of the urinary tract. **meconic a.**, white crystalline compound, $C_7H_4O_7$, from opium. **metaphosphoric a.**, a glassy solid, HPO_3, used as a test for albumin in urine. **mucic a.**, an acid, $C_6H_{10}O_8$, derivable from gums and sugars. **muriatic a.**, hydrochloric acid. **myristic a.**, a saturated fatty acid, $C_{14}H_{28}O_2$, from nutmeg. **nervonic a.**, an unsaturated fatty acid from nervone. **neuraminic a.**, a 9-carbon aminosugar acid, one of the sialic acids. **nicotinic acid**, niacin. **nitric a.**, colorless liquid, HNO_3, which fumes in moist air and has a characteristic pungent odor; used as a cauterizing agent. **nitrohydrochloric a.**, yellow, fuming mixture of nitric and hydrochloric acids. **nitrous a.**, an unstable compound, HNO_2, with which free amino groups react to form hydroxyl groups and liberate gaseous nitrogen. **nucleic a's**, substances which constitute the prosthetic groups of the nucleoproteins and contain phosphoric acid, sugars, and purine and pyrimidine bases. **nucleinic a.**, nucleic acid. **oleic a.**, an unsaturated fatty acid, $C_{17}H_{33}COOH$, found in animal and vegetable fats. **organic a.**, an acid containing the carboxyl group, COOH. **orthophosphoric a.**, phosphoric acid. **osmic a.**, a colorless or slightly yellow compound, OsO_4, used as a fixative in preparing histologic specimens. **oxalic a.**, a compound, $(COOH)_2$, found in various fruits and vegetables, and formed in metabolism of ascorbic acid in the body. **palmitic a.**, a saturated fatty acid, $C_{15}H_{31}COOH$, from animal and vegetable fats. **palmitoleic a.**, an unsaturated fatty acid, $C_{15}H_{29}COOH$, found in various oils. **pangamic a.**, an amino derivative of glucuronic acid, $C_{10}H_{19}O_8N$, one of the vitamins of the B complex. **pantothenic a.**, a vitamin of the B complex, $C_9H_{17}O_5N$. **pectic a.**, an acid, $C_{32}H_{48}O_{32}$, from pectin. **penicillic a.**, an antibiotic substance, $C_8H_{10}O_4$, isolated from cultures of certain species of organisms. **perchloric a.**, a colorless volatile liquid, $HClO_4$. **phenic a.**, phenol. **phenylcinchoninic a.**, cinchophen. **phenylpyruvic a.**, an intermediary product, $C_6H_5CH_2COCOOH$, in the metabolism of phenylalanine in the body. **phosphatidic a's**, compounds consisting of glycerol, two fatty acid molecules and phosphoric acid, first found in plants, but occurring also in animal tissues. **phosphoric a.**, a crystalline compound or clear, syrupy liquid, H_3PO_4, whose salts are called phosphates. **phosphorous a.**, a white, hygroscopic, crystalline compound, H_3PO_3, whose salts are called phosphites. **phytic a.**, the hexaphosphoric acid ester of inositol, found in many plants and microorganisms and in animal tissues. **picric a.**, trinitrophenol. **pimelic a.**, HOOC-$(CH_2)_5$COOH, formed in oxidation of unsaturated fats, and a possible precursor of biotin. **propionic a.**, a compound, CH_3CH_2-COOH, produced by oxidation of normal propyl alcohol or by action of certain bacteria on hexoses, pentoses, lactic acid, and glycerin. **pteroylglutamic a.**, folic acid. **pyroboric a.**, a diabasic acid, $H_2B_4O_7$, obtained by heating boric acid. **pyroligneous a.**, clear liquid from the destructive distillation of wood, etc. **pyrophosphoric a.**, crystalline acid, $H_4P_2O_7$, one of the forms of phosphoric acid. **pyruvic a.**, a compound, CH_3.CO.COOH, formed in the body in aerobic metabolism of carbohydrate; also formed by dry distillation of tartaric acid. **quinic a.**, crystalline compound, $C_7H_{12}O_6$, from cinchona. **ribonucleic a.**, a nucleic acid which on hydrolysis yields adenine, guanine, cytosine, uracil, ribose and phosphoric acid; *messenger RNA* is an RNA fraction which transfers information from DNA to the protein-forming system of the cell; *transfer RNA* is an RNA fraction which combines with one amino acid species, transferring it from activating enzyme to ribosome. **ribose nucleic a.**, ribonucleic acid. **rosolic a.**, a compound, $C_{20}H_{16}O_3$, used as an indicator and in manufacture of dyes. **salicylic a.**, a crystalline acid, $C_7H_6O_3$; bacteriostatic and keratolytic. **salicyluric a.**, a compound of glycol and salicylic acid, found in urine after administration of salicylic acid. **sarcolactic a.**, a dextrorotatory form of lactic acid, formed on muscular contraction. **shikimic a.**, a compound originally isolated from Japanese anise that is a precursor in the synthesis of different amino acids by various microorganisms. **stannic a.**, a vitreous acid of tin, H_2SnO_3, forming stannates. **stearic a.**, a saturated

fatty acid, $C_{17}H_{35}COOH$, from animal and vegetable fats. **succinic a.**, a compound, $COOH(CH_2)_2COOH$, formed in the aerobic metabolism of carbohydrate in the body. **sulfanilic a.**, a crystalline compound, C_6H_7-$NSO_3.H_2O$, used as a reagent. **sulfuric a.**, an oily, highly caustic, poisonous compound, H_2SO_4. **sulfurous a.**, a clear, colorless liquid, H_2SO_3. **tannic a.**, a substance obtained from bark and fruit of many plants; used as an astringent. **tartaric a.**, a compound with the molecular formula, $C_4H_6O_6$, used in preparing refrigerant drinks and effervescent powders. **taurocholic a.**, a bile acid, $C_{26}H_{45}$-NSO_7; when hydrolyzed, it splits into taurine and cholic acid. **thymic a.**, thymol. **thymonucleic a.**, a name applied to deoxyribonucleic acid derived from thymus gland. **trichloroacetic a.**, colorless, deliquescent crystals, $C_2HCl_3O_2$; germicidal, astringent and caustic. **triiodoethionic a.**, iophenoxic acid. **undecylenic a.**, an unsaturated fatty acid, $C_{11}H_{20}O_2$; antifungal agent. **uric a.**, a crystalline acid, $C_5H_4N_4O_3$, present in blood and urine, the chief end-product of nitrogen metabolism in man. **ursolic a.**, $C_{30}H_{48}O_3$, a compound found in the waxlike coatings of various leaves and fruits. **valerianic a.**, **valeric a.**, colorless, oily, pungent liquid, $C_5H_{10}O_2$. **xanthurenic a.**, $C_9H_5N(OH)_2COOH$, a metabolite of L-tryptophan, present in normal urine and in increased amounts in vitamin B_6 deficiency.

aciduminuria (as"id-am"ĭ-nu'rc-ah) excess of amino acid in the urine.

acidemia (as"ĭ-de'me-ah) abnormal acidity of the blood.

acid-fast (as'id-fast) not readily decolorized by acids after staining.

acidifiable (ah-sid"ĭ-fi'ah-bl) capable of being made acid.

acidifier (ah-sid"ĭ-fi'er) an agent that causes acidity; a substance used to increase gastric acidity.

acidify (ah-sid'ĭ-fi) to make sour; to convert into an acid.

acidimeter (as"ĭ-dim'ĕ-ter) instrument for performing acidimetry.

acidimetry (-ĕ-tre) determination of the amount of free acid in a liquid.

acidity (ah-sid'ĭ-te) the quality of being acid; the power to unite with positively charged ions or with basic substances.

acidocyte (ah-sid'o-sīt) an acidophilic cell (eosinophil).

acidocytopenia (as"ĭ-do-si"to-pe'ne-ah) decreased number of eosinophils in the blood.

acidocytosis (-si-to'sis) increased number of eosinophils in the blood.

Acidol (a'sĭ-dol) trademark for a preparation of betaine.

acidology (as"ĭ-dol'o-je) the science of surgical appliances.

acidophilic (as"ĭ-do-fil'ik) 1. easily stained with acid dyes. 2. growing best on acid media.

acidophilism (as"ĭ-dof'ĭ-lizm) the state produced by acidophil adenoma of the hypophysis, resulting in acromegaly.

acidosis (as"ĭ-do'sis) a state of increased

acidity of body tissues and fluids. adj., **acidot'ic. compensated a.**, a condition in which the compensatory mechanisms have returned the pH toward normal. **diabetic a.**, a metabolic acidosis produced by accumulation of ketones in uncontrolled diabetes. **hypercapnic a.**, respiratory acidosis. **hyperchloremic a.**, renal tubular acidosis. **metabolic a.**, a disturbance in which the acid-base status shifts toward the acid side because of changes in the fixed (nonvolatile) acids and bases. **nonrespiratory a.**, metabolic acidosis. **renal tubular a.**, a metabolic acidosis resulting from impairment of the reabsorption of bicarbonate by the renal tubules, the urine being alkaline. **respiratory a.**, a state due to excess retention of carbon dioxide in the body. **starvation a.**, a metabolic acidosis due to accumulation of ketones following a caloric deficit.

acidosteophyte (as″ĭ-dos′te-o-fīt″)   a sharp-pointed osteophyte.

acid-proof (as′id-pr<del></del>oof) acid-fast.

acidulated (ah-sid′u-lāt″ed) somewhat sour or acid.

acidulous (ah-sid′u-lus) moderately sour.

acidum (as′ĭ-dum) [L.] acid.

aciduric (as″ĭ-du′rik) capable of growing in extremely acid media.

acinesia (as″ĭ-ne′ze-ah) akinesia.

acinetic (as″ĭ-net′ik) 1. affected with akinesia. 2. diminishing muscular power.

aciniform (ah-sin′ĭ-form) grapelike.

acinitis (as″ĭ-ni′tis) inflammation of the acini of a gland.

acinose (as′ĭ-nōs) made up of acini.

acinous (as′ĭ-nus) acinose.

acinus (as′ĭ-nus), pl. *ac′ini* [L.] one of the smallest lobules of a compound gland.

acladiosis (ah-klad″e-o′sis) an ulcerative skin disease caused by a fungus of the genus Acladium.

Acladium (ah-kla′de-um) a genus of fungus sometimes infecting man.

aclasis (ak′lah-sis) pathologic continuity of structure, as in chondrodystrophy. **diaphyseal a.**, imperfect formation of bone in the cartilage between the diaphysis and epiphysis; dyschondroplasia.

aclastic (a-klas′tik) not refracting.

acleistocardia (ah-klīs″to-kar′de-ah) an open state of the foramen ovale.

aclinic (a-klin′ik) having no inclination.

aclusion (ah-kloo′zhun) imperfect occlusion of the teeth.

acme (ak′me) the critical stage or crisis of a disease.

acne (ak′ne) an affection of the skin with eruption of papules or pustules, more particularly acne vulgaris. **a. che′loidique**, keloid folliculitis. **a. conglоba′ta, conglobate a.**, a staphylococcal infection of the skin leading to formation of cutaneous and subcutaneous abscesses and keloidal scarring. **a. indura′ta**, acne vulgaris with deep-seated, destructive lesions. **keloid a.**, keloid folliculitis. **a. necrot′ica**, acne varioliformis. **a. papulo′sa**, acne vulgaris with the formation of papules. **a.**

rosa′cea, diffuse erythema with papules, pustules and telangiectases on the midthird of the face, with mild pruritus and tenderness, usually occurring in middle age. **a. varioli-for′mis**, a skin disease with reddish-brown, papulopustular umbilicated lesions, usually on the brow or scalp, leading to scarring. **a. vulga′ris**, a skin condition, usually occurring in adolescence, with comedones, papules, nodules and pustules on the face, neck and upper part of the trunk.

acnegenic (ak″ne-jen′ik) producing acne.

acneiform (ak-ne′ĭ-form) resembling acne.

acnitis (ak-ni′tis) a papulonecrotic tuberculid with lesions appearing on the face.

acnitrazole (ak-ni′trah-zōl) aminitrazole.

acoelomate (a-se′lo-māt)   without a coelom or body cavity.

A.C.O.G.   American College of Obstetricians and Gynecologists.

aconite (ak′o-nīt) dried tuberous root of *Aconitum napellus;* counterirritant and locally anesthetic.

aconitine (ah-kon′ĭ-tin) an alkaloid which is the active principle of aconite.

acorea (ah″ko-re′ah) absence of the pupil.

acoria (ah-ko′re-ah) insatiable appetite.

acormus (ah-kor′mus) a fetal monster with rudimentary trunk.

acouesthesia (ah-koo″es-the′ze-ah)   acoustic sensibility.

acoumeter (ah-koo′mĕ-ter)   instrument for measuring the hearing power.

acouphonia (ah-koo″o-fo′ne-ah) auscultatory percussion.

acousma (ah-koos′mah) the hearing of imaginary sounds.

acousmatagnosis (ah-koos″mat-ag-no′sis) inability to recognize sounds.

acousmatamnesia (-am-ne′ze-ah) inability to call up impressions of sounds.

acoustic (ah-koos′tik) relating to sound or hearing.

acoustics (ah-koos′tiks) the science of sound and hearing.

acoustogram (ah-koos′to-gram) the graphic tracing of the curves of sounds produced by motion of a joint.

A.C.P.   American College of Pathologists; American College of Physicians; Animal Care Panel, Inc.

acquired (ah-kwīrd′) incurred as a result of factors acting from or originating outside the organism; not inherited.

A.C.R. American College of Radiology.

acragnosia (ak″rag-no′ze-ah) lack of sensory recognition of a limb.

acral (a′kral) affecting the extremities.

acrania (ah-kra′ne-ah)   partial or complete absence of the cranium. adj., **acra′nial.**

acranius (a-kra′ne-us) fetal monster in which the cranium is absent or rudimentary.

acratia (ah-kra′she-ah) loss of strength or control; incontinence.

acridine (ak′rĭ-dēn) crystalline alkaloid, $C_{12}H_9N$, from anthracene.

acriflavine (ak″rĭ-fla′vin) deep orange, granular powder; antiseptic, germicide. **a. hydro-**

chloride, strong, reddish brown powder; wound disinfectant.

acrisia (ah-kri'se-ah) uncertainty about the nature of a disease.

acritical (a-krit″ĭ-kal) having no crisis.

acro- (ak'ro) word element [Gr.], *extreme; top; extremity.*

acroagnosis (ak″ro-ag-no'sis) acragnosia.

acroanesthesia (-an″es-the'ze-ah) anesthesia of the extremities.

acroarthritis (-ar-thri'tis) arthritis of the extremities.

acroasphyxia (-as-fik'se-ah) lack of circulation in the digits. **chronic a.,** acrocyanosis.

acroataxia (-ah-tak'se-ah) ataxia of the hands and fingers, and toes and feet.

acroblast (ak'ro-blast) the external layer of the mesoblast.

acrobrachycephaly (ak″ro-brak″e-sef'ah-le) abnormal height of the skull, with shortness of its anteroposterior dimension. adj., **acrobrachycephal'ic.**

acrobystiolith (-bis'te-o-lith″) a preputial calculus.

acrobystitis (-bis-ti'tis) inflammation of the prepuce.

acrocentric (-sen'trik) having the centromere toward one end of the replicating chromosome.

acrocephalia (-se-fa'le-ah) acrocephaly.

acrocephalic (-se-fal'ik) having a high, pointed head, with a vertical index of 77 or more.

acrocephalosyndactyly (-sef″ah-lo-sin-dak'tĭ-le) acrocephaly associated with webbing of the fingers or toes.

acrocephaly (-sef'ah-le) a high, pointed condition of the top of the skull.

acrochordon (-kor'don) pedunculated skin tag, occurring principally on neck, upper chest, and axillae in women of middle age or older.

acrocinesis (-si-ne'sis) acrokinesia.

acrocontracture (-kon-trak'tūr) contracture of an extremity.

acrocyanosis (-si″ah-no'sis) cyanosis and bluish or red discoloration of the digits.

acrodermatitis (-der″mah-ti'tis) inflammation of the skin of the hands and feet. **a. atroph'icans chron'ica, chronic atrophic a.,** chronic inflammation of the skin of the extremities, leading to atrophy of the cutis. **a. contin'ua, continuous a.,** a persistent dermatitis of the extremities due to infection or trauma, and resisting treatment. **enteropathic a.,** a familial disorder, occurring chiefly in infants, with localized eruption, and associated with disorders of the gastrointestinal tract. **Hallopeau's a.,** acrodermatitis continua.

acrodermatosis (-der″mah-to'sis) an eruption on the skin of the hands and feet.

acrodolichomelia (-dol″ĭ-ko-me'le-ah) abnormal length of hands and feet.

acrodynia (-din'e-ah) a condition characterized by extreme irritability and restlessness, with pain in the extremities and pink coloration of the hands and feet.

acroedema (-ĕ-de'mah) edema of the hand or foot.

acroesthesia (-es-the'ze-ah) 1. exaggerated sensitiveness. 2. pain in the extremities.

acrogeria (ak″ro-je're-ah) premature aging of the skin of the hands and feet.

acrognosis (ak″rog-no'sis) sensory recognition of a limb.

acrohyperhidrosis (ak″ro-hi″per-hĭ-dro'sis) excessive sweating of hands and feet.

acrohypothermy (-hi′po-ther″me) abnormal coldness of hands and feet.

acrokeratosis (-ker″ah-to'sis) a condition involving the skin of the extremities, with the appearance of horny growths.

acrokinesia (-ki-ne'se-ah) abnormal motility or movement of the extremities. adj., **acrokinet'ic.**

acrolein (ak-ro'le-in) a volatile liquid, C_3H_4O, from decomposition of glycerin.

acromacria (ak″ro-mak're-ah) acromegaly.

acromania (-ma'ne-ah) mania characterized by great motor activity.

acromastitis (-mas-ti'tis) thelitis.

acromegaly (-meg'ah-le) abnormal enlargement of facial features, hands and feet.

acromelalgia (-mel-al'je-ah) erythromelalgia.

acrometagenesis (-met″ah-jen'ĕ-sis) undue growth of the extremities.

acromicria (-mi'kre-ah) abnormal smallness of facial features, hands and feet.

acromio- (ah-kro'me-o) word element [Gr.], *acromion.*

acromioclavicular (ah-kro″me-o-klah-vik'u-lar) pertaining to acromion and clavicle.

acromiohumeral (-hu'mer-al) pertaining to acromion and humerus.

acromion (ah-kro'me-on) lateral extension of the spine of the scapula, forming the highest point of the shoulder. adj., **acro'mial.**

acromionectomy (ah-kro″me-on-ek'to-me) resection of the acromion.

acromiothoracic (ah-kro″me-o-tho-ras'ik) pertaining to acromion and thorax.

acromphalus (ah-krom'fah-lus) 1. bulging of the navel as the first stage of umbilical hernia. 2. the center of the navel.

acromyotonia (ak″ro-mi″o-to'ne-ah) myotonia of the extremities.

acronarcotic (-nar-kot'ik) acrid and narcotic.

acroneuropathy (-nu-rop'ah-the) a familial neuropathy affecting the distal parts of the extremities and producing anesthetic ulcers.

acroneurosis (-nu-ro'sis) any neurosis involving the extremities.

acronym (ak'ro-nim) a word formed by the initial letters of the principal components of a compound term, as *ACTH* from *Adreno-Corticotrophic Hormone.*

acronyx (ak'ro-niks) an ingrowing nail.

acro-osteolysis (ak″ro-os″te-ol'ĭ-sis) osteolysis involving the distal phalanges of fingers and toes.

acropachy (ak'ro-pak″e) clubbing of the fingers and toes.

acropachyderma (ak″ro-pak″e-der'mah) thickening of the skin over the face, scalp and extremities, together with deformities of the long bones.

acroparalysis (-pah-ral'ĭ-sis) paralysis of the extremities.

acroparesthesia (ak″ro-par″es-the′ze-ah) an abnormal sensation, such as tingling, numbness, pins and needles, in the digits.

acropathology (-pah-thol′o-je) pathology of the extremities.

acropathy (ak-rop′ah-the) any disease of the extremities.

acrophobia (ak″ro-fo′be-ah) morbid fear of heights.

acroposthitis (-pos-thi′tis) inflammation of the prepuce.

acroscleroderma (-skle″ro-der′mah) scleroderma of the fingers and toes.

acrosclerosis (-skle-ro′sis) scleroderma involving extremities and distal portions of head and face, accompanied by Raynaud's phenomenon.

acrose (ak′rōs) a sugar produced by the action of weak alkali on formaldehyde.

acrosome (ak′ro-sōm) the caplike investment of the anterior half of the head of a spermatozoon.

acrosphacelus (ak″ro-sfas′ĕ-lus) gangrene of the digits.

acrotism (ak′ro-tizm) defect or failure of the pulse. adj., **acrot′ic**.

acrotrophoneurosis (ak″ro-trof″o-nu-ro′sis) trophoneurotic disturbance of the extremities.

A.C.S. American Cancer Society; American Chemical Society; American College of Surgeons.

A.C.S.M. American College of Sports Medicine.

ACTH adrenocorticotropic hormone.

Actidil (ak′tī-dil) trademark for preparations of triprolidine.

actin (ak′tin) a protein occurring in filaments in muscle which, acting along with myosin particles, is responsible for the contraction and relaxation of muscle.

actinic (ak-tin′ik) producing chemical action; said of rays of light beyond the violet end of the spectrum.

actinism (ak′tī-nizm) the chemical property of light rays.

actinium (ak-tin′e-um) a chemical element (*see table*), at. no. 89, symbol Ac.

actino- (ak′tī-no)- word element [Gr.], *ray; radiation*.

actinobacillosis (ak″tī-no-bas″ī-lo′sis) infection due to actinobacilli.

Actinobacillus (-bah-sil′us) a genus of Schizomycetes (order Eubacteriales, family Brucellaceae) capable of infecting cattle, but rarely man. **A. ligniere′sii**, the causative agent of an actinomycosis-like disease of cattle and other domestic animals.

actinochemistry (-kem′is-tre) the chemistry of radiant energy.

actinocutitis (-ku-ti′tis) actinodermatitis.

actinodermatitis (-der″mah-ti′tis) dermatitis from exposure to actinic radiation.

actinogen (ak-tin′o-jen) any radioactive substance.

actinogenesis (ak″tī-no-jen′ĕ-sis) the formation or production of actinic rays.

actinogenic (-jen′ik) producing rays, especially actinic rays.

actinology (ak″tī-nol′o-je) 1. the study of radiant energy. 2. the science of the chemical effects of light.

actinolyte (ak-tin′o-līt) apparatus for concentrating the rays of electric light in phototherapy.

actinometer (ak″tī-nom′ĕ-ter) instrument for measuring the penetrating power of x-rays.

Actinomyces (ak″tī-no-mi′sēz) a genus of Schizomycetes (order Actinomycetales, family Actinomycetaceae). **A. bo′vis**, a gram-positive microorganism causing actinomycosis in cattle.

actinomyces (-mi′sēz) an organism of the genus Actinomyces. adj., **actinomycet′ic**.

Actinomycetaceae (-mi″se-ta′se-e) a family of Schizomycetes (order Actinomycetales), divided into two genera: Nocardia (aerobic forms) and Actinomyces (anaerobic forms).

Actinomycetales (-mi″se-ta′lēz) an order of Schizomycetes (families Actinomycetaceae, Actinoplanaceae, Mycobacteriaceae and Streptomycetaceae).

actinomycete (-mi′sēt) a moldlike microorganism occurring as elongated, frequently filamentous cells, with a branching tendency. adj., **actinomycet′ic**.

actinomycin (-mi′sin) an antibiotic from *Streptomyces antibioticus*.

actinomycoma (-mi-ko′mah) a tumor formed in actinomycosis.

actinomycosis (-mi-ko′sis) infection due to Actinomyces. adj., **actinomycot′ic**.

actinon (ak′tī-non) a radioactive isotope of radon, symbol An.

actinoneuritis (ak″tī-no-nu-ri′tis) neuritis caused by actinic radiation.

Actinoplanaceae (-plah-na′se-e) a family of Schizomycetes (order Actinomycetales).

Actinoplanes (-pla′nēz) a genus of Schizomycetes (order Actinomycetales, family Actinoplanaceae).

actinotherapy (-ther′ah-pe) treatment of disease by actinic radiation.

actinotoxemia (-toks-e′me-ah) toxemia from tissue destruction caused by actinic radiation.

actinotoxin (-tok′sin) a crude poison derived from alcoholic extracts of the tentacles of sea anemones.

action (ak′shun) the accomplishment of an effect, whether mechanical or chemical, or the effect so produced. adj., **ac′tive**. **cumulative a.**, the sudden and markedly increased action of a drug after administration of several doses. **reflex a.**, involuntary response to a stimulus conveyed to the nervous system and reflected to the periphery, passing below the level of consciousness. **specific dynamic a.**, specific chemical stimulation of cellular protoplasm produced by protein food independent of oxidation of the protein in the body.

activator (ak″tī-va′tor) a substance that makes another substance active or that renders an inactive enzyme capable of exerting its proper effect. **plasminogen a.**, a substance that activates plasminogen and converts it into plasmin. **tissue a.**, fibrinokinase.

activity (ak-tiv′ĭ-te) the quality or process of exerting energy or of accomplishing an effect.

displacement a., irrelevant activity produced by an excess of one of two conflicting drives in a person. **enzyme a.**, the catalytic effect exerted by an enzyme, expressed as units per milligram of enzyme (*specific activity*) or molecules of substrate transformed per minute per molecule of enzyme (*molecular activity*). **optical a.**, the ability of a chemical compound to rotate the plane of polarization of plane-polarized light.

actomyosin (ak″to-mi′o-sin) the system of actin filaments and myosin particles constituting muscle fibers and responsible for the contraction and relaxation of muscle.

acufilopressure (ak″u-fi′lo-presh″er) a combination of acupressure and ligation.

acumeter (ah-koo′mē-ter) acoumeter.

acuminate (ah-ku′mi-nāt) sharp-pointed.

acupressure (ak″u-presh′er) compression of a blood vessel by inserted needles.

acupuncture (-punk′tūr) therapeutic insertion of needles.

aous (a′kus) a needle or needle-like process.

acute (ah-kūt′) 1. sharp. 2. having severe symptoms and a short course.

acutenaculum (ak″u-tē-nak′u-lum) a needle holder.

acutorsion (-tor′shun) acupressure with twisting of a bleeding vessel.

acyanoblepsia (ah-si″ah-no-blep′se-ah) inability to distinguish blue tints.

acyanopsia (ah-si″ah-nop′se-ah) acyanoblepsia.

acyanotic (ah-si″ah-not′ik) not characterized or accompanied by cyanosis.

acyesis (ah″si-e′sis) 1. sterility in woman. 2. absence of pregnancy.

Acylanid (as″il-an′id) trademark for a preparation derived from a digitalis glycoside, lanatoside A.

acystia (a-sis′te-ah) congenital absence of bladder.

acystinervia (ah-sis″tī-ner′ve-ah) paralysis of bladder.

Acystosporidia (ah-sis″to-spo-rid′e-ah) an order of parasites related to Haemosporidia.

A.D. [L.] *au′ris dex′tra* (right ear).

ad [L.] preposition, *to*.

ad, [L.] adde *(add)*.

A.D.A. American Dental Association; American Diabetes Association; American Dietetics Association.

adactylia (a″dak-til′e-ah) congenital absence of fingers or toes. adj., **adac′tylous.**

adamantine (ad″ah-man′tin) pertaining to the enamel of the teeth.

adamantinoma (ad″ah-man″tī-no′mah) ameloblastoma.

adamantoblast (ad″ah-man′to-blast) an enamel cell.

adamantoblastoma (ad″ah-man″to-blas-to′-mah) ameloblastoma.

adamantoma (ad″ah-man-to′mah) ameloblastoma.

adaptation (ad″ap-ta′shun) adjustment, especially of the pupil to light, or of an organism to environmental conditions. **color a.**, 1. changes in visual perception of color with prolonged stimulation. 2. adjustment of vision to degree of brightness or color tone of illumination. **dark a.**, adaptation of the eye to vision in the dark or in reduced illumination.

adapter (ah-dap′ter) a device for connecting parts of surgical instruments or other apparatus.

adaptometer (ad″ap-tom′ĕ-ter) an instrument for measuring the time required for pupillary adaptation. **color a.**, an instrument to demonstrate adaptation of the eye to color or light.

adatom (ad′at-om) an atom that is adsorbed on a surface.

addict (ad′dikt) a person exhibiting addiction.

addiction (ah-dik′shun) physiologic or psychologic dependence on some agent (e.g. alcohol, drug), with a tendency to increase its use.

addictologist (ad″dik-tol′o-jist) a physician specializing in the study and treatment of addiction.

addisonism (ad′ĭ-son-izm″) symptoms seen in pulmonary tuberculosis, resembling Addison's disease.

adduct (ad-dukt′) to draw toward a center or median line.

adduction (ad-duk′shun) the act of adducting; the state of being adducted.

adductor (ad-duk′tor) that which adducts.

adelomorphous (ah-del″o-mor′fus) of indefinite form.

adelphotaxy (ah-del′fo-tak″se) assumption by cells of a definite arrangement.

Ademol (ad′e-mol) trademark for a preparation of flumethiazide.

adenalgia (ad″ĕ-nal′je-ah) pain in a gland.

adenase (ad′ĕ-nās) an enzyme found in spleen, pancreas and liver.

adenasthenia (ad″en-as-the′ne-ah) deficient glandular activity. **a. gas′trica,** deficient glandular secretion in the stomach.

adendric (ah-den′drik) without dendrons.

adenectomy (ad″ĕ-nek′to-me) excision of a gland.

adenectopia (ad″ĕ-nek-to′pe-ah) displacement of a gland.

adenemphraxis (ad″e-nem-frak′sis) obstruction of the duct of a gland.

adenia (a-de′ne-ah) lymphoma.

adeniform (ah-den′i-form) gland-shaped.

adenine (ad′ĕ-nīn) a white, crystalline base, $C_5H_5N_5$, found in plant and animal tissues; one of the decomposition products of nuclein.

adenitis (ad″ĕ-ni′tis) inflammation of a gland.

adenization (ad″ĕ-ni-za′shun) assumption of an abnormal glandlike appearance.

adeno- (ad′ĕ-no) word element [Gr.], *gland*.

adenoacanthoma (ad″e-no-ak″an-tho′mah) adenocarcinoma.

adenoameloblastoma (-ah-mel″o-blas-to′mah) ameloblastoma with formation of ductlike structures in place of or in addition to the typical odontogenic pattern.

adenoangiosarcoma (-an″je-o-sar-ko′mah) an angiosarcoma with glandular elements.

adenoblast (ad′ĕ-no-blast″) 1. a gland cell, secretory or excretory. 2. embryonic forerunner of gland tissue.

adenocancroid (ad″ĕ-no-kang′kroid) adenocarcinoma.

adenocarcinoma (ad″ĕ-no-kar″sĭ-no′mah) carcinoma with glandular elements; malignant carcinoma.

adenocele (ad′ĕ-no-sēl″) a cystic adenomatous tumor.

adenocellulitis (ad″ĕ-no-sel″u-li′tis) inflammation of a gland and the cellular tissue around it.

adenochondroma (-kon-dro′mah) adenoma blended with chondroma.

adenocyst (ad′ĕ-no-sist″) adenocystoma.

adenocystoma (ad″ĕ-no-sis-to′mah) adenoma blended with cystoma.

adenocyte (ad′ĕ-no-sīt″) a mature secretory cell of a gland.

adenodynia (ad″ĕ-no-din′e-ah) pain in a gland.

adenoepithelioma (-ep″ĭ-the″le-o′mah) a tumor composed of glandular and epithelial elements.

adenofibroma (-fi-bro′mah) adenoma blended with fibroma.

adenogenous (ad″ĕ-noj′ĕ-nus) originating from glandular tissue.

adenography (ad″ĕ-nog′rah-fe) anatomy, physiology, histology and pathology of glands.

adenohypersthenia (ad″ĕ-no-hi″per-sthe′ne-ah) excessive glandular activity.

adenohypophysis (-hi-pof′ĭ-sis) the anterior or glandular portion of the hypophysis cerebri.

adenoid (ad′ĕ-noid) 1. resembling a gland. 2. a hypertrophic mass of glandular tissue in the nasopharynx of children.

adenoidectomy (ad″ĕ-noid-ek′to-me) excision of adenoids.

adenoiditis (-i′tis) inflammation of an adenoid.

adenolipoma (ad″ĕ-no-lĭ-po′mah) a mixed adenoma and lipoma.

adenolipomatosis (-lip″o-mah-to′sis) the formation of numerous adenolipomas in the neck, axilla and groin.

adenology (ad″ĕ-nol′o-je) study or knowledge regarding glands.

adenolymphitis (ad″ĕ-no-lim-fi′tis) lymphadenitis.

adenolymphocele (-lim′fo-sēl) cyst of a lymph node.

adenolymphoma (-lim-fo′mah) adenoma of a lymph node.

adenoma (ad″ĕ-no′mah) an epithelial tumor composed of glandular tissue. **basophilic a.**, tumor of the basophilic cells of the anterior pituitary body. **chromophobe a.**, tumor of the chromophobe cells of the anterior pituitary body. **a. des′truens**, adenocarcinoma. **eosinophil a.**, tumor of the eosinophilic cells of the anterior pituitary body. **malignant a.**, adenocarcinoma. **a. seba′ceum**, a yellowish tumor on the face, containing a mass of yellowish glands. **a. sim′plex**, glandular hyperplasia.

adenomalacia (ad″ĕ-no-mah-la′she-ah) undue softness of a gland.

adenomatoid (ad″ĕ-no′mah-toid) resembling adenoma.

adenomatome (ad″e-no′mah-tōm) a scissors for removing adenoids.

adenomatosis (ad″ĕ-no″mah-to′sis) the formation of adenomas in glandular tissue.

adenomatous (ad″ĕ-no′mah-tus) pertaining to or resembling adenoma.

adenomere (ad′ĕ-no-mēr) the blind terminal portion of the glandular cavity of a developing gland, being the functional portion of the organ.

adenomyofibroma (ad″ĕ-no-mi″o-fi-bro′mah) a fibroma containing both glandular and muscular elements.

adenomyoma (-mi-o′mah) 1. adenomyosis. 2. a tumor made up of endometrium and muscle tissue, found in the uterus or uterine ligaments.

adenomyomatosis (-mi″o-mah-to′sis) the presence of multiple adenomyomas.

adenomyometritis (-mē-tri′tis) endometriosis.

adenomyosarcoma (-sar-ko′mah) adenosarcoma containing striated muscle.

adenomyosis (-mi-o′sis) invasion of the muscular wall of an organ (e.g. stomach, uterus) by glandular tissue.

adenomyositis (-mi″o-si′tis) endometriosis.

adenomyxoma (-mik-so′mah) a tumor composed of glandular and mucous tissue.

adenomyxosarcoma (-mik″so-sar-ko′mah) a sarcoma containing glandular elements.

adenoncus (ad″ĕ-nong′kus) a tumor or enlargement of a gland.

adenoneure (ad′ĕ-no-nūr″) a neuron controlling glandular action.

adenopathy (ad″ĕ-nop′ah-the) any disease of glands.

adenopharyngitis (ad″ĕ-no-far″in-ji′tis) inflammation of tonsils and pharynx.

adenophlegmon (-fleg′mon) phlegmonous inflammation of glands.

adenophthalmia (ad″ĕ-nof-thal′me-ah) inflammation of the meibomian glands.

adenosarcoma (ad″ĕ-no-sar-ko′mah) adenoma blended with sarcoma.

adenosarcorhabdomyoma (-sar″ko-rab″do-mi-o′mah) blended adenoma, sarcoma and rhabdomyoma.

adenosclerosis (-skle-ro′sis) hardening of a gland.

adenosine (ah-den′o-sēn) a nucleotide containing adenine, a pentose sugar and phosphoric acid. **a. diphosphate**, a compound containing two phosphoric acids, formed by hydrolysis of adenosine triphosphate, with release of one high-energy bond. **a. monophosphate**, adenosine containing only one phosphoric acid. **a. triphosphate**, a compound containing three phosphoric acids, with one low- and two high-energy bonds.

adenosis (ad″ĕ-no′sis) any disease of a gland.

adenotome (ad′ĕ-no-tōm″) an instrument for incising glands.

adenotomy (ad″ĕ-not′o-me) 1. anatomy of the glands. 2. incision of a gland.

adenotonsillectomy (ad″ĕ-no-ton″sil-lek′to-me) removal of the tonsils and adenoids.

adenotyphus (-ti′fus) typhus fever with lesions chiefly in the mesenteric glands.

adenovirus (-vi′rus) a virus causing infection of the upper respiratory tract, less virulent than the viruses causing influenza.

adermia (ah-der′me-ah) defect or absence of the skin.

adermogenesis (ah-der″mo-jen′ĕ-sis) imperfect development of skin.

ADH antidiuretic hormone.

adhesion (ad-he′zhun) 1. abnormal joining of parts to each other. 2. a structure by which parts abnormally cohere. **primary a.**, healing by first intention. **secondary a.**, healing by second intention.

adhesiotomy (ad-he″ze-ot′o-me) surgical division of adhesions.

A.D.I. American Documentation Institute.

adiactinic (a″di-ak-tin′ik) impervious to actinic rays.

adiadochokinesia (ah-di″ah-do″ko-ki-ne′ze-ah) inability to perform fine, rapidly repeated, coordinated movements.

adiaphoresis (ah-di″ah-fo-re′sis) deficiency of perspiration.

adiaphoria (ah-di″ah-fo′re-ah) nonresponse to stimuli as a result of previous similar stimuli.

adiapneustia (ah-di″ap-nūs′te-ah) defect or absence of perspiration.

adiastole (a-di-as′to-le) absence of diastole.

adiathermancy (ah-di″ah-ther′man-se) imperviousness to heat rays.

adicity (ah-dis′ĭ-te) valence.

adipectomy (ad″ĭ-pek′to-me) excision of adipose tissue.

adiphenine (ad″ĭ-fen′ēn) a drug used as a parasympathetic blocker or an antispasmodic.

adipic (ah-dip′ik) pertaining to fat.

adip(o)- (ad′ĭ po) word element [L.], *fat.*

adipocele (ad′ĭ-po-sēl″) a hernia containing fat.

adipocellular (ad″ĭ-po-sel′u-ler) composed of fat and connective tissue.

adipocere (ad′ĭ-po-sēr″) a waxy substance from bodies long dead.

adipofibroma (ad″ĭ-po-fi-bro′mah) a fibrous tumor with fatty elements.

adipogenous (ad″ĭ-poj′ĕ-nus) producing fat.

adipoid (ad′ĭ-poid) lipoid.

adipokinesis (ad″ĭ-po-ki-ne′sis) the mobilization of fat in the body. adj., **adipokinet′ic.**

adipokinin (-ki′nin) a factor from the anterior pituitary which accelerates mobilization of stored fat.

adipolysis (ad″ĭ-pol′ĭ-sis) the digestion of fats. adj., **adipolyt′ic.**

adipoma (ad″ĭ-po′mah) lipoma.

adiponecrosis (ad″ĭ-po-ne-kro′sis) necrosis of fatty tissue. **a. neonato′rum, a. subcuta′nea,** alteration of subcutaneous fat, thought to be caused by obstetric trauma, in newborn infants.

adipopexis (-pek′sis) the fixation or storing of fat. adj., **adipopec′tic.**

adipose (ad′ĭ-pōs) fatty.

adiposis (ad″ĭ-po′sis) a condition marked by deposits or degeneration of fatty tissue. **a. cerebra′lis,** fatness from cerebral pituitary disease. **a. doloro′sa,** a painful condition due to pressure on nerves caused by fatty deposits. **a. hepat′ica,** fatty degeneration of liver. **a. tubero′sa,** adiposis dolorosa in which the fatty degeneration occurs in nodular masses.

adipositis (ad″ĭ-po-si′tis) inflammation of adipose tissue.

adiposity (ad″ĭ-pos′ĭ-te) obesity.

adiposuria (ad″ĭ-po-su′re-ah) the occurrence of fat in the urine.

adipsia (a-dip′se-ah) abnormal avoidance of drinking.

aditus (ad′ĭ-tus), pl. *ad′itus* [L.] an entrance or opening; used in anatomic nomenclature for various passages in the body.

adjuvant (ad′joo-vant) 1. assisting or aiding. 2. a substance which aids another, such as an auxiliary remedy.

adnerval (ad-ner′val) adneural.

adneural (ad-nu′ral) toward a nerve.

adnexa (ad-nek′sah) [L., pl.] appendages; accessory organs, as of the eye *(adnex′a oc′-uli) or uterus (adnex′a u′teri).* adj., **adnex′al.**

adnexogenesis (ad-nek″so-jen′ĕ-sis) the embryonic development of the adnexa.

adnexopexy (-pek′se) surgical fixation of the oviduct and ovary.

adolescence (ad″o-les′ens) the period between the onset of puberty and beginning adulthood. adj., **adoles′cent.**

adoral (ad-o′ral) 1. situated near the mouth. 2. directed toward the mouth.

ADP adenosine diphosphate.

adren(o)- word element [L.], *adrenal gland.*

adrenal (ah-dre′nal) 1. near the kidney. 2. an adrenal gland.

adrenalectomy (ah-dre″nah-lek′to-me) excision of an adrenal gland.

Adrenalin (ah-dren′ah-lin) trademark for epinephrine.

adrenalinemia (-e′me-ah) presence of epinephrine in the blood.

adrenalinuria (-u′re-ah) presence of epinephrine in the urine.

adrenalism (ah-dren′ah-lizm) ill health due to adrenal dysfunction.

adrenalitis (ah-dre″nal-i′tis) inflammation of the adrenal glands.

adrenergic (ad″ren-er′jik) activated or transmitted by epinephrine; said of nerve fibers that liberate sympathin at a synapse when a nerve impulse passes, i.e. the sympathetic fibers.

adrenic (ah-dren′ik) pertaining to adrenal glands.

adrenocorticomimetic (ah-dre″no-kor″tĭ-ko-mi-met′ik) having effects similar to those of secretions of the adrenal cortex or its hormones.

adrenocorticotrophic (-trof′ik) adrenocorticotropic.

adrenocorticotrophin (-trof′in) adrenocorticotropin.

adrenocorticotropic (-trōp′ik) having a stimulating effect on the adrenal cortex.

adrenocorticotropin (-trōp′in) a substance which has a stimulating effect on the adrenal cortex, isolated from the anterior pituitary gland.

adrenoglomerulotropin (-glo-mer″u-lo-tro′pin) a hormone that stimulates production of aldosterone by the adrenal cortex.

adrenolytic (-lit′ik) antagonizing the action of epinephrine or of the adrenal gland.

adrenomegaly (-meg′ah-le) abnormal enlargement of the adrenal gland.

adrenopathy (ad″ren-op′ah-the) any disease of the adrenal glands.

Adrenosem (ah-dren′o-sem) trademark for preparations of carbazochrome.

adrenotoxin (ah-dre″no-tok′sin) an antibody produced by injecting an animal with adrenal tissue.

adrenotropism (ad″ren-ot′ro-pizm) predominance of the adrenal glands in the endocrine constitution. adj., **adrenotrop′ic.**

Adroyd (ad′roid) trademark for a preparation of oxymetholone.

ADS antidiuretic substance (hormone).

adsorb (ad-sorb′) to attract and retain other material on the surface.

adsorbent (ad-sorb′ent) 1. pertaining to or characterized by adsorption. 2. a substance that attracts other materials or particles to its surface. **gastrointestinal a.,** a substance, usually a powder, taken to adsorb gases, toxins and bacteria in the stomach and intestines.

adsorption (ad-sorp′shun) the action of a substance in attracting and holding other materials or particles on its surface.

adtorsion (ad-tor′shun) a turning inward of both eyes.

advancement (ad-vans′ment) detachment of a muscle, and reattachment at an advanced point, as done with an eye muscle for correction of strabismus. **capsular a.,** attachment of capsule of Tenon in front of its normal position.

adventitia (ad″ven-tish′e-ah) the outer coat of an organ or structure, especially the outer coat of an artery.

adventitious (ad″ven-tish′us) not normal to a part.

adynamia (ad″i-na′me-ah) lack of vital powers. adj., **adynam′ic.**

aec- for words beginning thus, see those beginning *ec-*.

Aedes (a-e′dēz) a genus of mosquitoes, including approximately 600 species. **A. aegyp′-ti,** the mosquito which transmits the causative organisms of yellow fever and dengue.

A.E.E.G.S. American Electroencephalographic Society.

aeg- for words beginning thus, see those beginning *eg-*.

A.E.L. American Electronics Laboratories.

aerenterectasia (a″er-en″ter-ek-ta′ze-ah) distention of the intestine with air or gas.

aeriform (ār′i-form, a-er′i-form) resembling air; gaseous.

aero- (a′er-o) word element [Gr.], *air; gas.*

Aerobacter (a″er-o-bak′ter) a genus of Schizomycetes (order Eubacteriales, family Enterobacteriaceae, tribe Escherichieae) which includes two species, *A. aero′genes* and *A. cloa′cae.*

aerobe (a′er-ōb) a microorganism that lives and grows in the presence of free oxygen. adj., **aero′bic. facultative a.,** a microorganism that can live in the presence of oxygen, but does not require it. **obligate a.,** one that cannot live without oxygen.

aerobiology (a″er-o-bi-ol′o-je) the study of the distribution of living organisms (microorganisms) by the air.

aerobion (a″er-o′be-on) an aerobe.

aerobiosis (a″er-o-bi-o′sis) life requiring free oxygen.

aerocele (a′er-o-sēl″) a tumor formed by air filling an adventitious pouch. **epidural a.,** a collection of air between the dura mater and the wall of the spinal column.

aerocolia (a″er-o-ko′le-ah) aerocoly.

aerocolpos (-kol′pos) distention of the vagina with gas.

aerocoly (a″er-o′ko-le) distention of the colon with gas.

aerodermectasia (a″er-o-der″mek-ta′ze-ah) subcutaneous or surgical emphysema.

aerodontalgia (-don-tal′je-ah) pain in the teeth due to lowered atmospheric pressure at high altitudes.

aerodontics (-don′tiks) the branch of dentistry concerned with effects on the teeth of high-altitude flying.

aerodromophobia (-dro″mo-fo′be-ah) morbid dread of traveling by air.

aerodynamics (-di-nam′iks) science of air or gases in motion.

aeroembolism (-em′bo-lizm) obstruction of a blood vessel by air or gas.

aeroemphysema (-em″fĭ-ze′mah) the presence of air or gas in body tissues.

aerogastrocolia (-gas″tro-ko′le-ah) air or gas in the stomach and colon.

aerogen (a′er-o-jen″) a gas-producing bacillus.

aerogenesis (a″er-o-jen′ĕ-sis) formation or production of gas. adj., **aerogen′ic.**

aerogram (a′er-o-gram″) roentgenogram of an organ after injection with air or gas.

aerohydrotherapy (a″er-o-hi″dro-ther′ah-pe) therapeutic use of air and water.

aeromammography (-mam-mog′rah-fe) roentgenography of the space behind the mammary gland after injection of air or other gas.

aeromedicine (-med′ĭ-sin) aviation medicine.

aerometer (a″er-om′ĕ-ter) instrument for estimating gaseous density.

aeromicrobe (a″er-o-mi′krōb) an aerobic microorganism.

Aeromonas (-mo′nas) a genus of Schizomycetes (order Pseudomonadales, suborder Pseudomonadineae, family Pseudomonadaceae).

aeroneurosis (-nu-ro′sis) a functional nervous disorder occurring in aviators.

aero-otitis (-o-ti′tis) barotitis. **a. me′dia,** inflammation of the middle ear due to changes in air pressure.

aeropathy (a″er-op′ah-the) decompression sickness.

aeroperitonia (a″er-o-per″ĭ-to-ne′ah) air or gas in the peritoneal cavity.

aerophagia (-fa′je-ah) habitual swallowing of air.

aerophilous (a″er-of′ĭ-lus) requiring air for proper growth.

aerophobia (a″er-o-fo′be-ah) 1. morbid dread of drafts of air. 2. morbid dread of being up in the air.

aerophore (a′er-o-fōr″) device for inflating the lungs of stillborn infants.

aerophyte (a′er-o-fīt″) a microorganism that lives upon air.

aeropiesotherapy (a″er-o-pi-e″so-ther′ah-pe) treatment by compressed or rarefied air.

Aeroplast (a′er-o-plast″) trademark for a vibesate.

aeroplethysmograph (a″er-o-plĕ-thiz′mo-graf) apparatus for graphically recording the expired air.

aeroscope (a′er-o-skōp″) instrument for testing the purity of air.

aerosinusitis (a″er-o-si″nus-i′tis) barosinusitis.

aerosol (a′er-o-sol″) a colloid system in which solid or liquid particles are suspended in a gas, especially a suspension of a drug or other substance to be dispensed in a fine spray or mist.

aerosolization (a″er-o-sol″i-za′shun) dispersion in a fine mist.

Aerosporin (-spor′in) trademark for a preparation of polymyxin B sulfate.

aerostatics (-stat′iks) science of air or gases at rest.

aerotaxis (-tak′sis) movement of a motile organism in response to the presence of molecular oxygen.

aerotherapy (-ther′ah-pe) treatment of disease by air.

aerothermotherapy (-ther″mo-ther′ah-pe) treatment with currents of hot air.

aerothorax (-tho′raks) pneumothorax.

aerotitis (-ti′tis) barotitis. **a. me′dia**, barotitis media.

aerotonometer (-to-nom′ĕ-ter) a device used in measuring the tension of the blood gases.

A.E.S. American Encephalographic Society; American Epidemiological Society.

aes-, aet- for words beginning thus, see also those beginning *es-, et-.*

Æsculapius (es″cu-la′pe-us) the god of healing in Roman mythology.

afebrile (a-feb′rīl) without fever.

affect (af′ekt) emotional tone or feeling.

affection (ah-fek′shun) morbid condition or diseased state.

affective (ah-fek′tiv) pertaining to emotional tone or feeling.

afferent (af′er-ent) conducting toward a center or specific site of reference.

affinity (ah-fin′ĭ-te) attraction; a tendency to seek out or unite with another object or substance. **chemical a.**, the force that unites atoms of different substances. **elective a.**, the force that causes union of a substance with one substance rather than another.

afibrinogenemia (a-fi″brin-o-jĕ-ne′me-ah) lack of fibrinogen in the circulating blood.

afterbrain (af′ter-brān″) metencephalon.

after-hearing (af″ter-hēr′ing) hearing of sounds after the stimulus has ceased.

after-image (-im′ij) a retinal impression remaining after cessation of the stimulus causing it.

after-pain (af′ter-pān″) a pain which follows expulsion of the placenta.

after-perception (af″ter-per-sep′shun) perception of after-sensations.

after-sensation (-sen-sa′shun) sensation persisting after cessation of the stimulus which caused it.

after-sound (af′ter-sownd″) sensation of a sound after cessation of the stimulus causing it.

after-taste (af′ter-tāst″) sensation of taste continuing after the stimulus has ceased.

Ag chemical symbol, *silver* [L. *argentum*].

A.G.A. American Geriatrics Association.

agalactia (ag″ah-lak′she-ah) absence or failure of secretion of milk.

agammaglobulinemia (a″gam-mah-glob″u-lin-e′me-ah) absence of gamma globulin in the blood. **Swiss type a.**, a lethal form with associated alymphocytosis and aplasia of the thymus gland, first recognized in Switzerland.

agamogenesis (ag″ah-mo-jen′ĕ-sis) reproduction by asexual process.

aganglionic (a-gang″gle-on′ik) lacking ganglion cells.

aganglionosis (a-gang″gle-on-o′sis) congenital absence of parasympathetic ganglion cells.

agar (ag′ar) dried hydrophilic, colloidal substance extracted from various species of red algae.

Agarbacterium (ag″ar-bak-te′re-um) a genus of Schizomycetes (order Eubacteriales, family Achromobacteraceae) which digest agar.

agastria (ah-gas′tre-ah) absence of the stomach.

agastric (ah-gas′trik) having no stomach.

agastroneuria (ah gas″tro nu′re ah) lack of nervous tonicity in the stomach.

age (āj) the duration, or the measure of time of the existence of a person or object. **achievement a.**, the age of a person expressed as the chronologic age of a normal person showing the same proficiency in study. **chronologic a.**, the actual measure of time elapsed since a person's birth. **mental a.**, the age level of mental ability of a person as gauged by standard intelligence tests.

agenesia (ah″jĕ-ne′ze-ah) 1. imperfect development. 2. sterility or impotence.

agenesis (a-jen′ĕ-sis) absence of an organ due to nonappearance of its primordium in the embryo.

agenitalism (a-jen′ĭ-tal-izm″) a eunuch-like condition due to lack of secretion of the testes.

agenosomia (ah-jen″o-so′me-ah) imperfect development of sexual organs.

agent (a′jĕnt) a person or substance by which something is accomplished. **alkylating a.**, a compound with two or more end (alkyl) groups that combine readily with other molecules. **chelating a.**, a compound which combines with metals to form weakly dissociated complexes in which the metal is part of a ring, and used to extract certain elements from a system. **chimpanzee coryza a.**, respiratory syncytial virus. **Eaton a.**, one of the pleuropneumonia-like organisms that cause primary atypical pneumonia. **levigating a.**, material used for moistening a solid before reducing it to a powder.

ageusia (ah-gu'ze-ah) absence of the sense of taste. adj., **ageu'sic.**

agger (aj'er), pl. *ag'geres* [L.] an elevation. **a. na'si,** an elevation at the anterior free margin of the middle turbinated bone.

agglutinable (ah-gloo'tĭ-nah-bl) capable of agglutination.

agglutinant (ah-gloo'tĭ-nant) 1. acting like glue. 2. a substance which promotes union of parts.

agglutination (ah-gloo"tĭ-na'shun) collection of separate particles into clumps or masses; especially the clumping together of bacteria by the action of certain antitoxins. adj., **agglutina'tive. group a.,** agglutination of an organism by an agglutinin specific for other organisms. **platelet a.,** clumping together of platelets due to action of antiplatelet agglutinins.

agglutinator (ah-gloo'tĭ-na"tor) an agglutinin.

agglutinin (ah-gloo'tĭ-nin) an antibody in serum which, when combined with its homologous antigen, causes the antigen elements to adhere to one another in clumps. **anti-Rh a.,** an agglutinin not normally present in human plasma, which may be produced in Rh-negative mothers carrying an Rh-positive fetus, or after transfusion of Rh-positive blood into an Rh-negative patient. **chief a.,** the specific immune agglutinin in the blood of an animal immunized against a disease or microorganism. **cold a.,** one which acts only at low temperature. **group a.,** one which has a specific action on certain organisms, but will agglutinate other species as well. **H. a.,** one produced by the motile strain of an organism. **immune a.,** a specific agglutinin found in the blood after recovery from the disease or injection of the microorganism. **incomplete a.,** one that is capable of uniting with only one antigenic site; called also *blocking antibody.* **leukocyte a.,** one that is directed against neutrophilic and other leukocytes. **major a.,** chief agglutinin. **minor a.,** partial agglutinin. **normal a.,** a specific agglutinin found in the blood of an animal or of man that has neither had the disease nor been injected with the causative organism. **O a.,** one produced by the nonmotile strain of an organism. **partial a.,** one present in agglutinative serum which acts on organisms closely related to the specific antigen, but in a lower dilution. **platelet a.,** one that is directed against platelets. **warm a.,** an incomplete antibody that sensitizes and reacts optimally with erythrocytes at 37°C.

agglutinogen (ag"loo-tin'o-jen) the substance in bacteria which stimulates the animal body to form agglutinin.

agglutinogenic (ah-gloo"tĭ-no-jen'ik) causing the formation of agglutinins.

agglutinoid (ah-gloo'tĭ-noid) an agglutinin in which the zymotoxic group is weakened or destroyed.

agglutinophilic (ah-gloo"tĭ-no-fil'ik) agglutinating easily.

agglutinophore (ah-gloo'tĭ-no-fōr") that part of an agglutinin which causes agglutination.

agglutinum (ah-gloo'tĭ-num) the agglutinable part of a bacillus.

aggregation (ag-re-ga'shun) 1. massing or clumping of materials together. 2. a clumped mass of material. **familial a.,** the occurrence of more cases of a given disorder in close relatives of a person with the disorder than in control families. **platelet a.,** a clumping together of platelets; also called *platelet clumping.*

aglaucopsia (ah"glaw-kop'se-ah) inability to distinguish green tints.

aglobulia (ah"glo-bu'le-ah) decrease in the proportion of blood corpuscles.

aglossia (ah-glos'e-ah) congenital absence of the tongue.

aglossostomia (ah"glos-o-sto'me-ah) developmental anomaly with absence of the tongue and the mouth opening.

aglucone (a-gloo'kōn) aglycone.

aglutition (ag"loo-tish'un) inability to swallow.

aglycemia (a"gli-se'me-ah) absence of sugar from the blood.

aglycone (a-gli'kōn) the noncarbohydrate portion of a glycoside molecule.

aglycosuric (ah-gli"ko-su'rik) free from glycosuria.

agmatology (ag"mah-tol'o-je) the sum of what is known about fractures.

agnathia (ag-na'the-ah) congenital absence of the lower jaw.

agnathus (ag'nah-thus) a fetal monster exhibiting agnathia.

agnogenic (ag"no-jen'ik) of unknown origin.

agnosia (ag-no'ze-ah) inability to recognize the import of sensory impressions. **acoustic a., auditory a.,** inability to recognize the significance of sounds. **finger a.,** loss of ability to indicate one's own or another's fingers. **tactile a.,** inability to recognize familiar objects by touch or feel. **time a.,** loss of comprehension of the succession and duration of events. **visual a.,** inability to recognize familiar objects by sight.

-agogue word element [Gr.], *something which leads or induces.*

agomphiasis (ah"gom-fi'ah-sis) loose state of the teeth.

agonad (ah-go'nad) an individual having no sex glands.

agonadal (ah-gon'ah-dal) having no sex glands; due to absence of sex glands.

agonal (ag'ŏ-nal) pertaining to death or extreme suffering.

agonist (ag'o-nist) a muscle which in moving a part is resisted by a muscle which relaxes.

agony (ag'o-ne) 1. death struggle. 2. extreme suffering.

agoraphobia (ag"o-rah-fo'be-ah) 1. morbid dread of open spaces. 2. dread of crowds of people.

-agra (ag'rah) word element [Gr.], *attack; seizure.*

agrammatism (a-gram'ah-tizm) inability to speak grammatically due to a disorder of the language center of the brain.

agranulocyte (a-gran'u-lo-sīt") a nongranular leukocyte.

agranulocytosis (a-gran″u-lo-si-to′sis) reduction in the number of granulocytes in peripheral blood, with sore throat, chills and fever, and necrotic ulceration of mucous membranes.

agranuloplastic (-plas′tik) able to form nongranular cells.

agranulosis (a-gran″u-lo′sis) agranulocytosis.

agraphia (a-graf′e-ah) loss of ability to express thoughts in writing. adj., **agraph′ic.**

agria (ag′re-ah) an obstinate pustular eruption.

Agrobacterium (ag″ro-bak-te′re-um) a genus of Schizomycetes (order Eubacteriales, family Rhizobiaceae) found in soil or in the roots or stems of plants.

A.G.S. American Geriatrics Society.

ague (a′gu) malaria.

A.H.A. American Heart Association; American Hospital Association.

AHG antihemophilic globulin (blood coagulation factor VIII).

A.H.P. Assistant House Physician.

A.H.S. Assistant House Surgeon

ahypnia (ah-hip′ne-ah) sleeplessness; insomnia.

A.I. artificial insemination.

A.I.C. Association des Infirmières Canadiennes.

aichmophobia (āk″mo-fo′be-ah) morbid dread of pointed instruments.

A.I.D. artificial insemination (donor semen).

A.I.H. American Institute of Homeopathy; artificial insemination (husband's semen)

A.I.H.A. American Industrial Hygiene Association.

ailurophobia (i-lu″ro fo′bc-ah) morbid fear of cats.

A.I.N. American Institute of Nutrition.

ainhum (ān′hum) a condition of unknown origin, occurring chiefly in dark-skinned races, leading to spontaneous amputation of the fourth or fifth toe.

air (ār) the gaseous mixture which makes up the atmosphere. **complemental a.,** the volume of air, in excess of normal, which can be taken into the lungs by forced inspiration. **factitious a.,** nitrous oxide. **reserve a.,** supplemental air **residual a.,** the volume of air remaining in the lungs after forced expiration. **supplemental a.,** the volume of air, in excess of normal, which can be expelled from the lungs by forced expiration. **tidal a.,** the volume of air inhaled and exhaled in quiet breathing.

airway (ār′wa) 1. the passage by which air enters and leaves the lungs. 2. a tube for securing unobstructed respiration during general anesthesia.

akaryocyte (ah-kar′e-o-sīt″) erythrocyte.

akatamathesia (ah-kat″ah-mah-the′ze-ah) inability to understand.

akathisia (ak″ah-the′ze-ah) a condition marked by motor restlessness and anxiety.

akinesia (a″ki-ne′ze-ah) abnormal absence or reduction of muscular movement. **a. al′-gera,** paralysis due to the intense pain of muscular movement.

akinesthesia (ah-kin″es-the′ze-ah) absence of movement sense.

Akineton (a″ki-ne′ton) trademark for preparations of biperiden.

Al chemical symbol, *aluminum.*

A.L.A. American Laryngological Association.

ala (a′lah), pl. *a′lae* [L.] a winglike process. adj., **a′late. a. mag′na,** the great wing of the sphenoid bone. **a. na′si,** the cartilaginous flap on the outer side of either nostril. **a. par′va,** the lesser wing of the sphenoid.

alalia (ah-la′le-ah) impairment of the ability to speak.

alanine (al′ah-nēn, al′ah-nin) a naturally occurring amino acid, $CH_3CH(NH_2)COOH$.

alar (a′lar) 1. pertaining to or like a wing. 2. pertaining to the axilla.

alastrim (ah-las′trim) a contagious eruptive fever resembling smallpox.

alba (al′bah) [L.] white.

Albamycin (al′bah-mi″sin) trademark for preparations of novobiocin.

albation (al-ba′shun) the act of bleaching or rendering white.

albedo (al-be′do) [L.] whiteness. **a. ret′inae,** paleness of the retina due to edema caused by transudation of fluid from the retinal capillaries.

albicans (al′bĭ-kans) [L.] white.

albinism (al′bĭ-nizm) congenital absence of normal pigmentation in the body (hair, skin, eyes).

albino (al-bi′no) a person affected with albinism,

albinuria (al″bĭ-nu′re-ah) whiteness of the urine.

albocinereous (al″bo-sĭ-ne′re-us) containing both white and gray matter.

albuginea (al″bu-jin′e-ah) 1. a tough, whitish layer of fibrous tissue investing a part or organ. 2. the tunica albuginea. **a. oc′uli,** sclera. **a. ova′rii,** the outer layer of the ovarian stroma. **a. pe′nis,** the outer envelope of the corpora cavernosa.

albumen (al-bu′men) albumin.

albumin (al-bu′min) one of a class of simple proteins which are soluble in water, coagulated by heat, and precipitated from solution on saturation with ammonium sulfate. **acid a.,** albumin altered by action of acid. **alkali a.,** albumin which has been treated with alkali. **circulating a.,** that found in the body fluids. **derived a.,** albumin altered by action of chemicals **egg a.,** the white of eggs. **iodinated serum a.,** radio-iodinated serum albumin. **native a.,** any normal albumin of the organism. **normal human serum a.,** a sterile solution of the serum albumin constituent from healthy donors. **radio-iodinated serum a.,** normal human serum albumin treated with iodine-131, used for measuring blood volume and cardiac output. **serum a.,** albumin of the blood. **a. tannate,** a yellowish astringent powder used in diarrhea in children. **vegetable a.,** albumin of vegetable tissue.

albuminate (al-bu′mĭ-nāt) a compound of albumin with a base.

albuminaturia (al-bu″mĭ-nah-tu′re-ah) excess of albuminates in the urine.

albuminemia (al-bu″mĭ-ne′me-ah) excess of albumin in the blood.

albuminiferous (-nif′er-us) yielding albumin.

albuminimeter (-nim′ĕ-ter) instrument for determining the proportion of albumin present.

albuminiparous (-nip′ah-rus) producing albumin.

albuminocholia (-no-ko′le-ah) presence of protein in the bile.

albuminogenous (al″bu-mĭ-noj′ĕ-nus) producing albumin.

albuminoid (al-bu′mĭ-noid) 1. resembling albumin. 2. an albumin-like substance; the term is sometimes applied to scleroproteins.

albuminolysin (al-bu″mĭ-nol′ĭ-sin) a lysin which splits up albumins.

albuminolysis (-nol′ĭ-sis) the splitting up of albumins.

albuminometer (-nom′ĕ-ter) a laboratory device for quantitative determination of albumin in a fluid, such as urine.

albuminoptysis (-nop′tĭ-sis) albumin in the sputum.

albuminorrhea (al-bu″mĭ-no-re′ah) excessive excretion of albumins.

albuminose (al-bu′mĭ-nōs) albumose.

albuminosis (al-bu″mĭ-no′sis) abnormal excess of albuminous elements.

albuminous (al-bu′mĭ-nus) charged with or resembling albumin.

albuminuretic (al-bu″min-u-ret′ik) 1. producing albuminuria. 2. a drug which produces albuminuria.

albuminuria (al-bu″mĭ-nu′re-ah) presence in the urine of serum albumin (protein) or serum globulin. **adventitious a.**, that not due to renal disease. **cardiac a.**, that caused by valvular disease. **false a.**, adventitious albuminuria. **orthostatic a.**, albuminuria on assuming the erect position.

Albumisol (al-bu′mĭ-sol) trademark for a preparation of normal human serum albumin.

albumoscope (al-bu′mo-skōp) an instrument for determining the presence of albumin in the urine.

albumose (al′bu-mōs) a primary product of the digestion of a protein; further digestion converts albumoses into peptones. **Bence Jones a.**, see under *protein*.

albumosemia (al″bu-mo-se′me-ah) albumose in the blood.

albumosuria (-su′re-ah) albumose in the urine. **Bence Jones a., myelopathic a.**, Bence Jones protein in the urine.

Alcaligenes (al″kah-lij′ĕ-nēz) a genus of Schizomycetes (order Eubacteriales, family Achromobacteraceae) found in the intestinal tract of vertebrates or in dairy products.

alcapton (al-kap′ton) a nitrogenous product occurring in urine.

alcaptonuria (al-kap″to-nu′re-ah) excretion in the urine of homogentisic acid and its oxidation products as a result of a genetic disorder of phenylalanine-tyrosine metabolism.

alcohol (al′ko-hol) 1. a colorless, volatile liquid, C_2H_6O, obtained by fermentation of carbohydrates by yeast. 2. a compound of a hydrocarbon with hydroxyl (OH). **absolute a.**, alcohol free from water and impurities. **benzyl a.**, a colorless liquid, $C_6H_5.CH_2.OH$, used as a local anesthetic. **cetyl a.**, a solid alcohol, $C_{16}H_{34}O$, used in making ointment bases. **denatured a.**, alcohol rendered unfit for human consumption. **ethyl a.**, ordinary alcohol ($CH_3.CH_2OH$). **isopropyl a.**, transparent, colorless, volatile liquid, $CH_3.CHOH.-CH_3$, used as surgical antiseptic and disinfectant and as a rubbing compound. **methyl a.**, methanol. **phenylethyl a.**, a colorless liquid, $C_8H_{10}O$, used as an antibacterial and preservative. **primary a.**, one containing the monovalent carbinol group, $-CH_2OH$. **rubbing a.**, a transparent, mobile, volatile liquid, applied topically to the skin. **secondary a.**, one containing the divalent group, $=CHOH$. **stearyl a.**, a mixture of solid alcohols, consisting chiefly of $CH_3(CH_2)_{16}CH_2OH$; used as an ingredient of various pharmaceutic or cosmetic preparations. **tertiary a.**, one containing the trivalent group, $≡COH$. **wood a.**, methanol.

alcoholase (al′ko-hol-ās″) an enzyme which converts lactic acid into alcohol.

alcoholemia (al″ko-hol-e′me-ah) alcohol in the blood.

alcoholic (al″ko-hol′ik) 1. containing or pertaining to alcohol. 2. a person addicted to alcohol.

alcoholism (al′ko-hol″izm) a morbid state caused by excessive consumption of alcohol, interfering with the patient's health and social or economic functioning.

alcoholize (al′ko-hol-īz″) 1. to treat with alcohol. 2. to transform into alcohol.

alcoholomania (al″ko-hol″o-ma′ne-ah) maniacal craving for alcohol.

alcoholometer (al″ko-hol-om′ĕ-ter) instrument for determining amount of alcohol present.

alcoholophilia (al″ko-hol″o-fil′e-ah) morbid appetite for alcoholic drink.

alcoholuria (al″ko-hol-u′re-ah) the presence of alcohol in the urine.

alcoholysis (al″ko-hol′ĭ-sis) decomposition of a compound due to the incorporation and splitting of alcohol.

Aldactazide (al-dak′tah-zīd) trademark for a preparation of spironolactone with hydrochlorothiazide.

Aldactone (al-dak′tōn) trademark for a preparation of spironolactone.

aldehyde (al′dĕ-hīd) a chemical compound derived from the primary alcohols by oxidation and containing the monovalent group $-CHO$. **acetic a.**, acetaldehyde. **cinnamic a.**, cinnamaldehyde. **formic a.**, formaldehyde.

aldosterone (al-dos′ter-ōn) the principal electrolyte-regulating steroid secreted by the adrenal cortex.

aldosteronism (al-dos′ter-ōn-izm″) an abnormality of electrolyte metabolism due to excessive secretion of aldosterone; it may be primary, or secondary in response to extraadrenal disease. **primary a.**, hypersecretion of aldosterone by the adrenal cortex, with excessive loss of potassium and generalized muscular weakness. **secondary a.**, abnormally high levels of aldosterone in the urine as the result of some other disease, such as cardiac failure or renal or hepatic disease.

aldosteronogenesis (al″do-stēr-o-no-jen′ĕ-sis) the production of aldosterone by the adrenal glands.

aldosteronoma (-stēr″ōn-o′mah) an aldosterone-secreting adrenal cortical tumor.

alecithal (ah-les′ĭ-thal) having no distinct yolk.

alemmal (ah-lem′al) having no neurilemma.

alethia (ah-le′the-ah) inability to forget.

aletocyte (ah-le′to-sīt) a wandering cell.

aleukemia (ah″lu-ke′me-ah) aleukemic leukemia.

aleukemic (ah″lu-ke′mik) characterized by aleukemia.

aleukemoid (ah″lu-ke′moid) resembling aleukemia.

aleukia (ah-lu′ke-ah) 1. aleukemia. 2. absence of blood plates.

aleukocytosis (ah-lu″ko-si-to′sis) diminished production of white corpuscles in the blood.

alexia (ah-lek′se-ah) visual aphasia or word blindness. **musical a.,** inability to read music.

alexic (ah-lek′sik) 1. pertaining to alexia. 2. having the properties of an alexin.

alexin (ah-lek′sin) complement.

aleydigism (ah-li′dig-izm) absence of secretion of the interstitial cells of Leydig.

Alflorone (al′flo-rōn) trademark for preparations of fludrocortisone.

alga (al′gah), pl. *al′gae* [L.] an individual organism belonging to the Algae.

Algae (al′je) a group of plants living in the water, including all seaweeds, and ranging in size from microscopic cells to fronds hundreds of feet long.

algefacient (al″jĕ-fa′shent) cooling or refrigerant.

algesia (al-je′ze-ah) sensitiveness to pain; hyperesthesia. adj., **alge′sic, alget′ic.**

algesimetry (al″jĕ-sim′ĕ-tre) measurement of sensitivity to pain.

algesthesis (al″jes-the′sis) a painful sensation.

-algia (al′je-ah) word element [Gr.], *pain.*

algicide (al′jĭ-sĭd) 1. destructive to algae. 2. an agent which destroys algae.

algid (al′jid) chilly; cold.

alginate (al′jĭ-nāt) a salt of alginic acid (*calcium, sodium* or *ammonium alginate*); used as foam, clot, or gauze for absorbable surgical dressings.

Alginobacter (al″jĭ-no-bak′ter) a genus of Schizomycetes (order Eubacteriales, family Enterobacteriaceae, tribe Escherichieae) found in soil.

Alginomonas (al″jĭ-no-mo′nas) a genus of Schizomycetes (order Pseudomonadales, suborder Pseudomonadineae, family Pseudomonadaceae) found on algae and in sea water and soil.

algo- (al′go) word element [Gr.], *pain; cold.*

algogenic (al″go-jen′ik) 1. causing pain. 2. lowering the temperature.

algology (al-gol′o-je) the scientific study of algae.

algometer (al-gom′ĕ-ter) device used in testing the sensitiveness of a part to pain.

algometry (al-gom′ĕ-tre) estimation of the sensitivity to painful stimuli.

algophobia (al″go-fo′be-ah) morbid dread of pain.

algopsychalia (-si-ka′le-ah) psychalgia.

algor (al′gor) chill or rigor; coldness. **a. mor′tis,** the cooling of the body after death, which proceeds at a definite rate, influenced by the environmental temperature and protection of the body.

Alidase (al′ĭ-dās) trademark for a preparation of hyaluronidase for injection.

alienia (ah″li-e′ne-ah) absence of the spleen.

alienism (āl′yen-izm) the study or treatment of mental disorders.

alienist (āl′yen-ist) one skilled in treating mental disorders.

aliform (al′ĭ-form) shaped like a wing.

aliment (al′ĭ-ment) food; nutritive material. adj., **alimen′tary.**

alimentation (al″ĭ-men-ta′shun) giving or receiving of nourishment. **rectal a.,** feeding by injection of nutriment into the rectum.

alimentology (-men-tol′o-je) the science of nutrition.

alimentotherapy (-men″to-ther′ah-pe) treatment by systematic feeding.

alinasal (-na′zal) pertaining to either ala of the nose.

aliphatic (-fat′ik) pertaining to or derived from fat; having an open-chain (carbohydrate) structure.

aliquot (al′ĭ-kwot) a number which will divide another without a remainder; e.g. 2 is an aliquot of 6.

alizarin (ah-liz′ah-rin) a red coloring principle, $C_{14}H_8O_4$, obtained from coal tar or madder.

alkalemia (al″kah-le′me-ah) abnormal alkalinity of the blood.

alkalescent (-les′ent) having a tendency to alkalinity.

alkali (al′kah-li) any one of a class of compounds which form salts with acids and soaps with fats. **caustic a.,** hydroxide of sodium or potassium in solid form.

alkalimeter (al″kah-lim′ĕ-ter) instrument for performing alkalimetry.

alkalimetry (-lim′ĕ-tre) measurement of alkalinity of a compound or of the alkali in a mixture.

alkaline (al′kah-līn) having the reactions of an alkali.

alkalinity (al″kah-lin′ĭ-te) 1. the quality of being alkaline. 2. the combining power of a base, expressed as the maximum number of equivalents of acid with which it reacts to form a salt.

alkalinuria (al″kah-lin-u′re-ah) an alkaline condition of the urine.

alkalipenia (al″kah-li-pe′ne-ah) abnormally low alkali reserve of the body.

alkalitherapy (-ther′ah-pe) treatment with alkalis.

alkalization (-za′shun) act of making alkaline.

alkaloid (al′kah-loid) any alkaline principle of organic origin. **animal a.,** alkaloid substance formed in decomposition of animal tis-

sues. **cadaveric a.**, **putrefactive a.**, a ptomaine.

alkalosis (al″kah-lo′sis) increased alkali
reserve (bicarbonate content) in the blood and
body tissues. adj., **alkalot′ic. compensated
a.**, a condition in which compensatory mechanisms have returned the pH toward normal.
hypokalemic a., a metabolic alkalosis due
to losses of potassium and associated with a
low serum potassium level. **metabolic a.**, a
disturbance in which the acid-base status
shifts toward the alkaline side because of
changes in the fixed (nonvolatile) acids and
bases. **respiratory a.**, a state due to excess
loss of carbon dioxide from the body.

alkapton (al-kap′tōn) alcapton.

alkaptonuria (al-kap″to-nu′re-ah) alcaptonuria.

alkavervir (al″kah-ver′vir) a mixture of
alkaloids extracted from *Veratrum viride*,
used to lower blood pressure.

alkyl (al′kil) a monovalent radical of the general formula C_nH_{2n+1}.

alkylate (al′kĭ-lāt) to treat with an alkylating
agent.

all(o)- (al′o) word element [Gr.], *other; deviating from normal.*

allachesthesia (al″ah-kes-the′ze-ah) allocheiria.

allantiasis (al″an-ti′ah-sis) botulism.

allantochorion (ah-lan″to-ko′re-on) the allantois and chorion as one structure.

allantoid (ah-lan′toid) 1. sausage-shaped. 2.
pertaining to the allantois.

allantoin (ah-lan′to-in) crystalline substance,
$C_4H_6N_4O_3$, from allantoic fluid and fetal urine.

allantoinuria (ah-lan″to-ĭ-nu′re-ah) allantoin
in the urine.

allantois (ah-lan′to-is) a ventral outgrowth of
the hindgut of the early embryo, which is a
conspicuous component of the developing
umbilical cord. adj., **allanto′ic.**

allele (ah-lēl′) one of two or more alternative
forms of a gene at the same site in a chromosome, which determine alternative characters
in inheritance. adj., **allel′ic. silent a.**, one
that produces no detectable effect.

allelomorph (ah-le′lo-morf) allele. adj., **al-
lelomor′phic.**

allelotaxis (ah-le″lo-tak′sis) development of
an organ from several embryonic structures.

allergen (al′ler-jen) a substance capable of
inducing hypersensitivity. adj., **allergen′ic.**

allergist (al′ler-jist) a physician specializing
in the diagnosis and treatment of allergic
conditions.

allergization (al″ler-ji-za′shun) active sensitization by introduction of allergens into the
body.

allergologist (al″ler-gol′o-jist) one who specializes in allergology.

allergology (-gol′o-je) the science dealing with
problems of hypersensitivity.

allergy (al′ler-je) hypersensitivity to a physical
or chemical agent. adj., **aller′gic.**

allesthesia (al″es-the′ze-ah) allocheiria.

allocheiria (al″o-ki′re-ah) reference of a sensa-

tion to the side opposite to that to which the
stimulus is applied.

allochezia (al″o-ke′ze-ah) discharge of non-
fecal matter by the anus, or of fecal matter
by an abnormal passage.

allochroism (-kro′izm) variation in color.

allochromasia (-kro-ma′ze-ah) change in color
of hair or skin.

allocinesia (-si-ne′ze-ah) performance of a
movement on the side of the body opposite
to that directed.

allodiploid (-dip′loid) 1. characterized by
allodiploidy. 2. an individual or cell characterized by allodiploidy.

allodiploidy (-dip′loi-de) the state of having
two sets of chromosomes derived from different ancestral species.

allodromy (al-lod′ro-me) disturbed rhythm of
the heart.

alloerotism (al″lo-er′o-tizm) direction of
libido toward others or toward objects outside one's self.

allolalia (-la′le-ah) any defect of speech of
central origin.

allomorphism (-mor′fizm) existence of the
same substance in different forms.

alloplasia (-pla′ze-ah) heteroplasia.

alloplastic (al′lo-plas″tik) pertaining to the
open, direct and unmodified expression of
impulses outwardly into the environment.

alloplasty (al′lo-plas″te) plastic repair of the
human body with other than human tissue.

alloploid (al′lo-ploid) 1. characterized by alloploidy. 2. an individual or cell characterized
by alloploidy.

alloploidy (al″lo-ploi′de) the state of having
any number of chromosome sets derived from
different ancestral species.

allopolyploid (-pol′e-ploid) 1. characterized by
allopolyploidy. 2. an individual or cell characterized by allopolyploidy.

allopolyploidy (-pol′e-ploi″de) the state of
having more than two sets of chromosomes
derived from different ancestral species.

allopsychic (-si′kik) pertaining to another's
mind or psyche.

allorhythmia (-rith′me-ah) irregularity of the
heart beat or pulse.

allorphine (al″lor-fēn) nalorphine.

allosome (al′lo-sōm) a chromosome which
differs from an ordinary chromosome.

allotherm (al′lo-therm) 1. poikilotherm. 2.
heterotherm.

allotriogeustia (al-lot″re-o-jōōs′te-ah) perverted sense of taste.

allotropic (al″lo-trop′ik) 1. exhibiting allotropism. 2. concerned with others; said of a type
of personality that is more preoccupied with
others than with itself.

allotropism (ah-lot′ro-pizm) existence of an
element in two or more distinct forms.

allotropy (ah-lot′ro-pe) 1. allotropism. 2. direction of one's interest more toward others
than toward one's self.

alloxan (ah-lok′san) a substance, $C_4H_2N_2O_4$,
first isolated from the oxidation products of
uric acid, capable of causing diabetes in ex-

perimental animals when administered orally or parenterally.

alloxantin (al″oks-an′tin) a derivative of alloxan.

alloxazine (ah-lok′sah-zēn) a compound, $C_{10}H_6N_4O_2$, allied to riboflavin.

alloxuremia (ah-lok″su-re′me-ah) presence of purine bases in the blood.

alloxuria (al″oks-u′re-ah) presence of purine bases in the urine.

alloy (al′oi) a mixture obtained by fusing metals together. **contour a.,** an alloy suitable for contour fillings.

allyl (al′il) a univalent radical, C_3H_5 or $CH_2.CHCH_2$, from garlic and other plants. **a. aldehyde,** acrolein. **a. sulfide,** a compound, $(C_3H_5)_2S$, used in cholera and phthisis.

allylguaicol (al″lil-gwi′ah-kol) eugenol.

almagacin (al″mah-ga′sin) a combination of gastric mucin, aluminum hydroxide gel and magnesium trisilicate, used as an antacid.

alochia (ah-lo′ke-ah) absence or suppression of the lochia.

aloe (al′o) dried juice of leaves of various species of Aloe, used in pharmaceutical preparations.

alogia (ah-lo′je-ah) inability to speak, due to a nerve lesion.

aloin (al′o-in) a mixture of active principles obtained from aloe, used as a cathartic.

alopecia (al″o-pe′she-ah) loss of hair from normally hairy areas of the body. **androgenetic a.,** hair loss, dependent on androgen secretion, in hereditarily predisposed persons. **a. arca′ta,** hair loss in sharply defined areas, usually the scalp. **a. cap′itis tota′lis,** loss of all the hair from the scalp. **a. cicatrisa′ta,** a disease marked by various sized and shaped patches of alopecia with atrophy of the scalp in the areas. **a. congenita′lis,** complete or partial absence of the hair at birth. **female-pattern a.,** loss of scalp hair in girls or women, analogous to male-pattern alopecia, but more benign. **a. heredita′ria,** hereditary baldness. **a. limina′ris,** hair loss at the hairline along the front and back edges of the scalp. **male-pattern a.,** loss of scalp hair genetically determined and androgen-dependent, beginning with frontal recession and progressing symmetrically to leave ultimately only a sparse peripheral rim of hair. **a. medicamento′sa,** hair loss due to ingestion of a drug. **a. symptomat′ica,** loss of hair due to systemic or psychogenic causes, or to stress. **a. tota′lis,** loss of hair from the entire scalp. **a. universa′lis,** loss of hair from the entire body.

aloxidone (al-ok″sĭ-di′ŏn) an anticonvulsant for petit mal epilepsy.

alpha (al′fah) first letter of Greek alphabet, α; used in names of chemical compounds to distinguish the first in a series of isomers, or to indicate position of substituting atoms or groups.

Alphadrol (al′fah-drol) trademark for a preparation of fluprednisolone.

alphaprodine (al″fah-pro′dēn) a chemical used to relieve pain and as a narcotic.

A.L.R.O.S. American Laryngological, Rhinological and Otological Society.

alseroxylon (al″ser-ok′sĭ-lon) a purified extract of *Rauwolfia serpentina*, used to reduce blood pressure and to slow heart rate, and as a tranquilizer.

alternation (awl″ter-na′shun) the regular succession of two opposing or different events in turn. **a. of generations,** alternate sexual and asexual reproduction, one generation reproducing sexually, the next asexually.

alum (al′um) a crystalline substance, ammonium alum, $AlNH_4(SO_4)_2.12H_2O$, or potassium alum, $AlK(SO_4)_2.12H_2O$; used as an astringent. **exsiccated a.,** a white odorless powder, $AlNH_4(SO_4)_2$ or $AlK(SO_4)_2$.

aluminosis (ah-loo″mĭ-no′sis) a lung disease of alum workers.

aluminum (ah-loo′mĭ-num) a chemical element (*see table*), at. no. 13, symbol Al. **a. chloride,** deliquescent, crystalline powder, $AlCl_3.6H_2O$, used topically as an astringent solution. **a. sulfate,** a compound, $Al_2(SO_4)_3$, used as an astringent solution.

Alurate (al′ūr-āt) trademark for a preparation of aprobarbital.

alveolalgia (al″ve-o-lal′je-ah) pain in the socket of an extracted tooth.

alveolectomy (-lek′to-me) surgical excision of part of the alveolar process.

alveolitis (al-ve″o-li′tis) inflammation of an alveolus.

alveoloclasia (-lo-kla′ze-ah) destruction or absorption of part of the alveolar process.

alveolodental (-lo-den′tal) pertaining to teeth and the alveolar process.

alveolotomy (al″ve-o-lot′o-me) incision of the alveolar process.

alveolus (al-ve′o-lus), pl. *alve′oli* [L.] a little hollow, as the socket of a tooth, a follicle or an acinar gland, or one of the thin-walled chambers of the lungs (*pulmonary alveoli*), surrounded by networks of capillaries through whose walls exchange of carbon dioxide and oxygen takes place. adj., **alve′olar. dental alveoli,** the cavities or sockets of either jaw, in which the roots of the teeth are embedded.

alveolysis (al″ve-ol′ĭ-sis) pyorrhea alveolaris.

alveus (al′ve-us), pl. *al′vei* [L.] a canal or trough.

Alvodine (al′vo-dīn) trademark for preparations of piminodine ethanesulfonate.

alymphia (ah-lim′fe-ah) absence or lack of lymph.

alymphocytosis (a-lim″fo-si-to′sis) deficiency of lymphocytes in the blood.

A.M. amperemeter; [L.] ante meridiem (*before noon*); meter angle.

Am chemical symbol, *americium*.

A.M.A. Aerospace Medical Association; American Medical Association; Australian Medical Association.

amacrine (am′ah-krīn) 1. without long processes. 2. a branched retinal structure, considered a modified nerve cell.

Amadil (am′ah-dil) trademark for a preparation of acetaminophen.

amalgam (ah-mal′gam) a compound of mercury with another metal. **emotional a.,** an unconscious attempt to bind, neutralize, deny or counteract anxiety.

amaranth (am′ah-ranth) a dark red-brown powder used as a coloring agent in pharmaceutical preparations.

amastia (ah-mas′te-ah) congenital absence of one or both mammary glands.

amaurosis (am″aw-ro′sis) loss of sight without apparent lesion of the eye, or from disease of the optic nerve or retina. adj., **amaurot′ic. a. fu′gax,** sudden temporary or fleeting blindness. **a. partia′lis fu′gax,** sudden transitory partial blindness.

ambenonium (am″be-no′ne-um) a chemical used as a cholinesterase inhibitor or to increase muscular strength in myasthenic patients.

ambidextrous (am″bĭ-deks′trus) using either hand for the performance of certain tasks.

ambilateral (-lat′er-al) pertaining to or affecting both sides.

ambilevous (-le′vus) awkward at using both hands.

ambiopia (am″be-o′pe-ah) diplopia.

ambisexual (am″bĭ-seks′u-al) pertaining to both sexes.

ambivalence (am-biv′ah-lens) simultaneous existence of conflicting emotional attitudes toward a goal, object or person. adj., **ambiv′alent.**

amblyacousia (am″ble-ah-ku′se-ah) dulness of hearing.

amblyaphia (-a′fe-ah) bluntness of the sense of touch.

amblygeustia (-gōōs′te-ah) dulness of the sense of taste.

Amblyomma (am″ble-om′mah) a genus of arthropods (family Ixodidae), comprising approximately 100 species, which are vectors of various disease-producing organisms. **A. america′num,** a species of ticks widely distributed in the United States and Central and South America; a vector of Rocky Mountain spotted fever. **A. cajennen′se,** a tick widely distributed in North, Central and South America; a vector of São Paulo fever. **A. macula′tum,** a tick widely distributed in the United States and Central and South America. **A. va′rium,** a species of Amblyomma, including the largest tick known.

amblyopia (-o′pe-ah) diminution of vision not due to organic defect or refractive errors. adj., **amblyop′ic. color a.,** dimness of color vision due to toxic or other influences. **a. ex anop′sia,** weakness of vision supposedly resulting from long disuse.

amblyoscope (am′ble-o-skōp″) an instrument for training an amblyopic eye to take part in vision.

ambo (am′bo) ambon.

amboceptor (am′bo-sep″tor) the body that is thought to join the complement to the animal or bacterial cell.

Ambodryl (am′bo-dril) trademark for preparations of bromodiphenhydramine.

ambon (am′bon) the edge of the socket in which the head of a long bone is lodged.

ambotoxoid (am″bo-tok′soid) a mixture of the soluble products of bacteria which have been lysed by a bacteriophage, with a filtrate from a culture of the organism.

ambulant (am′bu-lant) ambulatory.

ambulatory (am′bu-lah-tor″e) walking or able to walk; not confined to bed.

ambutonium (am″bu-to′ne-um) a chemical used as a parasympathetic blocker or an antispasmodic or to reduce gastric acid secretion.

ameba (ah-me′bah), pl. *ame′bae, ame′bas* [L.] a one-celled protozoan of the subphylum Sarcodina (phylum Protozoa). adj., **ame′bic.**

amebiasis (am″e-bi′ah-sis) infection with amebas, especially with *Entamoeba histolytica.*

amebicide (ah-me′bĭ-sīd) destructive to amebae.

amebiform (ah-me′bĭ-form) ameboid.

amebocyte (ah-me′bo-sīt) a cell showing ameboid movement.

ameboid (ah-me′boid) resembling an ameba.

ameboidism (ah-me′boid-izm) performance of ameba-like movements.

ameboma (am″e-bo′mah) a tumor-like mass caused by granulomatous reaction in the intestines in amebiasis.

amebula (ah-meb′u-lah) the spore of the malarial parasite in its ameba-like stage in the blood corpuscle.

ameburia (am″e-bu′re-ah) amebae in the urine.

amelia (ah-me′le-ah) developmental anomaly with absence of the limbs.

amelification (ah-mel′ĭ-fĭ-ka′shun) the development of enamel cells into enamel.

ameloblast (ah-mel′o-blast) a cell which takes part in forming dental enamel.

ameloblastoma (ah-mel″o-blas-to′mah) a locally invasive, highly destructive tumor of the jaw. **pituitary a.,** craniopharyngioma.

amelodentinal (am″ĕ-lo-den′tĭ-nal) pertaining to dental enamel and dentin.

amelogenesis (ah-mel″o-jen′ĕ-sis) formation of dental enamel. **a. imperfec′ta,** imperfect formation of enamel, resulting in brownish coloration and friability of the teeth.

amelogenic (am″ĕ-lo-jen′ik) forming enamel.

amelus (am′ĕ-lus) an individual exhibiting amelia.

amenorrhea (a-men″o-re′ah) absence of menstruation. adj., **amenorrhe′al. primary a.,** the condition in which onset of menstruation is delayed beyond the age of 17 years. **secondary a.,** cessation of menstruation after it has once been established at puberty.

amensalism (a-men′sal-izm) interaction between coexisting populations of different species, one of which is adversely affected and the other unaffected.

amentia (a-men′she-ah) lifelong intellectual retardation or subnormality, usually due to lack of development of adequate brain tissue. **nevoid a.,** amentia with nevus formation on face and scalp.

americium (am″er-ish′e-um) chemical element (*see table*), at. no. 95, symbol Am.

ametria (ah-me′tre-ah) congenital absence of the uterus.

ametrometer (am″ĕ-trom′ĕ-ter) instrument for measuring degree of ametropia.

ametropia (am″ĕ-tro′pe-ah) a condition of the eye in which parallel rays fail to come to a focus on the retina. adj., **ametrop′ic.**

amicrobic (ah″mi-kro′bic) not produced by microbes.

amicron (ah-mi′kron) a particle so small it cannot be seen with the ultramicroscope.

amidase (am′ĭ-dās) a deamidizing enzyme.

amide (am′ĭd) any compound derived from ammonia by substitution of an acid radical for hydrogen.

amido (am′ĭ-do) the monovalent radical NH_2 united with an acid radical.

amidopyrine (am″ĭ-do-pi′rēn) aminopyrine.

Amigen (am′ĭ-jen) trademark for protein hydrolysate preparation for intravenous injection.

amimia (a mim′e-ah) loss of ability to imitate or mimic or to use appropriate gestures, due to disorder of the language center of the brain.

amine (am′in, ah-mēn) an organic compound containing nitrogen. **catechol a.** see *catecholamine.*

aminitrozole (am″ĭ-ni′tro-zōl) a chemical used in treatment of trichomoniasis.

amino (am′ĭ no, ah mə′no) the monovalent radical NH_2, when not united with an acid radical.

amino-acidemia (am″ĭ-no-as″ĭ de′me ah) presence of amino acids in the blood.

amino-aciduria (-as″ĭ-du′re-ah) presence in the urine of amino acids.

aminoglutethimide (-gloo-teth′ĭ-mīd) a chemical used in treatment of most forms of epilepsy.

aminogram (am-i′no-gram) a graphic representation of the pattern of amino acids present in a substance, as determined quantitatively.

aminolysis (am″ĭ-nol′ĭ-sis) the splitting up of amines.

aminometradine (am″ĭ-no-met′rah-dēn) a chemical used to increase urine formation and in treatment of edema of heart failure.

aminometramide (-met′rah-mīd) aminometradine.

aminopentamide (-pen′tah-mīd) a chemical used for parasympathetic blockade and locally for dilatation of the pupil.

aminopherase (am″ĭ-nof′er-ās) an enzyme that effects transamination; transaminase.

aminophylline (am″ĭ-no-fil′in) a mixture of theophylline and ethylenediamine; diuretic, antispasmodic, coronary vasodilator, and myocardial and respiratory stimulant.

aminopolypeptidase (-pol″e-pep′ti-dās) an enzyme which splits off free amino groups from a polypeptide.

Aminopterin (am″in-op′ter-in) methotrexate.

aminopyrine (am″ĭ-no-pi′rēn) white or colorless, odorless crystals, $C_{13}H_{17}N_3O$; analgesic.

aminosis (am″ĭ-no′sis) excessive formation of amino acids in the body.

Aminosol (ah-me′no-sol) trademark for an amino acid preparation for intravenous injection.

aminotrate (am′ĭ-no-trāt″) trolnitrate.

aminuria (am″ĭ-nu′re-ah) presence of amines in the urine.

amisometradine (am-i″so-met′rah-dēn) a chemical used as diuretic.

amitosis (am″ĭ-to′sis) direct nuclear or cell division. adj., **amitot′ic.**

ammeter (am′me-ter) an instrument for measuring in amperes the strength of a current flowing in a circuit.

ammo-aciduria (am″o-as″ĭ-du′re-ah) presence of ammonia and amino acids in the urine.

ammonia (ah-mo′ne-ah) colorless gas with pungent odor and acrid taste, NH_3.

ammoniac (ah-mo′ne-ak) a fetid gum-resin; stimulant and expectorant.

ammoniate (ah-mo′ne-āt) to treat or combine with ammonia.

ammoniemia (ah-mo″ne-e′me-ah) presence of ammonia or its compounds in the blood.

ammonium (ah-mo′ne-um) hypothetical radical, NH_4, forming salts analogous to those of the alkaline metals. **a. acetate,** $CH_3.COO.NH_4$, diaphoretic, diuretic. **a. bromide,** crystalline compound, NH_4Br, used as a central nervous system depressant. **a. carbonate,** a mixture of NH_4HCO_3 (ammonium bicarbonate) and NH_4COONH_4 (ammonium carbamate). **a. chloride,** crystalline compound, NH_4Cl, used as a systemic acidifier and chloride replenisher. **ferric a. citrate,** a preparation of iron, ammonia and hydrated citric acid, used in treatment of iron deficiency anemia. **a. iodide,** NH_4I, resolvent and expectorant. **a. mandelate,** urinary antiseptic. **a. salicylate,** $C_6H_4.OH.COONH_4$, formerly used in administering salicylic acid.

ammoniuria (ah-mo″ne-u′re-ah) excess of ammonia in the urine.

ammonolysis (am″o-nol′ĭ-sis) decomposition of a compound due to the incorporation and splitting of ammonia.

ammonotelic (ah mo″no-tcl′ik) having ammonia as the chief excretory product of nitrogen metabolism.

amnalgesia (am″nal-je′ze-ah) abolition of pain and memory of a painful procedure by the use of drugs or hypnosis.

amnesia (am-ne′zhe-ah) pathologic impairment of memory. adj., **amnes′tic. anterograde a.,** loss of memory for events occurring subsequent to the episode precipitating the disorder. **auditory a.,** auditory aphasia. **retrograde a.,** loss of memory for events occurring prior to the episode precipitating the disorder. **visual a.,** alexia.

amniocentesis (am″ne-o-sen-te′sis) transabdominal or transcervical penetration of the uterus for aspiration of amniotic fluid.

amniochorial (-ko′re-al) pertaining to amnion and chorion.

amniogenesis (-jen′ĕ-sis) the development of the amnion.

amniography (am″ne-og′rah-fe) roentgenography of the gravid uterus.

amnion (am′ne-on) the innermost membrane

enclosing the developing fetus and the fluid in which it is bathed. adj., **amnion'ic, amniot'ic. a. nodo'sum,** a nodular condition of the fetal surface of the amnion, observed in oligohydramnios associated with absence of the kidneys of the fetus.

amnionitis (am″ne-o-ni′tis) inflammation of the amnion.

amniorrhea (-re′ah) escape of the liquor amnii.

amniorrhexis (-rek′sis) rupture of the amnion.

amnioscope (am′ne-o-skōp″) an instrument that, by passage through the abdominal wall into the amniotic cavity, permits direct visualization of the fetus in utero. **fiber optic a.,** an instrument in which the electromagnetic vibrations stimulating the sensation of sight are transmitted along bundles of flexible fibers having special optical qualities.

amniote (am′ne-ōt) any animal with amnion.

amniotome (am′ne-o-tōm″) instrument for cutting the fetal membrane.

amniotomy (am″ne-ot′o-me) surgical rupture of the fetal membranes.

amobarbital (am″o-bar′bĭ-tal) a hypnotic compound, $C_{11}H_{18}N_2O_3$, having a short to intermediate action. **a. sodium,** a sodium-containing compound, $C_{11}H_{17}N_2NaO_3$, for oral or parenteral administration.

amodiaquine (-di′ah-kwin) a chemical used to suppress malaria and to treat malaria due to *Plasmodium falciparum* or liver abscess due to ameba.

Amoeba (ah-me′bah) ameba.

Amoebobacter (ah-me″bo-bak′ter) a genus of Schizomycetes (order Pseudomonadales, suborder Rhodobacteriineae, family Thiorhadaceae).

amolanone (ah-mo′lah-nōn) a chemical used for parasympathetic blockade, relaxation of spasm of the urinary tract and as a topical anesthetic.

amorph (a′morf) an amorphic mutant gene.

amorphism (ah-mor′fizm) state of being amorphous.

amorphous (ah-mor′fus) having no definite form; shapeless.

amotio (ah-mo′she-o) [L.] a removing. **a. ret′inae,** detachment of the retina.

amp. ampere, ampule.

ampere (am′pēr) unit of electric current strength, the current yielded by one volt of electromotive force against one ohm of resistance.

amperemeter (am′pēr-me″ter) an instrument for measuring amperage.

Amphedroxyn (am″fe-drok′sin) trademark for a preparation of methamphetamine.

amphenidone (am-fen′ĭ-dōn) a chemical used as a tranquilizer.

amphetamine (am-fet′ah-mēn) a crystalline compound with a powerful stimulant action on the central nervous system, used as **a. phosphate,** $C_9H_{13}N.H_3PO_4$, or **a. sulfate,** $(C_9H_{13}N)_2.H_2SO_4$.

amphi- (am′fe) word element [Gr.], *both; on both sides.*

amphiarkyochrome (am″fe-ar′ke-o-krōm″) a nerve cell with peculiar staining qualities.

amphiarthrosis (am″fe-ar-thro′sis) a joint in which the surfaces are connected by disks of fibrocartilage, as between vertebrae.

amphiaster (am′fe-as″ter) diaster.

Amphibia (am-fib′e-ah) a class of animals living both on land and in water.

amphiblastula (am″fĭ-blas′tu-lah) a blastula resulting from unequal segmentation.

amphibolic (-bol′ik) 1. uncertain. 2. having both an anabolic and a catabolic function.

amphicelous (-se′lus) concave on either side or end.

amphicentric (-sen′trik) beginning and ending in the same vessel.

amphichroic (-kro′ik) affecting both red and blue litmus.

amphichromatic (-kro-mat′ik) amphichroic.

amphicrania (-kra′ne-ah) headache affecting both sides of the head.

amphicyte (am′fĭ-sīt) one of the cells forming the capsule surrounding a spinal ganglion.

amphicytula (am″fĭ-sit′u-lah) the ovum in its cytula stage.

amphidiarthrosis (-di″ar-thro′sis) a joint having the nature of both ginglymus and arthrodia, as that of the lower jaw.

amphigastrula (-gas′troo-lah) the gastrula resulting from unequal segmentation, the cells of the two hemispheres being of unequal size.

amphigonadism (-gon′ah-dizm) possession of both ovarian and testicular tissue.

amphimixis (-mik′sis) 1. intermingling of hereditary units of sperm and ovum in the fertilized ovum. 2. in psychiatry, association of libido or sexual energy with both urethral and genital regions.

amphimorula (-mor′u-lah) the morula resulting from unequal segmentation, the cells of the two hemispheres being of unequal size.

amphithymia (-thi′me-ah) a mental state characterized by both depression and elation.

amphitrichous (am-fit′rĭ-kus) having flagella at each end.

amphocyte (am′fo-sīt) a cell staining with either acid or basic dyes.

ampholyte (am′fo-līt) an organic or inorganic substance capable of acting as either an acid or a base.

amphophil (am′fo-fil) an amphophilic cell or element.

amphophilic (am″fo-fil′ik) staining with either acid or basic dyes.

amphoric (am-for′ik) pertaining to a bottle; resembling the sound made by blowing across the neck of a bottle.

amphoteric (am″fo-ter′ik) capable of acting as both an acid and a base; capable of neutralizing either bases or acids.

amphotericin (-ter′ĭ-sin) a name given to an antibiotic used in mycotic infections.

amphotericity (-ter-is′ĭ-te) the quality of being amphoteric; the power to unite with either positively or negatively charged ions, or with either basic or acid substances.

amphoterism (am-fo′ter-izm) the possession of both acid and basic properties.

amphotony (am-fot′o-ne) tonicity of the sympathetic and parasympathetic nervous systems.

amplitude (am'plĭ-tūd) largeness, fulness; widest range or extent. **a. of accommodation,** amount of accommodative power of the eye.

amprotropine (am"pro-tro'pēn) a chemical used for parasympathetic blockade and as an antispasmodic.

ampule (am'pūl) a small, hermetically sealed glass flask, e.g. one containing medication for parenteral administration.

ampulla (am-pul'ah), pl. *ampul'lae* [L.] a flask-like dilatation of a tubular structure, especially of the expanded ends of the semicircular canals of the ear. adj., **ampul'lar. a. chy'li,** receptaculum chyli. **a. duc'tus deferen'tis,** the enlarged and tortuous distal end of the ductus deferens. **Henle's a.,** ampulla ductus deferentis. **hepatopancreatic a.,** flask-like cavity in major duodenal papilla into which the common bile duct and pancreatic duct open. **ampul'lae lactif'erae,** sinus lactiferi. **Lieberkühn's a.,** the blind termination of lacteals in the villi of the intestines. **ampul'lae membrana'ceae,** the dilatations at one end of each of the three semicircular ducts. **ampul'lae os'seae,** the dilatations at one of the ends of the semicircular canals. **phrenic a.,** the dilatation at the lower end of the esophagus. **a. of rectum,** the dilated portion of the rectum just proximal to the anal canal. **a. of Thoma,** one of the small terminal expansions of an interlobar artery in the pulp of the spleen. **a. of uterine tube,** the longest and widest portion of the uterine tube, between the infundibulum and the isthmus of the tube. **a. of vas deferens,** ampulla ductus deferentis. **a. of Vater,** hepatopancreatic ampulla; the term "ampulla of Vater" is often mistakenly used instead of "papilla of Vater," or major duodenal papilla.

amputation (am"pu-ta'shun) removal of a limb or other appendage of the body. **Chopart's a.,** amputation of the foot by a midtarsal disarticulation. **congenital a.,** absence of a limb at birth, attributed to constriction of the part by an encircling band during intrauterine development. **consecutive a.,** an amputation during or after the period of suppuration. **a. in contiguity,** amputation at a joint. **a. in continuity,** amputation of a limb elsewhere than at a joint. **diaclastic a.,** amputation in which the bone is broken by an osteoclast and the soft tissues divided by an écraseur. **double-flap a.,** one in which two flaps are formed. **Dupuytren's a.,** amputation of the arm at the shoulder joint. **elliptical a.,** one in which the cut has an elliptical outline. **flap a.,** one in which flaps are made from soft tissues, the division being oblique. **flapless a.,** one in which flaps cannot be formed. **Gritti-Stokes a.,** amputation of the leg at the knee through condyles of the femur. **Hey's a.,** amputation of the foot between the tarsus and metatarsus. **interpelviabdominal a.,** amputation of the thigh with excision of the lateral portion of the pelvic girdle. **interscapulothoracic a.,** amputation

of the arm with excision of the lateral portion of the shoulder girdle. **intrauterine a.,** congenital amputation. **Larrey's a.,** double-flap amputation at the shoulder or hip joint. **Lisfranc's a.,** amputation of the foot between the metatarsus and tarsus. **Pirigoff's a.,** amputation of the foot at the ankle, through the malleoli of the tibia and fibula. **pulp a.,** pulpotomy. **racket a.,** one in which there is a single longitudinal incision continuous below with a spiral incision on either side of the limb. **root a.,** apicoectomy. **spontaneous a.,** loss of a part without surgical intervention. **Stokes's a.,** Gritti-Stokes amputation. **subperiosteal a.,** one in which the cut end of the bone is covered by periosteal flaps. **Syme's a.,** disarticulation of the foot with removal of both malleoli. **Teale's a.,** amputation with short and long rectangular flaps. **traumatic a.,** amputation of a part by accidental injury. **Tripier's a.,** amputation of the foot through the calcaneus.

A.M.R.L. Aerospace Medical Research Laboratories.

A.M.S. American Meteorological Society.

Amsustain (am'sus-tān) trademark for a preparation of dextroamphetamine.

amu, atomic mass unit.

amusia (ah-mu'ze-ah) loss of ability to produce *(motor amusia)* or to recognize *(sensory amusia)* musical sounds.

A.M.W.A. American Medical Women's Association; American Medical Writers' Association.

amydricaine (ah-mi'dri-kān) a chemical used as a surface or spinal anesthetic agent.

amyelia (a"mi-e'le-ah) absence of the spinal cord in a fetal monster.

amyelineuria (ah-mi"ē-lin-u're-ah) defective function of the spine.

amyelinic (ah-mi"ē-lin'ik) without myelin.

amyelonic (ah-mi"ē-lon'ik) 1. having no spinal cord. 2. having no marrow.

amyelotrophy (-lot'ro-fe) atrophy of spinal cord.

amyelus (ah-mi'ē-lus) a fetal monster with no spinal cord.

amygdala (ah-mig'dah-lah) 1. a tonsil. 2. a lobule of the cerebellum. 3. almond.

amygdalin (ah-mig'dah-lin) a glycoside from bitter almonds.

amygdaline (ah-mig'dah-līn) 1. like an almond. 2. pertaining to tonsils.

amygdalolith (ah-mig'dah-lo-lith") calculus in a tonsil.

amyl (am'il) the radical C_5H_{11}. **a. nitrite,** a clear, yellowish, inflammable liquid, $C_5H_{11}NO_2$, inhaled for relief of arterial spasm, convulsions and asthmatic paroxysms.

amyl(o)- (am'ĭ-lo) word element [Gr.], *starch.*

amylaceous (am"ĭ-la'shus) composed of or resembling starch.

amylase (am'ĭ-lās) an enzyme that catalyzes the hydrolysis of starch into simpler compounds.

amylene (am'ĭ-lēn) poisonous hydrocarbon, C_5H_{10}; dangerous anesthetic. **a. hydrate,** clear, colorless liquid, $C_5H_{12}O$, used as a vehicle in pharmacy.

amylobarbitone (am″ĭ-lo-bar′bĭ-tōn) amobarbital.

amylodextrin (-deks′trin) a compound formed during the change of starch into sugar.

amylogenesis (-jen′ĕ-sis) the formation of starch. adj., **amylogen′ic.**

amyloid (am′ĭ-loid) 1. starchlike; amylaceous. 2. an optically homogeneous, waxy, translucent glycoprotein which is deposited intercellularly in a variety of conditions.

amyloidosis (am″ĭ-loid-o′sis) intercellular deposit of amyloid in the tissues.

amylolysis (am″ĭ-lol′ĭ-sis) digestive change of starch into sugar.

amylolytic (am″ĭ-lo-lit′ik) effecting the digestion of starch.

amylopectinosis (-pek′tĭ-no″sis) a form of hepatic glycogen disease resulting from deficiency of glycogen "brancher" enzyme and associated with a form of cirrhosis of the liver.

amylophagia (-fa′je-ah) the eating of starch.

amylopsin (am″ĭ-lop′sin) a pancreatic enzyme which converts starch to maltose.

amylorrhea (am″ĭ-lo-re′ah) diarrhea with undigested starch in the stools.

amylorrhexis (-reks′is) the enzymatic splitting of starch.

amylose (am′ĭ-lōs) any carbohydrate other than a glucose or saccharose.

amylosis (am″ĭ-lo′sis) albuminoid degeneration.

amylosuria (am″ĭ-lo-su′re-ah) the presence of amylose in the urine.

amylum (am′ĭ-lum) [L.] starch.

amyluria (am″ĭ-lu′re-ah) presence of starch in the urine.

amyocardia (ah-mi″o-kar′de-ah) weakness of the heart muscle.

amyoplasia (ah-mi″o-pla′ze-ah) lack of muscle formation or development. **a. congen′ita,** generalized lack in the newborn of muscular development and growth, with contracture and deformity at most joints.

amyostasia (-sta′ze-ah) nervous tremor of the muscles.

amyosthenia (ah-mi″os-the′ne-ah) failure of muscular strength.

amyosthenic (ah-mi″os-then′ik) 1. characterized by amyosthenia. 2. an agent which diminishes muscular power.

amyotaxy (ah-mi′o-tak″se) muscular ataxia.

amyotonia (a-mi″o-to′ne-ah) atonic condition of the muscles. **a. congen′ita,** a rare congenital disease of children marked by general hypotonia of the muscles.

amyotrophia (ah-mi″o-tro′fe-ah) amyotrophy.

amyotrophy (ah″mi-ot′ro-fe) a painful condition with wasting and weakness of muscle, commonly involving the deltoid muscle. adj., **amyotroph′ic.**

Amytal (am′ĭ-tal) trademark for preparations of amobarbital.

amyxia (ah-mik′se-ah) absence of mucus.

amyxorrhea (a-mik″sŏ-re′ah) absence of mucous secretion.

An chemical symbol, *actinon.*

An. anisometropia; anode.

A.N.A. American Neurological Association; American Nurses' Association.

ana (an′ah) [Gr.] of each.

ana- (an′ah) word element [Gr.], *upward; again; backward; excessively.*

anabasis (ah-nab′ah-sis) the stage of increase in a disease. adj., **anabat′ic.**

anabiosis (an″ah-bi-o′sis) restoration of life processes after their apparent cessation; bringing back to consciousness. adj., **anabiot′ic.**

anabolergy (an″ah-bol′er-je) the work done in anabolism.

anabolin (ah-nab′o-lin) a product of constructive metabolism (anabolism).

anabolism (ah-nab′o-lizm) constructive metabolism; the process by which an organism converts simpler compounds into living, organized substance. adj., **anabol′ic.**

anacatharsis (an″ah-kah-thar′sis) violent and continued vomiting.

anachlorhydria (-klōr-hi′dre-ah) diminished hydrochloric acid in the gastric juice.

anacholia (-ko′le-ah) decreased secretion of bile.

anachoresis (-ko-re′sis) preferential collection or deposit of particles at a site, as of bacteria or metals that have localized out of the blood stream in areas of inflammation. adj., **anachoret′ic.**

anachronobiology (-kron″o-bi-ol′o-je) the study of the constructive effects (growth, development, maturation) of time on a living organism.

anacidity (-sid′ĭ-te) abnormal lack or deficiency of acid.

anaclisis (-kli′sis) the process of asexual drive becoming attached to and exploiting nonessential self-preservative trends such as eating and defecation.

anaclitic (-klit′ik) dependent upon another; characterized by libido depending on another instinct, such as hunger.

anacousia (-koo′ze-ah) anakusis.

anacroasia (-kro-a′ze-ah) inability to understand language, due to cerebral disease.

anacrotism (ah-nak′rŏ-tizm) the occurrence of one or more indentations on the ascending limb of the sphygmogram. adj., **anacrot′ic.**

anaculture (an′ah-kul″chur) a bacterial whole culture treated with formalin and incubated; used for prophylactic vaccination.

anadenia (an″ah-de′ne-ah) defect of glandular or absence of glands.

anadicrotism (-di′krŏ-tizm) the occurrence of two indentations on the ascending limb of the sphygmogram. adj., **anadicrot′ic.**

anadipsia (-dip′se-ah) intense thirst.

anadrenalism (-dre′nal-izm) absence or failure of adrenal function.

anaerobe (an-a′er-ōb) an organism that lives and grows in the absence of molecular oxygen. adj., **anaero′bic. facultative a.,** an organism that can live without molecular oxygen, but does not require its absence. **obligate a.,** an organism that cannot live in the presence of molecular oxygen.

anaerobion (an″a-er-o′be-on) anaerobe.

anaerobiosis (an-a″er-o-bi-o′sis) life without free oxygen. adj., **anaerobiot′ic.**

anaerogenic (-jen′ik) suppressing the formation of gas by gas-producing bacteria.

anaerophyte (an-a′er-o-fīt″) a vegetable anaerobic microorganism.

anaerosis (an″a-er-o′sis) interruption of the respiratory function.

anagen (an′ah-jen) the first phase of the hair cycle, during which synthesis of hair takes place.

anagenesis (an″ah-jen′ĕ-sis) regeneration of tissue.

anagocytic (an-ag″o-si′tik) retarding the growth of cells.

anakatadidymus (an″ah-kat″ah-did′ĭ-mus) a twin fetal monster, separate above and below, but united in the trunk.

anakusis (-ku′sis) deafness due to a nervous or central lesion.

anal (a′nal) relating to the anus.

analbuminemia (an″al-bu″mĭ-ne′me-ah) deficiency of serum albumins in the blood.

analeptic (an″ah-lep′tik) 1. restorative; cordial. 2. a restorative medicine.

Analexin (an″ah-lek′sin) trademark for preparations of phenyramidol.

analgesia (an″al-je′ze-ah) 1. absence of sensibility to pain. 2. reduction or abolition of the response to painful stimuli. **a. al′gera, a. dolor′sa,** acute pain with loss of sensibility in a part. **audio a.,** production of insensitivity to pain by the use of loud sound, particularly in dentistry. **continuous caudal a.,** continuous injection of an anesthetic solution into the sacral canal to relieve the pain of childbirth. **paretic a.,** loss of the sense of pain accompanied by partial paralysis.

analgesic (-je′sik) 1. relieving pain. 2. pertaining to analgesia. 3. a drug which relieves pain.

Analgesine (-je′sin) trademark for a preparation of antipyrine.

analgetic (-jet′ik) analgesic.

analgia (an-al′je-ah) painlessness. adj., **anal′gic.**

anallergic (an″ah-ler′jik) not causing allergy or sensitization.

analogous (ah-nal′o-gus) 1. serving a similar function, but not arising from common rudiments and not similar in basic plan and development. 2. having similar properties.

analogue (an′ah-log) 1. a part resembling another in function, but not in structure. 2. one of two or more chemical compounds having similar properties, but different atomic structure.

analogy (ah-nal′o-je) 1. resemblance in function between organs of different origin. 2. similarity in properties of two or more chemical compounds.

analysand (ah-nal′ĭ-sand) a person undergoing psychoanalysis.

analysis (ah-nal′ĭ-sis) 1. separation into component parts. 2. psychoanalysis. **bite a.,** occlusal analysis. **chromosome a.,** determination of the number and types of chromosomes in a cell. **gasometric a.,** analysis by measurement of the gas evolved. **gravimetric a.,** determination by weight of the quantity of the elements of a compound. **occlusal a.,** study of the relations of the occlusal surfaces of opposing teeth. **organic a.,** analysis of animal and vegetable tissues. **proximate a.,** determination of the simpler constituents of a substance. **qualitative a.,** determination of the nature of the constituents of a compound. **quantitative a.,** determination of the proportionate quantities of the constituents of a compound. **ultimate a.,** resolution of a substance into its component elements. **vector a.,** analysis of a moving force to determine both its magnitude and its direction, e.g. analysis of the scalar electrocardiogram to determine the magnitude and direction of the electromotive force for one complete cycle of the heart. **volumetric a.,** quantitative analysis by volume.

analyzer (an″ah-līz′er) the Nicol prism in a polarimeter.

anamnesis (an″am-ne′sis) the past history of a patient.

anamnestic (-nes′tik) 1. pertaining to anamnesis. 2. aiding the memory.

anamniotic (an″am-ne-ot′ik) having no amnion.

ananabolic (an″an-ah-bol′ik) characterized by absence of anabolism.

ananaphylaxis (an-an″ah-fī-lak′sis) antianaphylaxis.

anandria (an an′dre-ah) absence of male characteristics.

anangioplasia (an-an″je-o-pla′ze-ah) imperfect formation of blood vessels in a part. adj., **anangioplas′tic.**

anapeiratic (an″ah-pi-rat′ik) due to excessive use or overexercise.

anaphase (an′ah-fāz) the third stage of division of the nucleus in either meiosis or mitosis.

anaphia (an-a′fe-ah) lack or loss of the sense of touch.

anaphoresis (an″ah-fo-re′sis) diminished activity of the sweat glands.

anaphoria (-fo′re-ah) the tendency to tilt the head downward, with visual axes deviating upward, on looking straight ahead.

anaphrodisia (an″af-ro-diz′e-ah) absence or loss of sexual desire.

anaphrodisiac (-diz′e-ak) 1. repressing sexual desire. 2. a drug that represses sexual desire.

anaphylactin (an″ah-fi-lak′tin) a substance in the blood of animals that have survived intoxication which causes increased susceptibility to the same toxin.

anaphylactogen (-fi-lak′to-jen) a substance that produces anaphylaxis or anaphylactin.

anaphylactogenesis (-fi-lak″to-jen′ĕ-sis) the production of anaphylaxis. adj., **anaphylactogen′ic.**

anaphylatoxin (-fi″lah-tok′sin) the poisonous substance in anaphylaxis.

anaphylatoxis (-fi″lah-tok′sis) the reaction produced by an anaphylatoxin.

anaphylaxin (-fi-lak′sin) anaphylactin.

anaphylaxis (-fi-lak′sis) exaggerated reaction of an organism to a foreign protein or other substance to which it has previously become sensitized. adj., **anaphylac'tic. acquired a.**, that in which sensitization is known to have been produced by administration of a foreign protein. **active a.**, that produced by injection of a foreign protein. **antiserum a.**, passive anaphylaxis. **heterologous a.**, passive anaphylaxis induced by transfer of serum from an animal of a different species. **homologous a.**, passive anaphylaxis induced by transfer of serum from an animal of the same species. **indirect a.**, that induced by an animal's own protein modified in some way. **passive a.**, that resulting in a normal person from injection of serum of a sensitized person. **psychic a.**, liability to development of neurotic symptoms as a result of early psychic trauma. **reverse a.**, that following injection of antigen, succeeded by injection of antiserum.

anaplasia (an"ah-pla'ze-ah)   an irreversible alteration in adult cells toward more primitive (embryonic) cell types.

Anaplasma (-plaz'mah) a genus of Microtatobiotes (order Rickettsiales, family Anaplasmataceae) causing an infection in animals known as anaplasmosis, or gallsickness.

Anaplasmataceae (-plaz"mah-ta'se-e) a family of Microtatobiotes (order Rickettsiales).

anaplasty (an'ah-plas"te) plastic or restorative surgery. adj., **anaplas'tic.**

anaplerosis (an"ah-ple-ro'sis) surgical transplantation of tissue to fill a defect caused by disease or injury.

anapnograph (an-ap'no-graf)   device for registering speed and pressure of respired air current.

anapnoic (an"ap-no'ik) relieving dyspnea.

anapnometer (an"ap-nom'ē-ter) spirometer.

anapophysis (an"ah-pof'ĭ-sis)   an accessory vertebral process.

anaptic (an-ap'tik)   pertaining to or characterized by loss of the sense of touch.

anarithmia (an"ah-rith'me-ah)   inability to count, due to a lesion of the central nervous system.

anarthria (an-ar'thre-ah) lack of the faculty of speech because of impairment of speech organs and their innervation. **a. litera'lis**, stuttering.

anasarca (an"ah-sar'kah)   accumulation of great amounts of fluid in all the body tissues.

anastaltic (-stal'tik) styptic; highly astringent.

anastate (an'ah-stāt) any substance or condition characteristic of an anabolic process.

anastole (ah-nas'to-le) retraction, as of the lips of a wound.

anastomosis (ah-nas"to-mo'sis) 1. communication between two tubular organs. 2. surgical or pathologic formation of a connection between two normally distinct structures. adj., **anastomot'ic. arteriovenous a.**, anastomosis between an artery and a vein. **crucial a.**, an arterial anastomosis in the upper part of the thigh. **heterocladic a.**, one between branches of different arteries. **intestinal a.**, establishment of a communication between two formerly distant portions of the intestine.

anastral (an-as'tral)   of or pertaining to a mitotic figure.

anat. anatomy.

anatomic (an"ah-tom'ik)   pertaining to the structure of the body.

anatomical (-tom'e-kal)   pertaining to anatomy.

anatomist (ah-nat'o-mist) one skilled in anatomy.

anatomy (ah-nat'o-me)   the science dealing with the form and structure of living organisms. **applied a.**, consideration of anatomical facts in relation to physical diagnosis, surgery and other pertinent applications. **comparative a.**, description and comparison of the form and structure of different animals. **developmental a.**, embryology. **gross a.**, that dealing with structures visible with the unaided eye. **macroscopic a.**, gross anatomy. **microscopic a.**, histology. **morbid a.**, **pathologic a.**, anatomy of diseased tissues. **radiologic a.**, x-ray anatomy. **special a.**, anatomy devoted to study of a single type or species of organism. **topographic a.**, that devoted to determination of relative positions of various body parts. **veterinary a.**, the science dealing with the body form and structure of the principal domesticated animals. **x-ray a.**, study of organs and tissues based on their visualization by x-rays in both living and dead bodies.

anatoxin (an"ah-tok'sin) toxoid.

anatricrotism (-trik'ro-tizm)   the occurrence of three indentations on the ascending limb of the sphygmogram. adj., **anatricrot'ic.**

anatriptic (-trip'tik)   a medicine applied by rubbing.

anatrophic (-trof'ik) preventing atrophy.

anatropia (-tro'pe-ah) upward deviation of the visual axis of one eye when the other eye is fixing. adj., **anatrop'ic.**

anaxon (an-ak'son)   a nerve cell devoid of an axon.

anazoturia (an-az"o-tu're-ah)   decreased urea in the urine.

anchorage (ang'kŏ-rij) surgical fixation of a displaced viscus.

anchylo- (ang'kĭ-lo) for words beginning thus, see those beginning *ankylo-.*

ancipital (an-sip'ĭ-tal) two-edged.

anconad (ang'ko-nad)   toward the elbow or olecranon.

anconagra (ang"ko-nag'rah) gouty seizure of the elbow.

anconal (ang'ko-nal) pertaining to the elbow.

anconitis (an"ko-ni'tis) inflammation of the elbow joint.

ancylo- for words beginning thus, see also those beginning *ankylo-.*

Ancylostoma (an"sī-los'to-mah)   a genus of nematode parasites. **A. america'num**, *Necator americanus.* **A. brazilien'se**, a species parasitic in dogs and cats in tropical and subtropical regions; also reported in man. **A. cani'num**, the common hookworm of dogs and cats. **A. ceylon'icum**, a species infesting felines and canines in India. **A. duodena'le**, the common hookworm, parasitic in the small intestine.

ancylostomiasis (an"sī-los"to-mi'ah-sis)   infection by worms of the genus Ancylostoma or by other hookworms (*Necator americanus*).

Ancylostomidae (an″sī-lo-sto′mĭ-de) a family of nematode parasites having two ventrolateral cutting plates at the entrance to a large buccal capsule, and small teeth at its base; the hookworms.

ancyroid (an′sī-roid) anchor-shaped.

andr(o)- (an′dro) word element [Gr.], *male; masculine.*

andriatrics (an″dre-at′rĭks) the branch of medicine dealing with diseases of men.

audrin (an′drin) any one of the androgens of the testis.

androcyte (an′dro-sīt) spermatid.

androgen (an′dro-jen) any substance that stimulates male characteristics. adj., **androgen′ic.**

androgenicity (an″dro-jĕ-nis′ĭ-te) the quality of exerting a masculinizing effect.

android (an′droid) resembling a man.

andrology (an-drol′o-je) the science of man or human nature.

andromerogon (an″dro-mer′o-gon) an organism produced by andromerogony and containing only the paternal set of chromosomes.

andromerogony (-mer-og′o-ne) development of a portion of a fertilized ovum containing the male pronucleus only.

androphilic (-fil′ik) preferring man to animals.

androphobia (fo″be-ah) morbid dread of the male sex.

androphonomania (-fo″no-ma′ne-ah) a morbid impulse to homicide.

androstane (an′dro-stān) the hydrocarbon nucleus, $C_{19}H_{32}$, from which androgens are derived.

androstanediol (an″dro-stān′de-ol) an androgen, $C_{19}H_{32}O_2$, prepared by reducing androsterone.

androstene (an′dro-stēn) an unsaturated cyclic hydrocarbon, $C_{19}H_{30}$, forming the nucleus of testosterone and certain other androgens.

androstenediol (an″dro-stēn′de-ol) a crystalline androgenic steroid, $C_{19}H_{30}O_2$.

androsterone (an-dros′ter ōn) an androgenic hormone, $C_{19}H_{30}O_2$, occurring in urine or prepared synthetically.

-ane (ān) word termination denoting (1) a saturated open-chain hydrocarbon (C_nH_{2n+2}); (2) an organic compound in which hydrogen has replaced the hydroxyl group.

Anectine (an-ek′tin) trademark for preparations of succinylcholine.

anelectrode (an″e-lek′trōd) the positive pole of a battery.

anelectrotonus (an″e-lek-trot′ŏ-nus) lessened irritability of a nerve at the anode during passage of electric current.

anemia (ah-ne′me-ah) a state characterized by deficiency of either hemoglobin or erythrocytes in circulating blood. **achrestic a.,** anemia due to inability to utilize a necessary factor present in the body. **aplastic a.,** persistent anemia resistant to therapy and characterized by absence of regeneration of red blood cells. **Cooley's a.,** thalassemia. **Czerny's a.,** anemia in infants due to deficient nourish-

ment. **drepanocytic a., Dresbach's a.,** sickle cell anemia. **essential a.,** idiopathic anemia. **hemolytic a.,** anemia characterized by rapid destruction and later regeneration of red blood cells, due to infection, drugs or exposure to chemicals; it may also occur as a result of an autoimmune process. **hypochromic a.,** anemia in which the decrease in hemoglobin is proportionately much greater than the decrease in number of red blood cells. **hypoplastic a.,** anemia due to incapacity of blood-forming organs. **idiopathic a.,** that due to disease of the blood or the blood-producing organs. **Jaksch's a.,** infantile pseudoleukemia. **Lederer's a.,** acute anemia with megaloblastic blood cell regeneration, raised color index and high leukocyte count. **a. lymphat′ica.** Hodgkin's disease. **macrocytic a.,** anemia in which the red cells are much larger than normal. **Mediterranean a.,** thalassemia. **megaloblastic a.,** anemia characterized by the presence of megaloblasts in the bone marrow. **microcytic a.,** anemia characterized by decrease in size of the red cells. **miner's a.,** ancylostomiasis. **myelopathic a., myelophthisic a.,** anemia due to destruction or crowding out of hematopoietic tissues by space-occupying lesions. **normocytic a.,** anemia characterized by proportionate decrease in hemoglobin, packed red cell volume, and number of erythrocytes per cubic millimeter of blood. **pernicious a.,** megaloblastic anemia in adult life, considered due to lack of secretion by the gastric mucosa of a factor essential to proper blood formation. **primary a.,** that due to disease of the blood-forming organs. **secondary a.,** that due to some cause other than disease of the blood-forming organs. **sickle cell a.,** a genetically determined defect of hemoglobin synthesis associated with poor physical development and skeletal anomalies, occurring usually in Negroes. **spherocytic a.,** spherocytosis. **splenic a., a. splen′ica,** anemia with enlarged spleen. **symptomatic a.,** secondary anemia. **target cell a.,** thalassemia. **tunnel a.,** ancylostomiasis.

anemic (ah-ne′mik) pertaining to anemia.

anemometer (an″e-mom′e-ter) instrument for measuring velocity of wind.

anemophilous (an″em-of′ĭ-lus) fertilized by wind-borne pollen; said of certain flowers.

anemophobia (an″ĕ-mo-fo′be-ah) morbid fear of wind or draughts.

anemotrophy (an″em-ot′ro-fe) insufficient nourishment of the blood.

anencephalohemia (an″en-sef″ah-lo-he′me-ah) insufficient supply of blood to the brain.

anencephaly (an″en-sef′ah-le) developmental anomaly with absence of neural tissue in the cranium. adj., **anencephal′ic.**

anenzymia (an″en-zi′me-ah) absence of an enzyme normally present in the body. **a. catala′sea,** acatalasia.

anephrogenesis (a″nef-ro-jen′ĕ-sis) failure of embryonic development of kidney tissue.

anepia (an-e′pe-ah) inability to speak.

anergasia (an″er-ga′ze-ah) a behavioral disorder due to organic lesions of the central nervous system. adj., **anerga'sic.**

anergy (an'er-je) a total loss of reactivity. adj., **aner'gic.**

anerythrocyte (an"ĕ-rith'ro-sīt) an erythrocyte without hemoglobin.

anerythroplastic (an"e-rith'ro-plas"tik) not forming erythrocytes.

anerythropoiesis (an"e-rith"ro-poi-e'-sis) deficient production of erythrocytes.

anerythropsia (an"er-ī-throp'se-ah) inability to distinguish red colors.

anesthecinesia (an-es"the-sĭ-ne'ze-ah) combined sensory and motor paralysis.

anesthesia (an"es-the'ze-ah) absence of sensitivity to stimuli. **basal a.,** narcosis produced by preliminary medication so that the inhalation of anesthetic necessary to produce surgical anesthesia is greatly reduced. **block a.,** that produced by blocking transmission of impulses through a nerve. **bulbar a.,** anesthesia due to a lesion of the pons. **caudal a.,** caudal analgesia. **central a.,** anesthesia dependent on disease of the central nervous system. **cerebral a.,** that due to a cerebral lesion. **closed a.,** that produced by continuous rebreathing of a small amount of anesthetic gas in a closed system with an apparatus for removing carbon dioxide. **conduction a.,** regional anesthesia. **crossed a.,** loss of sensation on one side of the face and loss of pain and temperature sense on the opposite side of the body. **dissociated a., dissociation a.,** loss of perception of certain stimuli while that of others remains intact. **doll's head a.,** anesthesia of the head, neck and upper part of the chest. **a. doloro'sa,** tactile anesthesia with severe pain in the part, after occurrence of paralysis, seen in certain diseases of the spinal cord. **electric a.,** anesthesia induced by passage of an electric current. **frost a.,** abolition of feeling or sensation as a result of topical refrigeration produced by a jet of a highly volatile liquid. **gauntlet a.,** anesthesia from wrist to fingertips. **general a.,** a state of unconsciousness and insusceptibility to pain, produced by an anesthetic agent. **girdle a.,** a ring of anesthesia around the body. **gustatory a.,** ageusia. **infiltration a.,** local anesthesia produced by injection of the anesthetic solution directly into the tissues. **insufflation a.,** anesthesia produced by introduction of a gaseous mixture into the trachea through a slender tube. **intraoral a.,** that produced by injection of the agent in the tissues of the mouth. **local a.,** that confined to a limited area. **mental a.,** inability to recognize and identify sensory stimuli. **mixed a.,** that produced by use of more than one anesthetic agent. **muscular a.,** loss of the muscular sense. **olfactory a.,** anosmia. **open a.,** general inhalation anesthesia in which there is no rebreathing of the expired gases. **partial a.,** anesthesia with retention of some degree of sensibility. **peripheral a.,** anesthesia due to changes in the peripheral nerves. **rectal a.,** anesthesia produced by introduction of the anesthetic agent into the rectum.

refrigeration a., local anesthesia produced by chilling the part to near freezing temperature. **regional a.,** insensibility caused by interrupting the sensory nerve conductivity of any region of the body; it may be produced by (1) *field block,* encircling the operative field by means of injections of a local anesthetic; or (2) *nerve block,* making injections in close proximity to the nerves supplying the area. **segmental a.,** loss of sensation in a segment of the body due to lesion of a single nerve root. **spinal a.,** 1. anesthesia due to a spinal lesion. 2. anesthesia produced by injection of the agent beneath the membrane of the spinal cord. **splanchnic a.,** block anesthesia for visceral operation by injection of anesthetic agent into the region of the semilunar ganglia. **surgical a.,** that degree of anesthesia at which operation may safely be performed. **tactile a.,** loss of the sense of touch. **thermic a.,** loss of the heat sense. **topical a.,** that produced by application of a local anesthetic directly to the area involved. **twilight a.,** twilight sleep. **unilateral a.,** hemianesthesia. **visceral a.,** loss of visceral sensations.

anesthesimeter (an"es-thĕ-sim'ĕ-ter) 1. instrument for testing degree of anesthesia. 2. device for regulating the amount of anesthetic given.

Anesthesin (ah-nes'the-sin) trademark for a preparation of ethyl aminobenzoate.

anesthesiologist (an"es-the"ze-ol'o-jist) a specialist in anesthesiology.

anesthesiology (-ol'o-je) that branch of medicine concerned with administration of anesthetics and the condition of the patient while under anesthesia.

anesthesiophore (an"es-the'ze-o-fōr) the group of atoms in a molecule which produces the anesthetic action.

anesthetic (an"es-thet'ik) 1. lacking feeling or sensation. 2. an agent that produces anesthesia.

anesthetist (ah-nes'thĕ-tist) one who administers anesthetics.

anesthetization (ah-nes"thĕ-ti-za'shun) production of anesthesia.

anethole (an'ĕ-thōl) a colorless or faintly yellow liquid, $C_{10}H_{12}O$, used as a flavoring agent for drugs and to expel secretions from the air passages and to stimulate intestinal peristalsis.

anetoderma (ah-ne"to-der'mah) looseness and atrophy of the skin.

aneuploid (an'u-ploid) 1. characterized by aneuploidy. 2. an individual or cell characterized by aneuploidy.

aneuploidy (an"u-ploi'de) the state of having chromosomes in a number that is not an exact multiple of the haploid number.

aneuria (ah-nu're-ah) deficiency of nervous energy. adj., **aneu'ric.**

aneurin (ah-nu'rin) thiamine.

aneurysm (an'u-rizm) dilatation of a segment of a blood vessel, often involving the aorta or pulmonary artery. adj., **aneurys'mal. a. by anastomosis,** dilatation of a number of vessels, forming a pulsating tumor beneath the skin. **arteriovenous a.**, simultaneous rupture of an artery and vein, the blood being retained in the surrounding tissue. **Berard's a.**, varicose aneurysm whose sac is developed in tissues around the vein. **berry a.**, a small outpouching of the inner lining of a blood vessel, usually at an angle of bifurcation of the cerebral arteries. **cirsoid a.**, dilatation and tortuous lengthening of part of an artery. **compound a.**, one in which some of the layers of the wall of the vessel are ruptured and some merely dilated. **dissecting a.**, one in which rupture of the inner coat has permitted blood to escape between layers of the vessel wall. **false a.**, one in which all the coats are ruptured and the blood is retained in surrounding tissues. **fusiform a.**, a spindle-shaped aneurysm. **mixed a.**, compound aneurysm. **racemose a.**, cirsoid aneurysm. **sacculated a.**, a saclike aneurysm. **spurious a.**, false aneurysm. **varicose a.**, one formed by rupture of an aneurysm into a vein.

aneurysmectomy (an″u-riz-mek′to-me) excision of an aneurysm.

aneurysmoplasty (an″u-riz′mo-plas″te) plastic repair of an artery for aneurysm.

aneurysmorrhaphy (an″u-riz-mor′ah-fe) suture of an aneurysm.

aneurysmotomy (-mot′o-me) incision of an aneurysm.

anfractuosity (an-frak tu-os i-te) a cerebral sulcus.

anfractuous (an-frak′tu-us) convoluted; sinuous.

angi(o)- (an″je-o) word element [Gr.], *vessel (channel)*.

angiasthenia (an″je-as-the′ne-ah) loss of tone in the vascular system.

angiectasis (-ek′tah-sis) dilatation of a vessel.

angiectomy (-ek′to-me) excision of part of a blood or lymph vessel.

angiectopia (-ek-to′pe-ah) abnormal position or course of a vessel.

angiemphraxis (-em-frak′sis) obstruction of a vessel.

angiitis (-i′tis) inflammation of the coats of a vessel, chiefly blood or lymph vessels.

angina (an″ji-nah, an-ji′nah) any disease marked by spasmodic suffocative attacks. **agranulocytic a.**, agranulocytosis a. **cru′ris**, intermittent lameness with cyanosis of the affected limb; due to arterial obstruction. **intestinal a.**, generalized cramping abdominal pain occurring shortly after a meal and persisting for one to three hours, due to ischemia of the smooth muscle of the bowel. **a. laryn′gea**, laryngitis. **Ludwig's a.**, **a. ludovi′ci**, **a. lud′wigi**, purulent inflammation around the submaxillary gland. **a. parotid′ea**, mumps. **a. pec′toris**, a distinctive type of distress or pain due to deficiency of blood supply to the heart muscle. **Plaut's a.**, Vincent's angina. **streptococcus a.**, angina due to streptococci. **a. tonsilla′ris**, quinsy. **a. trachea′lis**, croup. **Vincent's a.**, inflammation of the gingivae and oral mucous membrane, with ulceration and membrane

formation and accompanied with pain on swallowing.

anginoid (an′ji-noid) resembling angina.

anginophobia (an″ji-no-fo′be-ah) morbid dread of angina pectoris.

anginose (an′ji-nōs) characterized by angina.

angioataxia (an″je-o-ah-tak′se-ah) irregular tension of the blood vessels.

angioblast (an′je-o-blast″) the earliest formative tissue from which blood cells and blood vessels arise. adj., **angioblast′ic**.

angioblastoma (an″je-o-blas-to′mah) hemangiosarcoma.

angiocardiogram (-kar′de-o-gram) the film produced by angiocardiography.

angiocardiography (-kar″de-og′rah-fe) radiography of the heart and great vessels after introduction of an opaque contrast medium into a blood vessel or one of the cardiac chambers.

angiocardiokinetic (-kar″de-o-ki-net′ik) pertaining to movements of heart and blood vessels.

angiocardiopathy (-kar″de-op′ah-the) disease of heart and blood vessels.

angiocarditis (-kar-di′tis) inflammation of heart and blood vessels.

angiocholecystitis (-ko″le-sis-ti′tis) inflammation of gallbladder and bile ducts.

angiocholitis (-ko-li′tis) inflammation of bile ducts.

angiochondroma (-kon-dro′mah) chondroma with excessive development of blood vessels.

angioclast (an′je-o-klast″) a forceps for compressing a bleeding artery.

Angiococcus (an″je-o-kok′us) a genus of Schizomycetes (order Myxobacterales, family Myxococcaceae).

angiodermatitis (-der″mah-ti′tis) inflammation of the vessels of the skin.

angiodiascopy (-di-as′ko-pe) visual inspection of blood vessels of the extremities.

angioendothelioma (-en″do-the″le-o′mah) hemangioendothelioma.

angiofibroma (-fi-bro′mah) angioma containing fibrous tissue.

angiogenesis (-jen′e-sis) development of blood vessels in the embryo.

angiogenic (-jen′ik) 1. pertaining to angiogenesis. 2. of vascular origin.

angioglioma (-gli-o′mah) a form of vascular glioma.

angiogram (an′je-o-gram) a roentgenogram of a blood vessel.

angiography (an″je-og′rah-fe) radiography of vessels of the body. (See also *arteriography; lymphangiography; phlebography.*)

angiohemophilia (an″je-o-he″mo-fil′e-ah) a congenital hemorrhagic diathesis with bleeding from the skin and mucosal surfaces, due to abnormal blood vessels with or without platelet defects or deficiencies of blood coagulation factor VIII or IX.

angiohyalinosis (-hi″ah-li-no′sis) hyaline degeneration of the muscular coat of blood vessels.

angiohypertonia (-hi″per-to′ne-ah) angiospasm.

angiohypotonia (an″je-o-hi″po-to′ne-ah) angioparalysis.

angioid (an′je-oid) resembling blood vessels.

angioinvasive (an″je-o-in-va′siv) tending to invade the walls of blood vessels.

angiokeratoma (-ker″ah-to′mah) angioma blended with keratoma of skin. **a. cor′poris diffu′sum,** a condition marked by dark purple lesions on the trunk, associated with cardiovascular disease, renal abnormalities and hypertension.

angiokinetic (-ki-net′ik) vasomotor.

angioleucitis (-lu-si′tis) inflammation of a lymph vessel.

angiolipoma (-lĭ-po′mah) angioma containing fatty tissue.

angiolith (an′je-o-lith″) a calcareous deposit in the wall of a blood vessel. adj., **angiolith′ic.**

angiology (an″je-ol′o-je) scientific study or description of the vessels (cardiovascular system).

angiolupoid (an″je-o-lu′poid) a tuberculous skin lesion consisting of small, oval red plaques.

angiolymphitis (-lim-fi′tis) lymphangitis.

angiolymphoma (-lim-fo′mah) tumor made up of lymph vessels.

angiolysis (an″je-ol′ĭ-sis) retrogression or obliteration of blood vessels, as in embryologic development.

angioma (an″je-o′mah) a tumor made up of blood or lymph vessels. adj., **angiom′atous. a. caverno′sum,** an erectile tumor. **hereditary hemorrhagic a.,** a condition marked by unexplained bleeding and angiomatous lesions of skin and mucous membrane. **a. serpigino′-sum,** skin disease marked by minute vascular points arranged in rings on the skin. **telangiectatic a.,** one made up of dilated blood vessels.

angiomalacia (an″je-o-mah-la′she-ah) softening of walls of the vessels.

angiomatosis (-mah-to′sis) the presence of multiple angiomas. **hemorrhagic familial a.,** hereditary hemorrhagic angioma. **a. of retina,** diseased retinal blood vessels with subretinal hemorrhages.

angiomegaly (-meg′ah-le) enlargement of blood vessels, especially a condition of the eyelid marked by great increase in its volume.

angiometer (an″je-om′ĕ-ter) instrument for measuring diameter and tension of blood vessels.

angiomyocardiac (an″je-o-mi″o-kar′de-ak) affecting blood vessels and heart muscle.

angiomyoma (-mi-o′mah) angioma blended with myoma.

angiomyoneuroma (-mi″o-nu-ro′mah) glomangioma.

angiomyosarcoma (-mi″o-sar-ko′mah) angioma blended with myoma and sarcoma.

angioneurectomy (-nu-rek′to-me) resection of all elements of the spermatic cord except the vas deferens with its artery and vein, for cure of enlarged prostate.

angioneuroma (-nu-ro′mah) glomangioma.

angioneuromyoma (-nu″ro-mi-o′mah) glomangioma.

angioneurosis (an″je-o-nu-ro′sis) angioparalysis, angiospasm or other neurosis primarily affecting blood vessels. adj., **angioneurot′ic.**

angionoma (-no′mah) ulceration of blood vessels.

angiopancreatitis (-pan″kre-ah-ti′tis) inflammation of the vascular tissue of the pancreas.

angioparalysis (-pah-ral′ĭ-sis) vasomotor paralysis of blood vessels.

angioparesis (-par′e-sis) vasomotor paresis.

angiopathy (an″je-op′ah-the) any disease of the vessels.

angioplany (an′je-o-plan″e) abnormality in position, course or structure of a vessel.

angioplasty (an′je-o-plas″te) plastic repair of blood vessels or lymphatic channels.

angiopoiesis (an″je-o-poi-e′sis) the formation of blood vessels. adj., **angiopoiet′ic.**

angiopressure (-presh′ūr) control of hemorrhage by application of hemostatic forceps.

angiopsathyrosis (-sath″ĭ-ro′sis) fragility of blood vessels.

angiorhigosis (-ri-go′sis) rigidity of blood vessels.

angiorrhaphy (an″je-or′ah-fe) suture of a blood vessel.

angiorrhexis (an″je-o-rek′sis) rupture of a blood vessel.

angiosarcoma (-sar-ko′mah) hemangiosarcoma.

angiosclerosis (-skle-ro′sis) hardening of the walls of blood vessels.

angioscope (an′je-o-skōp″) a microscope for observing the capillaries.

angioscotoma (an″je-o-sko-to′mah) a narrow linear defect in the visual field.

angioscotometry (-sko-tom′ĕ-tre) measurement of an angioscotoma.

angiosialitis (-si″ah-li′tis) inflammation of a salivary duct.

angiosis (an″je-o′sis) angiopathy.

angiospasm (an′je-o-spazm″) spasmodic contraction of the walls of a blood vessel. adj., **angiospas′tic.**

angiostaxis (an″je-o-stak′sis) hemorrhagic diathesis.

angiostenosis (-ste-no′sis) narrowing of the caliber of blood vessels.

angiosteosis (an″je-os″te-o′sis) calcification of a vessel.

angiostrongyliasis (an″je-o-stron″jĭ-li′ah-sis) infection by nematodes of the genus Angiostrongylus.

Angiostrongylus (-stron′jĭ-lus) a genus of nematode parasites. **A. cantonen′sis,** a species reported in cases of human meningoencephalitis in Hawaii and in other areas in the Pacific and in Asia. **A. vaso′rum,** a species of worms parasitic in the pulmonary arteries of dogs.

angiostrophy (an″je-os′tro-fe) twisting of a vessel for the arrest of hemorrhage.

angiosynizesis (an″je-o-sin″ĭ-ze′sis) collapse and subsequent adhesion of blood vessel walls.

angiotelectasis (-tel-ek′tah-sis) dilatation of blood vessels.

angiotensin (an″je-o-ten′sin) a vasopressor substance found in the blood.

angiotitis (-ti′tis) inflammation of the vessels of the ear.

angiotome (an′je-o-tōm″) one of the segments of the vascular system of the embryo.

angiotomy (an″je-ot′o-me) incision of a blood vessel or lymphatic channel.

angiotonase (an″je-o-to′nās) hypertensinase.

angiotonic (-ton′ik) increasing vascular tension.

angiotonin (-to′nin) angiotensin.

angiotribe (an′je-o-trīb″) a strong forceps for crushing tissue containing an artery, for the purpose of checking hemorrhage.

angiotripsy (an′je-o-trip″se) hemostasis by means of an angiotribe.

angiotrophic (an″je-o-trof′ik) pertaining to nutrition of vessels.

angiotrophoneurosis (-trof″-o-nu-ro′sis) a neurosis of the blood vessels with trophic disturbance.

angle (ang′gl) the space or figure formed by two diverging lines, measured as the number of degrees one would have to be moved to coincide with the other. **acromial a.,** that between head of humerus and clavicle. **alpha a.,** that formed by intersection of the visual axis with optic axis. **axial a.,** one whose formation depends partially on the axial wall of a tooth cavity. **cardiodiaphragmatic a.,** that formed by the junction of the shadows of the heart and diaphragm in posteroanterior roentgenograms of the heart. **cavity a′s,** the angles formed by the junction of two or more walls of a tooth cavity. **costovertebral a.,** the angle formed on either side of the vertebral column between the last rib and the lumbar vertebrae. **filtration a., a. of the iris,** the angle between the iris and cornea at the periphery of the anterior chamber of the eye, through which the aqueous readily permeates. **a. of jaw,** the junction of the lower edge with the posterior edge of the lower jaw. **kappa a.,** the angle between the pupillary axes. **line a.,** an angle formed by the junction of two planes; in dentistry, the junction of two surfaces of a tooth or of two walls of a tooth cavity. **Louis's a., Ludwig's a.,** that between manubrium and gladiolus. **meter a.,** angle formed by intersection of the visual axis and the perpendicular bisector of the line joining the centers of rotation of the two eyes when viewing a point one meter distant (*small meter angle*) or the angle formed by intersection of the visual axes of the two eyes in the midline at a distance of one meter (*large meter angle*). **optic a.,** visual angle. **point a.,** an angle formed by the junction of three planes; in dentistry, the junction of three surfaces of a tooth, or of three walls of a tooth cavity. **a. of pubis,** that between the pubic bones at the symphysis. **sternoclavicular a.,** that between the sternum and the clavicle. **tooth a.,** an angle formed by two or three surfaces of a tooth. **visual a.,** the angle between two lines passing from the extremities of an object seen, through the nodal point of the eye, to the corresponding extremities of the image of the object seen. **Y a.,** the angle between the radius fixus and the line joining the lambda and inion.

angstrom (ang′strom) a unit of linear measurement, equivalent to 0.1 millimicron (10^{-7} mm.); abbreviated A.

angulation (ang″gu-la′shun) formation of sharp obstructive bend, as in the intestine.

angulus (ang′gu-lus), pl. *an′guli* [L.] angle; used in names of anatomic structures or landmarks. **a. infectio′sus,** perlèche. **a. i′ridis** [BNA], the angle of the iris. **a. Ludovi′ci,** Louis's angle. **a. mandib′ulae** [BNA], the angle of the jaw. **a. ocu′li** [BNA], the canthus of the eye. **a. o′ris,** the corner of the mouth. **a. pu′bis** [BNA], the angle of the pubes. **a. ster′ni,** Louis's angle. **a. veno′sus,** the angle at the junction of the common jugular vein and the subclavian vein.

anhedonia (an-hem″ah-to-poi-e′sis) an-hematosis. adj., **anhematopoiet′ic.**

anhematopoiesis (an-hem″ah-to-poi-e′sis) an-hematosis. adj., **anhematopoiet′ic.**

anhematosis (an″hem-ah-to′sis) defective blood formation.

anhemolytic (an″he-mo-lit′ik) not destructive to blood cells.

anhidrosis (an″hǐ-dro′sis) absence of sweating.

anhidrotic (an″hǐ-drot′ik) 1. checking the flow of sweat. 2. an agent which suppresses perspiration.

anhydrase (an-hi′drās) an enzyme which catalyzes the removal of water from a compound. **carbonic a.,** an enzyme which catalyzes the decomposition of carbonic acid into carbon dioxide and water, facilitating transfer of carbon dioxide from tissues to blood and from blood to alveolar air.

anhydration (an″hi-dra′shun) the condition of not being hydrated.

anhydremia (an″hi-dre′me-ah) diminution of the fluid content of the blood.

anhydride (an-hi′drīd) compound derived from an acid by abstraction of a molecule of water. **chromic a.,** chromium trioxide, CrO_3; caustic.

anhydrochloric (an″hi-dro-klo′rik) characterized by absence of hydrochloric acid.

anhydromyelia (-mi-e′le-ah) deficiency of the fluid of the spinal cord.

anhydrous (an-hi′drus) containing no water.

anhypnosis (an″hip-no′sis) insomnia.

anianthinopsy (an″e-an″thǐ-nop′se) inability to distinguish violet tints.

anideus (ah-nid′e-us) a parasitic fetal monster consisting of a shapeless mass of flesh.

anidrosis (an″ǐ-dro′sis) anhidrosis.

anileridine (an″ǐ-ler′ǐ-dēn) a chemical used as a narcotic, analgesic or sedative.

anilide (an′ǐ-lid) any compound formed from aniline by substituting a radical for the hydrogen of NH_2.

aniline (an′ǐ-lin) an amine, $C_6H_5NH_2$, from coal tar and indigo.

anilinophil (an″ǐ-lin′o-fil) a cell which stains readily with aniline dyes. adj., **anilinoph′-ilous.**

anilism (an′ǐ-lizm) aniline poisoning.

anility (ah-nil'ĭ-te) the state of being like an old woman.

anima (an'ĭ-mah) Jung's term for the unconscious, or inner being, of the individual.

animal (an'ĭ-mal) a living organism having sensation and power of voluntary movement. **control a.**, an untreated animal otherwise identical in all respects to one that is used for purposes of experimentation, used for checking results of treatment. **Houssay a.**, an experimental animal deprived of both hypophysis (pituitary gland) and pancreas.

animalcule (an"ĭ-mal'kūl) a minute animal organism.

animation (an"ĭ-ma'shun) the quality of being full of life. **suspended a.**, temporary suspension or cessation of the vital functions.

anincretinosis (an"in-kre"tĭ-no'sis) a disorder due to defect of some internal secretion.

anion (an'ĭ-on) the element which in electrolysis passes to the positive pole.

aniridia (an"ĭ-rid'e-ah) congenital absence of the iris.

anis(o)- (an-i"so) word element [Gr.], *unequal.*

aniseikonia (an"ĭ-si-ko'ne-ah) inequality of the retinal images of the two eyes.

anisochromatic (an-i"so-kro-mat'ik) not of the same color throughout.

anisocoria (-ko're-ah) inequality in size of the pupils of both eyes.

anisocytosis (-si-to'sis) presence in the blood of erythrocytes showing abnormal variations in size.

anisodactylous (an"ĭ-so-dak'tĭ-lus) having digits of unequal lengths.

anisogamy (an"ĭ-sog'ah-me) conjugation of gametes differing in size and structure.

anisognathous (an"ĭ-sog'nah-thus) having jaws (maxilla and mandible) of unequal widths.

anisohypercytosis (an-i"so-hi"per-si-to'sis) increase in leukocytes, with abnormality in proportion of the various forms of neutrophils.

anisohypocytosis (-hi"po-si-to'sis) decrease in leukocytes, with abnormality in proportion of the various forms of neutrophils.

anisokaryosis (-kar"e-o'sis) inequality in the size of the nuclei of cells.

anisoleukocytosis (-lu"ko-si-to'sis) abnormality in proportion of various forms of leukocytes in the blood.

anisomastia (-mas'te-ah) inequality of the breasts.

anisomelia (-me'le-ah) inequality between paired limbs.

anisometropia (-mĕ-tro'pe-ah) inequality in refractive power of the two eyes, of considerable degree. adj., **anisometrop'ic.**

anisonormocytosis (-nor"mo-si-to'sis) normal number of leukocytes with abnormal proportion of various forms of neutrophils.

anisopiesis (-pi-e'sis) difference in blood pressure recorded in corresponding arteries on the right and left sides of the body.

anisopoikilocytosis (-poi"kĭ-lo-si-to'sis) the presence in the blood of erythrocytes of varying sizes and abnormal shapes.

anisorhythmia (-rith'me-ah) lack of synchronism in the rhythm of the atria and ventricles of the heart.

anisosphygmia (an-i"so-sfig'me-ah) difference in pulse rate recorded in corresponding arteries on the right and left sides of the body.

anisospore (an-i'so-spōr) a spore that unites with another to form an adult.

anisosthenic (an-i"sos-then'ik) not having equal power; said of muscles.

anisotonic (an-i"so-ton'ik) having different osmotic pressure; not isotonic.

anisotropic (-trop'ik) 1. having unlike properties in different directions. 2. doubly refracting, or having a double polarizing power.

anistotropy (an"i-sot'ro-pe) the quality of being anisotropic.

anisuria (an"i-su're-ah) alternating oliguria and polyuria.

ankle (ang'kl) the region of the joint between leg and foot; the tarsus.

ankyl(o)- (ang'kĭ-lo) word element [Gr.], *bent; crooked; in the form of a loop; adhesion.*

ankyloblepharon (ang"kĭ-lo-blef'ah-ron) fusion of the eyelids.

ankylocheilia (-ki'le-ah) adhesion of the lips.

ankyloglossia (-glos'e-ah) tongue-tie. **a. superior**, extensive adhesion of the tongue to the plate.

ankylopoietic (-poi-et'ik) producing ankylosis.

ankyloproctia (-prok'she-ah) stricture of the anus.

ankylosed (ang'kĭ-lōsd) affected with ankylosis.

ankylosis (ang"kĭ-lo'sis) abnormal immobility and consolidation of a joint. **extracapsular a., false a.**, that caused by rigidity of surrounding parts. **intracapsular a.**, that caused by rigidity of structures within the joint. **spurious a.**, extracapsular ankylosis. **true a.**, that in which motion is prevented by bony or fibrous union of the participating bones.

ankylotia (-lo'she-ah) closure of external meatus of ear.

ankylotome (ang-kil'o-tōm) knife for operating for tongue-tie.

ankyroid (ang'kĭ-roid) hooklike.

anlage (an'lah-geh) pl. *anla'gen* [Ger.] primordium.

anneal (an-nēl') to soften a material, as a metal, by controlled heating and cooling, to make its manipulation easier.

annectent (ah-nek'tent) connecting; joining together.

Annelida (an-nel'ĭ-dah) a phylum of metazoan invertebrates, the segmented worms, including leeches.

annular (an'u-lar) ring-shaped.

annulorrhaphy (an"u-lor'ah-fe) suture of a hernial ring or sac.

annulus (an'u-lus), p. *an'nuli* [L.] a small ring or encircling structure.

anococcygeal (a"no-kok-sij'e-al) pertaining to anus and coccyx.

anode (an'ōd) the electrode by which electric current enters a cell, apparatus or body. adj., **ano'dal.**

anodontia (an"o-don'she-ah) congenital absence of some or all of the teeth.

anodyne (an'o-dīn) 1. relieving pain. 2. a medicine that eases pain.

anodynia (an″o-din'e-ah) freedom from pain.

anoetic (-et'ik) not subject to conscious attention.

anoia (ah-noi'ah) idiocy.

anomalopia (ah-nom″ah-lo'pe-ah) a slight anomaly of visual perception. **color a.**, a minor deviation of color vision, without loss of ability to distinguish the four primary colors.

anomaloscope (ah-nom'ah-lo-skōp″) an apparatus used to detect anomalies of color vision.

anomaly (ah-nom'ah-le) deviation from normal. adj., **anom'alous. Alder's a.**, a condition in which the leukocytes, but mainly those of the myelocytic series, contain coarse, azurophilic granules. **Chediak-Higashi a.**, a hereditary disorder characterized by abnormalities in the nuclear structure of the leukocytes. **developmental a.**, absence, deformity or excess of body parts as the result of faulty development of the embryo. **Ebstein's a.**, a malformation of the tricuspid valve, usually associated with an atrial septal defect. **Pelger's nuclear a.**, a hereditary or acquired anomaly in the form of the nuclei of the leukocytes.

anomia (ah-no'me-ah) loss of power of naming objects or of recognizing names.

anoneme (an'o-nēm) a delicate filament extending from kinetoplast to cell wall.

anonychia (an″o-nik'e-ah) absence of the nails.

ano-opsia (an″o-op'se-ah) an upward strabismus.

Anopheles (ah-nof'ĕ-lēz) a widely distributed genus of mosquitoes, comprising over 300 species, many of which are important vectors of malaria.

anophthalmia (an″of-thal'me-ah) anophthalmos.

anophthalmos (an″of-thal'mos) congenital absence of the eyeballs.

anoplasty (a'no-plas″te) plastic repair of the anus.

anopsia (an-op'se-ah) 1. suppression of vision in one eye. 2. hypertropia.

anorchid (an-or'kid) a person with no testes or with undescended testes.

anorchism (an-or'kizm) congenital absence of one or both testes.

anorectic (an″o-rek'tik) 1. pertaining to anorexia. 2. an agent that diminishes the appetite for food.

anorectocolonic (a″no-rek″to-ko-lon'ik) pertaining to the anus, rectum and colon.

anorectum (-rek'tum) the distal portion of the alimentary tract, including the entire anal canal and the distal 2 cm. of the rectum. adj., **anorec'tal.**

anoretic (an″o-ret'ik) anorectic.

anorexia (-rek'se-ah) lack or loss of appetite for food. **a. nervo'sa**, loss of appetite due to emotional reasons.

anorexic (-rek'sik) anorectic.

anorexigenic (an″o-rek″sĭ-jen'ik) 1. producing anorexia. 2. an agent that diminishes or controls the appetite.

anorthography (an″or-thog'rah-fe) impairment of ability to write.

anorthopia (-tho'pe-ah) asymmetrical or distorted vision.

anorthosis (-tho'sis) absence of erectility.

anoscope (a'no-skōp) a speculum or endoscope used in direct visual examination of the anal canal.

anoscopy (a-nos'ko-pe) examination of the anal canal with an anoscope.

anosigmoidoscopy (a″no-sig″moi-dos'ko-pe) visual examination of the anus and sigmoid by means of a speculum. adj., **anosigmoidoscop'ic.**

anosmia (an-oz'me-ah) absence of the sense of smell. adj., **anos'mic, anosmat'ic.**

anosognosia (an″o-sog-no'zhe-ah) failure to recognize one's own disease or defect. adj., **anosogno'sic.**

anosphrasia (an″os-fra'ze-ah) anosmia.

anospinal (a″no-spi'nal) pertaining to anus and spinal cord.

anostosis (an″os-to'sis) defective formation of bone.

anotia (an-o'she-ah) developmental anomaly with absence of the ears.

anotus (an-o'tus) a fetus without ears.

anovaginal (a″no-vaj'ĭ-nal) pertaining to the anus and vagina.

anovarism (an-o'var-izm) absence of the ovaries.

anovesical (a″no-ves'ĭ-kal) pertaining to anus and bladder.

anovular (an-ov'u-lar) anovulatory.

anovulatory (an-ov'u-lah-tor″e) not associated with ovulation.

anoxemia (an″ok-se'me-ah) lack of sufficient oxygen in the blood. adj., **anoxe'mic.**

anoxia (an-ok'se-ah) absence or deficiency of oxygen, as reduction of oxygen in body tissues below physiologic levels. adj., **anox'ic. ambient a.**, diminished oxygen content of the surrounding atmosphere. **anemic a.**, reduction of oxygen in body tissues because of diminished oxygen-carrying capacity of the blood. **anoxic a.**, reduction of oxygen in body tissues due to interference with the oxygen supply. **histotoxic a.**, condition resulting from diminished ability of cells to utilize available oxygen. **stagnant a.**, a condition due to interference with the flow of blood and its transport of oxygen.

anoxybiosis (an-ok″se-bi-o'sis) anaerobiosis.

ansa (an'sah), pl. **an'sae** [L.] a looplike structure. **a. cervica'lis**, a loop in the neck formed by the descendens hypoglossi nerve. **Haller's a.**, the loop formed by the nerve connecting the facial and glossopharyngeal nerves. **a. of Henle**, Henle's loop. **a. hypoglos'si**, ansa cervicalis. **a. lenticula'ris**, a tract between the crusta and the lenticular nucleus. **an'sae nervo'rum spina'lium**, loops of spinal nerves joining the anterior spinal nerves. **a. peduncula'ris**, the portion of the brain to the ventral side of the thalamus. **a. of Reil**, ansa peduncularis. **a. sacra'lis**, the loop connecting the ganglion impar with the trunks of the sympathetic nerve. **a. subcla'via, a. of Vieussens,**

a small nerve extending between the middle and inferior cervical, or first dorsal, ganglia, and making a loop around the subclavian artery. **a. vitelli'na,** an embryonic vein from the yolk sac to the umbilical vein.

Ansolysen (an"so-li'sen) trademark for preparations of pentolinium.

ansotomy (an-sot'o-me) incision of the ansa lenticularis for treatment of tremor.

Antabuse (an'tah-būs) trademark for a preparation of disulfiram.

antacid (ant-as'id) 1. counteracting acidity. 2. an agent that counteracts acidity.

antagonist (an-tag'o-nist) an agent (muscle, drug) which exerts an action opposite to that of another.

antalgesic (ant"al-je'sik) analgesic.

antalgic (ant-al'jik) analgesic.

antalkaline (ant-al'kah-līn) counteracting alkalinity.

antaphrodisiac (ant"af-ro-diz'e-ak) an agent that allays the sexual impulse.

antazoline (ant-az'o-lēn) a chemical used as an antihistaminic.

ante (an'te) word element [L.], *before.*

ante- (an'te) word element [L.], *before* (in time or space).

antebrachium (an"te-bra'ke-um) the forearm. adj., **antebra'chial.**

antecedent (-se'dent) a precursor. **plasma thromboplastin a.,** factor XI.

antecurvature (-ker'vah-tūr) a slight anteflexion.

antefebrile (-feb'ríl) preceding fever.

anteflexion (-flek'shun) the bending of an organ so that its top is thrust forward.

antelocation (-lo-ka'shun) displacement of an organ forward.

antemetic (ant"e-met'ik) antiemetic.

ante mortem (an'te mor'tem) [L.] before death.

antemortem (an"te-mor'tem) performed or occurring before death.

antenna (an-ten'ah) one of the appendages on the head of arthropods.

Antepar (an'te-par) trademark for a preparation of piperazine citrate and piperazine phosphate.

antepartal (an"te-par'tal) occurring before childbirth.

ante partum (an'te par'tum) [L.] before parturition.

antepartum (an"te-par'tum) performed or occurring before parturition.

antephase (an'te-fāz) the portion of interphase immediately preceding mitosis, when energy is being produced and stored for mitosis and chromosome reproduction is taking place.

antephialtic (ant"ef-e-al'tik) preventing nightmare.

anteposition (an"te-po-zish'un) forward displacement, as of the uterus.

antepyretic (-pi-ret'ik) before the stage of fever.

anterior (an-te're-or) situated at or directed toward the front; opposite of posterior.

antero- (an'ter-o) word element [L.], *anterior; in front of.*

anteroclusion (an"ter-o-kloo'zhun) malrela-

tion of dental arches with the mandibular arch anterior to the maxillary arch.

anterograde (an'ter-o-grād") extending or moving forward.

anteroinferior (an"ter-o-in-fe're-or) situated in front and below.

anterolateral (-lat'er-al) situated in front and to one side.

anteromedian (-me'de-an) situated in front and on the middle line.

anteroposterior (-pos-te're-or) directed from the front toward the back.

anterosuperior (-su-pe're-or) situated in front and above.

anteversion (an"te-ver'zhun) the tipping forward of an entire organ.

anteverted (-vert'ed) tipped or bent forward.

anthelix (ant'he-liks) antihelix.

anthelmintic (ant"hel-min'tik) 1. destructive to worms. 2. an agent destructive to worms.

anthelone (ant-he'lōn) urogastrone.

anthemorrhagic (ant"hem-o-raj'ik) antihemorrhagic.

anthocyanin (an"tho-si'ah-nin) the red pigment of beet root.

anthophobia (-fo'be-ah) morbid dislike of flowers.

anthorisma (-riz'mah) a diffuse swelling.

anthracemia (an"thrah-se'me-ah) 1. asphyxia, as from carbon monoxide poisoning. 2. presence of *Bacillus anthracis* in the blood.

anthracene (an'thrah-sēn) crystalline hydrocarbon, $C_{14}H_{10}$, from coal tar.

anthracia (an-thra'se-ah) disease marked by formation of carbuncles.

anthracin (an'thrah-sin) a poisonous compound from cultures of the organism causing anthrax.

anthracoid (an'thrah-koid) resembling anthrax.

anthracometer (an"thrah-kom'ĕ-ter) instrument for measuring carbon dioxide in the air.

anthraconecrosis (an"thrah-ko-nĕ-kro'sis) degeneration of tissue into a black mass.

anthracosilicosis (-sil"ĭ-ko'sis) a lung disease due to inhalation of carbon dust and fine particles of silica.

anthracosis (an"thrah-ko'sis) a lung disease due to inhalation of carbon dust not containing silica.

anthracotherapy (an"thrah-ko-ther'ah-pe) treatment with charcoal.

anthralin (an'thrah-lin) a yellowish brown crystalline powder, $C_{14}H_{10}O_3$, used topically in eczema.

anthraquinone (an"thrah-kwin'ōn) a yellow substance, $C_{14}H_8O_2$, from anthracene.

anthrax (an'thraks) an infectious disease of cattle, horses, mules, sheep and goats, due to *Bacillus anthracis;* sometimes acquired by man through contact with infected animals or their byproducts, such as carcasses or skins. **acute a.,** a usually rapidly fatal form with high fever, death occurring in a day or two. **agricultural a.,** anthrax in man due to contact with the flesh of animals having the disease. **apoplectic a.,** fulminant anthrax, so called because the symptoms resemble those of cerebral apoplexy. **chronic a.**, a persistent form with local lesions confined to the tongue and throat. **cutaneous a.**, anthrax due to lodgment of the causative organisms in wounds or abrasions of the skin, producing swelling in various parts of the body. **fulminant a.**, a form characterized by sudden onset and rapidly fatal course. **industrial a.**, anthrax in man due to contact with wool, hair, hides or other material from infected animals. **localized a.**, cutaneous anthrax. **peracute a.**, fulminant anthrax. **pulmonary a.**, infection of the respiratory tract resulting from inhalation of dust or animal hair containing spores of *Bacillus anthracis*. **subacute a.**, a form of anthrax leading to death in three to five days or to complete recovery. **symptomatic a.**, blackleg.

anthropo- (an'thro-po) word element [Gr.], *man (human being)*.

anthropocentric (an"thro-po-sen'trik) with a human bias; considering man the center of the universe.

anthropogeny (an"thro-poj'ĕ-ne) development or evolution of man.

anthropoid (an'thro-poid) resembling a man.

Anthropoidea (an"thro-poi'de-ah) a suborder of Primates, including monkeys, apes and man, characterized by a larger and more complicated brain than the other suborders.

anthropokinetics (an"thro-po-ki-net'iks) study of the total human being in action, including biological and physical, psychologic and sociologic aspects.

anthropology (an"thro-pol'o-je) the science of the human race.

anthropometry (-pom'ĕ-tre) the measurement of human dimensions to obtain quantitative expression of the form of the body. adj., **anthropomet'ric.**

anthropomorphism (an"thro-po-mor'fizm) the attribution of human characteristics to non-human objects.

anthropophagy (an"thro-pof'ah-je) cannibalism.

anthropophilic (an"thro-po-fil'ik) preferring human beings to animals; said of certain mosquitoes.

anthropophobia (-fo'be-ah) morbid dread of society.

anthroposcopy (an"thro-pos'ko-pe) visual observation and description of physical traits not susceptible to exact measurement.

anthroposomatology (an"thro-po-so"mah-tol'o-je) sum of knowledge of the human body.

anthropozoonosis (-zo"o-no'sis) a disease of either animals or man that may be transmitted from one to the other.

anthydropic (ant"hi-drop'ik) relieving dropsy.

anthypnotic (ant"hip-not'ik) preventing sleep.

anthysteric (ant"his-ter'ik) relieving hysteria.

anti- (an'ti, an'te) word element [Gr.], *counteracting; effective against.*

antiabortifacient (an"ti-ah-bor"ti-fa'shent) 1. preventing abortion or promoting gestation. 2. an agent that prevents abortion or promotes successful gestation.

antiagglutinin (an"ti-ah-gloo'ti-nin) a substance that opposes the action of an agglutinin.

antialbumate (-al'bu-māt) a product of incomplete digestion of albumin.

antialbumin (-al-bu'min) a product of gastric digestion of albumin.

antialbumose (-al'bu-mōs) a product of gastric digestion of antialbumin.

antialexin (-ah-lek'sin) a substance which opposes the action of an alexin.

antiamboceptor (-am"bo-sep'tor) a substance which opposes the action of an amboceptor.

antiamebic (-ah-me'bik) 1. destroying or suppressing the growth of amebas. 2. an agent that destroys or suppresses the growth of amebas.

antiamylase (-am'ĭ-lās) a substance counteracting the action of amylase.

antianaphylactin (-an"ah-fi-lak'tin) an antibody which counteracts anaphylactin.

antianaphylaxis (-an"ah-fi-lak'sis) the state of desensitization to antigens.

antianemic (-ah-ne'mik) counteracting anemia.

antiantibody (-an'ti-bod"e) a substance which counteracts the effect of an antibody.

antiapoplectic (-ap"o-plek'tik) counteracting apoplexy.

antiarrhythmic (-ah-rith'mik) 1. preventing or alleviating cardiac arrhythmias. 2. an agent that prevents or alleviates cardiac arrhythmias.

antiarthritic (-ar-thrit'ik) 1. effective in treatment of arthritis. 2. an agent used in treatment of arthritis.

antibacterial (-bak-te're-al) 1. checking the growth of bacteria. 2. an agent that checks the growth of bacteria.

antibechic (-bek'ik) 1. relieving cough. 2. an agent that relieves cough.

antibiosis (-bi-o'sis) an association between two populations of organisms that is detrimental to one of them.

antibiotic (-bi-ot'ik) 1. destructive of life; pertaining to antibiosis. 2. a chemical compound produced by and obtained from certain living cells, especially lower plant cells, such as bacteria, yeasts, molds, or an equivalent synthetic compound, which is antagonistic to some other form of life, especially pathogenic or noxious organisms, being biostatic or biocidal.

antibiotin (-bi'o-tin) avidin.

antiblennorrhagic (-blen"o-raj'ik) preventing or relieving gonorrhea.

antibody (an'ti-bod"e) a protein produced in the body in response to stimulation by an antigen and reacting specifically with it. **anaphylactic a.**, a substance formed as a result of the first injection of a foreign protein and responsible for the anaphylactic symptoms following the second injection of the same protein. **blocking a.**, one which has the same specificity as one from another source, but which interferes with the action of the other because of dissimilar properties in regard to the expected mode of that action. **inhibiting a.**, blocking antibody. **neutralizing a.**, one which reduces or destroys infectivity of a homologous infectious agent by partial or complete destruction of the agent. **protective a.**, one responsible for immunity to an infectious agent observed in passive immunity. **sensitizing a.**, anaphylactic antibody.

antibrachium (an″tĭ-bra′ke-um) antebrachium, or forearm.

antibromic (-bro′mik) deodorant.

anticachectic (-kah-kek′tik) 1. preventing or relieving cachexia. 2. an agent that prevents or relieves cachexia.

anticalculous (-kal′ku-lus) suppressing the formation of calculi.

anticanitic (-kah-nit′ik) counteracting graying of the hair.

anticariogenic (-kār″e-o-jen′ik) effective in suppressing caries production.

anticarious (-ka′re-us) anticariogenic.

anticatarrhal (-kah-tahr′al) counteracting catarrh.

anticathode (-kath′ōd) the part of a vacuum tube opposite the cathode; the target.

anticheirotonus (-ki-rot′o-nus) spasmodic flexion of the thumb.

anticholagogue (-ko′lah-gog) an agent that inhibits secretion of bile. adj., **anticholagog′-ic.**

anticholinergic (-ko″lin-er′jik) blocking the passage of impulses through the parasympathetic nerves; parasympatholytic.

anticholinesterase (-ko″lin-es′ter-ās) a substance that inhibits the action of cholinesterase.

anticlinal (-kli′nal) sloping or inclined in opposite directions.

anticoagulant (-ko-ag′u-lant) 1. acting to prevent clotting of blood. 2. any substance which suppresses, delays or nullifies blood coagulation. **circulating a.**, a substance in the blood which inhibits normal blood clotting and causes a hemorrhagic syndrome.

anticoagulin (-ko-ag′u-lin) a substance that suppresses, delays or nullifies coagulation of the blood.

anticomplement (-kom′ple-ment) a substance that counteracts a complement.

anticonvulsant (-kon-vul′sant) 1. inhibiting convulsions. 2. an agent that suppresses convulsions.

anticonvulsive (-kon-vul′siv) anticonvulsant.

anticreatinine (-kre-at′ĭ-nin) a leukomaine derived from creatinine.

anticritical (-krit′ĭ-kal) preventing a crisis.

anticus (an-ti′kus) anterior.

anticytolysin (an″tĭ-si-tol′ĭ-sin) a substance that counteracts cytolysin.

anticytotoxin (-si″to-tok′sin) a substance that counteracts cytotoxin.

antidepressant (-de-pres′sant) 1. effective against depressive illness. 2. an agent effective against depressive illness.

antidepressive (-de-pres′siv) counteracting depression.

antidiarrheal (-di″ah-re′al) 1. counteracting diarrhea. 2. an agent that counteracts diarrhea.

antidinic (an″tĭ-din′ik) relieving giddiness or vertigo.

antidipsia (-dip′se-ah) aversion to the ingestion of fluids.

antidiuresis (-di″u-re′sis) the suppression of secretion of urine by the kidneys.

antidiuretic (-di″u-ret′ik) 1. pertaining to or causing suppression of urine. 2. an agent that causes suppression of urine.

antidote (an′tĭ-dōt) an agent that counteracts a poison. adj., **antido′tal. chemical a.**, one that changes the chemical nature of the poison. **mechanical a.**, one that prevents absorption of the poison. **physiologic a.**, one that counteracts the effects of the poison by producing other effects.

antidromic (an″tĭ-drom′ik) conducting impulses in a direction opposite to the normal.

antidysenteric (-dis″en-ter′ik) counteracting dysentery.

antiedemic (-e-dem′ik) 1. counteracting or relieving edema. 2. an agent that counteracts or relieves edema.

antiemetic (-e-met′ik) 1. useful in the treatment of vomiting. 2. an agent that relieves vomiting.

antienzyme (-en′zīm) a substance which counteracts an enzyme.

antiepileptic (-ep″ĭ-lep′tik) 1. combating epilepsy. 2. a remedy for epilepsy.

antiepithelial (-ep″ĭ-the′le-al) destructive to epithelial cells.

antiesterase (-es′ter-ās) an agent that counteracts the activity of esterolytic enzymes.

antifebrile (-feb′ril) counteracting fever.

antifebrin (-feb′rin) acetanilid.

antifertilizin (-fer″tĭ-li′zin) a substance on the surface of a spermatozoon that reacts with a substance on the surface of the ovum (fertilizin), thus binding the spermatozoon to the ovum.

antifibrinolysin (-fi″brĭ-no-li′sin) antiplasmin.

antifibrinolytic (-fi″brĭ-no-lit′ik) inhibiting fibrinolysis.

antifungal (-fung′gal) 1. checking the growth of fungi. 2. an agent that checks the growth of fungi.

antigalactic (-gah-lak′tik) diminishing secretion of milk.

antigen (an′tĭ-jen) a substance, usually a protein or protein-polysaccharide, which, foreign to the blood stream of an animal, stimulates formation of a specific antibody. adj., **antigen′ic. beef heart a.**, an antigen for the Wassermann reaction made by extracting fresh normal beef heart tissue with absolute alcohol. **carbohydrate a's**, numerous polysaccharides isolated from bacteria which function as specific haptens and as more or less complete antigens. **cholesterinized a.**, beef heart antigen to which has been added 0.4 per cent of cholesterol. **flagellar a.**, H antigen. **Forssman a.**, a heterophile antigen discovered in guinea pig tissues, which produced in rabbits antibodies that lysed sheep red blood cells in the presence of complement. **H a.** (Ger. *Hauch*, film), the antigen which occurs in the flagella of motile bacteria. **heterophile a.**, one capable of stimulating the production of antibodies that react with tissues from other animals or even plants. **isophile a.**, one occurring within a species, but not in all individuals of the species, e.g. human blood group antigens. **O a.** (Ger. *ohne Hauch*, without film), the antigen which occurs in the bodies of bacteria. **organ-specific a.**, a substance common to and a characteristic antigen for some organ or tissue in several or many different kinds of animals, without species specificity. **partial a.**, an antigen which does not produce antibody formation, but gives specific precipitation when mixed with the antibacterial immune serum. **V a., Vi a.**, an antigen contained in the sheath of a bacterium, as the typhoid bacillus, and giving greater virulence to the strain containing it.

antigenicity (an″tĭ-jĕ-nis′ĭ-te) ability of a substance to stimulate antibody formation.

antiglobulin (-glob′u-lin) a precipitin which precipitates globulin.

antigoitrogenic (-goi″tro-jen′ik) inhibiting the development of goiter.

antihallucinatory (-hal-lu′sĭ-nah-to″re) preventing occurrence of hallucinations.

antihelix (-he′liks) curved ridge opposite the helix of the ear.

antihelmintic (-hel-min′tik) anthelmintic.

antihemolysin (-he-mol′ĭ-sin) a substance which counteracts hemolysin.

antihemorrhagic (-hem″o-raj′ik) 1. exerting a hemostatic effect and counteracting hemorrhage. 2. an agent that prevents or checks hemorrhage.

antihidrotic (-hi-drot′ik) anhidrotic.

antihistamine (-his′tah-min) a substance capable of counteracting the pharmacologic effects of histamine by a mechanism other than the production of exactly opposite effects.

antihistaminic (-his″tah-min′ik) 1. counteracting the pharmacologic effects of histamine. 2. an antihistamine.

antihormone (-hor′mōn) a substance which counteracts a hormone.

antihydropic (-hi-drop′ik) effective in relieving or preventing dropsy.

antihypercholesterolemic (-hi″per-ko-les′ter-ol-e″mik) 1. effective against hypercholesterolemia. 2. an agent that prevents or relieves hypercholesterolemia.

antihypertensive (-ten′siv) 1. effective against hypertension. 2. an agent that prevents or relieves high blood pressure.

anti-icteric (an″te-ik″ter′ik) relieving icterus.

anti-immune (-ĭ-mūn′) preventing immunity.

anti-infective (-in-fek′tiv) 1. counteracting infection. 2. a substance that counteracts infection.

anti-isolysin (-i-sol′ĭ-sin) a substance that counteracts an isolysin.

antikenotoxin (an″tĭ-ke″no-tok′sin) a substance which counteracts the effect of kenotoxin.

antiketogenesis (-ke″to-jen′ĕ-sis) prevention of the formation of ketones (ketone bodies). adj., **antiketogenet′ic.**

antiketogenic (an″tĭ-ke″to-jen′ik) preventing or suppressing the development of ketones (ketone bodies) and preventing development of ketosis.

antilactase (-lak′tās) a substance that counteracts lactase.

antilethargic (-lĕ-thar′jik) hindering sleep.

antileukocytic (-lu″ko-sit′ik) destructive to white blood corpuscles (leukocytes).

anti-lewisite (-lu′ĭ-sīt) dimercaprol.

antilithic (-lith′ik) counteracting calculus formation.

antilobium (-lo′be-um) the tragus of the ear.

antilogia (-lo′je-ah) a combination of contradictory symptoms, rendering diagnosis uncertain.

antilysin (-li′sin) an antibody that inactivates a lysin.

antilysis (-li′sis) inhibition of lysis.

antilytic (-lit′ik) 1. pertaining to antilysis. 2. inhibiting or preventing lysis.

antimere (an′ti-mēr) one of the segments of the body bounded by planes at right angles to the long axis of the body.

antimetabolite (an″tĭ-mĕ-tab′o-līt) a substance exerting its desired effect perhaps by replacing or interfering with the utilization of an essential metabolite.

antimetropia (-mĕ-tro′pe-ah) hyperopia of one eye, with myopia in the other.

antimicrobic (-mi-kro′bik) checking the growth of microbes.

antimicrobiosis (-mi″kro-bi-o′sis) suppression of the growth of microorganisms.

antimongoloid (-mon′go-loid) opposite to that characteristic of Down's syndrome (mongolism), e.g. antimongoloid slant of the palpebral fissures.

antimony (an′tĭ-mo″ne) chemical element (*see table*), at. no. 51, symbol Sb. adj., **antimo′nial. a. potassium tartrate,** a compound used in treatment of parasitic infections, e.g. schistosomiasis or leishmaniasis. **a. sodium thioglycollate,** a remedy used in granuloma inguinale, **tartrated a.,** antimony potassium tartrate.

antimorphic (an″tĭ-mor′fik) in genetics, antagonizing or inhibiting normal activity (antimorphic mutant gene).

antimycotic (-mi-kot′ik) destructive to fungi.

antinarcotic (-nar-kot′ik) relieving narcotism.

antinauseant (-naw′ze-ant) 1. counteracting nausea. 2. an agent that counteracts nausea.

antineoplastic (-ne″o-plas′tik) inhibiting the maturation and proliferation of malignant cells.

antinephritic (-ne-frit′ik) serviceable in kidney diseases.

antineuralgic (-nu-ral′jik) relieving neuralgia.

antineuritic (-nu-rit′ik) relieving neuritis.

antinion (an-tin′e-on) frontal pole of the head.

antioncotic (an″tĭ-on-kot′ik) relieving swelling.

antiopsonin (-op′so-nin) a substance that counteracts opsonins.

antiovulatory (-ov′u-lah-to″re) suppressing ovulation.

antioxidant (-ok′sĭ-dant) a substance which

in small amount will inhibit the oxidation of other compounds.

antioxidation (an″tĭ-ok″sĭ-da′shun) prevention of oxidation.

antiparalytic (-par″ah-lit′ik) relieving paralytic symptoms.

antiparasitic (-par″ah-sit′ik) 1. destroying parasites. 2. an agent that destroys parasites.

antiparasympathomimetic (-par″ah-sim″pah-tho-mi-met′ik) parasympatholytic.

antipathic (-path′ik) opposite in nature.

antipediculotic (-pē-dik″u-lot′ik) 1. effective against lice and in treatment of pediculosis. 2. an agent effective against lice.

antipepsin (-pep′sin) an antienzyme that counteracts pepsin.

antipeptone (-pep′tōn) peptone derived from antialbumose by digestion.

antiperiodic (-pe″re-od′ik) serviceable against malarial or periodic recurrences.

antiperistalsis (-per″ĭ-stal′sis) adoral waves of contraction sometimes occurring normally in the lower ileum, competing with the normal aboral peristalsis and retarding passage of intestinal contents into the cecum. adj., **antiperistal′tic.**

antiphlogistic (-flo-jis′tik) 1. diminishing inflammation. 2. an agent that diminishes inflammation.

antiphthisic (-tiz′ik) antituberculotic.

antiplasmin (-plaz′min) a principle in the blood that inhibits plasmin.

antiplastic (-plas′tik) unfavorable to healing.

antipneumotoxin (-nu″mo-tok′sin) an antitoxin antagonistic to pneumotoxin.

antiprotease (-pro′te-ās) antiplasmin.

antiproteolysin (-pro″te-o-li′sin) antiplasmin.

antiprothrombin (-pro-throm′bin) a substance that retards the conversion of prothrombin into thrombin.

antiprotozoal (-pro″to-zo′al) antiprotozoan.

antiprotozoan (-pro″to-zo′an) effective against protozoa.

antipruritic (-proo-rit′ik) 1. preventing or relieving itching. 2. an agent that counteracts itching.

antipyic (-pi′ik) preventing suppuration.

antipyretic (-pi-ret′ik) 1. effective against fever. 2. an agent effective against fever.

antipyrine (-pi′rēn) a crystalline compound, $C_{11}H_{12}N_2O$, analgesic and antipyretic.

antipyrotic (-pi-rot′ik) 1. effective in the treatment of burns. 2. an agent used in the treatment of burns.

antirabic (-ra′bik) 1. used to prevent development of rabies. 2. an agent used to prevent rabies.

antiradiation (-ra″de-a′shun) capable of counteracting the effects of radiation; effective against radiation injury.

antirheumatic (-roo-mat′ik) counteracting rheumatism.

antirickettsial (-rĭ-ket′se-al) effective against rickettsiae.

antiscabious (-ska′be-us) counteracting scabies.

antiscorbutic (-skor-bu′tik) counteracting scurvy.

antisepsis (an″tĭ-sep′sis) prevention of sepsis by destruction of microorganisms and infective matter.

antiseptic (-sep′tik) 1. preventing sepsis. 2. a substance destructive to microorganisms.

antiserotonin (-ser″o-to′nin) a substance capable of antagonizing or inhibiting the action of serotonin. **benzyl a., Wooley's a.,** benanserin.

antiserum (-se′rum) a serum containing antibodies.

antisialagogue (-si-al′ah-gog) an agent that inhibits flow of saliva. adj., **antisialagog′ic.**

antisialic (-si-al′ik) checking the flow of saliva.

antispasmodic (-spaz-mod′ik) 1. preventing or relieving spasms. 2. an agent that prevents or relieves spasms.

antispastic (-spas′tik) antispasmodic.

antistalsis (-stal′sis) antiperistalsis.

Antistine (an-tis′tin) trademark for preparations of antazoline.

antistreptococcic (-strep″to-kok′sik) counteracting streptococcal infection.

antisudoral (-soo′dor-al) counteracting sweating.

antisympathetic (-sim″pah-thet′ik) 1. producing effects resembling those of interruption of the sympathetic nerve supply. 2. an agent that produces effects resembling those of interruption of the sympathetic nerve supply.

antisyphilitic (-sif″ĭ-lit′ik) counteracting syphilis.

antitabetic (-tah-bet′ik) counteracting tabes dorsalis.

antithenar (an″tĭ-the′nar) placed opposite to the palm or sole.

antithrombin (an″tĭ-throm′bin) a principle in the blood that inhibits thrombin.

antithromboplastin (-throm″bo-plas′tin) a substance that interferes with thromboplastin and inhibits coagulation of blood.

antitoxin (-tok′sin) a particular kind of antibody produced in the body in response to the presence of a toxin. adj., **antitox′ic. diphtheria a.,** preparation from the blood serum of plasma of healthy animals immunized against diphtheria toxin, used as a passive immunizing agent. **gas gangrene a.,** a sterile solution of antitoxic substances from blood of healthy animals immunized against gas-producing organisms of the genus Clostridium. **scarlet fever streptococcus a.,** sterile solution of antitoxic substances from blood serum of healthy animals immunized against toxin produced by the streptococcus considered the cause of scarlet fever. **tetanus a.,** preparation from the blood serum of plasma of healthy animals immunized against tetanus toxin, used as a passive immunizing agent.

antitragus (-tra′gus) a projection on the ear opposite the tragus.

antitrope (an″tĭ-trōp) one of two structures which are similar but oppositely oriented, like a right and a left glove. adj., **antitrop′ic.**

antitrypsin (an″ti-trip′sin) an antienzyme counteracting the action of trypsin. adj., **antitryp′tic.**

43   aortalgia

antitryptase (an″ti-trip′tās) antiplasmin.

antituberculotic (-tu-ber″ku-lot′ik) counteracting tuberculosis.

antitussive (-tus′siv) 1. effective against cough. 2. an agent that suppresses coughing.

antivenereal (-vē-ne′re-al) counteracting venereal disease.

antivenin (-ven′in) a material used in treatment of envenomation by a poisonous animal. **black widow spider a.**, an antitoxin to the venom of a black widow spider (*Latrodectus mactans*). **a. (Crotalidae) polyvalent,** serum produced by hyperimmunization of horses with venoms of fer-de-lance and Florida, Texas and tropical rattlers for treatment of envenomation by most pit vipers throughout the world.

antiviral (-vi′ral) 1. effective against viruses. 2. an agent effective against viruses.

antivirotic (-vi-rot′ik) antiviral.

antixerophthalmic (-ze″rof-thal′mik) counteracting xerophthalmia.

antixerotic (-ze-rot′ik) preventing dryness.

antizymotic (-zi-mot′ik) counteracting enzymes.

antodontalgic (ant″o-don-tal′jik) relieving toothache.

antorphine (an-tor′fēn) nalorphine.

antr(o)- (an′tro) word element [L.], *chamber; cavity;* often used with specific reference to the maxillary antrum or sinus.

antrectomy (an-trek′to-me) excision of an antrum.

Antrenyl (an′trĕ-nil) trademark for a preparation of oxyphenonium.

Antricola (an-trik′o-lah) a genus of arthropods (family Argasidae), primarily parasitic on birds.

antritis (an-tri′tis) inflammation of an antrum, especially of the antrum at Highmore.

antroatticotomy (an″tro-at″i-kot′o-me) atticoantrotomy.

antrocele (an′tro-sēl) accumulation of fluid in the maxillary antrum.

antrodynia (an″tro-din′e-ah) pain in the antrum.

antronasal (-na′zal) pertaining to maxillary antrum and nasal fossa.

antroscope (an′tro-skōp) instrument for inspecting antrum of Highmore.

antrostomy (an-tros′to-me) incision of an antrum with drainage.

antrotomy (an-trot′o-me) incision of an antrum.

antrotympanic (an″tro-tim-pan′ik) pertaining to tympanic antrum and tympanum.

antrotympanitis (-tim″pah-ni′tis) inflammation of tympanic antrum and tympanum.

antrum (an′trum), pl. *an′tra* [L.] a cavity or chamber. adj., **an′tral. a. of Highmore,** maxillary sinus. **mastoid a.,** an air space in the mastoid portion of the temporal bone communicating with the tympanic cavity and the mastoid cells. **a. maxilla′re, maxillary a.,** maxillary sinus. **pyloric a., a. pylor′icum,** the proximal, expanded portion of the pyloric part of the stomach. **tympanic a., a. tympan′-icum,** mastoid antrum.

Anturane (an′tu-rān) trademark for a preparation of sulfinpyrazone.

anuclear (a-nu′kle-ar) having no nucleus.

anulus (an′u-lus), pl. *an′uli* [L.] NA spelling of *annulus;* used in names of certain ringlike or encircling structures of the body.

anuresis (an″u-re′sis) complete suppression of urinary secretion by the kidneys. adj., **anuret′ic.**

anuria (ah-nu′re-ah) diminution of urinary secretion to 100 ml. or less in 24 hours. adj., **anu′ric.**

anus (a′nus) the opening of the rectum on the body surface. **imperforate a.,** congenital absence of the normal opening of the rectum.

anvil (an′vil) incus.

anxietas (ang-zi′e-tas) [L.] anxiety; unrest. **a. tibia′rum,** a condition of restlessness leading to constant change of position of the legs.

anxiety (ang-zi′ĕ-te) an exaggerated feeling of apprehension, uncertainty and fear. **acute a. attack,** an acute and dramatic burst of anxiety which is usually self limited, accompanied by the changes usually associated with intense fear. **conditioned a.,** that which originates or is increased as a consequence of earlier psychologic and emotional sensitization or conditioning. **destructive a.,** that which interferes with personal effectiveness or satisfaction. **a.-equivalent,** translation of anxiety into a kind of emotional activity, e.g., the experiencing or expression of angry feelings. **free-floating a.,** fear in the absence of known cause for anxiety. **neurotic a.,** that in which the apprehension is objectively out of proportion to any apparent cause. **a. panic,** acute anxiety attack. **separation a.,** apprehension due to removal of significant persons or familiar surroundings, common in infants six to 10 months old. **situational a.,** that in response to threats from external sources. **a.-tension state,** a less established pathologic entity than anxiety neurosis; a subacute phase, distinguished from anxiety neurosis as a chronic phase.

anydremia (an″i-dre′me-ah) anhydremia.

A.O.A. American Optometric Association; American Orthopaedic Association; American Orthopsychiatric Association; American Osteopathic Association

A.O.P.A. American Ortho-Psychiatric Association; American Orthotics and Prosthetics Association.

aorta (a-or′tah), pl. *aor′tae, aor′tas* [Gr.] great artery arising from left ventricle. **abdominal a.,** the part of the descending aorta below the diaphragm. **a. angus′ta,** narrowness of the aorta. **ascending a.,** the proximal segment of the aorta, from the orifice of the heart to the arch. **descending a.,** the distal segment of the aorta, extending from the arch to the point of bifurcation into the common iliac arteries. **thoracic a.,** the part of the descending aorta above the diaphragm.

aortal (a-or′tal) aortic.

aortalgia (a″or-tal′je-ah) pain in the region of the aorta.

aortarctia (a″or-tark'she-ah) narrowing of the aorta.

aortectasia (-tek-ta'ze-ah) dilatation of the aorta.

aortic (a-or'tik) pertaining to the aorta.

aortitis (a″or-ti'tis) inflammation of aorta.

aortoclasia (a-or″to-kla'ze-ah) rupture of the aorta.

aortogram (a-or'to-gram) the film produced by aortography.

aortography (a″or-tog'rah-fe) radiography of the aorta after introduction into it of a contrast material.

aortolith (a-or'to-lith) a calculus in the aorta.

aortomalacia (a-or″to-mah-la'she-ah) softening of the aorta.

aortopathy (a″or-top'ah-the) noninflammatory disease of the aorta.

aortorrhaphy (a″or-tor'ah-fe) suture of the aorta.

aortosclerosis (a-or″to-skle-ro'sis) sclerosis of the aorta.

aortostenosis (-ste-no'sis) narrowing of the aorta.

aortotomy (a″or-tot'o-me) incision of the aorta.

A.O.S. American Ophthalmological Society; American Otological Society.

A.O.T.A. American Occupational Therapy Association.

A.P.A. American Pharmaceutical Association; American Physiotherapy Association; American Psychiatric Association; American Psychoanalytic Association; American Psychological Association; American Psychopathological Association.

apallesthesia (ah-pal″es-the'ze-ah) loss of perception of the vibrations of a tuning fork placed against the body.

Apamide (ap'ah-mīd) trademark for a preparation of acetaminophen.

apancrea (ah-pan'kre-ah) absence of the pancreas.

apancreatic (ah-pan″kre-at'ik) 1. not pertaining to the pancreas. 2. due to absence of the pancreas.

apandria (ap-an'dre-ah) aversion to men.

apanthropy (ap-an'thro-pe) aversion to human society.

aparalytic (ah″par-ah-lit'ik) characterized by absence of paralysis.

aparthrosis (ap″ar-thro'sis) diarthrosis.

apathic (ah-path'ik) without sensation or feeling.

apathism (ap'ah-thizm) slowness of response to stimuli.

apathy (ap'ah-the) reactive absence of emotions. adj., **apathet'ic.**

APC abbreviation for acetylsalicylic acid, acetophenetidin and caffeine, used as an analgesic or antipyretic.

APE anterior pituitary extract.

apellous (ah-pel'us) skinless.

apepsia (ah-pep'se-ah) cessation or failure of digestive function. **a. nervo'sa,** anorexia nervosa.

aperient (ah-pe're-ent) 1. mildly cathartic. 2. a gentle purgative.

aperistalsis (ah″per-ī-stal'sis) absence of peristaltic action.

apertura (ap″er-tu'rah), pl. *apertu'rae* [L.] aperture.

aperture (ap'er-chūr) an opening. **numerical a.,** an expression of the measure of efficiency of a microscope objective.

apex (a'peks), pl. *a'pices* [L.] tip; the pointed end of a conical part. adj., **ap'ical. root a.,** the terminal end of the root of the tooth.

Apgar score (ap'gar) see under *score*.

A.Ph.A. American Pharmaceutical Association.

A.P.H.A. American Public Health Association.

aphacia (ah-fa'se-ah) aphakia.

aphagia (ah-fa'je-ah) loss of the power of swallowing.

aphagopraxia (ah-fa″go-prak'se-ah) inability to swallow.

aphakia (ah-fa'ke-ah) absence of the lens of an eye, occurring congenitally or as a result of trauma or surgery. adj., **apha'kic.**

aphalangia (ah″fah-lan'je-ah) absence of fingers or toes.

aphasia (ah-fa'zhe-ah) disturbance or loss of ability to comprehend, elaborate or express speech concepts. adj., **apha'sic. amnestic a.,** inability to remember words. **ataxic a.,** aphasia in which the patient knows what he wishes to say, but cannot utter the words. **auditory a.,** loss of ability to comprehend spoken language. **Broca's a.,** ataxic aphasia. **conduction a.,** aphasia due to lesion of path between sensory and motor speech centers. **gibberish a.,** aphasia with utterance of meaningless phrases. **jargon a.,** paraphasia. **mixed a.,** combined motor and sensory aphasia. **motor a.,** loss of ability to express one's thoughts in speech or writing. **motor a. of Broca,** loss of ability to express oneself in spoken words. **sensory a.,** inability to comprehend spoken (*auditory aphasia*) or written (*visual aphasia*) language. **total a.,** mixed aphasia. **visual a.,** loss of ability to comprehend written language.

aphasiologist (ah-fa″ze-ol'o-jist) a specialist in aphasiology.

aphasiology (ah-fa″ze-ol'o-je) scientific study of aphasia and specific neurologic lesions producing it.

aphemia (ah-fe'me-ah) loss of power of speech due to a central lesion.

aphephobia (af″ĕ-fo'be-ah) morbid dread of being touched.

aphonia (a-fo'ne-ah) loss of voice; inability to produce vocal sounds. **a. clerico'rum,** loss of voice from overuse, as by clergymen.

aphonic (a-fon'ik) 1. pertaining to aphonia. 2. without audible sound.

aphose (ah'fōz) any subjective visual sensation due to absence or interruption of light sensation.

aphosphorosis (ah-fos″fo-ro'sis) a condition caused by deficiency of phosphorus in the diet.

aphotic (a-fōt'ik) without light; totally dark.

aphrasia (ah-fra'ze-ah) inability to speak. **a. parano'ica,** stubborn and wilful silence.

aphrenia (ah-fre'ne-ah) 1. dementia. 2. unconsciousness.

aphrodisiac (af"ro-diz'e-ak) 1. arousing sexual desire. 2. a drug that arouses sexual desire.

aphtha (af'thah), pl. *aph'thae* [L.] a whitish spot. adj., **aph'thous. Bednar's a.**, whitish ulceration of the hard palate in young children. **cachectic aphthae**, aphthae formed beneath the tongue, with severe constitutional symptoms. **epizootic aphthae**, foot-and-mouth disease.

aphthosis (af-tho'sis) a condition marked by presence of aphthae.

aphylaxis (a"fi-lak'sis) absence of phylaxis or immunity. adj., **aphylac'tic.**

apicectomy (a"pi-sek'to-me) apicoectomy.

apicitis (-si'tis) inflammation of the apex of the lung or of the root of a tooth.

apicoectomy (-ko-ek'to-me) excision of the apical portion of the root of a tooth through an opening in overlying tissues of the jaw.

apicolysis (a"pi-kol'i-sis) collapse of the apex of the lung, with obliteration of the apical cavity.

apituitarism (ah"pi-tu'i-tar-izm") absence of a functioning pituitary gland.

A.P.L. anterior pituitary-like.

aplacental (a"plah-sen'tal) having no placenta.

aplanatic (ap"lah-nat'ik) correcting or not affected by spherical aberration.

aplasia (ah-pla'zhe-ah) absence of an organ due to failure of development of the embryonic primordium. adj., **aplas'tic. a. axia'lis extracortica'lis congen'ita**, congenital defect of axon formation on the surface of the cerebral cortex. **nuclear a.**, lack of formation or development of cranial nerve nuclei or of portions thereof. **a. pilo'rum intermit'tens**, spindle-shaped hairs.

A.P.M. Academy of Physical Medicine; Academy of Psychosomatic Medicine.

apnea (ap'ne-ah) 1. temporary cessation of breathing, 2. asphyxia. adj., **apne'ic.**

apneumia (ap-nu'me-ah) developmental anomaly with absence of the lungs.

apneusis (ap-nu'sis) sustained inspiratory effort, even to the point of asphyxia. adj., **apneu'stic.**

apo- (ap'o) word element [Gr.], *away from; separated.*

apoarteresis (ap"o-kar"ter-e'sis) suicide by persistent refusal of food.

apochromat (-kro'mat) an apochromatic objective.

apochromatic (-kro-mat'ik) free from chromatic aberration.

apocrine (ap'o-krin) concentrating secretory products at the free end of the secreting cell, from which they are thrown off, with the portion of the cell where they have accumulated (e.g. mammary gland).

apodia (ah-po'de-ah) developmental anomaly with absence of the feet.

apoenzyme (ap"o-en'zim) the protein component separable from certain enzymes, which requires presence of the appropriate coenzyme to be active.

apogee (ap'o-je) the state of greatest severity of a disease.

apolar (ah-po'lar) having neither poles nor processes; without polarity.

apolepsis (ap"o-lep'sis) suppression of a natural secretion.

apomorphine (-mor'fen) an alkaloid, $C_{17}H_{17}$-NO_2, from morphine. **a. hydrochloride**, a crystalline alkaloid, $C_{17}H_{17}NO_2.HCl.\frac{1}{2}H_2O$, a prompt and effective emetic.

aponeurectomy (-nu-rek'to-me) excision of an aponeurosis.

aponeurorrhaphy (-nu-ror'ah-fe) suture of an aponeurosis.

aponeurosis (-nu-ro'sis), pl. *aponeuro'ses* [Gr.] a sheetlike tendon attaching or investing muscles. adj., **aponeurot'ic.**

aponeurositis (-nu-ro-si'tis) inflammation of an aponeurosis.

aponeurotomy (-nu-rot'o-me) incision of an aponeurosis.

apophylaxis (-fi-lak'sis) decrease in the phylactic power of the blood. adj., **apophylac'tic.**

apophyseal (-fiz'e-al) pertaining to an apophysis.

apophysis (ah-pof'i-sis), pl. *apoph'yses* [Gr.] a process of a bone which has never been entirely distinct from the body of the bone.

apophysitis (ah-pof"i-zi'tis) inflammation of an apophysis.

apoplectiform (ap"o-plek'ti-form) apoplectoid.

apoplectoid (-plek'toid) resembling a stroke or seizure.

apoplexy (ap'o-plek"se) copious extravasation of blood into an organ; often used alone to designate such extravasations into the brain *(cerebral apoplexy)* after rupture of an intracranial blood vessel. adj., **apoplec'tic. adrenal a.**, sudden massive hemorrhage into the adrenal gland. **cerebral a.**, hemorrhage into the substance of the brain, sometimes causing paralysis, coma or death. **pituitary a.**, hemorrhagic necrosis of the pituitary gland, leading to massive degeneration. **renal a.**, rupture of the renal artery, with massive hemorrhage.

aposia (ah-po'ze-ah) absence of thirst.

apositia (ap"o-sish'e-ah) disgust or loathing of food. adj., **aposit'ic.**

apostasis (ah-pos'tah-sis) 1. an abscess. 2. an exfoliation.

apostema (ap"o-ste'ma) an abscess.

aposthia (ah-pos'the-ah) absence of the prepuce.

apothecary (ah-poth'e-ka're) a person who compounds and dispenses drugs.

apotripsis (ap"o-trip'sis) removal of a corneal opacity.

apozymase (ap"o-zi'mas) that portion of a zymase which requires the presence of a cozymase to become a complete zymase.

apparatus (ap"ah-ra'tus) 1. mechanical appliances used in diagnosis, therapy or experimentation. 2. the complex of parts which unite in any function. **Abbé-Zeiss a.**, a device for counting blood corpuscles. **absorption a.**, an apparatus used in gas analysis. **acoustic a.**,

auditory a., the organ of hearing. **Barcroft's a.**, a differential manometer for studying small samples of blood or other tissues. **Beckmann's a.**, an apparatus for determining molecular weight by lowering the freezing point or raising the boiling point of a solution. **ciliary a.**, the ciliary body. **Desault's a.**, Desault's bandage. **Fell-O'Dwyer a.**, a device used in artificial respiration and for prevention of collapse of the lung in chest operations. **Finsen's a.**, an arrangement for increasing the efficiency of ultraviolet irradiation applied locally in the treatment of disease. **Golgi a.**, an irregular complex of parallel membranes and vesicles in a cell, thought to play a role in its secretory activity. **Haldane's a.**, see under *chamber*. **juxtaglomerular a.**, juxtaglomerular cells. **Kirschner's a.**, an apparatus for applying skeletal traction in leg fractures. **lacrimal a.**, the lacrimal gland and ducts and associated structures. **Sayre's a.**, an apparatus for suspending a patient during the application of a plaster of Paris jacket. **segmental a.**, the brain stem. **sound-conducting a.**, the parts of the ear external to the cochlea. **sound-perceiving a.**, the cochlea and the auditory nerve, with its terminations and connections with the auditory nucleus and auditory center. **Soxhlet's a.**, an apparatus by which constituents can be extracted from solutions. **Tallerman's a.**, an apparatus for enclosing an extremity of the body in order to apply dry hot air to it. **vasomotor a.**, the neuromuscular mechanism controlling the constriction and dilation of blood vessels, and thus the amount of blood supplied to a part. **vocal a.**, the organs concerned in the production of voice sounds. **Wangensteen's a.**, a nasal suction apparatus connected with a duodenal tube for aspirating gas and fluid from stomach and intestine. **Zander a.**, a machine for giving passive exercise.

appendage (ah-pen'dij)   a less important portion of an organ, or an outgrowth, such as a tail. **epiploic a's**, appendices epiploicae.

appendectomy (ap"en-dek'to-me) excision of the vermiform appendix.

appendicectasis (ah-pen"dĭ-sek'tah-sis) dilatation of the vermiform appendix.

appendicectomy (-sek'to-me) appendectomy.

appendicitis (-sĭ'tis)   inflammation of the vermiform appendix.

appendicolithiasis (-ko-lĭ-thi'ah-sis) formation of calculi in the vermiform appendix.

appendicolysis (ah-pen"dĭ-kol'ĭ-sis) surgical separation of adhesions binding the appendix.

appendicopathy (-kop'ah-the) any disease of the vermiform appendix.

appendicosis (ah-pen"dĭ-ko'sis) a noninflammatory lesion of the appendix.

appendicostomy (ah-pen"dĭ-kos'to-me) fistulization of the vermiform appendix.

appendicular (ap"en-dik'u-lar) 1. pertaining to an appendix or appendage. 2. pertaining to the limbs.

appendix (ah-pen'diks), pl. *appen'dices* [L.]

1. a slender outgrowth or appendage. 2. the vermiform appendix. **auricular a.**, auricle (1). **ensiform a.**, xiphoid process. **appen'-dices epiplo'icae**, small fatty appendages of peritoneum studding the external surface of the colon. **vermiform a.**, **a. vermifor'mis**, a worm-shaped process of the cecum. **xiphoid a.**, see under *process*.

apperception (ap"er-sep'shun)   conscious perception of a sensory stimulus.

appestat (ap'pĕ-stat)   a center in the hypothalamus thought to control the appetite.

appetite (ap'ĕ-tīt) desire, chiefly desire for food.

appliance (ah-pli'ans)   something that is applied or otherwise used for achievement of a specific purpose. **prosthetic a.**, a device affixed to or implanted in the body to substitute for or assist the function of a defective or missing body part or organ.

apprehension (ap"re-hen'shun) 1. perception and understanding. 2. anticipatory fear or anxiety.

approximal (ah-prok'sĭ-mal)   close together.

apraxia (ah-prak'se-ah) impairment of ability to use objects correctly. **akinetic a.**, loss of ability to carry out spontaneous movement. **a. al'gera**, akinesia algera. **amnestic a.**, loss of ability to carry out a movement on command due to inability to remember the command. **cortical a.**, motor apraxia. **ideational a.**, sensory apraxia. **innervation a.**, **motor a.**, loss of ability to make proper use of an object. **sensory a.**, loss of ability to make proper use of an object due to lack of perception of its purpose.

Apresoline (ah-pres'o-lēn)   trademark for preparations of hydralazine.

aprobarbital (ap"ro-bar'bĭ-tal)   a crystalline powder, $C_{10}H_{14}N_2O_3$, used as a central nervous system depressant.

aproctia (ah-prok'she-ah) imperforation of the anus.

aprosexia (ap"ro-sek'se-ah)   inability to fix attention on any subject.

aprosopia (-so'pe-ah) developmental anomaly with partial or complete absence of the face.

aprosopus (ah-pros'o-pus) a fetal monster exhibiting aprosopia.

A.P.S.   American Pediatric Society; American Physiological Society; American Proctologic Society; American Psychological Society; American Psychosomatic Society.

apselaphesia (ap"sel-ah-fe'ze-ah) absence of the sense of touch.

apsithyria (ap"sĭ-thi're-ah) inability to whisper.

apsychia (ah-si'ke-ah) loss of consciousness.

apsychosis (ah"si-ko'sis) absence or loss of the function of thought.

A.P.T.A. American Physical Therapy Association.

aptyalism (ap-ti'ah-lizm) deficiency or absence of saliva.

apulmonism (ah-pul'mo-nizm) developmental anomaly with partial or complete absence of lung tissue.

apus (a'pus)   a fetal monster without feet.

apyknomorphous (ah″pik-no-mor′fus) not having the stainable cell elements placed compactly.

apyogenous (ah″pi-oj′ĕ-nus) not caused by pus.

apyretic (a″pi-ret′ik) without fever.

apyrexia (ah″pi-rek′se-ah) absence of fever.

apyrogenic (ah-pi″ro-jen′ik) not producing fever.

A.Q. achievement quotient.

aq. [L.] *aq′ua* (water). **aq. dest.**, *aq′ua destilla′-ta* (distilled water).

aqua (ak′wah) [L.] 1. water, H_2O. 2. a saturated solution of a volatile oil or other aromatic or volatile substance in purified water.

aquaphobia (ak″wah-fo′be-ah) morbid fear of water.

aqueduct (ak′we-dukt) any canal or passage. **cerebral a.**, a cavity of midbrain connecting the third and fourth ventricles and containing cerebrospinal fluid. **a. of cochlea,** foramen in temporal bone for a vein from the cochlea. **a. of Fallopius,** canal for facial nerve in petrous portion of temporal bone. **sylvian a., a. of Sylvius,** a canal connecting the third and fourth ventricles of brain. **ventricular a.,** aqueduct of Sylvius.

aqueous (a′kwe-us) 1. watery; prepared with water. 2. see under *humor.*

aquocapsulitis (ak″wo-kap″su-li′tis) serous inflammation of the iris.

Ar chemical symbol, *argon.*

A.R.A. American Rheumatism Association.

arachnephobia (ah-rak″ne-fo′be-ah) morbid dread of spiders.

arachnidism (ah-rak′nĭ-dizm) poisoning from spider bite.

arachnitis (ar″ak-ni′tis) arachnoiditis.

arachnodactyly (ah-rak″no-dak′tĭ-le) extreme length and slenderness of the fingers or toes.

arachnoid (ah-rak′noid) 1. resembling a spider's web. 2. the delicate membrane interposed between the dura mater and the pia mater, and with them constituting the meninges.

Arachnoidea (ar″ak noi′de-ah) a class of animals of the phylum Arthropoda, including 12 orders, comprising such forms as spiders, scorpions, ticks and mites.

arachnoiditis (ah-rak″noid-i′tis) inflammation of the arachnoid membrane.

arachnophobia (ah-rak″no-fo′be-ah) morbid fear of spiders.

arachnopia (-pi′ah) the pia mater and arachnoid membrane together.

Aralen (ar′ah-len) trademark for a preparation of chloroquine.

Aramine (ar′ah-min) trademark for a preparation of metaraminol.

araphia (ah-ra′fe-ah) failure of closure of the neural tube, the spinal cord developing as a flat plate. adj., **ara′phic.**

arbor (ar′bor), pl. *arbo′res* [L.] a tree. **a. vi′tae,** 1. treelike outlines seen on median section of cerebellum. 2. series of ridges within the cervix uteri.

arborescent (ar″bo-res′ent) branching like a tree.

arborization (ar″bor-i-za′shun) a collection of branches, as the branching terminus of a nerve-cell process.

arborvirus (ar″bor-vi′rus) see under *virus.*

arbovirus (ar″bo-vi′rus) arborvirus.

A.R.C. American Red Cross; anomalous retinal correspondence.

arc (ark) a part of the circumference of a circle, or a regularly curved line. **binaural a.,** the arc across the top of the head from one aural point to the other. **reflex a.,** the circuit traveled by impulses producing a reflex action: receptor organ, afferent nerve, nerve center, efferent nerve, effector organ in a muscle. **tungsten a.,** see under *lamp.*

arcate (ar′kāt) curved; bow-shaped.

arch (arch) a structure of bowlike or curved outline. **abdominothoracic a.,** the lower boundary of the front of the thorax. **a. of aorta,** the curving between the ascending aorta and the descending aorta, giving rise to the brachiocephalic trunk, the left common carotid and the left subclavian artery. **aortic a's,** a series of five pairs of arterial arches of the embryo in the region of the neck. **branchial a's,** four pairs of mesenchymal and later cartilaginous arches of the fetus in the region of the neck. **a's of Corti,** series of arches made up of rods of Corti. **costal a.,** the arch formed by the ribs. **dental a.,** the curving structure formed by the crowns of the teeth in their normal position, or by the residual ridge after loss of the teeth. **hemal a.,** arch formed by bodies of vertebrae, ribs and sternum. **hyoid a.,** the second branchial arch. **lingual a.,** a wire appliance which conforms to the lingual aspect of the dental arch, used to secure movement of the teeth in orthodontic work. **mandibular a.,** the first branchial arch, being the rudiment of the maxillary and mandibular regions. **maxillary a.,** 1. the palatal arch. 2. the superior dental arch. **nasal a.,** the arch formed by the nasal bones and the nasal processes of the maxilla. **neural a.,** vertebral arch. **oral a., palatal a.,** the arch formed by the roof of the mouth from the teeth on one side to those on the other. **palatomaxillary a.,** palatal arch. **palmar a.,** the arch of the radial and ulnar arteries in the palm of the hand. **pharyngeal a's,** branchial arches. **plantar a.,** arch formed by external plantar artery. **postaural a's,** branchial arches. **a. of pubis,** portion of pelvis formed by the rami of the ischia and the pubes on each side. **supraorbital a.,** curved margin of frontal bone forming upper boundary of orbit. **tarsal a's,** arches of palpebral arteries around the tarsal cartilages. **vertebral a's,** the structures formed by dorsad extension of the primitive vertebrae in the developing embryo, flanking the neural tube. **visceral a's,** branchial arches. **zygomatic a.,** arch formed by processes of zygomatic and temporal bones.

arch(i)- (ar′ke) word element [Gr.], *ancient; beginning; first; original.*

archamphiaster (ark-am′fe-as″ter) amphiaster forming polar globules.

Archangiaceae (ar-kan″je-a′se-e) a family of Schizomycetes (order Myxobacterales) found in the soil.

Archangium (ar-kan′je-um) a genus of Schizomycetes (order Myxobacterales, family Archangiaceae).

archebiosis (ar″ke-bi-o′sis) abiogenesis.

archegenesis (-jen′ĕ-sis) abiogenesis.

archencephalon (ark″en-sef′ah-lon) the primitive brain from which the midbrain and forebrain develop.

archenteron (ark-en′ter-on) the central cavity which is the provisional gut in the gastrula; the primitive digestive cavity of the embryo.

archeocyte (ar′ke-o-sīt″) a form of ameboid cell.

archeokinetic (ar″ke-o-ki-net′ik) relating to the primitive type of motor nerve mechanism as seen in the peripheral and ganglionic nervous systems.

archepyon (-pi′on) very thick pus.

archesporium (-spo′re-um) the cell giving rise to spore mother cells.

archetype (ar′ke-tīp) in psychology, a type unconsciously considered to be the universal standard or ideal.

archiblast (ar′kī-blast) cumulus oophorus. adj., **archiblas′tic.**

archiblastoma (ar″kī-blas-to′mah) tumor from the ectoderm.

archigaster (-gas′ter) archenteron.

archil (ar′kil) a violet-red stain obtained from the lichen *Roccella tinctoria.*

archinephron (ar″kī-nef′ron) the pronephros.

archineuron (-nu′ron) the neuron at which efferent impulse starts.

archipallium (-pal′e-um) that portion of the pallium which phylogenetically is the first to show the characteristic layering of the cellular elements.

archistome (ar′kī-stōm) the blastopore.

archuitis (ar-kī′tis) proctitis.

arciform (ar′sī-form) arcuate.

arctation (ark-ta′shun) narrowing of an opening or canal.

arcuate (ar′ku-āt) bent like a bow.

arcuation (ar″ku-a′shun) a bending or curvature.

arcus (ar′kus), pl. *ar′cus* [L.] arch; bow. **a. adipo′sus,** arcus senilis. **a. juveni′lis,** an opaque line partially encircling the margin of the cornea, occurring congenitally in children. **a. seni′lis,** an opaque line partially surrounding the margin of the cornea, usually occurring bilaterally in persons of 50 years or older as a result of lipoid degeneration.

area (a′re-ah), pl. *a′reae, areas* [L.] a limited space or plane surface. **association a's,** areas in the cerebral cortex that correlate the impressions received and start motor impulses in harmony with them. **auditory a.,** the auditory center. **Bamberger's a.,** an area of dullness in the left intercostal region, indicative of pericardial effusion. **Betz cell a.,** psychomotor area. **Broca's a.,** area subcallosa. **embryonic a.,** germinal area. **excitable a.,** the motor area of the cerebral cortex. **germinal a., a. germinati′va,** part of ovum where the

embryo is formed. **impression a.,** the surface of the oral structures that is recorded in an impression. **Kiesselbach's a.,** an area on the anterior part of the nasal septum above the intermaxillary bone, richly supplied with capillaries, and a common site of nosebleed. **Krönig's a.,** the area of resonance on the chest, due to the apices of the lungs. **a's of Langerhans,** islands of Langerhans. **motor a.,** ascending frontal and ascending parietal gyri. **a. opa′ca,** outer opaque part of area germinativa. **a. pellu′cida,** central clear part of area germinativa. **a. perfora′ta,** perforated space. **precentral a., psychomotor a.,** the area of the cerebral cortex concerned with the initiation of motor impulses. **silent a.,** an area of the brain in which pathologic conditions may occur without producing symptoms. **a. subcallo′sa, subcallosal a.,** area of gray matter between middle olfactory root and peduncle of corpus callosum. **a. vasculo′sa,** part of area opaca, where the blood vessels are first seen. **a. vitelli′na,** yolk area beyond the area vasculosa in mesoblastic eggs. **vocal a.,** the part of the glottis between the vocal cords.

arecoline (ah-rek′o-lin) a chemical used as a parasympathomimetic agent or veterinary anthelmintic.

areflexia (ah″re-flek′se-ah) absence of the reflexes.

arenoid (ar′ĕ-noid) resembling sand.

areola (ah-re′o-lah), pl. *are′olae* [L.] a colored zone surrounding a central area, e.g. the darkened area surrounding the nipple of the mammary gland. **Chaussier's a.,** the indurated area encircling a malignant pustule.

areolar (ah-re′o-lar) 1. containing minute spaces. 2. pertaining to an areola.

areometer (ar″e-om′ĕ-ter) hydrometer.

Arfonad (ar′fon-ad) trademark for a preparation of trimethaphan.

Argas (ar′gas) a genus of arthropods (family Argasidae) parasitic in poultry and other birds and sometimes man. **A. per′sicus,** the fowl tick, a species parasitic in chickens and turkeys.

Argasidae (ar-gas′ĭ-de) a family of arthropods (class Arachnoidea, order Acarina, suborder Ixodides) made up of the soft-bodied ticks.

argentaffin (ar-jen′tah-fin) staining readily with silver.

argentaffinoma (ar″jen-taf″fī-no′mah) a tumor arising from argentaffin cells, most frequently in the terminal ileum or the appendix.

argentation (-ta′shun) staining with silver.

argentic (ar-jen′tik) containing silver.

argentum (ar-jen′tum) [L.] silver (symbol Ag).

argilla (ar-jil′lah) kaolin.

arginase (ar′jī-nās) an enzyme of the liver that splits up arginine.

arginine (ar′jī-nin) an amino acid, $NH_2C-(NH)_2(CH_2)_3CHNH_2CO_2H$.

argininosuccinic-acidemia (ar″jī-ne″no-suk-sin″ik-as″ĭ-de′me-ah) presence in the blood of argininosuccinic acid.

argininosuccinic-aciduria (ar″jī-ne″no-suk-sin-ik-as″ī-du′re-ah) excretion in the urine of argininosuccinic acid, a feature of an inborn error of metabolism marked also by mental retardation.

argon (ar′gon) chemical element *(see table),* at. no. 18, symbol Ar.

argyria (ar-jĭ′re-ah) discoloration of skin and mucous membranes from excessive use of silver salts.

argyric (ar-jĭ′rik) pertaining to silver.

argyrism (ar′jĭ-rizm) argyria.

argyrophil (ar-jĭ′ro-fil) easily impregnated with silver.

argyrosis (ar″jĭ-ro′sis) argyria.

arhigosis (ah″rĭ-go′sis) inability to perceive cold.

arhinia (ah-rin′e-ah) developmental anomaly with absence of the nose.

arhythmia (ah-rith′me-ah) arrhythmia.

ariboflavinosis (a-ri″bo-fla″vĭ-no′sis) deficiency of riboflavin in the diet.

Aristocort (ah-ris′to-cort) trademark for a preparation of triamcinolone.

arithmomania (ah-rith″mo-ma′nc-ah) psychoneurotic compulsion to count objects, with concern for accuracy or significant numbers.

Arlidin (ar′lĭ-din) trademark for preparations of nylidrin.

arm (arm) 1. the upper extremity, from shoulder to elbow; often used to denote the entire extremity, from shoulder to wrist. 2. an armlike part, e.g. the portion of the chromatid extending in either direction from the centromere of a mitotic chromosome. **bird a.,** atrophy of the muscles of the forearm. **brawny a.,** a hard, swollen condition of the arm following mastectomy.

armamentarium (ar″mah-men-ta′re-um) the entire equipment of a practitioner, such as medicines, instruments, books.

armature (ar′mah-chūr) iron bar across end of a horseshoe magnet.

A.R.M.H. Academy of Religion and Mental Health.

Armillifer (ar-mil′lĭ-fer) a genus of wormlike parasites sometimes found in man and other vertebrates.

arnica (ar′nĭ-kah) dried flowerheads of *Arnica montana,* used in an alcoholic extract or tincture as a skin irritant.

A.R.N.M.D. Association for Research in Nervous and Mental Disease.

A.R.O. Association for Research in Ophthalmology.

aromatic (ar″o-mat′ik) 1. having a spicy fragrance. 2. a stimulant, spicy medicine. 3. pertaining to or derived from the benzene ring; having a closed-chain (carbohydrate) structure.

arrector (ah-rek′tor), pl. *arrecto′res* [L.] an erector muscle.

arrest (ah-rest′) sudden cessation or stoppage. **cardiac a.,** sudden cessation of beating of the heart. **epiphyseal a.,** arrest of the longitudinal growth of bone by surgical fusion of the epiphysis and diaphysis. **maturation a.,** interruption of the process of development, as of blood cells, before the final stage is reached.

arrhenic (ah-ren′ik) pertaining to arsenic.

arrheno- (ah-re′no) word element [Gr.], *male; masculine.*

arrhenoblastoma (ah-re″no-blas-to′mah) a rare ovarian tumor that causes development of masculine qualities.

arrhinia (ah-rin′e-ah) arhinia.

arrhythmia (ah-rith′me-ah) variation from the normal rhythm, especially of the heart beat. adj., **arrhyth′mic.**

A.R.R.S. American Roentgen Ray Society.

A.R.S. American Radium Society.

arsenate (ar′sĕ-nāt) a salt of arsenic acid.

arseniasis (ar″sĭ ni′ah sis) arsenical poisoning.

arsenic (ar′sĕ-nik) chemical element *(see table),* at. no. 33, symbol As. **a. trioxide, white a.,** white, odorless powder, As_2O_3; irritant and escharotic.

arsenical (ar-sen′ĭ-kal) 1. pertaining to arsenic. 2. a compound containing arsenic.

arsenoblast (ar-sen′o-blast) male element of sexual cell.

arsenotherapy (ar″sĕ-no-ther′ah-pe) treatment with arsenic and arsenical compounds.

arsine (ar′sēn) a toxic gas, $H_3As.$

arsphenamine (ars-fen′ah-min) a light yellow powder containing 30–32 per cent of arsenic; used intravenously in syphilis, yaws and other protozoan infections.

arsthinol (ars′thĭ-nol) an arsenical preparation used for the treatment of intestinal amebiasis and yaws.

A.R.T. Accredited Record Technicians.

Artane (ar′tān) trademark for preparations of trihexyphenidyl hydrochloride.

artefact (ar′te-fakt) artifact.

arterectomy (ar″ter-ek′to-me) excision of an artery.

arteria (ar-te′re-ah), pl. *arte′riae* [L.] artery. adj., **arte′rial. a. luso′ria,** an abnormally situated vessel in the region of the aortic arch.

arterialization (ar-te″re-al-ĭ-za′shun) the conversion of venous into arterial blood by the absorption of oxygen.

arteriarctia (-ark′she-ah) contraction of the lumen of an artery.

arteriasis (ar″tĕ-ri′ah-sis) degeneration of the walls of an artery.

arteriectasis (ar-te″re-ek′tah-sis) dilatation of an artery.

arteriectomy (-ek′to-me) excision of an artery.

arterio- (ar-te′re-o) word element [L., Gr.], *artery.*

arteriogram (ar-te′re-o-gram″) 1. a tracing of the arterial pulse. 2. a radiograph of an artery.

arteriography (ar-te″re-og′rah-fe) radiography of an artery or arterial system after injection of a contrast medium in the blood stream. **catheter a.,** radiography of vessels after introduction of contrast material through a catheter inserted into an artery. **selective a.,** radiography of a specific vessel which is opacified by medium introduced through a catheter passed through the aorta to the site of origin of the vessel.

arteriola (ar-te″re-o′lah), pl. *arterio′lae* [L.] arteriole. **arterio′lae rec′tae re′nis,** branches of the arteries of the kidney going to the medullary pyramids.

arteriol(o)- word element, *arteriole.*

arteriole (ar-te′re-ōl) a minute arterial branch. **postglomerular a.,** a branch of the renal vascular system that conveys blood away from a glomerulus. **precapillary a's,** terminal arterioles that end in capillaries. **preglomerular a.,** a branch of the renal vascular system that conveys blood to a renal glomerulus. **straight a's,** arteriolae rectae renis.

arteriolith (ar-te′re-o-lith″) a chalky concretion in an artery.

arteriology (ar-te″re-ol′o-je) sum of knowledge regarding the arteries.

arteriolonecrosis (ar-te″re-o″lo-ne-kro′sis) necrosis or destruction of arterioles.

arteriolosclerosis (-skle-ro′sis) thickening of the walls of the arterioles. adj., **arteriolosclerot′ic.**

arteriomalacia (ar-te″re-o″mah-la′she-ah) softening of the arterial wall.

arteriometer (ar-te″re-om′ĕ-ter) an instrument for measuring changes in the caliber of a beating artery.

arteriomotor (ar-te″re-o-mo′ter) causing dilation or constriction of arteries.

arteriomyomatosis (-mi″o-mah-to′sis) growth of muscular fibers in the walls of an artery, causing thickening.

arterionecrosis (-ne-kro′sis) necrosis of arteries.

arteriopathy (ar-te″re-op′ah-the) any disease of an artery. **hypertensive a.,** involvement of the smaller arteries and arterioles, associated with hypertension and characterized by hypertrophy of the medial coat of the vessels.

arterioplasty (ar-te′re-o-plas″te) plastic repair of an artery.

arteriopressor (ar-te″re-o-pres′or) increasing arterial blood pressure.

arteriorrhaphy (ar-te″re-or′ah-fe) suture of an artery.

arteriorrhexis (ar-te″re-o-rek′sis) rupture of an artery.

arteriosclerosis (-skle-ro′sis) thickening and loss of elasticity of arterial walls. adj., **arteriosclerot′ic. Mönckeberg's a.,** arteriosclerosis characterized by calcification of the middle coat of the artery. **a. oblit′erans,** arteriosclerosis in which proliferation of the intima has caused complete obliteration of the lumen of the artery. **peripheral a.,** arteriosclerosis of peripheral arteries. **senile a.,** arteriosclerosis occurring in old age.

arteriospasm (ar-te′re-o-spazm″) spasm of an artery.

arteriostenosis (ar-te″re-o-ste-no′sis) constriction of an artery.

arteriosympathectomy (-sim″pah-thek′to-me) periarterial sympathectomy.

arteriotomy (ar-te″re-ot′o-me) incision of an artery.

arteriotony (-ot′o-ne) blood pressure.

arteriovenous (ar-te″re-o-ve′nus) pertaining to both artery and vein.

arterioversion (ar-te″re-o-ver′zhun) eversion of the cut end of an artery to arrest hemorrhage.

arteritis (ar″ter-i′tis) inflammation of an artery. **a. defor′mans,** chronic endarteritis. **a. oblit′erans,** endarteritis obliterans. **rheumatic a.,** generalized inflammation of arterioles and arterial capillaries occurring in rheumatic fever. **temporal a.,** inflammation involving the temporal artery, with painful nodular swellings along the vessel. **a. verruco′sa,** arteritis marked by projections from the wall into the lumen of the blood vessel.

artery (ar′ter-e) a vessel in which blood flows away from the heart, in the systemic circulation carrying oxygenated blood. For named arteries of the body, *see table.* **end a.,** one which undergoes progressive branching without development of channels connecting with other arteries.

arthr(o)- word element [Gr.], *joint; articulation.*

arthragra (ar-thrag′rah) gouty pain in a joint.

arthral (ar′thral) pertaining to a joint.

arthralgia (ar-thral′je-ah) pain in a joint.

arthrectomy (ar-threk′to-me) excision of a joint.

arthritid (ar′thri-tid) a skin eruption of gouty origin.

arthritis (ar-thri′tis) inflammation of a joint. adj., **arthrit′ic. acute a.,** arthritis marked by pain, heat, redness and swelling. **acute rheumatic a.,** swelling, tenderness and redness of many joints of the body, often accompanying rheumatic fever. **atrophic a., a. defor′mans,** rheumatoid arthritis. **gonococcal a.,** severe pain and swelling of the joints resulting from infection by *Neisseria gonorrhoeae.* **hypertrophic a.,** arthritis deformans marked by hypertrophy of the cartilage at the edge of the joints; osteoarthritis. **infectious a., chronic a.,** rheumatoid arthritis. **juvenile rheumatoid a.,** a condition of acute onset in children, with swelling, tenderness and pain involving one or more of the larger joints. **proliferative a., rheumatoid a.,** a condition occurring in children with stiffness, tenderness and pain in various joints, leading to flexion deformities of knees, elbows, wrists and fingers; thought possibly to be due to derangement of the immunologic mechanism. **rheumatoid a., juvenile,** a condition occurring in children, with involvement of one or more joints, leading to impaired growth and development, with ankylosis and flexion contractures of the joints. **rheumatoid a., multiple,** rheumatoid arthritis involving many different joints. **rheumatoid a. of spine,** a condition occurring chiefly in young men, progressing from sacroiliac joints to spine and causing spinal ankylosis with scoliosis and exaggerated thoracic kyphosis. **suppurative a.,** inflammation of a joint with a serous, serofibrinous or purulent effusion and destruction of articular tissue.

arthritism (ar′thri-tizm) gouty or rheumatic diathesis.

COMMON NAME*	NA EQUIVALENT†	ORIGIN*	BRANCHES*	DISTRIBUTION
accompanying a. of sciatic nerve. see *sciatic a.*				
acromiothoracic a. see *thoracoacromial a.*				
alveolar a., inferior	a. alveolaris inferior	maxillary a.	dental, mylohyoid branches, mental a.	lower teeth, gums, mandible, lower lip, chin
alveolar a's, anterior superior	aa. alveolares superiores anteriores	infraorbital a.	dental branches	incisors and canine teeth of upper jaw, maxillary sinus
alveolar a., posterior superior	a. alveolaris superior posterior	maxillary a.	dental branches	molar and premolar teeth of upper jaw, maxillary sinus, buccinator muscle
angular a.	a. angularis	facial a.		lacrimal sac, inferior portion of orbicularis oculi, nose
aorta	aorta	left ventricle		
abdominal aorta	aorta abdominalis	lower portion of descending aorta, from aortic hiatus of diaphragm to bifurcation into common iliac a's	inferior phrenic, lumbar, median sacral, superior and inferior mesenteric, middle suprarenal, renal, and testicular or ovarian a's, celiac trunk	
arch of aorta	arcus aortae	continuation of ascending aorta	brachiocephalic trunk, left common carotid and left subclavian a's; continues as descending (thoracic) aorta	
ascending aorta	aorta ascendens	proximal portion of aorta, arising from left ventricle	right and left coronary a's; continues as arch of aorta	
descending aorta. see *thoracic aorta; abdominal aorta*	aorta descendens	continuation of arch of aorta		

* a. = artery; a's = (pl.) arteries.
† a. = [L.] arteria; aa. = [L. (pl.)] arteriae.

51

TABLE OF ARTERIES—*Continued*

COMMON NAME*	NA EQUIVALENT†	ORIGIN*	BRANCHES*	DISTRIBUTION
aorta (*continued*) thoracic aorta	aorta thoracica	proximal portion of descending aorta, continuing from arch of aorta to aortic hiatus of diaphragm	bronchial, esophageal, pericardiac and mediastinal branches, superior phrenic a's, posterior intercostal a's [III–XI], subcostal a's; continues as abdominal aorta	
appendicular a.	a. appendicularis	ileocolic a.		veriform appendix
arcuate a. of foot	a. arcuata pedis	dorsalis pedis a.	deep plantar branch and dorsal metatarsal a's	foot, including toes
arcuate a's of kidney	aa. arcuatae renis	interlobar a.	interlobar a's and straight arterioles of kidney	parenchyma of kidney
auditory a., internal. see *a. of labyrinth.*				
auricular a., deep	a. auricularis profunda	maxillary a.		skin of auditory meatus, tympanic membrane, temporomandibular joint
auricular a., posterior	a. auricularis posterior	external carotid a.	auricular and occipital branches, stylomastoid a.	middle ear, mastoid cells, auricle, parotid gland, digastric and other muscles
axillary a.	a. axillaris	continuation of subclavian a.	subscapular branches, and highest thoracic, thoracoacromial, lateral thoracic, subscapular, and anterior and posterior circumflex humeral a's	upper limb, including shoulder and axilla, and chest
basilar a.	a. basilaris	from junction of right and left vertebral a's	pontine branches, and anterior inferior cerebellar, labyrinthine, superior cerebellar and posterior cerebral a's	brain stem, internal ear, cerebellum, posterior part of cerebrum
brachial a.	a. brachialis	continuation of axillary a.	profunda brachii, superior and inferior ulnar collateral, radial and ulnar a's	shoulder, arm, forearm and hand
brachial a., deep. see *profunda brachii a.* brachial a., superficial	a. brachialis superficialis	variant brachial a., taking a more superficial course than usual	see *brachial a.*	see *brachial a.*

brachiocephalic trunk	truncus brachiocephalicus	arch of aorta	right common carotid and right, subclavian a's	right side of head and neck, right upper limb
buccal a.	a. buccalis	maxillary a.		buccinator muscle, mucous membrane of mouth
a. of bulb of penis	a. bulbi penis	internal pudendal a.		bulbourethral gland and bulb of penis
a. of bulb of urethra. see *a. of bulb of penis*				
a. of bulb of vestibule of vagina	a. bulbi vestibuli [vaginae]	internal pudendal a.		bulb of vestibule of vagina and greater vestibular glands
carotid a.	a. carotis communis	brachiocephalic (right), arch of aorta (left)	external and internal carotid a's	see *carotid a., external* and *carotid a., internal*
carotid a., external	a. carotis externa	common carotid a.	superior thyroid ascending pharyngeal, lingual, facial, sternocleidomastoid, occipital, posterior auricular, superficial temporal and maxillary a's	neck, face, skull
carotid a., internal	a. carotis interna	common carotid a.	caroticotympanic branches, and ophthalmic, posterior communicating, anterior choroid, anterior cerebral and middle cerebral a's	middle ear, brain, hypophysis, orbit, choroid plexus of lateral ventricle
caudal a. see *sacral a., median*				
celiac trunk	truncus celiacus	abdominal aorta	left gastric, common hepatic and splenic a's	esophagus, stomach, duodenum, spleen, pancreas, liver, gallbladder
central a. of retina	a. centralis retinae	ophthalmic a.		retina
cerebellar a., inferior, anterior	a. cerebelli inferior anterior	basilar a.	a. of labyrinth	lower anterior cerebellar cortex, inner ear
cerebellar a., inferior, posterior	a. cerebelli inferior posterior	vertebral a.		lower part of cerebellum, medulla, choroid plexus of fourth ventricle
cerebellar a., superior	a. cerebelli superior	basilar a.		upper part of cerebellum, midbrain, pineal body choroid plexus of third ventricle
cerebral a., anterior	a. cerebri anterior	internal carotid a.	cortical (orbital, frontal, parietal) and central branches and anterior communicating a.	orbital, frontal and parietal cortex and corpus callosum

TABLE OF ARTERIES — *Continued*

COMMON NAME*	NA EQUIVALENT†	ORIGIN*	BRANCHES*	DISTRIBUTION
cerebral a., middle	a. cerebri media	internal carotid a.	cortical (orbital, frontal, parietal, temporal) and central (striate) branches	orbital, frontal, parietal and temporal cortex, and basal ganglia
cerebral a., posterior	a. cerebri posterior	terminal bifurcation of basilar a.	cortical (temporal, occipital, parieto-occipital), central and choroid branches	occipital and temporal lobes, basal ganglia, choroid plexus of lateral ventricle, thalamus, midbrain
cervical a., ascending	a. cervicalis ascendens	inferior thyroid a.	spinal branches	muscles of neck, vertebrae, vertebral canal
cervical a., deep	a. cervicalis profunda	costocervical trunk		deep neck muscles
cervical a., transverse	a. transversa colli	subclavian a.	deep and superficial branches	trapezius, muscles and lymph nodes of neck, rhomboid and latissimus dorsi muscles
choroid a., anterior	a. choroidea anterior	internal carotid a.		choroid plexus of lateral ventricle, hippocampus, fimbria
ciliary a's, anterior	aa. ciliares anteriores	ophthalmic and lacrimal a's	episcleral and anterior conjunctival a's	iris, conjunctiva
ciliary a's, posterior, long	aa. ciliares posteriores longae	ophthalmic a.		iris, ciliary processes
ciliary a's, posterior, short	aa. ciliares posteriores breves	ophthalmic a.		choroid coat of eye
circumflex femoral a., lateral	a. circumflexa femoris lateralis	profunda femoris a.	ascending, descending and transverse branches	hip joint, thigh muscles
circumflex femoral a., medial	a. circumflexa femoris medialis	profunda femoris a.	deep, ascending, transverse and acetabular branches	hip joint, thigh muscles
circumflex humeral a., anterior	a. circumflexa humeri anterior	axillary a.		shoulder joint and head of humerus, long tendon of biceps, tendon of pectoralis major muscle
circumflex humeral a., posterior	a. circumflexa humeri posterior	axillary a.		deltoid, shoulder joint, teres minor and triceps muscles
circumflex iliac a., deep	a. circumflexa ilium profunda	external iliac a.	ascending branch	psoas, iliacus, sartorius, tensor fasciae latae, and oblique and transverse abdominal muscles, and adjacent skin

circumflex iliac a., superficial	a. circumflexa ilium superficialis	inguinal nodes, skin of thigh and abdomen
circumflex a. of scapula	a. circumflexa scapulae	subscapular muscle, shoulder joint, teres major and minor muscles
coccygeal a. see *sacral a., median*		
colic a., left	a. colica sinistra	descending colon
colic a., middle	a. colica media	transverse colon
colic a., right	a. colica dextra	ascending colon
colic a., right, inferior. see *ileocolic a.*		
colic a., superior accessory. see *colic a., middle*		
collateral a., middle	a. collateralis media	profunda brachii a
collateral a., radial	a. collateralis radialis	profunda brachii a
collateral a., inferior ulnar	a. collateralis ulnaris inferior	brachial a.
collateral a., superior ulnar	a. collateralis ulnaris superior	brachial a.
communicating a., anterior	a. communicans anterior cerebri	anterior cerebral a.
communicating a., posterior	a. communicans posterior cerebri	internal carotid and posterior cerebral a's
conjunctival a's, anterior	aa. conjunctivales anteriores	anterior ciliary a's
conjunctival a's, posterior	aa. conjunctivales posteriores	medial palpebral a.
coronary a., left	a. coronaria sinistra	left aortic sinus; anterior interventricular and circumflex branches
coronary a., right	a. coronaria dextra	right aortic sinus; posterior interventricular branch
costocervical trunk	truncus costocervicalis	subclavian a.	deep cervical and highest intercostal a's
cremasteric a.	a. cremasterica	inferior epigastric a.	cremaster muscle, coverings of spermatic cord

TABLE OF ARTERIES – *Continued*

COMMON NAME*	NA EQUIVALENT†	ORIGIN*	BRANCHES*	DISTRIBUTION
cystic a.	a. cystica	right branch of hepatic a., proper		gallbladder
deep brachial. see *profunda brachii a.*				
deep a. of clitoris	a. profunda clitoridis	internal pudendal a.		clitoris
deep a. of penis	a. profunda penis	internal pudendal a.		corpus cavernosum penis
deep femoral a. see *profunda femoris a.*				
deep lingual a. see *profunda linguae a.*				
deferential a. see *a. of ductus deferens*				
dental a's, anterior superior. see *alveolar a's, anterior superior*				
dental a., inferior. see *alveolar a., inferior*				
dental a., posterior superior. see *alveolar a., posterior superior*				
diaphragmatic a..inferior. see *phrenic a., inferior*				
diaphragmatic a's, superior. see *phrenic a's, superior*				
digital a's, collateral. see *digital a's, palmar, proper*				
digital a's, palmar, common	aa. digitales palmares communes	superficial palmar arch	proper palmar digital a's	fingers
digital a's, palmar, proper	aa. digitales palmares propriae	common palmar digital a's		fingers

56

digital a's, plantar, common	aa. digitales plantares communes			toes
digital a's, plantar, proper	aa. digitales plantares propriae	common plantar digital a's	proper plantar digital a's	toes
digital a's of foot, common. see *metatarsal a's, plantar*				
digital a's of foot, dorsal	aa. digitales dorsales pedis	dorsal metatarsal a's		dorsum of toes
digital a's of hand, dorsal	aa. digitales dorsales manus	dorsal metacarpal a's		dorsum of fingers
dorsal a. of clitoris	a. dorsalis clitoridis	internal pudendal a.		clitoris
dorsal a. of foot. see *dorsalis pedis a.*				
dorsal a. of nose	a. dorsalis nasi	ophthalmic a.		skin of dorsum of nose
dorsal a. of penis	a. dorsalis penis	internal pudendal a.		glans, corona and prepuce of penis
dorsalis pedis a.	a. dorsalis pedis	continuation of anterior tibial a.	lateral and medial tarsal, and arcuate a's	foot, including toes
a. of ductus deferens	a. ductus deferentis	umbilical a.	ureteric branches	ureter, bladder, ductus deferens, seminal vesicles
duodenal a. see *pancreaticoduodenal a., inferior*				
epigastric a., external. see *circumflex iliac a., deep*				
epigastric a., inferior	a. epigastrica inferior	external iliac a.	pubic branch, cremasteric a., a. of round ligament of uterus	cremaster and abdominal muscles, peritoneum
epigastric a., superficial	a. epigastrica superficialis	femoral a.		skin of abdomen, inguinal lymph nodes
epigastric a., superior	a. epigastrica superior	internal thoracic a.		abdominal muscles, diaphragm, skin, peritoneum
episcleral a's	aa. episclerales	anterior ciliary a.		iris, ciliary processes
ethmoidal a., anterior	a. ethmoidalis anterior	ophthalmic a.	anterior meningeal a.	dura mater, nose, frontal sinus, skin, anterior ethmoidal cells
ethmoidal a., posterior	a. ethmoidalis posterior	ophthalmic a.		posterior ethmoidal cells, dura mater, nose

TABLE OF ARTERIES—Continued

COMMON NAME*	NA EQUIVALENT†	ORIGIN*	BRANCHES*	DISTRIBUTION
facial a.	a. facialis	external carotid a.	ascending palatine, submental, inferior and superior labial and angular a's; tonsillar and glandular branches	face, tonsil, palate, submandibular gland
facial a., deep. see *maxillary a.*				
facial a., transverse	a. transversa faciei	superficial temporal a.		parotid gland, masseter muscle, skin of face
fallopian a. see *uterine a.*				
femoral a.	a. femoralis	continuation of external iliac a.	superficial epigastric, superficial circumflex iliac, external pudendal, profunda femoris and descending geniculate a's	lower abdominal wall, external genitalia, lower limb
femoral a., deep. see *profunda femoris a.*				
fibular a. see *peroneal a.*				
frontal a. see *supratrochlear a.*				
funicular a. see *testicular a.*				
gastric a., left	a. gastrica sinistra	celiac trunk	esophageal branches	esophagus, lesser curvature of stomach
gastric a., right	a. gastrica dextra	common hepatic a.		lesser curvature of stomach
gastric a's, short	aa. gastricae breves	splenic a.		upper part of stomach
gastroduodenal a.	a. gastroduodenalis	common hepatic a.	superior pancreaticoduodenal and right gastroepiploic a's	stomach, duodenum, pancreas, greater omentum
gastroepiploic a., left	a. gastroepiploica sinistra	splenic a.	epiploic branches	stomach, greater omentum
gastroepiploic a., right	a. gastroepiploica dextra	gastroduodenal a.	epiploic branches	stomach, greater omentum
genicular a.,	a. genus descendens	femoral a.	saphenous and articular branches	knee joint, skin of upper and medial part of leg
genicular a., inferior, lateral	a. genus inferior lateralis	popliteal a.		knee joint
genicular a., inferior, medial	a. genus inferior medialis	popliteal a.		knee joint

58

Term	Latin	Origin	Branches	Distribution
genicular a., middle	a. genus media	popliteal a.		knee joint, cruciate ligaments, patellar synovial and alar folds
genicular a., superior, lateral	a. genus superior lateralis	popliteal a.		knee joint, femur, patella, contiguous muscles
genicular a., superior medial	a. genus superior medialis	popliteal a.		knee joint, femur, patella, contiguous muscles
gluteal a., inferior	a. glutea inferior	internal iliac a.	sciatic a.	buttock, back of thigh
gluteal a., superior	a. glutea superior	internal iliac a.	superficial and deep branches	various muscles and other structures of hip and buttocks
helicine a's of penis	aa. helicinae penis	deep and dorsal aa. of penis		erectile tissue of penis
hemorrhoidal a., inferior. see *rectal a., inferior.* hemorrhoidal a., middle. see *rectal a., middle.* hemorrhoidal a., superior. see *rectal a., superior*				
hepatic a., common	a. hepatica communis	celiac trunk	right gastric, gastroduodenal, proper hepatic a's	stomach, pancreas, duodenum, liver, gallbladder, greater omentum
hepatic a., proper	a. hepatica propria	common hepatic a.	right and left branches	liver, gallbladder
hyaloid a.	a. hyaloidea	fetal ophthalmic a.		fetal lens and vitreous body
hypogastric a. see *iliac a., internal*				
ileal a's	aa. ilei	superior mesenteric a.		ileum
ileocolic a.	a. ileocolica	superior mesenteric a.	appendicular a.	ileum, cecum, vermiform appendix, ascending colon
iliac a., common	a. iliaca communis	abdominal aorta	internal and external iliac a's	pelvis, abdominal wall, lower limb
iliac a., external	a. iliaca externa	common iliac a.	inferior epigastric, deep circumflex iliac a's	abdominal wall, external genitalia, lower limb
iliac a., internal	a. iliaca interna	continuation of common iliac a.	iliolumbar, obturator, superior gluteal, inferior gluteal, umbilical, inferior vesical, uterine, middle rectal and internal pudendal a's	wall and viscera of pelvis, buttock, reproductive organs, medial aspect of thigh
iliolumbar a.	a. iliolumbalis	internal iliac a.	iliac and lumbar branches, lateral sacral a's	pelvic muscles and hip bones, fifth lumbar vertebra, sacrum
infraorbital a.	a. infraorbitalis	maxillary a.	anterior superior alveolar a's	maxilla, maxillary sinus, upper teeth, lower eyelid, cheek, side of nose

TABLE OF ARTERIES – *Continued*

COMMON NAME°	NA EQUIVALENT†	ORIGIN*	BRANCHES*	DISTRIBUTION
innominate a. see *brachiocephalic trunk*				
intercostal a., highest	a. intercostalis suprema	costocervical trunk	posterior intercostal a's I and II	first and second intercostal spaces, vertebral column, back muscles
intercostal a's, posterior, I and II	aa. intercostales posteriores [I et II]	highest intercostal a.	dorsal and spinal branches	first and second intercostal spaces, back muscles, vertebral column
intercostal a's, posterior, III–XI	aa. intercostales posteriores [III–XI]	thoracic aorta	dorsal, lateral, and lateral cutaneous branches	body wall of thorax
interlobar a's of kidney	aa. interlobares renis	renal a.	arcuate a's of kidney	lobes of kidney
interlobular a's of kidney	aa. interlobulares renis	arcuate a's of kidney		renal glomeruli
interlobular a's of liver	aa. interlobulares hepatis	right or left branch of proper hepatic a.		between lobules of liver
interosseous a., anterior	a. interossea anterior	posterior or common interosseous a.	median a.	flexor digitorum profundus and flexor pollicis longus muscles, radius, ulna
interosseous a., common	a. interossea communis	ulnar a.	anterior and posterior interosseous a's	deep structures of forearm
interosseous a., posterior	a. interossea posterior	common interosseous a.	recurrent interosseous a.	superficial and deep muscles on back of forearm
interosseous a., recurrent	a. interossea recurrens	posterior or common interosseous a.		back of elbow joint
intestinal a's	aa. intestinales	vessels arising from superior mesenteric a. and supplying intestines; they include pancreaticoduodenal, jejunal, iliac, ileocolic and colic a's		
jejunal a's	aa. jejunales	superior mesenteric a.		jejunum
labial a., inferior	a. labialis inferior	facial a.		lower lip
labial a., superior	a. labialis superior	facial a.	septal and alar branches	upper lip and nose
a. of labyrinth	a. labyrinthi	basilar or anterior inferior cerebellar a.	vestibular and cochlear branches	internal ear

lacrimal a.	a. lacrimalis	ophthalmic a.	lateral palpebral a.	lacrimal gland, eyelids, conjunctiva
laryngeal a., inferior	a. laryngea inferior	inferior thyroid a.		larynx, upper part of trachea, esophagus
laryngeal a., superior	a. laryngea superior	superior thyroid a.		larynx
lingual a.	a. lingualis	external carotid a.	suprahyoid, sublingual, dorsal lingual, profunda linguae a's	tongue, sublingual gland, tonsil, epiglottis
lingual a., deep. see *profunda linguae a.*				
lumbar a's	aa. lumbales	abdominal aorta	dorsal and spinal branches	abdominal wall, vertebrae, lumbar muscles, renal capsule
lumbar a., lowest	a. lumbalis ima	middle sacral a.		sacrum, gluteus maximus muscle
malleolar a., anterior, lateral	a. malleolaris anterior lateralis	anterior tibial a.		ankle joint
malleolar a., anterior, medial	a. malleolaris anterior medialis	anterior tibia. a.		ankle joint
mammary a., external. see *thoracic a., lateral*				
mammary a., internal. see *thoracic a., internal*				
mandibular a. see *alveolar a., inferior*				
masseteric a.	a. masseterica	maxillary a.		masseter muscle
maxillary a.	a. maxillaris	external carotid a.	pterygoid branches; deep auricular, anterior tympanic, inferior alveolar, middle meningeal, masseteric, deep temporal, buccal, posterior superior alveolar, infraorbital, descending palatine, and sphenopalatine a's, and a. of pterygoid canal	both jaws, teeth, muscles of mastication, ear, meninges, nose, paranasal sinuses, palate
maxillary a., external. see *facial a.*				
maxillary a., internal. see *maxillary a.*				
median a.	a. mediana	anterior interosseous a.		median nerve, muscles of front of forearm
meningeal a., anterior	a. meningea anterior	anterior ethmoidal a.		dura mater of anterior cranial fossa

COMMON NAME*	NA EQUIVALENT†	ORIGIN*	BRANCHES*	DISTRIBUTION
meningeal a's, middle	a. meningea media	maxillary a.	frontal, parietal, anastomotic, accessory meningeal, and petrous branches, and superior tympanic a.	cranial bones, dura mater of brain
meningeal a's, posterior	a. meningea posterior	ascending pharyngeal a.		bones and dura mater of posterior cranial fossa
mental a.	a. mentalis	inferior alveolar a.		skin and muscles of chin
mesenteric a's, inferior	a. mesenterica inferior	abdominal aorta	left colic, sigmoid and superior rectal a's	descending colon, rectum
mesenteric a's, superior	a. mesenterica superior	abdominal aorta	inferior pancreaticoduodenal, jejunal, ileal, ileocolic, right colic and middle colic a's	small intestine, proximal half of colon
metacarpal a's, dorsal	aa. metacarpeae dorsales	dorsal carpal rete and radial a.	dorsal digital a's	dorsum of fingers
metacarpal a's, palmar	aa. metacarpeae palmares	deep palmar arch		lumbrical and interosseous muscles, bones of fingers
metatarsal a's, dorsal	aa. metatarseae dorsales	arcuate a. of foot	dorsal digital a's	dorsum of foot, including toes
metatarsal a's, plantar	aa. metatarseae plantares	plantar arch	perforating branches, common and proper plantar digital a's	plantar surface of toes
musculophrenic a.	a. musculophrenica	internal thoracic a.		diaphragm, abdominal and thoracic walls
nasal a's, posterior lateral and septal	aa. nasales posteriores laterales et septi	sphenopalatine a.		structures bounding nasal cavity, nasal septum, adjacent sinuses
nutrient a's of humerus	aa. nutriciae humeri	brachial and deep brachial a's		substance of humerus
obturator a.	a. obturatoria	internal iliac a.	pubic, acetabular, anterior and posterior branches	pelvic muscles, hip joint
obturator a., accessory	a. obturatoria accessoria	name given to obturator a. when it arises from inferior epigastric instead of internal iliac a.		
occipital a.	a. occipitalis	external carotid a.	auricular, meningeal, mastoid, descending, occipital and sternocleidomastoid branches	muscles of neck and scalp, meninges, mastoid cells

ophthalmic a.	a. ophthalmica	internal carotid a.	lacrimal and supraorbital a's, central a. of retina, ciliary, posterior and anterior ethmoidal, palpebral, supratrochlear and dorsal nasal a's	eye, orbit, adjacent facial structures
ovarian a.	a. ovarica	abdominal aorta	ureteric branches	ureter, ovary, uterine tube
palatine a., ascending	a. palatina ascendens	facial a.		soft palate, portions of wall of pharynx, tonsil, auditory tube
palatine a., descending	a. palatina descendens	maxillary a.	greater and lesser palatine a's	palate, tonsil
palatine a., greater	a. palatina major	descending palatine a.		hard palate
palatine a's, lesser	aa. palatinae minores	descending palatine a.		soft palate and tonsil
palpebral a's, lateral	aa. palpebrales laterales	lacrimal a.		eyelids, conjunctiva
palpebral a's, medial	aa. palpebrales mediales	ophthalmic a.	posterior conjunctival a's	eyelids
pancreaticoduodenal a., inferior	a. pancreaticoduodenalis inferior	superior mesenteric a.		pancreas, duodenum
pancreaticoduodenal a., superior	a. pancreaticoduodenalis superior	gastroduodenal a.		pancreas, duodenum
perforating a's	aa. perforantes	profunda femoris a.		adductor, hamstring and gluteal muscles, femur
pericardiacophrenic a.	a. pericardiacophrenica	internal thoracic a.		pericardium, diaphragm, pleura
perineal a.	a. perinealis	internal pudendal a.		perineum, skin of external genitalia
peroneal a.	a. peronea	posterior tibial a.	perforating, communicating, calcaneal, and lateral and medial malleolar branches, calcaneal rete	lateral side and back of ankle, deep calf muscles
pharyngeal a., ascending	a. pharyngea ascendens	external carotid a.	posterior meningeal, pharyngeal, inferior tympanic a's	pharynx, soft palate, ear, meninges, cranial nerves, capitis muscles
phrenic a., great. see phrenic a., inferior				
phrenic a., inferior	a. phrenica inferior	abdominal aorta	superior suprarenal a's	diaphragm, suprarenal gland
phrenic a's, superior	aa. phrenicae superiores	thoracic aorta		upper surface of vertebral portion of diaphragm
plantar a., lateral	a. plantaris lateralis	posterior tibial a.	plantar arch, plantar metatarsal a's	sole of foot, toes
plantar a., medial	a. plantaris medialis	posterior tibial a.	deep and superficial branches	muscles and joints of foot, skin of medial aspect of sole and toes

TABLE OF ARTERIES—*Continued*

COMMON NAME*	NA EQUIVALENT†	ORIGIN*	BRANCHES*	DISTRIBUTION
popliteal a.	a. poplitea	continuation of femoral a.	lateral and medial superior genicular, middle genicular, sural, lateral and medial inferior genicular, anterior and posterior tibial a's; genicular articular rete, patellar rete	knee and calf
princeps pollicis a. principal a. of thumb. see *princeps pollicis a.*	a. princeps pollicis	radial a.	radialis indicis a.	sides and palmar aspect of thumb
profunda brachii a.	a. profunda brachii	brachial a.	nutrient to humerus, deltoid branch, middle and radial collateral a's	humerus, muscles and skin of arm
profunda femoris a.	a. profunda femoris	femoral a.	medial and lateral circumflex femoral a's, perforating a's	thigh muscles, hip joint, gluteal muscles, femur
profunda linguae a. a. of pterygoid canal pudendal a's, external	a. profunda linguae a canalis pterygoidei aa. pudendae externae	termination of lingual a. maxillary a. femoral a.	anterior scrotal or anterior labial branches, inguinal branches posterior scrotal or posterior labial branches	side and tip of tongue roof of pharynx, auditory tube external genitalia, medial thigh muscles
pudendal a, internal	a. pudenda interna	internal iliac a.	inferior rectal, perineal, urethral a's, a. of bulb of penis or vestibule, deep a. of penis or clitoris, dorsal a. of penis or clitoris	external genitalia, anal canal, perineum
pulmonary trunk	truncus pulmonalis	right ventricle	right and left pulmonary a's	conveys unaerated blood toward lungs
pulmonary a., left	a. pulmonalis sinistra	pulmonary trunk	numerous branches named according to segments of lung to which they distribute unaerated blood	left lung
pulmonary a., right	a. pulmonalis dextra	pulmonary trunk	numerous branches named according to segments of lung to which they distribute unaerated blood	right lung

64

radial a.	a. radialis	brachial a.	palmar carpal, superficial palmar and dorsal carpal branches; recurrent radial a., princeps pollicis a., deep palmar arch	forearm, wrist, hand
radial a., collateral. see collateral a., radial				
radial a. of index finger. see radialis indicis a.				
radiate a's of kidney. see interlobular a's of kidney				
ranine a. see profunda linguae a.				
radialis indicis a.	a. radialis indicis	princeps pollicis a.		both sides of index finger
rectal a., inferior	a. rectalis inferior	internal pudendal a.		rectum, levator ani and external sphincter muscles, overlying skin
rectal a., middle	a. rectalis media	internal iliac a.		rectum, vagina
rectal a., superior	a. rectalis superior	inferior mesenteric a.		rectum
recurrent a., radial	a. recurrens radialis	radial a.		brachioradialis and brachialis muscles, elbow joint
recurrent a., tibial, anterior	a. recurrens tibialis anterior	anterior tibial a.		anterior tibial muscle and long extensor muscle of toes; knee joint, skin of lower leg
recurrent a., tibial, posterior	a. recurrens tibialis posterior	anterior tibial a.		knee joint, tibiofibular joint
recurrent a., ulnar	a. recurrens ulnaris	ulnar a.	anterior and posterior branches	elbow joint, adjacent skin, and muscles
renal a.	a. renalis	abdominal aorta	ureteric branches, inferior suprarenal a., interlobar a's	kidney, suprarenal gland, ureter
a. of round ligament of uterus	a. ligamenti teretis uteri	inferior epigastric a.		round ligament of uterus
sacral a's, lateral	aa. sacrales laterales	iliolumbar a.	spinal branches	structures about coccyx and sacrum
sacral a., median	a. sacralis mediana	central continuation of abdominal aorta, beyond origin of common iliac a's	lowest lumbar a.	sacrum, coccyx, rectum

TABLE OF ARTERIES—Continued

COMMON NAME*	NA EQUIVALENT†	ORIGIN*	BRANCHES*	DISTRIBUTION
scapular a., transverse. see *suprascapular a.*				
sciatic a.	a. comitans nervi ischiadici	inferior gluteal a.		accompanies sciatic nerve
sigmoid a's	aa. sigmoideae	inferior mesenteric a.		sigmoid colon
spermatic a., external. see *cremasteric a.*				
sphenopalatine a.	a. sphenopalatina	maxillary a.	posterior lateral nasal a's and a's of septum	structures adjoining nasal cavity, nasopharynx
spinal a., anterior	a. spinalis anterior	vertebral a.		anterior portion of spinal cord
spinal a., posterior	a. spinalis posterior	vertebral a.		posterior portion of spinal cord
splenic a.	a. lienalis	celiac trunk	pancreatic and splenic branches; left gastroepiploic and short gastric a's	spleen, pancreas, stomach, greater omentum
straight arterioles of kidney	arteriolae rectae renis	arcuate a's of kidney		renal pyramids
stylomastoid a.	a. stylomastoidea	posterior auricular a.	mastoid and stapedial branches, posterior tympanic a.	tympanic cavity walls, mastoid cells, stapedius
subclavian a.	a. subclavia	brachiocephalic trunk (right), arch of aorta (left)	vertebral, internal thoracic a's, thyrocervical and costocervical trunks	neck, thoracic wall, spinal cord, brain, meninges, upper limb
subcostal a.	a. subcostalis	thoracic aorta	dorsal and spinal branches	upper abdominal wall
sublingual a.	a. sublingualis	lingual a.		sublingual gland, side of tongue, floor of mouth
submental a.	a. submentalis	facial a.		tissues under chin
subscapular a.	a. subscapularis	axillary a.	thoracodorsal and circumflex scapular a's	scapular region
supraorbital a.	a. supraorbitalis	ophthalmic a.		forehead, superior muscles of orbit, upper eyelid, frontal sinus
suprarenal a., inferior	a. suprarenalis inferior	renal a.		suprarenal gland
suprarenal a., middle	a. suprarenalis media	abdominal aorta		suprarenal gland
suprarenal a's, superior	aa. suprarenales superiores	inferior phrenic a.		suprarenal gland

suprascapular a.	a. suprascapularis	thyrocervical trunk	acromial branch	clavicle and scapula, shoulder joint, muscles
supratrochlear a.	a. supratrochlearis	ophthalmic a.		anterior part of scalp
sural a's	aa. surales	popliteal a.		muscles of popliteal fossa and calf, adjacent skin
sylvian a. see *cerebral a., middle*				
tarsal a., lateral	a. tarsea lateralis	dorsalis pedis a.		muscles and joints of tarsus
tarsal a's, medial	aa. tarseae mediales	dorsalis pedis a.		skin and joints of medial aspect of foot
temporal a's, deep	aa. temporales profundae	maxillary a.		temporal muscle, pericranium, subjacent bone
temporal a., middle	a. temporalis media	superficial temporal a.		temporal muscle
temporal a., superficial	a. temporalis superficialis	external carotid a.	parotid, anterior auricular, frontal and parietal branches; transverse facial, zygomatico-orbital, middle temporal a's	parotid gland, auricle, scalp, skin of face, masseter muscle
testicular a.	a. testicularis	abdominal aorta	ureteric branches	ureter, epididymis, testis
thoracic a., highest	a. thoracica suprema	axillary a.		intercostal, serratus anterior, pectoralis major and minor muscles
thoracic a., internal	a. thoracica interna	subclavian a.	mediastinal, thymic, bronchial, sternal, perforating, lateral costal and anterior intercostal branches; pericardiacophrenic, musculophrenic, superior epigastric a's	anterior thoracic wall, mediastinal structures, diaphragm
thoracic a., lateral	a. thoracica lateralis	axillary a.	mammary branches	pectoral muscles, mammary gland
thoracoacromial a.	a. thoracoacromialis	axillary a.	clavicular, pectoral, deltoid and acromial branches	pectoral, deltoid, subclavian muscles, acromion
thoracodorsal a.	a. thoracodorsalis	subscapular a.		subscapular and teres major and minor muscles
thyrocervical trunk	truncus thyrocervicalis	subclavian a.	inferior thyroid, suprascapular and transverse cervical a's	deep neck, including thyroid gland, scapular region
thyroid a., inferior	a. thyroidea inferior	thyrocervical trunk	pharyngeal, esophageal, tracheal and glandular branches; inferior laryngeal, ascending cervical a's	larynx, esophagus, trachea, neck muscles, thyroid gland
thyroid a., lowest. see *thyroidea ima a.*				

COMMON NAME*	NA EQUIVALENT†	ORIGIN*	BRANCHES*	DISTRIBUTION
thyroid a., superior	a. thyroidea superior	external carotid a.	hyoid, sternocleidomastoid, superior laryngeal, cricothyroid muscular and glandular branches	hyoid muscles, larynx, thyroid gland, pharynx
thyroidea ima a.	a. thyroidea ima	arch of aorta, brachiocephalic trunk or right common carotid a.		thyroid gland
tibial a., anterior	a. tibialis anterior	popliteal a.	posterior and anterior tibial recurrent a's, lateral and medial anterior malleolar a's, lateral and medial malleolar rete	leg, ankle, foot
tibial a., posterior	a. tibialis	popliteal a.	fibular circumflex branch; peroneal, medial plantar, lateral plantar a's	leg, foot, including heel
transverse a. of face. see *facial a., transverse*				
transverse a. of neck. see *cervical a., transverse*				
transverse a. of scapula. see *suprascapular a.*				
tympanic a., anterior	a. tympanica anterior	maxillary a.		lining membrane of tympanic cavity
tympanic a., inferior	a. tympanica inferior	ascending pharyngeal a.		medial wall of tympanic cavity
tympanic a., posterior	a. tympanica posterior	stylomastoid a.		posterior part of tympanic membrane, secondary tympanic membrane
tympanic a., superior	a. tympanica superior	middle meningeal a.		tensor tympani muscle lining membrane of meatus
ulnar a.	a. ulnaris	brachial a.	palmar carpal, dorsal carpal and deep palmar branches; ulnar recurrent and common interosseous a's; superficial palmar arch	membrane of meatus forearm, wrist, hand

68

Term	Latin	Origin	Branches	Distribution
ulnar a., collateral, inferior. see *collateral a., ulnar, inferior*				
ulnar a., collateral, superior. see *collateral a., ulnar, superior*				
umbilical a.	a. umbilicalis	internal iliac a.	a. of ductus deferens, superior vesical a's	
urethral a.	a. urethralis	internal pudendal a.		ductus deferens, seminal vesicles, testes, urinary bladder, ureter urethra
uterine a.	a. uterina	internal iliac a.	ovarian and tubal branches; vaginal a.	uterus, vagina, round ligament of uterus, uterine tube, ovary
vaginal a.	a. vaginalis	uterine a.		vagina, fundus of bladder
vertebral a.	a. vertebralis	subclavian a.	spinal and meningeal branches; posterior inferior cerebellar, basilar, anterior and posterior spinal a's	muscles of neck, vertebrae, spinal cord, cerebellum, cerebrum
vesical a., inferior	a. vesicalis inferior	internal iliac a.		bladder, prostate, seminal vesicles
vesical a's, superior	aa. vesicales superiores	umbilical a.		bladder, urachus, ureter
zygomatico-orbital a.	a. zygomaticoorbitalis	superficial temporal a.		orbicularis oculi muscle

Arthrobacter (ar″thro-bak′ter) a genus of Schizomycetes (order Eubacteriales, family Corynebacteriaceae) found in the soil.

arthrocace (ar-throk′ah-se) ulceration of a joint or joints.

arthrocele (ar′thro-sēl) a joint swelling.

arthrocentesis (ar″thro-sen-te′sis) puncture of a joint cavity with aspiration of fluid.

arthrochalasis (-kal′ah-sis) abnormal relaxation or flaccidity of a joint. **a. mul′tiplex congen′ita,** overflaccidity of multiple joints, not associated with hyperelasticity of the skin.

arthrochondritis (-kon-dri′tis) inflammation of cartilages of a joint.

arthroclasia (-kla′ze-ah) manipulation of a joint.

arthrodesis (-de′sis) surgical fusion of a joint.

arthrodia (ar-thro′de-ah) a synovial joint which allows a gliding motion.

arthrodynia (-din′e-ah) arthralgia.

arthrodysplasia (-dis-pla′ze-ah) any abnormality of joint development.

arthroempyesis (-em″pi-e′sis) suppuration within a joint.

arthroendoscopy (-en-dos′ko-pe) inspection of the interior of a joint with an endoscope.

arthrography (ar-throg′rah-fe) radiography of a joint. **air a.,** pneumoarthrography.

arthrogryposis (ar″thro-grī-po′sis) 1. persistent flexure of a joint. 2. tetanoid spasm.

arthrokleisis (-kli′sis) ankylosis.

arthrolith (ar′thro-lith) calculous deposit within a joint.

arthrology (ar-throl′o-je) scientific study or description of the joints.

arthrolysis (ar-throl′ĭ-sis) mobilization of an ankylosed joint.

arthrometer (ar-throm′ē-ter) instrument for measuring the angles of movements of joints.

Arthromitaceae (ar″thro-mi-ta′se-e) a family of Schizomycetes (order Caryophanales) found in the intestinal tract of insects and crustaceans.

Arthromitus (ar″throm-ī′tus) a genus of Schizomycetes (order Caryophanales, family Arthromitaceae).

arthroneuralgia (ar″thro-nu-ral′je-ah) neuralgia of a joint.

arthronosos (-no′sos) any disease of a joint.

arthropathy (ar-throp′ah-the) any joint disease. **Charcot's a., neurogenic a.,** osteoarthritis with joint enlargement due to trophic disturbance, affecting ankle, knee, hip, spine or hand. **osteopulmonary a.,** clubbing of fingers and toes, and enlargement of ends of the long bones, in cardiac or pulmonary disease.

arthrophyma (ar″thro-fi′mah) a joint swelling.

arthrophyte (ar′thro-fīt) abnormal growth in a joint cavity.

arthroplasty (ar′thro-plas″te) plastic repair of a joint.

arthropod (ar′thro-pod) an individual of the phylum Arthropoda.

Arthropoda (ar-throp′o-dah) a phylum of the animal kingdom including bilaterally symmetrical animals with segmented bodies bearing jointed appendages; embracing the largest number of known animals, with at least 740,000 species, divided into 12 classes.

arthropyosis (ar″thro-pi-o′sis) formation of pus in a joint cavity.

arthrosclerosis (-skle-ro′sis) stiffening or hardening of the joints.

arthrosis (ar-thro′sis) 1. an articulation. 2. disease of a joint.

arthrosteitis (ar″thros-te-i′tis) inflammation of the bony structures of a joint.

arthrostomy (ar-thros′to-me) incision of a joint with drainage.

arthrosynovitis (ar″thro-sin″o-vi′tis) inflammation of the synovial membrane of a joint.

arthrotomy (ar-throt′o-mc) incision of a joint.

arthroxesis (ar-throk′se-sis) scraping of joints.

artiad (ar′te-ad) an element of an even-numbered valency.

articular (ar-tik′u-lar) pertaining to a joint.

articulare (ar-tik″u-la′re) the point of intersection of the dorsal contours of the articular process of the mandible and the temporal bone.

articulate (ar-tik′u-lāt) 1. to unite by joints; to join. 2. united by joints. 3. capable of expressing one's self orally.

articulatio (ar-tik′u-la′she-o), pl. *articulatio′-nes* [L.] an articulation or joint.

articulation (-la′shun) 1. the place of union or junction between two or more bones of the skeleton. 2. enunciation of words and sentences.

articulator (ar-tik′u-la″tor) a device for effecting a jointlike union. **dental a.,** a device which simulates movements of the temporo-mandibular joints or mandible, used in dentistry.

articulo (ar-tik′u-lo) [L., *articulus*] at the moment, or crisis. **a. mor′tis,** at the point or moment of death.

artifact (ar′tĭ-fakt) a structure or appearance that is not natural, but is due to manipulation (man-made).

aryl (ar′il) prefix, *a radical belonging to the aromatic series.*

arytenoid (ar″ĭ-te′noid) shaped like a jug or pitcher.

arytenoidectomy (ar″ĭ-te-noid-ek′to-me) excision of an arytenoid cartilage.

arytenoiditis (-i′tis) inflammation of arytenoid muscle or cartilage.

arytenoidopexy (ar″ĭ-te-noi′do-pek″se) surgical fixation of arytenoid cartilage or muscle.

As chemical symbol, arsenic

As. astigmatism.

A.S. [L.] *au′ris sinis′tra* (left ear).

ASA acetylsalicylic acid (aspirin).

A.S.A. American Society of Anesthesiologists; American Standards Association; American Stomatological Association; American Surgical Association.

A.S.A.I.O. American Society for Artificial Internal Organs.

A.S.B. American Society of Bacteriologists.

asbestiform (as-bes′tĭ-form) resembling asbestos.

asbestos (as-bes′tos) fibrous magnesium and calcium silicate.

asbestosis (as″bes-to′sis) a lung disease due to asbestos fibers.

ascariasis (as″kah-ri′ah-sis) infection with Ascaris.

ascaricide (as-kar′ĭ-sīd) a drug destructive to ascarids. adj., **ascarici′dal.**

ascarid (as′kah-rid) an organism (worm) of the genus Ascaris.

Ascaris (as′kah-ris) a genus of nematode parasites found in the intestines of man and other vertebrates. **A. lumbricoi′des,** a species widely distributed about the world. **A. su′is,** a species morphologically similar to *A. lumbricoides,* but commonly found in pigs.

ascaris (as′kah-ris), pl. *ascar′ides* [L.] an ascarid.

Ascarops (as′kah-rops) a genus of parasitic worms. **A. strongyli′na,** a thick, nonbursate stomach worm parasitic in swine.

A.S.C.H. American Society of Clinical Hypnosis.

A.S.C.I. American Society for Clinical Investigation.

ascites (ah-si′tēz) abnormal accumulation of fluid in the peritoneal cavity. adj., **ascit′ic. chylous a.,** presence of milky fluid containing globules of fat in peritoneal cavity owing to rupture of the thoracic duct or to extravasation through its wall.

A.S.C.L.T. American Society of Clinical Laboratory Technicians.

Ascomycetes (as″ko-mi-se′tēz) a genus of fungi.

ascorbate (as-kor′bāt) a derivative of ascorbic acid.

ascospore (as′ko-spōr) a spore contained or produced in an ascus.

A.S.C.P. American Society of Clinical Pathologists.

ascus (as′kus) the spore case of certain fungi.

-ase (ās) suffix used in forming the name of an enzyme, affixed to the name of the substrate (luciferase) or to a term indicating the general nature of the substrate (proteinase), the type of reaction effected (hydrolase) or a combination of these (transaminase).

asemasia (as″e-ma′ze-ah) loss of the power of communication by words, gestures or signals.

asemia (ah-se′me-ah) inability to make or comprehend signs or tokens of communication.

asepsis (a-sep′sis) absence of septic matter; freedom from infection or infectious material. adj., **asep′tic.**

asepticize (a-sep′tĭ-sīz) to free from pathogenic material.

asexual (a-seks′u-al) without sex; not pertaining to sex.

asexualization (a-seks″u-al-i-za′shun) castration.

A.S.G. American Society for Genetics.

A.S.H. American Society of Hematology.

A.S.H.A. American School Health Association; American Speech and Hearing Association.

A.S.H.I. Association for the Study of Human Infertility.

A.S.H.P. American Society of Hospital Pharmacists.

asialia (ah″si-a′le-ah) aptyalism.

asiderosis (ah″sid-er-o′sis) deficiency of iron reserve of the body.

A.S.I.I. American Science Information Institute.

A.S.I.M. American Society of Internal Medicine.

-asis, word element, *state; condition.*

asitia (ah-sish′e-ah) loathing of food.

asonia (ah-so′ne-ah) tone deafness.

A.S.P. American Society of Parasitologists.

aspect (as′pekt) 1. that part of a surface viewed from a particular direction. 2. the look or appearance. **dorsal a.,** that surface of a body viewed from the back or from above. **ventral a.,** that surface of a body viewed from the front or from below.

aspergilloma (as″per-jil-lo′mah) a tumor-like mass formed by growth of the fungus, frequently observed in the lungs in aspergillosis.

aspergillosis (-lo′sis) infection caused by Aspergillus.

Aspergillus (as″per-jil′us) a genus of fungi (molds), several species of which are endoparasitic and probably pathogenic. **A. fumiga′tus,** a species causing a respiratory disease in young ducklings.

aspermia (ah-sper′me-ah) absence of seminal fluid or spermatozoa.

asphalgesia (as″fal-je′ze-ah) a burning sensation felt on touching certain articles.

asphyxia (as-fik′se-ah) apparent or actual cessation of life due to interruption of effective gaseous exchange in the lungs. adj., **asphyx′ial. a. carbon′ica,** suffocation from the inhalation of coal gas or water gas. **fetal a.,** a prenatal condition due to deprivation in the fetus of oxygen. **a. liv′ida,** asphyxia in which the skin is cyanotic. **local a.,** acroasphyxia. **a. neonato′rum,** failure of supply or utilization of oxygen in the newborn infant. **traumatic a.,** discoloration of the head and neck as a result of sudden or severe compression of the trunk.

asphyxiate (as-fik′se-āt) to deprive of oxygen for utilization by the tissues.

aspidium (as-pid′e-um) the dried rhizome and stipes of a genus of plants known as male fern.

aspirate (as′pĭ-rāt) to withdraw fluid by negative pressure, or suction.

aspiration (as″pĭ-ra′shun) withdrawal of fluid by the aspirator.

aspirator (as″pĭ-ra′tor) an instrument for evacuating fluid by suction.

aspirin (as′pĭ-rin) a white crystalline compound, $C_9H_8O_4$; analgesic, antipyretic and antirheumatic. **aluminum a.,** combination of aspirin and aluminum oxide; analgesic and antipyretic.

asplenia (ah-sple′ne-ah) absence of the spleen.

asporogenic (as″po-ro-jen′ik) not producing spores.

asporous (as-spo′rus) having no true spores.

A.S.R.T. American Society of Radiologic Technologists.

assay (as-sa′) 1. to examine or analyze. 2. an analysis. **biological a.,** determination of the potency of a drug or other substance by comparing the effects it has on animals with those of a reference standard. **microbiological a.**, the assay of nutrient or other substances by their effect on living microorganisms.

assimilation (ah-sim″ĭ-la′shun) 1. conversion of absorbed material into the substance of the absorbing body. 2. psychologically, absorption of new experiences into existing psychologic make-up.

association (ah-so″se-a′shun) 1. close relation in time or space. 2. in psychiatry, the continuing development and expansion of ideas. **a. center,** center of cerebral cortex not itself functionally differentiated, but connected with other centers by association fibers or tracts. **clang a.,** association of words or ideas because of similarity in sound. **free a.,** oral expression of one's ideas as they arrive spontaneously; a method used in psychoanalysis.

assortment (ah-sort′ment) the genetic consequence of the random distribution of nonhomologous chromosomes to daughter cells in meiosis.

A.S.S.S. American Society for the Study of Sterility.

astasia (as-ta′zhe-ah) motor incoordination with inability to stand. adj., **astat′ic. a.-aba′-sia,** hysterical inability or refusal to stand or walk because of fear of falling.

astatine (as′tah-tēn) chemical element (see table), at. no. 85, symbol At.

asteatosis (as″te-ah-to′sis) deficiency or absence of sebaceous secretion.

aster (as′ter) a cluster of raylike filaments extending from each daughter centriole at the beginning of division of the nucleus of a cell.

astereognosis (ah-ster″e-og-no′sis) inability to recognize familiar objects by feeling their shape.

asterion (as-te′re-on) the junction of occipital, parietal and temporal bones.

asterixis (as″ter-ik′sis) a motor disturbance marked by intermittency of sustained contraction of groups of muscles; called *liver flap* because of its occurrence in coma associated with liver disease, but observed also in other conditions.

asternal (a-ster′nal) not joined to the sternum.

asternia (ah-ster′ne-ah) developmental anomaly with absence of the sternum.

asteroid (as′ter-oid) star-shaped.

Asterol (as′ter-ol) trademark for preparations of diamthazole.

asthen(o)- word element, *weak; weakness.*

asthenia (as-the′ne-ah) debility; loss of strength. adj., **asthen′ic. neurocirculatory a.,** a neurosis characterized by easy fatigability, breathlessness, and pain in the region of the heart. **tropical anhidrotic a.,** a condition due to generalized anhidrosis in conditions of high temperature, characterized by a tendency to overfatigability, irritability, anorexia, inability to concentrate, and drowsiness, with headache and vertigo.

asthenocoria (as″thě-no-ko′re-ah) sluggishness of the pupillary light reflex.

asthenometer (as″thě-nom′ě-ter) device used in measuring muscular asthenia.

asthenope (as′thě-nōp) a person with asthenopia.

asthenopia (as″thě-no′pe-ah) impairment of vision, with pain in eyes, back of head, and neck. adj., **asthenop′ic. accommodative a.,** asthenopia due to strain of ciliary muscle. **muscular a.,** asthenopia due to weakness of external ocular muscles.

asthenospermia (as″thě-no-sper′me-ah) reduced motility of spermatozoa in the semen.

asthma (az′mah) a term applied loosely to a condition of difficult breathing; used specifically to designate a condition in which episodes of bronchospasm in a patient with a personal or family history of allergy alternate with symptom-free periods. adj., **asthmat′-ic. cardiac a.,** a term applied to breathing difficulties due to pulmonary edema in heart disease. **Heberden's a.,** angina pectoris. **thymic a.,** laryngismus stridulus.

astigmatism (ah-stig′mah-tizm) ametropia caused by differences in curvature in different meridians of the refractive surfaces of the eye. adj., **astigmat′ic. compound a.,** that in which the two principal meridians are both hyperopic (*compound hyperopic astigmatism*) or myopic (*compound myopic astigmatism*), but in varying degrees. **corneal a.,** that due to the presence of toric curvatures on the anterior or posterior surface of the cornea. **hyperopic a.,** that in which the light rays are brought to a focus behind the retina. **irregular a.,** that in which the refraction varies even in one principal meridian, making correction by lenses impossible. **lenticular a.,** astigmatism due to defect of the crystalline lens. **mixed a.,** that in which one principal meridian is hyperopic and the other myopic. **myopic a.,** that in which the light rays are brought to a focus in front of the retina. **regular a.,** that in which the refraction changes gradually in power from one principal meridian of the eye to the other, the two meridians always being at right angles; the condition is further classified as being *against the rule* when the meridian of greatest refractive power tends toward the horizontal, *with the rule* when it tends toward the vertical, and *oblique* when it lies 45 degrees from the horizontal and vertical.

astigmia (ah-stig′me-ah) astigmatism.

astigmometer (as″tig-mom′ě-ter) apparatus used in measuring astigmatism.

A.S.T.M.H. American Society of Tropical Medicine and Hygiene.

astomia (ah-sto′me-ah) congenital atresia of the mouth. adj., **asto′matous.**

astomus (ah-sto′mus) a fetal monster exhibiting astomia.

ASTRA Applied Space Technology–Regional Advancement, an information service sponsored by NASA and conducted by the Midwest Research Institute.

astragalectomy (ah-strag″ah-lek′to-me) excision of the astragalus.

astragalus (ah-strag'ah-lus) talus. adj., **astrag'alar.**

astraphobia (as"trah-fo'be-ah) morbid fear of lightning.

astringent (ah-strin'jent) 1. causing contraction and arresting discharges. 2. an agent that arrests discharges.

astroblast (as'tro-blast) a cell that develops into an astrocyte.

astroblastoma (as"tro-blas-to'mah) a rare, malignant tumor of the nervous system.

astrocyte (as'tro-sīt) 1. a star-shaped cell of the neuroglia. 2. a bone corpuscle.

astrocytoma (as"tro-si-to'mah) a tumor of the central nervous system, usually slowly growing, consisting of astrocytes.

astroglia (as-trog'le-ah) neuroglia tissue made up of astrocytes.

astronaut (as'tro-nawt) a traveler in outer space.

astrosphere (as'tro-sfer) a structure made up of a group of radiating fibrillae which converge toward the centrosome and continue in the centrosphere of a cell.

asymbolia (ah"sim-bo'le-ah) loss of ability to understand symbols, as words, figures, gestures, signs. **pain a.,** absence of the usual psychologic reaction to pain.

asymphytous (ah-sim'fī-tus) separate or distinct; not grown together.

asymptomatic (a"simp-to-mat'ik) showing no symptoms.

asynchronism (a-sin'kro-nizm) occurrence at different times.

asynclitism (ah-sin'klī-tizm) oblique presentation of the head in parturition.

asyndesis (ah-sin'dē-sis) disorder of thinking in which related elements of a thought cannot be welded together in a whole.

asynechia (ah"sī-nek'e-ah) absence of continuity of structure.

asynergia (a"sin-er'je-ah) failure of cooperation among muscle groups that is necessary for execution of movement.

asynesia (ah"sī-ne'ze-ah) dullness of intellect.

asynovia (ah"sī-no've-ah) absence or insufficiency of synovia.

asyntaxia (a"sin-tak'se-ah) lack of proper and orderly embryonic development.

asystole (a-sis'to-le) imperfect or incomplete systole. adj., **asystol'ic.**

At chemical symbol, *astatine.*

at. atmosphere; atomic.

Atabrine (at'ah-brin, at'ah-brēn) trademark for quinacrine.

atactic (ah-tak'tik) pertaining to or characterized by ataxia; marked by incoordination or irregularity.

atactiform (ah-tak'tī-form) resembling ataxia.

atactilia (ah"tak-til'e-ah) loss of the sense of touch.

ataractic (at"ah-rak'tik) 1. pertaining to or characterized by ataraxia. 2. an agent that induces ataraxia.

ataralgesia (at"ar-al-je'ze-ah) combined sedation and analgesia intended to abolish mental distress and pain attendant on surgical procedures.

Atarax (at'ah-raks) trademark for preparations of hydroxyzine hydrochloride.

ataraxia (at"ah-rak'se-ah) a state of detached serenity without depression of mental faculties or impairment of consciousness.

ataraxic (-rak'sik) ataractic.

atavism (at'ah-vizm) inheritance of characters from remote ancestors. adj., **atavis'tic.**

ataxaphasia (ah-tak"sah-fa'ze-ah) ability to utter words, but not sentences.

ataxia (ah-tak'se-ah) incoordination occurring in the absence of apraxia, paresis, rigidity, spasticity or involuntary movement. adj., **atac'tic, atax'ic. Friedreich's a., hereditary a.,** the spinal form of hereditary sclerosis. **locomotor a.,** tabes dorsalis. **a.-telangiectasia,** a heredofamilial, progressive ataxia, associated with oculocutaneous telangiectasia, sinopulmonary disease with frequent respiratory infections and abnormal eye movements.

ataxiamnesic (ah-tak"se-am-ne'sik) characterized by ataxia and amnesia.

ataxophemia (ah-tak"so-fe'me-ah) lack of coordination of speech muscles.

ataxy (ah-tak'se) ataxia.

atel(o)- (at'e-lo) word element [Gr.], *incomplete, imperfectly developed.*

atelectasis (at"ē-lek'tah-sis) incomplete expansion or collapse of pulmonary alveoli, or of a segment, lobe or lobes of a lung. adj., **atelectat'ic. acquired a.,** compression or collapse of previously expanded pulmonary alveoli attending some underlying disease of the lungs. **congenital a.,** that present at *(primary atelectasis)* or immediately after birth *(secondary atelectasis).* **primary a.,** that in which the alveoli have never been expanded with air. **secondary a.,** that in which resorption of the contained air has led to collapse of the alveoli.

atelia (ah-te'le-ah) incompleteness; imperfection due to failure to develop completely. adj., **ateliot'ic.**

ateliosis (ah-te"le-o'sis) a condition characterized by failure to develop completely. adj., **ateliot'ic.**

atelocardia (at"ē-lo kar'de-ah) imperfect development of the heart.

atelocephalous (-sef'ah-lus) having an incomplete skull.

atelocephaly (-sef'ah-le) imperfect development of the skull. adj., **atelocephal'ic.**

atelocheilia (-ki'le-ah) imperfect development of the lip.

ateloglossia (-glos'e-ah) imperfect development of the tongue.

atelomyelia (-mi-e'le-ah) imperfect development of the spinal cord.

atelorhachidia (-rah-kid'e-ah) imperfect development of the vertebral column.

atelostomia (-sto'me-ah) imperfect development of the mouth.

athelia (ah-the'le-ah) congenital absence of the nipples.

athermic (ah-ther'mik) without rise of temperature.

athermosystaltic (ah-ther″mo-sis-tal′tik) not contracting under the action of cold or heat.

atherogenesis (ath″er-o-jen′ĕ-sis) formation of atheromatous lesions in arterial walls. adj., **atherogen′ic.**

atheroma (ath″er-o′mah) an abnormal mass of fatty or lipid material, as a sebaceous cyst or a discrete deposit in an arterial wall. adj., **atherom′atous.**

atheromatosis (ath″er-o-mah-to′sis) the presence of multiple atheromas.

atheronecrosis (-ne-kro′sis) necrosis accompanying atherosclerosis.

atherosclerosis (-skle-ro′sis) a condition characterized by degeneration and hardening of the walls of arteries and sometimes valves of the heart.

atherosis (ath″er-o′sis) atheromatosis.

athetoid (ath′ĕ-toid) 1. resembling athetosis. 2. affected with athetosis.

athetosis (ath″ĕ-to′sis) repetitive involuntary, slow, gross movements.

Athiorhodaceae (ah-thi″o-ro-da′se-e) a family of Schizomycetes (order Pseudomonadales, suborder Rhodobacteriineae) including two genera, Rhodopseudomonas and Rhodospirillum.

athrepsia (ah-threp′se-ah) marasmus. adj., **athrep′tic.**

athrombia (ah-throm′be-ah) defective clotting of the blood.

athymia (ah-thi′me-ah) 1. dementia. 2. absence of functioning thymus tissue.

athymism (ah-thi′mizm) the condition induced by removal of the thymus.

athyreosis (ah-thi″re-o′sis) athyria. adj., **athyreot′ic.**

athyria (ah-thi′re-ah) absence of functioning thyroid tissue.

atlantad (at-lan′tad) toward the atlas.

atlantal (at-lan′tal) pertaining to the atlas.

atlas (at′las) the uppermost segment of the backbone.

atloaxoid (at″lo-ak′soid) pertaining to atlas and axis.

atlodymus (at-lod′ĭ-mus) a fetal monster with two heads and one body.

atmiatrics (at″me-at′riks) treatment by medicated vapors.

atmocausis (at″mo-kaw′sis) treatment by superheated steam.

atmos (at′mos) a unit of air pressure, being the pressure of 760 mm. of mercury on one square centimeter.

atmosphere (at′mos-fēr) 1. the entire gaseous envelope surrounding the earth, extending to an altitude of 10 miles and including the troposphere, tropopause and stratosphere. 2. a unit of pressure, equivalent to that on a surface at sea level, being about 15 pounds per square inch, or equivalent to that of a column of mercury 760 mm. high. adj., **atmospher′ic.**

at. no. atomic number.

atocia (ah-to′se-ah) sterility in the female.

atom (at′om) an ultimate particle of a chemical element. adj., **atom′ic.**

atomization (at″om-ī-za′shun) dispersal of a bulk of liquid in a fine spray.

atomizer (at′om-īz″er) an instrument for dispensing liquid in a fine spray.

atonia (ah-to′ne-ah) atony.

atony (at′o-ne) absence or lack of normal tone. adj., **aton′ic.**

atopen (at′o-pen) an allergen.

atopic (ah-top′ik) 1. displaced. 2. pertaining to allergy.

atopognosia (ah-top″og-no′ze-ah) inability to correctly locate a sensation.

atopy (at′o-pe) hypersensitivity due to hereditary influences.

atoxic (ah-tok′sik) not poisonous; not due to a poison.

atoxigenic (a-tok″sī-jen′ik) not producing or elaborating toxins.

ATP adenosine triphosphate.

atraumatic (a″traw-mat′ik) not producing injury or damage.

atresia (ah-tre′zhe-ah) absence of a normal opening. adj., **atret′ic. aortic a.,** absence of the opening from the left ventricle of the heart into the aorta. **follicular a., a. follic′uli,** absence of an opening in an ovarian follicle which retains a blighted ovum. **tricuspid a.,** absence of the opening between the right atrium and right ventricle.

atria (a′tre-ah) plural of *atrium.*

atrichia (ah-trik′e-ah) absence of hair.

atrichosis (at″rī-ko′sis) complete congenital lack of hair.

atrichous (ah-trik′us) 1. having no hair. 2. having no flagella.

atriomegaly (a″tre-o-meg′ah-le) abnormal enlargement of an atrium of the heart.

atrionector (-nek′tor) the sinoatrial node.

atrioseptopexy (-sep″to-pek″se) surgical correction of a defect in the interatrial septum.

atrioseptoplasty (-sep′to-plas″te) plastic repair of the interatrial septum.

atrioventricular (-ven-trik′u-lar) pertaining to the atrium and ventricle.

atrium (a′tre-um), pl. *a′tria* [L.] an external chamber, or entrance hall, especially the upper chamber *(a′trium cor′dis)* on either side of the heart, transmitting to the ventricle of the same side blood received *(left a′trium)* from the pulmonary veins and *(right a′trium)* from the venae cavae. adj., **a′trial.**

atrophia (ah-tro′fe-ah) [L.] atrophy.

atrophoderma (at″ro-fo-der′mah) atrophy of the skin.

atrophy (at′ro-fe) decrease in size of a normally developed organ or tissue; wasting. adj., **atroph′ic. acute yellow a.,** atrophy and yellow discoloration of liver, with jaundice. **Aran-Duchenne a.,** myelopathic muscular atrophy. **bone a.,** resorption of bone evident in both external form and internal density. **disuse a.,** atrophy of a tissue or organ as a result of its inactivity or diminished function. **Duchenne-Aran a.,** myelopathic muscular atrophy. **eccentric a.,** atrophy with dilatation of the organ. **Fuchs's a.,** peripheral atrophy of the optic nerve. **Leber's a.,** hereditary atrophy of the optic nerve. **myelopathic muscular a.,**

progressive muscular wasting due to degeneration of cells of the anterior horns of the spinal cord, beginning usually in the small muscles of the hands, but in some cases (scapulohumeral type) in those of the upper arm and shoulder, and progressing slowly to the muscles of the lower extremity. **pathologic a.**, decrease in size of an organ or tissue beyond the range of normal variability. **physiologic a.**, that occurring as part of the normal aging process. **progressive neuromuscular a.**, **progressive neuropathic (peroneal) muscular a.**, muscular atrophy due to degeneration of the cells of the posterior columns of the spinal cord and of the peripheral nerves, beginning in the muscles supplied by the peroneal nerves, and progressing slowly to involve the muscles of the hands and arms.

atropine (at'ro-pēn) a parasympatholytic alkaloid obtained from plants or produced synthetically. **a. sulfate**, a soluble compound of atropine, with similar uses.

A.T.S. American Thoracic Society; American Trudeau Society; antitetanus serum.

attack (ah-tak') an episode or the onset of illness. **vagal a.**, a sinking sensation with dyspnea, attributed to vasomotor spasm.

attic (at'ik) part of the cavity of the middle ear, just above the tympanic canal of the facial nerve.

atticoantrotomy (at"tĭ-ko-an-trot'o-me) surgical exposure of the attic and mastoid antrum.

atticotomy (at"ĭ-kot'o-me) incision into the attic.

attitude (at'ĭ-tūd) 1. a posture or position of the body; in obstetrics, the position of the child in the uterus. 2. a pattern of mental views established by cumulative prior experience.

atto- word element designating an amount 10^{-18} the size of the unit to which it is joined; symbol a.

attraction (ah-trak'shun) the force or influence by which one object is drawn toward another. **capillary a.**, the force which causes a liquid to rise in a fine-caliber tube.

at. wt. atomic weight.

atypia (a-tip'e-ah) deviation from the normal or typical state.

Au chemical symbol, *gold* (L. *aurum*).

A.U. 1. Angstrom unit. 2. (L. *aures unitas*), both ears together; (L. *auris uterque*), each ear.

audi(o)- word element, *hearing.*

audile (aw'dil) pertaining to hearing.

audioanalgesia (aw"de-o-an"al-je'ze-ah) reduction or abolition of pain by listening to recorded music to which has been added a background of white sound.

audiogenic (-jen'ik) produced by sound.

audiogram (aw'de-o-gram") a graphic record of the findings by audiometry.

audiologist (aw"de-ol'o-jist) an expert in audiology.

audiology (-ol'o-je) the science concerned with the sense of hearing.

audiometer (-om'ĕ-ter) apparatus used in audiometry.

audiometrician (aw"de-o-mĕ-trish'an) a specialist in audiometry.

audiometry (aw"de-om'ĕ-tre) measurement of the acuity of hearing for the various frequencies of sound waves.

audiosurgery (aw"de-o-ser'jer-e) surgery of the ear.

audition (aw-dish'un) perception of sound; hearing. **chromatic a.**, chromesthesia.

auditory (aw'dĭ-to"re) pertaining to the ear or the sense of hearing.

augnathus (awg-nath'us) a fetal monster with double lower jaw.

aula (aw'lah) forward part of third ventricle.

aura (aw'rah) a peculiar sensation forerunning the appearance of more definite symptoms. **epileptic a.**, a peculiar sensation preceding an attack of epilepsy.

aural (aw'ral) 1. pertaining to the ear. 2. pertaining to an aura.

aurantiasis (aw"ran-ti'ah-sis) yellowness of skin caused by intake of large amounts of food containing carotene.

Aureomycin (aw"re-o-mi'sin) trademark for chlortetracycline.

auriasis (aw-ri'ah-sis) chrysiasis.

auric (aw'rik) pertaining to gold.

auricle (aw'rĭ-kl) 1. the flap of the ear. 2. the ear-shaped appendage of either atrium of the heart, sometimes incorrectly used to designate the entire atrium.

auricula (aw-rik'u-lah), pl. *auric'ulae* [L.] auricle.

auricular (aw-rik'u-lar) pertaining to an auricle or ear.

auriculare (aw-rik"u-la're) a point at the top of the opening of the external auditory meatus.

auricularis (aw-rik"u-la'ris) [L.] pertaining to the ear.

auriculotemporal (aw-rik"u-lo-tem'po-ral) pertaining to the ear and the temporal bone.

auriculoventricular (-ven-trik'u-lar) atrioventricular.

auripuncture (aw'rĭ-punk"chūr) puncture of membrana tympani.

auris (aw'ris), pl. *au'res* [L.] ear.

auriscope (aw'rĭ-skōp) instrument for examining the ear.

auristillae (aw"ris-til'e), pl. of *auristil'la* [L.] ear drops.

aurotherapy (aw"ro-ther'ah-pe) use of gold salts in treatment of disease.

aurothioglucose (-thi"o-gloo'kōs) a gold preparation used in treating rheumatoid arthritis.

aurothioglycanide (-thi"o-gli'kah-nīd) a gold preparation used in treating rheumatic arthritis.

aurothioglycolanilide (-thi"o-gli"kol-an'ĭ-līd) aurothioglycanide.

aurum (aw'rum) [L.] gold (symbol Au).

auscultate (aws-kult') auscultate.

auscultate (aws'kul-tāt) to examine by auscultation.

auscultation (aws"kul-ta'shun) listening to sounds produced within the body by various organs as they perform their functions. **direct a., immediate a.**, listening to sounds produced within the body with the unaided ear, without interposition of an instrument. **mediate a.**, that performed by use of an instrument to transmit the sound to the examiner's ear.

auscultatory (aws-kul'tah-to"re) pertaining to auscultation.

aut(o)- word element [Gr.], *self.*

autacoid (aw'tah-koid) an organic substance produced in one organ and carried by the blood to other organs, on which it acts like a drug; any internal secretion.

autarcesis (aw-tar'se-sis) normal ability of body cells to resist infection. adj., **autarcet'-ic.**

autism (aw'tizm) morbid self-absorption with extreme withdrawal and failure to relate to other persons. **early infantile a.**, an emotional illness characterized by early failure to relate emotionally to parents and others. adj., **autis'tic.**

autoagglutination (aw"to-ah-gloo"ti-na'shun) clumping together of a person's cells due to a substance present in his own serum.

autoagglutinin (-ah-gloo'ti-nin) a factor in serum capable of causing clumping together of the subject's own cellular elements.

autoamputation (-am"pu-ta'shun) spontaneous detachment from the body and elimination of an appendage or an abnormal growth, such as a polyp.

autoantibody (-an'ti-bod"e) an antibody or antibody-like factor supposedly directed against components native to the tissues of the organism in which it is found.

autoantigen (-an'ti-jen) a substance that stimulates production of antibody in the organism in which it occurs.

autoantitoxin (-an"ti-tok'sin) antitoxin produced by the body itself.

autocatalysis (-kah-tal'i-sis) 1. catalysis in which a product of the reaction hastens or intensifies the catalysis. 2. the process in mitosis by which a chromosome brings about the synthesis of an exact replica immediately beside itself.

autochthonous (aw-tok'tho-nus) originating in the same area in which it is found.

autocinesis (aw"to-si-ne'sis) autokinesis.

autoclasis (aw-tok'lah-sis) destruction of a part by influences within itself.

autoclave (aw'to-klāv) a self-locking apparatus for the sterilization of materials by steam under pressure.

autocytolysin (aw"to-si-tol'i-sin) autolysin.

autocytolysis (-si-tol'i-sis) autolysis.

autodigestion (-di-jes'chun) dissolution of tissue by its own secretions.

autodiploid (-dip'loid) 1. characterized by autodiploidy. 2. an individual or cell characterized by autodiploidy.

autodiploidy (-dip'loi-de) the state of having two sets of chromosomes as the result of doubling of the haploid set.

autoecholalia (-ek"o-la'le-ah) insane repetition of one's own words.

autoecic (aw-te'sik) living always upon the same organism.

autoeczematization (aw"to-ek-zem"ah-ti-za'-shun) the spread, at first locally and later more generally, of lesions from an originally circumscribed focus of eczema.

autoeroticism (-ē-rot'i-sizm) autoerotism.

autoerotism (-er'o-tizm) direction of a person's libido toward himself. adj., **autoerot'ic.**

autogamy (aw-tog'ah-me) 1. self-fertilization; fertilization by union of two chromatin masses derived from the same primary nucleus within a cell. 2. conjugation of closely related cells.

autogenesis (aw"to-jen'ě-sis) 1. spontaneous generation. 2. origination within the organism. adj., **autogenet'ic, autog'enous.**

autograft (aw'to-graft) a graft transferred from one part of the patient's body to another part.

autographism (aw-tog'rah-fizm) dermographia.

autohemagglutination (aw"to-hem"ah-gloo"-ti-na'shun) agglutination of erythrocytes by a factor produced in the subject's own body.

autohemagglutinin (-hem"ah-gloo'ti-nin) a substance produced in a person's body that causes agglutination of his own erythrocytes.

autohemolysin (-he-mol'i-sin) a hemolysin produced in the body of an animal which causes destruction of its own red blood corpuscles.

autohemolysis (-he-mol'i-sis) hemolysis of the blood corpuscles of an individual by his own serum.

autohemotherapy (-he"mo-ther'ah-pe) treatment by administration of the patient's own blood.

autohormonoclasis (-hor"mōn-ok'lah-sis) inactivation of the hormone of a gland in the presence of activity of the gland.

autohypnosis (-hip-no'sis) self-induced hypnotic state.

autoimmunization (-im"mu-ni-za'shun) production in an organism of reactivity to its own tissues.

autoinoculation (-in-ok"u-la'shun) inoculation with a virus from one's own body.

autointoxication (-in-tok"si-ka'shun) poisoning by uneliminated material (toxins) formed within the body.

autoisolysin (-i-sol'i-sin) a substance that lyses the corpuscles of the individual in which it is formed and also those of other individuals of the same species.

autokeratoplasty (-ker'ah-to-plas"te) corneal grafting with tissue from the other eye.

autokinesis (-ki-ne'sis) voluntary motion. adj., **autokinet'ic.**

autolesion (-le'zhun) a self-inflicted injury.

autologous (aw-tol'o-gus) related to self; belonging to the same organism.

autolysate (aw-tol'i-sāt) a specific substance produced by autolysis.

autolysin (aw-tol'i-sin) a lysin originating in an organism and capable of destroying its own cells and tissues.

autolysis (aw-tol'i-sis) the disintegration of cells or tissues by endogenous enzymes. adj., **autolyt'ic.**

automatic (aw″to-mat′ik) spontaneous; done involuntarily.

automatism (aw-tom′ah-tizm) mechanical, repetitive motor behavior performed unconsciously. **command a.**, uncritical response to commands, as in hypnosis and certain mental states.

automysophobia (aw″to-mi″so-fo′be-ah) morbid dread of personal uncleanness.

autonomic (-nom′ik) not subject to voluntary control.

autonomotropic (-nom″o-trop′ik) having an affinity for the autonomic nervous system.

autopathy (aw-top′ah-the) a disease without apparent external causation.

autopepsia (aw″to-pep′se-ah) digestion of stomach wall by its own secretion.

autophagy (aw-tof′ah-je) eating or biting of one's own flesh.

autophilia (aw″to-fil′e-ah) pathologic self-esteem; narcissism.

autophobia (-fo′be-ah) morbid dread of solitude.

autophonomania (-fo″no-ma′ne-ah) suicidal mania.

autophony (aw-tof′o-ne) the sensation of abnormal loudness of one's own voice.

autoplasmotherapy (aw″to-plaz″mo-ther′ah-pe) therapeutic injection of one's own blood plasma.

autoplastic (aw′to-plas″tik) pertaining to the indirect modification and adaptation of impulses prior to their outward expression.

autoplasty (aw′to-plas″te) plastic repair of diseased or injured parts with tissue from another region of the body.

autoploid (aw′to-ploid) 1. characterized by autoploidy. 2. an individual or cell characterized by autoploidy.

autoploidy (aw″to-ploi′de) the state of having two or more chromosome sets as the result of redoubling of the haploid set.

autopolymer (-pol′ĭ-mer) a material which polymerizes on addition of an activator and a catalyst, without the use of heat.

autopolyploid (-pol′ĭ-ploid) 1. characterized by autopolyploidy. 2. an individual or cell characterized by autopolyploidy.

autopolyploidy (-pol″ĭ-ploi′de) the state of having more than two chromosome sets as the result of redoubling of the haploid set.

autoprecipitin (-pre-sip′ĭ-tin) a substance which precipitates the serum of the animal in which it was developed.

autoprothrombin (-pro-throm′bin) an activation product of prothrombin.

autopsy (aw′top-se) necropsy.

autopsychic (aw″to-si′kik) pertaining to one's ideas concerning his own personality.

autoradiogram (-ra′de-o-gram) the film produced by autoradiography.

autoradiography (-ra″de-og′rah-fe) the recording, on specially sensitized film, of radiation emitted by the tissue itself, especially after purposeful introduction into it of radioactive material.

autoregulation (-reg″u-la′shun) control of certain phenomena by factors inherent in a situation; usually restricted to circulatory physiology. **a. of blood flow,** regulation by an organ of its blood supply in accordance with its needs.

autoreinfusion (aw″to-re″in-fu′zhun) autotransfusion (2).

autoscopy (aw-tos′ko-pe) the visual hallucination of one's self.

autosensitization (aw″to-sen″sĭ-ti-za′shun) development of sensitivity to one's own serum or tissues.

autosepticemia (-sep″tĭ-se′me-ah) septicemia from poisons developed within the body.

autoserodiagnosis (-se″ro-di″ag-no′sis) diagnostic use of autoserum.

autoserotherapy (-ther′ah-pe) treatment by autoserum.

autoserum (aw″to-se′rum) serum prepared from the patient's own blood.

autosite (aw′to-sīt) a fetal monster capable of independent life, on or in which a parasitic twin lives.

autosome (aw′to-sōm) one of the 22 pairs of chromosomes in man not concerned with determination of the sex of the subject.

autosplenectomy (aw″to-sple-nek′to-me) extirpation of the spleen by progressive fibrosis and shrinkage.

autostimulation (-stim″u-la′shun) stimulation of an animal with antigenic material from its own tissues.

autosuggestion (-sug-jes′chun) suggestion arising in one's self.

autotomography (-to-mog′rah-fe) a method of body section roentgenography involving movement of the patient instead of the x-ray tube. adj., **autotomograph′ic.**

autotopagnosia (-top-ag-no′se-ah) inability to orient correctly different parts of the body.

autotoxin (-tok′sin) a toxin developed within the body.

autotransformer (-trans-for′mer) a transformer which has part of its turns common to both primary and secondary circuits.

autotransfusion (-trans-fu′zhun) 1. the forcing of blood into vital parts by bandaging or elevating the limbs. 2. reinfusion of a patient's own blood.

autotransplantation (-trans″plan-ta′shun) transfer of tissue from one part of the body to another part.

autotroph (aw′to-trōf) an autotrophic organism.

autotrophic (aw″to-trof′ik) capable of synthesizing necessary nutrients if water, carbon dioxide, inorganic salts and a source of energy are available.

autovaccination (-vak″sĭ-na′shun) injection of autovaccine.

autovaccine (-vak′sēn) a vaccine prepared from the patient's own tissues or secretions.

autoxidation (aw″tok-sĭ-da′shun) the spontaneous reaction of a compound with molecular oxygen at room temperature.

auxanography (awk″sah-nog′rah-fe) determination of the best medium for bacterial cultivation.

auxanology (-nol′o-je) the science of growth.

auxesis (awk-se'sis) increase in size; growth. adj., **auxet'ic.**

auxilytic (awk"sī-lit'ik) increasing the lytic or destructive power.

auxin (awk'sin) a chemical substance present in plants which is capable of accelerating the growth of cells.

auxiometer (awk"se-om'ĕ-ter) an apparatus for measuring the power of lenses.

auxocardia (awk"so-kar'de-ah) 1. diastole. 2. enlargement of the heart.

auxochrome (awk'so-krōm) a substituent atom or group of atoms in a molecule which increases the intensity of absorption of light by a chromophore. adj., **auxochro'mic.**

auxocyte (awk'so-sīt) an oocyte, spermatocyte or sporocyte in the early stages of development.

auxodrome (awk'so-drōm) the course of growth of a child as plotted on a specially devised graph.

auxology (awk-sol'o-je) the science of the growth of organisms.

auxotherapy (awk"so-ther'ah-pe) substitution therapy.

auxotroph (awk'so-trōf) an auxotrophic organism.

auxotrophic (awk"so-trof'ik) requiring a growth factor; used especially with reference to a mutation that causes such a requirement.

A.V. atrioventricular.

av., avoir. avoirdupois.

avascular (a-vas'ku-lar) not vascular; bloodless.

avascularization (a-vas"ku-lar-i-za'shun) expulsion of blood, as by bandaging.

Avertin (ah-ver'tin) trademark for tribromoethanol.

avidin (av'ĭ-din) a protein in egg white which combines with biotin to render the latter inactive.

avirulence (a-vir'u-lens) lack of strength or virulence; lack of competence of an infectious agent to produce pathogenic effects. adj., **avir'ulent.**

avitaminosis (a-vi"tah-mĭ-no'sis) disease due to deficiency of vitamins in the diet. adj., **avitaminot'ic.**

avoidance (ah-void'ance) a conscious or unconscious reaction defensively intended to escape anxiety, conflict, danger, fear or pain. **phobic a.,** avoidance of an external phobic object.

avoirdupois (av'er-dŭ-poiz") a common system of weight used in English-speaking countries.

avulsion (ah-vul'shun) the tearing away of a structure or part. **phrenic a.,** extraction of a portion of the phrenic nerve.

ax. axis.

axiation (ak"se-a'shun) establishment of an axis; development of polarity in an organ or other structure.

axifugal (ak-sif'u-gal) directed away from an axis or axon.

axilla (ak-sil'ah) the armpit.

axillary (ak'sĭ-ler"e) of or pertaining to the armpit.

axio- (ak'se-o) word element [L., Gr.] denoting relation to an axis; in dentistry, used in special reference to the long axis of a tooth.

axioplasm (ak'se-o-plazm") the amorphous material of an axon in which the nerve fibers are buried.

axipetal (ak-sip'ĕ-tal) directed toward an axis or axon.

axis (ak'sis) 1. straight line through a center. 2. the second cervical vertebra. adj., **ax'ial, ax'ile. basibregmatic a.,** the vertical line from the basion to the bregma. **basicranial a.,** line from basion to gonion. **basifacial a.,** line from gonion to subnasal point. **binauricular a.,** line joining the two auricular points. **brain a.,** the brain stem. **celiac a.,** a thick branch from the abdominal aorta. **cerebrospinal a.,** the central nervous system. **dorsoventral a.,** one passing from the back to the belly surface of the body. **electrical a. of heart,** the resultant of the electromotive forces within the heart at any instant. **facial a.,** basifacial axis. **frontal a.,** imaginary line running from right to left through center of eyeball. **a. of heart,** a line passing through the center of the base of the heart and the apex. **neural a.,** cerebrospinal axis. **optic a.,** 1. a straight line joining the central points of curvature of the corneal (anterior pole) and scleral (posterior pole) spheres of the eye. 2. the visual axis. **sagittal a.,** imaginary line extending through the eye from before backward. **visual a.,** line from point of vision of retina to the object of vision.

axis cylinder (ak"sis-sil'in-der) axon.

axite (ak'sīt) a terminal filament of an axon.

axodendrite (ak"so-den'drīt) a nonmedullated side-fibril of an axon.

axofugal (ak-sof'u-gal) axifugal.

axolemma (ak"so-lem'ah) the limiting membrane surrounding the cytoplasm of the axon.

axolysis (ak-sol'ĭ-sis) degeneration of an axon.

axon (ak'son) the long outgrowth of the body of a nerve cell which conducts impulses from the body toward the next neuron.

axone (ak'sōn) axon.

axoneme (ak'so-nēm) a slender axial filament, such as the axial thread of a chromosome, or that forming the central core of a flagellum or cilium.

axoneure (ak'so-nūr) axoneuron.

axoneuron (ak"so-nu'ron) a nerve cell of the cerebrospinal system.

axonometer (ak"so-nom'ĕ-ter) apparatus for determination of cylindrical axis of a lens.

axonotmesis (ak"son-ot-me'sis) damage to nerve fibers causing complete peripheral degeneration, but not disturbing the epineurium and intimate supporting structures of the nerve, so that regeneration of fibers occurs, with spontaneous recovery.

axopetal (ak-sop'ĕ-tal) axipetal.

axophage (ak'so-fāj) a glia cell occurring in excavations in the myelin in myelitis.

axoplasm (ak'so-plazm) axioplasm.

axopodium (ak"so-po'de-um) a more or less permanent type of pseudopodium, long and needle-like, characterized by an axial rod, composed of a bundle of fibrils inserted near the center of the body of the cell.

axospongium (ak″so-spun′je-um) the network structure of the substance of an axon.

axostyle (ak′so-stīl) a supporting structure embedded along the longitudinal axis in the cytoplasm of a parasitic flagellate (Mastigophora).

Az. azote (nitrogen).

azacyclonol (a″zah-si′klo-nol) a chemical used as a tranquilizer.

azaleine (ah-za′le-in) fuchsin.

azamethonium (a″zah-mĕ-tho′ne-um) a chemical used for ganglionic blockade and to reduce blood pressure.

azapetine (a″zah-pet′ēn) a chemical used for sympathetic blockade and to dilate peripheral blood vessels.

azaserine (a″zah-ser′ēn) an agent used in treatment of acute leukemia.

azeotropy (a″ze-ot′ro-pe) absence of change in composition of a mixture of substances when it is boiled under pressure. adj., **azeotrop′ic.**

azobenzene (az″o-ben′zēn) a derivative, $C_{12}H_{10}N_2$, from nitrobenzene.

azoic (ah-zo′ik) destitute of living organisms.

azolitmin (az″o-lit′min) a red coloring principle from litmus.

azoospermia (a″zo-o-sper′me-ah) absence of spermatozoa in the semen.

azosulfamide (az″o-sul′fah-mīd) an agent used to treat infection.

azotation (az″o-ta′shun) the absorption of nitrogen from the air.

azote (a′zōt) nitrogen.

azotemia (az″o-te′me-ah) presence of nitrogenous compounds in the blood; uremia. adj., **azote′mic.**

azotenesis (-tĕ-ne′sis) a disease due to excess nitrogen in the system.

azotification (az-o″ti-fi-ka′shun) fixation of atmospheric nitrogen.

azotize (az′o-tīz) to charge with nitrogen.

Azotobacter (ah-zo′to-bak″ter) a genus of Schizomycetes (order Eubacteriales, family Azotobacteraceae).

Azotobacteraceae (ah-zo″to-bak″tĕ-ra′se-e) a family of Schizomycetes (order Eubacteriales) widely distributed in the soil.

azotometer (az″o-tom′ĕ-ter) instrument for measuring urea in urine.

Azotomonas (a-zo″to-mo′nas) a genus of Schizomycetes (order Pseudomonadales, suborder Pseudomonadineae, family Pseudomonadaceae) found in the soil.

azotorrhea (az″o-to-re′ah) discharge of abnormal quantities of nitrogenous matter in the stools.

azoturia (-tu′re-ah) excess of urea in the urine.

Azulfidine (a-zul′fi-dēn) trademark for a preparation of salicylazosulfapyridine.

azure (azh′ūr) a methyl thionin dye.

azuresin (azh″u-rez′in) a complex combination of azure A dye and carbacrylic cationic exchange resin used as a diagnostic aid in detection of gastric secretion.

azurophil (azh-u′ro-fil) an element which stains easily with azure dye.

azurophilia (azh″u-ro-fil′e-ah) a condition in which the blood contains cells having azurophilic granules.

azurophilic (-fil′ik) staining easily with azure dyes.

azygogram (az′ĭ-go-gram) the film obtained by azygography.

azygography (az″ĭ-gog′rah-fe) radiography of the azygous venous system. adj., **azygograph′ic.**

azygos (az′ĭ-gos) any unpaired part.

azygous (az′ĭ-gus) having no fellow; unpaired.

azymia (a-zim′e-ah) absence of enzyme.

azymic (ah-zim′ik) not giving rise to fermentation.

azymous (ah-zi′mus) azymic.

B

B chemical symbol, *boron.*

B. Bacillus; base.

B.A. Bachelor of Arts; bucco-axial.

Ba chemical symbol, *barium.*

Babesia (ba-be′ze-ah) a genus of protozoan parasites.

babesiosis (ba-be″ze-o′sis) infection with Babesia.

baby (ba′be) an infant (birth to two years). **blue baby,** an infant born with cyanosis due to a congenital heart lesion or to congenital atelectasis. **"cloud b.,"** an apparently well infant who, because of viruses and bacteria in the respiratory tract or elsewhere, is able to contaminate the surrounding atmosphere and thus be responsible for nursery epidemics of staphylococcal infection.

bacca (bak′ah) a berry; a berry-like fruit.

baccate (bak′āt) berry-shaped.

bacciform (bak′sĭ-form) berry-shaped.

Bacillaceae (bas″il-la′se-e) a family of Schizomycetes (order Eubacteriales).

bacillary (bas′i-la″re) pertaining to bacilli or to rodlike structures.

bacillemia (bas″i-le′me-ah) presence of bacilli in the blood.

bacilli (bah-sil′i) plural of *bacillus.*

bacillicidal (bah-sil″i-si′dal) destructive to bacilli.

bacillicide (bah-sil′i-sīd) an agent that destroys bacilli.

bacilliculture (bah-sil″i-kul″tūr) the propagation of bacilli.

bacilliform (bah-sil′ĭ-form) shaped like a bacillus.

bacillogenous (bas″ĭ-loj′ĕ-nus) caused by bacilli.

bacillophobia (bah-sil″o-pho′be-ah)   morbid dread of microbes.

bacillosis (bas″ĭ-lo′sis) infection with bacilli.

bacillotherapy (bah-sil″o-ther′ah-pe) treatment with bacilli or bacteria.

bacilluria (bas″ĭ-lu′re-ah) bacilli in the urine.

Bacillus (bah-sil′lus) a genus of Schizomycetes (family Bacillaceae, order Eubacteriales) separated into 25 species, three of which are pathogenic. **B. an′thracis,** the causative agent of anthrax. **B. co′li,** Escherichia coli. **B. dysente′riae,** Shigella dysenteriae. **B. enterit′idis,** Salmonella enteritidis. **B. lep′rae,** Mycobacterium leprae. **B. mal′lei,** Actinobacillus mallei. **B. pneumo′niae,** Klebsiella pneumoniae. **B. pseudomal′lei,** Pseudomonas pseudomallei. **B. pyocya′neus,** Pseudomonas aeruginosa. **B. tet′ani,** Clostridium tetani. **B. ty′phi, B. typho′sus,** Salmonella typhosa. **B. welch′ii,** Clostridium perfringens.

bacillus (bah-sil′us), pl. bacil′li [L.] 1. a rod-shaped bacterium; any spore-forming, rod-shaped microorganism of the order Eubacteriales. 2. an organism of the genus Bacillus. **Bang's b.,** Brucella abortus. **Battey bacilli,** unclassified mycobacteria that may produce tuberculosis-like disease in man. **Bordet-Gengou b.,** Bordetella pertussis. **colon b.,** Escherichia coli. **Ducrey's b.,** Haemophilus ducreyi. **Fick's b.,** Proteus vulgaris. **Flexner's b.,** Shigella flexneri. **Friedländer's b.,** Klebsiella pneumoniae. **Gärtner's b.,** Salmonella enteritidis. **Hansen's b.,** Mycobacterium leprae. **Johne's b.,** Mycobacterium paratuberculosis. **Klebs-Löffler b.,** Corynebacterium diphtheriae. **Koch-Weeks b.,** Haemophilus aegyptius. **Morax-Axenfeld b.,** Haemophilus duplex. **Morgan's b.,** Proteus morgani. **Nocard's b.,** Salmonella typhimurium. **Pfeiffer's b.,** Haemophilus influenzae. **Sonne-Duval b.,** Shigella sonnei. **tubercle b.,** Mycobacterium tuberculosis. **typhoid b.,** Salmonella typhosa.

bacitracin (bas″ĭ-tra′sin) an antibiotic substance produced in ordinary culture mediums by an aerobic, gram-positive, spore-forming bacillus found in a contaminated wound, and named for the patient, Margaret Tracey; useful in a wide range of infections, applied topically or given intramuscularly. **zinc b.,** the zinc salt of bacitracin, used in an ointment as a topical antibacterial agent.

backbone (bak′bōn) the rigid column formed by the vertebrae.

back-cross (bak′kros) a mating between a heterozygote and a homozygote. **double back-cross,** the mating between a double heterozygote and a homozygote.

backflow (bak′flo) abnormal backward flow of fluids; regurgitation. **pyelovenous b.,** drainage from the renal pelvis into the venous system occurring under certain conditions of back pressure.

Bact. Bacterium.

bacter(io)- word element [Gr.], bacteria.

bacteremia (bak″ter-e′me-ah) presence of bacteria in the blood.

bacteria (bak-te′re-ah) plural of bacterium. adj., **bacte′rial.**

bactericidal (bak-tēr″ĭ-si′dal) destructive to bacteria.

bactericide (bak-tēr′ĭ-sīd) an agent which destroys bacteria.

bacterid (bak′ter-id) a skin condition due to hypersensitivity to a bacterial infection.

bacteriemia (bak-ter″e-e′me-ah) bacteremia.

bacterioagglutinin (bak-te″re-o-ah-gloo′tĭ-nin) an agglutinin formed by action of bacteria.

bacteriochlorin (-klo′rin) a compound found in photosynthetic bacteria which catalyzes the photoreduction of carbon dioxide.

bacteriocholia (-ko′le-ah) the presence of bacteria in the biliary tract.

bacteriocidin (-si′din) a bactericidal substance present in the blood.

bacterioclasis (bak-te″re-ok′lah-sis) the breaking up of bacteria into fragments.

bacteriodiagnosis (bak-te″re-o-di″ag-no′sis) diagnosis by bacteriologic examination of tissues or fluids.

bacteriogenic (-jen′ik) caused by bacteria.

bacterioid (bak-te′re-oid) resembling a bacterium.

bacteriologist (bak-te″re-ol′o-jist) an expert in the study of bacteria.

bacteriology (-ol′o-je) the scientific study of bacteria. adj., **bacteriolog′ic.**

bacteriolysin (-ol′ĭ-sin) a substance formed in the blood as a result of infection, and capable of destroying the bacteria causing the infection.

bacteriolysis (-ol′ĭ-sis) the destruction of bacteria. adj., **bacteriolyt′ic.**

bacterio-opsonin (bak-te″re-o-op-so′nin) a substance that has an opsonic action on bacteria.

bacteriopexia (-pek′se-ah) the fixation of bacteria by histiocytes.

bacteriophage (bak-te′re-o-fāj″) a bacterial virus. adj., **bacteriopha′gic.**

bacteriophagia (bak-te″re-o-fa′je-ah) destruction of bacteria by a cell or an organism.

bacteriophobia (-fo′be-ah) morbid fear of bacteria.

bacterioprecipitins (-pre-sip′ĭ-tins) precipitins occurring in the serum treated with bacteria.

bacterioprotein (-pro′te-in) a toxalbumin formed by bacteria.

bacteriosis (bak-te″re-o′sis) a bacterial disease.

bacteriostatic (bak-te″re-o-stat′ik) arresting the growth of bacteria.

bacteriotherapy (-ther′ah-pe) the cure of disease by introducing bacteria into the system.

bacteriotoxin (-tok′sin) a toxin destructive to bacteria. adj., **bacteriotox′ic.**

bacteriotrypsin (-trip′sin) an enzyme produced by Vibrio comma.

Bacterium (bak-te′re-um) a former name for a genus of Schizomycetes (order Eubacteriales). **B. aerog′enes,** Aerobacter aerogenes. **B. aerugino′sum,** Pseudomonas aeruginosa. **B. chol′erae su′is,** Salmonella choleraesuis.

B. co'li, *Escherichia coli.* **B. pes'tis bubon'-icae,** *Pasteurella pestis.* **B. son'nei,** *Shigella sonnei.* **B. tularen'se,** *Pasteurella tularensis.* **B. typho'sum,** *Salmonella typhosa.*

bacterium (bak-te're-um), pl. *bacte'ria* [L., Gr.] a nonspore-forming or nonmotile, rod-shaped microorganism; applied loosely to any microorganism of the order Eubacteriales.

bacteriuria (bak-te″re-u're-ah) bacteria in the urine.

bacteroid (bak'ter-oid) 1. resembling a bacterium. 2. a structurally modified bacterium.

Bacteroidaceae (bak″tē-roi-da'se-e) a family of Schizomycetes (order Eubacteriales).

Bacteroides (bak″tē-roi-dēz) a genus of Schizomycetes (order Eubacteriales, family Bacteroidaceae).

bacteroides (bak″tē-roi'dēz) 1. a highly pleomorphic, rod-shaped microorganism. 2. a microorganism of the genus Bacteroides.

bacteruria (bak″ter-u're-ah) bacteriuria.

Bactoscilla (bak″tos-sil'lah) a genus of Schizomycetes (order Beggiatoales, family Vitreoscillaceae).

baculiform (bah-ku'lĭ-form) rod-shaped.

baculum (bak'u-lum) a heterotopic bone developed in the fibrous septum of the penis, found in all insectivores, bats, rodents and carnivores, and in primates except man.

bag (bag) 1. a sac or pouch. 2. an inflatable rubber pouch for inserting in a part, for the purpose of dilating it. **Barnes's b.,** a lyre-shaped rubber bag for dilating the uterine cervix. **colostomy b.,** a receptacle worn over the stoma by a colostomy patient, to receive the fecal discharge. **Douglas b.,** a receptacle for the collection of expired air, permitting measurement of respiratory gases. **Lyster b.,** a large rubber-lined bag for holding water supplies in camps. **micturition b.,** a receptacle used for urine by ambulatory patients with urinary incontinence. **Politzer b.,** a soft bag of rubber for inflating the eustachian tube. **Voorhees b.,** a rubber bag to be inflated with water to dilate the uterine cervix. **b. of waters,** the membranes enclosing the liquor amnii and the developing fetus in utero.

bagassosis (bag″ah so'sis) a lung disease due to inhalation of dust from the residue of cane after extraction of sugar (bagasse).

BAL, dimercaprol (British anti-lewisite).

balance (bal'ans) 1. an instrument for weighing. 2. harmonious adjustment of different elements or parts. **acid-base b.,** the proportion of acid and base required to keep the blood neutral. **analytical b.,** a laboratory device for accurately measuring weight, sensitive to variations of the order of 0.05 to 0.1 mg. **inhibition-action b.,** the balance maintained in every person between emotional feelings and response to them. **microchemical b.,** a laboratory device for determining weight, sensitive to variations of the order of 0.001 mg. **semimicro b.,** a device for determining weight, sensitive to variations of 0.01 mg. **water b.,** the fairly accurate and uniform balance between intake and output of water by the body.

balaneutics (bal″ah-nu'tiks) the science of giving baths.

balanic (bah-lan'ik) pertaining to the glans penis or glans clitoridis.

balanitis (bal″ah-ni'tis) inflammation of the glans penis. **gangrenous b.,** infection of the glans penis by a combination of microorganisms, leading to its ulceration and rapid destruction. **phagedenic b.,** gangrenous balanitis.

balanoblennorrhea (bal″ah-no-blen″o-re'ah) gonorrheal balanitis.

balanoplasty (bal'ah-no-plas″te) plastic repair of the glans penis.

balanoposthitis (bal″ah-no-pos-thi'tis) inflammation of glans penis and prepuce.

balanopreputial (-pre-pu'she-al) pertaining to glans penis and prepuce.

balanorrhagia (-ra'je-ah) gonorrheal balanitis.

balantidiasis (bal″an-tĭ-di'ah-sis) infection with organisms of the genus Balantidium.

Balantidium (bal″an-tid'e-um) a genus of ciliated protozoa, including many species found in the intestine in vertebrates and invertebrates. **B. co'li,** a species found in the large intestine of man, causing diarrhea and secondary complications. **B. su'is,** a species occurring in pigs, often considered the same species as *B. coli.*

Balarsen (bah-lar'sen) trademark for preparations of arsthinol.

ball (bawl) a globular structure, or sphere. **Bichat's fat b.,** sucking pad.

ballism (bal'izm) quick jerking or shaking movements seen in chorea.

ballistocardiogram (bah-lis″to-kar'de-o-gram″) the record produced by ballistocardiography.

ballistocardiograph (-kar'de-o-graf″) the apparatus used in ballistocardiography.

ballistocardiography (-kar″de-og'rah-fe) graphic recording of forces imparted to the body by cardiac ejection of blood.

ballistophobia (-fo'be-ah) morbid dread of missiles.

ballottement (bah-lot'maw) [Fr.] a diagnostic maneuver, involving pressure on an organ, as the uterus or kidney, and noting the impact when it rebounds.

balm (bahm) 1. a balsam. 2. a soothing or healing medicine. **mountain b.,** eriodictyon.

balneology (bal″ne-ol'o-je) the science dealing with baths and bathing.

balneotherapeutics (bal″ne-o-ther″ah-pu'tiks) scientific study of the use of baths in the treatment of disease.

balneotherapy (-ther'ah-pe) use of baths in the treatment of disease.

bals. balsam.

balsam (bawl'sam) a semifluid, fragrant, resinous vegetable juice. adj., **balsam'ic. friar's b.,** compound tincture of benzoin. **gurjun b.,** an oleoresin obtained from trees of the genus Dipterocarpus, in India. **b. of Peru, Peruvian b.,** a dark brown viscid liquid obtained from *Myroxylon pereirae;* used as a dressing for wounds and in treatment of certain skin conditions. **tolu b.,** brown, plastic solid obtained from *Myroxylon balsamum;* used as a vehicle for cough mixtures.

bancroftosis (ban″krof-to′sis) infestation with *Wuchereria bancrofti.*

band (band) a strip which constricts or binds a part. **A b.**, a doubly refractile (anisotropic) band on a myofibril of striated muscle. **coronary b.**, see under *cushion.* **I b.**, a singly refractile (isotropic) band on a myofibril of striated muscle. **iliotibial b.**, part of fascia lata forming a sheath for the tensor fasciae femoris. **matrix b.**, a piece of metal fitted around a tooth to supply a missing wall of a cavity or to support the tooth during packing of amalgam into the cavity. **phonatory b's**, vocal cords. **retention b.**, muscle of Treitz. **zinc b.**, a band on a myofibril of striated muscle at the center of the I band.

bandage (ban′dij) a strip or piece of gauze or other fabric for wrapping any part or member. **Barton's b.**, a double figure-of-8 bandage for fracture of the lower jaw. **capeline b.**, a bandage applied like a cap or hood to the head or shoulder or to a stump. **demigauntlet b.**, a bandage that covers the hand, but leaves the fingers uncovered. **Desault's b.**, a bandage for a fractured clavicle. **Esmarch's b.**, an India rubber bandage applied to a limb from the distal part upward, to expel blood from the part to be operated on. **figure-of-8 b.**, a bandage in which the turns cross each other like the figure 8. **gauntlet b.**, a bandage which covers the hand and fingers like a glove. **Gibney b.**, a bandage of overlapping strips of adhesive applied over the sides and backs of the foot and leg to hold the foot in slight varus. **Gibson's b.**, **Hamilton's b.**, a bandage for fracture of the lower jaw. **plaster b.**, a bandage stiffened with a paste of plaster of Paris. **pressure b.**, a bandage for applying pressure. **Priessnitz b.**, see under *compress.* **protective b.**, a bandage for covering a part or keeping dressings in place. **roller b.**, a simple, continuous strip, to be applied spirally or circularly. **scultetus b.**, a many-tailed bandage with overlapping ends. **spica b.**, a spiral bandage folded regularly on itself like the letter **V**. **suspensory b.**, a bandage for supporting the scrotum. **T b.**, a bandage shaped like the letter **T**. **Velpeau b.**, one used in immobilization of certain fractures about the upper end of the humerus and shoulder joint, binding the arm and shoulder to the chest.

bank (bank) a place of storage for such materials as blood *(blood bank),* or for other human tissue *(bone bank, eye bank, skin bank,* etc.) to be used in reparative surgery.

Banthine (ban′thīn) trademark for preparations of methantheline bromide.

bantingism (ban′ting-izm) treatment of corpulence by diet.

bar (bahr) 1. a structure that hinders or impedes. 2. a unit used in measuring pressure, equivalent to that of a column of mercury about 750 mm. high per square centimeter. **median b.**, a fibrotic formation across the neck of the prostate gland, producing obstruction of the urethra. **Mercier's b.**, a ridge

on the wall of the urinary bladder, extending between the ureteral orifices.

baragnosis (bar″ag-no′sis) impairment of ability to perceive differences in weight or pressure.

barbital (bahr′bĭ-tahl) a long-acting barbiturate. **b. sodium, soluble b.**, white, odorless, bitter powder, more soluble than barbital, used similarly.

barbituism (bahr-bit′ū-izm) barbiturism.

barbiturate (bahr-bit′u-rāt) a derivative of barbituric acid; such compounds are frequently used for their hypnotic potency.

barbiturism (bahr-bit′ū-rizm) a toxic condition produced by use of barbital and its derivatives.

barbotage (bahr″bo-tahzh′) [Fr.] repeated alternate injection and withdrawal of fluid with a syringe, as in gastric lavage or administration of an anesthetic agent into the subarachnoid space.

baresthesia (bar″es-the′ze-ah) sensibility for weight or pressure.

baresthesiometer (bar″es-the″ze-om′ĕ-ter) instrument for estimating sense of weight or pressure.

barium (ba′re-um) chemical element *(see table),* at. no. 56, symbol Ba. **b. chloride,** poisonous white, odorless crystals, $BaCl_2$.$2H_2O$; used as a purgative in veterinary medicine. **b. sulfate,** fine, white, bulky powder, $BaSO_4$; used as an opaque medium for x-ray examination of the alimentary tract.

bark (bahrk) the tough external layer of a woody stem or trunk. **cinchona b., Jesuit's b., Peruvian b.**, cinchona.

baroceptor (bar″o-sep′tor) baroreceptor.

barodontalgia (bar″o-don-tal′je-ah) aerodontalgia.

barognosis (bar″og-no′sis) the faculty by which weight is recognized.

barograph (bar′o-graf) a self-registering barometer.

barometer (bah-rom′ĕ-ter) an instrument indicating the atmospheric pressure. **aneroid b.**, one containing no mercury or other fluid, making use of a chamber in which the air is partially exhausted.

barometrograph (bar″o-met′ro-graf) a self-registering barometer.

baro-otitis (bar″o-o-ti′tis) barotitis.

barophilic (-fil′ik) growing best under high atmospheric pressure.

baroreceptor (-re-sep′tor) a sensory nerve terminal which is stimulated by changes in pressure.

baroscope (bar′o-skōp) a delicate or highly sensitive form of barometer.

barosinusitis (bar″o-si″nu-si′tis) pain in the sinus due to rapid changes in atmospheric air pressure.

barotaxis (-tak′sis) the orientation of living organisms in response to pressure.

barotitis (-ti′tis) a morbid condition due to exposure to differing atmospheric pressures. **b. me′dia,** a symptom complex due to difference between atmospheric pressure of the environment and air pressure in the internal ear.

barotrauma (bar″o-traw′mah) injury due to pressure, as to structures of the ear, in high-altitude flyers, owing to differences between atmospheric and intratympanic pressures.

Barr body (bahr bod′e) sex chromatin; observed in cells of the normal female, considered to be the remnant of the inactive X chromosome.

bartholinitis (bar″to-lin-i′tis) inflammation of Bartholin's glands.

Bartonella (bar″to-nel′lah) a genus of Microtatobiotes (order Rickettsiales, family Bartonellaceae).

Bartonellaceae (-nel-la′se-e) a family of Microtatobiotes (order Rickettsiales) occurring as pathogenic parasites in the erythrocytes of man and other animals.

bartonellemia (-nel-le′me-ah) presence in the blood of organisms of the genus Bartonella.

bartonelliasis (-nel-li′ah-sis) bartonellosis.

bartonellosis (-nel-lo′sis) infection by microorganisms of the genus Bartonella.

baruria (bah-ru′re-ah) high specific gravity of urine.

baryesthesia (bar″e-es-the′ze-ah) baresthesia.

baryglossia (-glos′e-ah) barylalia.

barylalia (-la′le-ah) indistinct, thick speech, resulting from a lesion of the central nervous system.

baryphonia (-fo′ne-ah) deepness and hoarseness of the voice.

barytron (bar″i-tron) an electrical particle lighter than a proton, but heavier than an electron.

basad (ba′sad) toward a basal aspect.

basal (ba′sal) pertaining to a base; fundamental; in physiology, pertaining to the lowest possible level.

Basaljel (ba′sal-jel) trademark for basic aluminum carbonate gel.

base (bās) 1. the foundation on which a thing is constructed or compounded. 2. a substance that yields hydroxyl ions and reacts with an acid to form a salt and water. **acrylic resin b.**, a denture base of an acrylic resin. **denture b.**, the material in which the teeth of a denture are set and which rests on the supporting tissues when the denture is in place in the mouth. **hexone b's**, bases containing six atoms of carbon, including arginine, lysine and histadine. **ointment b.**, a vehicle for medicinal substances intended for external application to the body. **record b.**, **temporary b.**, **trial b.**, baseplate.

baseosis (ba″se-o′sis) alkalosis.

baseplate (bās′plāt) a sheet of plastic material used in making trial plates for artificial dentures.

basial (ba′se-al) pertaining to the basion.

basic (ba′sik) 1. pertaining to a base. 2. capable of uniting with negatively charged ions or with acid substances.

basicity (ba-sis′i-te) the quality of being basic; the power to unite with negatively charged ions or with acid substances.

basidium (bah-sid′e-um), pl. *basid′ia* [L.] the clublike spore-producing organ of certain of the higher fungi.

basihyoid (ba″se-hi′oid) the body of the hyoid bone.

basilad (bas′i-lad) toward the base.

basilar (bas′i-lar) pertaining to the base.

basilateral (ba″si-lat′er-al) pertaining to the base and side.

basilemma (-lem′ah) 1. basement membrane. 2. neuroglia.

basiloma (bas″i-lo′mah) a basal cell carcinoma.

basion (ba′se-on) the midpoint of the anterior border of the foramen magnum.

basiotripsy (ba″se-o-trip″se) cranioclasis.

basiphobia (ba″sē-fo′be-ah) morbid dread of walking.

basis (ba′sis) a foundation or base; especially the principal ingredient of a medication (prescription).

basisphenoid (ba″sē-sfe′noid) an embryonic bone which becomes the back part of the body of the sphenoid.

basocyte (ba′so sīt) a cell staining readily with alkaline dyes; a basophilic leukocyte.

basocytopenia (ba″so-si″to-pe′ne-ah) deficiency of basophilic leukocytes of the blood.

basocytosis (-si-to′sis) excess of basophilic leukocytes of the blood.

baso-erythrocyte (-ē-rith′ro-sīt) an erythrocyte containing basophil granules.

basopenia (-pe′ne-ah) basocytopenia.

basophil (ba′so-fil) 1. a cell or other element staining readily with basic dyes. 2. a medium-sized leukocyte with a two-lobed nucleus, and cytoplasm containing large granules that stain a deep blue, normally constituting 0.5 per cent of the leukocytes of the blood.

basophile (ba′so-fil) 1. basophil. 2. basophilic.

basophilia (ba″so-fil′e-ah) 1. degeneration of erythrocytes with formation of basophilic granules (blue dots). 2. abnormal increase in the basophilic leukocytes of the blood.

basophilic (-fil′ik) staining readily with alkaline dyes.

basophilism (ba-sof′i-lizm) abnormal increase of basophilic cells. **pituitary b.**, Cushing's syndrome, including vascular hypertension, hirsutism, adiposity and osteoporosis.

basoplasm (ba′so-plazm) the portion of the cytoplasm which stains easily with alkaline dyes.

bath (bath) 1. an apparatus for the immersion of an object in a fluid medium. 2. application of water or other medium to the human body for cleansing or therapeutic purposes, especially immersion in a solution of a considerable portion or a particular part of the body. **contrast b.**, alternate immersion of a part in hot water and ice water. **cool b.**, one in water from 60 to 75°F. **douche b.**, application of water to the body in a jet. **graduated b.**, one in which the temperature of the water is gradually lowered. **half b.**, a bath of the hips and lower part of the body. **hip b.**, sitz bath. **hot b.**, one in water from 98 to 112°F. **needle b.**, a shower bath in which the water is projected in a fine, needle-like spray. **sitz b.**, immersion of only the hips and buttocks. **temperate b.**, one in water 75 to 85°F. **tepid b.**, one in water 85 to 92°F. **warm b.,** one in water 90 to 104°F. **whirlpool b.,** one in which the water is kept in constant motion by mechanical means.

bathmotropism (bath-mot′ro-pizm) influence on the excitability of muscle tissue. adj. **bathmotrop′ic.**

bathochromy (bath″o-kro′me) a shift of the absorption band toward lower frequencies (longer wavelengths) with deepening of color from yellow to black.

bathophobia (-fo′be-ah) morbid dread of depths or of looking down from a high place, with fear of falling.

bathrocephaly (bath″ro-sef′ah-le) external bulging of the squamous portion of the occipital bone, producing a steplike deformity of the skull.

bathy- (bath′e) word element [Gr.], *deep.*

bathyanesthesia (bath″e-an″es-the′ze-ah) loss of deep sensibility.

bathyesthesia (-es-the′ze-ah) deep sensibility; the sensibility in the parts of the body beneath the surface.

bathygastry (bath″ē-gas′″tre) gastroptosis.

bathyhyperesthesia (bath″ē-hi″per-es-the′ze-ah) abnormally increased sensitiveness of deep body structures.

bathyhypesthesia (-hīp″es-the′ze-ah) abnormally diminished sensitiveness of deep body structures.

bathypnea (-ne′ah) deep breathing.

batophobia (bat″o-fo′be-ah) morbid dread of high objects.

battery (bat′er-e) a series of cells affording galvanic currents. **constant b.,** see under *cell.* **galvanic b.,** apparatus for generating galvanic electricity. **storage b.,** an apparatus for storing electricity.

Bayer 205 (ba′er) suramin sodium.

baytinal (ba′ti-nal) a thiobarbiturate used as an intravenous anesthetic agent.

B.C. bone conduction; buccocervical.

BCG Bacille Calmette-Guérin (vaccine for prevention of tuberculosis).

Be chemical symbol, *beryllium.*

beaker (bēk′er) a round laboratory vessel of various materials, usually with parallel sides and often with a pouring spout, of a capacity ranging from 1 to hundreds of milliliters.

beat (bēt) a throb, as of the heart or pulse. **apex b.,** the beat felt over the apex of the heart, usually in the fifth left intercostal space. **ectopic b.,** a heart beat originating at some point other than the sinoatrial node. **forced b.,** an extrasystole produced by artificial stimulation of the heart. **premature b.,** an extrasystole.

bechic (bek′ik) 1. relieving a cough. 2. an agent for relief of cough.

bed (bed) a supporting structure, especially a structure for supporting the body during sleep. **fracture b.,** a bed for the use of patients with broken bones. **Gatch b.,** a bed fitted with jointed springs, which may be adjusted to various positions. **Klondike b.,** one arranged to protect the patient from drafts in outdoor sleeping. **nail b.,** the surface covered by the nail of a finger or toe.

bedpan (bed′pan) a shallow vessel used for defecation or urination by patients confined to bed.

bedsonia (bed-so′ne-ah), pl. *bedso′niae* [L.] an infectious agent of the group causing psittacosis, lymphogranuloma venereum and trachoma.

beeswax (bēz′waks) wax from honeycomb. **bleached b.,** white wax. **unbleached b.,** yellow wax.

Beggiatoa (bej″je-ah-to′ah) a genus of Schizomycetes (order Beggiatoales, family Beggiatoaceae) growing in water.

Beggiatoaceae (-to-a′ce-e) a family of Schizomycetes (order Beggiatoales).

Beggiatoales (-to-a′lēz) an order of Schizomycetes.

behavior (be-hāv′yer) the externally observable activity of a person. **automatic b.,** that which takes place outside of conscious awareness.

behaviorism (be-hāv′yer-izm) the theory that the proper subject of psychologic study is personal behavior.

bejel (bej′el) a nonvenereal disease similar to yaws, occurring in the Middle East and caused by an organism indistinguishable from *Treponema pallidum.*

belemnoid (be-lem′noid) 1. dart-shaped. 2. the styloid process.

belladonna (bel″ah-don′ah) a plant which is the source of the alkaloids hyoscyamine and atropine, to which its properties are due.

belly (bel′e) 1. the abdomen. 2. the prominent, fleshy part of a bulging muscle.

belonoid (bel′o-noid) needle-shaped.

bemegride (bem′e-grīd) a drug used as a respiratory stimulant and as an antagonist in the treatment of barbiturate poisoning.

bemidone (bem′ĭ-dōn) a narcotic agent.

benactyzine (ben-ak′tĭ-zēn) an agent used in parasympathetic blockade and as an ataractic.

Benadryl (ben′ah-dril) trademark for diphenhydramine.

benanserin (ben-an′ser-in) an agent used as a serotonin antagonist.

bend (bend) a bent structure, or flexure. **varolian b.,** the third cerebral flexure in the developing fetus.

bendroflumethiazide (ben″dro-floo″mĕ-thi′ah-zīd) an agent used as a diuretic and antihypertensive.

bends (bendz) pain in muscles and joints caused by exposure to sudden reduction of air pressure.

Beneckea (be-nek′e-ah) a genus of Schizomycetes (order Eubacteriales, family Achromobacteraceae) found in salt and fresh water and in soil.

Benemid (ben′ē-mid) trademark for probenecid.

benign (be-nīn′) not recurrent or tending to progress.

Benoquin (ben′o-kwin) trademark for a preparation of monobenzone.

benoxinate (ben-ok′sĭ-nāt) an agent used as a surface anesthetic for the eye.

bentonite (ben′to-nīt) a fine, odorless powder

used in preparing pharmaceutical agents for external use.

benzaldehyde (ben-zal′dĕ-hīd)   a colorless, strongly refractive liquid, C_7H_6O, used chiefly as a flavoring agent.

benzalin (ben′zah-lin) nigrosin.

benzalkonium chloride (ben″zal-ko′ne-um klo′rĭd) a mixture of alkyldimethyl-benzylammonium chlorides; disinfectant and germicide.

benzcurine (benz′ku-rēn) gallamine.

Benzedrex (ben′zĕ-dreks) trademark for an inhalant used in shrinking nasal mucosa.

Benzedrine (ben′zĕ-drēn) trademark for amphetamine.

benzene (ben′zēn) a liquid hydrocarbon, C_6H_6, from coal tar.

benzestrol (ben-zes′trol) an estrogenic compound, $C_{20}H_{26}O_2$.

benzethonium (ben″zĕ-tho′ne-um) an ammonium derivative used as a local anti-infective.

benzhexol (benz hek′sol) trihexyphenidyl.

benzhydramine (-hi′drah-mēn) diphenhydramine.

benzidine (ben′zĭ-dēn) a compound, NH_2.-C_6H_4.$C_6H_4NH_2$, used as a test for blood.

benzin (ben′zin) a liquid obtained from petroleum, a solvent for rubber, fats, oils, etc.

benzoate (ben′zo-āt) a salt of benzoic acid.

benzoated (ben′zo-āt″ed) charged with benzoic acid.

benzocaine (ben′zo-kān) a crystalline compound, $C_9H_{11}NO_2$, used topically as a local anesthetic.

benzoin (ben′zo-in, ben-zo′in) the balsamic resin from *Styrax benzoin;* antiseptic and expectorant, applied locally and administered orally or by inhalation.

benzol (ben′zol) benzene.

benzomethamine (ben″zo-meth′ah-mēn) an agent used to produce parasympathetic blockade and to reduce hydrochloric acid secretion in the stomach.

benzonatate (ben-zo′nah-tat) an agent used as an antitussive.

benzononatine (ben-zo″no-na′tin) benzonatate.

benzoquinonium (ben″zo-kwĭ-no′ne-um) an ammonium derivative used as a relaxant for skeletal muscle.

benzpyrinium (benz″pi-rin′e-um) a pyridium derivative used as a parasympathomimetic agent and to relieve paralytic ileus.

benztropine (benz′tro-pēn) an agent used to produce parasympathetic blockade, as an antihistaminic and to reduce the tremors of parkinsonism.

benzyl (ben′zil) the hydrocarbon radical, C_7H_7. **b. benzoate**, a clear, oily liquid, $C_{14}H_{12}O_2$, used externally for scabies and pediculosis.

benzylpenicillin (ben″zil-pen-ĭ-sil′in) penicillin G.

beriberi (ber″e-ber′e) an endemic form of polyneuritis, due to an unbalanced diet, with a deficiency of vitamin B_1.

berkelium (ber-ke′le-um) chemical element (*see table*), at. no. 97, symbol Bk.

Berubigen (be-roo′bĭ-jen) trademark for preparations of vitamin B_{12}.

berylliosis (bĕ-ril″e-o′sis) a morbid condition caused by exposure to fumes or finely divided dust of beryllium salts, involving lungs, skin, subcutaneous tissues, lymph nodes, liver and other organs.

beryllium (bĕ-ril′le-um) chemical element (*see table*), at. no. 4, symbol Be.

beta (ba′tah) second letter of the Greek alphabet, β; used in names of chemical compounds to distinguish one of two or more isomers or to indicate position of substituting atoms or groups.

betacism (ba′tah-sizm) excessive use of *b* sound in speaking.

Betadine (ba′tah-dēn) trademark for preparations of povidone-iodine.

betaine (be′tah-in) an agent used as a lipotropic agent and in hydrochloride form as a substitute for hydrochloric acid in achlorhydria.

Betalin (ba′tah-lin) trademark for preparations of vitamin B complex.

betamethasone (ba″tah-meth′ah-sōn) a crystalline adrenocortical steroid, $C_{22}H_{29}FO_5$.

betanaphthol (-naf′thol) pale, crystalline powder with faint, phenol-like odor, $C_{10}H_8O$; intestinal antiseptic and vermifuge.

Betaprone (ba′tah-prōn) trademark for a preparation of betapropiolactone.

betapropiolactone (ba″tah-pro″pe-o-lak′tōn) an agent used for sterilization of human arterial grafts.

betatron (ba′tah-tron) an apparatus for accelerating electrons to millions of electron volts by magnetic induction.

Betaxin (be-tak′sin) trademark for preparations of thiamine hydrochloride.

betazole (ba′tah-zōl) a pyrazole derivative used in place of histamine to stimulate gastric acid secretion.

bethanechol (bĕ-tha′ne-kol) a choline derivative used as a parasympathetic agent and in treatment of abdominal distention or urinary retention.

bev billion electron volts (3.82×10^{-11} gram calorie, or 1.6×10^{-3} erg).

Bevidox (bev′ĭ-doks) trademark for a solution of vitamin B_{12}.

bezoar (be′zōr) a mass formed in the stomach by compaction of repeatedly ingested material that does not pass into the intestine.

BFP biological false-positive reaction; a positive finding in serologic tests for syphilis when syphilis does not exist.

Bi chemical symbol, *bismuth.*

bi- (bi) word element [L.], *two.*

biarticular (bi″ar-tik′u-lar) affecting two joints.

bibasic (bi-ba′sik) doubly basic.

bibliotherapy (bib″le-o-ther′ah-pe) use of books and reading in treatment of nervous disorders.

bicameral (bi-kam′er-al) having two chambers or cavities.

bicapsular (-kap′su-lar) having two capsules.

bicarbonate (-kar′bon-āt) a salt containing two equivalents of carbonic acid and one of a basic substance. **blood b., plasma b.,** the bicarbonate of the blood plasma, an index of the alkali reserve.

bicaudal (bi-kaw'dal) having two tails.

bicaudate (-kaw'dāt) bicaudal.

bicellular (-sel'u-lar) · made up of two cells.

bicephalus (-sef'ah-lus) a two-headed monster.

biceps (bi'seps) a muscle having two heads.

bichloride (bi-klo'rīd) a chloride containing two equivalents of chlorine.

biciliate (-sil'e-āt) having two cilia.

bicipital (-sip'ĭ-tal) having two heads; pertaining to a biceps muscle.

biconcave (-kon'kāv) having two concave surfaces.

bicontaminated (bi″kon-tam'ĭ-nāt″ed) infected by two different types of organisms.

biconvex (bi-kon'veks) having two convex surfaces.

bicornate (-kor'nāt) bicornuate.

bicornuate (-kor'nu-āt) having two horns or cornua.

bicoronial (bi″kŏ-ro'ne-al) pertaining to the two coronas.

bicorporate (bi-kor'po-rāt) having two bodies.

bicoudate (-koo'dāt) twice bent; said of catheters.

bicuspid (-kus'pid) 1. having two cusps. 2. a premolar tooth.

bicuspidate (-kus'pĭ-dāt) having two cusps or projections.

b.i.d. [L.] *bis in di'e* (twice a day).

bidermoma (bi″der-mo'mah) a teratoid growth containing two germ layers.

biduous (bid'u-us) lasting two days.

bifid (bi'fid) cleft into two parts.

biforate (bi-fo'rāt) having two perforations or foramina.

bifurcate (-fer'kāt) divided into two branches.

bifurcation (bi″fer-ka'shun) 1. division into two branches. 2. the point at which division into two branches occurs.

bighead (big'hed) 1. a condition of young rams characterized by edematous swelling of the head, due to *Clostridium novyi*. 2. thickening of the face and ears in white sheep, due to photosensitivity after ingestion of certain plants. 3. hydrocephalus in mink.

bilateral (bi-lat'er-al) having or pertaining to two sides.

bile (bīl) the secretion of the liver, serving both a digestive and an excretory function. adj., **bil'iary.**

Bilharzia (bil-har'ze-ah) an early name for flukes of the genus now called Schistosoma.

bilharziasis (bil″har-zi'ah-sis) infection with organisms of the genus now called Schistosoma (formerly Bilharzia); schistosomiasis.

bili- (bil'ĭ) word element [L.], *bile*.

bilicyanin (bil″ĭ-si'ah-nin) a blue pigment derived by oxidation from biliverdin.

bilifulvin (-ful'vin) bilirubin.

bilifuscin (-fus'in) one of a class of compounds related to bile pigments, but produced in constructive metabolism in the body; chiefly responsible for color of the feces.

biligenesis (-jen'ĕ-sis) production of bile. adj., **biligenet'ic.**

biligenic (-jen'ik) producing bile.

bilin (bi'lin) the main constituent of the bile, composed chiefly of the sodium salts of normal bile acids.

bilirachia (bil″ĭ-ra'ke-ah) presence of bile pigments in spinal fluid.

bilirubin (-roo'bin) a pigment produced by degradation of hemoglobin and found in blood serum; classified as *indirect* ("free" or unconjugated) while en route to the liver from its site of formation by reticuloendothelial cells, and *direct* (bilirubin diglucuronide) after its conjugation in the liver.

bilirubinemia (-roo″bī-ne'me-ah) presence of bilirubin in the blood.

bilirubinuria (-roo″bī-nu're-ah) presence of bilirubin in the urine.

biliuria (bil″e-u're-ah) presence of bile acids in the urine.

biliverdin (bil″ĭ-ver'din) one of the substances formed by degradation of heme and secreted in bile.

bilobate (bi-lo'bāt) having two lobes.

bilobular (-lob'u-lar) having two lobules.

bilocular (-lok'u-lar) having two compartments.

bimanual (-man'u-al) with both hands.

bimastoid (-mas'toid) pertaining to both mastoid processes.

binary (bi'nah-re) made up of two elements, or of two radicals which act as elements.

binaural (bi-naw'ral, bin-aw'ral) pertaining to both ears.

binauricular (bin″aw-rik'u-lar) pertaining to both auricles.

binder (bīnd'er) a band to be worn snugly around the abdomen.

binocular (bin-ok'u-lar) pertaining to both eyes.

binomial (bi-no'me-al) composed of two names or terms.

binotic (bin-ot'ik) binaural.

binovular (bin-ov'u-lar) derived from two ova.

binucleate (bi-nu'kle-āt) having two nuclei.

binucleation (bi″nu-kle-a'shun) formation of two nuclei within a cell without division of the cytoplasm into two daughter cells.

binucleolate (bi-nu'kle-o-lāt) having two nucleoli.

bio- (bi'o) word element [Gr.], *life; living.*

bio-assay (bi″o-as-sa') biological assay.

bioastronautics (-as″tro-naw'tiks) scientific study of effects of space and interplanetary travel on biological systems.

biocatalyst (-kat'ah-list) an enzyme.

biochemistry (-kem'is-tre) the study of chemical reactions occurring in living organisms.

biocidal (-si'dal) causing the death of living organisms.

bioclimatologist (-kli″mah-tol'o-jist) one skilled in bioclimatology.

bioclimatology (-tol'o-je) scientific study of effects on living organisms of conditions of natural environment (rainfall, daylight, temperature, etc.) prevailing in specific regions of the earth.

biocolloid (bi″o-kol'oid) a colloid from animal or vegetable tissue.

biocycle (-si'kl) the sequence of certain rhythmically repeated phenomena observed in living organisms.

biodegradable (bi″o-de-grād′ah-bl) susceptible of degradation by biological processes, as by bacterial or other enzymatic action.

Bio-des (bi′o-des) trademark for a preparation of diethylstilbestrol.

biodetritus (bi″o-de-tri′tus) detritus produced by disintegration and decomposition of once-living material.

biodynamics (-di-nam′iks) the doctrine or science of living force.

bioelectricity (-e″lek-tris′ĭ-te) electrical phenomena apparent in living cells.

bioflavonoid (-flă′vo noid) a generic term for a group of compounds widely distributed in plants and concerned with maintenance of a normal state of the walls of small blood vessels.

biogen (bi′o-jen) a hypothetical unit of living matter, made up of one or more molecules and having the power of growth and division.

biogenesis (bi″o-jen′ĕ-sis) the origination of living organisms only from organisms already living.

biogeography (-je-og′rah-fe) the scientific study of the geographic distribution of living organisms.

biokinetics (-ki-net′iks) the science of movement of living organisms.

biol. biology (biological).

biological (-loj′ĭ-kal) a medicinal preparation made from living organisms and their products: serums, vaccines, antigens and antitoxins.

biologist (bi-ol′o-jist) a specialist in biology.

biology (bi-ol′o-je) scientific study of living organisms. adj., **biolog′ical. molecular b.,** study of the relation between genes and the functional characteristics they determine, or of molecular structures and events underlying biological processes. **radiation b.,** scientific study of effects of ionizing radiation on living organisms.

bioluminescence (bi″o-lu″mĭ-nes′ens) emission of light by an organism as a consequence of the oxidation of some substrate in the presence of an enzyme.

biolysis (bi-ol′ĭ-sis) decomposition of organic matter by living organisms.

biolytic (bi″o-lit′ik) 1 pertaining to biolysis. 2. destructive to life.

biomass (bi′o-mas) the entire assemblage of living organisms of a particular region, considered collectively.

biomathematics (bi″o-math″ĕ-mat′iks) mathematics as applied to the phenomena of living things.

biome (bi′ōm) a large, distinct, easily differentiated community of organisms arising as a result of complex interactions of physical and biotic environmental factors.

biomechanics (bi″o-mĕ-kan′iks) the science of mechanics as applied to the living body.

biometeorologist (-me″te-or-ol′o-jist) one skilled in biometeorology.

biometeorology (-ol′o-je) scientific study of effects on living organisms of the extra-organic aspects (temperature, humidity, barometric pressure, rate of air flow, and air ionization) of the physical environment, whether natural or artificially created, and also their effects in closed ecological systems, as in satellites or submarines.

biometer (bi-om′ĕ-ter) instrument for measuring carbon dioxide given off by living tissue.

biometrics (bi″o-met′riks) biometry.

biometry (bi-om′ĕ-tre) the application of statistical methods to biological facts.

biomicroscope (bi″o-mi′kro-skōp) a microscope for examining living tissue.

biomicroscopy (-mi-kros′ko-pe) observation by microscope of living cell or tissue in its functional state.

biomutation (-mu-ta′shun) the modification produced in an organism when injected into the animal body.

bion (bi′on) an individual living organism.

bionecrosis (bi″o-ne-kro′sis) necrobiosis.

bionergy (bi-on′er-je) the vital energy which underlies all organic life.

bionics (bi-on′iks) scientific study of functions, characteristics and phenomena observed in the living world and application of knowledge gained therefrom in the world of machines.

bionomics (bi″o-nom′iks) ecology.

bionomy (bi-on′o-me) the science of the laws of life.

bionucleonics (bi″o-nu″kle-on′iks) scientific study of biological applications of radioactive and rare stable isotopes.

biophore (bi′o-fōr) early name for one of the submicroscopic particles in a cell which manifest specific functions.

biophylactic (bi″o-fi-lak′tik) guarding or preserving life.

biophysics (-fiz′iks) the physics of vital processes.

biophysiology (-fiz″e-ol′o-je) portion of biology including organogeny, morphology and physiology.

bioplasia (-pla′ze-ah) the storing up of food energy in the form of growth.

bioplasm (bi′o-plazm) the more vital or essential part of protoplasm. adj., **bioplas′mic.**

bioplast (bi′o-plast) 1. an independently existing mass of living substance. 2. a living cell.

bioplastic (bi″o-plas′tik) aiding in growth.

biopoiesis (-poi-e′sis) the origin of life from inorganic matter.

biopsy (bi′op-se) examination of tissue removed from the living body, sometimes designated according to means of removal, or site or type of tissue removed for study, as *cervical, excision, liver, needle, sternal biopsy.* **aspiration b.,** needle biopsy. **endoscopic b.,** examination of tissue removed from the interior of the body by an instrument inserted through an endoscope. **excision b.,** biopsy of tissue removed from the body by excision. **fractional b.,** histologic study of only fragments of a growth which have been removed for the purpose before excision of the lesion in its entirety. **needle b.,** biopsy of tissue obtained from an internal organ by means of a hollow needle inserted through the body wall.

punch b., biopsy of material obtained from the body tissues by a punch. **sponge b.**, examination of material (particles of tissue and tissue juices) absorbed in a sponge rubbed over a lesion or over mucous membrane, the entire sponge being stained and sectioned. **sternal b.**, examination of bone marrow of the sternum removed by puncture or aspiration.

biorheology (bi″o-re-ol′o-je) study of deformation and flow of matter in living systems and in materials directly derived from them.

bios (bi′os) any one of a group of growth factors for single-celled organisms such as yeast.

bioscopy (bi-os′ko-pe) examination with respect to viability or to the extinction of life.

biose (bi′ōs) a disaccharide.

bioset (bi′o-set) a grouping of biological components.

biospectrometry (bi″o-spek-trom′ĕ-tre) the spectrometry of matter in living tissue.

biospectroscopy (-spek-tros′ko-pe) the spectroscopy of living tissue.

biosphere (bi′o-sfēr) the regions of the known universe in which the environment supports the existence of living organisms.

biostatic (bi″o-stat′ik) inhibiting the growth and reproduction of living organisms.

biostatistics (-stah-tis′tiks) collected numerical data relating to living organisms.

biosynthesis (-sin′thĕ-sis) creation of a compound by physiologic processes in a living organism.

biotaxis (-tak′sis) 1. the selecting and arranging powers of living cells. 2. systematic classification of organisms.

biotaxy (-tak′se) biotaxis (1).

biotelemetry (-tel-em′ĕ-tre) registration and measurement of certain vital phenomena occurring in living organisms remote from the measuring device.

biotherapy (-ther′ah-pe) treatment by means of living organisms and their products, including vaccines, immune serum, blood transfusion.

biotic (bi-ot′ik) pertaining to living organisms.

biotics (bi-ot′iks) the science of the qualities of living organisms.

biotin (bi′o-tin) a member of the vitamin B complex, $C_{10}H_{16}O_3N_2S$, required by or occurring in all forms of life.

biotomy (bi-ot′o-me) vivisection.

biotoxication (bi″o-tok″sĭ-ka′shun) intoxication due to a poison derived from a living organism.

biotoxicology (-tok″sĭ-kol′o-je) scientific study of poisons produced by living organisms, their cause, detection and effects, and treatment of conditions produced by them.

biotoxin (-tok′sin) a poisonous substance produced by and derived from a living organism (plant or animal).

biotransformation (-trans″for-ma′shun) conversion of a material by natural processes occurring in a living organism.

biotrepy (bi-ot′rĕ-pe) study of the body by means of its reactions to chemical substances.

biotripsis (bi″o-trip′sis) wearing away of the skin.

biotropism (bi-ot′ro-pizm) increase in the virulence of an organism as a result of therapeutic procedures.

biotype (bi′o-tīp) a group of individuals having the same fundamental constitution.

biovular (bi-ov′u-lar) binovular.

bipara (bip′ah-rah) a woman who has had two pregnancies which resulted in viable offspring; para II.

biparental (bi″pah-ren′tal) derived from two parents, male and female.

biparous (bip′ah-rus) producing two at a birth.

bipenniform (bi-pen′ĭ-form) doubly feather-shaped.

biperiden (-per′ĭ-den) an agent used to produce parasympathetic blockade and to reduce tremors of parkinsonism.

bipolar (-po′lar) 1. having two poles. 2. pertaining to both poles.

bipotentiality (bi″po-ten″she-al′ĭ-te) ability to develop in either of two different ways.

biramous (bi-ra′mus) having two branches.

birefractive (bi″re-frak′tiv) doubly refractive.

birefringence (bi″re-frin′jens) the quality of transmitting light unequally in different directions. adj., **birefrin′gent. flow b.**, that exhibited only when the substance is in solution and flowing. **form b.**, that produced by regular orientation of tiny particles in a substance or object, differing in refractive index from the surrounding medium.

birth (berth) a coming into being; act or process of being born. **complete b.**, entire separation of the infant from the maternal body (after cutting of the umbilical cord). **multiple b.**, the birth of two or more offspring produced in the same gestation period. **premature b.**, expulsion of the fetus from the uterus before termination of the normal gestation period, but after independent existence has become a possibility.

birthmark (berth′mark) a congenital blemish or spot on the skin. **physiologic b.**, a small, irregular, bluish red patch in the occipital region, frequently present at birth and commonly persisting.

bisacodyl (bis-ak′o-dil) a drug used as a laxative.

bisacromial (bis″ah-kro′me-al) pertaining to the two acromial processes.

bisalbuminemia (bis″al-bu″mĭ-ne′me-ah) congenital anomaly with two electrophoretically distinct albumins in the serum.

bisection (bi-sek′shun) division into two parts.

bisexual (-seks′u-al) having both active (male) and passive (female) sexual interests and characteristics.

bisferious (bis-fe′re-us) dicrotic; having two beats.

bishydroxycoumarin (bis″hi-drok″se-koo′mah-rin) a white crystalline powder, $C_{19}H_{12}O_6$; anticoagulant.

bisiliac (bis-il′e-ak) pertaining to the two ilia.

bis in die (bis in de′a) [L.] twice a day.

bismuth (biz′muth) chemical element (*see table*), at. no. 83, symbol Bi. **b. glycolylarsanilate**, glycobiarsol. **b. potassium tartrate**, a white, granular powder, used in treatment of syphilis. **b. sodium triglycollamate**, a double salt of sodium bismuthyl triglycollamate and disodium triglycollamate, used as a suppressant for lupus erythematosus and in treatment of chronic syphilis. **b. subcarbonate,** a basic salt, Bi_2O_3, used topically in lotions and ointments, and internally as an astringent, protective and adsorbent. **b. subgallate,** bright yellow, amorphous powder, applied locally in skin diseases. **b. subnitrate,** a white, slightly hygroscopic powder, sometimes used as a gastrointestinal astringent. **b. subsalicylate,** white microcrystalline powder; antisyphilitic and gastrointestinal protective. **b. white,** bismuth subnitrate.

bismuthosis (biz″muth-o′sis) the absorption of bismuth and its deposits in the tissues.

bistephanic (bi″stĕ-fan′ik) pertaining to the two stephania.

bistoury (bis′too-re) a long, narrow surgical knife.

Bistrimate (bis′trī-māt) trademark for a preparation of bismuth sodium triglycollamate.

bistrimin (bis′trī-min) phenyltoloxamine.

bisulfate (bi-sul′fāt) an acid sulfate; one with twice the proportion of acid found in a normal sulfate.

bite (bīt) 1. seizure with the teeth. 2. a wound or puncture made by an insect. 3. in dentistry, the occlusion of the teeth, or an imprint of the teeth or gums in some plastic material, used in making artificial dentures. **close b., closed b.,** occlusion in which the lower incisors lie behind, or lingual to, the upper incisors, extending nearly or quite to the gingival margin when the jaw is closed. **cross b.,** crossbite. **end-to-end b.,** occlusion in which the incisors of both jaws meet along their cutting edge when the jaw is closed. **open b.,** occlusion in which the labial teeth cannot be brought together because of occlusal interference of the buccal teeth. **over-b.,** overbite, a condition in which the upper incisor teeth overlap the lower ones when the jaws are closed.

bite-block (bīt′blok) occlusion rim.

bitelock (bīt′lok) a dental device for retaining bite rims in the same relation outside the mouth which they occupied in the mouth.

bitemporal (bi-tem′po-ral) pertaining to both temples or temporal bones.

biteplate (bīt′plāt) an appliance worn in the palate as a diagnostic or therapeutic adjunct in orthodontics or prosthodontics.

bite-rim (bīt′rim) a rim of wax placed on the base plate in an arch such as is described by the teeth as a guide for placing the artificial teeth.

bitewing (bīt′wing) a film used in making roentgenograms of the teeth, having a flange to be held between the jaws and permitting production of images of both the upper and lower teeth.

bitrochanteric (bi-tro″kan-ter′ik) pertaining to both trochanters.

bitumen (bī-too′men) a natural or artificial solid or dry petroleum product.

bituminosis (bī-too″mī-no′sis) a form of pneumoconiosis due to dust from soft coal.

biuret (bi′u-ret) a crystalline urea derivative,

$C_2O_2N_3H_5$, used in testing for urea and proteins.

bivalent (bi-va′lent, biv′ah-lent) having a valency of two.

biventral (bi-ven′tral) having two bellies.

bizygomatic (-zi″go-mat′ik) pertaining to the two zygomatic bones.

Bk chemical symbol, *berkelium.*

black (blak) reflecting no light or true color; of the darkest hue. **ivory b.,** animal charcoal.

blackhead (blak′hed) 1. comedo. 2. infectious enterohepatitis, a disease of fowl due to a protozoan parasite and commonly characterized by cyanosis of the head.

blackleg (blak′leg) an infection of domestic animals due to *Clostridium chauvoei.*

blackout (blak′owt) loss of vision and momentary lapse of consciousness due to diminished circulation to the brain and the retina.

bladder (blad′er) a membranous sac, especially that into which urine drains through the ureters. **chyle b.,** receptaculum chyli. **cord b.,** defective bladder function due to a lesion in the central nervous system. **irritable b.,** sensitivity of bladder marked by constant desire to urinate. **sacculated b.,** bladder with pouches between the hypertrophied muscular fibers. **urinary b.,** the musculomembranous sac in the anterior part of the pelvic cavity that serves as a reservoir for urine.

blast (blast) the wave of air pressure produced by the detonation of high-explosive bombs or shells or by other explosions; it causes pulmonary concussion and hemorrhage (*lung blast, blast chest*), laceration of abdominal viscera, ruptured ear drums and effects on the nervous system.

blastema (blas-te′mah) 1. the primitive substance from which cells are formed. 2. a group of cells that give rise to a new individual or to an organ or part.

blast (blast) word element [Gr.], *immature cell.*

blast(o)- (blas′to) word element [Gr.], *a bud or sprout.*

Blastocaulis (blas″to-kaw′lis) a genus of Schizomycetes (order Hyphomicrobiales, family Pasteuriaceae).

blastocoele (blas′to-sēl) the fluid-filled central segmentation cavity of the blastula. adj., **blastocoe′lic.**

blastocyst (blas′to-sist) the thin-walled cystic blastula produced in development of many mammals, including man.

blastocyte (blas′to-sīt) an undifferentiated embryonic cell.

blastocytoma (blas″to-si-to′mah) a tumor composed of undifferentiated embryonic tissue.

blastoderm (blas′to-derm) 1. the cellular cap at the animal pole of yolk-rich eggs. 2. the disk consisting of the primary germ layers.

blastodisk (blas′to-disk) the convex structure formed by the blastomeres at the animal pole of an ovum undergoing incomplete cleavage.

blastogenesis (blas″to-jen′ĕ-sis) 1. reproduction by budding. 2. transmission of characters by germ plasm.

blastolysis (blas-tol′ĭ-sis) destruction of the germ substance. adj., **blastolyt′ic.**

blastoma (blas-to'mah) 1. a true tumor. 2. blastocytoma. adj., **blasto'matous.**

blastomatosis (blas"to-mah-to'sis) the presence of numerous blastomas.

blastomere (blas'to-mēr) one of the cells produced by cleavage of a fertilized ovum.

Blastomyces (blas"to-mi'sēz) a genus of fungi. **B. brasilien'sis,** the fungus which causes South American blastomycosis. **B. dermatit'-idis,** the fungus which causes North American blastomycosis.

blastomycosis (-mi-ko'sis) infection with Blastomyces. **North American b.,** infection due to *Blastomyces dermatitidis,* predominantly involving the skin (cutaneous), lungs (pulmonary) or bones and other organs as well (systemic). **South American b.,** infection due to *Blastomyces brasiliensis,* involving the skin, respiratory system and other organs.

blastospore (blas'to-spōr) a spore formed by budding from a hypha.

blastozooid (blas"to-zo'oid) an organism that develops from a blastema, i.e. by asexual reproduction.

blastula (blas'tu-lah) the developing ovum subsequent to the morula stage, when it has a fluid-filled central segmentation cavity.

blastulation (blas"tu-la'shun) the formation of the blastula.

bleb (bleb) a blister.

bleeding (blēd'ing) 1. the escape of blood, as from an injured vessel. 2. the purposeful withdrawal of blood from a vessel of the body. **implantation b.,** that occurring at the time of implantation of the fertilized ovum in the uterine wall. **occult b.,** escape of blood in such small quantity that it can be detected only by chemical tests. **placentation b.,** escape of blood from uterine vessels being eroded and tapped by the developing placenta during the early weeks of pregnancy.

blennadenitis (blen"ad-ē-ni'tis) inflammation of mucous glands.

blennogenic (blen"o-jen'ik) producing mucus.

blennoid (blen'oid) resembling mucus.

blennorrhagia (blen"o-ra'je-ah) blennorrhea.

blennorrhea (-re'ah) 1. free discharge of mucus. 2. gonorrhea. adj., **blennorrhe'al.**

blennostasis (blen-nos'tah-sis) diminution of mucous secretion. adj., **blennostat'ic.**

blennothorax (blen"o-tho'raks) mucus in the chest.

blennuria (blen-u're-ah) mucus in the urine.

blephar(o)- (blef'ah-ro) word element [Gr.], *eyelid; eyelash.*

blepharadenitis (blef"ar-ad"ē-ni'tis) blepharoadenitis.

blepharal (blef'ar-al) pertaining to the eyelids.

blepharectomy (blef"ar-ek'to-me) excision of an eyelid.

blepharism (blef'ah-rizm) spasm of the eyelid.

blepharitis (blef"ah-ri'tis) inflammation of the edges of the lid margins. **angular b.,** inflammation involving the outer angle or, less frequently, the inner angle of the eyelids. **squamous b.,** seborrhea of lid margins, with formation of little plates of dried secretion on the eyelashes. **ulcerative b.,** a condition

characterized by loss of eyelashes and appearance of small ulcerated pockets on the lid margin.

blepharo-adenitis (blef"ah-ro-ad"ē-ni'tis) inflammation of the meibomian glands of the eyelids.

blepharo-atheroma (-ath"er-o'mah) encysted tumor of an eyelid.

blepharochalasis (-kal'ah-sis) acquired atrophy of the skin of the upper eyelid.

blepharoconjunctivitis (-kon-junk"tī-vi'tis) inflammation of eyelids and conjunctiva.

blepharoncus (blef"ar-ong'kus) a tumor on the eyelid.

blepharophimosis (blef"ah-ro-fi-mo'sis) diminution in the overall size of the opening between the eyelids.

blepharoplast (blef'ah-ro-plast") a body in a cell giving rise to a flagellum.

blepharoplasty (blef'ah-ro-plas"te) plastic repair of an eyelid.

blepharoplegia (blef"ah-ro-ple'je-ah) paralysis of an eyelid.

blepharoptosis (blef"ar-op-to'sis) drooping of an upper eyelid.

blepharopyorrhea (blef"ah-ro-pi"ŏ-re'ah) purulent ophthalmia.

blepharorrhaphy (blef"ah-ror'ah-fe) suture of an eyelid.

blepharospasm (blef'ah-ro-spazm") spasm of the orbicular muscle of the eyelids.

blepharostat (blef'ah-ro-stat") an instrument for holding the eyelids apart.

blepharostenosis (blef"ah-ro-ste-no'sis) blepharophimosis.

blepharosynechia (-sī-nek'e-ah) growing together of the eyelids.

blepharotomy (blef"ah-rot'o-me) incision of an eyelid.

blindness (blīnd'nes) lack or loss of visual perception. **color b.,** popular term for any deviation from normal perception of color. **day b.,** defective vision in conditions of bright illumination. **epidemic b.,** a form of avian leukosis with blindness and misshapen pupil or irregular depigmentation of the iris in one or both eyes. **flight b.,** blackout. **letter b.,** inability to recognize individual letters. **mind b.,** psychic blindness. **moon b.,** periodic ophthalmia. **night b.,** defective vision in conditions of diminished illumination. **note b.,** inability to read musical notes because of a brain lesion. **object b.,** inability to recognize objects on sight due to a brain lesion. **psychic b.,** failure of proper interpretation of visual stimuli due to a brain lesion. **snow b.,** defect of vision caused by exposure to the glare of sun upon snow. **text b., word b.,** visual aphasia.

blister (blis'ter) a collection of serous, bloody or watery fluid under the skin. **fever b.,** coldsore.

bloat (blōt) 1. a disorder of ruminants characterized by distention of the stomach with gas. 2. enteritis in young rabbits, accompanied by gaseous distention of the abdomen.

block (blok) 1. an obstruction or stoppage. 2. regional anesthesia. **bundle-branch b.,** see under *heart block.* **field b.,** production of anesthesia in an area by injection of an anesthetic agent at points around its perimeter. **heart b.,** see *heart block.* **mental b.,** obstruction to thought or memory, particularly that produced by emotional factors. **nerve b.,** interruption of transmission of impulses by injection of an anesthetic agent in close proximity to a nerve. **paravertebral b.,** infiltration of the stellate ganglion with procaine hydrochloride.

Blockain (blok′ăn) trademark for a preparation of propoxycaine hydrochloride.

blocking (blok′ing) 1. interruption of an afferent nerve pathway, as by injection of an anesthetic. 2. repression of an idea from consciousness due to mental conflict.

blood (blud) the fluid which circulates through the heart, arteries and veins. **aerated b., arterial b.,** that which carries oxygen to the tissues through the systemic arteries. **central b.,** blood from the pulmonary venous system; sometimes applied to blood obtained from chambers of the heart or from bone marrow. **cord b.,** that contained in umbilical vessels at time of delivery of the fetus. **defibrinated b.,** blood incapable of clotting because the fibrin has been removed. **occult b.,** that which has escaped from tissues in such small amounts as to be detectible only by chemical tests. **peripheral b.,** that circulating through vessels remote from the heart. **splanchnic b.,** that circulating in thoracic, abdominal and pelvic viscera, further distinguished on the basis of specific organ, e.g. pulmonary, hepatic, splenic. **venous b.,** blood that has given up its oxygen to the tissues and is carrying carbon dioxide back through the systemic veins, to be exchanged in the lungs. **whole b.,** that from which none of the elements has been removed.

blood type (blud′tīp) 1. the phenotype of erythrocytes defined by one or more antigenic determinants controlled by allelic genes. 2. any characteristic, function or trait of a cellular or fluid component of blood, regarded as the expression (phenotype) of the actions and interactions of dominant genes, and useful in medicolegal and other studies of human inheritance.

blowpipe (blo′pīp) a tube through which a current of air is forced upon a flame to concentrate and intensify the heat.

B.L.R.O.A. British Laryngological, Rhinological, and Otological Association.

blue (blu) 1. the color of the visible spectrum with wavelength of 467–481 mμ, lying between green and violet. 2. a dye of blue color. **Berlin b.,** ferric ferrocyanide. **Evans b.,** an odorless green, bluish green or brown powder, used as a diagnostic aid in estimation of blood volume. **indigo b.,** a neutral tasteless, insoluble, dark blue powder, $C_{16}H_{10}N_2O_2$. **methylene b.,** a synthetic organic compound, in dark green crystals or lustrous crystalline powder, used as an antidote in cyanide poisoning. **Prussian b.,** ferric ferrocyanide. **toluidine b.,** a stain used to demonstrate basophilic and metachromatic substances.

Blutene (bloo′tēn) trademark for a preparation of tolonium.

B.M.A. British Medical Association.

B.M.R. basal metabolic rate.

BNA Basle Nomina Anatomica, a system of anatomic nomenclature adopted at the annual meeting of the German Anatomic Society in 1895.

B.O.A. British Orthopaedic Association.

body (bod′e) 1. a mass of matter. 2. the trunk of a vertebrate animal, considered apart from the limbs. **acetone b's,** ketone bodies. **alloxur b's,** purine bases. **amylaceous b's,** corpora amylacea. **Arantius b.,** a small tubercle at the middle of the free edge of each of the three cusps of the aortic and pulmonary valves. **Aschoff's b's,** microscopic foci of fibrinoid degeneration and granulomatous inflammation, characteristically found in various tissues in rheumatic fever. **asteroid b.,** an irregularly star-shaped inclusion body found in the giant cells in sarcoidosis and other diseases. **Auer's b's,** rod-shaped bodies in the lymphocytes in leukemia. **Babes-Ernst b's,** metachromatic granules. **Barr b.,** a mass of chromatin situated at the periphery of the nucleus of cells of normal females, but not observed in those of normal males, derived from an inactive X chromosome. **bigeminal b.,** one of the embryonic structures which develop into the corpora quadrigemina. **Cabot's ring b's,** loops or figures-of-8 seen in stained erythrocytes in anemia. **carotid b's,** masses of chromaffin cells located on the wall of each internal carotid artery. **cavernous b's,** corpora cavernosa. **cell b.,** the portion of a cell containing the nucleus independent of any projections the cell may have. **chromaffin b.,** paraganglion. **ciliary b.,** the thickened part of the vascular tunic of the eye, connecting choroid and iris. **crescent b., demilune b.,** achromocyte. **dentate b., denticulate b.,** dentate nucleus. **Döhle's inclusion b's,** bodies staining less darkly than the nuclei, seen in neutrophil leukocytes in scarlet fever and other infections. **elementary b.,** 1. a blood platelet. 2. an inclusion body. **fimbriate b.,** corpus fimbriatum. **foreign b.,** a mass of material which is not normal to the place where it is found. **geniculate b.,** corpus geniculatum. **geniculate b's, lateral,** two forebrain eminences, one on each side, marking the termination of the optic tract. **geniculate b's, medial,** two forebrain eminences, one on each side of the midbrain, concerned with hearing. **Gordon's b's,** bodies found in the lesions of Hodgkin's disease. **Hassall's b's,** see under *corpuscle.* **Heinz b's, Heinz-Ehrlich b's,** intracorpuscular structures resulting from oxidative injury to and polymerization of denatured hemoglobin. **Highmore's b.,** mediastinum testis. **Howell b's, Howell-Jolly b's,** small, round or oval bodies seen in erythrocytes when stains are added to fresh blood. **hyaloid b.,** vitreous humor. **immune b.,** amboceptor. **inclusion b's,** particles contained within the cell. **intermediary b.,** amboceptor. **ketone b's,** intermediate products of fat metabolism, including acetone, acetoacetic acid and beta-oxybutyric acid. **Langerhans b's,** islands of Langerhans. **Laveran's b's,** plasmodia of malaria. **Leishman-Donovan b's,** oval bodies found in the spleen in chronic dysentery, adynamic fever and malarial cachexia. **Lieutaud's b.,** the trigone of the bladder. **malpighian b,** malpighian corpuscle. **mamillary b's,** two small eminences on the inferior surface of the forebrain behind the site of attachment of the stalk of the hypophysis. **metachromatic b's,** see under *granule.* **Negri b's,** oval or round bodies in the nerve cells of animals dead of hydrophobia. **Nissl b's,** Nissl substance. **olivary b's,** oval prominences on the sides of the anterior pyramids of the medulla oblongata. **pacchionian b's,** small eminences of arachnoid tissue under the dura mater of the brain. **parabasal b.,** a structure usually closely associated with the nucleus of a protozoan and connected with the basal granule. **parolivary b's,** gray masses on dorsal and mesial surfaces of the dentate nucleus. **pineal b.,** a small, conical structure attached by a stalk to the posterior wall of the third ventricle. **pituitary b.,** hypophysis cerebri. **polar b's,** rudimentary ova produced by mitosis in the development of a mature, functional ovum. **psammoma b.,** a spherical, laminated mass of calcareous material occurring in both benign and malignant epithelial and connective-tissue tumors, and sometimes associated with chronic inflammation. **quadrigeminal b's,** corpora quadrigemina. **restiform b.,** lateral column of medulla oblongata extending to cerebellum. **Rosenmüller's b.,** parovarium. **Russell's b's,** small vacuolated bodies seen in cancer. **Seidelin b's,** bodies found in the red corpuscles in yellow fever. **Spengler's immune b's,** immune bodies extracted from the red blood corpuscles of animals immunized against tuberculosis. **spongy b.,** corpus spongiosum. **striate b's,** corpora striata. **suprarenal b.,** adrenal gland. **thyroid b.,** see *thyroid.* **tigroid b's,** Nissl substance. **trachoma b's,** minute bodies in the epithelial cells of the conjunctiva in trachoma. **vitelline b.,** yolk nucleus. **vitreous b.,** the gelatinous mass filling the posterior four fifths of the eyeball, behind the diaphragm formed by the lens and ciliary body. **wolffian b.,** mesonephros.

B.O.E.A. ethyl biscoumacetate.

boil (boil) furuncle. **Delhi b., Natal b., Oriental b.,** cutaneous leishmaniasis.

bolometer (bo-lom'ĕ-ter) 1. an instrument for measuring the force of the heart beat. 2. an instrument for measuring minute degrees of radiant heat.

boloscope (bo'lo-skōp) an apparatus for locating metallic foreign bodies in the tissues.

bolus (bo'lus) a rounded mass, such as (*a*) a large pill, (*b*) a quantity of food entering the esophagus at one swallow, (*c*) a quantity of opaque medium introduced into an artery at one time in arteriography, (*d*) a cushion used in bolstering the position of a patient for

radiography, or (*e*) a rounded pad used to apply pressure to a wound. **alimentary b.,** the mass of food, made ready by mastication, which enters the esophagus at one swallow.

bond (bond) the linkage between atoms or radicals of a chemical compound, or the symbol representing this linkage and indicating the valence of the atoms or radicals, as H.O.H or H – O – H; Ca:O or Ca = O; HC:CH or HC≡CH.

bone (bōn) 1. the hard, tough, elastic material which forms the skeleton of vertebrate animals, composed principally of calcium salts. 2. one of the individual segments of which the vertebrate skeleton is composed, in the adult human body numbering 206. (*See the table for regional listing and alphabetical listing of common names of various bones of the body.*) **ankle b.,** talus. **basiotic b.,** a small bone in the fetus between the basilar process and the basisphenoid. **brittle b's,** fragilitas ossium. **cancellous b.,** bone containing many empty spaces, the calcified matrix being arranged in trabeculae rather than lamellae. **carpal b.,** one of the eight bones composing the carpus. **cartilage b.,** bone which replaces a provisional cartilaginous model. **cavalry b.,** bony formation in the adductor magnus femoris. **cheek b.,** zygoma. **coffin b.,** the third phalanx of the horse's hoof. **compact b.,** bone containing no empty spaces, being made up of lamellae which fit closely together. **ear b's,** the incus, malleus and stapes. **exercise b.,** a bony growth in muscle due to exercise or pressure. **flat b.,** one of greater width and length than thickness, often consisting of two layers of compact bone separated by a layer of cancellous bone and usually bent or curved. **haunch b.,** ilium. **heel b.,** calcaneus. **hip b.,** the bone to which the legs are attached. **incisive b.,** a separate bone in the upper jaw of the fetus which later fuses with the maxilla on either side. **innominate b.,** coxa. **jaw b.,** mandible or maxilla, especially the mandible. **jugal b.,** zygoma. **lingual b.,** hyoid. **long b.,** one whose length far exceeds its breadth and thickness. **malar b.,** zygoma. **marble b's,** osteopetrosis. **mastoid b.,** the mastoid process of the temporal bone. **membrane b.,** bone which develops directly within sheets of mesenchyme. **metacarpal b.,** one of the five bones composing the metacarpus. **metatarsal b.,** one of the five bones composing the metatarsus. **pelvic b.,** coxa. **petrous b.,** the petrous portion of the temporal bone. **pneumatic b.,** bone that contains air-filled spaces. **premaxillary b.,** incisive bone. **pterygoid b.,** pterygoid process. **pubic b.,** pubis. **pyramidal b.,** triquetrum. **rider's b.,** cavalry bone. **semilunar b.,** lunate. **sesamoid b's,** small bones embedded in tendons or joint capsules, occurring mainly in hands and feet. **shin b.,** tibia. **short b.,** one of approximately equal length, width and thickness. **solid b.,** compact bone. **spongy b.,** cancellous bone. **squamous b.,** the upper forepart of the temporal bone, forming an upright plate. **supraoccipital b.,** the part of

TABLE OF BONES, LISTED BY REGIONS OF THE BODY

REGION	NAME	TOTAL NUMBER
Axial skeleton		
Skull		21
	(eight paired — 16)	
	inferior nasal concha	
	lacrimal	
	maxilla	
	nasal	
	palatine	
	parietal	
	temporal	
	zygomatic	
	(five unpaired — 5)	
	ethmoid	
	frontal	
	occipital	
	sphenoid	
	vomer	
Ossicles of each ear	incus	6
	malleus	
	stapes	
Lower jaw	mandible	1
Neck	hyoid	1
Vertebral column		26
	cervical vertebrae (7)	
	(atlas)	
	(axis)	
	thoracic vertebrae (12)	
	lumbar vertebrae (5)	
	sacrum (5 fused)	
	coccyx (4–5 fused)	
Chest		
	sternum	1
	ribs (12 pairs)	24

REGION	NAME	TOTAL NUMBER
Upper limb (×2)		64
Shoulder	scapula	
	clavicle	
Upper arm	humerus	
Lower arm	radius	
	ulna	
	carpal (8)	
Wrist	(capitate)	
	(hamate)	
	(lunate)	
	(pisiform)	
	(scaphoid)	
	(trapezium)	
	(trapezoid)	
	(triquetral)	
Hand	metacarpal (5)	
Fingers	phalanges (14)	
Lower limb (×2)		62
Pelvis	os coxa (1)	
	(ilium)	
	(ischium)	
	(pubis)	
Thigh	femur	
Knee	patella	
Leg	tibia	
	fibula	
	tarsal (7)	
Ankle	(calcaneus)	
	(cuboid)	
	(cuneiform, medial)	
	(cuneiform, intermediate)	
	(cuneiform, lateral)	
	(navicular)	
	(talus)	
Foot	metatarsal (5)	
Toes	phalanges (14)	

TABLE OF BONES

COMMON NAME*	NA EQUIVALENT†	REGION	DESCRIPTION	ARTICULATIONS
astragalus. see *talus*				
atlas	atlas	neck	first cervical vertebra, ring of bone supporting the skull	with occipital b. and axis
axis	axis	neck	second cervical vertebra, with thick process (dens) around which first cervical vertebra pivots	with atlas above and third cervical vertebra below
calcaneus	calcaneus	foot	the "heel bone," of irregularly cuboidal shape, largest of the tarsal bones	with talus and cuboid b.
capitate b.	o. capitatum	wrist	third from thumb side of 4 bones of distal row of carpal b's.	with second, third and fourth metacarpal b's, and hamate, lunate, trapezoid and scaphoid b's
carpal b's	oss. carpi	wrist	see *capitate, hamate, lunate, pisiform, scaphoid, trapezium, trapezoid and triquetral* (b.)	
clavicle	clavicula	shoulder	elongated, slender, curved bone (collar bone) lying horizontally at root of neck, in upper part of thorax	with sternum and ipsilateral scapula and cartilage of first rib
coccyx	o. coccygis	lower back	triangular bone formed usually by fusion of last 4 (sometimes 3 or 5) (coccygeal) vertebrae	with sacrum
concha, inferior nasal	concha nasalis inferior	skull	thin, rough plate of bone attached by one edge to side of each nasal cavity, the free edge curling downward	with ethmoid and ipsilateral lacrimal and palatine b's and maxilla
cuboid b.	o. cuboideum	foot	pyramidal bone, on lateral side of foot, in front of calcaneus	with calcaneus, lateral cuneiform b., fourth and fifth metatarsal b's, occasionally with navicular b.
cuneiform b., intermediate	o. cuneiforme intermedium	foot	smallest of 3 cuneiform b's, located between medial and lateral cuneiform b's	with navicular, medial and lateral cuneiform b's and second metatarsal b.
cuneiform b., lateral	o. cuneiforme laterale	foot	wedge-shaped bone at lateral side of foot, intermediate in size between medial and intermediate cuneiform b's	with cuboid, navicular, intermediate cuneiform b's and second, third and fourth metatarsal b's

94

*b. = bone; b's = (pl.) bones.
†o. = os; oss. = (L. pl.) ossa.

cuneiform b., medial	o. cuneiforme mediale	foot	largest of 3 cuneiform b's, at medial side of foot
epistropheus. see *axis*			
ethmoid b.	o. ethmoidale	skull	unpaired bone in front of sphenoid b. and below frontal b., forming part of nasal septum and superior and medial conchae of nose	with sphenoid and frontal b's, vomer, and both lacrimal, nasal and palatine b's, maxillae and inferior nasal conchae
fabella		knee	sesamoid b. in lateral head of gastrocnemius muscle	
femur	femur	thigh	longest, strongest, heaviest bone of the body (thigh b.)	proximally with hip b., distally with patella and tibia
fibula	fibula	leg	lateral and smaller of 2 bones of leg	proximally with tibia, distally with tibia and talus
frontal b.	o. frontale	skull	unpaired bone constituting anterior part of skull	with ethmoid and sphenoid b's, and both parietal, nasal, lacrimal and zygomatic b's and maxillae
hamate b.	o. hamatum	wrist	most medial of 4 bones of distal row of carpal b's	with fourth and fifth metacarpal b's and lunate, capitate and triquetral b's
hip b.	o. coxae	pelvis and hip	broadest bone of skeleton, composed orginally of 3 bones which become fused together in acetabulum: *ilium*, broad, flaring, uppermost portion; *ischium*, thick, three-sided part behind and below acetabulum and behind obturator foramen; *os pubis*, consisting of body (expanded anterior portion), inferior ramus (extending backward and fusing with ramus of ischium) and superior ramus (extending from body to acetabulum)	with femur, anteriorly with its fellow (at symphysis pubis), posteriorly with sacrum
humerus	humerus	arm	long bone of upper arm	proximally with scapula, distally with radius and ulna
hyoid b.	o. hyoideum	neck	U-shaped bone at root of tongue, between mandible and larynx	none; attached by ligaments and muscles to skull and larynx
ilium	o. ilium	pelvis	see *hip b.*	
incus	incus	ear	middle ossicle of chain in the middle ear, so named because of its resemblance to an anvil	with malleus and stapes
innominate b. see *hip b.*			
ischium	o. ischii	pelvis	see *hip b.*	
lacrimal b.	o. lacrimale	skull	thin, uneven scale of bone near rim of medial wall of each orbit	with ethmoid and frontal b's, and ipsilateral inferior nasal concha and maxilla

TABLE OF BONES—Continued

COMMON NAME*	NA EQUIVALENT†	REGION	DESCRIPTION	ARTICULATIONS
lunate b.	o. lunatum	wrist	second from thumb side of 4 bones of proximal row of carpus	with radius, and capitate, hamate, scaphoid and triquetral b's
malleus	malleus	ear	most lateral ossicle of chain in middle ear, so named because of its resemblance to a hammer	with incus; fibrous attachment to tympanic membrane
mandible	mandibula	lower jaw	horseshoe-shaped bone carrying lower teeth	with temporal b's
maxilla	maxilla	skull (upper jaw)	paired bone, below orbit and at either side of nasal cavity, carrying upper teeth	with ethmoid and frontal b's, vomer, fellow maxilla, and ipsilateral inferior nasal concha and lacrimal, nasal, palatine and zygomatic b's
maxilla, inferior. see *mandible* maxilla, superior. see *maxilla*				
metacarpal b's	oss. metacarpalia	hand	five miniature long bones of hand proper, slightly concave on palmar surface	first—trapezium and proximal phalanx of thumb; second—third metacarpal b., trapezium, trapezoid, capitate and proximal phalanx of index finger (second digit); third—second and fourth metacarpal b's, capitate and proximal phalanx of middle finger (third digit); fourth—third and fifth metacarpal b's, capitate, hamate and proximal phalanx of ring finger (fourth digit); fifth—fourth metacarpal b., hamate b. and proximal phalanx of little finger (fifth digit)
metatarsal b's	oss. metatarsalia	foot	five miniature long bones of foot, concave on plantar and slightly convex on dorsal surface	first—medial cuneiform b., proximal phalanx of great toe, and occasionally with second metatarsal b.; second—medial, intermediate and lateral cuneiform b's, third and occasionally with first metatarsal b. and proximal phalanx of second toe; third—lateral cuneiform b., second and fourth metatarsal b's and proximal phalanx of third toe; fourth—lateral cuneiform b., cuboid b., third and fifth metatarsal b's and proximal phalanx of fourth toe; fifth—cuboid b., fourth metatarsal b. and proximal phalanx of fifth toe

Term	Location	Description
multangulum majus. see *trapezium*; *trapezoid*		
nasal b.	skull	paired bone, the two uniting in median plane to form bridge of nose; with frontal and ethmoid b's, fellow of opposite side and ipsilateral maxilla
o. nasale		
navicular b.	foot	bone at medial side of tarsus, between talus and cuneiform b's; with talus and 3 cuneiform b's, occasionally with cuboid b.
o. naviculare		
occipital b.	skull	unpaired bone constituting back and part of base of skull; with sphenoid b. and atlas and both parietal and temporal b's
o. occipitale		
os magnum. see *capitate b.*		
palatine b.	skull	paired bone, the two forming posterior portion of bony palate; with ethmoid and sphenoid b's, vomer, fellow of opposite side, and ipsilateral inferior nasal concha and maxilla
o. palatinum		
parietal b.	skull	paired bone between frontal and occipital b's, forming superior and lateral parts of skull; with frontal, occipital, sphenoid, fellow parietal and ipsilateral temporal b's
o. parietale		
patella	knee	small, irregularly rectangular compressed (sesamoid) bone over anterior aspect of knee (kneecap); with femur
patella		
phalanges (proximal middle and distal phalanges)	fingers and toes	miniature long bones, two only in thumb and great toe, three in each of other fingers and toes; proximal phalanx of each digit with corresponding metacarpal or metatarsal b., and phalanx distal to it; other phalanges with phalanges proximal and distal (if any) to them
oss. digitorum (phalanx proximalis, phalanx media and phalanx distalis)		
pisiform b.	wrist	medial and palmar of 4 bones of proximal row of carpal b's; with triquetral b.
o. pisiforme		
pubic b.	pelvis	see *hip b's*
o. pubis		
radius	forearm	lateral and shorter of 2 bones of forearm; proximally with humerus and ulna, distally with ulna and lunate and scaphoid b's
radius		
ribs	chest	12 pairs of thin, narrow, curved long bones, forming posterior and lateral walls of chest; all posteriorly with thoracic vertebrae; upper 7 pairs (true ribs) with sternum; lower 5 pairs (false ribs) by costal cartilages, with rib above or lowest 2 — floating ribs) unattached anteriorly
costae		
sacrum	lower back	wedge-shaped bone formed usually by fusion of 5 vertebrae below lumbar vertebrae; with fifth lumbar vertebra above, coccyx below, and with ilium at each side
o. sacrum		
scaphoid	wrist	most lateral of 4 bones of proximal row of carpal b's; with radius, trapezium and trapezoid, capitate and lunate b's
o. scaphoideum		

TABLE OF BONES—*Continued*

COMMON NAME*	NA EQUIVALENT†	REGION	DESCRIPTION	ARTICULATIONS
scapula	scapula	shoulder	wide, thin, triangular bone (shoulder blade) opposite second to seventh ribs in upper part of back	with ipsilateral clavicle and humerus
sesamoid b's	oss. sesamoidea	chiefly hands and feet	small, flat, round bones related to joints between phalanges or between digits and metacarpal or metatarsal b's; include also 2 at knee (fabella and patella)	
sphenoid b.	o. sphenoidale	base of skull	unpaired, irregularly shaped bone, constituting part of sides and base of skull and part of lateral wall of orbit	with frontal, occipital and ethmoid b's, vomer and both parietal, temporal, palatine and zygomatic b's
stapes	stapes	ear	most medial ossicle of chain in middle ear, so named because of its resemblance to a stirrup	with incus; ligamentous attachment to vestibuli
sternum	sternum	chest	elongated flat bone, forming anterior wall of chest, consisting of 3 segments: *manubrium* (topmost segment), *body* (in youth composed of 4 separate segments joined by cartilage) and *xiphoid process* (lowermost segment)	with both clavicles and upper 7 pairs of ribs
talus	talus	ankle	the "ankle bone," second largest of tarsal b's	with tibia, fibula, calcaneus and navicular b.
tarsal b's	oss. tarsi	ankle and foot	see *calcaneus, cuboid, intermediate, lateral* and *medial cuneiform b's, navicular b.* and *talus*	
temporal b.	o. temporale	skull	irregularly shaped bone, one on either side, forming part of side and base of skull, and containing middle and inner ear	with occipital, sphenoid, mandible, and ipsilateral parietal and zygomatic b's
tibia	tibia	leg	medial and larger of 2 bones of lower leg (shin b.)	proximally with femur and fibula, distally with talus and fibula
trapezium	o. trapezium	wrist	most lateral of 4 bones of distal row of carpal b's	with first and second metacarpal b's and trapezoid and scaphoid b's
trapezoid b.	o. trapezoideum	wrist	second from thumb side of 4 bones of distal row of carpal b's	with second metacarpal b. and capitate, trapezium and scaphoid b's
triquetral b.	o. triquetrum	wrist	third from thumb side of 4 bones of proximal row of carpal b's	with hamate, lunate and pisiform b's and articular disk

turbinate b., inferior.
see *concha, infe-*
rior, nasal

ulna	ulna	forearm	medial and longer of 2 bones of forearm

proximally with humerus and radius, distally
with radius and articular disk

vertebrae (cervical, thoracic [dorsal], lumbar, sacral and coccygeal)	vertebrae (vertebrae cervicales, vertebrae thoracicae, vertebrae lumbales, vertebrae sacrales, vertebrae coccygeae)	back	separate segments of vertebral column; about 33 in the child; uppermost 24 remain separate as true, movable vertebrae; the next 5 fuse to form the sacrum; the lowermost 3-5 fuse to form the coccyx

each first cervical (atlas) and fifth lumbar,
each vertebra articulates with adjoining
vertebrae above and below; the first cervical
articulates with the occipital b. and second
cervical vertebra (axis); the fifth lumbar
with the fourth lumbar vertebra and sacrum; the thoracic vertebrae articulate also
with the heads of the ribs

vomer	vomer	skull	thin bone forming posterior and posteroinferior part of nasal septum

with ethmoid and sphenoid b's and both maxillae and palatine b's

zygomatic b.	o. zygomaticum	skull	bone forming hard part of cheek and lower, lateral portion of rim of each orbit

with frontal and sphenoid b's and ipsilateral
maxilla and temporal b.

99

the occipital bone behind the foramen magnum, distinct in early childhood. **sutural b's,** variable and irregularly shaped bones in the sutures between the bones of the skull. **tarsal b.,** one of the seven bones composing the tarsus. **thigh b.,** femur. **triangular b.,** triquetral. **turbinated b.,** see *concha nasalis.* **tympanic b.,** the part of the temporal bone surrounding the middle ear. **unciform b.,** hamate. **wormian b's,** sutural bones.

bonelet (bōn′let) an ossicle, or small bone.

Bonine (bo′nēn) trademark for preparations of meclizine hydrochloride.

Boophilus (bo-of′i-lus) a genus of ticks (family Ixodidae) primarily parasitic on cattle. **B. annula′tus,** a species which formerly transmitted the organism causing cattle fever, but which has now been eradicated from the United States. **B. bo′vis,** the medium of transmission of the microbe of Texas cattle fever. **B. decolora′tus,** a species found in South Africa. **B. mi′croplus,** a species closely related to *B. annulatus* and still found in the United States, Mexico, and Central and South America.

boot (boot) a covering for the foot. **Gibney b.,** an adhesive tape support used in treatment of sprains and other painful conditions of the ankle, the tape being applied in a basket-weave fashion with strips placed alternately under the sole of the foot and around the back of the leg.

borate (bo′rāt) a salt of boric acid.

borax (bo′raks) sodium borate.

borborygmus (bor″bor-ig′mus) the sound of flatus in the intestines.

Bordetella (bor″dĕ-tel′lah) a genus of Schizomycetes (order Eubacteriales, family Brucellaceae). **B. bronchisep′tica,** a common cause of bronchopneumonia in small animals. **B. parapertus′sis,** the causative agent of parapertussis. **B. pertus′sis,** the causative agent of whooping cough (pertussis).

borism (bo′rizm) poisoning by a boron compound.

boron (bo′ron) chemical element *(see table),* at. no. 5, symbol B.

Borrelia (bo-rel′e-ah) a genus of Schizomycetes (order Spirochaetales, family Treponemataceae). **B. anseri′na,** a species transmitted by arthropods and causing a fatal disease in chickens, turkeys and pheasants. **B. recurren′tis,** the causative agent of relapsing fever, transmitted by the human body louse. **B. vincen′tii,** a species occurring in large numbers with a fusiform bacillus in Vincent's angina.

boss (bos) a rounded eminence.

bosselated (bos′ĕ-lāt″ed) covered with bosses.

bot (bot) the larva of a botfly or gadfly; different species characteristically infect different species of animals.

Bothriocephalus (both″re-o-sef′ah-lus) Diphyllobothrium.

botryoid (bot′re-oid) shaped like a bunch of grapes.

botryotherapy (bot″re-o-ther′ah-pe) the grape cure.

bottle (bot′l) a hollow vessel with a narrow mouth or neck, and no handles. **wash b.,** a laboratory vessel of glass, designed with two tubes which permit the inflow and discharge of a wash liquid.

botuliform (bot-u′li-form) sausage-shaped.

botulin (bot′u-lin) a toxin sometimes found in imperfectly preserved or canned meats and vegetables.

botulism (bot′u-lizm) poisoning by toxins produced by *Clostridium botulinum.*

bougie (boo′zhe) a long instrument for introduction, usually through a natural orifice, into a body channel such as the esophagus or urethra for the purpose of dilating its lumen. **armed b.,** a bougie with a piece of caustic attached to its end. **bulbous b.,** a bougie with a bulb-shaped tip. **filiform b.,** a bougie of very small diameter. **soluble b.,** bougie composed of a substance that becomes fluid at body temperature.

bougienage (boo″zhĕ-nahzh′) passage of a bougie.

bouquet (boo-ka′) a structure resembling a cluster of flowers.

bourbonal (boor′bo-nal) ethyl vanillin.

bouton (boo-taw′) [Fr.] a knoblike swelling or enlargement. **b. de Biskra, b. d'orient,** cutaneous leishmaniasis. **b's terminaux,** knoblike terminal enlargements on the end of unmyelinated nerve fibers in relation to dendrites of another cell.

bowel (bow′el) the intestine.

bowlegs (bo′legz) a deformity in which the space between the knees is abnormally large.

B.P. 1. blood pressure; boiling point; buccopulpal. 2. British Pharmacopoeia, a publication of the General Medical Council, describing and establishing standards for medicines, preparations, materials and articles used in the practice of medicine, surgery or midwifery.

B.P.A. British Paediatric Association.

Br chemical symbol, *bromine.*

brachi(o)- (bra′ke-o) word element [L., Gr.], *arm.*

brachial (bra′ke-al) pertaining to the arm.

brachialgia (bra″ke-al′je-ah) pain in the arm.

brachiation (-a′shun) locomotion in a position of suspension by means of the hands and arms, as by monkeys swinging from branch to branch.

brachiocephalic (-o-sĕ-fal′ik) pertaining to arm and head.

brachiocrural (-kroo′ral) pertaining to arm and leg.

brachiocubital (-ku′bĭ-tal) pertaining to arm and forearm.

brachiocyllosis (-sil-lo′sis) crookedness of the arm.

brachium (bra′ke-um), pl. *bra′chia* [L.] the arm. **b. cerebel′li,** brachium conjunctivum. **b. collic′uli inferio′ris,** fibers of the auditory pathway connecting the inferior quadrigeminal body to the medial geniculate body. **b. collic′uli superio′ris,** fibers connecting the optic tract and lateral geniculate body with the superior quadrigeminal body. **b. conjunc-ti′vum** [BNA], the superior peduncle of the cerebellum, a fibrous band extending from each hemisphere of the cerebellum upward over the pons, the two joining to form the sides and part of the roof of the fourth ventricle. **b. op'ticum,** one of the processes extending from the corpora quadrigemina to the optic thalamus. **b. pon'tis** [BNA], the brachium of the pons; the middle peduncle of the cerebellum.

brachy- (brak'e) word element [Gr.], *short.*

brachybasia (brak″e-ba′ze-ah) a slow, shuffling, short-stepped gait.

brachycardia (-kar'de-ah) bradycardia.

brachycephalia (-sĕ-fa'lc-ah) brachycephaly.

brachycephalic (-sĕ-fal'ik) having a cephalic index over 80.

brachycephaly (-sef'ah-le) anteroposterior shortening and increased height of the skull.

brachycheilia (-ki'le-ah) shortness of the lip.

brachydactylia (-dak-til'e-ah) abnormal shortness of fingers and toes.

brachygnathia (brak″ig-na'the-ah) abnormal shortness of the mandible.

brachymetacarpalism (brak″e-met″ah-kar'pal-izm) brachymetacarpia.

brachymetacarpia (-met″ah-kar'pe-ah) abnormal shortness of the metacarpal bones.

brachymetatarsia (-met″ah-tar'se-ah) abnormal shortness of the metatarsal bones.

brachymetropia (-mĕ-tro'pe-ah) myopia. adj., **brachymetrop'ic.**

brachyphalangia (fah·lan'je·ah) abnormal shortness of one of the phalanges.

brachytherapy (-ther'ah-pe) treatment with ionizing radiation whose source is applied to the surface of the body or located a short distance from the area being treated.

brachyuranic (-u-ran'ik) having a short palate.

brady- (brad'e) word element [Gr.], *slow.*

bradyacusia (brad″e-ah-ku'ze-ah) dullness of hearing.

bradyarthria (-ar'thre-ah) abnormal slowness in vocal articulation.

bradycardia (-kar'de-ah) abnormal slowness of the heart rate and pulse. adj., **bradycar'diac.**

bradycinesia (-si-ne'ze-ah) bradykinesia.

bradydiastolia (-di″as-to'le-ah) abnormal prolongation of the diastole.

bradyecoia (-e-koi'ah) partial deafness.

bradyesthesia (-es-the'ze-ah) dullness of perception.

bradygenesis (-jen'ĕ-sis) abnormal lengthening of certain stages in embryonic development.

bradyglossia (-glos'e-ah) abnormal slowness of utterance.

bradykinesia (-ki-ne'ze-ah) abnormal slowness of movement. adj., **bradykinet'ic.**

bradykinin (-ki'nin) a kinin composed of a chain of amino acids liberated by the action of trypsin or certain snake venoms on a globulin of blood plasma.

bradylalia (-la'le-ah) slow utterance due to a central lesion.

bradylexia (-lek'se-ah) abnormal slowness in reading.

bradylogia (-lo'je-ah) abnormal slowness of speech.

bradymenorrhea (-men″o-re'ah) menstruation of unusually long duration.

bradypepsia (-pep'se-ah) abnormally slow digestion.

bradyphagia (-fa'je-ah) abnormal slowness of eating.

bradyphasia (-fa'ze-ah) slow utterance of speech.

bradyphemia (-fe'me-ah) slowness of speech.

bradyphrasia (-fra'ze-ah) slowness of speech due to mental defect.

bradypnea (-ne'ah) abnormal slowness of breathing.

bradyspermatism (-sper'mah-tizm) abnormally slow ejaculation of semen.

bradysphygmia (-sfig'me-ah) abnormal slowness of the pulse.

bradystalsis (-stal'sis) delayed or slow peristalsis.

bradytocia (-to'she-ah) slow parturition.

bradyuria (-u're-ah) slow discharge of urine.

brain (brān) the mass of nerve tissue occupying the large cavity of the skull, comprising forebrain, midbrain and hindbrain, and giving rise to the 12 pairs of cranial nerves; sometimes used popularly to designate only the cerebrum as the organ of the mind.

brainstem (brān'stem) the stemlike portion of the brain, made up of diencephalon, midbrain, pons and medulla oblongata.

brainwashing (brān-wash'ing) mental conditioning of a captive designed to secure attitudes conformable to the wishes of the captors.

branchial (brang'ke-al) pertaining to, or resembling, gills.

branchiogenic (brang″ke-o-jen'ik) derived from a branchial cleft.

branchiomerism (brang″ke-om'er-izm) metameric division of the entoderm.

brash (brash) a burning sensation in the stomach. **weaning b.,** diarrhea in infants occurring as a result of weaning.

breast (brest) the modified structure on the upper anterior thorax, containing the glandular elements that secrete milk for nourishment of the infant. **chicken b.,** congenital chondrosternal prominence. **funnel b.,** congenital chondrosternal depression. **pigeon b.,** congenital chondrosternal prominence.

breath (breth) the air taken in and expelled by the expansion and contraction of the thorax. **liver b.,** hepatic fetor.

breathing (brēth'ing) the alternate inspiration and expiration of air into and out of the lungs. **glossopharyngeal b.,** respiration unaided by the primary or ordinary accessory muscles of respiration, the air being "swallowed" rapidly into the lungs by use of the tongue and muscles of the pharynx.

breech (brēch) the buttock.

breeze (brēz) a gently moving current of air. **static b.,** the current of air from a static electric machine when in operation.

bregma (breg'mah) junction of coronal and sagittal sutures. adj., **bregmat'ic.**

bretylium (bre-til'e-um) an ammonium derivative used as a sympathetic nerve blockade and as an antihypertensive.

Brevibacteriaceae (brev″ĭ-bak-te″re-a′se-e) a family of Schizomycetes (order Eubacteriales).

Brevibacterium (-bak-te′re-um) a genus of Schizomycetes (order Eubacteriales, family Brevibacteriaceae).

brevicollis (-kol′is) shortness of the neck.

Brevital (brev′ĭ-tal) trademark for a preparation of methohexital.

bridge (brij) a structure joining two other parts or organs, especially a structure bearing one or more artificial teeth, attached to natural teeth in the jaw. **cantilever b.**, a dental bridge attached at one end to a natural tooth or root, the other end resting unattached in a depression in a tooth. **cytoplasmic b.**, a band of protoplasm joining two adjacent blastomeres. **extension b.**, a bridge having an artificial tooth attached beyond the point of anchorage of the bridge. **Gaskell's b.**, bundle of His. **intercellular b's**, processes of cell substance connecting adjoining cells. **b. of Varolius**, pons varolii. **Wheatstone's b.**, an instrument for measuring electric resistance.

bridgework (brij′werk) a partial denture retained by attachments other than clasps. **fixed b.**, a partial denture retained with crowns or inlays cemented to the natural teeth. **removable b.**, a partial denture retained by attachments which permit its removal.

brim (brim) the edge of the superior strait of the pelvis.

brisement (brēz-maw′) [Fr.] a crushing. **b. forcé**, the forcible breaking up of a bony ankylosis.

Bristamin (bris′tah-min) trademark for a preparation of phenyltoloxamine.

broach (brōch) a fine barbed instrument for dressing a tooth canal or extracting the pulp.

bromate (bro′māt) a salt of bromic acid.

bromated (bro′māt-ed) charged with bromine.

bromatology (bro″mah-tol′o-je) the science of foods and diet.

bromatotherapy (bro″mah-to-ther′ah-pe) dietotherapy.

bromatoxism (bro″mah-tok′sizm) poisoning by food.

bromethol (bro-meth′ol) tribromoethanol solution.

bromhidrosis (bro″mĭ-dro′sis) the secretion of foul-smelling perspiration.

bromide (bro′mīd) a binary compound of bromine.

bromidrosis (bro″mĭ-dro′sis) bromhidrosis.

bromine (bro′mēn) chemical element (see table), at. no. 35, symbol Br.

bromism (bro′mizm) poisoning by bromine.

bromisovalum (brōm″i-so-val′um) a urea derivative used as a sedative and hypnotic.

bromochlorotrifluoroethane (bro″mo-klo″-ro-tri-flu″o-ro-eth′ān) halothane.

bromoderma (-der′mah) skin eruption due to use of bromides.

bromodiphenhydramine (-di″fen-hi′drah-min) an ethyldimethylamine derivative used as an antihistaminic.

bromohyperhidrosis (-hi″per-hĭ-dro′-sis) excessive fetid perspiration.

bromo-iodism (bro″mo-i′o-dizm) poisoning by bromides and iodides.

bromomania (-ma′ne-ah) mania induced by misuse of bromides.

bromomenorrhea (-men″o-re′ah) profuse, foul-smelling menstruation.

bromophenol (-fe′nol) a violet-colored, strong-smelling liquid, C_6H_4BrOH.

brompheniramine (brōm″fen-ir′ah-mēn) a pyridine derivative used as an antihistaminic.

bromsaligenin (brōm″sal-ĭ-jen′in) a drug used as an antispasmodic.

Bromsulphalein (brom-sul′fah-lin) trademark for a preparation of sulfobromophthalein.

bromum (bro′mum) [L.] bromine.

Bromural (brōm-u′ral) trademark for preparations of bromisovalum.

bronchadenitis (brongk″ad-ĕ-ni′tis) inflammation of the bronchial glands.

bronchi (brong′ki) plural of bronchus.

bronchial (brong′ke-al) pertaining to the bronchi.

bronchiarctia (brong″ke-ark′she-ah) stenosis of the bronchi.

bronchiectasis (-ek′tah-sis) chronic dilatation of one or more bronchi.

bronchiloquy (brong-kil′o-kwe) high-pitched pectoriloquy due to lung consolidation.

bronchiocele (brong′ke-o-sēl″) dilatation or swelling of a bronchiole.

bronchiocrisis (brong″ke-o-kri′sis) bronchial crisis.

bronchiogenic (-jen′ik) bronchogenic.

bronchiole (brong′ke-ōl) one of the successively smaller channels into which the segmental bronchi divide within the pulmonary segments. **respiratory b.**, one of the final branches of the bronchioles, communicating directly with the alveolar ducts.

bronchiolectasis (brong″ke-o-lek′tah-sis) chronic dilatation of bronchioles.

bronchiolitis (-li′tis) inflammation of the bronchioles.

bronchiolus (brong-ki′o-lus), pl. bronchi′oli [L.] bronchiole.

bronchiospasm (brong′ke-o-spazm″) spasmodic narrowing of the bronchi.

bronchiostenosis (brong″ke-o-ste-no′sis) bronchostenosis.

bronchismus (brong-kiz′mus) bronchial spasm.

bronchitis (brong-ki′tis) inflammation of the bronchi. adj., **bronchit′ic. catarrhal b.**, a form with profuse mucopurulent discharge. **fibrinous b.**, bronchitis with formation of fibrinous casts. **b. oblit′erans**, bronchitis in which the smaller bronchi become filled with fibrous exudate. **plastic b.**, fibrinous bronchitis. **putrid b.**, chronic bronchitis with offensive sputum.

broncho-adenitis (brong″ko-ad″ĕ-ni′tis) bronchadenitis.

broncho-alveolitis (-al″ve-o-li′tis) bronchopneumonia.

bronchobiliary (-bil′e-a″re) pertaining to or communicating with a bronchus and the biliary tract.

bronchoblastomycosis (-blas″to-mi-ko′sis) blastomycosis of the lungs.

bronchoblennorrhea (brong"ko-blen"o-re'ah) chronic bronchitis with copious thick sputum.

bronchocavernous (-kav'er-nus) both bronchial and cavernous.

bronchocele (brong'ko-sēl) 1. localized dilatation of a bronchus. 2. goiter.

bronchoclysis (brong-kok'lĭ-sis) instillation of a medicated solution into the bronchi.

bronchoconstriction (brong"ko-kon-strik'-shun) bronchostenosis.

bronchoconstrictor (-kon-strik'tor) 1. narrowing the lumina of the air passages of the lungs. 2. an agent which causes constriction of the bronchi.

bronchodilatation (-dil"ah-ta'shun) dilatation of a bronchus.

bronchodilator (-di-la'tor) 1. expanding the lumina of the air passages of the lungs. 2. an agent which causes dilatation of the bronchi.

bronchoegophony (-e-gof'o-ne) egobronchophony.

bronchoesophageal (-e-sof"ah-je'al) pertaining to or communicating with a bronchus and the esophagus.

bronchoesophagology (-e-sof"ah-gol'o-je) the branch of medicine concerned with air passages (bronchi) and esophagus.

bronchoesophagoscopy (-e-sof"ah-gos'ko-pe) instrumental examination of the bronchi and esophagus.

bronchogenic (-jen'ik) originating in the bronchi.

bronchogram (brong'ko-gram) the film obtained at bronchography.

bronchography (brong-kog'rah-fe) radiography of the lungs after instillation of an opaque medium in the bronchi.

broncholith (brong'ko-lith) bronchial calculus.

broncholithiasis (brong"ko-lĭ-thi'ah-sis) formation of calculi in the bronchi.

bronchologic (brong"ko-loj'ik) pertaining to bronchology.

bronchology (brong-kol'o-je) the study of diseases of the bronchial tree.

bronchomoniliasis (brong"ko-mo"nĭ-li'ah-sis) infection of the bronchi with Monilia (Candida).

bronchomotor (-mo'tor) affecting the caliber of the bronchi.

bronchopathy (brong-kop'ah-the) disease of the bronchi.

bronchophony (brong-kof'o-ne) the sound of the voice as heard through the stethoscope applied over a healthy bronchus.

bronchoplasty (brong'ko-plas"te) plastic repair of a bronchus.

bronchoplegia (brong"ko-ple'je-ah) paralysis of the bronchial tubes.

bronchopleural (-ploor'al) pertaining to a bronchus and the pleura, or communicating with a bronchus and the pleural cavity.

bronchopneumonia (-nu-mo'ne-ah) inflammation of the bronchi and lungs.

bronchopneumopathy (-nu-mop'ah-the) noninflammatory disease of bronchi and lung tissue.

bronchopulmonary (-pul'mo-ner"e) pertaining to bronchi and lungs.

bronchorrhagia (brong"ko-ra'je-ah) hemorrhage from the bronchi.

bronchorrhaphy (brong-kor'ah-fe) suture of a bronchus.

bronchorrhea (brong"ko-re'ah) bronchitis with profuse expectoration.

bronchoscope (brong'ko-skōp) an endoscope especially designed for passage through the trachea to permit inspection of the interior of the tracheobronchial tree.

bronchoscopy (brong-kos'ko-pe) inspection of the interior of the tracheobronchial tree with a bronchoscope.

bronchosinusitis (brong"ko-si"nus-i'tis) coexisting infection of paranasal sinuses and lower respiratory passages.

bronchospasm (brong'ko-spazm) bronchial spasm.

bronchospirography (brong"ko-spi-rog'rah-fe) the graphic recording of breathing in one lung or lobe.

bronchospirometry (-spi-rom'ĕ-tre) determination of the function of the lungs by measurement of tidal volume, vital capacity, maximum breathing capacity and oxygen consumption. **differential b.,** measurement of the function of each lung separately.

bronchostaxis (-stak'sis) bleeding from the bronchial wall.

bronchostenosis (-ste-no'sis) stenosis of bronchi.

bronchostomy (brong-kos'to-me) the surgical creation of an opening through the chest wall into the bronchus.

bronchotetany (brong"ko-tet'ah-ne) spasm of the bronchi, causing dyspnea.

bronchotomy (brong-kot'o-me) incision of a bronchus.

bronchotracheal (brong"ko-tra'ke-al) pertaining to bronchi and trachea.

bronchovesicular (-vē-sik'u-ler) bronchial and vesicular.

bronchus (brong'kus), pl. *bron'chi* [L.] one of the larger passages conveying air to (right or left principal bronchus) and within the lungs (lobar and segmental bronchi).

brontophobia (bron"to-fo'be-ah) morbid fear of thunder.

brown (brown) 1. the color produced by the mixture of red and yellow. 2. a dye which stains objects brown. **Bismarck b.,** a brown aniline dye used in staining specimens for microscopic study.

Broxolin (brok'so-lin) trademark for a preparation of glycobiarsol.

B.R.S. British Roentgen Society.

Brucella (broo-sel'lah) a genus of Schizomycetes (order Eubacteriales, family Brucellaceae). **B. abor'tus,** the causative agent of contagious abortion in cattle and the commonest cause of brucellosis in man. **B. bronchisep'tica,** *Bordetella bronchiseptica.* **B. meliten'sis,** the causative agent of classic Malta fever (undulant fever). **B. o'vis,** the causative agent of an infectious disease in sheep. **B. su'is,** a species found in swine which is capable of producing severe disease in man.

brucella (broo-sel'ah), pl. *brucel'lae,* an organism of the genus Brucella.

Brucellaceae (broo″sel-la'se-e) a family of Schizomycetes (order Eubacteriales).

brucellar (broo-sel'ar) pertaining to brucellae.

brucellemia (broo″sel-le'me-ah) the presence of brucellae in the blood.

brucellergen (broo sel'er-jen) an antigen obtained from Brucella; used in testing for brucella infection.

brucellosis (broo″sel-lo'sis) an infectious, widespread disease affecting cattle, swine, goats and other domestic and wild animals, and transmissible to man, caused by various species of Brucella.

Brugia (broo'je-ah) a genus of nematode parasites of the superfamily Filarioidea. **B. mala'yi,** a species morphologically distinguishable from *Wuchereria bancrofti,* also found in cases of elephantiasis.

bruise (brooz) a large, blotchy, superficial discoloration due to hemorrhage into the tissues from ruptured vessels (ecchymosis).

bruit (brōōt) [Fr.] a sound or murmur, especially an abnormal one. **aneurysmal b.,** blowing sound heard over an aneurysm. **placental b.,** auscultatory sound heard over the placenta in pregnancy.

bruxism (bruk'sizm) grinding of the teeth.

B.S. Bachelor of Science.

BSA bovine serum albumin.

B.T.U., B.Th.U. British thermal unit.

B.U. Bodansky unit.

buba (boo'bah) yaws.

bubo (bu'bo) a tender, enlarged lymph node, resulting from absorption of infective material and occurring in various diseases, e.g. lymphogranuloma venereum, plague, syphilis, gonorrhea, chancroid. **climatic b.,** lymphogranuloma venereum. **indolent b.,** a syphilitic bubo with no tendency to break down. **inguinal b.,** painful swelling of the inguinal lymph nodes, which sometimes become matted together. **parotid b.,** parotitis. **pestilential b.,** plague. **sympathetic b.,** bubo due to friction and injury. **tropical b.,** lymphogranuloma venereum. **venereal b.,** venereal lymphogranuloma.

bubonalgia (bu″bo-nal'je-ah) pain in the groin.

bubonic (bu-bon'ik) pertaining to buboes.

bubonocele (bu-bon'o-sēl) incomplete inguinal hernia.

bucardia (bu-kar'de-ah) cor bovinum.

buccal (buk'al) pertaining to the mouth, especially to the inner surface of the cheeks.

bucco- (buk'ko) word element [L.] denoting relationship to the cheek.

bucco-axial (buk″o-ak'se-al) pertaining to or formed by the buccal and axial walls of a tooth cavity.

buccoclination (-kli-na'shun) deviation of a posterior tooth from the vertical, in the direction of the cheek.

buccocclusion (-kloo'zhun) malocclusion in which the dental arch or a quadrant or group of teeth is buccal to the normal.

buccoversion (-ver'zhun) position of a tooth lying buccally to the line of occlusion.

buclizine (bu'klī-zēn) a diethylene diamine derivative used as an antihistaminic.

bucnemia (buk-ne'me-ah) inflammatory disease of the leg.

bud (bud) 1. a small protuberance on a plant from which growth occurs. 2. a structure resembling the bud of a plant, especially a protuberance in the embryo from which an organ or part develops. **end b.,** the compact mass of cells remaining from the primitive knot and streak, located at the caudal end of the embryo. **limb b.,** one of the four lateral swellings appearing in vertebrate embryos, which develop into the two pairs of limbs. **tail b.,** 1. the primordium of the caudal appendage. 2. end bud. **taste b's,** end-organs in the tongue receiving stimuli which give rise to the sense of taste. **ureteric b.,** a hollow bud arising from the mesonephric duct, which develops into the ureter. **b. of urethra,** the enlarged proximal part of the corpus spongiosum.

budding (bud'ing) gemmation.

buffer (buf'er) a substance which, by its presence in solution, increases the amount of acid or alkali necessary to produce unit change in pH.

bulb (bulb) 1. any rounded mass. 2. the oblongata. adj., **bul'bar. b. of aorta,** the enlargement of the aorta at its point of origin from the heart. **auditory b.,** the membranous labyrinth and cochlea. **b. of corpus cavernosum,** enlarged muscular and proximal part of the cavernous body. **dental b.,** the dentinal papilla. **end b.,** 1. the bulbous peripheral extremity of a sensory nerve. 2. end bud. **gustatory b's,** taste buds. **hair b.,** the bulbous expansion at the lower end of a hair root. **Krause's b's.,** see under *corpuscle.* **medullary b.,** medulla oblongata. **olfactory b.,** the bulblike extremity of the olfactory nerve on the under surface of each anterior lobe of the cerebrum. **taste b's,** taste buds. **b. of urethra,** the proximal part of the corpus spongiosum. **b. of vestibule, vestibulovaginal b.,** bulbus vestibuli vaginae.

bulbiform (bul'bī-form) bulb-shaped.

bulbitis (bul-bi'tis) inflammation of the bulb of the urethra.

bulbonuclear (bul″bo-nu'kle-ar) pertaining to medulla oblongata and its nuclei.

bulbourethral (-u-re'thral) pertaining to the bulb of the urethra.

bulbous (bul'bus) resembling a bulb.

bulbus (bul'bus), pl. *bul'bi* [L.] bulb. **b. aor'tae,** bulb of the aorta. **b. carot'icus,** carotid sinus. **b. oc'uli,** the bulb, or globe, of the eye. **b. olfacto'rius,** olfactory bulb. **b. ure'thrae,** bulb of the urethra. **b. vestib'uli vagi'nae,** one of two masses of erectile tissue, situated one on either side of the vaginal orifice.

bulimia (bu-lim'e-ah) insatiable hunger. adj., **bulim'ic.**

bulla (bul'ah), pl. *bul'lae* [L.] a circumscribed, fluid-containing, elevated lesion of the skin, more than 5 mm. in diameter. adj., **bul'late, bul'lous.**

bumblefoot (bum'bl-foot) infection associated with localized bulbous swelling of the footpad in chickens or turkeys.

button

B.U.N. blood urea nitrogen.

bunch (bunch) traumatic swelling of a bone in horses.

bundle (bun'dl) a collection of units. **atrioventricular b., auriculoventricular b.,** bundle of His. **ground b.,** either portion of the anterolateral tract of the spinal cord. **b. of His,** a muscular band connecting the atria with the ventricles of the heart. **Keith's b.,** bundle of fibers in the wall of the atrium of the heart between the venae cavae. **Schultze's b.,** interfascicular fasciculus. **sinoatrial b.,** Keith's bundle. **Thorel's b.,** a bundle of muscle fibers in the heart connecting the sinoatrial and atrioventricular nodes. **b. of Vicq d'Azyr,** a bundle of white fibers around the base of the anterior nucleus of the optic thalamus.

bunion (bun'yun) a deformity of the foot with bony enlargement of the medial side of the head of the first metatarsal bone, formation of a bursal sac over the enlargement, and lateral angulation of the great toe (hallux valgus). **tailor's b.,** chronic inflammation and enlargement of the head of the fifth metatarsal bone.

bunionectomy (bun″yun-ek'to-me) excision of a bunion.

bunionette (bun″yun-et′) bony enlargement of the lateral side of the head of the fifth metatarsal bone, usually with an overlying bursal sac and medial angulation of the little toe.

Bunostomum (bu″no-sto'mum) a genus of hookworm parasitic in cattle.

buphthalmos (būf-thal'mos) abnormal distention and enlargement of the eyeball in infancy.

bur (ber) a form of drill used for creating openings in bone or similar hard material.

buret (bu-ret′) a glass tube with a capacity of the order of 25 to 100 ml. and graduation intervals of 0.05 to 0.1 ml., with stopcock attachment, used to deliver an accurately measured quantity of liquid.

burette (bu-ret′) buret.

burn (bern) injury to tissues caused by exposure to high temperatures or to energy which ordinarily stimulates the sensation of heat. **thermal b.,** injury resulting from either wet or dry heat; three degrees of injury are recognized: (1) mild epidermal damage, with reactive hyperemia, (2) severe epidermal damage, with formation of vesicles or bullae; (3) damage to or complete destruction of the corium.

burner (bern'er) an apparatus for producing a flame for heating purposes. **Argand b.,** one with an inner tube by which air is supplied to the flame, to increase combustion. **Bunsen b.,** one with air holes at the botton of the tube, admitting so much air that all the carbon is burned, giving an intensely hot and only slightly luminous flame.

burnishing (ber'nish-ing) a dental procedure related to polishing and abrading, used to reduce the height or thickness of a surface.

bursa (ber'sah), pl. *bur′sae, bursas* [L.] a sac or a saclike cavity. adj., **bur′sal. b. anseri′na,** one under the insertion of the sartorius and gracilis muscles. **Boyer's b.,** one beneath hyoid bone. **Calori's b.,** one between the trachea and the arch of the aorta. **Fleischmann's b.,** one beneath the tongue. **gluteal b.,** one beneath the gluteus maximus muscle. **His's b.,** the dilatation at the end of the archenteron. **iliac b.,** one at the point of insertion of the iliopsoas muscle into the lesser trochanter. **Luschka's b.,** bursa pharyngea (1). **b. muco′sa,** any membranous sac that secretes synovia. **omental b., b. omenta′lis,** the lesser sac of the peritoneum. **b. pharyn′gea, pharyngeal b.,** 1. a recess in the pharynx of the fetus and newborn. 2. a cyst in the pharyngeal tonsil. **popliteal b.,** one in the popliteal space beneath the tendon of the semimembranosus and the tendon of the inner head of the gastrocnemius. **prepatellar b.,** one over the patella. **synovial b.,** bursa mucosa.

bursalogy (ber sal'o-je) the study of bursas.

bursectomy (ber-sek'to-me) excision of a bursa.

bursitis (ber-si'tis) inflammation of a bursa. **Duplay's b.,** inflammation of the bursa beneath the deltoid muscle. **Thornwaldt's b.,** chronic inflammation of the pharyngeal bursa.

bursolith (ber'so-lith) a calculus in a bursa.

bursopathy (ber-sop'ah-the) any disease of a bursa.

bursotomy (ber sot'o me) incision of a bursa.

busulfan (bu-sul'fan) an agent used to suppress chronic myelogenous leukemia.

butabarbital (bu″tah-bar'bĭ-tal) a short to intermediate-acting barbiturate. **sodium b.,** a white, bitter powder, $C_{10}H_{15}N_2NaO_3$.

butacaine sulfate (bu″tah-kān sul'fāt) a colorless, odorless, crystalline powder; used instead of cocaine for surface anesthesia in the eye and on mucous membranes.

butamben (bu-tam'ben) butylaminobenzoate.

butamin (bu'tah-min) tutocaine.

butane (bu'tān) an anesthetic hydrocarbon, C_4H_{10}.

Butazolidin (bu″tah-zol'ĭ-din) trademark for a preparation of phenylbutazone.

Butesin (bu-te'sin) trademark for a preparation of butyl aminobenzoate.

butethamine (bu teth'ah-mēn) an agent used as a local anesthetic.

Butisol (bu'tĭ-sol) trademark for preparations of butabarbital.

butter (but'er) oily mass procured by churning cream, or a substance of similar consistency. **b. of antimony,** antimony trichloride. **cacao b.,** the fixed oil or fat from cacao. **nutmeg b.,** a soft, unctuous solid with the odor and taste of nutmeg, formed by cooling the oil expressed from steamed, bruised nutmegs. **b. of tin,** stannic chloride. **b. of zinc,** zinc chloride.

buttock (but'ok) either of the two fleshy masses formed by the gluteus muscles, on the posterior aspect of the lower trunk.

button (but'on) a small round structure, resembling the device used for fastening garments. **Biskra b.,** cutaneous leishmaniasis. **Jaboulay's b.,** a device used for lateral intestinal anastomosis. **Murphy's b.,** a metallic device used for connecting the ends of a divided intestine.

butyl (bu'til) a hydrocarbon radical, C_4H_9. **b. aminobenzoate,** a white crystalline powder, $C_{11}H_{15}NO$, used as a topical anesthetic. **b. chloride,** a drug used as a veterinary anthelmintic.

butylene (bu'tĭ-lēn) .a gaseous hydrocarbon, C_4H_8.

butyraceous (bu"tĭ-ra'shus) resembling butter.

butyrate (bu'tĭ-rāt) a salt of butyric acid.

Butyribacterium (bu-ti"re-bak-te're-um) a genus of Schizomycetes (order Eubacteriales, family Propionibacteriaceae), occurring as parasites in the intestinal tract.

butyrin (bu'tĭ-rin) a yellowish fat, C_3H_5-$(C_4H_7O_2)_3$, the chief constituent of butter.

butyroid (bu'tĭ-roid) resembling butter.

butyrometer (bu"tĭ-rom'ĕ-ter) an apparatus for estimating the butter fat of milk.

butyrous (bu'tĭ-rus) resembling butter.

byssaceous (bis-sa'shus) composed of fine, flaxlike threads.

byssinosis (bis"ĭ-no'sis) a lung disease due to inhalation of cotton dust.

C

C chemical symbol, *carbon.*

C. Celsius.

c. cathode (cathodal); cervical; clonus; closure; congius (gallon); contact; contraction; cubic; current; cylinder.

C.A. chronologic age.

Ca chemical symbol, *calcium.*

Ca. cathode.

cacanthrax (kak-an'thraks) malignant anthrax.

cacao (kah-ka'o) cocoa.

cacation (kah-ka'shun) defecation.

cacatory (kak'ah-to"re) marked by severe diarrhea.

cacesthesia (kak"es-the'ze-ah) disordered sensibility.

caché (kash-a') a lead cone used for applying a radioactive substance.

cachet (kah-sha') a wafer or capsule for medicines.

cachexia (kah-kek'se-ah) a state of malnutrition, emaciation and debility. adj., **cachec'-tic. c. hypophysiopri'va,** the symptoms resulting from removal of the hypophysis cerebri. **lymphatic c.,** Hodgkin's disease. **malarial c.,** chronic malaria. **pachydermic c.,** myxedema. **pituitary c.,** that due to diminution or absence of pituitary function. **c. strumipri'va, c. thyreopri'va,** a disordered state resulting from removal of the thyroid. **thyroid c.,** exophthalmic goiter.

cachinnation (kak"ĭ-na'shun) excessive or hysteric laughter.

cacodyl (kak'o-dil) poisonous arsenical compound, $As(CH_3)_2$.

cacodylate (kak'o-dil"āt) a salt of cacodylic acid.

cacogenics (kak"o-jen'iks) race deterioration. adj., **cacogen'ic.**

cacogeusia (-gu'se-ah) a bad taste.

cacomelia (-me'le-ah) congenital deformity of a limb.

cacoplastic (-plas'tik) susceptible of imperfect organization only.

cacorhythmic (-rith'mik) marked by irregularity of rhythm.

cacosmia (kak-oz'me-ah) foul odor; stench.

cacothenics (kak"o-then'iks) degeneration of the race from bad environment and unsanitary surroundings.

cacothymia (kak"o-thi'me-ah) depression of spirits with morbid ill temper.

cacotrophy (kak-ot'ro-fe) ill-nourished condition.

cacumen (kah-ku'men) pl. *cacu'mina* [L.] 1. the top of a plant. 2. part of cerebellum below the declivis.

cadaver (kah-dav'er) a dead body. adj., **cadav'-eric, cadav'erous.**

cadaverine (kah-dav'er-in) pentamethylenediamine.

cadmium (kad'me-um) chemical element *(see table),* at. no. 48, symbol Cd. **c. sulfide,** a light yellow or orange powder used in treatment of seborrheic dermatitis of the scalp.

caduceus (kah-du'se-us) the wand of Hermes or Mercury; used as a symbol of the medical profession and as the emblem of the Medical Corps of the U. S. Army.

cae- for words beginning thus, see also those beginning *ce-.*

caelotherapy (se"lo-ther'ah-pe) the therapeutic use of religion and religious symbols.

caffea (kaf'e-ah) coffee.

caffeine (kaf'ēn, kaf'e-in) a central nervous system stimulant, $C_8H_{10}N_4O_2$. **citrated c.,** white, odorless powder, mixture of caffeine and citric acid. **c. sodium benzoate,** a mixture of equal parts of anhydrous caffeine and sodium benzoate, used as a central nervous system stimulant.

caffeinism (kaf'ēn-izm) morbid state induced by excessive use of coffee.

cage (kāj) a box or enclosure. **thoracic c.,** the bony structure enclosing the thorax, consisting of the ribs, vertebral column and sternum.

cainotophobia (ki-no"to-fo'be-ah) morbid dread of anything new.

Cal. large calorie (kilogram calorie).

cal. small calorie (gram calorie).

calamine (kal'ah-mīn) a mixture of zinc and ferric oxides, used topically in lotions and ointments.

calamus (kal'ah-mus) 1. a reed or reedlike structure. 2. the peeled, dried rhizome of *Acorus calamus;* mild aromatic. **c. scripto'-**

rius, the pointed lower portion of the floor of the fourth ventricle.

calcaneitis (kal-ka″ne-i′tis) inflammation of the calcaneus.

calcaneo-apophysitis (kal-ka″ne-o-ah-pof″ĭ-si′tis) inflammation of the posterior part of the calcaneus, marked by pain and swelling.

calcaneodynia (-din′e-ah) pain in the heel.

calcaneotibial (-tib′e-al) pertaining to calcaneus and tibia.

calcaneum (kal-ka′ne-um) calcaneus.

calcaneus (kal-ka′ne-us) 1. os calcis. 2. talipes calcaneus. adj., **calca′neal, calca′nean.**

calcar (kal′kar) 1. a spur. 2. hippocampus minor. adj., **cal′carine. c. femora′le,** the plate of strong tissue which strengthens the neck of the femur.

calcareous (kal-kār′e-us) containing lime.

calcariuria (kal-kār″e-u′re-ah) presence of lime salts in the urine.

calcemia (kal-se′me-ah) excessive calcium in the blood.

calcibilia (kal″sĭ-bil′e-ah) presence of calcium in the bile.

calcic (kal′sik) 1. pertaining to lime. 2. pertaining to calcium.

calcicosis (kal″sĭ-ko′sis) lung disease due to inhalation of marble dust.

calciferol (kal-sif″er-ol) a white, odorless, crystalline compound, $C_{28}H_{44}O$; an oil-soluble, antirachitic vitamin.

calcific (kal-sif′ik) forming lime.

calcification (kal″sĭ-fĭ-ka′shun) the deposit of calcium salts in a tissue. **Mönckeberg's c.,** see under *arteriosclerosis.*

calcine (kal′sīn) to reduce to a dry powder.

calcinosis (kal″sĭ no′sis) a condition characterized by abnormal deposition of calcium salts in the tissues. **c. circumscrip′ta,** a condition marked by calcifications occurring only in subcutaneous fat. **c. universa′lis,** calcinosis in which calcifications appear in other connective tissues, as well as in subcutaneous fat.

calciokinesis (kal″se-o-ki-ne′sis) mobilization of calcium stored in the body. adj., **calciokinet′ic.**

calciorrhachia (-ra′ke-ah) calcium in the cerebrospinal fluid.

calcipenia (kal″sĭ-pe′ne-ah) deficiency of calcium in the system.

calcipexy (kal′sĭ pek″se) fixation of calcium in the tissues. adj., **calcipec′tic, calcipex′ic.**

calciphilia (kal″sĭ-fil′e-ah) a tendency to calcification.

calciphylaxis (-fi-lak′sis) the formation of calcified tissue in response to administration of a challenging agent after induction of a hypersensitive state. adj., **calciphylac′tic.**

calciprivia (-priv′e-ah) deprivation or loss of calcium. adj., **calcipri′vic.**

calcitonin (-to′nin) a polypeptide, thought to be a secretion of the thyroid gland, which lowers both calcium and phosphate in the plasma.

calcium (kal′se-um) chemical element *(see table),* at. no. 20, symbol Ca; an important component of the body. **c. aminosalicylate,**

an antibacterial compound, $C_{14}H_{12}CaN_2O_6$, used in tuberculosis. **c. bromide,** hydrated salt containing 84–94 per cent calcium bromide; used in asthma and convulsive disorders. **c. carbonate, precipitated,** white, microcrystalline powder, $CaCO_3$, used as an antacid. **c. chloride,** a deliquescent compound, $CaCl_2$·$2H_2O$, used as an electrolyte replenisher. **c. cyclamate,** an odorless, white, crystalline compound, $C_{12}H_{24}CaN_2O_6S_2$·$2H_2O$, used as a noncaloric sweetener. **c. disodium edatate, c. disodium edathamil,** chemical name calcium disodium(ethylenedinitrilo)tetraacetate; used as an antidote in poisoning by lead and other metals. **c. gluconate,** $C_{12}H_{22}CaO_{14}$, used to replenish calcium in the body. **c. glycerophosphate,** fine, white, odorless powder, $C_3H_7CaPO_6$; used in bone diseases. **c. hydroxide,** an astringent compound, $Ca(OH)_2$, used topically in solution or lotions. **c. hypophosphite,** $Ca(PH_2O_2)_2$, formerly used in tuberculosis and neurasthenia. **c. iodobehenate,** white or yellowish, unctuous powder; used in administering iodides. **c. lactate,** white, almost odorless compound, $C_6H_{10}CaO_6$·$5H_2O$; electrolyte replenisher. **c. levulinate,** white, bitter powder, $C_{10}H_{14}CaO_6$·$2H_2O$, more soluble than calcium gluconate. **c. mandelate,** white, odorless powder, $C_{16}H_{14}CaO_6$; urinary antiseptic. **c. oxide,** lime. **c. pantothenate,** calcium salt of the dextrorotatory isomer of pantothenic acid, used as a growth-promoting vitamin. **c. phosphate, dibasic,** a white, odorless powder, $CaHPO_4$, used to replenish calcium in the body. **c. phosphate, tribasic,** $Ca_3(PO_4)_2$; antacid and source of calcium. **c. sulfate,** a compound of calcium and sulfate (SO_4), existing as $CaSO_4$, $CaSO_4$·$^1/_2H_2O$ (plaster of Paris), or $CaSO_4$·$2H_2O$; dry calcium sulfate has been used as an absorbent dressing for ulcers and wounds; plaster of Paris is used in dressings to support or immobilize parts.

calciuria (kal″se-u′re-ah) calcium in the urine.

calcoglobule (kal″ko-glob′ūl) a globule of calcium deposited in developing dentin.

calcoid (kal′koid) a tumor of the tooth pulp.

calcospherite (kal″ko-sfēr′īt) a small calcareous body found in tumors, nerve tissue, etc.

calculifragous (kal″ku-lif′rah-gus) breaking up calculi.

calculogenesis (-lo-jen′ĕ-sis) the formation of calculi.

calculosis (-lo′sis) a condition characterized by the presence of calculi.

calculus (kal′ku-lus), pl. *cal′culi* [L.] a small hard mass formed chiefly in hollow organs of the body or their passages. adj., **cal′culary, cal′culous. biliary c.,** a gallstone. **dendritic c.,** an irregular, branching calculus formed in the kidney pelvis and calices. **dental c.,** an adherent, calcified mass of bacteria, fungi, desquamated epithelial cells and food debris, formed on the surface of teeth and dental appliances. **fusible c.,** urinary calculus made up of phosphate of ammonium, calcium and magnesium. **lacrimal c.,** one in a lacrimal gland or duct. **renal c.,** one in the kidney. **salivary c.,** one in a salivary gland or duct.

urinary c., one in any part of the urinary tract.
vesical c., one in the urinary bladder.

calefacient (kal″ĕ-fa′shent) causing a sensation of warmth.

calf (kaf) the fleshy back part of the leg below the knee.

caliber (kal′ĭ-ber) the diameter of the opening of a canal or tube.

calibrator (kal″ĭ-bra′ter) a device for measuring the caliber of a canal or tube.

calicectasis (-sek′tah-sis) dilatation of a calix of the kidney.

calicectomy (-sek′to-me) excision of a calix of the kidney.

caliculus (kah-lik′u-lus) a small, bud- or cup-shaped structure.

callectasis (kal″e-ek′tah-sis) dilatation of the calix of the kidney.

californium (kal″ĭ-fôr′ne-um) chemical element *(see table)*, at. no. 98, symbol Cf.

calipers (kal′ĭ-perz) a two-bladed instrument used in taking measurements.

calisthenics (kal″is-then′iks) systematic exercise for attaining strength and gracefulness.

calix (ka′liks), pl. *cal′ices* [L.] a cuplike structure, such as one of the recesses of the kidney pelvis receiving the summits of the renal pyramids. adj., **calice′al.**

Calliphora (kal-lif′o-rah) a genus of flies, the blowflies.

callosity (kah-los′ĭ-te) a callus (1).

callosum (kah-lo′sum) corpus callosum. adj., **callo′sal.**

callous (kal′us) of the nature of a callus.

callus (kal′us) 1. an acquired, localized area of thickening of the stratum corneum, resulting from continued physical trauma. 2. fibrous tissue formed by condensation of granulation tissue at the site of fracture, in which fibrocartilage and hyaline cartilage form, sealing the ends of the bone together (*provisional callus*) and being ultimately replaced by mature bone (*permanent callus*).

calmative (kal′mah-tiv, kah′mah-tiv) 1. having a calming or sedative effect. 2. an agent which has a calming or sedative effect.

calomel (kal′o-mel) a heavy, white, impalpable powder, Hg_2Cl; used as a cathartic.

calor (kal′er) [L.] heat.

caloricity (kal″o-ris′ĭ-te) the power of the body of developing heat.

calorie (kal′o-re) a unit of measurement of heat. **15°c.,** the amount of heat required to raise the temperature of 1 gm. of water from 14.5°C. to 15.5°C. **gram c.,** small calorie. **International Table c., I.T. c.,** a unit of heat, equivalent to 4.1868 joules. **kilogram c., large c.,** the calorie used in metabolic studies, being the amount of heat required to raise the temperature of 1 kg. of water 1 degree Celsius (C.). **mean c.,** one one-hundredth of the amount of heat required to raise the temperature of 1 gm. of water from 0 to 100°C. **small c.,** the amount of heat required to raise the temperature of 1 gm. of water 1 degree Celsius (C.). **standard c.,** small calorie. **thermochemical c.,** a unit of heat, equivalent to 4.184 joules.

calorifacient (kah-lor″ĭ-fa′shent) heat-producing.

calorific (kal″o-rif′ik) producing heat.

calorigenetic (kah-lor″ĭ-jĕ-net′ik) calorigenic.

calorigenic (kah-lor″ĭ-jen′ik) 1. generating heat. 2. increasing the rate of oxidation of tissue cells.

calorimeter (kal″o-rim′ĕ-ter) a laboratory device for the rapid measurement of the heat evolved in any system.

calorimetry (-rim′ĕ-tre) measurement of the actual heat eliminated or stored in any system.

caloripuncture (kah-lor′ĭ-punk″tūr) ignipuncture.

caloritropic (-trop″ik) thermotropic.

calory (kal′o rc) calorie.

calvaria (kal-va′re-ah) the domelike superior portion of the cranium, comprising superior portions of the frontal, parietal and occipital bones.

calvarium (kal-va′re-um) calvaria.

calx (kalks) 1. lime. 2. the heel. **c. chlora′ta,** chlorinated lime. **c. sulfura′ta,** sulfurated lime.

calyculus (kah-lik′u-lus), pl. *calyc′uli* [L.] caliculus.

Calymmatobacterium (kah-lim″mah-to-bak-te′re-um) a genus of Schizomycetes (order Eubacteriales, family Brucellaceae).

calyx (ka′liks) calix.

camera (kam′er-ah), pl. *cam′erae* [L.] a cavity or chamber. **c. bul′bi, c. oc′uli,** one of the chambers of the eye.

Camoquin (kam″o-kwin) trademark for a preparation of amodiaquine.

camphor (kam′fer) a ketone derived from *Cinnamomum camphora* or produced synthetically, used locally as an analgesic and antipruritic agent. **monobromated c.,** colorless crystals or powder with mild characteristic odor and taste, $C_{10}H_{15}BrO$; sedative.

camphorate (kam′fer-āt) to combine with camphor.

campimeter (kam-pim′ĕ-ter) an instrument for measuring the field of vision.

campimetry (kam-pim′ĕ-tre) perimetry.

camptocormia (kamp″to-kor′me-ah) forward flexion of the trunk.

camptodactylia (-dak-til′e-ah) a clawlike condition of the hand or foot.

camptospasm (kamp′to-spazm) camptocormia.

canal (kah-nal′) any passage or duct in the body. **Alcock's c.,** a sheath of the obturator fascia containing the internal pudendal artery. **alimentary c.,** the digestive tube from mouth to anus. **anal c.,** the most distal portion of the alimentary tract, from the pectinate line to the anal verge. **arachnoid c.,** space beneath arachnoid membrane of brain transmitting great veins of Galen. **c. of Arantius,** ductus venosus. **archenteric c.,** neurenteric canal. **archinephric c.,** the duct of the primitive kidney. **Arnold's c.,** a passage in the petrous portion of the temporal bone for the auricular branch of the pneumogastric nerve. **arterial c.,** ductus arteriosus. **atrioventricular c.,** the common canal connecting the primitive atrium and ventricle; it sometimes persists as a congenital anomaly. **Bernard's c.**, the accessory duct of the pancreas. **Bichat's c.**, small subarachnoid passage for cerebral veins. **birth c.**, the canal through which the fetus passes in birth. **Braune's c.**, the uterine cavity and vagina after the os is fully dilated. **Braun's c.**, neurenteric canal. **bullular c.**, canal of Petit. **caroticotympanic c's**, short canals from carotid canal to the tympanum, transmitting branches of carotid plexus. **carotid c.**, one in petrous portion of temporal bone, transmitting internal carotid artery. **cervical c.**, the canal of the cervix uteri. **c. of Cloquet**, hyaloid canal. **cochlear c.**, the space between Reissner's membrane and the basilar membrane. **Corti's c.**, the passage made by the arches of Corti. **crural c.**, femoral canal. **c. of Cuvier**, ductus venosus. **dentinal c's**, the minute canals in dentin. **digestive c.**, alimentary tract. **Dorello's c.**, a canal in the tip of the temporal bone. **fallopian c.**, aqueduct of Fallopius. **femoral c.**, medial part of the femoral sheath lateral to the base of the lacunar ligament. **c. of Ferrein**, the canal between the free edges of the eyelid when closed. **c's of Fontana**, ring-shaped series of spaces in the sclera in front of its attachment to the iris. **c. of Gartner**, the remains in the female of the main part of the wolffian duct of the embryo. **haversian c.**, one of the anastomosing channels of the haversian system in compact bone, containing blood and lymph vessels, nerves and marrow. **hepatic c.**, hepatic duct or any of its smaller branches. **Hirschfeld's c's**, interdental canals. **c. of Huguier**, small canal between squamous and petrous portions of temporal bone, transmitting chorda tympani nerve. **Hunter's c.**, a triangular canal in the adductor magnus of the thigh, transmitting femoral artery and vein and long saphenous nerve. **Huschke's c.**, canal formed by union of tubercles of tympanic ring. **hyaloid c.**, canal running through vitreous body, transmitting hyaloid artery of fetus. **incisor c.**, canal opening into the mouth by an opening behind the incisor teeth of upper jaw. **infraorbital c.**, small canal running obliquely through floor of orbit, transmitting infraorbital artery and nerve. **inguinal c.**, a space at the lower margin on either side between the layers composing the abdominal wall, through which passes the round ligament in the female, and the spermatic cord in the male. **interdental c's**, channels in the alveolar process of the mandible between the roots of the central and lateral incisors. **Jacobson's c.**, tympanic canal. **c. of Loewenberg**, portion of cochlear canal above membrane of Corti. **medullary c.**, the cavity of a long bone, containing the marrow. **Müller's c.**, see under *duct*. **nasal c.**, canal in posterior part of nasal bone, transmitting nasal nerves. **nasopalatine c.**, incisor canal. **neural c.**, the canal in the epiblast of the embryo forming the cerebrospinal cavity. **neurenteric c.**, a temporary communication in the embryo between the cavities of the yolk sac and the amnion. **c. of Nuck**, a tubular process of peritoneum projecting into inguinal canal of female fetus. **nutrient c. of bone**, haversian canal. **omphalomesenteric c.**, omphalomesenteric duct. **parturient c.**, birth canal. **perivascular c.**, a lymph space about a blood vessel. **c. of Petit**, a small channel surrounding the lens of the eye. **portal c.**, space in capsule of Glisson of liver, transmitting branches of hepatic artery, portal vein and hepatic duct. **pterygoid c.**, vidian canal. **pterygopalatine c.**, one in sphenoid and palate bones, transmitting vessels and nerves. **pulp c.**, the hollow part of the root of a tooth, containing the pulp. **Recklinghausen's c's.**, 1. small lymph channels in the connective tissue, regarded as the end-branches of the lymphatics. 2. the canals of the cornea. **root c.**, pulp canal. **c. of Rosenthal**, the spiral canal of the modiolus of the ear. **sacculocochlear c.**, the canal connecting the saccule and cochlea. **sacral c.**, continuation of vertebral canal in the sacrum. **Saviotti's c's**, artificially formed slits between glandular cells of the pancreas. **Schlemm's c.**, venous sinus of sclera. **semicircular c's**, long canals of the labyrinth of the ear. **spermatic c.**, inguinal canal. **spinal c.**, the canal through the vertebrae, transmitting the spinal cord. **spiral c.**, the canal of the cochlea enclosing the scala vestibuli, scala media and scala tympani. **Stilling's c.**, hyaloid canal. **tarsal c.**, the canal under the head of the abductor hallucis. **tubotympanal c.**, a tube in the developing embryo from which the tympanum and eustachian tube are formed. **tympanic c.**, one in petrous portion of temporal bone, transmitting Jacobson's nerve. **uterine c.**, the cavity of the uterus. **vertebral c.**, spinal canal. **vidian c.**, one in sphenoid bone, transmitting vidian artery and nerve. **Volkmann's c's**, canals in subperiosteal layer of bones communicating with haversian canals. **vomerobasilar c.**, canal formed at junction of vomer and sphenoid bone. **c. of Wirsung**, pancreatic duct. **zygomaticotemporal c.**, zygomaticotemporal foramen.

canaliculus (kan″ah-lik′u-lus), pl. *canalic′uli* [L.] a small canal or channel. adj., **canalic′ular. bile canaliculi**, fine tubular channels forming a three-dimensional network within the parenchyma of the liver. **dental canaliculi**, minute channels in dentin, extending from the pulp cavity to the overlying cement and enamel. **haversian canaliculi**, minute passages in bones connecting with the haversian canals. **lacrimal c.**, the short passage in an eyelid, beginning at the lacrimal point and draining tears from the lacrimal lake to the lacrimal sac. **mastoid c.**, a small channel in the temporal bone transmitting the tympanic branch of the vagus nerve. **tympanic c.**, a small opening in the floor of the petrosal fossa for transmitting the tympanic branch of the glossopharyngeal nerve and a small blood vessel.

canalis (kah-nal'is), pl. *cana'les* [L.] a canal or channel.

canalization (kan"al-i-za'shun) the formation of canals in a mass of tissue by the anastomosis and progressive dilation of organizing capillary channels.

canaloplasty (kah-nal'o-plas"te) plastic reconstruction of a passage, as of the external auditory meatus.

canavanine (kah-nav'ah-nin) a naturally occurring amino acid, isolated from soybean meal.

cancellate (kan'sel-lāt) having a lattice-like structure.

cancellus (kan-sel'us), pl. *cancel'li* [L.] the lattice-like structure in bone. adj., **can'cellous.**

cancer (kan'ser) a malignant tumor. **can'cerous. black c.,** melanoma. **chimneysweeps' c.,** epithelioma of the scrotum. **c. en cuirasse,** cancer about the skin of the thorax. **epithelial c.,** epithelioma. **smokers' c.,** epithelioma of lip from irritation of a pipe. **soot c.,** epithelioma of the scrotum.

canceremia (kan"ser-e'me-ah) the presence of cancer cells in the blood.

cancericidal (-ĭ-si'dal) destructive to cancer cells.

cancerism (kan'ser-izm) tendency to cancer.

cancerogenic (kan"ser-o-jen'ik) carcinogenic.

cancerology (kan"ser-ol'o-je) the study of cancer.

cancerophobia (kan"ser-o-fo'be-ah) carcinophobia.

cancriform (kang'krĭ-form) resembling cancer.

cancroid (kang'kroid) 1. cancer-like. 2. a skin cancer of a low grade of malignancy.

cancrum (kang'krum) [L.] canker. **c. o'ris,** gangrenous stomatitis. **c. puden'di,** noma.

Candida (kan'dĭ-dah) a genus of yeastlike fungi which produce mycelia, but not ascospores. **C. al'bicans,** a species which causes human infection.

candidemia (kan"dĭ-de'me-ah) presence in the blood of fungi of the genus Candida.

candidiasis (-di'ah-sis) infection by fungi of the genus Candida.

candle (kan'dl) a unit of luminous intensity equal to the intensity of light from a ⁷/₈-inch sperm candle burning at the rate of 120 grains an hour. **international c.,** a unit equal to the intensity of light from 5 square millimeters of platinum at the temperature of solidification.

canities (kah-nish'e-ēz) diffuse graying of the hair.

canker (kang'ker) an ulceration, especially of the lip or oral mucosa.

Cannabis (kan'ah-bis) a genus of plants, hemp. **C. in'dica,** an Asiatic variety of common hemp; preferred for medicinal use. **C. sati'va,** the common hemp; narcotic and antispasmodic.

cannabism (kan'ah-bizm) habitual use of hemp derivatives as intoxicants.

cannula (kan'u-lah) a small tubular instrument for insertion into the body. **Bellocq's c.,** an instrument for plugging the posterior nares.

cannulate (kan'u-lāt) to penetrate with a cannula, which may be left in place.

cannulation (kan"u-la'shun) introduction of a cannula into a tubelike organ or body cavity.

cantharides (kan-thar'ĭ-dēz) dried insects of the species *Cantharis vesicatoria;* irritant and vesicant.

cantharidin (kan-thar'ĭ-din) crystalline active principle, $C_{20}H_{24}O_8$, from cantharides.

cantharidism (kan-thar'ĭ-dizm) morbid effect of overuse of cantharides.

canthectomy (kan-thek'to-me) excision of a canthus.

canthitis (kan-thi'tis) inflammation of a canthus.

cantholysis (kan-thol'ĭ-sis) surgical section of a canthus and canthal ligament.

canthoplasty (kan'tho-plas"te) plastic repair of a canthus.

canthorrhaphy (kan-thor'ah-fe) suture of a canthus.

canthotomy (kan-thot'o-me) incision of a canthus.

canthus (kan'thus), pl. *can'thi* [L.] the angular junction of the eyelids at either corner of the eyes. adj., **can'thal.**

Cantil (kan'til) trademark for a preparation of mepenzolate bromide.

caoutchouc (koo'chook) India rubber or gum elastic; used in dentistry and surgery.

C.A.P. College of American Pathologists.

cap (kap) a structure covering the end or head of something. **duodenal c.,** pileus ventriculi. **enamel c.,** the enamel organ when it covers the top of the dental papilla like a cap. **skull c.,** calvaria.

capacitance (kah-pas'ĭ-tans) the property of taking and holding an electric charge.

capacitor (kah-pas'ĭ-tor) a device for holding and storing charges of electricity.

capacity (kah-pas'ĭ-te) the power of receiving and holding, usually expressed numerically as the measure of such ability. **functional residual c.,** the amount of gas remaining in the lung at the resting expiratory level. **heat c.,** thermal capacity. **inspiratory c.,** the maximal amount of gas that can be inspired from the resting expiratory level. **thermal c.,** the amount of heat absorbed by a body in being raised 1 degree C. **total lung c.,** the amount of gas contained in the lung at the end of a maximal inspiration. **vital c.,** a measure of the volume of air which can be expelled by the lungs after maximal expiration and maximal inspiration.

capelet (kap'ĕ-let) a swelling on the point of a horse's hock or on its elbow.

capillarectasia (kap"ĭ-lār"ek-ta'ze-ah) dilatation of capillaries.

Capillaria (kap"il-la're-ah) a genus of nematode parasites. **C. hepat'ica,** a species parasitic in animals, including man.

capillariomotor (kap"ĭ-lār"e-o-mo'tor) pertaining to control of the caliber of the capillaries.

capillaritis (kap"ĭ-lār-i'tis) inflammation of the capillaries.

capillarity (kap"ĭ-lār'ĭ-te) the action by which

the surface of a liquid where it is in contact with a solid, as in a capillary tube, is elevated or depressed.

capillary (kap′ĭ-ler″e) 1. hairlike. 2. one of the minute blood vessels interposed between arterioles and venules, or a similar channel conveying lymph.

capillus (kah-pil′us), pl. *capil′li* [L.] a hair.

capitate (kap′ĭ-tāt) head-shaped.

capitatum (kap″ĭ-ta′tum) the capitate bone.

capitellum (kap″ĭ-tel′um) capitulum.

capitonnage (kap″ĭ-to-nahzh′) [Fr.], closure of a cyst by approximating the opposing surfaces of the cavity.

capitular (kah-pit′u-ler) pertaining to the head of a bone.

capitulum (kah-pit′u-lum), pl. *capit′ula* [L.] a small boss on the surface of a bone, as on the humerus.

Capla (kap′lah) trademark for a preparation of mebutamate.

capnohepatography (kap″no-hep″ah-tog′rah-fe) radiography of the liver after intravenous injection of carbon dioxide gas.

capotement (kah-pōt-maw′) [Fr.] a splashing sound heard in dilatation of the stomach.

cappa (kap′ah) a layer of gray matter of the quadrigeminal body.

capping (kap′ing) the provision of a protective or obstructive covering. **pulp c.,** the covering of an exposed dental pulp with some material to provide protection against external influences.

Capsebon (kap′se-bon) trademark for a suspension of cadmium sulfide.

capsicum (kap′sĭ-kum) dried ripe fruit of species of *Capsicum frutescens;* powerful local stimulant.

capsitis (kap-si′tis) capsulitis.

capsotomy (kap-sot′o-me) capsulotomy.

capsula (kap′su-lah), pl. *cap′sulae* [L.] capsule.

capsulation (kap″su-la′shun) enclosure in a capsule.

capsule (kap′sūl) an enclosing structure, as (1) a membrane or saclike structure enclosing an organ or part; (2) a small, soluble container for medicine; (3) the envelope surrounding certain bacteria. adj., **cap′sular. articular c.,** a fibrous structure uniting the ends of bones forming a diarthrodial joint. **auditory c.,** the cartilaginous structure in the embryo which becomes the external ear. **bacterial c.,** a gelatinous envelope surrounding a bacterial cell which is associated with the virulence of pathogenic bacteria; usually polysaccharide, but sometimes polypeptide. **Bonnet's c.,** Tenon's capsule. **Bowman's c.,** malpighian capsule. **c's of the brain,** two layers of white matter in the substance of the brain. **cartilage c.,** a basophilic zone of cartilage matrix bordering on a lacuna and its enclosed cartilage cells. **dental c.,** periodontium. **external c.,** the layer of white fibers forming the outer border of the corpus striatum. **Gerota's c.,** the fascia surrounding the kidney. **Glisson's c.,** sheath of connective tissue inclosing hepatic artery, hepatic duct and portal vein. **c. of heart,** pericardium. **internal c.,** a broad band of

white matter separating the lentiform nucleus from the thalamus and caudate nucleus. **joint c.,** the capsular ligament of a joint. **c. of lens,** transparent sac enclosing lens of eye. **malpighian c.,** a two-layered cellular envelope enclosing the tuft of capillaries constituting the glomerulus of the kidney. **nasal c.,** the cartilaginous pouch in the embryo from which the nose develops. **optic c.,** the embryonic structure from which the sclera develops. **renal c.,** the fibrous or the fatty material enveloping the kidney, the inner fibrous layer being continuous with the lining of the renal sinus. **sodium iodide I-131 c's,** capsules containing radioactive iodine as sodium iodide, used in tests of thyroid disease and in treatment of neoplasms. **suprarenal c.,** adrenal gland. **Tenon's c.,** the connective tissue enclosing the eyeball.

capsulectomy (kap″su-lek′to-me) excision of a capsule, as of the capsule of the kidney or of the crystalline lens.

capsulitis (kap″su-li′tis) inflammation of a capsule.

capsulolenticular (kap″su-lo-len-tik′u-ler) pertaining to the capsule and lens.

capsuloma (kap″su-lo′mah) a capsular tumor of the kidney.

capsuloplasty (kap′su-lo-plas″te) plastic repair of a joint capsule.

capsulorrhaphy (kap″su-lor′ah-fe) suture of a joint capsule.

capsulotomy (kap″su-lot′o-me) incision of a capsule, as that of the lens or of a joint.

captodiamine (kap″to-di′ah-mēn) a dimethylethylamine derivative used as an antihistaminic and sedative.

captodramin (kap″to-dram′in) captodiamine.

caput (kap′ut), pl. *cap′ita* [L.] the head or headlike object or part. **c. co′li,** the cecum. **c. gallinag′inis,** the verumontanum. **c. medu′-sae,** the pattern presented by congested cutaneous veins about the umbilicus in obstruction of the portal vein. **c. obsti′pum,** torticollis. **c. succeda′neum,** edema sometimes occurring in and under the fetal scalp during labor.

C.A.R. Canadian Association of Radiologists.

caramel (kar′ah-mel) a concentrated solution obtained by heating sugar or glucose until it is a uniform dark brown mass, used as a coloring agent

caramiphen (kah-ram′ĭ-fen) an agent used in parasympathetic blockade, as an antispasmodic and in treatment of parkinsonism.

caraway (kar′ah-wa) dried ripe fruit of *Carum carvi,* used as a flavoring agent.

carbachol (kar′bah-kol) white or yellowish crystals, $C_6H_{15}ClN_2O_2$; parasympathomimetic (cholinergic) agent.

carbamide (kar-bam′ĭd) urea in anhydrous, lyophilized, sterile powder form; injected intravenously in dextrose or invert sugar solution to induce diuresis.

carbaminohemoglobin (kar-bam″ĭ-no-he″mo-glo′bin) a combination of carbon dioxide and free amino groups of hemoglobin.

carbamylcholine chloride (kar″bah-mil-ko′-lēn klo′rĭd) carbachol.

carbarsone (kar′bar-sōn) an arsenical compound, $C_7H_9AsN_2O_4$; used in amebic dysentery.

carbasus (kar′bah-sus) gauze. **c. absor′bens,** absorbent gauze. **c. absor′bens adhe′siva,** adhesive absorbent gauze. **c. absor′bens steri′lis,** sterile absorbent gauze.

carbazochrome salicylate (kar-baz′o-krōm sal′-ĭ-sil″āt) a salicylate complex used as a hemostatic agent for capillary bleeding.

carbetapentane (kar-ba″tah-pen′tān) a carboxylate derivative used as an antitussive agent.

carbethyl salicylate (kar-beth′il sal′ĭ-sil″āt) salicylic ethyl ester carbonate, used as an analgesic and antiarthritic agent.

carbinol (kar′bĭ-nol) methanol.

carbinoxamine (kar″bin-ok′sah-mēn) a pyridine derivative used as an antihistaminic.

carbo (kar′bo) [L.] carbon; charcoal. **c. anima′-lis,** animal charcoal. **c. lig′ni,** charcoal.

Carbocaine (kar′bo-kān) trademark for preparations of mepivacaine hydrochloride.

carbocholine (kar″bo-ko′lēn) carbachol.

carbohemia (-he′me-ah) incomplete oxidation of the blood.

carbohemoglobin (-he″mo-glo′bin) a combination of carbon dioxide and hemoglobin.

carbohydrase (-hi′drās) an enzyme which catalyzes the hydrolysis of carbohydrates.

carbohydrate (-hi′drāt) a compound of carbon, hydrogen and oxygen, the latter two in the proportion of water.

carbolfuchsin (kar″bol-fŏŏk′sin) staining fluid containing carbolic acid and fuchsin.

carbolism (kar′bo-lizm) phenol poisoning.

carbolize (kar′bo-līz) to impregnate with phenol.

carboluria (kar″bo-lu′re-ah) phenol in the urine.

carbometer (kar-bom′ĕ-ter) an instrument for determining the proportion of carbon dioxide exhaled with the breath.

carbon (kar′bon) chemical element *(see table)*, at. no. 6, symbol C. **c. dioxide,** odorless, colorless gas, CO_2, used with oxygen to stimulate respiration and in solid form as an escharotic. **c. monoxide,** an odorless gas, CO, formed by incomplete combustion of carbon; rapidly fatal because it forms a stable compound with hemoglobin. **c. tetrachloride,** clear, colorless, mobile liquid; anthelmintic and insecticide.

carbonate (kar′bon-āt) a salt of carbonic acid.

carbonemia (kar″bo-ne′me-ah) excess of carbon dioxide in the blood.

carbonize (kar′bo-nīz) to convert into charcoal or carbon.

carbonometry (kar″bo-nom′ĕ-tre) measurement of carbon dioxide.

carbonuria (-u′re-ah) excretion of urine containing carbon dioxide or other carbon compounds.

carbonyl (kar′bo-nil) the divalent radical, =CO.

Carbo-resin (kar′bo-rez″in) trademark for a mixture of carbacrylamine resins.

Carboxydomonas (kar-bok″se-do-mo′nas) a genus of Schizomycetes (order Pseudomonadales, suborder Pseudomonadineae, family Methanomonadaceae).

carboxyhemoglobin (kar-bok″se-he″mo-glo′-bin) a combination of carbon monoxide and hemoglobin.

carboxyl (kar-bok′sil) the monovalent radical, −COOH, found in nearly all organic acids.

carboxylase (kar-bok′sĭ-lās) an enzyme which splits carbon dioxide from carboxyl groups.

carboxylesterase (kar-bok″sil-es′ter-ās) an enzyme that catalyzes the hydrolysis of the esters of carboxylic acids.

carboxymyoglobin (kar-bok″se-mi″o-glo′bin) a compound formed from myoglobin on exposure to carbon monoxide.

carboxypeptidase (-pep′tĭ-dās) an exopeptidase that acts only on the peptide linkage of a terminal amino acid containing a free carboxyl group.

carboxypolypeptidase (-pol″e-pep′-tĭ-dās) an enzyme which causes splitting off of a free carboxyl group from a polypeptide.

carbromal (kar-bro′mal) white, odorless, crystalline powder, $C_7H_{13}BrN_2O_2$; nerve sedative and somnifacient.

carbuncle (kar′bung-kl) a deeply situated staphylococcal infection producing multiple adjacent draining skin sinuses. adj., **carbunc′-ular. malignant c.,** malignant anthrax. **renal c.,** a massive parenchymal suppuration due to bacterial metastasis following vascular thrombosis or infarction of the kidney.

carbunculosis (kar-bung″ku-lo′sis) formation of numerous carbuncles.

Carcholin (kar′ko-lin) trademark for a preparation of carbachol.

carcinectomy (kar″sī-nek′to-me) excision of a cancer.

carcinogen (kar-sin′o-jen) a substance which causes cancer. adj., **carcinogen′ic.**

carcinogenesis (kar″sī-no-jen′ē-sis) production of cancer.

carcinogenicity (-jĕ-nis′ĭ-te) the ability to produce cancer.

carcinoid (kar′sĭ-noid) resembling cancer.

carcinolysis (kar″sī-nol′ĭ-sis) destruction of cancer cells. adj., **carcinolyt′ic.**

carcinoma (kar″sī-no′mah) a malignant tumor made up of connective tissue enclosing epithelial cells. **alveolar c.,** carcinoma in which the cells appear in groups, enclosed in connective tissue. **basal cell c.,** a cutaneous cancer of relatively low-grade malignancy, arising from the basal layers of the epidermis. **bronchogenic c.,** carcinoma of the lung. **chorionic c.,** choriocarcinoma. **colloid c.,** carcinoma in which the cells have undergone colloid degeneration. **cylindrical cell c.,** carcinoma in which the cells are cylindrical or nearly so. **embryonal c.,** seminoma. **epidermoid c.,** squamous cell carcinoma. **gelatinous c.,** colloid carcinoma. **giant cell c.,** carcinoma containing many giant cells. **hair matrix c.,** basal cell carcinoma. **c. in si′tu,** carcinoma which has not invaded adjoining tissues, but is still confined to its site of origin. **prickle cell c.,** squamous cell carcinoma. **c. sarcomato′des,** carcinosarcoma. **scirrhous c.,** carcinoma with a hard structure composed of connective tissue alveoli filled with masses of cells which have no vessels or interstitial substance. **c. sim'plex,** carcinoma in which the relative proportion between the stroma and the cells is normal. **squamous cell c.,** a rapidly growing and readily metastasizing carcinoma originating in the epidermis, particularly the prickle cell layer. **sweat gland c.,** a rare skin tumor arising from the sweat glands, having a metastatic tendency between that of basal cell and that of squamous cell carcinoma.

carcinomatosis (kar″si-no″mah-to'sis) the development of multiple carcinomas.

carcinomatous (kar″si-no'mah-tus) of or pertaining to carcinoma or cancer.

carcinophilia (kar″si-no-fil'e-ah) special affinity for cancerous tissue. adj., **carcinophil'ic.**

carcinophobia (-fo'be-ah) morbid dread of cancer.

carcinosarcoma (-sar-ko'mah) carcinoma sarcomatodes.

carcinosis (kar″si-no'sis) dissemination of a cancer. **miliary c.,** that marked by development of numerous nodules resembling miliary tuberculosis.

cardamom (kar'dah-mom) fruit of *Elettaria cardamomum,* source of a seed and oil used as flavoring agents.

cardi(o)- (kar'de-o) word element [Gr.], *heart.*

cardia (kar'de-ah) the upper orifice of the stomach.

cardiac (kar'de-ak) pertaining to the heart or to the upper orifice of the stomach.

cardialgia (kar″de-al'je-ah) pain in the epigastrium.

cardianeuria (-ah-nu'rc-ah) deficiency of tone in the heart.

cardiant (kar'de-ant) 1. affecting the heart. 2. a medicine affecting the heart.

cardiataxia (kar″de-ah-tak'se-ah) incoordination of heart movements.

cardiectasis (-ek'tah-sis) dilatation of the heart.

cardio-accelerator (kar″de-o-ak-sel'er-a″tor) an agent which quickens the heart's action.

cardio-angiology (-an″je-ol'o-je) study of the heart and blood vessels.

cardio-aortic (-a-or'tik) pertaining to heart and aorta.

cardio-arterial (-ar-te're-al) pertaining to heart and arteries.

cardiocele (kar'de-o-sel″) hernial protrusion of the heart through the diaphragm.

cardiocentesis (kar″de-o-sen-te'sis) surgical puncture of the heart.

cardiochalasia (-kah-la'ze-ah) relaxation or incompetence of the cardiac orifice of the stomach.

cardiocinetic (-si-net'ik) cardiokinetic.

cardiocirrhosis (-sir-ro'sis) cirrhosis of the liver associated with heart disease.

cardioclasis (kar″de-ok'lah-sis) rupture of the heart.

cardiodiaphragmatic (kar″de-o-di″ah-fragmat'ik) pertaining to the heart and the diaphragm.

cardiodilator (-di'la-tor) an instrument for dilating the cardia.

cardiodiosis (kar″de-o-di-o'sis) dilatation of the cardia.

cardiodynamics (-di-nam'iks) study of the forces involved in the heart's action.

cardiodynia (-din'e-ah) pain in the region of the heart.

cardiogenesis (-jen'ĕ-sis) development of the heart in the embryo.

cardiogenic (-jen'ik) originating in the heart.

Cardiografin (-gra'fin) trademark for a solution of methylglucamine diatrizoate.

cardiogram (kar'de-o-gram″) a record produced by cardiography. **apex c.,** the record produced by apex cardiography. **precordial c.,** kinetocardiogram. **ultrasound c.,** echocardiogram.

cardiograph (kar'de-o-graf″) an instrument for recording the heart movements. adj., **cardiograph'ic.**

cardiography (kar″de-og'rah-fe) the graphic recording of a physical or functional aspect of the heart, e.g. electrocardiography, kinetocardiography, phonocardiography, vibrocardiography. **apex c.,** graphic recording of low-frequency pulsations at the anterior chest wall over the apex of the heart. **ultrasonic c.,** echocardiography.

Cardio-green (kar″de-o-grēn) trademark for a preparation of indocyanine green.

cardiohepatic (-hĕ-pat'ik) pertaining to heart and liver.

cardio-inhibitor (-in-hib'ĭ-ter) an agent which restrains the heart's action.

cardiokinetic (-ki-net'ik) 1. exciting or stimulating the heart. 2. an agent that excites or stimulates the heart.

cardiolith (kar'de-o-lith) a calculus in the heart.

cardiologist (kar″de-ol'o-jist) a specialist in the study and treatment of heart disease.

cardiology (-ol'o-je) study of the heart and its functions.

cardiolysin (-ol'ĭ-sin) a lysin which acts on the heart muscle.

cardiolysis (-ol'ĭ-sis) the separation of adhesions constricting the heart.

cardiomalacia (kar″de-o-mah-la'she-ah) softening of the heart substance.

cardiomegaly (-meg'ah-le) hypertrophy of the heart.

cardiometer (kar″de om'ĕ tor) instrument for estimating the power of the heart's action.

cardiomotility (kar″de-o-mo-til'ĭ-te) motility of the heart.

cardiomyoliposis (-mi″o-li-po'sis) fatty degeneration of the heart muscle.

cardiomyopathy (-mi-op'ah-the) a subacute or chronic disorder of heart muscle, often with endocardial and sometimes pericardial involvement.

cardionector (-nek'tor) a structure that regulates the heart beat, i.e. the sinoatrial node or the bundle of His.

cardionephric (-nef'rik) pertaining to heart and kidney.

cardioneural (-nu'ral) pertaining to heart and nervous system.

cardioneurosis (-nu-ro'sis) functional neurosis marked by cardiac symptoms.

cardio-omentopexy (kar″de-o-o-men′to-pek″se) suture of a portion of the omentum to the heart.

cardiopalmus (-pal′mus) palpitation of the heart.

cardiopathy (kar″de-op′ah-thc) a morbid condition of the heart.

cardiopericardiopexy (kar″de-o-per″ĭ-kar′de-o-pek″se) surgical establishment of adhesive pericarditis, for relief of coronary disease.

cardiopericarditis (-per″ĭ-kar-di′tis) inflammation of heart and pericardium.

cardiophobia (-fo′be-ah) morbid dread of heart disease.

cardiophone (kar′de-o-fōn″) an instrument for making audible the sound of the heart muscle.

cardioplasty (kar′de-o-plas″te) plastic repair of the opening between the esophagus and the stomach.

cardioplegia (kar″de-o-ple′je-ah) interruption of myocardial contraction, as by use of chemical compounds or cold in cardiac surgery.

cardiopneumatic (-nu-mat′ik) pertaining to the heart and the lungs.

cardiopneumograph (-nu′mo-graf) a machine for registering cardiopneumatic movements.

cardioptosis (-to′sis) downward displacement of the heart.

cardiopulmonary (-pul′mo-ner″e) pertaining to the heart and lungs.

cardiopuncture (-punk′tūr) cardiocentesis.

cardiopyloric (-pi-lor′ik) pertaining to cardia and pylorus.

cardiorenal (-re′nal) pertaining to heart and kidneys.

cardiorrhaphy (kar″de-or′ah-fe) suture of the heart.

cardiorrhexis (kar″de-o-rek′sis) rupture of the heart.

cardiosclerosis (-skle-ro′sis) fibroid induration of the heart.

cardioscope (kar′de-o-skōp″) cardiophone.

cardiospasm (kar′de-o-spazm″) spasm of the cardiac sphincter of the stomach.

cardiosphygmograph (kar″de-o-sfig′mo-graf) instrument for recording movements of heart and pulse.

cardiosplenopexy (-splen′o-pek″se) suture of splenic parenchyma to the denuded surface of the heart for revascularization of the myocardium.

cardiosymphysis (-sim′fĭ-sis) obliteration of the pericardial sac by adhesions.

cardiotachometer (-tah-kom′ĕ-ter) an instrument which records the heart rate continuously for hours or days.

cardiotachometry (-tah-kom′ĕ-tre) continuous recording of the heart rate for long periods of time.

cardiotherapy (-ther′ah-pe) the treatment of diseases of the heart.

cardiotomy (kar″de-ot′o-me) surgical incision of the heart.

cardiotonic (kar″de-o-ton′ik) having a tonic effect on the heart.

cardiotopometry (-to-pom′ĕ-tre) measurement of the area of cardiac dullness.

cardiotoxic (-tok′sik) poisonous to the heart.

cardiotrophotherapy (kar″de-o-trof″o-ther′-ah-pe) metabolic treatment of heart disorders.

cardiovalvular (-val′vu-lar) pertaining to the valves of the heart.

cardiovalvulotome (-val′vu-lo-tōm″) an instrument for incising the mitral valve.

cardiovascular (-vas′ku-lar) pertaining to heart and blood vessels.

cardiovasology (-vas-ol′o-je) cardioangiology.

carditis (kar-di′tis) inflammation of the heart; myocarditis.

cardivalvulitis (kar″dī-val″vu-li′tis) inflammation of the heart valves.

Cardrase (kar′drās) trademark for a preparation of ethoxzolamide.

care (kār) attention to the needs of a patient or requirements of a situation. **nursing c.,** see *nursing.* **tender loving c.,** that designed to meet fully the emotional and physical needs of a patient, especially of an infant.

caries (ka′re-ēz) decay, as of bone or teeth. adj., **ca′rious. dental c.,** a destructive process causing decalcification of the tooth enamel and leading to continued destruction of enamel and dentin, and cavitation of the tooth. **dry c.,** caries sicca. **c. fungo′sa,** tuberculosis of bone. **necrotic c.,** form in which pieces of the bone lie in a suppurating cavity. **c. sic′ca,** a form of bone decay unaccompanied by enlargement, swelling or abscess formation in surrounding tissues, often caused by *Mycobacterium tuberculosis.*

carina (kah-ri′nah), pl. *cari′nae* [L.] a ridgelike structure. **c. tra′cheae,** a downward and backward projection of the lowest tracheal cartilage, forming a ridge between the openings of the right and left principal bronchi. **c. urethra′lis vagi′nae,** the median ridge on the anterior wall of the vagina.

cariogenic (kār″e-o-jen′ik) conducive to caries.

cariogenicity (-je-nis′ĭ-te) the quality of being conducive to caries.

carisoprodol (kar″i-so′pro-dol) a drug used as an analgesic and skeletal muscle relaxant.

carminative (kar-min′ah-tive) 1. relieving flatulence. 2. an agent that relieves flatulence.

carmine (kar′min, kar′mīn) a crimson pigment. **indigo c.,** sodium indigotindisulfonate.

carminophilic (kar″mĭ-no-fil′ik) stainable with carmine.

carnophobia (kar″no-fo′be-ah) aversion to meat diet.

caro (ka′ro), pl. *car′nes* [L.] flesh, or muscular tissue.

carotenase (kar-ot′ĕ-nās) an enzyme which converts carotene into vitamin A.

carotene (kar′o-tēn) a lipochrome or coloring matter from carrots, tomatoes and other vegetables, egg yolk, milk fat and other substances; in the body it can be converted into vitamin A.

carotenemia (kar″o-tĕ-ne′me-ah) presence of carotene in the blood.

carotenoid (kah-rot′ĕ-noid) 1. resembling carotene. 2. a compound resembling carotene.

carotenosis (kar″o-tĕ-no′sis) deposition of carotene in tissues, especially the skin.

caroticotympanic   (kah-rot″ĭ-ko-tim-pan'ik)
  pertaining to carotid canal and tympanum.
carotid (kah-rot'id) see *Table of Arteries*, and
  under *body, canal* and *sinus.*
carotidynia (kah-rot″ĭ-din'e-ah) pain caused
  by pressure on the common carotid artery.
carotin (kar'o-tin) carotene.
carotinase (kar-ot'ĭ-nās) carotenase.
carpal (kar'pal) pertaining to the carpus.
carpectomy (kar-pek'to-me) excision of a carpal bone.
carphology (kar-fol'o-je) picking at the bed-
  clothes; a sign of great exhaustion.
carpitis (kar-pi'tis) inflammation of the synovial membranes of the bones of the carpus
  of domestic animals.
carpometacarpal (kar″po-met″ah-kar'pal) pertaining to carpus and metacarpus.
carpoptosis (-to'sis) wrist drop.
carpus (kar'pus) the eight bones composing
  the articulation between the hand and the
  forearm; the wrist.
carrier (kār'e-er) an agent by which something
  is carried, especially an individual harboring
  pathogenic microorganisms and capable of
  transmitting them to others. **chronic c.,** one
  who has recovered from the disease or, though
  he has never had the disease, carries the
  organisms in his body. **contact c.,** one who has
  been exposed to an infection, and, although
  healthy, may act as a carrier of the infection.
  convalescent c., one convalescent from a disease who may still carry its causative organisms. **gamete c.,** one who transmits a parasitic disease by parasites undergoing intracapsular conjugation in his body. **healthy c.,**
  a person who has never had the disease, but
  carries the infecting organism in his body.
  hemophiliac c., the female transmitter of
  classic sex-linked hemophilia, who may show
  only a coagulation factor deficiency. **incu-
  batory c.,** one in the incubation period of an
  infectious disease, who will soon manifest
  the symptoms.
cart (kart)   a wheeled vehicle for conveying
  materials in hospital, e.g. patients themselves
  or supplies and equipment used in performing
  bedside procedures. **crash c.,** resuscitation
  cart. **dressing c.,** one containing all supplies
  and equipment that may be necessary for
  changing dressings of surgical or injured
  patients. **medicine c.,** one for transporting
  medications to patients. **resuscitation c.,** one
  containing all equipment necessary for initiating emergency resuscitation at a patient's
  bedside.
cartilage (kar'tĭ-lij) the gristle or white elastic
  substance attached to articular bone surfaces and forming parts of the skeleton. **alar
  c's,** the cartilages of the wings of the nose.
  aortic c., the second costal cartilage on the
  right side. **arthrodial c., articular c.,** that
  lining the articular surfaces of bones. **arytenoid c's,** two pyramid-shaped cartilages
  of the larynx. **central c.,** an opacity in the
  center of the crystalline lens. **connecting c.,**
  that connecting the surfaces of an immovable

joint. **corniculate c.,** a small nodule of cartilage at the apex of each arytenoid cartilage.
  costal c's, cartilages between true ribs
  and the sternum. **cricoid c.,** the lowest cartilage of the larynx. **cuneiform c.,** a small
  elongated piece of cartilage on either side,
  in front of the arytenoid cartilages. **dentinal
  c.,** the substance remaining after the lime
  salts of dentin have been dissolved in an
  acid. **diarthrodial c.,** articular cartilage.
  elastic c., cartilage whose matrix contains
  yellow elastic fibers. **ensiform c.,** xiphoid
  process. **epactal c's,** one or more small
  cartilages in the lateral wall of the nose.
  floating c., a detached portion of semilunar
  cartilage in the knee joint. **hyaline c.,** cartilage with a glassy, translucent appearance,
  the matrix and embedded collagenous fibers
  having the same index of refraction. **interosseous c.,** connecting cartilage. **investing
  c.,** articular cartilage. **Jacobson's c.,** hyaline
  cartilage supporting Jacobson's organ. **mandibular c., Meckel's c.,** ventral segment of
  first branchial arch of embryo. **ossifying c.,**
  temporary cartilage. **palpebral c's,** tarsal
  cartilages. **parachordal c.,** one of the two
  cartilages beside the occipital part of
  notochord of the embryo. **permanent c.,**
  cartilage which does not normally become
  ossified. **precursory c.,** temporary cartilage. **Reichert's c.,** cartilage of the hyoid
  arch of the embryo, developing into styloid
  process and adjacent structures. **reticular c.,**
  elastic cartilage. **c. of Santorini,** corniculate
  cartilage. **semilunar c.,** one of the two interarticular cartilages of the knee joint. **sesamoid c's,** small cartilages such as those in the
  side of the wing of the nose. **slipping rib c.,**
  a loosened or deformed cartilage whose slipping over an adjacent rib cartilage may produce discomfort or pain. **stratified c.,** fibrocartilage. **tarsal c's,** the cartilaginous portion
  of the eyelids. **temporary c.,** cartilage that is
  normally destined to become changed into
  bone. **thyroid c.,** the shield-shaped cartilage
  of the larynx **tympanomandibular c.,**
  Meckel's cartilage. **c. of Wrisberg,** cuneiform cartilage. **xiphoid c.,** xiphoid process.
  Y c., Y-shaped cartilage within the acetabulum, joining ilium, ischium and os pubis.
  yellow c., elastic cartilage.
cartilaginoid (kar″tĭ-laj'ĭ-noid)   resembling
  cartilage.
cartilaginous (-laj'ĭ-nus) consisting of cartilage.
cartilago (kar″tĭ-lah'go), pl. *cartilag'ines* [L.]
  cartilage.
caruncle (kar'ung-kl) a small fleshy eminence,
  often abnormal. **hymenal c's,** mucosal tags
  at the vaginal orifice supposedly relics of the
  ruptured hymen. **lacrimal c.,** red eminence
  at medial angle of eye. **Morgagni's c., morgagnian c.,** the middle lobe of the prostate.
  myrtiform c's, hymenal caruncles. **sublingual c.,** an eminence on either side of the
  frenulum of the tongue, on which the major
  sublingual duct and the submandibular duct

open. **urethral c.,** a polypoid growth usually near the meatus of the urethra in females, sometimes causing difficulty in voiding.

caruncula (kah-rung'ku-la), pl. *carun'culae* [L.] caruncle.

carver (kar'ver) a tool for producing and perfecting anatomic form in artificial teeth and dental restorations.

caryo- (kār'e-o) for words beginning thus, see also those beginning *karyo-.*

Caryophanaceae (ka″re-o-fah-na'se-e) a family of Schizomycetes (order Caryophanales).

Caryophanales (-fah-na'lēz) an order of Schizomycetes found in water and in decomposing organic materials, and in the intestines of arthropods and vertebrates.

Caryophanon (ka″re-o'fah-non) a genus of Schizomycetes (order Caryophanales, family Caryophanaceae).

cascara (kas-kār'ah) husk, bark. **c. sagra'da,** dried bark of *Rhamnus purshiana,* used as a stimulant cathartic.

case (kās) 1. a particular instance of a disease. 2. an apparatus for enclosing something. **index c.,** the case of the original patient (propositus or proband) that stimulates investigation of other members of the family to discover a possible genetic factor in the condition. **trial c.,** a box containing + and − spherical and + and − cylindrical lenses, arranged in pairs, a trial spectacle frame and various other devices used in testing vision.

casease (ka'se-ās) a bacterial enzyme capable of dissolving albumin.

caseation (ka″se-a'shun) the conversion of tissue by degeneration into a dry, amorphous mass like cheese.

casebook (kās'book) a book in which a physician enters the records of his cases.

casein (ka'se-in) the phosphoprotein found in milk. **vegetable c.,** legumin.

caseinogen (ka″se-in'o-jen) the precursor of casein.

caseous (ka'se-us) cheeselike.

cassette (ka-set') [Fr.] a light-proof housing for x-ray film, containing front and back intensifying screens, between which the film is placed.

cast (kast) an object molded to shape, as (1) a mass of molded plastic material produced by effusion into a body passage, especially such masses in the urine, named according to the constituents, as epithelial, fatty, hyaline, mucous, waxy, etc.; or (2) a rigid dressing molded to the body while pliable, and hardening to give a firm support. **dental c.,** the facsimile of oral structures obtained by pouring plaster into an impression made of the mouth. **hanging c.,** one applied to the arm in fracture of the shaft of the humerus, suspended by a sling looped around the neck. **quarter c.,** a cut in the quarter of a horse's hoof. **tube c.,** a mass of plastic material formed in a renal tubule.

castrate (kas'trāt) 1. to subject to excision of

the gonads. 2. an individual whose gonads have been removed.

castration (kas-tra'shun) excision of the gonads, especially in the male, rendering the individual incapable of reproduction. **female c.,** oophorectomy. **male c.,** orchiectomy. **parasitic c.,** destruction of gonadal tissue by endoparasitic organisms.

casualty (kaz'u-al-te) 1. an accidental or other injury. 2. a person suffering accidental or other injury.

casuistics (kaz″u-is'tiks) the recording and study of cases of disease.

catabasis (kah-tab'ah-sis) the stage of decline of a disease. adj., **catabat'ic.**

catabiosis (kat″ah-bi-o'sis) the natural decline of vital phenomena in a cell. adj., **catabiot'-ic.**

catabolergy (-bol'er-je) the energy used in catabolism.

catabolin (kah-tab'o-lin) a product of destructive metabolism (catabolism).

catabolism (kah-tab'o-lizm) destructive metabolism; the process by which an organism reconverts living, organized substance into simpler compounds, with release of energy for its use. adj., **catabol'ic.**

catabolite (kah-tab'o-līt) a compound produced in catabolism.

catachronobiology (kat″ah-kron″o-bi-ol'o-je) the study of the deleterious effects of time on a living system.

catacrotism (kah-tak'ro-tizm) the occurrence of one or more indentations on the descending limb of the sphygmogram. adj., **catacrot'ic.**

catadicrotism (kat″ah-di'kro-tizm) the occurrence of two indentations on the descending limb of the sphygmogram. adj., **catadicrot'-ic.**

catadioptric (-di-op'trik) pertaining to both refraction and reflection of light.

catagen (kat'ah-jen) the transitional (second) phase of the hair cycle, with cessation of proliferation of the cells of the matrix and formation of a bulbous enlargement at the base of the hair.

catagenesis (kat″ah-jen'ē-sis) involution.

catalase (kat'ah-lās) a crystalline enzyme which specifically catalyzes the decomposition of hydrogen peroxide and is found in almost all cells except certain bacteria. adj., **catalat'ic.**

catalepsy (kat'ah-lep″se) a condition in which the entire body or limbs remain passively in any position in which they are placed. adj., **catalep'tic.**

cataleptiform (kat″ah-lep'tĭ-form) resembling catalepsy.

cataleptoid (-lep'toid) resembling catalepsy.

catalysis (kah-tal'ĭ-sis) influence on a chemical reaction by small quantities of a substance which does not enter into the reaction, but persists unchanged. adj., **catalyt'ic. negative c.,** inhibition of a chemical reaction by a catalyst. **positive c.,** acceleration of a chemical reaction by a catalyst.

catalyst (kat'ah-list) a substance capable of

promoting or altering the speed of a chemical reaction, but one that does not take part in it.

catalyze (kat′ah-līz) to promote the occurrence or influence the velocity of a chemical reaction.

catalyzer (kat′ah-līz″er) catalyst.

catamenia (kat″ah-me′ne-ah) menstruation. adj., **catame′nial.**

catamnesis (kat″am-ne′sis) the medical history of a patient from the date on which he sought medical attention.

cataphasia (kat″ah-fa′ze-ah) speech disorder with constant repetition of a word or phrase.

cataphora (kah-taf′ŏ-rah) state resembling sleep, with loss of feeling and voice.

cataphoresis (kat″ah-fo-re′sis) introduction of medicine through the unbroken skin, by means of an electric current.

cataphoria (-fo′re-ah) the tendency to tilt the head upward, the visual axes deviating downward on looking straight ahead. adj., **cataphor′ic.**

cataphrenia (-fre′ne-ah) mental debility of the dementia type which tends to recovery. adj., **cataphren′ic.**

cataphylaxis (-fi-lak′sis) movement of leukocytes and antibodies to the site of an infection. adj., **cataphylac′tic.**

cataplasia (-pla′ze-ah) atrophy with tissues reverting to earlier conditions.

cataplexy (kat′ah-plek″se) a sudden, temporary loss of muscular tone, causing collapse. adj., **cataplec′tic.**

cataract (kat′ah-rakt) opacification of the lens or its capsule, sufficient to interfere with vision of the eye. adj., **catarac′tous. after-c.,** secondary cataract. **anterior polar c.,** a congenital cataract with opacity of the anterior pole of the capsule and underlying lens fibers. **anterior pyramidal c.,** anterior capsular opacity projecting forward into the aqueous humor. **atopic c.,** that resulting from allergy, often associated with atopic eczema and asthma. **blue c., blue dot c.,** a condition marked by small punctate opacities of a delicate bluish tint throughout the nucleus and cortex of the lens. **capsular c.,** opacification of the capsule of the lens, often associated with degeneration of subcapsular lens fibers. **coronary c.,** one in which club-shaped opacities are arranged in a ring or crown, the center of the lens and extreme periphery remaining transparent. **cortical c.,** opacification involving lens fibers just beneath the capsule and beginning at the periphery of the lens. **cupuliform c.,** opacification of the capsule and subcapsular cortical fibers at the posterior pole of the lens. **hypermature c.,** one in which the entire lens has become opaque and the cortex liquid, allowing the lens nucleus to sink downward by gravity. **lamellar c.,** one due to opacity of some of the layers between the cortex and nucleus, the remaining layers being transparent. **lenticular c.,** one occurring in the lens proper. **mature c.,** one in which the whole lens substance is involved. **membranous c.,** a cataract made up

of the remains of the capsule of the lens. **morgagnian c.,** a fluid cataract with a hard nucleus. **nuclear c.,** sclerosis of the central, older portion of the lens, causing increase in the refractive index of the lens and myopia. **polar c.,** opacity confined to the anterior or posterior pole of the lens. **pyramidal c.,** conoid opacity at the anterior pole, the apex extending forward. **secondary c.,** a condition sometimes following extracapsular extraction of a cataractous lens, due to density of the capsular remains or proliferation of the capsular epithelium. **senile c.,** the cataract of old persons. **siliculose c., siliquose c.,** cataract with atrophy of the lens, leaving a calcareous deposit in the capsule. **snowflake c.,** flaky, chalky deposits in the lens in young diabetics. **toxic c.,** that due to exposure to a toxic drug, e.g. naphthalene. **traumatic c.,** opacification of the lens due to injury to the eye. **zonular c.,** a condition with a strong hereditary tendency, with opacification of a circumscribed layer of lens fibers over the central portion of the lens.

cataracta (kat″ah-rak′tah) cataract. **c. brunes′-cens,** nuclear cataract, with deposition of pigments producing a dark brown color. **c. ceru′lea,** blue dot cataract.

catarrh (kah-tahr′) inflammation of a mucous membrane with free discharge. adj., **catarr′-hal.**

catarrhine (kat′ah rīn) characterized by nostrils that are close together and directed downward.

catastate (kat′ah-stāt) catabolite.

catathymia (kat″ah-thi′me-ah) a psychic disorder marked by perseveration.

catatonia (-to′ne-ah) a form of schizophrenia marked by conspicuous motor disturbances (retardation and stupor, or excessive activity and excitement). adj., **cataton′ic.**

catatricrotism (-tri′kro-tizm) the occurrence of three indentations in the descending limb of the sphygmogram. adj., **catatricrot′-ic.**

catatropia (-tro′pe-ah) downward turning of the visual axis.

cataxia (kah-tak′se-ah) the breaking up of bacterial associations.

catechol (kat′ĕ-kol) a compound, 1,2-dihydroxybenzene, $C_6H_6O_2$.

catecholamine (kat″ĕ-kol-am′in) a compound of catechol and an amine, having a sympathomimetic action.

catelectrotonus (kat″e-lek-trot′o-nus) increase of nerve irritability near the cathode.

Catenabacterium (kah-te″nah-bak-te′re-um) a genus of Schizomycetes (order Eubacteriales, family Lactobacillaceae, tribe Lactobacilleae) found in the intestinal tract.

catgut (kat′gut) absorbable suture material prepared from collagen from healthy mammals.

catharsis (kah-thar′sis) a purging or cleansing, especially the emotional reliving of past (repressed) events as a means of releasing tension and anxiety.

cathartic (kah-thar'tik) 1. promoting defecation. 2. an agent that promotes defecation; sometimes classified according to increasing intensity of their action as laxatives, purgatives and drastics. **bulk c.,** an indigestible hydrophilic colloid that lubricates the feces and also increases motor activity of the intestines by adding to the bulk of their contents. **lubricant c.,** one that acts by softening the feces and reducing friction between them and the intestinal wall. **saline c.,** one that increases fluidity of intestinal contents by retention of water by osmotic forces, and indirectly increases motor activity. **stimulant c.,** one that directly increases motor activity of the intestinal tract.

cathepsin (kah-thep'sin) an intracellular protein-splitting enzyme which acts in an essentially neutral medium.

catheter (kath'ĕ-ter) a tubular instrument for passage through body channels, chiefly for discharging fluids from a cavity. **Bozeman's c.,** a double-current uterine catheter. **cardiac c.,** a long, fine catheter especially designed for passage through a peripheral blood vessel into the chambers of the heart, under roentgenologic control. **elbowed c.,** a catheter bent at an angle near the beak. **eustachian c.,** an instrument for dilating the eustachian tube. **faucial c.,** eustachian catheter. **female c.,** short catheter for female bladder. **Gouley's c.,** a solid, curved instrument grooved on its lower aspect, for passing over a guide through a stricture into the bladder. **indwelling c.,** one which is held in position in the urethra. **Itard's c.,** a variety of eustachian catheter. **lobster-tail c.,** one with three joints at the tip. **Mercier's c.,** a flexible catheter elbowed at the end. **Nélaton's c.,** a catheter of soft rubber. **Pezzer's c.,** a self-retaining catheter with a bulbous extremity. **Phillips's c.,** a urethral catheter with a woven filiform guide. **prostatic c.,** one with a short angular tip. **railway c.,** a straight elastic catheter with open end to be introduced with a filiform guide in cases of stricture. **Schrötter's c.,** a hard-rubber catheter of varying caliber, used for dilating laryngeal strictures. **self-retaining c.,** a catheter constructed so that it remains in the bladder, effecting constant drainage. **two-way c.,** a double-channel catheter used in irrigation. **vertebrated c.,** one made in small sections fitted together so as to be flexible. **winged c.,** one with two projections on the end to retain it in the bladder.

catheterization (kath″ĕ-ter-i-za'shun) passage of a catheter into a body channel or cavity. **cardiac c.,** introduction of a catheter into the interior of the heart by way of a vein or an artery, or by direct needle puncture.

catheterize (kath'ĕ-ter-īz″) to introduce a catheter into a body cavity, usually into the urinary bladder for the withdrawal of urine.

cathexis (kah-thek'sis) attachment of psychic or emotional energy to an object or idea. adj., **cathec'tic.**

cathode (kath'ōd) the electrode by which an electric current leaves a cell, apparatus or body. adj., **cath'odal.**

cathodic (kah-thod'ik) 1. pertaining to a cathode. 2. efferent, or centrifugal.

Cathomycin (kath'o-mi″sin) trademark for preparations of novobiocin.

cation (kat'i-on) an electropositive element.

catoptrophobia (kat″op-tro-fo'be-ah) a morbid dread of mirrors.

cauda (kaw'dah), pl. *cau'dae* [L.] a tail or tail-like appendage. adj., **cau'dal. c. cerebel'li,** vermiform process of cerebellum. **c. equi'na,** the sheaf of roots of the lower spinal nerves descending from their point of attachment to the spinal cord to the site of emergence of the nerves from the spinal canal.

caudad (kaw'dad) toward a cauda or toward the posterior or distal end.

caudal (kaw'dal) pertaining to a cauda or to the posterior or distal end.

caudate (kaw'dāt) having a tail.

caudatum (kaw-da'tum) the caudate nucleus.

caul (kawl) part of the amnion which sometimes envelops the head of the fetus at birth.

Caulobacter (kaw″lo-bak'ter) a genus of Schizomycetes (order Pseudomonadales, suborder Pseudomonadineae, family Caulobacteraceae).

Caulobacteraceae (-bak″ter-a'se-e) a family of Schizomycetes (order Pseudomonadales, suborder Pseudomonadineae).

caumesthesia (kaw″mes-the'ze-ah) a condition in which, with a low temperature, a patient experiences a sense of burning heat.

causalgia (kaw-zal'je-ah) intense, burning superficial pain.

caustic (kaws'tik) 1. burning or escharotic. 2. a burning or escharotic compound. **Lugol's c.,** one part each of iodine and potassium iodide, with two parts of water. **lunar c.,** silver nitrate. **mitigated c.,** silver nitrate diluted with potassium nitrate.

cauterant (kaw'ter-ant) a caustic material or application.

cauterization (kaw″ter-i-za'shun) application of a caustic or of a hot instrument.

cautery (kaw'ter-e) 1. application of a caustic, or of a burning substance or instrument, for the destruction of tissue. 2. a hot instrument or caustic substance used to destroy tissue. **actual c.,** burning by a hot iron, moxa or lens. **cold c.,** application of carbon dioxide. **galvanic c.,** galvanocautery. **potential c.,** application of an escharotic. **virtual c.,** potential cautery.

caverniloquy (kav″er-nil'o-kwe) low-pitched pectoriloquy indicative of a cavity.

cavernitis (-ni'tis) inflammation of the corpus cavernosum.

cavernoma (-no'mah) hemangioma.

cavernositis (-no-si'tis) cavernitis.

cavernostomy (-nos'to-me) open drainage of a tuberculous cavity of the lung.

cavernous (kav'er-nus) pertaining to a hollow, or containing hollow spaces.

cavitas (kav'ĭ-tas), pl. *cavita'tes* [L.] cavity.

cavitation (kav"ĭ-ta'shun) the formation of a cavity, or empty place.

cavitis (ka-vi'tis) inflammation of a vena cava.

cavity (kav'ĭ-te) a hollow or space, especially a space within the body or one of its organs; in dentistry, the lesion produced by caries. **abdominal c.,** the part of the body cavity between the diaphragm above and the pelvis below. **amniotic c.,** the cavity of the amnion. **buccal c.,** the part of the oral cavity between the cheek and the posterior teeth on either side of the dental arch. **cleavage c.,** the blastocoele. **complex c.,** a carious lesion that involves three or more surfaces of a tooth in its prepared state. **compound c.,** a carious lesion that involves two surfaces of a tooth in its prepared state. **cotyloid c.,** acetabulum. **cranial c.,** the space enclosed by the bones of the cranium. **dental c.,** the defect (lesion) produced by destruction of enamel and dentin in a tooth affected by caries. **glenoid c.,** cavity in head of scapula for articulation with humerus. **medullary c.,** the cavity of a bone that contains the bone marrow (medulla ossium). **nasal c.,** the mucosa-lined cavity at either side of the nasal septum, within the nose. **nerve c.,** pulp cavity. **oral c.,** the cavity of the mouth, bounded by the jaw bones and associated structures (muscles and mucosa). **pericardial c.,** the potential space between the epicardium and the parietal layer of the serous pericardium. **peritoneal c.,** the potential space between the parietal and the visceral peritoneum. **pleural c.,** the potential space between the parietal and the visceral pleura. **pleuroperitoneal c.,** the temporarily continuous coelomic cavity in the embryo that is later partitioned by the developing diaphragm. **prepared c.,** a lesion from which all carious tissue has been removed, preparatory to restoration of the tooth by filling material. **pulp c.,** the pulp-filled central chamber in the crown of a tooth. **Rosenmüller's c.,** depression in pharynx on either side of openings of eustachian tubes. **segmentation c.,** blastocoele. **serous c.,** any cavity, like that enclosed by the peritoneum or pleura, not communicating with the outside of the body, the lining membrane of which secretes a watery fluid. **sigmoid c.,** either of two depressions in head of ulna for articulation with the humerus and the radius. **simple c.,** a carious lesion whose preparation involves only one surface of the tooth. **somatic c.,** coelom. **somite c.,** myocoele. **yolk c.,** the open space within the developing ovum of some animals.

cavum (ka'vum), pl. *ca'va* [L.] cavity.

cavus (ka'vus) [L.] hollow.

CBC complete blood cell count.

cc. cubic centimeter.

CCA chimpanzee coryza agent (respiratory syncytial virus).

c.cm. cubic centimeter.

C.D. curative dose.

Cd chemical symbol, *cadmium.*

Cd. caudal.

C.D.₅₀ median curative dose.

Ce chemical symbol, *cerium.*

ceasmic (se-as'mik) characterized by the persistence, after birth, of embryonic fissures.

cebocephalia (se"bo-sĕ-fa'le-ah) monkey-like deformity of the head, with eyes close together and nose flat.

cebocephalus (-sef'ah-lus) a fetal monster exhibiting cebocephalia.

cecal (se'kal) pertaining to the cecum.

cecectomy (se-sek'to-me) excision of the cecum.

cecitis (se-si'tis) inflammation of the cecum.

ceco- (se'ko) word element [L.], *cecum.*

cecocoloplicopexy (se"ko-ko"lo-pli'ko-pek"se) fixation of cecum and ascending colon to posterior abdominal wall, by means of parietal peritoneum, to prevent torsion.

cecocolostomy (-ko-los'to-me) anastomosis of cecum to a formerly remote portion of the colon.

cecofixation (-fik-sa'shun) cecopexy.

cecoileostomy (-il"e-os'to-me) ileocecostomy.

Cecon (se'kon) trademark for preparations of ascorbic acid.

cecopexy (se'ko-pek"se) fixation of the cecum to the abdominal wall.

cecoplication (se"ko-pli-ka'shun) 1. cecopexy. 2. closure of cecostomy.

cecorectal (-rek'tal) pertaining to cecum and rectum.

cecorrhaphy (se-kor'ah-fe) suture of the cecum.

cecosigmoidostomy (se"ko-sig"moid-os'to-me) anastomosis of the cecum to the sigmoid colon.

cecostomy (se-kos'to-me) fistulization of the cecum.

cecotomy (se-kot'o-me) incision of the cecum.

cecum (se'kum) the proximal part of the large intestine just distal to the ileum.

Cel. Celsius.

Cedilanid (se"dĭ-lan'id) trademark for a preparation of a crystalline digitalis glycoside (lanatoside C) in tablet form.

-cele (sēl) word element [Gr.], *hernia.*

celi(o)- (se'le-o) word element [Gr.], *abdomen; through the abdominal wall.*

celiac (se'le-ak) pertaining to the abdomen.

celialgia (se"le-al'je-ah) pain in the abdomen.

celiectasia (-ek-ta'ze-ah) excessive size of the abdominal cavity.

celiectomy (-ek'to-me) 1. excision of the celiac branches of the vagus nerve. 2. excision of an abdominal organ.

celiocentesis (se"le-o-sen-te'sis) puncture of the abdomen.

celioma (se"le-o'mah) a tumor of the abdomen.

celiomyalgia (se"le-o-mi-al'je-ah) pain in the abdominal muscles.

celiomyositis (-mi"o-si'tis) inflammation of the abdominal muscles.

celioncus (se"le-ong'kus) a tumor of the abdomen.

celioparacentesis (se"le-o-par"ah-sen-te'sis) puncture of the abdomen.

celiopathy (se"le-op'ah-the) any abdominal disease.

celiopyosis (se"le-o-pi-o'sis) suppuration in the abdominal cavity.

celiorrhaphy (se″le-or′ah-fe) suture of the abdominal wall.

celioscope (se′le-o-skōp″) peritoneoscope.

celioscopy (se″le-os′ko-pe) peritoneoscopy.

celiosite (se′le-o-sīt″) an abdominal parasite.

celiothelioma (se″le-o-the″le-o′mah) mesothelioma.

celiotomy (se″le-ot′o-me) opening of the abdominal cavity through an incision in its wall; laparotomy. **vaginal c.,** incision into the abdominal cavity through the vagina.

celitis (se-li′tis) any abdominal inflammation.

cell (sel) 1. a small cavity or compartment. 2. a definite unit in the organization of living substance, consisting of a small mass of protoplasm with a nucleus and surrounded by a membrane (the plasma, or cell, membrane). **acid c's,** delomorphous cells. **adelomorphous c's,** transparent columnar cells lining the glands of the stomach, believed to secrete pepsinogen. **air c.,** one containing air, as in the lungs or auditory tube. **amacrine c's,** branched retinal structures, regarded as modified nerve cells. **ameboid c.,** a cell which changes its form and moves about. **Anitschkow's c.,** a cell with peculiar nuclear structure, occurring normally in the heart and heart valves. **antipodal c's,** a group of four cells in the early embryo. **apolar c.,** a nerve cell without processes. **argentaffin c's,** cells containing cytoplasmic granules capable of reducing silver compounds, located throughout the gastrointestinal tract, chiefly in basilar portions of gastric glands and the crypts of Lieberkühn. **band c.,** a cell of the granulocytic series with a nucleus resembling a curved or coiled band, but not segmented into lobes connected by a filament. **basal c.,** an early keratinocyte, present in the basal layer of the epidermis. **basket c.,** a neuron of the cerebral cortex whose fibers form basket works around the body of another cell. **beaker c.,** goblet cell. **Betz c's,** large pyramidal ganglion cells forming a layer of the gray matter of the brain. **bipolar c.,** a nerve cell with two processes. **blast c.,** the least differentiated blood cell type. **blood c.,** one of the formed elements of the blood. **bone c.,** a nucleated cell in the lacunae of bone. **bristle c's,** ciliary cells in distribution of the auditory nerve. **Buhot c.,** one with an acentric nucleus and protoplasm containing numerous vacuoles in the middle of which is usually a small dark inclusion, found in bone marrow in all typical cases of gargoylism. **cameloid c.,** elliptocyte. **cartilage c's,** connective tissue cells in the cartilage capsules. **central c.,** adelomorphous cell. **chromaffin c's,** cells whose cytoplasm shows fine brown granules when stained with potassium bichromate, occurring in the adrenal medulla and in scattered groups in various organs and throughout the body. **ciliated c.,** a cell provided with cilia. **Claudius's c's,** large cells near the organ of Corti. **cleavage c.,** one of the cells derived from the fertilized ovum by mitosis; a blastomere. **column c., columnar c.,** a neuron in the posterior column of the spinal cord. **Corti's c's,** the hair cells in outer surface of organ of Corti. **crescent c.,** sickle cell. **daughter c.,** a cell formed by division of a mother cell. **decidual c.,** one of the cells from the mucous membrane of the uterus after impregnation. **Deiters' c's,** 1. specialized cells associated with Corti's cells in the inner ear. 2. branching cells constituting the reticulum of neuroglia. **delomorphous c's,** large cells in the glands of the stomach, believed to secrete the acid of the gastric juice. **demilune c's,** granular protoplasmic cells in mucous glands between the mucous cells and the basement membrane. **Dorothy Reed c's,** Sternberg-Reed cells. **Edelmann's c.,** kinetocyte. **embryonal c's,** small round cells composing embryonal tissue. **enamel c.,** ameloblast. **endothelial c's,** cells composing endothelium. **epithelial c's,** cells composing epithelium. **fat c's,** connective tissue cells filled with oil. **Ferrata c.,** promonocyte. **fiber c.,** one of the elongated cells composing a fiber, especially if still nuclear. **flagellate c.,** one with long cilia. **floor c's,** cells of the floor of the arch of Corti. **foam c.,** a cell containing vacuoles. **formative c's,** embryonal cells. **ganglion c.,** a large nerve cell, especially one of those of the spinal ganglia. **Gaucher's c.,** a large cell characteristic of Gaucher's disease, with eccentrically placed nuclei and fine wavy fibrils parallel to the long axis of the cell. **germ c.,** one which, under suitable conditions, will contribute to the formation of a new individual of the species. **germ c., primordial,** the earliest recognizable precursor in the embryo of an ovum or spermatozoon. **c's of Giannuzzi,** demilune cells. **giant c.,** large, multinucleated cell. **gitter c's,** honeycomb-like cells filled with granules of fat. **glia c's,** Deiters' cells. (2). **goblet c.,** an epithelial cell bulged out like a goblet by contained mucin. **Golgi's c's,** nerve cells with short processes in the posterior horns of the spinal cord. **granular c.,** one containing granules, such as a keratinocyte in the stratum granulosum of the epidermis, when it contains a dense collection of darkly staining granules. **granulosa c.,** a cell of the ovary which secretes follicular hormone. **gustatory c's,** taste cells. **hair c's,** epithelial cells with hairlike processes. **Hargraves' cell,** L.E. cell. **HeLa c's,** cells of the first continuously cultured carcinoma strain, descended from a human cervical carcinoma. **Hensen's c's,** cylindrical cells outside the outer hair cells in the organ of Corti. **Hofbauer c's,** large chromophilic cells in the chorionic villi which are probably clasmatocytes. **Hortega c.,** one of the cells of the microglia. **Hürthle c's,** large eosinophilic cells sometimes found in the thyroid gland. **interstitial c's,** the cells of the connective tissue of the ovary or testis which furnish the internal secretion of those structures. **juxtaglomerular c's,** specialized cells, containing secretory granules, located in the tunica media of the afferent glomerular arterioles. **Kupffer's c's,** large star-shaped or pyramidal cells along the walls of the venous capillaries of the liver. **Langerhans' c's,** 1. star-shaped cells in the germinative layer of the epidermis. 2. spindle-shaped cells in the acini of the pancreas. **L.E. c.,** a mature neutrophilic polymorphonuclear leukocyte with a large phagocytic vacuole containing partially digested and lysed nuclear material, characteristic of lupus erythematosus. **Leydig's c's,** interstitial cells of the testis. **Lipschütz c.,** centrocyte. **lutein c's,** the enlarged follicular cells of the ovary seen after rupture of an ovarian follicle. **lymph c.,** lymph corpuscle. **lymphoid c.,** a mononuclear cell in lymphoid tissue which ultimately is concerned with humoral or cellular immunologic reactivity. **malpighian c.,** keratinocyte. **marrow c's,** large cells characteristic of true marrow. **mast c.,** a connective tissue cell capable of elaborating basophilic, metachromatic cytoplasmic granules that contain histamine, heparin and, in some species, serotonin. **mastoid c's,** hollow spaces of various size and shape in the mastoid process of the temporal bone, communicating with the tympanic antrum and lined with a continuation of its mucous membrane. **mossy c's,** neuroglia cells having a large body with numerous branching processes. **mother c.,** a cell that divides to form new cells. **mucous c's,** cells which secrete mucus. **mulberry c.,** 1. a vacuolated plasma cell. 2. a rounded cell with centrally placed nuclei and coarse cytoplasmic vacuoles around the outside, developing at the periphery of a retrogressing corpus luteum. **myeloid c.,** myeloplax. **myeloma c.,** a cell found in bone marrow and sometimes in peripheral blood in multiple myeloma. **nerve c.,** any cell of a nerve, nerve center or ganglion. **nuclear c.,** nerve cell consisting of a nucleus surrounded by branching protoplasm. **oxyntic c's,** delomorphous cells. **Paget c's,** degenerated cells found in the epidermis in Paget's disease of the nipple. **parietal c's,** delomorphous cells. **peptic c's,** adelomorphous cells. **pheochrome c's,** cells of the embryonic suprarenal body staining dark with chromium salts. **Pick's c's,** round, oval or polyhedral cells with foamy, lipid-containing cytoplasm found in the bone marrow and spleen in Niemann-Pick disease. **pigment c's,** cells containing granules of pigment. **plasma c.,** plasmocyte. **polar c's,** polar bodies. **polychromatic c's, polychromatophil c's,** immature erythrocytes staining with both acid and basic stains in a diffuse mixture of blue-gray and pink. **pregnancy c's,** peculiar cells observed in the anterior pituitary in pregnant women. **prickle c.,** a dividing keratinocyte in the stratum germinativum of the epidermis, with delicate radiating processes connecting with other similar cells. **primordial germ c's,** the earliest germ cells, at first located outside the gonad. **prop c's,** Hensen's cells. **Purkinje's c's,** large branched cells of the middle layer of the brain. **reticulum c.,** one of the primitive mesenchymal cells forming the framework of

lymph nodes, bone marrow and spleen, which may differentiate into myeloblast, lymphoblast or monoblast. **Rieder c.,** an immature cell observed in leukemia, whose nucleus has several wide and deep indentations suggesting lobulation. **Rouget c's,** contractile cells on the walls of capillaries. **scavenger c.,** a cell which absorbs and removes irritant products. **segmented c.,** any cell containing specific granules and having the nucleus segmented into lobes, connected by a slender, threadlike structure or filament. **Sertoli's c's,** cells developing into spermatoblasts. **Sézary c.,** a reticular lymphocyte having a large convoluted or folded nucleus with a narrow rim of cytoplasm that may contain vacuoles. **sickle c.,** a crescentic or sickle-shaped erythrocyte. **signet c.,** a globular, vacuolated cell, with the flattened nucleus pushed to the periphery, producing resemblance to a signet ring. **Smee c.,** an apparatus for producing galvanic electricity. **smudge c's,** disrupted leukocytes appearing during preparation of peripheral blood smears. **sperm c.,** 1. a spermatozoon. 2. a spermatoblast. **spider c's,** Deiters' cells (2). **squamous c's,** epithelial cells which are flat, like scales, **stab c., staff c.,** band cell. **stem c.,** a generalized mother cell whose descendants specialize, often in different directions. **Sternberg's giant c's, Sternberg-Reed c's,** giant, polyploid mesenchymal cells with hyperlobulated nuclei and multiple large nucleoli characteristic of Hodgkin's disease. **stipple c.,** a red blood cell containing granules that take a basic or bluish stain with Wright's stain. **target c.,** an abnormally thin erythrocyte showing, when stained, a dark center and a peripheral ring of hemoglobin, separated by a pale, unstained zone containing less hemoglobin. **tart c.,** a histiocyte or monocytoid reticuloendothelial cell containing a second, characteristic nucleus, usually in the cytoplasm filling the concavity of the major nucleus. **taste c's,** cells in taste buds associated with the nerves of taste. **tendon c's,** peculiar cells occurring in white fibrous tissue. **Touton c's,** large cells containing lipoid material found in the lesions of xanthoma. **Türk c.,** a nongranular mononuclear cell observed in the peripheral blood during severe anemias, chronic infections and leukemoid reactions. **Tzauck c.,** a degenerated epithelial cell caused by acantholysis and observed in pemphigus. **Unna's plasma c.,** plasmocyte. **vasofactive c., vasoformative c.,** a cell that joins with other cells to form blood vessels. **visual c's,** the neuroepithelial elements of the retina. **wandering c's,** mononuclear phagocytic cells which are components of the reticuloendothelial system. **zymogenic c's,** cells at the bottom of the gastric glands that contain black secretory granules.

cella (sel'ah), pl. *cel'lae* [L.] cell.

Cellfalcicula (sel"fal-sik'u-lah)   a genus of Schizomycetes (order Pseudomonadales, suborder Pseudomonadineae, family Spirillaceae).

celloidin (sĕ-loi'din) a collodion prepared for use in microscopic work.

cellula (sel'u-lah), pl. *cel'lulae* [L.] cell.

cellular (sel'u-ler) composed of cells.

cellularity (sel"u-lar'ĭ-te) the state of a tissue or organ relative to its constituent cells.

cellulase (sel'u-lās) an enzyme that hydrolyzes cellulose to cellobiose, secreted by bacteria and by fungi which destroy wood.

cellule (sel'ūl) a minute cell.

cellulicidal (sel"u-lĭ-si'dal) destroying cells.

cellulifugal (-lif'u-gal) directed away from a cell body.

cellulipetal (-lip'ĕ-tal) directed toward a cell body.

cellulitis (-li'tis) a spreading, diffuse, edematous and sometimes suppurative inflammation in solid tissues. **dissecting c.**, inflammation with suppuration spreading between layers of the involved tissue. **gangrenous c.**, that leading to death of the tissue followed by bacterial invasion and putrefaction. **gaseous c.**, inflammation due to a gas-producing organism and presence of gas in the tissues. **pelvic c.**, parametritis. **purulent c.**, that characterized by presence of pus.

cellulofibrous (-lo-fi'brus) partly cellular and partly fibrous.

celluloid (sel'u-loid) a plastic compound of pyroxylin and camphor.

Cellulomonas (sel"u-lo-mo'nas) a genus of Schizomycetes (order Eubacteriales, family Corynebacteriaceae) found in soil.

celluloneuritis (-nu-ri'tis) inflammation of nerve cells.

cellulose (sel'u-lōs) the structural form of polysaccharides in plants, acting as a support for plant tissues. **absorbable c., oxidized c.**, an absorbable oxidation product of cellulose, applied locally to stop bleeding. **c. tetranitrate**, $(C_{12}H_{16}N_4O_{18})_n$, the principal constituent of pyroxylin.

celology (se-lol'o-je) the study of hernias.

celom (se'lom) coelom.

Celontin (se-lon'tin) trademark for a preparation of methsuximide.

celoschisis (se-los'kĭ-sis) fissure of the abdominal wall.

celoscope (se'lo-skōp) endoscope.

celosomia (se"lo-so'me-ah) a developmental anomaly characterized by fissure or absence of the sternum, with hernial protrusion of the viscera.

celosomus (-so'mus) a fetal monster exhibiting celosomia.

celothelioma (-the"le-o'mah) mesothelioma.

celotomy (se-lot'o-me) kelotomy.

celozoic (se"lo-zo'ik) inhabiting the intestinal canal of the body; said of parasites.

cement (se-ment') a substance supporting or connecting other structures, or in which they may be embedded. **dental c.**, cementum. **muscle c.**, the myoglia. **nerve c.**, the neuroglia.

cementicle (se-men'tĭ-kl) a small, discrete globular mass of dentin in the region of a tooth root.

cementoblast (se-men'to-blast) a large cuboid-al cell active in the formation of cementum.

cementoblastoma (se-men"to-blas-to'mah) an odontogenic fibroma whose cells are developing into cementoblasts and in which there is only a small proportion of calcified tissue.

cementoclasia (-kla'se-ah) destruction by disease of the cementum of a tooth root.

cementocyte (se-men'to-sīt) a cell found in lacunae of cellular cementum, frequently having long processes radiating from the cell body toward the periodontal surface of the cementum.

cementogenesis (se-men"to-jen'ĕ-sis) development of cementum on the root dentin of a tooth.

cementoma (se"men-to'mah) an odontogenic fibroma in which the cells have developed into cementoblasts and which consists largely of cementum.

cementosis (-to'sis) proliferation of cementum.

cementum (se-men'tum) calcified tissue of mesodermal origin covering the root of a tooth.

cenesthesia (sen"es-the'ze-ah) the sense or feeling of consciousness. adj., **cenesthe'sic, cenesthet'ic.**

ceno- (se'no) word element [Gr.], *new; empty;* or denoting relationship to a common feature or characteristic.

cenophobia (se"no-fo'be-ah) cenotophobia.

cenopsychic (-si'kik) of recent appearance in mental development.

cenosis (se-no'sis) a morbid discharge. adj., **cenot'ic.**

cenosite (se'no-sīt) a parasite able to live apart from its host.

cenotophobia (se-no"to-fo'be-ah) morbid fear of new things or new ideas.

cenotype (sen'o-tīp) the original from which other types have arisen.

censor (sen'sor) 1. a member of a committee on ethics or for critical examination of a medical or other society. 2. the psychic influence which prevents unconscious thoughts and wishes coming into consciousness.

Cent. centigrade.

center (sen'ter) a point from which a process starts, especially a plexus or ganglion giving off nerves which control a function. **accelerating c.**, one in the medulla which accelerates action of the heart. **arm c.**, one controlling arm movements. **association c.**, one controlling associated movements. **auditory c.**, one in the first temporosphenoidal convolution, concerned with the sense of hearing. **Broca's c.**, speech center. **cardio-inhibitory c.**, one in the medulla which depresses heart action. **ciliospinal c.**, one in the lower cervical part of the cord controlling dilatation of the pupil. **deglutition c.**, swallowing center. **epiotic c.**, the center of ossification in the mastoid portion of the temporal bone. **facial c.**, one in the frontal convolutions, controlling face movements. **germinal c.**, the area in lymphoid tissue where mitotic figures are observed, differentiation and formation of lymphocytes occur and elements related to antibody synthesis are found. **gustatory c.**, one supposed to control taste. **health c.**, a community health organization for creating health work and coordinating the efforts of all health agencies. **heat-regulating c.**, the center for the control of body temperature. **Kronecker's c.**, cardioinhibitory center. **leg c.**, one in the upper portion of the ascending frontal convolution. **motor c.**, nerve center controlling motion. **nerve c.**, an aggregation, in brain or spinal cord, of cell bodies of neurons. **olfactory c.**, one in the cortex near the front end of the uncinate gyrus, concerned with the sense of smell. **c. of ossification**, the place in bones at which ossification begins. **pneumotaxic c.**, a special group of cells in the midbrain which is responsible for periodic inhibition of the respiratory center. **psychocortical c's**, centers of the cerebral cortex concerned in mental operations. **reflex c.**, a nerve center at which afferent sensory impressions are converted into efferent motor impulses. **respiratory c.**, a special group of cells in the medulla, from which impulses pass to diaphragm and rib muscles, resulting in their regular and coordinated contraction. **Setschenow's c's**, reflex inhibitory centers in medulla oblongata and spinal cord. **spasm c.**, one in the medulla, at its junction with the pons. **speech c.**, one in the third left frontal convolution, concerned with the power of speech. **swallowing c.**, one on the floor of the fourth ventricle concerned with deglutition. **trophic c.**, one regulating nutrition. **vasomotor c.**, one in the medulla concerned with the dilation and constriction of blood vessels. **visual c.**, in the occipital lobe, especially in the cuneus. **Wernicke's c.**, the speech center in the cortex of the left temporo-occipital convolution. **word c.**, one concerned with the recognition of words, different areas being involved for recognition of written and of spoken words.

centesimal (sen-tes'ĭ-mal) divided into hundredths.

centesis (sen-te'sis) word element [Gr.], *puncture and aspiration of.*

centi- (sen'tĭ) word element [L.], *hundred;* used in naming units of measurement to indicate a submultiple (10^{-2}) of the unit designated by the root with which it is combined; symbol c.

centigrade (sen'tĭ-grād) having 100 gradations (steps or degrees), as the Celsius temperature scale (thermometer).

centigram (sen'tĭ-gram) one hundredth of a gram; abbreviated cg.

centiliter (sen'tĭ-le"ter) one hundredth of a liter; abbreviated cl.

centimeter (sen'tĭ-me"ter) one hundredth of a meter; abbreviated cm. **cubic c.**, a unit of mass, being that of a cube each side of which measures 1 cm.; abbreviated c.cm., cm.³, cu. cm. or cc.

centinormal (sen"tĭ-nor'mal) one hundredth of normal strength.

centipoise (sen'tĭ-poiz) one hundredth of a poise.

centiunit (sen"tĭ-u'nit) one hundredth part of a unit (10^{-2}).

centrad (sen'trad) toward a center.

central (sen'tral) pertaining to a center; located at the midpoint.

centraphose (sen'trah-fōz) a subjective sensation of darkness.

centrencephalic (sen"tren-se-fal'ik) pertaining to the center of the encephalon.

centric (sen'trik) pertaining to a center.

centriciput (sen-tris'ĭ-put) the head, excluding occiput and sinciput.

centrifugal (sen-trif'u-gal) moving away from a center.

centrifugation (sen-trif"u-ga'shun) the process of separating materials from solution by rotating vessels containing the solution at high speed.

centrifuge (sen'trĭ-fūj) 1. to rotate, in a suitable container, at extremely high speed, to cause the deposition of solids in solution. 2. a laboratory device for subjecting substances in solution to relative centrifugal force up to 25,000 times gravity. **microscope c.**, a high-speed centrifuge with a built-in microscope permitting a specimen to be viewed under centrifugal force.

centrilobular (sen"trĭ-lob'u-lar) pertaining to the central portion of a lobule.

centriole (sen'tre-ōl) a minute cell within the centrosome.

centripetal (sen-trip'ĕ-tal) moving toward a center.

centro- (sen'tro) word element [L., Gr.] indicating relation to a center or to a central location.

centrocyte (sen'tro-sit) a cell containing in its protoplasm granules which stain with hematoxylin.

centrokinesia (sen"tro-ki-ne'se-ah) movement originating from central stimulation. adj., **centrokinet'ic.**

centrolecithal (-les'ĭ-thal) having the yolk in the center.

centromere (sen'tro-mēr) the clear region at the point of junction of the arms of a replicating chromosome.

centrosclerosis (sen"tro-skle-ro'sis) osteosclerosis of the marrow cavity of a bone.

centrosome (sen'tro-sōm) a specially differentiated region of cytoplasm near the nucleus of a cell.

centrosphere (sen'tro-sfēr) a clear, homogeneous zone surrounding the centrosome of a cell.

centrostaltic (sen"tro-stal'tik) pertaining to a center of motion.

centrum (sen'trum), pl. *cen'tra* [L.] a center. **c. commu'ne**, the solar plexus.

cephal(o)- (sef'ah-lo) word element [Gr.], *head.*

cephalad (sef'ah-lad) toward the head.

cephalalgia (sef"al-al'je-ah) pain in the head; headache.

cephaledema (-ĕ-de'mah) edema of the head.

cephalemia (-e'me-ah) congestion of the head or brain.

cephalhematocele (-he-mat'o-sēl) a collection of blood under the pericranium, communicating with the dural sinuses.

cephalhematoma (sef″al-he″mah-to′mah) a localized effusion of blood beneath the periosteum of the skull of a newborn infant, due to disruption of the vessels during birth.

cephalhydrocele (-hi′dro-sēl) a serous or watery accumulation under the pericranium.

cephalic (sē-fal′ik) pertaining to the head.

cephalin (sef′ah-lin) 1. a monaminomonophosphatide in brain tissue, nerve tissue and yolk of egg. 2. a crude phospholipid usually extracted from brain tissue, used as a clotting agent in blood coagulation work.

cephalitis (sef″ah-li′tis) encephalitis.

cephalocele (sē-fal′o-sēl) protrusion of a part of the cranial contents.

cephalocentesis (sef″ah-lo-sen-te′sis) surgical puncture of the head.

cephalodynia (-din′e-ah) pain in the head.

cephalogaster (-gas′ter) the anterior portion of the enteric canal of the embryo.

cephalogyric (-ji′rik) pertaining to turning motions of the head.

cephalohematoma (-he″mah-to′mah) cephalhematoma.

cephalohemometer (-he-mom′ĕ-ter) an instrument for measuring intracranial blood pressure.

cephaloma (sef″ah-lo′mah) a soft or encephaloid tumor.

cephalomelus (sef″ah-lom′e-lus) a double monster with a limb attached to the head.

cephalomeningitis (sef″ah-lo-men″in-ji′tis) inflammation of the meninges of the brain.

cephalometer (sef″ah-lom′ĕ-ter) an instrument for measuring the head.

cephalometry (sef″ah-lom′ĕ-tre) determination of dimensions of the head and face.

cephalomotor (sef″ah-lo-mo′tor) pertaining to motions of the head.

cephalomyia (-mi′yah) estrus.

cephalonia (sef″ah-lo′ne-ah) idiocy with enlargement of the head and sclerosis of the brain.

cephalont (sef′ah-lont) a stage in a developing protozoan in which it is attached to the individual host cell.

cephalopathy (sef″ah-lop′ah-the) any disease of the head.

cephalopelvic (sef″ah-lo-pel′vik) pertaining to the fetal head and maternal pelvis.

cephalothoracic (-tho-ras′ik) pertaining to head and thorax.

cephalothoracopagus (-tho″rah-kop′ah-gus) a double fetal monster joined at head and thorax.

cephalotomy (sef″ah-lot′o-me) craniotomy.

cephalotractor (sef″ah-lo-trak′tor) obstetrical forceps.

cephalotribe (sef′ah-lo-trīb″) instrument for crushing the fetal head.

cephalotripsy (sef′ah-lo-trip″se) the crushing of the fetal head.

cephalotropic (sef″ah-lo-trop′ik) having an affinity for brain tissue.

cephalotrypesis (-tri-pe′sis) trephination of the skull.

ceptor (sep′tor) 1. a receptor or intermediary

body. 2. a nerve process which receives impulses from an adjoining neuron.

cera (se′rah) [L.] wax. **c. al′ba,** white wax. **c. fla′va,** yellow wax.

ceramics (sē-ram′iks) the modeling and processing of objects made of clay or similar materials. **dental c.,** the use of porcelain and similar materials in restorative dentistry.

cerasin (ser′ah-sin) substance from cherry and plum tree gums, said to be a carbohydrate charged with a lime salt.

cerasine (ser′ah-sin) a cerebroside occurring in brain tissue.

cerate (sēr′āt) an unctuous substance for external application, compounded with fat or wax, or both.

ceratin (ser′ah-tin) keratin.

ceratitis (ser″ah-ti′tis) keratitis.

cerato- (ser′ah-to) for words beginning thus, see also those beginning *kerato-*.

ceratonosus (ser″ah-ton′o-sus) any disease of the cornea.

Ceratophyllus (ser-ah-tof′ĭ-lus) a genus of fleas.

ceratum (se-ra′tum) [L.] cerate.

cercaria (ser-ka′re-ah), pl. *cerca′riae* [Gr.] the final, free-swimming larval stage of a trematode parasite.

cerclage (ser-klahzh′) [Fr.] encirclement with a ring or loop, as for correction of an incompetent cervix uteri or fixation of adjacent ends of a fractured bone.

cercus (ser′kus) a bristle-like structure.

cerebellar (ser″ĕ-bel′ar) pertaining to the cerebellum.

cerebellifugal (ser″ĕ-bel-lif′u-gal) conducting away from the cerebellum.

cerebellipetal (-lip′ĕ-tal) conducting toward the cerebellum.

cerebellitis (-li′tis) inflammation of the cerebellum.

cerebellospinal (ser″ĕ-bel′o-spi′nal) pertaining to cerebellum and spinal cord.

cerebellum (ser″ĕ-bel′um) that part of the hindbrain lying dorsal to the pons and medulla oblongata, comprising a median portion (the vermis) and a cerebellar hemisphere on each side.

cerebral (ser′ĕ-bral, sē-re′bral) pertaining to the cerebrum.

cerebralgia (ser″ĕ-bral′je-ah) pain in the head.

cerebrasthenia (-bras-the′ne-ah) asthenia complicated with brain disorders.

cerebration (-bra′shun) functional activity of the brain. **unconscious c.,** mental action of which the person is unconscious.

cerebrifugal (-brif′u-gal) conducting away from the cerebrum.

cerebripetal (-brip′ĕ-tal) conducting toward the cerebrum.

cerebritis (-bri′tis) inflammation of the cerebrum.

cerebroid (ser′ĕ-broid) resembling brain substance.

cerebrology (ser″ĕ-brol′o-je) the scientific study of the brain.

cerebroma (ser"ĕ-bro'mah) abnormal mass of brain tissue outside the cranium.

cerebromalacia (ser"ĕ-bro-mah-la'she-ah) abnormal softness of the brain.

cerebromeningitis (-men"in-ji'tis) inflammation of the brain and its covering membranes.

cerebropathia (-path'e-ah) [L.] cerebropathy. **c. psy'chica toxe'mica,** Korsakoff's psychosis.

cerebropathy (ser"ĕ-brop'ah-the) any brain disease.

cerebrophysiology (ser"ĕ-bro-fiz"e-ol'o-je) physiology of the brain.

cerebropontile (-pon'tīl) pertaining to cerebrum and pons.

cerebropsychosis (-si-ko'sis) any cerebral disorder characterized by mental aberration.

cerebrosclerosis (-skle-ro'sis) abnormal hardness of the brain.

cerebrose (scr'ĕ brōs) a compound derived from brain substance, $C_6H_{12}O_6$.

cerebroside (sĕ-re'bro-sīd) a compound of a nitrogenous base, a long-chain fatty acid and a sugar, found chiefly in nerve tissue.

cerebrosis (ser"ĕ-bro'sis) any brain disease.

cerebrospinal (ser"ĕ-bro-spi'nal) pertaining to brain and spinal cord.

cerebrospinant (-spi'nant) an agent which affects brain and cord.

cerebrotomy (ser"ĕ-brot'o-me) anatomy or dissection of the brain.

cerebrotonia (ser"ĕ-bro-to'ne-ah) a psychic type characterized by predominance of restraint, inhibition and desire for concealment; considered typical of an ectomorph.

cerebrum (ser'ĕ-brum) the mass of nerve tissue whose broad, convex surface is closely related to the internal aspect of the calvaria, composed of the cerebral hemispheres, each made up of a frontal, temporal, parietal and occipital lobe, and constituting part of the forebrain.

cerium (se're-um) chemical element *(see table),* at. no 58, symbol Ce. **c. oxalate,** a mixture of the oxalates of cerium, neodymium, praseodymium, lanthanum and other associated elements; antemetic.

Cer-o-cillin (ser'o-sil"lin) trademark for preparations of penicillin O for parenteral administration.

cerolysin (se-rol'ĭ-sin) a lysin which decomposes wax.

ceroma (se-ro'ma) a tumor that has undergone waxy degeneration.

ceroplasty (se'ro-plas"te) the making of anatomical models in wax.

ceruloplasmin (sĕ-roo"lo-plaz'min) an alpha globulin of the blood, being the form in which most of the plasma copper is transported.

cerumen (sĕ-roo'men) a waxy secretion of the glands of the external ear canal. adj., **ceru'minal, ceru'minous.**

ceruminolysis (sĕ-roo"mĭ-nol'ĭ-sis) dissolution or disintegration of cerumen in the external auditory canal. adj., **ceruminolyt'ic.**

ceruminosis (-no'sis) excessive secretion of cerumen.

cervic(o)- (ser'vĭ-ko) word element [L.], *neck; cervix.*

cervical (ser'vĭ-kal) pertaining to the neck or to the cervix.

cervicectomy (ser"vĭ-sek'to-me) trachelectomy.

cerviciplex (ser-vis'ĭ-pleks) the cervical plexus.

cervicitis (ser"vĭ-si'tis) inflammation of the cervix uteri.

cervicocolpitis (ser"vĭ-ko-kol-pi'tis) inflammation of the cervix uteri and vagina.

cervicofacial (-fa'shal) pertaining to neck and face.

cervicoplasty (ser'vĭ-ko-plas"te) plastic surgery on the neck.

cervicovesical (ser"vĭ-ko-ves'ĭ-kal) relating to cervix uteri and bladder.

Cervilaxin (ser"vĭ-lak'sin) trademark for a preparation of relaxin.

cervix (ser'viks), pl. *cer'vices* [L.] a neck or necklike part, especially the lower, narrow portion of the uterus between the isthmus and the opening of the uterus into the vagina. **incompetent c.,** one that is abnormally prone to dilate before termination of the normal period of gestation, resulting in premature expulsion of the fetus. **c. u'teri,** the narrow lower end of the uterus. **c. ves'icae,** the neck of the bladder.

cesarotomy (se"zar-ot'o-me) abdominal hysterotomy.

cesium (se'ze-um) chemical element *(see table),* at. no. 55, symbol Cs.

cesticidal (ses"tĭ-si'dal) destructive to the platyhelminths, or cestodes.

cestode (ses'tōd) a tapeworm; an organism of the class Cestoidea.

cestodology (ses"to-dol'o-je) the scientific study of cestodes.

cestoid (ses'toid) resembling a tapeworm.

Cestoidea (ses-toi'de-ah) a class of animals of the phylum Platyhelminthes, characterized by a noncellular cuticular layer covering their bodies and generally having a segmented body with a special holdfast segment to the anterior end; the tapeworms.

cetylpyridinium (se"til-pi"rĭ-din'e-um) a pyridinium derivative used as a local anti-infective.

Cevalin (se'vah-lin) trademark for preparations of ascorbic acid.

Cevex (se'veks) trademark for a liquid preparation of ascorbic acid.

Ce-vi-sol (se'vi-sol) trademark for a preparation of ascorbic acid.

C.F. carbolfuchsin.

Cf chemical symbol, *californium.*

CFT complement fixation test.

cg. centigram.

C.G.S. centimeter-gram-second, the metric units of linear measurement, weight and time.

C.H.A. Catholic Hospital Association.

chalazion (kah-la'ze-on) a small tumor produced by chronic inflammation of one or more of the meibomian glands.

chalcosis (kal-ko'sis) copper deposits in tissue.

chalicosis (kal"ĭ-ko'sis) lung disease from inhalation of stony particles.

chalk (chawk) a noncrystalline form of calcium

carbonate. **prepared c.**, a native form of calcium carbonate freed from its impurities by elutriation.

chalone (kal′ōn) colyone.

chalybeate (kah-lib′e-āt) impregnated with iron.

chamaecephalic (kam″e-sĕ-fal′ik) having a low, flat head, with a vertical index of 70 or less.

chamber (chām′ber) an enclosed space. **air c.**, in dentistry, a recess in the palatal surface of the base of an upper denture to help retain it by creating a partial vacuum. **anterior c.**, the part of the aqueous-containing space of the eyeball between the cornea and iris. **aqueous c.**, the aqueous-containing space in the eyeball, between the cornea and lens. **counting c.**, a shallow glass chamber specially ruled to facilitate the counting of discrete particles in the sample under study. **Haldane's c.**, an airtight chamber for the analysis of respiratory gases. **hyperbaric c.**, an enclosed space in which gas (oxygen) can be raised to greater than atmospheric pressure. **ionization c.**, an enclosure containing two or more electrodes between which an electric current may be passed when the enclosed gas is ionized by radiation; used for determining the intensity of roentgen and other rays. **posterior c.**, that part of the aqueous-containing space of the eyeball between the iris and the lens. **pulp c.**, the natural cavity in the central portion of the tooth crown occupied by the dental pulp. **suction c.**, **vacuum c.**, air chamber. **vitreous c.**, the vitreous-containing space in the eyeball, bounded anteriorly by the lens and ciliary body and posteriorly by the posterior wall of the eyeball.

chancre (shang′ker) primary lesion of syphilis. **hard c.**, **hunterian c.**, true chancre. **noninfecting c.**, chancroid. **c. re′dux**, chancre developing on the scar of a healed primary chancre. **simple c.**, **soft c.**, chancroid. **true c.**, the true primary lesion of syphilis, caused by *Treponema pallidum* and followed by constitutional syphilis.

chancroid (shang′kroid) a soft, nonsyphilitic venereal sore. **phagedenic c.**, chancroid with a tendency to slough. **serpiginous c.**, phagedenic chancroid spreading in curved lines.

chancrous (shang′krus) of the nature of chancre.

chappa (chap′ah) a disease of South Africa resembling syphilis or yaws.

character (kar′ak-ter) 1. a separate and distinct trait exhibited by an individual. 2. the sum of observable attributes of a material or of an individual. **dominant c.**, one which can develop through the agency of a single gene. **mendelian c's**, in genetics, the separate and distinct traits exhibited by an animal or plant and dependent on the genetic constitution of the organism. **primary sex c.**, one directly concerned in the reproductive function of the individual. **recessive c.**, one which must be carried in the gene from each parent to become apparent in the offspring.

secondary sex c., one typical of the sex, but not directly concerned in the reproductive function of the individual. **sex-linked c.**, one transmitted by a gene carried in the sex chromosome and appearing only in individuals of one sex.

charcoal (char′kōl) carbon prepared by burning organic material. **activated c.**, residue of destructive distillation of various organic materials, treated to increase its adsorptive power; used in gas masks, in emergency treatment of poisoning by certain drugs, and also as a decolorizer. **purified animal c.**, charcoal prepared from bone and purified by removal of materials dissolved by hot hydrochloric acid and water; adsorbent and decolorizer.

chart (chart) a record of data in graphic or tabular form. **genealogical c.**, a graph showing various descendants of a common ancestor, used to indicate those affected by a genetically determined disease. **reading c.**, a chart with material printed in gradually increasing type sizes, used in testing acuity of near vision. **Snellen's c.**, a chart printed with block letters in gradually decreasing sizes, used in testing distance vision.

chauffage (sho-fahzh′) [Fr.] application of a low-heated cautery near a part.

Ch.B. [L.] *Chirur′giae Baccalau′reus* (Bachelor of Surgery).

ChE cholinesterase.

check-bite (chek′bīt) a sheet of hard wax or modeling compound placed between the teeth and used to check occlusion of the teeth.

cheek (chēk) a fleshy, rounded protuberance, especially the fleshy portion of either side of the face. **cleft c.**, a developmental anomaly characterized by an abnormal fissure.

cheil(o)- (ki′lo) word element [Gr.], *lip*.

cheilectropion (ki″lek-tro′pe-on) eversion of the lip.

cheilitis (ki-li′tis) inflammation of a lip. **actinic c.**, **c. actin′ica**, involvement of the lips after exposure to actinic rays, with pain and swelling, and development of a scaly crust on the vermilion border.

cheilognathopalatoschisis (ki″lo-na″tho-pal″ah-tos′ki-sis) cleft of the lip, upper jaw and hard and soft palates.

cheiloncus (ki-long′kus) a tumor of the lip.

cheiloplasty (ki′lo-plas″te) plastic repair of a lip.

Cheilopoda (ki-lop′o-dah) Chilopoda.

cheilopodiasis (ki″lo-po-di′ah-sis) chilopodiasis.

cheilorrhaphy (ki-lor′ah-fe) suture of the lip.

cheiloschisis (ki-los′ki-sis) harelip.

cheilosis (ki-lo′sis) a fissured condition of the lips and angles of the mouth.

cheilostomatoplasty (ki″lo-sto-mat′o-plas″te) plastic repair of lip and mouth.

cheilotomy (ki-lot′o-me) incision of the lip.

cheir(o)- (ki′ro) word element [Gr.], *hand*. See also words beginning *chio(o)-*.

cheiralgia (ki-ral′je-ah) pain in the hand.

cheirarthritis (ki″rar-thri′tis) inflammation of the joints of the hand and fingers.

cheirokinesthesia (ki″ro-kin″es-the′ze-ah) the subjective perception of movements of the hand, especially in writing.

cheiromegaly (-meg′ah-le) abnormal enlargement of the hands and fingers.

cheiroplasty (ki′ro-plas″te) plastic surgery on the hand.

cheiropompholyx (ki″ro-pom′fo-liks) a skin disease with peculiar vesicles on the palms and soles.

cheiroscope (ki′ro-skōp) an instrument used in the training of binocular vision.

cheirospasm (ki′ro-spazm) writers' cramp.

chelate (ke′lāt) to combine with a metal in weakly dissociated complexes in which the metal is part of a ring; by extension, applied to a chemical compound in which a metallic ion is sequestered and firmly bound into a ring within the chelating molecule.

Chel-iron (kēl′i-ron) trademark for preparations of ferrocholinate.

cheloid (ke′loid) keloid.

chem. chemical; chemist; chemistry.

chem(o)- (ke′mo, kem′o) word element [Gr.], chemical; chemistry.

chemexfoliation (kem′eks-fo′le-a″shun) removal of epidermis and part of dermis by chemicals applied to the body surface.

chemical (kem′i-kal) 1. pertaining to chemistry. 2. a substance produced by the forces or operations of chemistry.

chemicocautery (kem″i-ko-kaw′ter-e) cauterization by chemical means.

chemioogenesis (-jen′e-sis) initiation of segmentation of an ovum by chemical means.

chemiluminescence (kem′i-lu″mi-nes′ens) chemoluminescence.

cheminosis (-no′sis) a disease due to chemical agents.

chemism (kem′izm) chemical activity.

chemist (kem′ist) an expert in chemistry.

chemistry (kem′is-tre) the science of the composition of matter. **colloid c.**, the scientific study of colloids. **inorganic c.**, the scientific study of compounds not containing carbon. **organic c.**, the scientific study of carbon-containing compounds.

chemoantigen (ke″mo-an′ti-jen) a chemical compound capable of acting as an antigen.

chemoautotroph (-aw′to-trōf) a chemoautotrophic microorganism.

chemoautotrophic (-aw″to-trof′ik) a term applied to bacteria which can synthesize their cell constituents from carbon dioxide by means of energy derived from inorganic reactions.

chemobiotic (-bi-ot′ik) a compound of a chemotherapeutic agent and an antibiotic.

chemodectoma (-dek-to′mah) any tumor of the chemoreceptor system, e.g. a carotid body tumor.

chemokinesis (-ki-ne′sis) increased activity of an organism caused by a chemical substance.

chemoluminescence (-loo″mi-nes′ens) light produced by the oxidation of a chemical compound.

chemolysis (ke-mol′i-sis) chemical decomposition.

chemomorphosis (ke″mo-mor-fo′sis) change of form from chemical action.

chemopallidectomy (-pal″i-dek′to-me) destruction of tissue of the globus pallidus by a chemical agent.

chemoprophylaxis (-pro″fi-lak′sis) prevention of disease by chemical means.

chemopsychiatry (-si-ki′ah-tre) the treatment of mental and emotional disorders by the use of drugs.

chemoreceptor (-re-sep′tor) a receptor organ sensitive to stimulation by chemical substances.

chemoreflex (-re′fleks) a reflex resulting from chemical action.

chemosensitive (-sen′si-tiv) sensitive to chemical stimuli.

chemoserotherapy (se″ro-ther′ah-pe) treatment of infection by means of drugs and serum.

chemosis (ke-mo′sis) edema of conjunctiva of the eye. adj., **chemot′ic.**

chemosterilant (ke″mo-ster′i-lant) a chemical compound which upon ingestion causes sterility of an organism.

chemosurgery (-ser′jer-e) removal of malignant, gangrenous or infected tissue after its fixation in situ by chemical means.

chemosynthesis (-sin′the-sis) the building up of chemical compounds under the influence of chemical stimulation, specifically the formation of carbohydrates from carbon dioxide and water as a result of energy derived from chemical reactions. adj., **chemosynthet′ic.**

chemotaxis (-tak′sis) taxis in response to the influence of chemical stimulation. adj., **chemotac′tic.**

chemotherapy (-ther′ah-pe) treatment by chemical substances having a specific effect on the microorganisms causing disease without injuring the patient.

chemotropism (ke-mot′ro-pizm) tropism in response to the influence of chemical stimulation. adj., **chemotrop′ic.**

chemurgy (kem′er-je) the application of chemistry to the arts.

cherubism (cher′u-bizm) a facial appearance produced by fibrous dysplasia of the jaws.

chest (chest) the part of the body enclosed by the ribs and sternum, especially its anterior aspect. **flail c.**, one whose wall moves paradoxically with respiration, owing to multiple fractures of the ribs. **funnel c.**, congenital chondrosternal depression. **pigeon c.**, congenital chondrosternal prominence.

chiasm (ki′azm) a crossing or decussation. **optic c.**, structure in the forebrain formed by junction of fibers of the optic nerves.

chiasma (ki-az′mah) chiasm. **c. formation**, the cytologic basis of genetic recombination, or crossing over.

chickenpox (chik′en-poks) an acute communicable childhood disease, caused by a virus, with mild constitutional symptoms and a maculopapular vesicular skin eruption.

chigger (chig'er) the six-legged red larva of the mite *Eutrombicula alfreddugsi*, known as harvest mite and red bug; its bite produces a wheal on the skin which is accompanied by intense itching.

chigoe (chig'o) *Tunga penetrans.*

chilblain (chil'blān) a localized painful erythematous condition due to exposure to cold.

child (chīld) the human young, from infancy to puberty.

childbed (chīld'bed) the puerperal state or period.

chill (chil) a sensation of cold, with convulsive shaking of the body.

Chilomastix (ki"lo-mas'tiks) a genus of parasitic protozoa. **C. mesnil'i,** a species sometimes found in the human intestine.

Chilopoda (ki-lop'o-dah) a class of the phylum Arthropoda, including the centipedes.

chimera (ki-me'rah) an organism whose body contains different cell populations derived from different zygotes of the same or different species, occurring spontaneously or produced artificially. **heterologous c.,** one in which the foreign cells are derived from an organism of a different species. **homologous c.,** one in which the foreign cells are derived from an organism of the same species, but of a different genotype. **isologous c.,** one in which the foreign cells are derived from a different organism having the identical genotype, as from an identical twin. **radiation c.,** an organism which has been subjected to heavy radiation and later received injection of cells from nonirradiated donors.

chimerism (ki'mer-izm) presence in an organism of cells derived from different zygotes of the same or different species.

chin (chin) the anterior prominence of the lower jaw; the mentum.

chiniofon (kin'e-o-fon) a bitter, slightly odorous, canary yellow powder; amebicide.

chionablepsia (ki"o-nah-blep'se-ah) snow blindness.

chir(o)- (ki'ro) word element [Gr.], *hand*. See also words beginning *cheir(o)-*

chirognostic (ki"rog-nos'tik) able to distinguish right from left.

chiroplasty (ki'ro-plas"te) plastic repair of the hand.

chiropodalgia (ki"ro-po-dal'je-ah) pain in the hands and feet.

chiropodist (ki-rop'o-dist) podiatrist.

chiropody (ki-rop'o-de) podiatry.

chiropractic (ki"ro-prak'tik) a system of treating disease by manipulation of the vertebral column.

chiropractor (-prak'tor) a specialist in chiropractic.

chirospasm (ki'ro-spazm) writers' cramp.

chirurgenic (ki"rur-jen'ik) induced by or occurring as the result of a surgical procedure.

chirurgery (ki-rur'jur-e) surgery.

chitin (ki'tin) a nitrogen-containing polysaccharide constituting the shells of crustaceae and the structural substance of insects and fungi.

Chlamydia (klah-mid'e-ah) a genus of Microtatobiotes (order Rickettsiales, family Chlamydiaceae). **C. oculogenita'lis,** the agent causing inclusion conjunctivitis. **C. tracho'matis,** the causative agent of trachoma.

Chlamydiaceae (klah-mid"e-a'se-e) a family of Microtatobiotes (order Rickettsiales) parasitic in warm-blooded animals.

Chlamydobacteriaceae (klah-mi"do-bak-te"-re-a'se-e) a family of Schizomycetes (order Chlamydobacteriales).

Chlamydobacteriales (-bak-te"re-a'lēz) an order of Schizomycetes.

chlamydospore (klam'i-do-spor") 1. the reproductive organ of certain fungi, so called because of its being enclosed by two envelopes. 2. a spore that is covered.

chloasma (klo-az'mah) hyperpigmentation in circumscribed areas of the skin; melanoderma. **c. gravida'rum,** chloasma occurring in pregnancy. **c. hepat'icum,** discoloration of the skin allegedly due to disorder of the liver. **c. uteri'num,** chloasma occurring during menstruation, in pregnancy or at the time of the menopause.

chlophedianol (klo"fe-di'ah-nol) a chlorobenzhydrol used as an antitussive.

chloracne (klor-ak'ne) an acneiform eruption, caused by chlorine.

chloral (klo'ral) an oily liquid, $Cl_3C.CHO$. **c. hydrate,** a crystalline compound, $CCl_3CH(OH)_2$, produced by hydration of chloral; used as a hypnotic.

chloralism (klo'ral-izm) poisoning from habitual use of chloral.

chloramphenicol (klor"am-fen'i-kol) a broad-spectrum antibiotic with specific therapeutic activity against rickettsias and many different bacteria.

chloranemia (klo"rah-ne'me-ah) idiopathic hypochromic anemia.

chlorate (klo'rāt) a salt of chloric acid.

chlorbutol (klor'bu-tol) chlorobutanol.

chlorcyclizine (klor-si'kli-zēn) a white, odorless or almost odorless powder used as an antihistaminic.

chlordiazepoxide (klor"di-a"ze-pok'sīd) a tranquilizing drug.

chloremia (klo-re'me-ah) 1. the presence of excessive chlorides in the blood. 2. chlorosis.

chloretic (klo-ret'ik) an agent which accelerates the flow of bile.

Chloretone (klo're-tōn) trademark for a preparation of chlorobutanol.

chlorguanide (klor-gwan'īd) proguanil.

chlorhydria (klor-hi'dre-ah) excess of hydrochloric acid in the stomach.

chloride (klo'rīd) a binary compound of chlorine.

chloridemia (klo"rī-de'me-ah) chlorides in the blood.

chloridimeter (-dim'ĕ-ter) an instrument used in chloridimetry.

chloridimetry (-dim'ĕ-tre) measurement of the chloride content of a fluid.

chloriduria (-du're-ah) excess of chlorides in the urine.

chlorinated (klo'rī-nat"ed) charged with chlorine.

chlorine (klo'rēn) chemical element *(see table)*, at. no. 17, symbol Cl.

chlorinum (klo-ri'num) chlorine.

chlorisondamine (klor"i-son'dah-mēn) an isoindoline derivative used to produce ganglionic blockade and to reduce blood pressure.

chlorite (klo'rīt) a salt of chlorous acid; disinfectant and bleaching agent.

chlormerodrin (klor-mer'o-drin) a mercurial diuretic, $C_5H_{11}ClHgN_2O_2$.

chlormezanone (-mez'ah-nōn) an agent used as a muscle relaxant and tranquilizer.

chloro-anemia (klo"ro-ah-ne'me-ah) chlorosis.

Chlorobacteriaceae (-bak-te"re-a'se-e) a family of Schizomycetes (order Pseudomonadales, suborder Rhodobacteriineae).

Chlorobacterium (-bak-te're-um) a genus of Schizomycetes (order Pseudomonadales, suborder Rhodobacteriineae, family Chlorobacteriaceae).

Chlorobium (klo-ro'be-um) a genus of Schizomycetes (order Pseudomonadales, suborder Rhodobacteriineae, family Chlorobacteriaceae).

chloroblast (klo'ro-blast) an erythroblast.

chlorobutanol (klo"ro-bu'tah-nol) colorless or white crystals, $CCl_3(CH_3)_2C.OH$; used as a preservative and as a hypnotic.

Chlorochromatium (-kro-ma'te-um) a genus of Schizomycetes (order Pseudomonadales, suborder Rhodobacteriineae, family Chlorobacteriaceae).

chloroform (klo'ro-form) a colorless, mobile liquid, $CHCl_3$, with ethereal odor and sweet taste; solvent, anesthetic and counterirritant.

chloroformism (klo'ro-form"izm) ill effects of excessive use of chloroform.

chloroleukemia (klo"ro-lu-ke'me-ah) myelogenous leukemia in which no specific tumor masses are observed at autopsy, but the body organs and fluids show a definite green color.

chlorolymphosarcoma (-lim"fo-sar-ko'mah) chloroma.

chloroma (klo-ro'mah) a malignant, green-colored tumor arising from myeloid tissue.

Chloromycetin (klo"ro-mi-se'tin) trademark for preparations of chloramphenicol.

chloromyeloma (-mi"ĕ-lo'mah) chloroma with multiple growths in bone marrow.

chloropenia (-pe'ne-ah) deficiency in chlorine. adj., **chlorope'nic.**

chloropexia (-pek'se-ah) the fixation of chlorine in the body.

chlorophane (klo'ro-fān) a green-yellow pigment from the retina.

chlorophenol (klo"ro-fe'nol) a combination of chlorine and phenol.

chlorophenothane (-fe'no-thān) a compound of DDT used in a lotion as an insecticide in pediculosis and scabies.

chlorophyll (klo'ro-fil) the green photosynthetic pigment contained in many vegetable organisms.

chloroplast (klo'ro-plast) the photosynthetic unit of a plant cell, containing all the chlorophyll.

chloroprivic (klo"ro-pri'vik) relating to lack or loss of chlorides.

chloroprocaine (-pro'kān) an aminobenzoate derivative used as a local or epidural anesthetic.

chloropsia (klo-rop'se-ah) defect of vision in which objects appear green.

chloroquine (klo'ro-kwin) an antimalarial compound, used also in amebic abscess and lupus erythematosus.

chlorosarcoma (klo"ro-sar-ko'mah) chloroma.

chlorosis (klo-ro'sis) a disorder, generally of pubescent females, characterized by greenish yellow discoloration of the skin and hypochromic erythrocytes. adj., **chlorot'ic. Egyptian c., tropical c.,** ancylostomiasis.

chlorothen (klo'ro then) a pyridine derivative used as an antihistaminic.

chlorothiazide (klo"ro-thi'ah-zīd) an odorless, crystalline powder, $C_7H_5ClN_3O_4S$; used as a diuretic and antihypertensive.

chlorothymol (-thi'mol) a white, crystalline compound, $C_{10}H_{13}C_{10}$; used as an antibacterial.

chlorotrianisene (-tri-an'ĭ-sēn) an estrogenic compound, $C_{23}H_{21}ClO_3$.

chlorpheniramine (klor"fen-ir'ah-mēn) a pyridine derivative used as an antihistaminic.

chlorphenoxamine (-ok'sah-mēn) an agent used as an antihistaminic and to reduce muscular rigidity.

chlorpromazine (klor-pro'mah-zēn) a phenothiazine derivative used as a tranquilizer and antiemetic, and to potentiate analgesics.

chlorpropamide (-pro'pah-mīd) an orally effective antidiabetic agent.

chlorprophenpyridamine (klor"pro-fen-pi-rid'-ah-mēn) chlorpheniramine.

chlorquinaldol (klor-kwin'al-dol) a bactericide and fungicide for application to the skin.

chlortetracycline (klor"tet-rah-si'klēn) an antibiotic isolated from *Streptomyces aureofaciens*, effective against a wide range of organisms.

chlorthalidone (klor-thal'ĭ-dōn) a phthalimidine derivative used as a diuretic and antihypertensive.

Chlor-trimeton (-tri'mĕ-ton) trademark for preparations of chlorpheniramine.

chloruresis (klor"u-re'sis) excretion of chlorides in the urine. adj., **chloruret'ic.**

chloruria (klo-ru're-ah) excess chlorides in the urine.

chlorzoxazone (-zok'sah-zōn) a drug used as a skeletal muscle relaxant.

Ch.M. [L.] *Chirur'giae ma'gister* (Master of Surgery).

choana (ko-a'nah), pl. *choa'nae* [L.] the posterior cavity of the nose.

Choanotaenia (ko-a"no-te'ne-ah) a genus of tapeworm.

chokes (chōks) a burning sensation in the substernal region, with uncontrollable coughing, occurring during decompression.

chol(o)- (ko'lo) word element [Gr.], *bile*.

cholagogue (ko'lah-gog) an agent that stimulates gallbladder contraction. adj., **cholagog'-ic.**

cholaligenic (ko-lal"ĭ-jen'ik) forming cholalic acid from cholesterol.

Cholan (ko'lan) trademark for preparations of dehydrocholic acid.

cholangeitis (ko-lan″je-i′tis) inflammation of the bile ducts.

cholangiogastrostomy (ko-lan″je-o-gas-tros′to-me) anastomosis of a bile duct to the stomach.

cholangiogram (ko-lan′je-o-gram″) the film obtained by cholangiography.

cholangiography (ko-lan″je-og′rah-fe) radiography of the bile ducts.

cholangiohepatoma (ko-lan″je-o-hep″ah-to′mah) a tumor containing abnormally mixed masses of liver cell cords and bile ducts.

cholangiole (ko-lan′je-ōl) one of the fine terminal elements of the bile duct system. adj., **cholangi′olar.**

cholangiolitis (ko-lan″je-o-li′tis) inflammation of the cholangioles.

cholangioma (-o′mah) a tumor of the bile ducts.

cholangiostomy (ko″lan-je-os′to-me) incision of a bile duct with drainage.

cholangiotomy (-ot′o-me) incision of a bile duct.

cholangitis (ko″lan-ji′tis) inflammation of a bile duct.

cholate (ko′lāt) a salt or ester of cholic acid.

chole- (ko′le) word element [Gr.], *bile.*

cholecalciferol (ko″le-kal-sif′er-ol) an oil-soluble antirachitic vitamin.

cholecyanin (-si′ah-nin) bilicyanin.

cholecyst (ko′le-sist) gallbladder.

cholecystagogue (ko″le-sis′tah-gog) an agent which promotes evacuation of the gallbladder.

cholecystalgia (-sis-tal′je-ah) biliary colic.

cholecystectasia (-sis″tek-ta′ze-ah) distention of the gallbladder.

cholecystectomy (-sis-tek′to-me) excision of the gallbladder.

cholecystenteric (-sis″ten-ter′ik) pertaining to or communicating with the gallbladder and intestine.

cholecystenterostomy (-sis″ten-ter-os′to-me) formation of a new communication between the gallbladder and the intestine.

cholecystic (-sis′tik) pertaining to the gallbladder.

cholecystitis (-sis-ti′tis) inflammation of the gallbladder.

cholecystocholangiogram (-sis″to-ko-lan′je-o-gram) a roentgenogram of the gallbladder and bile ducts.

cholecystoduodenostomy (-du″o-dē-nos′to-me) formation of an opening between gallbladder and duodenum.

cholecystogastrostomy (-gas-tros′to-me) formation of an opening between gallbladder and stomach.

cholecystogram (ko″le-sis′to-gram) a roentgenogram of the gallbladder.

cholecystography (-sis-tog′rah-fe) roentgenography of the gallbladder.

cholecystojejunostomy (-sis″to-je-ju-nos′to-me) formation of an opening between gallbladder and jejunum.

cholecystokinetic (-ki-net′ik) stimulating contraction of the gallbladder.

cholecystokinin (-kin′in) a hormone secreted in the small intestine, which stimulates contraction of the gallbladder.

cholecystolithiasis (ko″le-sis″to-li-thi′ah-sis) presence of stones in the gallbladder.

cholecystopathy (-sis-top′ah-the) disease of the gallbladder.

cholecystorrhaphy (-sis-tor′ah-fe) suture of the gallbladder.

cholecystostomy (-sis-tos′to-me) incision of the gallbladder with drainage.

cholecystotomy (-sis-tot′o-me) incision of the gallbladder.

choledochal (kol′e-dok-al) pertaining to the common bile duct.

choledochectomy (kol″e-do-kek′to-me) excision of part of the common bile duct.

choledochitis (-ki′tis) inflammation of the common bile duct.

choledocho- word element [Gr.], *common bile duct.*

choledochoduodenostomy (ko-led″ō-ko-du″o-dē-nos′to-me) anastomosis of common bile duct to duodenum.

choledochoenterostomy (-en″ter-os′to-me) anastomosis of common bile duct to intestine.

choledochogastrostomy (-gas-tros′to-me) anastomosis of common bile duct to stomach.

choledochojejunostomy (-je-ju-nos′to-me) anastomosis of common bile duct to the jejunum.

choledocholithiasis (-li-thi′ah-sis) calculi in the common bile duct.

choledocholithotomy (-li-thot′o-me) incision of common bile duct for removal of stone.

choledocholithotripsy (-lith′o-trip″se) crushing of a gallstone in the common bile duct.

choledochoplasty (ko-led′o-ko-plas″te) plastic repair of the common bile duct.

choledochorrhaphy (ko-led″o-kor′ah-fe) suture of the common bile duct.

choledochostomy (-kos′to-me) incision of the common bile duct with drainage.

choledochotomy (-kot′o-me) incision of the common bile duct.

Choledyl (kōl′ĕ-dil) trademark for a preparation of oxtriphylline.

cholehemia (ko″le-he′me-ah) bile in the blood.

choleic (ko-le′ik) pertaining to the bile.

cholelith (ko′lē-lith) gallstone.

cholelithiasis (ko″le-lī-thi′ah-sis) the presence of gallstones. adj., **cholelith′ic.**

cholelithotomy (-lī-thot′o-me) incision of the biliary tract for removal of gallstones.

cholelithotripsy (-lith′o-trip″se) crushing of a gallstone.

cholelithotrity (lī-thot′rī-te) cholelithotripsy.

cholemesis (ko-lem′ĕ-sis) vomiting of bile.

cholemia (ko-le′me-ah) bile or bile pigment in the blood. adj., **chole′mic.**

cholemimetry (ko″le-mim′ĕ-tre) measurement of bile pigment in the blood.

cholepathia (-path′e-ah) disease of the biliary tract. **c. spas′tica,** spasmodic contraction of bile ducts.

choleperitoneum (-per″ī-to-ne′um) bile in the peritoneum.

cholepyrrhin (-pir′in) bilirubin.

cholera (kol′er-ah) a condition marked by diarrhea and vomiting; Asiatic cholera. **Asiatic c.,** an acute infectious disease, chiefly epidemic, caused by *Vibrio comma* and characterized by a high mortality. **bilious c.,** a gastrointestinal infection characterized by violent and painful vomiting and by copious bilious stools. **chicken c.,** pasteurellosis in chickens. **dry c.,** cholera sicca. **epidemic c.,** Asiatic cholera. **European c.,** bilious cholera. **fowl c.,** an infectious disease caused by pasteurellae and occurring in all species of domestic poultry and in other birds throughout the world. **c. ful'minans,** cholera sicca. **hog c.,** an acute, highly infectious disease of swine, caused by a virus and having a high mortality rate. **c. infan'tum,** a noncontagious diarrhea occurring in infants; formerly common in the summer months. **malignant c.,** Asiatic cholera. **c. mor'bus,** a popular name for an acute gastroenteritis with diarrhea, cramps and vomiting. **c. nos'tras,** bilious cholera. **pandemic c.,** Asiatic cholera. **c. sic'-ca, c. sid'erans,** cholera in which death occurs before diarrhea has appeared. **simple c.,** bilious cholera. **spasmodic c.,** Asiatic cholera. **sporadic c.,** bilious cholera. **summer c.,** cholera morbus.

choleraic (kol″ĕ-ra'ik) pertaining to cholera.

cholerase (kol'er-ās) an enzyme from *Vibrio comma.*

choleresis (ko-ler'ĕ-sis) output of bile by the liver.

choleretic (ko″ler-et'ik) 1. increasing the output of bile by the liver. 2. an agent that stimulates an increase in the output of bile by the liver

choleriform (ko-ler'ĭ-form) resembling cholera.

cholerine (kol'er-ēn) a relatively mild form of cholera.

cholerophobia (kol″er-o-fo'be-ah) morbid fear of cholera.

cholerrhagia (ko″lĕ-ra'je-ah) an excessive flow of bile.

cholerythrin (ko-ler'ĭ-thrin) bilirubin.

cholestasis (ko″le-sta'sis) retention and accumulation of bile in the liver, due to factors within *(intrahepatic cholestasis)* or outside the liver *(extrahepatic cholestasis).* adj., **cholestat'ic.**

cholesteatoma (ko″le-ste″ah to'mah) a cystic mass with a lining of stratified squamous epithelium filled with desquamating debris frequently including cholesterol; sometimes associated with chronic infection of the middle ear *(cholesteatoma tympani).*

cholesterase (ko-les'ter-ās) an enzyme which splits up cholesterol.

cholesteremia (ko-les″ter-e'me-ah) cholesterolemia.

cholesterin (ko-les'ter-in) cholesterol.

cholesterinemia (ko-les″ter-in-e'me-ah) cholesterolemia.

cholesterinuria (-u're-ah) cholesteroluria.

cholesteroderma (ko-les″ter-o-der'mah) xanthoderma.

cholesterol (ko-les'ter-ol) the principal animal sterol, $C_{27}H_{46}O$, found in small amounts in many tissues, usually in the free state.

cholesterolemia (ko-les″ter-ol-e'me-ah) cholesterol in the blood.

cholesterolosis (-o'sis) cholesterosis.

cholesteroluria (ko-les″ter-ol-u're-ah) cholesterol in the urine.

cholesterosis (ko-les″ter-o'sis) deposition of cholesterol in abnormal quantities. **c. cu'tis,** xanthomatosis.

choletherapy (ko″le-ther'ah-pe) use of bile as a medicine.

choleuria (-u're-ah) choluria.

choleverdin (-ver'din) bilicyanin.

choline (ko'lēn) a colorless base, $C_5H_{15}O_2N$, occurring in the body in combined form in phospholipids or acetylcholine; essential in nutrition of many animals and useful in preventing and curing certain liver disorders.

choline-acetylase (ko″lēn-ah-set'ĭ-lās) an enzyme which brings about the synthesis of acetylcholine.

cholinergic (ko″lin-er'jik) activated or transmitted by acetylcholine; applied to nerve fibers that liberate acetylcholine at a synapse when a nerve impulse passes, i.e. the parasympathetic fibers.

cholinesterase (-es'ter ās) an esterase present in all body tissues which hydrolyzes acetylcholine into choline and acetic acid.

cholinolytic (ko″lin-o-lit'ik) 1. blocking the action of acetylcholine or of cholinergic substances. 2. an agent that blocks the action of acetylcholine or of cholinergic substances.

cholinomimetic (-mi-met'ik) having an action similar to that of choline.

cholochrome (ko'lo-krōm) a biliary pigment.

Cholografin (ko″lo-gra'fin) trademark for preparations of iodipamide.

cholohemothorax (he″mo-tho'raks) bile and blood in the thorax.

chololithiasis (li-tho-li'ah-sis) cholelithiasis.

cholorrhea (-re'ah) profuse secretion of bile.

choloscopy (ko-los'ko-pe) examination of the biliary tract.

cholothorax (ko″lo-tho'raks) a pleural effusion containing bile.

choluria (ko-lu're-ah) bile in the urine. adj., **cholu'ric.**

chondr(o)- (kon'dro) word element [Gr.], *cartilage.*

chondral (kon'dral) pertaining to cartilage.

chondralgia (kon-dral'je-ah) pain in a cartilage.

chondrectomy (kon-drek'to-me) excision of a cartilage.

chondric (kon'drik) pertaining to cartilage.

chondrification (kon″drĭ-fi-ka'shun) development of cartilage.

chondrin (kon'drin) a cartilage proteid.

chondrio- (kon'dre-o) word element [Gr.], *cartilage; granule.*

chondriocont (kon'dre-o-kont″) a rod-shaped or filamentous chondriosome.

chondriome (kon'dre-ōm) the entire complement of chondriosomes in a cell.

chondriosome (kon'dre-o-sōm″) one of the particles constantly found in protoplasm, distinguishable by their greater degree of refractivity.

chondritis (kon-dri'tis) inflammation of a cartilage.

chondroadenoma (kon″dro-ad″ĕ-no′mah) adenoma containing cartilaginous elements.

chondroangioma (-an″je-o′mah) angioma containing cartilaginous elements.

chondroblast (kon′dro-blast) an immature cartilage-producing cell.

chondroblastoma (kon″dro-blas-to′mah) a benign tumor arising from young chondroblasts in the epiphysis of a bone.

chondrocalcinosis (-kal″sĭ-no′sis) a condition resembling gout, resulting from calcification of the articular plate of a joint.

chondroclast (kon′dro-klast) a giant cell concerned in absorption and removal of cartilage.

Chondrococcus (kon″dro-kok′kus) a genus of Schizomycetes (order Myxobacterales, family Myxococcaceae).

chondroconia (-ko′ne-ah) reddish granules found in myelocytes.

chondrocostal (-kos′tal) pertaining to ribs and costal cartilages.

chondrocranium (-kra′ne-um) the embryonic skull from the seventh week to the middle of the third month, when it is a unified cartilaginous mass without clear boundaries indicating the limits of future bones.

chondrocyte (kon′dro-sīt) a mature cartilage-producing cell.

chondrodermatitis (kon″dro-der″mah-ti′tis) an inflammatory process involving cartilage and skin.

chondrodynia (-din′e-ah) pain in a cartilage.

chondrodysplasia (-dis-pla′ze-ah) dyschondroplasia.

chondrodystrophia (-dis-tro′fe-ah) chondrodystrophy. **c. feta′lis,** achondroplasia.

chondrodystrophy (-dis′tro-fe) a disorder of cartilage formation.

chondroendothelioma (-en″do-the″le-o′mah) an endothelioma containing cartilage tissue.

chondroepiphysitis (-ep″ĭ-fiz-i′tis) inflammation of epiphyses and cartilages.

chondrofibroma (-fi-bro′mah) a chondroma with fibrous elements.

chondrogen (kon′dro-jen) the base of cartilage.

chondrogenesis (kon″dro-jen′ĕ-sis) formation of cartilage.

chondrogenic (-jen′ik) giving rise to or forming cartilage.

chondroid (kon′droid) resembling cartilage.

chondroitin (kon-dro′ĭ-tin) a compound, $C_{18}H_{27}NO_{14}$, formed in decomposition of chondroitic acid.

chondroituria (kon″dro-i-tu′re-ah) chondroitic acid in the urine.

chondrolipoma (-li-po′mah) a tumor containing cartilaginous and fatty tissue.

chondrology (kon-drol′o-je) the study of cartilages.

chondrolysis (kon-drol′ĭ-sis) dissolution of cartilage.

chondroma (kon-dro′mah) a cartilaginous tumor. **joint c.,** a mass of cartilage in the synovial membrane of a joint. **c. sarcomato′sum,** chondrosarcoma. **synovial c.,** a cartilaginous body formed in a synovial membrane.

chondromalacia (kon″dro-mah-la′she-ah) abnormal softening of cartilage.

chondromatosis (-mah-to′sis) formation of multiple chondromas. **synovial c.,** a rare condition in which cartilage is formed in the synovial membrane of joints, tendon sheaths or bursae, sometimes becoming detached and producing a number of loose bodies.

chondrometaplasia (-met″ah-pla′ze-ah) a condition characterized by metaplastic activity of the chondroblasts.

chondromitome (-mi′tōm) paranucleus.

chondromucin (-mu′sin) a compound of chondroitic acid and mucin forming the intercellular substance of cartilage.

chondromucoid (-mu′koid) chondromucin.

Chondromyces (-mi′sēz) a genus of Schizomycetes (order Myxobacterales, family Polyangiaceae).

chondromyoma (-mi-o′mah) myoma with cartilaginous elements.

chondromyxoma (-mik-so′mah) myxoma with cartilaginous elements.

chondromyxosarcoma (-mik″so-sar-ko′mah) a sarcoma containing cartilaginous and mucous tissue.

chondro-osseous (-os′e-us) composed of cartilage and bone.

chondro-osteodystrophy (-os″te-o-dis′tro-fe) 1. eccentro-osteochondrodysplasia. 2. lipochondrodystrophy.

chondropathology (-pah-thol′o-je) pathology of the cartilages.

chondropathy (kon-drop′ah-the) disease of cartilage.

chondrophyte (kon′dro-fīt) a cartilaginous growth on a bone.

chondroplasia (kon″dro-pla′ze-ah) the formation of cartilage by specialized cells (chondrocytes).

chondroplast (kon′dro-plast) chondroblast.

chondroplasty (kon′dro-plas″te) plastic repair of cartilage.

chondroporosis (kon″dro-po-ro′sis) the formation of sinuses or spaces in cartilage.

chondroprotein (-pro′te-in) a protein occurring in cartilage.

chondrosarcoma (-sar-ko′ma) sarcoma with cartilaginous elements.

chondrosis (kon-dro′sis) the formation of cartilage.

chondrosteoma (kon″dros-te-o′mah) osteoma with cartilaginous elements.

chondrosternal (kon″dro-ster′nal) pertaining to costal cartilages and sternum.

chondrosternoplasty (-ster′no-plas″te) repair of established congenital chondrosternal depression with fixed deformity of the gladiolus and costal cartilages.

chondrotomy (kon-drot′o mc) incision of a cartilage.

chondroxiphoid (kon″dro-zi′foid) pertaining to the ensiform cartilage.

chondrus (kon′drus) sun-bleached plant of *Chondrus crispus* or *Gigartina mamillosa;* used as a protective agent for the skin.

chonechondrosternon (ko″ne-kon″dro-ster′non) congenital chondrosternal depression.

chord (kord) cord.

chorda (kor'dah), pl. *chor'dae* [L.] a cord or sinew. adj., **chor'dal. c. dorsa'lis,** notochord. **c. gubernac'ulum,** a portion of the gubernaculum testis or of the round ligament of the uterus that develops in the inguinal crest and adjoining body wall. **c. mag'na,** tendo calcaneus. **chor'dae tendin'eae,** tendinous strings joining the papillary muscles of the heart with the valves. **c. umbilica'lis,** umbilical cord. **c. voca'lis,** vocal cord. **chor'dae willis'ii,** Willis's cords.

Chordata (kor-da'tah) a phylum of the animal kingdom made up of organisms distinguished by having a notochord and gill slits.

chordate (kor'dāt) an individual of the phylum Chordata.

chordee (kor'de) downward deflection of the penis, due to a congenital anomaly or to infection.

chorditis (kor-di'tis) inflammation of vocal or spermatic cords.

chordoma (kor-do'mah) a tumor developed from embryonic remains of the notochord.

chordoskeleton (kor″do-skel'ĕ-ton) the part of the skeleton formed about the notochord.

chordotomy (kor-dot'o-me) surgical division of a nerve tract of the spinal cord.

chorea (ko-re'ah) a nervous disease with involuntary and irregular movements. adj., **chore'ic. chronic c.,** Huntington's chorea. **c. gravida'rum,** a rare form of chorea seen in pregnancy. **hereditary c., Huntington's c.,** a progressive hereditary affection, marked by irregular movements, speech disturbance and dementia. **c. insa'niens,** a grave form of chorea associated with mania, and usually ending fatally. **limp c.,** chorea accompanied by extreme muscular weakness. **maniacal c.,** chorea insaniens. **mimetic c.,** chorea caused by imitation. **Sydenham's c.,** ordinary and uncomplicated chorea.

choreiform (ko-re'ĭ-form) resembling chorea.

choreoathetosis (ko″re-o-ath″ĕ-to'sis) a morbid condition characterized by choreic and athetoid movements.

choreophrasia (-fra'ze-ah) meaningless repetition of words or phrases.

chorioadenoma (-ad″e-no'mah) adenoma of the chorion.

chorioallantois (-ah-lan'to-is) an extraembryonic sac of some vertebrate embryos, formed by fusion of the chorion and allantois. adj., **chorioallanto'ic.**

chorioamnionitis (-am″ne-o-ni'tis) bacterial infection of the fetal membranes.

chorioangioma (-an″je-o'mah) hydatidiform mole.

choriocapillaris (-kap″ĭ-la'ris) the second or capillary layer of the choroid.

choriocarcinoma (-kar″si-no'mah) a tumor formed from malignant proliferation of the epithelium of the chorionic villi.

choriocele (ko're-o-sēl″) protrusion of the chorion through an aperture.

chorioepithelioma (ko″re-o-ep″ĭ-the″le-o'mah) choriocarcinoma.

choriogenesis (ko″re-o-jen'ĕ-sis) the development of the chorion.

chorioid (ko're-oid) choroid.

chorioma (ko″re-o'mah) choriocarcinoma.

choriomeningitis (ko″re-o-men″in-ji'tis) inflammation of the meninges and choroid plexus. **lymphocytic c.,** a specific viral infection of meninges and choroid plexus with an increased number of lymphocytes in the cerebrospinal fluid and infiltrating the membranes. **pseudolymphocytic c.,** a benign, aseptic lymphocytic meningitis, with virus in the cerebrospinal fluid, and with severe headache, drowsiness, irritability and vomiting.

chorion (ko're-on) the outermost of the fetal membranes. **c. frondo'sum,** the part of chorion covered by villi. **c. lae've,** the smooth, membranous part of the chorion. **shaggy c.,** chorion frondosum.

chorionitis (ko″re-o-ni'tis) scleroderma.

Chorioptes (ko″re-op'tēz) a genus of mites infesting domestic animals and causing a kind of mange.

chorioretinitis (ko″re-o-ret″ĭ-ni'tis) inflammation of choroid and retina.

chorioretinopathy (-ret″ĭ-nop'ah-the) a noninflammatory process involving both choroid and retina.

chorista (ko-ris'tah) an error of development characterized by separation.

choristoma (ko″ris-to'mah) a mass of histologically normal tissue in an abnormal location.

choroid (ko'roid) the vascular coat of the eye, between the sclera and the retina. adj., **choroid'al.**

choroidea (ko-roi'de-ah) choroid.

choroideremia (ko-roi″der-e'me-ah) absence of the choroid.

choroiditis (ko″roi-di'tis) inflammation of the choroid.

choroidocyclitis (ko-roi″do-sik-li'tis) inflammation of choroid and ciliary processes.

choroido-iritis (-i-ri'tis) inflammation of choroid and iris.

choroidoretinitis (-ret″ĭ-ni'tis) inflammation of choroid and retina.

chrom(o)- (kro'mo) word element [Gr.], *color.*

chromaffin (kro-maf'in) staining strongly with chrome salts.

chromaffinity (kro″mah-fin'ĭ-te) the property of staining strongly with chrome salts.

chromaffinoblastoma (kro-maf″ĭ-no-blas'to'mah) a tumor containing embryonic chromaffin cells.

chromaffinoma (kro-maf″ĭ-no'mah) pheochromocytoma.

chromaffinopathy (kro-maf″ĭ-nop'ah-the) a disease of the chromaffin system.

chromagogue (kro'mah-gog) tending to eliminate pigments.

chromaphil (kro'mah-fil) chromaffin.

chromat(o)- (kro'mah-to) word element [Gr.], *color; chromatin.*

chromate (kro'māt) a salt of chromic acid.

chromatid (kro'mah-tid) either of the two long, thin, parallel strands held together at one spot (the centromere), constituting a replicating chromosome in a dividing cell.

chromatin (kro'mah-tin) the DNA-containing chromosomal substance of the nucleus of a cell. **sex c.,** a mass of chromatin situated at the periphery of the nucleus, which is present in normal females, but not in normal males.

chromatin-negative (-neg'ah-tiv) lacking sex chromatin; characteristic of the nuclei of cells in a normal male.

chromatinolysis (kro"mah-tĭ-nol'ĭ-sis) chromatolysis.

chromatinorrhexis (kro-mat"ĭ-no-rek'sis) splitting up of chromatin.

chromatin-positive (kro'mah-tin-poz'ĭ-tiv) containing sex chromatin; characteristic of the nuclei of cells in a normal female.

chromatism (kro'mah-tizm) abnormal pigmentation.

Chromatium (kro-ma'te-um) a genus of Schizomycetes (order Pseudomonadales, suborder Rhodobacteriineae, family Thiorhodaceae).

chromatodysopia (kro"mah-to-dis-o'pe-ah) imperfect perception of colors.

chromatogenous (kro"mah-toj'ĕ-nus) producing color or coloring matter.

chromatogram (kro-mat'o-gram) the record produced by chromatography.

chromatography (kro"mah-tog'rah-fe) chemical analysis by determining reactions apparent on adsorption of the substance on different materials contained in a vertical glass tube. **electric c.,** electrochromatography. **paper c.,** chromatography using paper treated with various chemicals instead of an adsorption column.

chromatokinesis (kro"mah-to-ki-ne'sis) movement of chromatin during the life and division of a cell.

chromatolysis (kro"mah-tol'ĭ-sis) 1. disintegration of the chromatin of cell nuclei. 2. disappearance of the Nissl substance of a nerve cell as the result of a noxious influence.

chromatometer (-tom'ĕ-ter) instrument for measuring color or color perception.

chromatopathy (-top'ah-the) a skin disease marked by disorder of pigmentation.

chromatophil (kro-mat'o-fil) a cell or structure which stains easily. adj., **chromatophil'ic.**

chromatophore (kro-mat'o-fōr) a pigment-containing cell.

chromatopsia (kro"mah-top'se-ah) perversion of color vision, in which objects are seen as abnormally colored.

chromatoptometry (-top-tom'ĕ-tre) measurement of color perception.

chromatosis (kro"mah-to'sis) abnormal deposition of pigment, as in the skin.

chromaturia (-tu're-ah) abnormal coloration of the urine.

chromesthesia (kro"mes-the'ze-ah) association of color sensations with sensations of taste, hearing and smell.

chromhidrosis (krōm-hĭ-dro'sis) secretion of colored sweat.

chromicize (kro'mĭ-sīz) to treat with chromium.

chromidiosis (kro-mid"e-o'sis) outflow of chromatin from the nucleus to the cytoplasm of a cell.

chromidium (kro-mid'e-um), pl. *chromid'ia,* a grain of extranuclear chromatin in the cytoplasm of a cell.

chromidrosis (kro"mĭ-dro'sis) chromhidrosis.

chromium (kro'me-um) chemical element *(see table),* at. no. 24, symbol Cr. **c. oxide,** a substance used in dentistry as a polishing agent, especially for stainless steel.

Chromobacterium (kro"mo-bak-te're-um) a genus of Schizomycetes (order Eubacteriales, family Rhizobiaceae).

chromoblast (kro'mo-blast) an embryonic cell which develops into a pigment cell.

chromoblastomycosis (kro"mo-blas"to-mi-ko'sis) a chronic fungus infection of the skin, producing wartlike nodules or papillomas which may or may not ulcerate.

chromocrinia (-krin'e-ah) secretion or excretion of coloring matter.

chromocyte (kro'mo-sīt) a colored cell.

chromocytometer (kro"mo-si-tom'ĕ-ter) an instrument for measuring the hemoglobin of the red blood corpuscles.

chromodacryorrhea (-dak"re-o-re'ah) the shedding of colored tears.

chromodermatosis (-der"mah-to'sis) any skin disease with pigmentation.

chromoflavine (-fla'vin) acriflavine.

chromogen (kro'mo-jen) a precursor of coloring matter.

chromogene (kro'mo-jēn) a gene located on a chromosome.

chromogenesis (kro"mo-jen'ĕ-sis) the formation of color or pigment.

chromogenic (-jen'ik) producing color or pigment.

chromolipoid (-lip'oid) lipochrome.

chromolysis (kro-mol'ĭ-sis) chromatolysis.

chromoma (kro-mo'mah) a malignant tumor supposed to be derived from chromatophore cells.

chromomere (kro'mo-mēr) 1. a beadlike granule of chromatin found in a chromosome. 2. granulomere.

chromometer (kro-mom'ĕ-ter) instrument for chromometry.

chromometry (kro-mom'ĕ-tre) measurement of coloring matter.

chromomycosis (kro"mo-mi-ko'sis) chromoblastomycosis.

chromonema (-ne'mah) the threadlike structure of a chromosome.

chromoparic (-par'ik) producing color.

chromopectic (-pek'tik) pertaining to, characterized by or promoting chromopexy.

chromopexic (-pek'sik) chromopectic.

chromopexy (kro'mo-pek"se) the fixation of pigment, especially by the liver in the formation of bilirubin.

chromophage (kro'mo-fāj) pigmentophage.

chromophane (kro'mo-fān) a retinal pigment

chromophil (kro'mo-fil) any easily stainable structure. adj., **chromophil'ic.**

chromophobia (kro"mo-fo'be-ah) 1. the quality of staining poorly with dyes. 2. morbid aversion to colors. adj., **chromopho'bic.**

chromophore (kro"mo-fōr) a configuration in an unsaturated organic molecule containing a group with one or more multiple bonds, which acts to shift the absorption of light into lower frequencies (longer wavelengths).

chromophoric (kro"mo-fōr'ik) bearing color.

chromophose (kro'mo-fōs) a subjective sensation of color.

chromophytosis (kro"mo-fi-to'sis) skin discoloration due to a vegetable parasite.

chromoplasm (kro'mo-plazm) the easily staining portion of a cell nucleus.

chromoplastid (kro"mo-plas'tid) a protoplasmic pigment granule.

chromoprotein (-pro'te-in) a conjugated protein which contains a colored prosthetic group.

chromopsia (kro-mop'se-ah) chromatopsia.

chromoptometer (kro"mop-tom'ĕ-ter) instrument for measuring color perception.

chromoradiometer (kro"mo-ra"de-om'ĕ-ter) an instrument for measuring x-ray dosage.

chromoscopy (kro-mos'ko-pe) diagnosis of renal function by color of the urine after administration of dyes.

chromosome (kro'mo-sōm) in animal cells, a structure in the nucleus containing a linear thread of DNA which transmits genetic information and is associated with RNA and histones; during cell division the material composing the chromosome is compactly coiled, making it visible with appropriate staining and permitting its movement in the cell with minimal entanglement; each organism of a species is normally characterized by the same number of chromosomes in its somatic cells, 46 being the number normally present in man, including the two (X and Y) which determine the sex of the organism. 2. in bacterial genetics, a closed circle of double-stranded DNA which contains the genetic material of the cell and is attached to the cell membrane; the bulk of this material forms a compact bacterial nucleus (called also nuclear body or nucleotoid). **accessory c.**, an unpaired chromosome. **bivalent c.**, a pair of chromosomes temporarily united. **heterotypical c.**, allosome. **gametic c.**, one in a haploid cell (gamete) consisting of a double strand of DNA. **homologous c's**, chromosomes which are identical in size and shape, have identical chromomeres along their length, and contain similar genes, which synapse during meiosis and separate, one going to either pole. **Philadelphia c.**, an abnormal chromosome observed in the leukocytes of patients with chronic granulocytic leukemia. **sex c.**, the chromosome responsible for determination of the sex of the individual which develops from a zygote. **somatic c.**, one in a diploid (tissue) cell of the body. **X c.**, an accessory chromosome carried in both the sperm and ovum, being the female-determining factor. **Y c.**, an accessory chromosome occurring only in the sperm, being the male-determining factor.

chromotoxic (kro"mo-tok'sik) due to toxic action on hemoglobin.

chromotropic (-trop'ik) attracting color or pigment.

chron(o) (kron'o) word element [Gr.], *time.*

chronaxia (kro-nak'se-ah) chronaxy.

chronaxie (kro'nak-se) chronaxy.

chronaximeter (kro"nak-sim'ĕ-ter) an instrument for measuring chronaxy.

chronaxy (kro'nak-se) the time required for excitation of a neural element by a definite stimulus; the minimum time at which a current just double the rheobase will excite contraction.

chronic (kron'ik) persisting for a long time; applied to a morbid state, designating one showing little change or extremely slow progression over a long period.

chronobiology (kron"o-bi-ol'o-je) the study of the duration of life.

chronognosis (kron"og-no'sis) perception of the lapse of time.

chronograph (kron'o-graf) an instrument for recording small intervals of time.

chronoscope (kron'o-skōp) an instrument for measuring small intervals of time.

chronotaraxis (kron"o-tar-ak'sis) disorientation in relation to time.

chronotropic (-trop'ik) affecting the time or rate.

chronotropism (kro-not'ro-pizm) interference with regularity of a periodical movement, such as the heart's action.

chrotoplast (kro'to-plast) a skin cell.

chrys(o)- (kris'o) word element [Gr.], *gold.*

chrysarobin (kris"ah-ro'bin) a mixture of neutral principles derived from goa powder; used in treatment of various skin diseases.

chrysiasis (krī-si'ah-sis) deposition of gold in living tissue.

chrysocreatinine (kris"o-kre-at'ĭ-nin) a leucomaine from muscle.

chrysoderma (-der'mah) permanent pigmentation of the skin due to gold deposit.

Chrysomyia (-mi'yah) a genus of flies whose larvae may be secondary invaders of wounds or internal parasites of man.

chrysophoresis (-fo-re'sis) the distribution to various parts of the body of particles of gold administered therapeutically, by macrophages and polymorphonuclear leukocytes.

Chrysops (kris'ops) a genus of flies of worldwide distribution; commonly known as deerflies, they are important vectors of various organisms, e.g. *Pasteurella tularensis* and *Loa loa.*

chrysotherapy (kris"o-ther'ah-pe) treatment with gold salts.

chthonophagia (thon"o-fa'je-ah) geophagy.

chylangioma (ki-lan"je-o'mah) tumor of intestinal lymph vessels filled with chyle.

chyle (kil) the product of intestinal digestion absorbed into the lymphatic system through the lacteals and conveyed through the thoracic duct to empty into the venous system at the root of the neck.

chylectasia (ki"lek-ta'ze-ah) dilatation of a chylous vessel.

chylemia (ki-le'me-ah) chylous material in the blood.

chylidrosis (ki"lī-dro'sis) chylous perspiration.

chylifacient (-fa'shent) forming chyle.

chylifaction (ki″li-fak′shun) chylification. adj., **chylifac′tive.**

chyliferous (ki-lif′er-us) conveying chyle.

chylification (ki″li-fi-ka′shun) formation of chyle.

chyliform (ki′li-form) resembling, but not containing, chyle.

chylocele (ki′lo-sēl) distention of the tunica vaginalis testis with effused chyle.

chylocyst (ki′lo-sist) receptaculum chyli.

chyloderma (ki″lo-der′mah) lymph scrotum.

chylology (ki-lol′o-je) the study of chyle.

chylomediastinum (ki″lo-me″de-as-ti′num) effused chyle in the mediastinum.

chylomicron (-mi′kron) a minute particle consisting of triglyceride, phospholipid, cholesterol and a protein, found in blood plasma after intestinal digestion of a fatty meal.

chylomicronemia (-mi″kro-ne′me-ah) the presence of chylomicrons in the blood.

chylopericardium (-per″i-kar′de-um) effused chyle in the pericardium.

chyloperitoneum (-per″i-to-ne′um) effused chyle in the peritoneal cavity.

chylophoric (-for′ik) conveying chyle.

chylopneumothorax (-nu″mo-tho′raks) effused chyle and air in a pleural cavity.

chylopoiesis (-poi-e′sis) the formation of chyle. adj., **chylopoiet′ic.**

chylothorax (-tho′raks) effused chyle in the pleural cavity.

chylous (ki′lus) of the nature of or containing chyle.

chyluria (ki-lu′re-ah) chyle in the urine.

Chymar (ki′mar) trademark for preparations of chymotrypsin.

chymase (ki′mās) an enzyme of the gastric juice which hastens the action of the pancreatic juice.

chyme (kīm) the gruel-like material produced in the stomach by enzymatic and mechanical action on ingested food and discharged through the pylorus into the duodenum.

chymification (ki″mi-fi-ka′shun) conversion of food into chyme.

chymosin (ki-mo′sin) rennin.

chymotrypsin (ki″mo-trip′sin) an endopeptidase with action similar to that of trypsin, produced in the intestine by activation of chymotrypsinogen; a product crystallized from an extract of the pancreas of the ox is used clinically.

chymotrypsinogen (-trip-sin′o-jen) the inactive precursor of chymotrypsin, the form in which it is secreted by the pancreas.

Ci abbreviation for *curie* recommended by the International Commission on Radiological Units and Measurements.

C.I. color index.

cib. [L.] *ci′bus* (food).

cicatrectomy (sik″ah-trek′to-me) excision of a cicatrix.

cicatricial (sik″ah-trish′al) pertaining to a cicatrix.

cicatrix (sik′ah-triks, si-ka′triks) the mark or fibrous tissue left after the healing of a wound. **vicious c.,** one causing deformity.

cicatrization (sik″ah-tri-za′shun) the formation of permanent fibrous tissue in the healing of a wound.

-cide (sīd) word element [L.], *destruction or killing* (homicide); *an agent which kills or destroys* (germicide). adj., **-ci′dal.**

cilia (sil′e-ah) [L.] 1. plural of cilium. 2. eyelashes.

ciliariscope (sil″e-ar′i-skōp) instrument for examining ciliary region of eye.

ciliarotomy (sil″e-ar-ot′o-me) surgical division of the ciliary zone.

ciliary (sil′e-er″e) pertaining to the eye or the eyelashes.

ciliate (sil′e-āt) a protozoan of the subphylum Ciliophora, characterized by the presence of cilia throughout its life.

ciliated (sil′e-āt″ed) provided with cilia.

ciliectomy (sil″e-ek′to-me) excision of the roots of the eyelashes.

Ciliophora (sil″e-of′o-rah) a subphylum of Protozoa, including two major groups, the ciliates and suctorians, and distinguished from the other subphyla by the presence of cilia at some stage in the existence of the member organisms.

cilioretinal (sil″e-o-ret′i-nal) pertaining to ciliary body and retina.

cilium (sil′e-um), pl. *cil′ia* [L.] a hair or slender hairlike process, e.g. the fine projections from the surfaces of ciliated cells.

Cillobacterium (sil″lo-bak-te′re-um) a genus of Schizomycetes (order Eubacteriales, family Lactobacillaceae, tribe Lactobacilleae) found in the intestinal tract and occasionally associated with purulent infections.

cillosis (sil-lo′sis) spasmodic quivering of the eyelid.

cimbia (sim′be-ah) a white band running across the ventral surface of the crus cerebri.

Cimex (si′meks) a genus of arthropods (order Hemiptera), including blood-sucking insects — the bedbugs and allied forms. **C. lectula′rius,** the common bedbug; other species are limited to tropical and subtropical areas and feed on other animals as well as man.

cinchona (sin-ko′nah) dried bark of stem or root of various species of Cinchona.

cinchonine (sin′ko-nēn) an alkaloid obtained from cinchona. **c. sulfate,** the sulfate of cinchonine, $(C_{19}H_{22}N_2O)_2 \cdot H_2SO_4 \cdot 2H_2O$.

cinchonism (sin′ko-nizm) poisoning from cinchona bark or its alkaloids.

cinchophen (sin′ko-fen) a compound with antipyretic properties; used in the treatment of gout.

cineangiocardiography (sin″e-an″je-o-kar″de-og′rah-fe) the photographic recording of fluoroscopic images of the heart and great vessels by motion picture techniques.

cineangiography (-an″je-og′rah-fe) the photographic recording of fluoroscopic images of the blood vessels by motion picture techniques.

cinedensigraphy (sin″e-den-sig′rah-fe) graphic recording of movements of interal body structures by means of roentgen rays and radiosensitive cells.

cinefluorography (-floo″or-og′rah-fe) photoggraphy, by motion picture techniques, of the shadow images appearing on the fluoroscopic screen.

cinematics (sin″e-mat′iks) kinematics.

cinematography (sin″ē-mah-tog′rah-fe) the taking of motion pictures.

cinematoradiography (sin″e-mah-to-ra″de-og′rah-fe) the recording of x-ray images by motion picture techniques; cinefluorography.

cinemicrography (sin″ē-mi-krog′rah-fe) the making of motion pictures of a small object through the lens system of a microscope.

cineol (sin′e-ol) eucalyptol.

cineplasty (sin′e-plas″te) kineplasty.

cineradiography (sin″e-ra″de-og′rah-fe) the photographic recording by motion picture techniques of x-ray images.

cinerea (sĭ-ne′re-ah) the gray matter of the nervous system. adj., **cine′real.**

cineritious (sin″ē-rish′us) ashen gray in color.

cineroentgenofluorography (sin″e-rent″gen-o-floo″or-og′rah-fe) cineradiography.

cinesi- for words beginning thus, see those beginning *kinesi-*.

cineto- for words beginning thus, see those beginning *kineto-*.

cingulectomy (sing″gu-lek′to-me) bilateral extirpation of the anterior half of the gyrus cinguli.

cingulum (sing′gu-lum), pl. *cin′gula* [L.] a bundle of association fibers partly encircling the corpus callosum not far from the median plane, interrelating the cingulate and hippocampal gyri.

cingulumotomy (sing″gu-lum-ot′o-me) the creation of lesions in the cingulum of the frontal lobe for relief of intractable pain.

cinnamon (sin′ah-mun) the dried bark of *Cinnamomum loureirii;* cordial, carminative and flavoring agent.

C.I.O.M.S. Council for International Organizations of Medical Sciences.

cionectomy (si″o-nek′to-me) uvulectomy.

cionitis (-ni′tis) uvulitis.

cionotomy (-not′o-me) uvulotomy.

circadian (ser″kah-de′an) denoting a period of about 24 hours.

circle (ser′kl) a round figure, structure or part. **Berry's c's,** charts with circles on them for testing stereoscopic vision. **defensive c.,** the coexistence of two conditions which tend to have an antagonistic or inhibiting effect on each other. **diffusion c.,** a confused image formed on the retina when the retina is not at the focus of the eye. **Haller's c's,** arterial and venous circles within the eye. **Minsky's c.,** a device for the graphic recording of eye lesions. **sensory c.,** a body area within which it is impossible to distinguish separately the impressions arising from two sites of stimulation. **Weber's c's,** circles on the skin delineating the distance at which two simultaneously applied points can be separately distinguished. **c. of Willis,** a loop of vessels near the base of the brain.

circulation (ser″ku-la′shun) movement in a circle, returning to the point of origin, as the circulation of the blood. **allantoic c.,** umbilical circulation. **chorionic c.,** the fetal part of the placental circulation. **collateral c.,** that carried on through secondary channels after obstruction of the principal channel supplying the part. **extracorporeal c.,** circulation of blood outside the body, as through an artificial kidney or a heart-lung apparatus. **fetal c.,** the flow of blood within the fetal vessels. **first c.,** primitive circulation. **hypophyseoportal c.,** the flow of blood from the capillaries of the median eminence of the hypothalamus to the sinusoidal capillaries of the anterior lobe of the hypophysis. **intervillous c.,** the maternal part of the placental circulation. **lesser c.,** pulmonary circulation. **omphalomesenteric c.,** vitelline circulation. **placental c.,** the dual circulation in the placenta during pregnancy, the maternal and fetal blood streams being separated by membrane barriers across which molecular diffusion takes place. **portal c.,** a general term denoting the circulation of blood through larger vessels from the capillaries of one organ to those of another; applied especially to the passage of blood from the gastrointestinal tract and spleen through the portal vein to the liver. **primitive c.,** that by which the earliest nutriment and oxygen are conveyed to the developing embryo. **pulmonary c.,** the flow of blood from the right ventricle through the pulmonary artery to the lungs, where carbon dioxide is exchanged for oxygen, and back through the pulmonary vein to the left atrium. **sinusoidal c.,** that occurring through the sinusoids of an organ. **systemic c.,** the flow of blood from the left ventricle through the aorta, carrying oxygen and nutrient material to all the tissues of the body, and returning through the superior and inferior venae cavae to the right atrium. **umbilical c.,** the circulation between the fetus and placenta through the umbilical cord. **vitelline c.,** that in the paired vitelline arteries and veins between the embryo and the yolk sac.

circulatory (ser′ku-lah-tor″e) pertaining to circulation.

circulus (ser′ku-lus), pl. *cir′culi* [L.] a circle.

circum- (ser′kum) word element [L.] around.

circumcision (ser″kum-sizh′un) excision of the foreskin. **female c.,** incision of the fold of skin over the glans clitoridis.

circumolusion (-kloo′zhun) compression of an artery by a wire and pin.

circumcorneal (-kōr′ne-al) surrounding the cornea.

circumduction (-duk′shun) circular movement of a limb or of the eye.

circumflex (ser′kum-fleks) having a winding course.

circuminsular (ser″kum-in′su-lar) surrounding the island of Reil.

circumintestinal (-in-tes′tĭ-nal) surrounding the intestine.

circumlental (-len′tal) surrounding the lens.

circumnuclear (-nu′kle-ar) surrounding a nucleus.

circumocular (-ok′u-ler) surrounding the eye.

circumpolarization (ser″kum-po″ler-i-za′shun) the rotation of polarized light.

circumrenal (-re′nal) around the kidney.

circumstantiality (-stan″she-al′ĭ-te) thinking or conversation characterized by unnecessary elaboration of trivial details.

cirrhonosus (sĭ-ron′o-sus) a fetal disease marked by a golden-yellow color of the pleura.

cirrhosis (sĭ-ro′sis) interstitial inflammation of an organ, particularly the liver. adj., **cirrhot′ic. atrophic c.**, cirrhosis marked by shriveling and shrinkage in size of liver. **biliary c.**, cirrhosis of liver from chronic retention of bile. **Budd's c.**, chronic enlargement of the liver from intestinal intoxication. **Cruveilhier-Baumgarten c.**, congenital cirrhosis of the liver. **fatty c.**, form in which liver cells become infiltrated with fat. **glissonian c.**, perihepatitis. **hypertrophic c.**, a form marked by enlargement of the liver. **Laennec's c.**, atrophic cirrhosis of the liver. **portal c.**, a degenerative and inflammatory disease of the liver leading to obstruction of the portal circulation. **Todd's c.**, hypertrophic cirrhosis of the liver.

cirrus (sir′us), pl. *cir′ri* [L.] a specialized structure of certain protozoa, composed of fused cilia from several rows, serving in locomotion and obtaining food, and as sensory organs.

cirsectomy (ser-sek′to-me) excision of a varicose vein.

cirsenchysis (ser-sen′kĭ-sis) therapeutic injection of a varicose vein.

cirsocele (ser′so-sēl) varicocele.

cirsodesis (ser-sod′ĕ-sis) ligation of a varicose vein.

cirsoid (ser′soid) resembling a varix.

cirsomphalos (ser-som′fah-los) varicose state of the navel.

cirsotomy (ser-sot′o-me) incision of a varicosity.

cistern (sis′tern) a closed space serving as a reservoir for fluid, e.g. one of the enlarged spaces of the body containing lymph or other fluid. **c. of Pecquet** (pek-ka′), receptaculum chyli.

cisterna (sis-ter′nah), pl. *cister′nae* [L.] cistern. adj., **cister′nal.**

cistron (sis′tron) a gene regarded as a hereditary unit of function.

citrate (sit′rāt, si′trāt) a salt of citric acid.

citrated (sit′rāt-ed) treated with a salt of citric acid, e.g. sodium citrate.

citrinin (sit′rĭ-nin) a bacteriostatic derivative of *Penicillium citrinum.*

citrulline (sit-rul′lēn) an alpha-amino acid.

citrullinuria (cit-rul″lĭ-nu′re-ah) presence in the urine of large amounts of citrulline.

cittosis (sit-to′sis) pica.

Cl chemical symbol, *chlorine.*

cl. centiliter.

clamp (klamp) a surgical device for compressing a part or structure. **Michel's c's**, metal clips for closing the edges of a wound. **rubber dam c's**, metallic rings that fit snugly about the teeth and secure the dam in the mouth.

clapotement (klah-pōt-maw′) [Fr.] a splashing sound, as in succussion.

clarificant (klah-rif′ĭ-kant) a substance which clears a liquid of turbidity.

clasmatocyte (klaz-mat′o-sīt) a macrophage.

clasmatodendrosis (klaz-mat″o-den-dro′sis) breaking up of the protoplasmic expansions of astrocytes.

clasmatosis (klaz″mah-to′sis) the breaking off of parts of a cell.

class (klas) 1. a taxonomic category subordinate to a phylum and superior to an order. 2. a group of variables all of which show a value falling between certain limits.

classification (klas″sĭ-fĭ-ka′shun) systematic arrangement of a number of similar entities on the basis of certain differing characteristics. **Denver c.**, an arrangement of the chromosomes of man, the autosomes being arranged in seven groups as nearly as possible in descending order of length and numbered 1 to 22. **Lancefield c.**, the classification of hemolytic streptococci into groups on the basis of serologic action.

clastic (klas′tik) undergoing or causing division.

clastothrix (klas′to-thriks) brittleness of the hair.

Clathrochloris (klath″ro-klo′ris) a genus of Schizomycetes (order Pseudomonadales, suborder Rhodobacteriineae, family Chlorobacteriaceae).

claudicant (klaw′dĭ-kant) 1. pertaining to or characterized by claudication. 2. a patient with intermittent claudication.

claudication (klaw″dĭ-ka′shun) limping; lameness. **intermittent c.**, angina cruris.

claustrophilia (klaws″tro-fil′e-ah) an abnormal desire to be in a closed room or space.

claustrophobia (-fo′be-ah) morbid fear of closed places.

claustrum (klaws′trum), pl. *claus′tra* [L.] a thin layer of gray substance on the lateral surface of the external capsule.

clava (kla′vah) an enlargement of the funiculus gracilis in the oblongata.

clavacin (klav′ah-sin) an antibiotic substance isolated from cultures of *Aspergillus clavatus.*

Claviceps (klav′ĭ-seps) a genus of fungi. **C. purpu′rea**, the fungus which produces ergot.

clavicle (klav′ĭ-kl) the shoulder bone.

clavicotomy (klav″ĭ-kot′o-me) cutting of the clavicle.

clavicula (klah-vik′u-lah), pl. *clavic′ulae* [L.] clavicle.

claviformin (klav″ĭ-for′min) an antibacterial substance derived from cultures of *Aspergillus claviforme.*

clavus (kla′vus) a corn. **c. hyster′icus**, a sensation as if a nail were being driven into the head.

clawfoot (klaw′foot) atrophy and distortion of the foot.

clawhand (klaw′hand) atrophy and distortion of the hand.

clearance (klēr′ans) the process of clearing, or of extracting a substance from solution, especially a numerical expression of the volume of solution so cleared per unit time. **inulin c.,** an expression of the renal efficiency in eliminating inulin from the blood. **urea c.,** the removal of urea from the blood by renal elimination, the minute volume of blood so cleared of urea being taken as indicative of renal function.

cleavage (klēv'ij)   1. division into distinct parts.   2. the early successive splitting of a fertilized ovum into smaller cells (blastomeres) by mitosis. **complete c.,** holoblastic cleavage. **determinate c.,** that which follows a precise pattern, each blastomere having an unalterable fate. **equatorial c.,** that which occurs in a plane passing through the equator of the egg. **holoblastic c.,** that involving the entire fertilized ovum. **incomplete c.,** meroblastic cleavage. **indeterminate c.,** that which follows a less rigid pattern, the blastomeres having more capabilities than they usually show. **latitudinal c.,** that in planes passing at right angles to the egg axis. **meridional c.,** that in planes passing through the egg axis. **meroblastic c.,** that involving only the protoplasmic portions of the fertilized ovum. **partial c.,** meroblastic cleavage.

cleft (kleft)   a fissure. **branchial c's,** a series of openings in the early embryo, separating the branchial arches. **visceral c's,** branchial clefts.

cleid(o)- (kli'do)   word element [Gr.], *clavicle.*

cleidagra (kli-dag'rah)   gouty pain in the clavicle.

cleidocranialiasis (kli"do-kra"ne-al-i'ah-sis)   cleidocranial dysostosis.

cleidomastoid (-mas'toid)   pertaining to clavicle and mastoid.

cleidorrhexis (-rek'sis)   fracture of a clavicle of the fetus in difficult labor.

cleidotomy (kli-dot'o-me)   division of the clavicle of the fetus in difficult labor.

cleisagra (kli-sag'rah)   cleidagra.

clemizole (klem'ĭ-zōl)   a drug used as an antiallergic and antihistaminic.

clier (kli'er)   a glandular swelling in cattle.

climacteric (kli-mak'ter-ik, kli"mak-ter'ik)   the combined phenomena accompanying cessation of the reproductive function in the female or diminution of testicular activity in the male.

climatology (kli"mah-tol'o-je)   scientific study of natural environmental conditions (e.g. rainfall, temperature) prevailing in specific regions of the earth.

climatotherapy (kli"mah-to-ther'ah-pe)   treatment of disease by change of climate.

climax (kli'maks)   the period of greatest intensity, as in the course of a disease.

clinic (klin'ik)   1. medical instruction based on observation of patients.   2. an establishment where patients are admitted for special study and treatment by a group of physicians practicing medicine together. **ambulant c.,** one for patients not confined to the bed. **dry c.,** a clinical lecture with case histories, but without patients present.

clinical (klin'ĭ-kl)   pertaining to the sickbed or to a patient.

clinician (kli-nish'an)   an expert clinical teacher or practitioner.

clinicogenetic (klin"ĭ-ko-jĕ-net'ik)   pertaining to the clinical manifestations of a chromosomal (genetic) abnormality.

clinicopathologic (-path'o-loj-ik)   relating to the clinical and pathologic manifestations of disease.

clinocephalism (kli"no-sef'ah-lizm)   congenital flatness or concavity of the vertex of the head.

clinodactyly (-dak'til-e)   permanent deviation or deflection of one or more fingers.

clinoid (kli'noid)   bed-shaped.

clinomania (kli"no-ma'ne-ah)   a morbid inclination to remain lying down or to stay in bed.

clinometer (kli-nom'ĕ-ter)   an instrument for measuring the paralysis of the ocular muscles as shown by torsion of the eyeballs.

cliseometer (klis"e-om'ĕ-ter)   instrument for measuring the angles between the axis of the body and that of the pelvis.

Clistin (klis'tin)   trademark for preparations of carbinoxamine maleate.

clithrophobia (klith"ro-fo'be-ah)   intense dread of being locked in.

clition (klit'e-on)   the midpoint of the anterior border of the clivus.

clitoridectomy (klit"o-rĭ-dek'to-me)   excision of the clitoris.

clitoriditis (-di'tis)   inflammation of the clitoris.

clitoridotomy (-dot'o-me)   incision of the clitoris.

clitoris (klit'o-ris)   a female organ homologous with the penis.

clitorism (klit'o-rizm)   hypertrophy of the clitoris.

clitoritis (klit"o-ri'tis)   inflammation of the clitoris.

clivus (kli'vus), pl. *cli'vi* [L.]   a sloping surface, especially the surface of the posterior cranial fossa sloping downward from the pituitary fossa.

clo (klo)   a unit of insulation, being the amount provided by man's normal, everyday clothing, representing that of ¼-inch thickness of wool.

cloaca (klo-a'kah), pl. *cloa'cae* [L.]   the common chamber in vertebrates below placental mammals into which fecal, urinary and reproductive elements pass before expulsion from the body; it is also a temporary feature in embryonic development of other species.

clock (klok)   a device for measuring time. **biological c.,** the physiologic mechanism which governs the rhythmic occurrence of certain biochemical, physiologic and behavioral phenomena in living organisms.

clone (klōn)   1. the asexual progeny of a single cell.   2. a strain of cells descended in culture from a single cell.

clonic (klon'ik)   pertaining to or characterized by clonus.

clonicity (klo-nis'ĭ-te)   the condition of being clonic.

clonicotonic (klon"ĭ-ko-ton'ik)   both clonic and tonic.

clonism (klon'izm) a succession of clonic spasms.

clonograph (klon'o-graf) an instrument for recording spasmodic movements.

clonorchiasis (klon"or-ki'ah-sis) infestation with Clonorchis.

Clonorchis (klo-nor'kis) a genus of Asiatic liver flukes.

clonospasm (klon'o-spazm) clonic spasm.

Clonothrix (klo'no-thriks) a genus of Schizomycetes (order Chlamydobacteriales, family Crenotrichaceae).

clonus (klo'nus) spasm in which rigidity and relaxation succeed each other. **ankle c., foot c.,** a series of convulsive movements of the ankle, induced by suddenly pushing up the foot while the leg is extended. **toe c.,** rhythmic contraction of the great toe, induced by sudden passive extension of its first phalanx. **wrist c.,** spasmodic contraction of the hand muscles, induced by forcibly bending the hand backward.

Clopane (klo'pān) trademark for preparations of cyclopentamine.

Clostridium (klo-strid'e-um) a genus of Schizomycetes (order Eubacteriales, family Bacillaceae). **C. bifermen'tans,** a species common in feces, sewage and soil and associated with gas gangrene. **C. botuli'num,** the agent causing botulism in man. **C. histolyt'icum,** a species found in feces and soil. **C. kluy'veri,** a species used in study of both microbial synthesis and microbial oxidation of fatty acids. **C. no'vyi,** a species which is an important cause of gas gangrene. **C. oedemat'iens,** *C. novyi.* **C. perfrin'gens,** the most common causative agent of gas gangrene. **C. sporog'enes,** a species widespread in nature, reportedly associated with pathogenic anaerobes in gangrenous infections. **C. ter'tium,** a species found in feces, sewage and soil and present in some gangrenous infections. **C. tet'ani,** a common inhabitant of soil and human and horse intestines, and the cause of tetanus in man and domestic animals. **C. welch'ii,** *C. perfringens.*

clostridium (klo-strid'i-um), pl. *clostrid'ia* [Gr.] an individual of the genus Clostridium.

clot (klot) a semisolidified mass of coagulum, as of blood or lymph. **agony c.,** one formed in the heart during the death agony. **antemortem c.,** one formed in the heart or in a large vessel before death. **blood c.,** one formed of blood, either in or out of the body. **chicken fat c.,** a yellow-colored blood clot looking like a mass of chicken fat. **currant jelly c.,** a reddish fibrin clot of a jelly-like consistency. **distal c.,** one formed in a vessel on the distal side of a ligature. **external c.,** one formed outside a blood vessel. **heart c.,** one formed within the heart. **internal c.,** one formed by solidification of blood within a vessel. **laminated c.,** one formed in layers filling the interior of an aneurysm. **marantic c.,** a blood clot due to enfeebled circulation and general malnutrition. **muscle c.,** one formed in the coagulation of muscle plasm. **passive c.,** one formed in the sac of an aneurysm as a result of cessation of the circulation through the aneurysm. **plastic c.,** one formed from the intima of an artery at the point of ligation, forming a permanent obstruction of the artery. **postmortem c.,** one formed in the heart or in a large blood vessel after death. **proximal c.,** one formed in a vessel on the proximal side of a ligature. **stratified c.,** a thrombus made up of layers of different colors.

clubbing (klub'ing) proliferation of soft tissue about the terminal phalanges of fingers or toes, without osseous change.

clubfoot (klub'foot) a congenital deformity of the foot.

clubhand (klub'hand) deformity of the hand, resembling that of the foot in clubfoot.

cluneal (kloo'ne-al) pertaining to the buttocks.

clunis (kloo'nis), pl. *clu'nes* [L.] buttock.

clysis (kli'sis) infusion of fluid into tissue or a body cavity, as an enema.

clyster (klis'ter) an enema.

C.M. [L.] *Chirur'giae ma'gister* (Master in Surgery).

Cm chemical symbol, *curium.*

cm. centimeter.

C.M.A. Canadian Medical Association.

C.M.B. Central Midwives Board.

c./min. cycles per minute.

c. mm. cubic millimeter.

CN symbol, *cyanogen.*

C.N.A. Canadian Nurses' Association.

cnemial (ne'me-al) pertaining to the tibia, or skin.

C.N.S. central nervous system; Congress of Neurological Surgeons.

Co chemical symbol, *cobalt.*

C.O.A. Canadian Orthopaedic Association.

CoA coenzyme A.

coacervate (ko-as'er-vāt) a collection of less fully hydrated particles of a colloid system, with less solvent bound to them than they had before.

coacervation (ko-as"er-va'shun) the formation of coacervates in a colloid system.

coadaptation (ko"ad-ap-ta'shun) the mutual, correlated, adaptive changes in two interdependent organs.

coagglutination (ko"ah-gloo"tī-na'-shun) agglutination by an antigen and the homologous antibody of the corpuscles of another animal.

coagglutinin (ko"ah-gloo'tī-nin) partial agglutinin.

coagulant (ko-ag'u-lant) 1. causing coagulation. 2. an agent which causes coagulation.

coagulase (ko-ag'u-lās) an enzyme that accelerates the formation of blood clots, but is not involved in coagulation of blood in vivo.

coagulate (ko-ag'u-lāt) to form into a coagulum, or clot.

coagulation (ko-ag"u-la'shun) formation of a clot. **blood c.,** the process by which a clot is formed in whole blood or plasma, considered divisible into three stages: (1) formation of intrinsic and extrinsic thromboplastin; (2) formation of thrombin; (3) formation of fibrin. **electric c.,** destruction of tissue by application of a bipolar current delivered by a needle point.

coagulative (ko-ag′u-la″tiv) associated with coagulation.

coagulin (ko-ag′u-lin) 1. thromboplastin. 2. an antibody (precipitin) that coagulates its antigen.

coagulinoid (ko-ag′u-lin-oid″) a coagulin whose activity has been destroyed by heat.

coagulometer (ko-ag″u-lom″ĕ-ter) an apparatus for determining coagulation time of the blood.

coagulum (ko-ag′u-lum), pl. *coag′ula* [L.] a clot. **closing c.**, a fibrinous and cellular mass closing the original point of entry of the implanting blastocyst into the endometrium.

coalescence (ko″ah-les′ens) a fusion or growing together.

coapt (ko′apt) to fit or bring together.

coaptation (ko″ap-ta′shun) a fitting together or adjustment of parts.

coarctate (ko-ark′tāt) to press close together, constrict.

coarctation (ko″ark-ta′shun) stricture or narrowing.

coarctotomy (-tot′o-me) the cutting of a stricture.

coat (kōt) a layer of substance covering or enveloping another. **buffy c.**, the thin yellowish layer of leukocytes overlying the packed erythrocytes in centrifuged blood.

cobalamin (ko-bal′ah-min) a cobalt-containing complex common to all members of the vitamin B₁₂ group.

cobalt (ko′bawlt) chemical element *(see table)*, at. no. 27, symbol Co.

coca (ko′kah) the plant *Erythroxylon coca*, and its leaves.

cocaine (ko-kān′, ko′kān) an alkaloid, C₁₇H₂₁NO₄, obtained from leaves of various species of Erythroxylon or produced synthetically; used as a local anesthetic. **c. hydrochloride**, the hydrochloride of cocaine, C₁₇H₂₁NO₄.HCl.

cocainism (ko′kān-izm) poisoning due to cocaine.

cocainize (ko-kān′īz) to treat with cocaine.

cocarboxylase (ko″kar-bok′sĭ-lās) a coenzyme of carboxylase acting with the latter in splitting pyruvic acid.

cocarcinogenesis (ko-kar″sĭ-no-jen′ĕ-sis) the development of cancer only in preconditioned cells as a result of conditions favorable to its growth.

cocci (kok′si) plural of *coccus*.

Coccidia (kok-sid′e-ah) a group of sporozoa commonly parasitic in epithelial cells of the intestinal tract, including two genera, *Eimeria* and *Isospora*, sometimes found in domestic animals and man.

coccidial (kok-sid′e-al) pertaining to or caused by Coccidium.

Coccidioides (kok-sid″e-oi′dēz) a genus of pathogenic fungi. **C. immit′is**, a species causing skin and lung lesions.

coccidioidin (kok-sid″e-oi′din) a sterile preparation from cultures of the organism used in a test for infection by *Coccidioides immitis*.

coccidioidomycosis (-oi″do-mi-ko′sis) infection with Coccidioides.

coccidioidosis (kok-sid″e-oi-do′sis) coccidioidomycosis.

coccidiosis (-o′sis) infection by organisms of the group Coccidia.

Coccidium (kok-sid′e-um) a class of protozoans.

coccinella (kok″sĭ-nel′ah) [L.] cochineal.

coccobacillus (kok″o-bah-sil′us) an oval bacterial cell intermediate between the coccus and bacillus forms. adj., **coccobac′illary**.

coccobacteria (-bak-te′re-ah) spheroidal or rodlike bacteria.

coccogenous (kok-oj′ĕ-nus) produced by cocci.

coccoid (kok′oid) resembling a coccus.

cocculin (kok′u-lin) picrotoxin

coccus (kok′us), pl. *coc′ci* [L.] a bacterium which is spherical in form. adj., **coc′cal**.

coccyalgia (kok″se-al′je-ah) coccygodynia.

coccycephalus (-sef′ah-lus) a fetal monster whose head is beak-shaped.

coccydynia (kok″sĭ-din′e-ah) coccygodynia.

coccygectomy (-jek′to-me) excision of the coccyx.

coccygodynia (kok″sĭ-go-din′e-ah) pain in the coccyx.

coccygotomy (kok″sĭ-got′o-me) coccygectomy.

coccyx (kok′siks) os coccygis. adj., **coccyg′eal**.

cochineal (koch′ĭ-nēl) dried female insects of *Coccus cacti*, enclosing young larvae; used as a coloring agent or dye.

cochlea (kok′le-ah) spiral cavity of the internal ear. adj., **coch′lear**.

Cochlearia (kok″le a′re ah) genus of plants including horseradish and scurvy grass.

cochleariform (-ar′ĭ-form) spoon-shaped.

cochleitis (-i′tis) inflammation of the cochlea.

cochleovestibular (kok″le-o-ves-tib′u-ler) pertaining to cochlea and vestibule of the ear.

Cochliomyia (-mi′yah) a genus of flies whose larvae burrow into the skin. **C. hominivor′ax**, the American screwworm fly, which deposits its eggs in the wounds of animals.

cocillana (ko″sil-yah′nah) bark of *Guarea rusbyi*, a tree of South America; emetic and expectorant.

cocoa (ko′ko) powder prepared from roasted, cured kernels of ripe seeds of *Theobroma cacao*, used as a flavoring agent.

coconscious (ko-kon′shus) not in the field of the conscious, yet capable of being remembered.

coconsciousness (ko-kon′shus-nes) consciousness secondary to the main stream of consciousness.

cocontraction (ko″kon-trak′shun) coordination of antagonist muscles.

coetolabile (kok″to-la′bil) capable of being altered by heating.

coetoprecipitin (-pre-sip′ĭ-tin) a precipitin produced by injecting a heated serum or other antigen.

coetostabile (-sta′bil) incapable of being altered by heating.

code (kōd) 1. a set of rules for regulating conduct. 2. a system by which information can be communicated. **genetic c.**, the system by which information is transferred from genetic material to proteins, the pattern of nucleotides in the nucleic acids being thought to determine each amino acid in the chain making up each protein.

codeine (ko'dēn) an alkaloid, $C_{18}H_{21}NO_3.H_2O$, obtained from opium or prepared from morphine by methylation; analgesic and antitussive. **c. phosphate,** $C_{18}H_{21}NO_3.H_3PO_4.$- $\frac{1}{2}H_2O$. **c. sulfate,** $(C_{18}H_{21}NO_3)_2.H_2SO_4.3H_2O$.

codon (ko'don) the specific pattern of nucleotides (perhaps three) in the genetic material which corresponds to a particular amino acid in the genetic code.

coe- for words beginning thus, see also those beginning *ce-*.

coefficient (ko″ĕ-fish'ent) ·a number by which one value is to be multiplied in order to give another value, or a number which indicates the range of an effect produced under certain conditions. **c. of absorption,** the volume of a gas absorbed by a unit volume of a liquid at 0°C. and a pressure of 760 mm. Hg. **Baumann's c.,** ratio of the ethereal to the total sulfates in the urine. **biological c.,** the amount of potential energy consumed by the body at rest. **Bouchard's c.,** the ratio between the amount of urine and the total solids of the urine. **c. of conductivity,** the quantity of heat that passes in a unit of time through a unit thickness of a substance when the difference in temperature is 1 degree C. **c. of expansion,** a number indicating the amount a substance expands when heated 1 degree C. **Falta's c.,** the percentage of ingested sugar eliminated from the system. **isotonic c.,** the quantity of salt which should be added to distilled water to prevent destruction of the erythrocytes when it is added to blood. **lethal c.,** that concentration of a disinfectant that will kill bacteria at a temperature of 20–25°C. in the shortest time. **c. of partage,** the ratio between the amount of an acid absorbed by ether from an aqueous solution of the acid and the amount of the acid that remains behind in the solution. **urotoxic c.,** the quantity of toxic matter produced in the urine in 24 hours by 1 kg. of the poison. **Yvon's c.,** the ratio between the quantity of urea and the phosphates of the urine.

-coele (sēl) word element [Gr.], *cavity; space.*

Coelenterata (se-len″ter-a'tah) a phylum of invertebrates which includes the hydras, jellyfish, sea anemones and corals.

coelenterate (se-len'ter-āt) 1. pertaining or belonging to the Coelenterata. 2. an individual member of the phylum Coelenterata.

coeloblastula (se″lo-blas'tu-lah) the common type of blastula, consisting of a hollow sphere composed of blastomeres.

coelom (se'lom) the body cavity, especially the cavity of a simple animal organism or that between the somatic mesoderm and the splanchnic mesoderm in the developing embryo. adj., **coelom'ic.**

coelosomy (se″lo-so'me) a developmental anomaly characterized by protrusion of the viscera from and their presence outside the body cavity.

coenurosis (se″nu-ro'sis) infection of sheep with the larva of *Coenurus cerebralis.*

coenzyme (ko-en'zīm) an organic molecule, usually containing phosphorus and some vitamins, sometimes separable from certain enzymes, which is required for the activation of an apoenzyme. **c. A,** a substance essential for the metabolism of carbohydrates and fats and for the formation of acetylcholine. **c. I,** diphosphopyridine nucleotide. **c. II,** triphosphopyridine nucleotide.

coeur (ker) [Fr.] heart. **c. en sabot** (on sä-bo') a heart whose shape on a radiograph resembles that of a wooden shoe; noted in tetralogy of Fallot.

cofactor (ko-fak-tor) an element or principle whose presence is necessary for the functioning of another.

coferment (ko-fer'ment) coenzyme.

coffee (kof'e) the dried seeds of *Coffea arabica,* or the decoction prepared from them.

coffeeism (kof'e-in-izm″) caffeinism.

Cogentin (ko-jen'tin) trademark for preparations of benztropine.

cognition (kog-nish'un) the processes involved in knowing.

cohesion (ko-he'zhun) the clinging together of separate particles in a single mass.

coil (koil) a winding structure or spiral; called also *helix.* **induction c.,** coil for producing electricity by induction. **Leiter's c.,** a coiled metallic tube used in warming or cooling a part. **resistance c.,** coil of wire placed in electric circuit to increase resistance. **Ruhmkorff c.,** a powerful induction coil.

coilonychia (koi″lo-nik'e-ah) koilonychia.

coition (ko-ish'un) coitus.

coitophobia (ko″i-to-fo'be-ah) morbid fear of coitus.

coitus (ko'i-tus) sexual congress per vaginam between male and female; usually applied to the mating process in human beings. **c. incomple'tus, c. interrup'tus,** coitus in which the penis is withdrawn from the vagina before ejaculation. **c. reserva'tus,** coitus in which ejaculation of semen is intentionally suppressed.

colalgia (ko-lal'je-ah) pain in the colon.

colation (ko-la'shun) the process of straining.

colchicine (kol'chĭ-sēn) a poisonous alkaloid, $C_{22}H_{25}O N_6$, from *Colchicum autumnale;* used in treatment of gout.

cold (kōld) 1. absence of heat. 2. a condition attributed to exposure to low temperature, characterized by lacrimation, coryza and other symptoms referable to the upper respiratory tract. **common c.,** a condition of suspected viral causation, with inflammation of the nasopharynx and variable degrees of malaise. **rose c.,** coryza and lacrimation due to hypersensitivity to pollen of roses.

coldsore (kold'sor) a lesion caused by the virus of herpes simplex, usually on the lips, chin or cheeks.

colectomy (ko-lek'to-me) excision of the colon.

coleocystitis (ko″le-o-sis-ti'tis) inflammation of the vagina and bladder.

Coleomitus (ko″le-o-mi'tus) a genus of Schizomycetes (order Caryophanales, family Arthromitaceae).

coleotomy (ko″le-ot′o-me) incision into the vagina.

Colesiota (ko-le″se-o′tah) a genus of Microtatobiotes (order Rickettsiales, family Chlamydiaceae). **C. conjuncti′vae,** a species causing infectious ophthalmia in sheep.

Colettsia (ko-let′se-ah) a genus of Microtatobiotes (order Rickettsiales, family Chlamydiaceae). **C. pe′coris,** a parasitic microorganism found in the conjunctiva of domestic animals.

colibacillemia (ko″li-bas″ĭ-le′me-ah) the presence of Escherichia coli in the blood.

colibacillosis (-lo′sis) infection with Escherichia coli. **c. gravida′rum,** severe pyelitis during pregnancy caused by Escherichia coli.

colibacilluria (-lu′re-ah) the presence of Escherichia coli in the urine.

colibacillus (ko″lĕ-bah-sil′us) Escherichia coli.

colic (kol′ik) acute paroxysmal abdominal pain. **appendicular c.,** pain in the vermiform appendix. **biliary c.,** that caused by spasm or obstruction of the biliary tract. **Devonshire c.,** lead colic. **gallstone c.,** that caused by calculi in the biliary tract. **hepatic c.,** biliary colic. **lead c.,** colic from lead poisoning. **menstrual c.,** the pain of menstruation. **mucous c.,** mucous colitis. **ovarian c.,** pain in the ovaries. **painter's c.,** lead colic. **renal c.,** colic caused by renal calculus. **salivary c.,** pain in the salivary duct and gland with swelling. **sand c.,** indigestion in horses and cattle from the presence of sand taken in with food or drink. **uterine c.,** colicky paroxysmal pains at the menstrual period.

colica (kol′ĭ-kah) [L.] colic.

colicin (kol′ĭ-sin) an antibiotic produced by Escherichia coli and affecting other strains of the same species.

colicolitis (ko″lĭ-ko-li′tis) colitis caused by Escherichia coli.

colicoplegia (-ple′je-ah) combined lead colic and lead paralysis.

colicystitis (ko″lĭ-sis-ti′tis) cystitis due to Escherichia coli.

colicystopyelitis (-sis″to-pi″ĕ-li′tis) inflammation of the bladder and renal pelvis due to Escherichia coli.

coliform (kol′ĭ-form) resembling Escherichia coli.

colilysin (ko-lil′ĭ-sin) a lysin formed by Escherichia coli.

colinephritis (ko″lĭ-ne-fri′tis) nephritis due to Escherichia coli.

coliplication (-pli-ka′shun) coloplication.

colipuncture (-punk″tūr) colocentesis.

colipyelitis (-pi″ĕ-li′tis) pyelitis caused by Escherichia coli.

colipyuria (-pi-u′re-ah) pus in the urine due to infection with Escherichia coli.

colisepsis (-sep′sis) infection with Escherichia coli.

colistimethate (ko-lis″tĭ-meth′āt) a colistin derivative used in the treatment of urinary tract infections.

colistin (ko-lis′tin) an antibiotic substance

produced by a microorganism in the soil, related chemically to polymyxin. **c. sulfate,** a water-soluble salt of colistin, effective against several gram-negative bacilli, but not against Proteus.

colitides (ko-lit′ĭ-dēz) inflammatory disorders of the colon considered collectively.

colitis (ko-li′tis) pl. colit′ides, inflammation of the colon. **amebic c.,** colitis caused by ameba. **mucous c.,** a disease of the mucous membrane of the colon, with colic, diarrhea and passage of membranous threads in stools.

colitoxemia (ko″li-tok-se′me-ah) toxemia due to Escherichia coli.

colitoxicosis (-tok″si-ko′sis) intoxication caused by Escherichia coli.

colitoxin (-tok′sin) a toxin from Escherichia coli.

coliuria (ko″le-u′re-ah) presence of Escherichia coli in the urine.

collagen (kol′ah-jen) a scleroprotein present in connective tissue of the body. adj. **collag′enous.**

collagenase (kol-laj′ĕ-nās) an enzyme that catalyzes the digestion of collagen.

collagenation (kol-laj″ĕ-na′shun) the appearance of collagen in developing cartilage.

collagenic (kol″ah-jen′ik) 1. producing collagen. 2. pertaining to collagen.

collagenoblast (kol-laj′ĕ-no-blast″) an immature collagen-producing cell.

collagenocyte (kol-laj′ĕ-no-sīt″) a mature collagen-producing cell.

collagenogenic (kol-laj″ĕ-no-jen′ik) producing collagen.

collagenolysis (-li′sis) dissolution or digestion of collagen. adj. **collagenolyt′ic.**

collagenosis (kol″ah-jĕ-no′sis) a disease characterized by areas of collagenous degeneration.

collapse (kŏ-laps′) 1. to break down or flatten. 2. a state of extreme prostration.

collapsotherapy (kŏ-lap″so-ther′ah-pe) collapse therapy.

collemia (kŏ-le′me-ah) a glutinous condition of the blood.

colliculectomy (kŏ-lik″u-lek′to-me) excision of the verumontanum.

colliculitis (-li′tis) inflammation about the verumontanum.

colliculus (kŏ-lik′u-lus), pl. collic′uli [L.] a small elevation. **c. semina′lis,** an elevation in the wall of the prostatic part of the male urethra, the urethral crest; the orifices of the prostatic utricle and ejaculatory ducts are situated on it.

collimation (kol″ĭ-ma′shun) in microscopy, the process of making light rays parallel; the adjustment of two or more optical axes with respect to each other.

colliquation (-kwa′shun) liquefactive degeneration of tissue.

colliquative (kŏ-lik′wah-tiv) characterized by excessive liquid discharge, or by liquefaction of tissue.

collodiaphyseal (kol″o-di″ah-fiz′e-al) pertaining to the neck and shaft of a long bone, especially the femur.

collodion (kŏ-lo'de-on) pyroxylin dissolved in ether and alcohol. **flexible c.,** a mixture of collodion, camphor and castor oil, applied locally as a protectant. **salicylic acid c.,** flexible collodion containing salicylic acid, used topically as a heterolytic.

colloid (kol'oid) 1. resembling glue. 2. a state of matter composed of single large molecules or aggregations of smaller molecules (disperse particles, 1 to 100 mμ in diameter) of solid, liquid or gas, in a continuous medium (disperse medium), which also may be solid, liquid or gas.

colloidin (kŏ-loi'din) a jelly-like principle produced in colloid degeneration.

colloidoclasia (kŏ loi''do-kla'ze-ah) breaking up of the physical equilibrium of the colloid of the body, producing anaphylactic crises (colloidoclastic shock).

colloidopexy (kŏ-loi'do-pek''se) 1. metabolic fixation of colloids in the organism. 2. phagocytosis of small colloid particles.

colloma (kŏ-lo'mah) colloid cancer.

collonema (kol''o-ne'mah) myxoma.

collopexia (-pek'se-ah) fixation of the neck of the uterus.

collum (kol'um) pl. col'la [L.] the neck, or a neckline part. **c. distor'tum,** torticollis. **c. val'gum,** coxa valga.

collutory (kol'u-to''re) mouthwash or gargle.

collyrium (kŏ-lir'e-um) pl. collyr'ia [L.] eyewash.

colo- (ko'lo) word element [Gr.], colon.

coloboma (kol''o-bo'mah) a developmental anomaly resulting from failure of closure of the embryonic ocular cleft, affecting choroid, ciliary body, eyelid (palpebral coloboma, coloboma palpebra'le), iris (coloboma i'ridis), lens (coloboma len'tis), optic nerve or retina. **bridge c.,** coloboma of the iris in which a strip of iris tissue bridges over the fissure. **c. of choroid,** fissure in the choroid coat due to persistence of a fetal fissure. **Fuchs's c.,** a small, crescent-shaped defect of the choroid at the lower edge of the optic disk. **c. lob'uli,** a congenital fissure of the ear lobe.

colocecostomy (ko''lo-se-kos'to-me) cecocolostomy.

colocentesis (-sen-te'sis) surgical puncture of the colon.

colocholecystostomy (-ko''le-sis-tos'to-me) cholecystocolotomy.

coloclysis (ko-lok'li-sis) irrigation of the colon.

coloclyster (ko''lo-klis'ter) an enema introduced into the colon.

colocolic (-ko'lik) pertaining to two separate portions of the colon.

colocolostomy (-ko-los'to-me) anastomosis between two previously remote portions of the colon.

colocutaneous (-ku-ta'ne-us) pertaining to the colon and skin, or communicating with the colon and the cutaneous surface of the body.

colocynth (kol'o-sinth) dried pulp of unripe but full-grown fruit of Citrullus colocynthis; hydragogue cathartic.

colocynthin (kol''o-sin'thin) strongly purgative principle from colocynth.

coloenteritis (ko''lo-en''ter-i'tis) enterocolitis.

colofixation (-fik-sa'shun) fixation of the colon in cases of ptosis.

Cologel (kol'o-jel) trademark for a preparation of methylcellulose.

coloileal (ko''lo-il'e-al) pertaining to or communicating with the colon and ileum.

colon (ko'lon) the part of the large intestine extending from the cecum to the rectum. adj., **colon'ic. ascending c.,** the portion of the right colon which passes cephalad from the cecum to the right colic flexure. **descending c.,** the portion of the left colon which passes caudad from the left colic flexure to the sigmoid colon. **left c.,** the distal portion of the large intestine, developed embryonically from the hindgut and functioning in the storage and elimination from the body of nonabsorbable residue of ingested material. **right c.,** the proximal portion of the large intestine, developed embryonically from the terminal portion of the midgut and functioning in absorption of ingested material. **sigmoid c.,** that portion of the left colon situated in the pelvis and extending from the descending colon to the rectum. **transverse c.,** that portion of the large intestine passing transversely across the upper part of the abdomen, between the right and left colic flexures.

colonalgia (ko''lon-al'je-ah) pain in the colon.

colonitis (ko''lon-i'tis) inflammation of the colon.

colonometer (kŏl''o-nom'ē-ter) an instrument for counting colonies of bacteria.

colonopathy (ko''lon-op'ah-the) disease of the colon.

colonopexy (ko'lon-o-pek''se) sigmoidopexy.

colonorrhagia (ko''lon-o-ra'je-ah) hemorrhage from the colon.

colonorrhea (-re'ah) a mucous discharge from the colon.

colonoscopy (ko''lon-os'ko-pe) endoscopic examination of the colon, frequently done with the instrument passed through the abdominal wall (transabdominal colonoscopy).

colony (kol'o-ne) a discrete group of organisms, as a collection of bacteria in a culture.

colopexy (ko'lo-pek''se) sigmoidopexy.

colophony (ko-lof'o-ne) rosin.

coloplication (ko''lo-pli-ka'shun) operation of taking a reef in the colon.

coloproctectomy (-prok-tek'to-me) surgical removal of the colon and rectum.

coloproctitis (-prok-ti'tis) inflammation of colon and rectum.

coloproctostomy (-prok-tos'to-me) anastomosis of the colon to the rectum.

coloptosis (ko''lop-to'sis) downward displacement of the colon.

colopuncture (ko''lo-punk''tur) colocentesis.

color (kul'er) 1. a property of a surface or substance due to absorption of certain light rays and reflection of others within the range of wavelengths (roughly 370–760 mμ) adequate to excite the retinal receptors. 2. radiant energy within the range of adequate chromatic stimuli of the retina, i.e. between the infra-red and ultraviolet. 3. a sensory impression of one of the rainbow hues. **complementary c's**, a pair of colors the sensory mechanisms for which are so linked that when they are mixed on the color wheel they cancel each other out, leaving neutral gray. **confusion c's**, different colors which are liable to be mistakenly matched by persons with defective color vision, and hence are used for detecting different types of color vision defects. **primary c's**, (a) according to the Newton theory, the seven rainbow hues: violet, indigo, blue, green, yellow, orange, red; (b) in painting and printing, blue, yellow, red; (c) according to the Helmholz theory, red, green, blue. **pure c.**, one whose stimulus consists of homogeneous wavelengths, with little or no admixture of wavelengths of other hues.

coloration (kul″er-a′shun) the state of being colored. **protective c.**, coloration of the body blending with the environmental background, to make the organism less visible to predators. **warning c.**, brilliant, conspicuous coloration of poisonous or unpalatable animals, as a warning to potential predators.

colorectitis (ko″lo-rek-ti′tis) inflammation of colon and rectum.

colorectostomy (-rek-tos′to-me) coloproctostomy.

colorectum (-rek′tum) the distal 10 inches (25 cm.) of the bowel, including the distal portion of the colon and the rectum, regarded as a specific organ. adj., **colorec′tal.**

colorimeter (kul″er-im′ē-ter) an instrument for measuring pigments.

colorrhaphy (ko-lor′ah-fe) suture of the colon.

colosigmoidostomy (ko″lo-sig″moid-os′to-me) anastomosis of a formerly remote portion of the colon to the sigmoid.

colostomy (ko-los′to-me) formation of an artificial opening into the colon. **dry c.**, that performed in the left colon, the discharge from the stoma consisting of soft or formed fecal matter. **ileotransverse c.**, anastomosis of the ileum to the transverse colon, with exclusion of the cecum and ascending colon from the intestinal tract. **wet c.**, 1. colostomy of the right colon, the discharge from the stoma being liquid. 2. colostomy combined with ureterocolostomy, so that urine also is discharged through the stoma.

colostrorrhea (ko-los″tro re′ah) unusually free secretion of colostrum.

colostrum (ko-los′trum) the first milk secreted by the female mammal before or after birth of the young.

colotomy (ko-lot′o-me) incision of the colon. **Littre's c.**, incision into the colon in the inguinal region.

colotyphoid (ko″lo-ti′foid) typhoid with follicular ulceration of the colon.

colovaginal (-vaj′ĭ-nal) pertaining to or communicating with the colon and vagina.

colovesical (-ves′ĭ-kal) pertaining to or communicating with the colon and urinary bladder.

colp(o)- (kol′po) word element [Gr.], *vagina.*

colpalgia (kol-pal′je-ah) pain in the vagina.

colpatresia (kol″pah-tre′ze-ah) atresia of the vagina.

colpectasia (kol″pek-ta′ze-ah) dilatation of the vagina.

colpectomy (kol-pek′to-me) excision of the vagina.

colpeurysis (kol-pu′rī-sis) operative dilatation of the vagina.

colpitis (kol-pi′tis) inflammation of the vaginal mucosa.

colpocele (kol′po-sēl) vaginal hernia.

colpocleisis (kol″po-kli′sis) surgical closure of the vagina.

colpocystitis (-sis-ti′tis) inflammation of vagina and bladder.

colpocystocele (-sis′to-sēl) protrusion of a fold of the vagina into the bladder.

colpocytogram (-si′to-gram) differential listing of cells observed in smears from the vaginal mucosa.

colpocytology (-si-tol′o-je) the quantitative and differential study of cells exfoliated from the epithelium of the vagina.

colpodynia (-din′e-ah) pain in the vagina.

colpohyperplasia (-hi″per-pla′ze-ah) excessive growth of the mucous membrane of the vagina.

colpomicroscope (-mi′kro-skōp) an instrument for examining stained tissues of the cervix in situ.

colpomicroscopy (-mi-kros′ko-pe) microscopic examination of the stained tissues of the cervix in situ.

colpoperineoplasty (-per″ĭ-ne′o-plas″te) plastic repair of vagina and perineum.

colpoperineorrhaphy (-per″ĭ-ne-or′ah-fe) suture of vagina and perineum.

colpopexy (kol′po-pek″se) fixation of the vagina.

colpoplasty (-plas″te) plastic repair of the vagina.

colpopoiesis (kol″po-poi-e′sis) formation of a vagina by plastic operation.

colpoptosis (kol″pop-to′sis) prolapse of the vagina.

colporrhagia (kol″po-ra′je-ah) hemorrhage from the vagina.

colporrhaphy (kol-por′ah-fe) suture of the vagina.

colporrhexis (kol″po-rek′sis) laceration of the vagina.

colposcope (kol′po-skop) a speculum for examining the vagina.

colposcopy (kol-pos′ko-pe) examination of the vagina.

colpospasm (kol′po-spazm) vaginal spasm.

colpostenosis (kol″po-ste-no′sis) narrowing of the vagina.

colpostenotomy (-ste-not′o-me) a cutting operation for stricture of the vagina.

colpotomy (kol-pot′o-me) incision of the vagina.

colpoxerosis (kol″po-ze-ro′sis) abnormal dryness of vulva and vagina.

colt-ill (kōlt′il) infectious catarrhal fever of young horses.

columbium (ko-lum′be-um) niobium.

columella (kol″u-mel'ah), pl. *columel'lae* [L.] a little column. **c. coch'leae, c. modi'olus,** modiolus. **c. na'si,** the fleshy external termination of the septum of the nose.

column (kol'um) a supporting part. **anterior c.,** layer of white matter in either half of spinal cord between the anterior horn and the anterior median fissure. **Bertini c's,** cortical substance between the pyramids of the kidney. **Burdach's c.,** posteroexternal column. **Clarke's c.,** nucleus dorsalis. **direct cerebellar c.,** a tract outside the lateral pyramidal tract. **enamel c.,** one of the long prismatic bodies which make up the substance of the enamel. **fat c's,** columns of adipose tissue extending from subcutaneous tissue to hair follicles and sweat glands. **c. of Goll,** fasciculus gracilis. **c. of Gowers,** a mass of fibers in front of the direct cerebellar column. **lateral c.,** layer of white matter in either half of the spinal cord between the posterior horn and nerve roots and the anterior horn and nerve roots. **c. of Lissauer,** a column of white matter between the posterior cornu and the periphery of the spinal cord. **c. of Morgagni,** folds of mucous membrane seen at the junction of the rectum with the anus. **posterior c.,** a mass of white matter in the spinal cord on either side between the posterior horns and the posterior median fissure. **posteroexternal c.,** the outer wider portion of the posterior column of the cord. **renal c's,** extensions of the cortical substance of the kidney between contiguous renal pyramids. **respiratory c.,** solitary fasciculus. **c. of Sertoli,** an elongated cell in the seminiferous tubule supporting spermatogenic cells. **spinal c.,** vertebral column. **c. of Spitzka-Lissauer,** a group of nerve fibers of cord in front of and behind the posterior horns. **c. of Türck,** the anterior or direct pyramidal tract of the spinal cord. **vertebral c.,** the rigid structure in the midline of the back, composed of the vertebrae.

columna (ko-lum'nah), pl. *colum'nae* [L.] a pillar or column.

columning (kol'um-ing) support of the prolapsed uterus by means of tampons.

Coly-mycin (kol'e-mi″sin) trademark for preparations of colistimethate.

colyone (ko'le-ōn) a substance formed in one organ which, when carried by the blood to another organ, decreases functional activity in the latter. adj., **colyon'ic.**

colypeptic (ko″le-pep'tik) hindering or delaying digestion.

colyphrenia (-fre'ne-ah) abnormal slowness of mental processes.

colyseptic (-sep'tik) antiseptic.

coma (ko'mah) 1. a state of profound unconsciousness from which the patient cannot be aroused, even by powerful stimuli. 2. a comet-shaped image caused by light passing obliquely through a lens. **alcoholic c.,** coma from alcoholism. **apoplectic c.,** that due to apoplexy. **diabetic c.,** the coma produced by severe diabetic acidosis. **Kussmaul's c.,** coma with acetone in urine from diabetes. **trance c.,** lethargy produced by hypnosis. **uremic c.,** that due to uremia. **c. vigil,** stupor with delirium, wakefulness and semiconsciousness.

comatose (ko'mah-tōs) affected with coma.

comedo (kom'ē-do), pl. *comedo'nes,* an abnormal mass of keratin and sebum within the dilated orifice of a hair follicle.

comes (ko'mēz), pl. *com'ites* [L.] an accompanying structure, as an artery which accompanies a nerve trunk.

comfortization (kum″for-tĭ-za'shun) the scientific application of physiologic principles to promote comfort in potentially stressful situations.

commensal (kŏ-men'sal) the organism or species that benefits by a symbiotic relationship with another organism or species without harming it.

commensalism (kŏ-men'sal-izm) the biological association of two individuals or populations of different species, one of which is benefited and the other unaffected by the relationship.

comminution (kom″ĭ-nu'shun) a breaking into small fragments.

commissura (kom″ĭ-su'rah), pl. *commissu'rae* [L.] commissure. **c. bre'vis,** the posterior part of the inferior vermiform process of the cerebellum. **c. cerebel'li,** pons. **c. mag'na,** corpus callosum.

commissure (kom'ĭ-shūr) a connecting band of tissue, e.g. at the junction of the upper and the lower lips, or connecting the cusps of the cardiac valves. **anterior c.,** a cord of white fibers in front of crura of fornix. **arcuate c.,** the posterior optic commissure. **Gudden's c.,** arcuate commissure. **Meynert's c.,** commissure of nerve fibers extending from floor of third ventricle through optic tracts to subthalamic body. **middle c.,** band of gray matter joining optic thalami. **optic c.,** the crossing of the two optic nerves. **posterior c.,** a white band joining the optic thalami posteriorly.

commissurorrhaphy (kom″ĭ-shūr-or'ah-fe) suture of connecting bands of a commissure, to lessen the size of the orifice.

commissurotomy (-ot'o-me) splitting or incision at the junction of the connecting bands of a commissure, to increase the size of the orifice, as in one of the valves of the heart.

communicans (kŏ-mu'nĭ-kans) [L.] communicating.

community (kŏ-mu'nĭ-te) a body of individuals living in a defined area or having a common interest or organization. **biotic c.,** an assemblage of populations living in a defined area.

commutator (kom'u-ta″ter) a device for reversing electric currents.

compathy (kom'pah-the) sharing of emotional feelings with another person.

Compazine (kom'pah-zēn) trademark for preparations of prochlorperazine.

compensation (kom″pen-sa'shun) a mental mechanism operating beyond conscious awareness by which an individual attempts to make up for real or fancied deficiencies. **dosage c.,** in genetics, the mechanism by which the effect of the two X chromosomes of the normal female is rendered identical to that of the one X chromosome of the normal male.

complaint (kom-plānt') any feature of his condition for which a patient seeks medical relief. **chief c., principal c.,** the feature of his condition on which the patient places most emphasis or which led him to seek medical advice.

complement (kom'plĕ-ment) a substance in normal blood serum which with specific amboceptor causes lysis of cells, destruction of bacteria and other phenomena.

complementation (kom″plĕ-men-ta'shun) a relation such that the members of a pair or set have no environment in common. **interallelic c.,** intragenic complementation. **intergenic c.,** the essentially full restoration of wild-type function in a cis-trans test when two mutations, in transposition, are located in different cistrons (genes). **intracistronic c., intragenic c.,** the partial restoration of function sometimes seen in the cis-trans test when the two mutations are located at different sites within the same cistron.

complementoid (kom″plĕ-men'toid) a complement whose activity has been destroyed by heating.

complementophil (-men'to-fil) having an affinity for a complement.

complex (kom'pleks) 1. a combination of various things, like or unlike. 2. a group of associated ideas having a strong emotional tone. 3. that portion of an electrocardiographic tracing which represents the systole of an atrium or ventricle. **anomalous c.,** an electrocardiographic complex which varies from the normal type. **auricular c.,** the portion of the electrocardiogram produced by auricular (atrial) activity. **Cain c.,** rivalry between siblings. **calcarine c.,** hippocampus minor. **castration c.,** an unconscious dread of castration. **Clerambault-Kandinsky c.,** a mental state in which the patient thinks his mind is controlled by some outside influence. **Diana c.,** a psychic complex in which a woman wishes she were a man. **Eisenmenger c.,** defects of the interventricular septum with dilatation of the pulmonary artery and dextrolocation of the aorta. **Electra c.,** a series of symptoms attributed to suppressed sexual desire of a daughter for her father, with hostility toward the mother. **father c.,** Electra complex. **Golgi c.,** see under *apparatus*. **inferiority c.,** an abnormal feeling of inferiority, producing timidity or, as a compensation, exaggerated aggressiveness. **Jocasta c.,** Oedipus complex. **Lutembacher's c.,** see under *disease*. **mother c., Oedipus c.,** a series of symptoms attributed to suppressed sexual desire of a son for his mother, with hostility toward the father. **sex c.,** the correlation between the internal secretions and the sex function. **symptom c.,** syndrome. **ventricular c.,** the portion of the electrocardiogram produced by ventricular activity.

compliance (kom-pli'ans) the quality of yielding to pressure or force without disruption, or an expression of the measure of ability to do so, as an expression of the distensibility of an air- or fluid-filled organ, e.g. lung or urinary bladder, in terms of unit of volume per unit of pressure.

complication (kom″pli-ka'shun) a disease concurrent with another disease.

compos mentis (kom″pos men'tis) [L.] of sound mind.

compound (kom'pownd) 1. made up of diverse elements or ingredients. 2. a substance made up of different elements. **acyclic c.,** an organic compound which contains no ring structure of the atoms. **aliphatic c.,** acyclic compound. **c. E,** cortisone. **c. F,** cortisol. **heterocyclic c.,** an organic compound which contains rings made up of more than one kind of atom. **inorganic c.,** a compound of chemical elements containing no carbon atoms. **organic c.,** a compound of chemical elements containing carbon atoms. **organometallic c.,** one in which carbon is linked to a metal. **quaternary ammonium c.,** tetraethylammonium. **saturated c.,** a chemical compound in which all the valences of the elements composing it are satisfied. **unsaturated c.,** a chemical compound in which not all the valences of the elements composing it are satisfied.

compress (kom'pres) a square of gauze or similar dressing, for application of pressure or medication to a restricted area. **cribriform c.,** one perforated with holes. **fenestrated c.,** one with an opening for discharge of secretions. **graduated c.,** one consisting of layers of gradually decreasing size. **Priessnitz c.,** a cold wet compress.

compression (kom-presh'un) act of pressing upon or together; the state of being pressed together.

compressor (kom-pres'er) that which causes compression.

compulsion (kom-pul'shun) an overwhelming urge to perform an irrational act or ritual. **repetition c.,** the unconscious need to repeat earlier experiences, relationships or patterns of reaction. adj., **compul'sive.**

conarium (ko-na're-um) the pineal gland.

conation (ko-na'shun) the conscious tendency to act.

conative (kon'ah-tiv) pertaining to the basic strivings of a person, as expressed in his behavior and actions.

concave (kon'kāv) rounded and somewhat depressed or hollowed out.

concavity (kon-kav'ĭ-te) a depression or hollowed surface.

concavoconcave (kon-ka″vo-kon'kāv) concave on two surfaces.

concavoconvex (-kon'veks) having one concave and one convex surface.

concentration (kon″sen-tra'shun) 1. increase in strength by evaporation. 2. medicine which has been strengthened by evaporation of its nonactive parts. 3. the relative content of a contained or dissolved substance in a solution. **hydrogen ion c.,** an expression of the degree of acidity or alkalinity (pH) of a solution.

conception (kon-sep'shun) 1. the union of male and female gametes, marking the beginning of a new organism. 2. an impression or idea.

conceptus (-sep'tus) the developing product of conception (embryo: fetus with enveloping membranes) within the uterus.

concha (kong'kah), pl. *con'chae* [L.] a shell-shaped structure. **c. of auricle,** the hollow of the auricle of the extended ear, bounded anteriorly by the tragus and posteriorly by the anthelix. **c. bullo'sa,** a cystic distention of the middle nasal concha. **ethmoidal c., inferior,** nasal concha, middle. **ethmoidal c., superior,** nasal concha, superior. **ethmoidal c., supreme,** nasal concha, supreme. **nasal c., inferior,** a bone forming the lower part of the lateral wall of the nasal cavity. **nasal c., middle,** the lower of two bony plates projecting from the inner wall of the ethmoid labyrinth and separating the superior from the middle meatus of the nose. **nasal c., superior,** the upper of two bony plates projecting from the inner wall of the ethmoid labyrinth and forming the upper boundary of the superior meatus of the nose. **nasal c., supreme,** a third thin bony plate occasionally found projecting from the inner wall of the ethmoid labyrinth, above the two usually found. **c. santori'ni,** nasal concha, supreme. **sphenoidal c.,** a thin curved plate of bone at the anterior and lower part of the body of the sphenoid bone, on either side, forming part of the roof of the nasal cavity.

conchitis (kong-ki'tis) inflammation of a concha.

conchotomy (-kot'o-me) incision of a concha.

conclination (kon"kli-na'shun) inward rotation of the upper pole of the vertical meridian of each eye.

concordance (kon-kor'dans) in genetics, the occurrence of a given trait in both members of a twin pair.

concrescence (-kres'ens) a growing together of parts originally separate.

concretion (-kre'shun) a hardened mass; calculus.

concussion (-kush'un) violent shock or jarring. **c. of the brain,** vertigo, nausea, loss of consciousness, weak pulse and slow respiration, from severe head injury. **c. of the labyrinth,** deafness, vertigo and tinnitus, from head injury.

condensation (kon"den-sa'shun) 1. pathologic hardening of a part, with or without diminution in size. 2. the unconscious union of concepts to produce a new idea or mental picture.

condenser (kon-den'ser) 1. a vessel or apparatus for condensing gases or vapors. 2. device for illuminating microscopic objects. 3. an apparatus for concentrating energy or matter. **Abbé's c.,** as originally designed, a two-lens condenser combination placed below the stage of a microscope.

condom (kon'dum) a rubber sheath to be worn over the penis in coitus.

conductance (kon-duk'tans) ability to conduct or transmit, as electricity or other energy or material; in studies of respiration, an expression of the amount of air reaching the alveoli per unit of time per unit of pressure, the reciprocal of resistance.

conduction (kon-duk'shun) conveyance of energy, as of heat, sound or electricity. **aerial c., air c.,** conduction of sound waves to the organ of hearing through the air. **aerotympanal c.,** conduction of sound waves to the ear through the air and the tympanum. **bone c.,** conduction of sound waves to the inner ear through the bones of the skull. **saltatory c.,** the passage of a potential from node to node of a nerve fiber, rather than along the membrane.

conductivity (kon"duk-tiv'ĭ-te) capacity for conduction.

condylarthrosis (kon"dil-ar-thro'sis) articulation in which a bony eminence is lodged in a joint cavity.

condyle (kon'dĭl) rounded eminence at articular end of bone. adj., **con'dylar.**

condylectomy (kon"dil-ek'to-me) excision of a condyle.

condylion (kon-dil'e-on) point at lateral tip of the mandibular condyle.

condyloid (kon'dĭ-loid) resembling a condyle.

condyloma (kon"dĭ-lo'mah) an elevated lesion of the skin. adj., **condylo'matous. c. acumina'tum,** a papilloma of viral origin, sometimes occurring on skin or mucous surfaces of external genital organs. **flat c., c. la'tum,** a wide, flat, syphilitic condyloma with yellowish discharge.

condylotomy (-lot'o-me) transection of a condyle.

condylus (kon'dĭ-lus), pl. *con'dyli* [L.] condyle.

cone (kōn) a solid figure or body having a circular base and tapering to a point, especially one of the conelike structures of the retina. **ether c.,** a cone-shaped device used over the face in administration of ether for anesthesia. **c. of light,** the triangular light reflex on the membrana tympani. **retinal c's,** minute percipient organs near the outermost layer of the retina. **sarcoplasmic c.,** the conical mass of sarcoplasm at each end of the nucleus of a smooth or cardiac muscle fiber. **twin c's,** cone cells of the retina in which two cells are blended.

confabulation (kon-fab"u-la'shun) the recitation of imaginary experiences to fill gaps in memory.

confection (-fek'shun) a medicated sweetmeat, conserve or electuary. **c. of senna,** a mild laxative containing powdered senna leaf, with other ingredients.

conference (kon'fer-ens) a meeting devoted to consideration of a specific problem or problems. **clinicopathologic c.,** a meeting devoted to consideration of the history and clinical, laboratory and pathologic findings in a particular case, in an effort to establish the diagnosis.

configuration (kon-fig"u-ra'shun) arrangement; form. **atomic c.,** a specific arrangement of particles forming the nucleus of an atom.

confinement (kon-fīn′ment) restraint within doors, especially at childbirth.

conflict (kon′flikt) a painful state of consciousness caused by presence of opposing impulses or desires and failure to resolve them.

conformation (kon″for-ma′shun) the particular shape of an entity, such as the shape a molecule assumes.

conformator (kon′for-ma′tor) instrument for determining outlines of skull.

confusion (kon-fu′zhun) disturbed orientation in regard to time, place or person, sometimes accompanied by disordered consciousness.

congener (kon′jē-ner) something closely related to another thing, as a chemical compound closely related to another in composition and exerting similar or antagonistic effects. adj., **congen′erous.**

congenital (kon-jen′ĭ-tal) present at and existing from the time of birth.

congestin (-jes′tin) a toxic congestion-producing substance derived from the tentacles of sea anemones.

congestion (-jes′chun) abnormal accumulation of blood in a part. **passive c.**, congestion due to lack of vital power or to obstruction to escape of blood from the part. **venous c.**, passive congestion.

congestive (-jes′tiv) associated with congestion.

conglobate (-glo′bāt) aggregated in one mass.

conglobation (kon″glo-ba′shun) the lumping together of particles in a mass.

conglutin (kon-gloo′tin) a proteid from the lupines, peas, beans and almonds.

conglutinant (-gloo′tĭ-nant) promoting union, as of the lips of a wound.

conglutination (-gloo″tĭ-na′shun) union or adherence of parts.

coniasis (ko-ni′ah-sis) presence of dustlike concretions, as in the biliary tract.

coniofibrosis (ko″ne-o-fi-bro′sis) pneumoconiosis with connective tissue growth in the lungs.

coniosis (ko″ne-o′sis) a diseased state due to inhalation of dust.

coniotoxicosis (ko″ne-o-tok″sĭ-ko′sis) pneumoconiosis in which the irritant affects the tissues directly

conization (ko″ni-za′shun) excision of a cone of tissue, as of the endocervical mucous membrane.

conjugata (kon″ju-ga′tah) the conjugate diameter of the pelvis. **c. ve′ra**, the true conjugate diameter of the pelvis.

conjugate (kon′ju-gāt) 1. joined or in pairs. 2. the conjugate diameter of the pelvis.

conjugation (kon″ju-ga′shun) a joining; a method of reproduction in protozoa, with temporary union of two individuals during which a daughter nucleus from each enters and fuses with a daughter nucleus of the other, and the organisms then separate as two fertilized cells.

conjunctiva (kon″junk-ti′vah) the delicate membrane lining the eyelids and covering the eyeball. adj., **conjuncti′val.**

conjunctivitis (kon-junk″tĭ-vi′tis) inflammation of the conjunctiva. **allergic c., anaphy-**

lactic c., hay fever. **granular c.**, trachoma. **phlyctenular c.**, conjunctivitis marked by small vesicles surrounded by a reddened zone. **spring c., vernal c.**, congestion of the conjunctiva, with mucoid secretion, due to allergy to an agent present in the spring.

conjunctivoma (kon-junk″tĭ-vo′mah) a tumor of conjunctival tissue.

conjunctivoplasty (kon″junk-ti′vo-plas″te) plastic repair of the conjunctiva.

connector (kun-nek′tor) a device which joins together two separate parts or structures, e.g. the bilateral parts of a removable partial denture.

connexus (ko-nek′sus) a connection or connecting structure.

conoid (ko′noid) cone-shaped.

consanguinity (kon″sang-gwin′ĭ-te) blood relationship.

conscience (kon′shens) the moral, self-critical part of oneself; the conscious superego.

conscious (kon′shus) capable of responding to sensory stimuli and having subjective experiences.

consciousness (kon′shus-nes) responsiveness of the mind to impressions made by the senses. **double c.**, coexistence of two or more distinct mental states.

conservative (kon-ser′vah-tiv) aimed at elimination of a morbid process with preservation of as much tissue and function as possible.

consolidation (-sol″ĭ-da′shun) the process of becoming solidified, or more dense.

constant (kon′stant) 1. not subject to variation. 2. a value that does not change. **Avogadro's c.**, a value representing the number of particles, real or imaginary, in 1 gram mole of any substance having a chemical formula; often stated to be 6.02246×10^{23}.

constellation (kon″stē-la′shun) a group of emotional ideas which have not become repressed.

constipated (kon′stĭ-pāt″ed) affected with constipation

constipation (kon″stĭ-pa′shun) a condition characterized by abnormally infrequent and difficult evacuation of feces.

constitution (-tu′shun) 1. the make-up or functional habit of the body. 2. the order in which the atoms of a molecule are joined together.

constitutional (-tu′shun-al) affecting the whole body.

constriction (kon-strik′shun) a narrowing or compression.

constrictor (-strik′tor) that which causes constriction.

consultant (-sul′tant) a physician or surgeon whose opinion on diagnosis or treatment is sought by the physician originally attending a patient.

consultation (kon″sul-ta′shun) deliberation of two or more physicians about diagnosis or treatment in a particular case.

consumption (kon-sump′shun) 1. the act of consuming, or the process of being consumed. 2. wasting of the body; pulmonary tuberculosis. **lux′us c.**, ingestion of food in excess of body needs.

contact (kon'takt) 1. mutual touching of two bodies. 2. the completion of an electric circuit. 3. a person who has been sufficiently near an infected person to have been exposed to the transfer of infectious material. **balancing c.,** the contact between the upper and lower teeth on the side opposite the working contact. **complete c.,** contact of the entire adjoining surfaces of two teeth. **direct c., immediate c.,** contact of a healthy person with a diseased person, whereby a contagious disease may be communicated. **indirect c., mediate c.,** contact of a healthy person with objects which may have been contaminated by an infected person. **occlusal c.,** contact between the upper and lower teeth when the jaws are closed. **proximal c., proximate c.,** touching of the proximal surfaces of two adjoining teeth. **weak c.,** contact in which adjoining surfaces of two teeth barely touch. **working c.,** that between the upper and lower teeth on the side toward which the mandible has been moved.

contactant (kon-tak'tant) a substance that touches or may touch the surface of the body.

contactology (kon"tak-tol'o-je) the specialized field of knowledge related to the prescription and use of contact lenses.

contagion (kon-ta'jun) 1. the spread of disease from one person to another. 2. a disease which spreads from one person to another. 3. the living organism (germ or virus) by which disease is spread from one person to another. **direct c., immediate c.,** communication of disease by direct contact with a sick person. **emotional c.,** the intuitive communication of an emotion from a significant adult to an infant or child; the "contagion" of emotional reactions. **mediate c.,** communication of disease from a sick to a well person through an intervening object or person. **psychic c.,** communication of a nervous disorder through mental influence.

contagiosity (-ta"je-os'ĭ-te) the quality of being contagious.

contagious (-ta'jus) readily transmitted by direct or indirect contact.

contagium (-ta'je-um) morbific matter that may spread disease. **c. vi'vum,** a living organism that causes disease.

content (kon'tent) that which is contained within a thing. **latent c.,** the part of a dream which is hidden in the unconsciousness. **manifest c.,** the part of a dream which is remembered after awakening.

continence (kon'ti-nens) ability to exercise voluntary control over natural impulses. adj., **con'tinent.**

contra-angle (kon"trah-ang'gl) an angulation by which the working point of an instrument is brought close to the long axis of its shaft.

contra-aperture (-ap'er-tūr) a second opening made in an abscess to facilitate the discharge of matter.

contraception (-sep'shun) prevention of fertilization of the ovum and development of a new individual.

contraceptive (kon"trah-sep'tiv) 1. diminishing the likelihood of or preventing conception. 2. an agent that diminishes the likelihood of or prevents conception. **intrauterine c.,** a device used within the uterus to prevent pregnancy. **oral c.,** a chemical compound taken orally in order to block ovulation and prevent the occurrence of pregnancy.

contractile (kon-trak'til) contracting under the proper stimulus.

contractility (kon"trak-til'ĭ-te) a capacity for movement, one of the fundamental properties of protoplasm; the ability to contract.

contraction (kon-trak'shun) a drawing together; a shortening or shrinkage. **carpopedal c.,** a kind of tetany in infants, with flexing of the fingers, toes, elbows and knees, and a general tendency to convulsions. **cicatricial c.,** drawing together of the tissues in wound healing, with formation of a cicatrix. **clonic c.,** muscular contraction alternating with relaxation. **closing c.,** muscular contraction at the anode or cathode at the instant the electric circuit is closed. **Dupuytren's c.,** see under *contracture.* **front-tap c.,** contraction of gastrocnemius on tapping muscles of front of leg. **Hicks c's,** painless contractions of the uterus during pregnancy, gradually increasing in frequency and intensity after the thirtieth week. **hourglass c.,** contraction of an organ, as the stomach or uterus, at the middle. **idiomuscular c.,** contraction not produced by nervous stimulus, peculiar to degenerated muscles. **isometric c.,** contraction in which tension is developed, but length of the muscle is not changed. **isotonic c.,** contraction in which the muscle is shortened, but the same tonus is maintained. **opening c.,** muscular contraction at the anode or cathode at the instant the electric circuit is opened. **paradoxic c.,** contraction of a muscle, caused by the passive approximation of its extremities. **postural c.,** the state of muscular tension and contraction which just suffices to maintain the posture of the body. **rheumatic c.,** tetany. **tetanic c.,** sustained muscular contraction with alternating relaxation. **tonic c.,** tetanic contraction. **Volkmann's c.,** see under *contracture.* **Westphal's c.,** involuntary (reflex) muscular contraction seen in paralysis agitans and various spinal affections.

contracture (-trak'tūr) an abnormal condition of shortening and distortion. **Dupuytren's c.,** flexion deformity of the fingers and toes. **ischemic c.,** muscular contracture and degeneration due to interference with the circulation from pressure. **organic c.,** permanent and continuous contracture. **Volkmann's c.,** contraction of the fingers and sometimes of the wrist, with loss of power, after severe injury or improper use of a tourniquet.

contrafissure (kon"trah-fish'er) a fracture in a part opposite the site of the blow.

contraincision (-in-sizh'un) a counteropening.

contraindication (-in"dĭ-ka'shun) a condition

which forbids use of a particular treatment.

contrainsular (kon"trah-in'su-lar) counteracting insular secretion (insulin).

contralateral (-lat'er-al) pertaining to or situated on the opposite side.

contrasexual (-seks'u-al) pertaining to or characteristic of the opposite sex.

contravolitional (-vo-lish'un-al) done in opposition to the will.

contrecoup (kon"truh-koo') [Fr.] injury produced at a site by a blow on the opposite side of the part or on a remote part.

control (kon-trōl') 1. the governing or limitation of certain objects or events. 2. a standard against which experimental observations may be evaluated. **birth c.**, the practice of contraception.

contrusion (kon-troo'shun) crowding of the teeth.

contuse (kon-tūz') to bruise; to wound by beating.

contusion (kon-too'zhun) injury to tissues caused by blunt force which did not disrupt or lacerate their surface; a bruise.

conus (ko'nus), pl. co'ni [L.] a cone. 2. posterior staphyloma of the myopic eye. **c. arterio'sus,** the anterosuperior portion of the right ventricle of the heart, at the entrance to the pulmonary trunk. **c. medulla'ris,** the conical extremity of the spinal cord, at the level of the upper lumbar vertebrae. **c. termina'lis,** conus medullaris. **co'ni vasculo'si,** conical masses in the globus major of the epididymis.

convalescence (kon"vah-les'ens) the stage of recovery from an illness, operation or accidental injury.

convalescent (-les'ent) 1. pertaining to or characterized by convalescence. 2. a patient who is recovering from a disease, operation or accidental injury.

convection (kon-vek'shun) the act of conveying or transmission, specifically transmission of heat in a liquid or gas by circulation of heated particles.

convergence (-ver'jens) a moving together, or inclination toward a common point. adj., **conver'gent. negative c.,** a divergence of the visual axes. **positive c.,** inward deviation of the visual axis.

conversion (-ver'zhun) 1. the transformation of emotions into physical manifestations. 2. manipulative correction of malposition of a fetal part during labor. **autonomic c.,** conversion into an autonomic expression of repressed emotional conflict. **behavior c.,** the expression in neurotic behavior of a psychic conflict in acting-out.

convertin (-ver'tin) a substance in blood which alters prothrombin to thrombin.

convex (kon'veks) rounded and somewhat elevated.

convexoconcave (kon-vek"so-kon'kāv) having one convex and one concave surface.

convexoconvex (-kon'veks) convex on two surfaces.

convolution (kon"vo-lu'shun) an irregularity or elevation caused by the infolding of a structure upon itself. **Broca's c.,** inferior

frontal gyrus. **Heschl's c.,** anterior transverse temporal gyrus.

convulsion (kon-vul'shun) involuntary spasm or contraction of muscles. **epileptiform c.,** convulsion marked by loss of consciousness. **mimetic c., mimic c.,** chronic spasm of facial muscles. **puerperal c.,** convulsion just before or after childbirth. **salaam c.,** nodding spasm. **tetanic c.,** tonic convulsion without loss of consciousness. **uremic c.,** convulsion due to retention in the blood of matters that should be eliminated by the kidney.

convulsive (-vul'siv) of the nature of a convulsion.

Cooperia (koo-pe're-ah) a genus of parasitic worms.

cooperid (koo'per-id) a parasitic worm of the genus Cooperia.

cope (kōp) a plate of metal to be placed over the root of a tooth which is to be crowned.

coping (kōp'ing) a thin, metal covering or cap, such as the plate of metal applied over the root of a tooth prior to attaching an artificial crown.

copiopia (ko"pe-o'pe-ah) eyestrain.

copodyskinesia (ko"po-dis"ki-ne'ze-ah) difficulty of movement due to fatigue from habitual performance of a particular action.

copper (kop'er) chemical element (see table), at. no. 29, symbol Cu. **c. aceto-arsenite,** Paris green. **c. sulfate,** cupric sulfate.

coprecipitin (ko"pre-sip'ĭ-tin) a precipitin which acts on two or more organisms.

copremesis (kop-rem'ĕ-sis) the vomiting of fecal matter.

copremia (kŏ-pre'me-ah) toxemia from chronic constipation.

coprohematology (kop"ro-he"mah-tol'o-je) study of the blood content of the feces.

coprolalia (-la'le-ah) the utterance of obscene words, especially words relating to feces.

coprolith (kop'ro-lith) hard fecal concretion in the intestine.

coprology (kop-rol'o-je) the study of the feces.

coproma (kop-ro'mah) a large tumor-like accumulation of fecal matter in the rectum.

coprophagia (kop"ro-fa'je-ah) eating of filth or feces.

coprophilia (-fil'e-ah) a psychopathologic interest in filth, especially in feces and defecation. adj., **coprophil'ic.**

coprophobia (-fo'be-ah) fear of feces.

coproporphyria (-por-fir'e-ah) increased formation and excretion of coproporphyrin.

coproporphyrin (-por'fĭ-rin) a porphyrin found in feces and urine.

coproporphyrinogen (-por"fĭ-rin'o-jen) the fully reduced, colorless compound giving rise to coproporphyrin by oxidation.

coproporphyrinuria (-por"fĭ-rin-u're-ah) the presence of coproporphyrin in the urine.

coprostasis (kop-ros'tah-sis) fecal impaction.

coprozoa (kop"ro-zo'ah) protozoa found in fecal matter outside the body, but not inhabiting the intestines.

coprozoic (-zo'ik) living in fecal matter.

copula (kop'u-lah) amboceptor.

copulation (kop"u-la'shun) sexual congress or

coitus; usually applied to the mating process in lower animals.

cor (kor) [L.] heart. **c. adipo′sum,** fatty heart. **c. bilocula′re,** a heart with only two chambers. **c. bovi′num,** a greatly enlarged heart, usually associated with aortic insufficiency. **c. hirsu′tum,** cor villosum. **c. pseudotrilocula′re biatria′tum,** a congenital anomaly in which the heart functions as a three-chambered heart, the blood passing from the right to the left atrium and thence to the left ventricle and aorta. **c. pulmona′le,** heart disease secondary to disease of the lungs or of their blood vessels. **c. tomento′sum,** cor villosum. **c. triatria′tum,** a heart with three atria, the pulmonary veins entering a separate chamber above and behind the left atrium, communicating with it through one or several openings across a membrane. **c. trilocula′re biatria′tum,** a three-chambered heart with two atria, the interventricular septum being deficient or lacking. **c. trilocula′re biventricula′re,** a three-chambered heart with two ventricles, the interatrial septum being deficient or lacking. **c. villo′sum,** a roughened state of the pericardium, due to an exudate on its surface, occurring in pericarditis and giving it a hairy appearance.

coracidium (kor″ah-sid′e-um), pl. *coracid′ia* [L.] a free-swimming or free-crawling embryo of the broad fish tapeworm *Diphyllobothrium latum.*

coraco-acromial (kor″ah-ko-ah-kro′me-al) pertaining to acromion and coracoid process.

coracoid (kor′ah-koid) like a crow's beak.

Coramine (ko′rah-min) trademark for preparations of nikethamide.

cord (kord) any long, cylindrical and flexible body or organ. **Braun's c's,** strings of cells which have been observed in the kidney of the early embryo. **dental c.,** a cordlike mass of cells from which the enamel organ develops. **Ferrein's c's,** the lower, or true, vocal cords. **ganglionated c.,** the main trunk of the sympathetic nervous system. **genital c.,** a structure in the embryo formed by the union of the two wolffian and the two müllerian ducts. **gubernacular c.,** gubernaculum testis. **lumbosacral c.,** a nerve trunk from the branches of the fourth and fifth lumbar nerves; it extends to the sacral plexus. **nerve c.,** any nerve trunk or bundle of nerve fibers. **oblique c.,** the oblique ligament. **psalterial c.,** stria vascularis. **sexual c's,** the seminiferous tubules during the early fetal stage. **spermatic c.,** the structure extending from the abdominal inguinal ring to the testis, comprising the pampiniform plexus, nerves, ductus deferens, testicular artery and other vessels. **spinal c.,** that part of the central nervous system lodged in the vertebral canal, extending from the foramen magnum to about the level of the third lumbar vertebra. **umbilical c.,** the structure connecting the fetus and placenta, and containing the channels through which fetal blood passes to and from the placenta. **vocal c's,** the thyroarytenoid ligaments of the larynx; the superior pair being called the

false, and the inferior pair the *true,* vocal cords. **Weitbrecht's c.,** the annular ligament of the elbow. **Wilde's c's,** the transverse striae of the corpus callosum. **Willis's c's,** transverse bands crossing the superior longitudinal sinus.

cordal (kor′dal) pertaining to a cord; used specifically in referring to the vocal cords.

cordate (kor′dāt) heart-shaped.

cordectomy (kor-dek′to-me) excision of a cord, as of a vocal cord.

cordiform (kor′dĭ-form) heart-shaped.

corditis (kor-di′tis) inflammation of the spermatic cord.

cordopexy (kor′do-pek″sc) surgical fixation of a vocal cord.

cordotomy (kor-dot′o-me) chordotomy.

Cordran (kor′dran) trademark for preparations of flurandrenolone.

core(o)- (kor′e, kor′o) word element [Gr.], *pupil of eye.*

coreclisis (kor″e-kli′sis) iridencleisis.

corectasis (kor-ek′tah-sis) morbid dilatation of the pupil.

corectome (ko-rek′tōm) cutting instrument for iridectomy.

corectomedialysis (ko-rek″to-me″de-al′ĭ-sis) coredialysis.

corectomy (ko-rek′to-me) iridectomy.

corectopia (kor″ek-to′pe-ah) abnormal location of the pupil of the eye.

coredialysis (ko″re-di-al′ĭ-sis) creation of an artificial pupil by detaching the iris from the ciliary ligament.

corediastasis (-di-as′tah-sis) dilatation of the pupil.

corelysis (ko-rel′ĭ-sis) operative destruction of the pupil; especially detachment of adhesions of iris to cornea or lens.

coremorphosis (ko″re-mor-fo′sis) coreoplasty.

corenclisis (ko″ren-kli′sis) iridencleisis.

coreometer (ko″re-om′ĕ-ter) device for measuring the pupil.

coreometry (-om′ĕ-tre) measurement of the pupil.

coreoplasty (ko′re-o-plas″te) creation of an artificial pupil.

corepressor (ko″re-pres′sor) a small nodule which combines with an aporepressor to form the substance that controls the synthesis of an enzyme.

coretomy (ko-ret′o-me) iridotomy.

corium (ko′re-um) the fibrous inner layer of the skin, the true skin, derived from the embryonic mesoderm, varying from 1/50 to 1/8 inch in thickness, well supplied with nerves and blood vessels and containing the hair roots and sebaceous and sweat glands; on the palms and soles it bears ridges whose arrangement in whorls and loops is peculiar to the individual.

corn (korn) a circumscribed, conical, horny mass resulting from compression and consolidation of epidermal cells caused by pressure or friction *(hard corn).* **soft c.,** a painful thickening of the skin between two toes, often being moist and macerated.

cornea (kŏr′ne-ah) the transparent anterior

part of the eye. adj. **cor'neal. conical c.,** keratoconus.

corneitis (kor"ne-i'tis) inflammation of the cornea.

corneo-iritis (kor"ne-o-i-ri'tis) inflammation of cornea and iris.

corneosclera (-skle'rah) the cornea and sclera regarded as one organ.

corneous (kor'ne-us) hornlike.

corniculum (kor-nik'u-lum) [L.] a little horn.

cornification (kor"ni-fi-ka'shun) the process of becoming horny.

cornu (kor'nu), pl. cor'nua [L.] 1. a hornlike excresence or projection. 2. an anatomic structure which appears horn-shaped, especially in section. **c. ammo'nis,** hippocampus. **c. cuta'neum, c. huma'num,** a horny excrescence on human skin.

cornual (kor'nu-al) pertaining to a horn, especially to the horns of the spinal cord.

corona (ko-ro'nah), pl. coro'nae [L.] a crown; used in anatomic nomenclature to designate a crownlike eminence or encircling structure. adj., **coro'nal. c. den'tis,** the crown of a tooth. **c. glan'dis pe'nis,** rim around proximal part of glans penis. **c. radia'ta,** 1. the widely spread fibers radiating from the internal capsule to the various gyri of the cerebral hemisphere. 2. an investing layer of radially elongated follicle cells surrounding the zona pellucida. **c. ven'eris,** zone of syphilitic sores on the forehead.

coronad (kor'o-nad) toward the crown of the head.

coronarism (kor'o-nar-izm") spasm of the coronary arteries.

coronaritis (kor"o-nar-i'tis) inflammation of the coronary arteries.

coronary (kor'o-ner"e) encircling in the manner of a crown; a term applied to vessels, ligaments, etc.

coroscopy (ko-ros'ko-pe) skiascopy.

corotomy (ko-rot'o-me) iridotomy.

corpulency (kor'pu-len-se) undue fatness; obesity.

corpus (kor'pus), pl. cor'pora [L.] body. **c. adipo'sum buc'cae,** sucking pad. **cor'pora albican'tia,** two small protuberances at the base of the brain. **cor'pora amyla'cea,** starchlike masses in neuroglia, prostate, etc. **c. aran'tii,** Arantius' body. **c. bigem'inum,** optic lobe. **c. callo'sum,** the great commissure of the cerebrum. **c. caverno'sum,** either of the two erectile columns of the dorsum of the penis or clitoris. **c. cilia're,** ciliary body. **c. denta'tum,** dentate nucleus. **c. fimbria'tum,** band of white matter bordering the lateral edge of the lower cornu of the lateral ventricle. **cor'pora fla'va,** waxy bodies in the central nervous system. **c. genicula'tum,** one of a pair of tubercles on the lower part of the optic thalami. **c. hemorrhag'icum,** 1. a blood clot in a corpus luteum. 2. the stage of a corpus luteum when it contains clotted blood. **c. highmoria'num,** mediastinum testis. **c. interpeduncula're,** a small mass of gray matter just in front of the pons varolii, between the peduncles. **c. lu'teum,** yellow mass formed in the graafian follicle after discharge of the ovum. **c. pyramida'le,** pyramid of the medulla. **cor'pora quadrigem'ina,** four oval bodies behind the third ventricle. **c. restifor'me,** either of the two columns of the oblongata extending to the cerebrum and the cord. **c. stria'tum,** a gray mass on the floor of either lateral ventricle. **c. subthalam'icum,** subthalamus **c. vit'reum,** the vitreous body of the eye. **c. wolffia'num,** wolffian body.

corpuscle (kor'pusl) any small mass, organ or body. adj., **corpus'cular. amylaceous c's,** corpora amylacea. **Bizzozero's c's,** thrombocytes. **blood c's,** formed bodies in the blood. **Burckhardt's c's,** yellowish bodies found in trachoma secretion. **cancroid c's,** the small nodules of epithelioma of the skin. **cartilage c's.,** see under cell. **cement c.,** cementocyte. **chorea c's,** round hyaline bodies in the sheaths of the vessels of the corpora striata in chorea. **chromophil c.,** Nissl's body. **chyle c.,** a lymphocyte found in chyle. **colloid o's,** corpora amylacea. **colostrum c's,** large granular cells in colostrum. **concentric c's,** Hassall's corpuscles. **corneal c's,** star-shaped corpuscles within the corneal spaces. **c. of Donné,** colostrum corpuscles. **Drysdale's c's,** transparent microscopic cells in the fluid of ovarian cysts. **Eichhorst's c's,** microcytes in pernicious anemia. **genital c's,** special nerve endings in the external genitals. **ghost c.,** phantom corpuscle. **Gluge's c's,** granular corpuscles in diseased nerve tissue. **Golgi's c's,** spindle-shaped corpuscles at the junction of tendon and muscular fibers. **Grandry's c's,** Merkel's corpuscles. **Hassall's c's,** nucleated cells in the thymus gland. **Hayem's elementary c's,** blood platelets. **Krause's c's,** round bodies constituting nerve endings in mucous membrane of mouth, nose, eyes and genitals. **Leber's c's,** Hassall's corpuscles. **Lostorfer's c's,** granular bodies from the blood in syphilis. **lymph c's,** leukocytes from lymph. **lymphoid c's,** lymphocytes in tissues. **malpighian c.,** the funnel-like structure constituting the beginning of the structural unit of the kidney (nephron) and comprising the malpighian capsule and its partially enclosed glomerulus. **Meissner's c's,** tactile corpuscles. **Merkel's c's,** tactile corpuscles in the submucosa of the tongue and mouth. **Miescher's c's,** Rainey's corpuscles. **muscle c.,** a muscle nucleus. **nerve c's,** sheath cells between the neurilemma and medullary sheath. **Norris's c's,** colorless, transparent disks, invisible in the blood serum. **Nunn's c's,** epithelial cells in ovarian cysts that have undergone fatty degeneration. **Pacini's c's, pacinian c's,** oval bodies surrounding certain cutaneous nerve endings. **phantom c.,** an achromocyte. **Purkinje's c's,** large, branched nerve cells composing the middle layer of the cortex of the cerebellum. **pus c's,** leukocytes, chiefly polymorphonuclear, found in greatly increased numbers in some bacterial infections. **Rainey's c's,** encapsulated, spore-bearing bodies found in the muscles of various animals. **red blood c.**, erythrocyte. **shadow c.**, phantom corpuscle. **tactile c's**, oval or round bodies connected with nerve fibers in the papillae of the corium. **thymus c's**, Hassall's corpuscles. **Traube's c's**, decolorized erythrocytes. **c's of Vater**, pacinian corpuscles. **Virchow's c's**, corneal corpuscles. **Wagner's c's**, oval bodies at the termination of certain nerve fibers. **white blood c.**, leukocyte. **Zimmermann's c.**, 1. a blood platelet. 2. a phantom corpuscle.

corpusculum (kor-pus'ku-lum), pl. *corpus'cula* [L.] corpuscle.

correction (kŏ-rek'shun) a setting right, c.g. the provision of specific lenses for improvement of vision, or an arbitrary adjustment made in values or devices in performance of experimental procedures.

correlation (kor″ĕ-la'shun) the union of afferent impulses within a nerve center to bring about an appropriate response.

correspondence (kor″ĕ-spon'dens) the condition of being in agreement or conformity. **anomalous retinal c.**, a condition in which disparate points on the retinas of the two eyes come to be associated sensorially. **harmonious retinal c.**, the condition in which the corresponding points on the retinas of the two eyes are associated sensorially. **retinal c.**, the state concerned with the impingement of image-producing stimuli on the retinas of the two eyes.

corrosive (kŏ-ro'siv) having a caustic and locally destructive effect.

Cortate (kor'tāt) trademark for preparations of desoxycorticosterone acetate.

Cort-dome (kort'dōm) trademark for preparations of hydrocortisone.

Cortef (kor'tef) trademark for preparations of hydrocortisone.

cortex (kor'teks), pl. *cor'tices* [L.] an outer layer, as (1) the bark of the trunk or root of a tree; (2) the separable rind of a fruit; (3) the outer layer of an organ or other structure, as distinguished from its inner substance. adj., **cor'tical. adrenal c.**, the thick parenchymatous layer enclosing the medulla of the adrenal gland. **cerebellar c.**, the superficial gray matter of the cerebellum. **cerebral c., c. cer'ebri**, the convoluted layer of gray substance covering each cerebral hemisphere. **c. len'tis**, the softer, external part of the lens of the eye. **provisional c.**, the cortex of the fetal adrenal gland that undergoes involution in early fetal life. **renal c.**, the smooth-textured outer layer of the kidney, extending in columns between the pyramids constituting the renal medulla.

cortexone (kor-tek'sōn) desoxycorticosterone.

cortiadrenal (kor″te-ad-re'nal) pertaining to the adrenal cortex.

corticate (kor'tĭ-kāt) having a cortex or bark.

corticectomy (kor″tĭ-sek'to-me) excision of an area of cortex of an organ, as of a scar or microgyrus of the cerebral cortex in treatment of focal epilepsy.

corticifugal (-sif'u-gal) corticoefferent.

corticipetal (-sip'ĕ-tal) corticoafferent.

corticoadrenal (kor″tĭ-ko-ah-dre'nal) pertaining to the adrenal cortex.

corticoafferent (-af'er-ent) conveying impulses toward the cerebral cortex.

corticoefferent (-ef'er-ent) conveying impulses away from the cerebral cortex.

corticofugal (kor″tĭ-kof'u-gal) corticoefferent.

corticoid (kor'tĭ-koid) a hormone of the adrenal cortex, or other natural or synthetic compound with similar activity.

corticopeduncular (kor″tĭ-ko-pe-dung'ku-ler) pertaining to cortex and peduncles of the brain.

corticopleuritis (-ploo-ri'tis) inflammation of the cortical pleura.

corticospinal (-spi'nal) pertaining to cerebral cortex and spinal cord.

corticosteroid (-ste'roid) a steroidal compound in urine which has biological properties resembling those of adrenal cortical extract.

corticosterone (-stēr'ōn) a compound isolated from adrenal cortex that maintains life in adrenalectomized animals, having several other activities attributed to adrenal cortex.

corticosuprarenoma (-su″prah-re-no'mah) a tumor derived from adrenal cortex.

corticotrophic (-trof'ik) adrenocorticotropic.

corticotrophin (-tro'fin) corticotropin.

corticotropic (-trop'ik) adrenocorticotropic.

corticotropin (-tro'pin) 1. adrenocorticotropin. 2. a pharmaceutical preparation from the anterior lobe of the pituitary gland of mammals, containing principles that exert an influence on the adrenal cortex.

cortisol (kor'tĭ-sol) an adrenal cortical hormone, 17-hydroxycorticosterone, or hydrocortisone, whose effects closely simulate those of cortisone.

cortisone (kor'tĭ-sōn) a carbohydrate-regulating hormone from the adrenal cortex which is concerned in gluconeogenesis. **c. acetate**, a white, crystalline powder, $C_{23}H_{36}O_6$; adrenocortical steroid.

Cortogen (kor'to-jen) trademark for preparations of cortisone.

Cortone (kor'tōn) trademark for preparations of cortisone.

Cortrophin (kor-tro'fin) trademark for preparations of corticotropin.

corundum (kŏ-run'dum) native aluminum oxide, Al_2O_3, used in dentistry as an abrasive and polishing agent.

coruscation (kor″us-ka'shun) the sensation as of a flash of light before the eyes.

corybantism (kor″ĭ-ban'tism) delirium with hallucinations.

Corynebacteriaceae (ko-ri″ne-bak-te″re-a'se-e) a family of Schizomycetes (order Eubacteriales).

Corynebacterium (-bak-te're-um) a genus of Schizomycetes (order Eubacteriales, family Corynebacteriaceae). **C. diphthe'riae**, the causative agent of diphtheria. **C. pseudodiph-therit'icum**, a nonpathogenic microorganism present in the upper respiratory tract.

coryza (ko-ri'zah) profuse discharge from the mucous membrane of the nose.

coryzavirus (ko-ri″zah-vi'rus) one of a group

of viral agents isolated from patients with the common cold.

C.O.S. Canadian Ophthalmological Society; Clinical Orthopaedic Society.

cosmetic (koz-met′ik) 1. improving the appearance. 2. an agent or substance used to improve the appearance.

cost(o) (kos′to) word element [L.], *rib*.

costa (kos′tah), pl. *cos′tae* [L.] 1. a rib. 2. a thin, firm, rodlike structure running along the base of the undulating membrane of certain flagellates. adj., **cos′tal. c. fluc′tuans dec′ima,** Stiller's sign.

costectomy (kos-tek′to-me) excision of a rib.

costive (kos′tiv) constipated.

costiveness (kos′tiv-nes) constipation.

costocervical (kos″to-ser′vĭ-kal) pertaining to ribs and neck.

costochondral (-kon′dral) pertaining to a rib and its cartilage.

costoclavicular (-klah-vik′u-ler) pertaining to ribs and clavicle.

costocoracoid (-kor′ah-koid) pertaining to ribs and coracoid process.

costogenic (-jen′ik) arising from defect of the bone marrow of the ribs.

costopneumopexy (-nu′mo-pek″se) fixation of the lung to a rib.

costoscapularis (-skap″u-la′ris) the serratus anterior muscle.

costosternal (-ster′nal) pertaining to ribs and sternum.

costosternoplasty (-ster′no-plas″te) plastic repair of congenital chondrosternal depression, the sternum being straightened and supported with a segment of rib.

costotomy (kos-tot′o-me) transection of a rib.

costotransverse (kos″to-trans-vers′) lying between the ribs and the transverse processes of the vertebrae.

costotransversectomy (-trans″ver-sek′to-me) resection of the head of a rib and the transverse process of the vertebra.

costovertebral (-ver′tĕ-bral) pertaining to a rib and a vertebra.

Cothera (ko-ther′ah) trademark for preparations of dimethoxanate hydrochloride.

cotton (kot′un) a textile material derived from the seeds of cultivated varieties of *Gossypium*. **absorbent c.,** purified cotton. **collodion c.,** pyroxylin. **purified c.,** cotton freed from impurities, deprived of fatty matter, bleached and sterilized in its final container.

co-twin (ko′twin) one of two individuals produced at the same gestation and born at the same time.

cotyledon (kot″ĭ-le′don) any subdivision of the uterine surface of the placenta.

cotyloid (kot′ĭ-loid) cup-shaped.

couching (kowch′ing) displacement of the lens in cataract.

cough (kof) sudden noisy expulsion of air from lungs. **dry c.,** cough without expectoration. **ear c.,** reflex cough produced by disease of the ear. **hacking c.,** a short, frequent and feeble cough. **productive c.,** cough attended with expectoration of material from the bronchi. **reflex c.,** cough due to irritation of some

remote organ. **stomach c.,** cough caused by reflex irritation from stomach disorder. **wet c.,** productive cough. **whooping c.,** pertussis.

coulomb (koo′lom) the unit of electrical quantity.

Coumadin (koo′mah-din) trademark for preparations of warfarin sodium.

coumarin (koo′mah-rin) colorless, prismatic crystals, $C_9H_6O_2$, used as a flavoring agent.

count (kownt) ascertainment of the number of individual units (e.g. blood corpuscles, cells) in a given series or quantity of solution. **Addis c.,** a count of the cells in 10 cc. of urinary sediment as a means of calculating total urinary sediment in a 12-hour specimen. **blood cell c.,** determination of the number of formed elements in a measured volume of blood, usually a cubic millimeter (as of red cells, white cells and platelets). **differential blood cell c.,** determination of the proportion of each kind of leukocyte. **direct platelet c.,** estimation of the number of platelets per cubic millimeter of blood directly from whole blood. **filament-nonfilament c.,** determination of the number of filamentous and nonfilamentous leukocytes in a blood specimen. **indirect platelet c.,** the count of the total number of platelets per cubic millimeter of blood by counting the platelets on a stained blood film. **Schilling's c.,** a differential blood cell count in which the leukocytes are divided into four groups.

counter (kown′ter) an apparatus for determining the number of units in any collection. **Coulter c.,** an automatic photoelectric instrument used in enumeration of formed elements in the peripheral blood. **Geiger c., Geiger-Müller c.,** a device for electrically determining the number of ionized particles emitted by a substance. **scintillation c.,** a device for indicating the emission of ionizing particles, permitting determination of the concentration of radioactive isotopes in the body.

counterextension (kown″ter-eks-ten′shun) traction in a proximal direction coincident with traction in opposition to it

counterirritant (-ir′ĭ-tant) 1. producing counterirritation. 2. an agent which produces counterirritation

counterirritation (-ir″ĭ-ta′shun) superficial irritation intended to relieve some other irritation.

counteropening (-o″pen-ing) a second opening, as in an abscess, made to facilitate drainage.

counterpoison (kown′ter-poi″zon) a poison given to counteract another poison.

counterpuncture (kown′ter-punk″tūr) a puncture made opposite to another.

counterstain (kown′ter-stān) a stain applied to render effects of another stain more discernible.

countertraction (kown′ter-trak″shun) traction opposed to another traction; used in reduction of fractures.

countertransference (kown″ter-trans-fer′ens) displacement of feelings and projection of needs and conflicts of the therapist onto the patient in psychotherapy.

coup (koo) [Fr.] stroke. **c. de fouet** (koo duh fwa) ["stroke of the whip"] rupture of the plantaris muscle accompanied by a sharp disabling pain. **c. de sabre** (koo duh sahb) a linear, circumscribed lesion of scleroderma on the forehead or scalp, so called because of its resemblance to the scar of a saber wound. **c. de sang** (koo duh sang) congestion of the brain. **c. sur coup** (koo sur koo) ["blow on blow"] administration of a drug in small doses at short intervals to secure rapid, complete or continuous action.

coupling (kup′ling) in genetics, occurrence in a double heterozygote on the same chromosome of the two mutant alleles of interest.

coverglass (kuv′er-glas) a small plate of optical glass of controlled thickness, used over material placed on a slide for microscopic study.

coverslip (kuv′er-slip) a small plate of plastic or other transparent substance used over material placed on a slide for microscopic study.

Cowdria (kow′dre-ah) a genus of Microtatobiotes (order Rickettsiales, family Rickettsiaceae, tribe Ehrlichieae).

cowperitis (kow″per-i′tis) inflammation of Cowper's glands.

cowpox (kow′poks) a mild eruptive disease in cows, due to a virus and communicable to man.

coxa (kok′sah), pl. *cox′ae* [L.] the hip, or hip joint. **c. mag′na,** overgrowth of the head and neck of the femur causing prominence of the hip. **c. pla′na,** flattening of the head of the femur resulting from osteochondrosis of its epiphysis. **c. val′ga,** deformity of the hip joint with increase in the angle of inclination between the neck and shaft of the femur. **c. va′ra,** deformity of the hip joint with decrease in the angle of inclination between the neck and shaft of the femur.

coxalgia (kok-sal′je-ah) hip joint disease.

coxarthropathy (koks″ar-throp′ah-the) hip joint disease.

Coxiella (kok″se-el′ah) a genus of Microtatobiotes (order Rickettsiales, family Rickettsiaceae, tribe Rickettsieae). **C. burnet′ii,** the causative agent of Q fever.

coxitis (kok-si′tis) inflammation of the hip joint.

coxodynia (kok″so-din′e-ah) pain in the hip.

coxofemoral (-fem′o-ral) pertaining to hip and thigh.

coxotomy (kok-sot′o-me) incision of the hip joint.

coxotuberculosis (kok″so-tu-ber″ku-lo′sis) tuberculosis of the hip joint.

cozymase (ko-zi′mās) a coenzyme in yeast, muscle and blood serum.

c.p. candle power.

c.p.m. counts per minute, an expression of the particles emitted after administration of a radioactive material such as I¹³¹.

c.p.s. cycles per second.

Cr chemical symbol, *chromium.*

cradle (kra′dl) frame for placing over the body of a patient, under the bed coverings, for application of heat or for protecting injured parts. **electric c., heat c.,** a frame with wiring for light bulbs, for application of heat to the patient's body.

Craigia (kra′ge-ah) a genus of ameboid protozoans parasitic in the intestine and causing dysentery.

craigiasis (kra-gi′ah-sis) infection with Craigia.

cramp (kramp) a painful spasmodic muscular contraction. **heat c.,** spasm accompanied by pain, weak pulse and dilated pupils; seen in workers in intense heat. **intermittent c.,** tetany. **recumbency c's,** cramping in muscles of legs and feet occurring while resting or during light sleep. **writers' c.,** spasm and neuralgia of fingers, hand and forearm, due to excessive writing.

crani(o)- (kra′ne-o) word element [L.], *skull.*

cranial (kra′ne-al) pertaining to the cranium.

craniectomy (kra″ne-ek′to-me) excision of a segment of the skull.

craniocele (kra′ne-o-sēl″) protrusion of part of the brain through the skull.

craniocerebral (kra″ne-o-ser′e-bral) pertaining to skull and brain.

cranioclasis (kra″ne-ok′lah-sis) crushing of the fetal skull in difficult labor.

cranioclast (kra′ne-o-klast″) instrument for crushing the fetal skull in utero.

cranioclasty (-klas″te) cranioclasis.

craniocleidodysostosis (kra″ne-o-kli″do-dis″-os-to′sis) cleidocranial dysostosis.

craniodidymus (-did′ĭ-mus) a fetal monster with two heads.

craniofenestria (-fē-nes′tre-ah) defective development of the fetal skull, with areas in which no bone is formed.

craniograph (kra′ne-o-graf″) an instrument for outlining the skull.

craniolacunia (kra″ne-o-lah-ku′ne-ah) defective development of the fetal skull, with depressed areas on the inner surface of the bones.

craniology (kra″ne-ol′o-je) the scientific study of skulls.

craniomalacia (kra″ne-o-mah-la′she-ah) abnormal softness of the bones of the skull.

craniometer (kra″ne-om′ē-ter) instrument for measuring the head.

craniometry (-om′ē-tre) measurement of the skull and facial bones.

craniopagus (-op′ah-gus) a double fetal monster joined at the head.

craniopathy (-op′ah-the) any disease of the skull. **metabolic c.,** frontal internal hyperostosis.

craniopharyngeal (kra″ne-o-fah-rin′je-al) pertaining to cranium and pharynx.

craniopharyngioma (-fah-rin″je-o′mah) a tumor arising from the remnants of the craniopharyngeal duct.

cranioplasty (kra′ne-o-plas″te) plastic repair of the skull.

craniopuncture (-punk″tūr) exploratory puncture of the brain.

craniorachischisis (kra″ne-o-rah-kis′kĭ-sis) congenital fissure of skull and spinal column.

craniosacral (-sa′kral) pertaining to skull and sacrum.

cranioschisis (kra″ne-os′kĭ-sis) congenital fissure of the skull.

craniosclerosis (kra″ne-o-skle-ro′sis) abnormal calcification and thickening of the cranial bones.

cranioscopy (kra″ne-os′ko-pe) diagnostic examination of the head.

craniospinal (kra″ne-o-spi′nal) pertaining to skull and the spine.

craniostenosis (-ste-no′sis) narrowness of the skull due to premature closure of the cranial sutures.

craniostosis (kra″ne-os-to′sis) premature closure of the cranial sutures.

craniosynostosis (kra″ne-o-sin″os-to′sis) premature closure of the sutures of the skull.

craniotabes (-ta′bēz) reduction in mineralization of the skull, with abnormal softness of the bone and widening of the sutures and fontanels, occurring chiefly in rickets.

craniotome (kra′ne-o-tōm″) cutting instrument used in craniotomy.

craniotomy (kra″ne-ot′o-me) opening of the skull, as for surgery on the brain or decompression of the fetal head in difficult labor.

craniotympanic (kra″ne-o-tim-pan′ik) pertaining to skull and tympanum.

cranium (kra′ne-um), pl. *cra′nia* [L.] the skeleton of the head, exclusive of the mandible and facial bones.

crater (kra′ter) an excavated area with surrounding wall, such as is caused by ulceration.

craterization (kra″ter-i-za′shun) excision of bone tissue to create a crater-like depression.

cravat (krah-vat′) a triangular bandage.

cream (krēm) the butter-fat–containing fraction of cow's milk which separates on standing or by centrifugation, or a substance that resembles it in consistency. **cold c.,** a preparation of spermaceti, white wax, mineral oil, sodium borate and purified water, applied topically to skin, and sometimes used as a vehicle for medications. **leukocytic c.,** the reddish gray layer observed above the packed red cells in centrifuged blood. **c. of tartar,** potassium bitartrate.

Creamalin (krēm′ah-lin) trademark for preparations of aluminum hydroxide gel.

creatinase (kre-at′ĭ-nās) an enzyme that catalyzes the decomposition of creatine.

creatine (kre′ah-tin) a crystallizable nitrogenous compound synthesized in the body.

creatinemia (kre″ah-tĭ-ne′me-ah) excessive creatine in the blood.

creatinine (kre-at′ĭ-nin) a waste product formed from creatine and phosphocreatine.

creatinuria (kre-at″ĭ-nu′re-ah) the presence of creatine in the urine.

creatorrhea (kre″ah-to-re′ah) the presence of muscle fibers in the feces.

creatotoxism (-tok′sizm) meat poisoning.

cremasteric (kre″mas-ter′ik) pertaining to the cremaster muscle.

crenated (kre′nāt-ed) having a notched or scalloped border.

crenation (kre-na′shun) the production of indentations in the surface of a cell, due to withdrawal of moisture from the cytoplasm, and giving it a notched appearance.

crenocyte (kre′no-sīt) a crenated erythrocyte.

crenocytosis (kre″no-si-to′sis) crenated erythrocytes in the blood.

crenotherapy (-ther′ah-pe) treatment by use of mineral waters.

Crenothrix (kre′no-thriks) a genus of Schizomycetes (order Chlamydobacteriales, family Crenotrichaceae).

Crenotrichaceae (kre″no-trĭ-ka′se-e) a family of Schizomycetes (order Chlamydobacteriales).

creosote (kre′o-sōt) a mixture of phenols from wood tar; used as a disinfectant. **c. carbonate,** a clear, viscid liquid, a mixture of carbonates of various constituents of creosote.

crepitant (krep′ĭ-tant) having a dry, crackling sound.

crepitation (krep″ĭ-ta′shun) a dry, crackling sound or sensation, such as that produced by the grating of the ends of a fractured bone.

crepitus (krep′ĭ-tus) 1. crepitation. 2. a crepitant rale. **c. re′dux,** the return of crepitus, forerunning recovery in pneumonia.

crescent (kres′ent) a structure shaped like a new moon. adj., **crescen′tic. Giannuzzi's c's,** crescentic cell masses on the basement membrane of the acini of the mucous glands. **myopic c.,** a crescentic staphyloma in the fundus of the eye in myopia. **sublingual c.,** the crescent-shaped area on the floor of the mouth, bounded by the lingual wall of the mandible and the base of the tongue.

cresol (kre′sol) a phenol from coal or wood tar; a preparation consisting of a mixture of isomeric cresol from coal tar or petroleum is used as a disinfectant.

cresomania (kre″so-ma′ne-ah) abnormal delusions of possessing great wealth.

cresoxydiol (kres ok″se-di′ol) mephenesin.

cresoxypropanediol (-pro-pan′de-ol) mephenesin.

crest (krest) a projection, or projecting structure or ridge, especially one surmounting a bone or its border. **ampullar c.,** the most prominent part of a localized thickening of the membrane lining the ampullae of the semicircular ducts. **cross c.,** a ridge of enamel extending across the face of a tooth. **dental c.,** the maxillary ridge passing along the alveolar processes of the fetal maxillary bones. **frontal c.,** a median ridge on the internal surface of the frontal bone. **iliac c.,** the thickened, expanded upper border of the ilium. **lacrimal c., anterior,** the lateral margin of the groove on the posterior border of the frontal process of the maxilla. **lacrimal c., posterior,** a vertical ridge dividing the lateral or orbital surface of the lacrimal bone into two parts. **nasal c.,** a ridge on the internal border of the nasal bone. **neural c.,** a cellular band dorsolateral to the neural tube that gives origin to the cerebrospinal ganglia. **obturator c.,** a strong ridge forming the inferior border of the superior ramus of the pubic bone. **occipital c., external,** a ridge sometimes extending on the external surface of the occipital bone from the external protuberance toward the foramen magnum. **occipital c., internal,** a median ridge on the internal surface of the occipital bone, extending from the midpoint of the cruciform eminence toward the foramen magnum. **palatine c.,** a ridge sometimes seen on the inferior surface of the horizontal plate of the palatine bone. **pubic c.,** the thick, rough anterior border of the body of the pubic bone. **sacral c., intermediate,** either of two indefinite ridges just medial to the dorsal sacral foramina. **sacral c., lateral,** either of two series of tubercles lateral to the dorsal sacral foramina. **sacral c., median,** a median ridge on the dorsal surface of the sacrum. **sphenoidal c.,** a median ridge on the anterior surface of the body of the sphenoid bone. **supramastoid c.,** ridge on temporal bone above auditory meatus. **supraventricular c.,** a ridge on the inner wall of the right ventricle, marking off the conus arteriosus. **temporal c.,** a ridge on the frontal bone. **c. of tibia,** the prominent ridge on the front of the tibia. **turbinated c.,** a horizontal ridge on the internal surface of the palate bone. **urethral c.,** an elevation along the posterior wall of the urethra. **c. of vestibule,** a ridge between the spherical and elliptical recesses of the vestibule, dividing posteriorly to bound the cochlear recess.

cretin (kre'tin)   a patient exhibiting cretinism.

cretinism (kre'tĭ-nizm)   arrested physical and mental development with dystrophy of bones and soft tissues, due to congenital lack of thyroid secretion. **athyreotic c.,** cretinism due to thyroid aplasia or destruction of the thyroid of the fetus in utero. **athyrotic c.,** that due to failure of development of the thyroid gland. **endemic c.,** that occurring in children born in areas where goiter is endemic. **sporadic c.,** cretinism in one not descended from cretins or living in a region where the condition prevails. **sporadic goitrous c.,** a genetically determined condition in which enlargement of the thyroid gland is associated with deficiency in the supply of circulating thyroid hormone.

cretinoid (kre'tĭ-noid)   resembling a cretin.

cretinous (kre'tĭ-nus)   affected with cretinism.

crevice (krev'is)   a fissure. **gingival c.,** the space between the cervical enamel of a tooth and the overlying unattached gingiva.

crevicular (krĕ-vik'u-lar)   pertaining to the gingival crevice.

cribration (krī-bra'shun)   the quality of being cribriform.

cribriform (krib'rĭ-form)   perforated like a sieve.

cribrum (kri'brum), pl. *cri'bra* [L.]   lamina cribrosa of the ethmoid bone.

cricoarytenoid (kri"ko-ar"ĭ-te'noid)   pertaining to cricoid and arytenoid cartilages.

cricoid (kri'koid)   shaped like a signet ring.

cricoidectomy (kri"koi-dek'to-me)   excision of the cricoid cartilage.

cricoidynia (-din'e-ah)   pain in the cricoid cartilage.

cricopharyngeal (kri"ko-fah-rin'je-al)   pertaining to cricoid cartilage and pharynx.

cricothyreotomy (-thi"re-ot'o-me)   incision through the cricoid and thyroid cartilages.

cricotomy (kri-kot'o-me)   incision of the cricoid cartilage.

cricotracheotomy (kri"ko-tra"ke-ot'o-me)   incision of the trachea through the cricoid cartilage.

criminosis (krim"ĭ-no'sis)   a neurosis marked by criminal behavior.

crinogenic (kri"no-jen'ik, krin"o-jen'ik)   causing secretion in a gland.

crinosin (kri'no-sin)   a substance in hairlike filaments, derived from brain tissue.

crisis (kri'sis), pl. *cri'ses* [L.]   1. the turning point of a disease. 2. a paroxysmal attack of pain, especially in tabes dorsalis. **aplastic c.,** sudden temporary disappearance of erythroblasts from bone marrow, occurring in certain hemolytic states and sometimes during infections in children. **blood c.,** a sudden temporary appearance of great numbers of nucleated red cells in the blood. **bronchial c.,** paroxysms of dyspnea in tabes dorsalis. **clitoris c.,** attacks of sexual excitement in women with tabes dorsalis. **deglobulinization c.,** a condition occurring in congenital spherocytic anemia, with sudden onset of fever, abdominal pain and vomiting, associated with reticulocytopenia, leukopenia, thrombocytopenia, erythroblastopenia and return of serum bilirubin to normal. **Dietl's c.,** an attack of intense lumbar pain with nausea and vomiting from floating kidney. **gastric c.,** paroxysms of intense pain in abdomen in tabes dorsalis. **genital c. of newborn,** estrinization of vaginal mucosa and hyperplasia of the breast, influenced by transplacentally acquired estrogens. **hemoclastic c.,** temporary leukopenia, with relative lymphocytosis, lowered blood pressure, and changes in blood coagulability; a form of anaphylactic shock. **nephralgic c.,** paroxysmal pain in the kidney region in tabes dorsalis. **nitritoid c.,** redness of the face, dyspnea and precordial pain following the injection of arsphenamine. **rectal c.,** severe pain in rectum in tabes dorsalis. **tabetic c.,** a painful paroxysm occurring in tabes dorsalis. **vesical c.,** paroxysms of pain in bladder in tabes dorsalis.

crista (kris'tah), pl. *cris'tae* [L.]   crest. **cris'tae cu'tis,** ridges of the skin produced by the projecting papillae of the corium on the palm of the hand or sole of the foot, producing a fingerprint or footprint characteristic of the individual; called also *dermal ridges*. **c. gal'li,** a thick, triangular process projecting upward from the cribriform plate of the ethmoid bone.

Cristispira (kris"tĭ-spi'rah)   a genus of Schizomycetes (order Spirochaetales, family Spirochaetaceae) found in the intestinal tracts of molluscs.

C.R.N.A. Certified Registered Nurse Anesthetist.

cross (kros)   a mating between organisms having different genes determining particular traits of inheritance. **dihybrid c.,** one in which the parents have different genes determining two particular traits. **monohybrid c.,** one in which the parents have different genes involving only one particular trait. **polyhybrid c.,** one in which the parents have different genes determining more than three particular traits. **trihybrid c.,** one in which the parents have different genes determining three particular traits.

crossbite (kros'bīt)   a condition in which mandibular teeth are in buccal version to the maxillary teeth.

crossing over (kros'ing o'ver)   the exchange of segments between homologous chromosomes, permitting new combinations of genes.

crossmatching (kros-mach'ing)   a procedure vital in blood transfusions, testing for agglutination of donor red cells by recipient's serum, and of recipient's red cells by donor serum.

crossway (kros'wa)   a place of crossing over. **sensory c.,** posterior part of internal capsule of the brain.

crotamiton (kro″tah-mi'ton)   a compound used in the treatment of scabies.

crotaphion (kro-taf'e-on)   cranial point at tip of great wing of sphenoid bone.

crotchet (kroch'et)   a hook used in extracting the fetus after craniotomy.

crotonism (kro'ton-izm)   poisoning by croton oil.

croup (kroop)   laryngeal spasm, dyspnea, difficult respiration, often with a local membranous deposit. adj., **croup'ous. catarrhal c.,** simple inflammation of larynx with formation of membrane. **false c., spasmodic c.,** spasm of laryngeal muscles with slight inflammation.

crown (krown)   a crown-shaped structure, especially the exposed or enamel-covered part of a tooth. **anatomic c.,** the enamel-covered portion of a tooth. **artificial c.,** a metal, porcelain or plastic reproduction of a crown affixed to the remaining natural structure of a tooth. **clinical c.,** the portion of a tooth exposed beyond the margin of the gum. **physiologic c.,** the portion of a tooth distal to the gingival crevice or to the margin of the gingiva.

crowning (krown'ing)   the appearance of the fetal scalp at the vaginal orifice in childbirth.

crucial (kroo'shal)   1. cross-shaped. 2. decisive.

cruciate (kroo'she-āt)   shaped like a cross.

crucible (kroo'sĭ-bl)   a laboratory vessel in which samples under study can be subjected to high temperatures.

cruciform (kroo'sĭ-form)   cross-shaped.

crupper (krup'er)   the rump of a horse.

crus (krus), pl. **cru'ra** [L.]   a leg or leglike structure. adj., **cru'ral. cru'ra cerebel'li,** peduncles of cerebellum. **c. cer'ebri,** a structure comprising fiber tracts descending from the cerebral cortex to form the longitudinal fascicles of the pons. **crura of diaphragm,**

two pillars which connect the diaphragm to the spinal column. **crura of fornix,** two flattened bands of white substance that unite to form the body of the fornix.

crust (krust)   the dried residue of exudate from an erosive or ulcerative skin lesion, or from the intact skin. **milk c.,** crusta lactea.

crusta (krus'tah), pl. **crus'tae** [L.]   1. any crust. 2. part of crus cerebri below the substantia nigra. **c. lac'tea,** a thick coating of dried exudate on the scalp of a nursing infant. **c. petro'sa,** cementum of a tooth. **c. phlogis'-tica,** buffy coat.

Crustacea (krus-ta'she-ah)   a class of animals including the lobsters, crabs, shrimps, wood lice, water fleas.

crutch (kruch)   a staff extending from the armpit to the ground, with a crosspiece at the top fitting under the arm and a crossbar for the hand, used to support the weight of the body in walking.

crux (kruks), pl. **cru'ces** [L.] cross. **c. of heart,** the intersection of the walls separating the right and left sides and the upper and lower chambers of the heart. **cru'ces pilo'rum,** crosslike figures formed by the pattern of hair growth, the hairs lying in opposite directions.

cry(o)- (kri'o)   word element [Gr.], cold.

cryalgesia (kri″al-je'ze-ah)   pain on application of cold.

cryanesthesia (kri″an-es-the'ze-ah)   loss of power of perceiving cold.

cryesthesia (kri″es the'ze-ah)   abnormal sensitiveness to cold.

crymoanesthesia (kri″mo-an″es-the'ze-ah)   anesthesia produced by refrigeration.

crymodynia (-din'e-ah)   cryalgesia.

crymophilic (-fil'ik)   cryophilic.

crymophylactic (-fi-lak'tik)   resistant to cold.

crymotherapy (-ther'ah-pe)   cryotherapy.

cryo-aerotherapy (kri″o-a″er-o-ther'ah-pe)   treatment by cold air.

cryobiology (-bi-ol'o-je)   the science dealing with the effect of low temperatures on biological systems.

cryocardioplegia (kar″de-o-ple'je-ah)   cessation of contraction of the myocardium produced by application of cold during cardiac surgery.

cryocautery (-kaw'ter-e)   cold cautery.

cryocrit (kri'o krit)   the percentage of the total volume of blood serum or plasma occupied by cryoprecipitates after centrifugation.

cryofibrinogen (kri″o-fi-brin'o-jen)   a blood protein resembling fibrinogen that precipitates from plasma on cooling.

cryofibrinogenemia (-fi-brin″o-jen-e'me-ah)   the presence of cryofibrinogens in the blood.

cryogammaglobulin (-gam″mah-glob'u-lin)   a gamma globulin readily precipitated from plasma on cooling.

cryogenic (-jen'ik)   producing low temperatures.

cryoglobulin (-glob'u-lin)   a serum globulin that precipitates, gels or crystallizes spontaneously at low temperatures.

cryoglobulinemia (kri″o-glob″u-lin-e′me-ah) presence in the blood of cryoglobulins.

cryometer (kri-om′ĕ-ter) a thermometer for measuring very low temperature.

cryopathy (kri-op′ah-the) morbid condition caused by cold.

cryophilic (kri″o-fil′ik) preferring low temperatures; psychrophilic.

cryoprecipitate (-pre-sip′ĭ-tāt) any precipitate that results from cooling.

cryoprotein (-pro′te-in) a blood protein that precipitates on cooling.

cryoscope (kri′o-skōp) an instrument for performing cryoscopy.

cryoscopy (kri-os′ko-pe) examination of fluids based on the principle that the freezing point of a solution varies according to the amount and nature of the solute. adj., **cryoscop′ic.**

cryostat (kri′o-stat) a device interposed in a cooling system by which temperature is automatically maintained between certain levels.

cryosurgery (kri″o-ser′jer-e) the destruction of tissue by application of extreme cold.

cryotherapy (-ther′ah-pe) the therapeutic use of cold.

cryotolerant (-tol′er-ant) able to withstand very low temperatures.

crypt (kript) a follicle or pit. **alveolar c.,** the bony compartment surrounding a developing tooth. **anal c's,** small recesses in the rectal mucosa, arranged circumferentially about the proximal margin of the anal canal and opening superiorly. **dental c.,** the space occupied by a developing tooth. **enamel c.,** a space bounded by dental ledges on either side and usually by the enamel organ, and filled with mesenchyma. **c's of Fuchs, c's of iris,** pitlike depressions in the iris, in the region of the circulosus arteriosus minor. **c's of Lieberkühn,** simple tubular glands opening on the surface of the intestinal mucous membrane. **Luschka's c's,** peculiar outpouchings of the mucosa of the gallbladder. **c's of Morgagni,** anal crypts. **synovial c.,** a pouch in the synovial membrane of a joint. **c's of tongue,** deep, irregular invaginations from the surface of the lingual tonsil.

crypta (krip′tah), pl. *cryp″tae* [L.] crypt.

crypt(o)- (krip′to) word element [Gr.], *concealed; pertaining to a crypt.*

cryptectomy (krip-tek′to-me) excision or obliteration of a crypt.

cryptenamine (krip-ten′ah-mīn) a mixture of alkaloids from an extract of *Veratrum viride,* used to lower blood pressure.

cryptesthesia (krip″tes-the′ze-ah) subconscious perception of occurrences not ordinarily perceptible to the senses.

cryptitis (krip-ti′tis) inflammation of the mucous membrane of the anal crypts.

cryptocephalus (krip″to-sef′ah-lus) a fetal monster with an inconspicuous head.

cryptococcosis (-kok-o′sis) infection by fungi of the genus Cryptococcus.

Cryptococcus (-kok′us) a genus of fungi. **C. neofor′mans,** a species of yeastlike fungi of worldwide distribution, causing infection in man.

cryptodidymus (krip″to-did′ĭ-mus) a twin monster, one fetus being enclosed within the body of the other.

cryptogam (krip′to-gam) one of the lower plants that have no true flowers, but propagate by spores.

cryptogenetic (krip″to-jĕ-net′ik) of obscure or doubtful origin.

cryptogenic (-jen′ik) cryptogenetic.

cryptoglioma (-gli-o′mah) one stage of glioma in which presence of the growth is masked.

cryptoleukemia (-lu-ke′me-ah) leukemia without abnormal cells in the blood.

cryptolith (krip′to-lith) a concretion in a crypt.

cryptomenorrhea (krip″to-men″o-re′ah) suppression of menstruation.

cryptomerorachischisis (-me″ro-rah-kis′kĭ-sis) spina bifida occulta.

cryptomnesia (krip″tom-ne′ze-ah) subconscious memory. adj., **cryptomne′sic.**

cryptoneurous (krip″to-nu′rus) having no distinct nervous system.

cryptophthalmos (krip″tof-thal′mos) congenital absence of the fissure between the eyelids, the eyeball being rudimentary or absent.

cryptoplasmic (krip″to-plaz′mik) occurring in a concealed form.

cryptopodia (-po′de-ah) swelling of the lower leg and foot, covering all but the sole of the foot.

cryptopyic (-pi′ik) attended by concealed suppuration.

cryptorchid (krip-tor′kid) a person with undescended testes.

cryptorchidectomy (krip″tor-kĭ-dek′to-me) excision of an undescended testis.

cryptorchidism (krip-tor′kĭ-dizm) cryptorchism.

cryptorchidopexy (krip-tor′kĭ-do-pek″se) fixation of an undescended testis in the scrotum.

cryptorchism (krip-tor′kizm) retention of one or both of the testes in the abdominal cavity.

cryptorrhea (krip″to-re′ah) abnormal activity of an organ of internal secretion.

cryptorrheic (-re′ik) cryptorrhetic.

cryptorrhetic (-ret′ik) pertaining to internal secretions.

cryptoscope (krip′to-skōp) fluoroscope.

cryptotoxic (krip″to-tok′sik) having hidden toxic properties.

cryptoxanthin (-zan′thin) a pigment in egg yolk, green grass and yellow corn which can be converted in the body into vitamin A.

cryptozygous (-zi′gus) having the calvaria wider than the face, so that the zygomatic arches are concealed when the head is viewed from above.

crystal (kris′tal) a naturally produced angular solid of definite form. adj., **crys′talline. blood c's,** hematoidin crystals in the blood. **Böttcher's c's,** microscopic crystals seen on adding a drop of solution of ammonium phosphate to a drop of prostatic fluid. **Charcot-Leyden c's,** minute crystals in sputum in asthma and bronchitis. **Charcot-Neumann c's,** minute crystals of spermine phosphate. **Charcot-Robin c's,** crystals formed in leukemic blood. **coffin-lid c's,** knife-rest crystals.

dumbbell c's, crystals of calcium oxalate occurring in urine. **hedgehog c's,** wedge-shaped spiny crystals of uric acid. **knife-rest c's,** peculiar notched crystals of triple phosphate in urine. **rock c.,** a variety of quartz used in making spectacle lenses. **Teichmann's c's,** crystals of hemin.

crystalbumin (kris″tal-bu′min) albumin found in water extract of the crystalline lens.

crystalfibrin (-fi′brin) an extractive from the crystalline lens.

crystallin (kris′tah-lin) globulin from the lens of the eye.

crystallization (kris″tah li za′shun) formation of crystals.

crystalloid (kris′tah-loid) 1. resembling a crystal. 2. a noncolloid substance.

crystalloiditis (kris″tah-loi-di′tis) inflammation of the crystalline lens.

crystallophobia (kris″tah-lo-fo′be-ah) morbid fear of glass or glass objects.

crystalluria (kris″tah-lu′re-ah) the presence of crystals in the urine, causing irritation of the kidney.

crystalluridrosis (kris″tah-lu″rĭ dro′sis) crystallization on the skin of urinary elements from the perspiration.

Crysticillin (kris″ti-sil′in) trademark for aqueous preparations of penicillin G procaine.

Crystodigin (kris″to-dij′in) trademark for preparations of crystalline digitoxin.

Crystoids (kris′toidz) trademark for anthelmintic pills of hexylresorcinol.

C.S. current strength.

Cs chemical symbol, *cesium.*

C.S.A.A. Child Study Association of America.

C.S.F. cerebrospinal fluid.

C.S.G.B.I. Cardiac Society of Great Britain and Ireland.

C.S.M. cerebrospinal meningitis.

C.T.A. Canadian Tuberculosis Association.

Ctenocephalides (te″no-se-fal′i-dēs) a genus of fleas commonly found on carnivores. **C. ca′nis, C. fe′lis,** species found on dogs and cats, which also bite human beings.

Cu chemical symbol, *copper* (L. *cuprum*).

cu. cubic.

cubit (ku′bit) a unit of linear measure, based on the distance from the elbow to the tip of the middle finger, and ranging from 46 to 53 cm.

cubitus (ku′bĭ-tus) the forearm. adj., **cu′bital**

cuboid (ku′boid) resembling a cube.

cucumber (ku′kum-ber) the fruit of various species of *Cucumis*. **bitter c.,** colocynth.

cuff (kuf) a small, bandlike structure encircling a part or object. **musculotendinous c.,** one formed by intermingled muscle and tendon fibers. **rotator c.,** a musculotendinous structure encircling and giving strength to the shoulder joint.

cuffing (kuf′ing) formation of a cufflike surrounding border, as of leukocytes about a blood vessel observed in certain infections.

cuirass (kwe-ras′) a covering for the chest. **tabetic c.,** an area of diminished sense of touch encircling the chest of a patient with tabes dorsalis.

cul-de-sac (kul-dē-sak′) [Fr.] a blind pouch. **Douglas' c.,** pouch between the anterior wall of the rectum and the posterior wall of the uterus.

culdocentesis (kul″do-sen-te′sis) transvaginal puncture of Douglas' cul-de-sac for aspiration of blood or pus.

culdoscope (kul′do-skōp) an endoscope used in culdoscopy.

culdoscopy (kul-dos′ko-pe) direct examination of uterus and adnexa through an endoscope passed through the wall of the vagina posterior to the cervix.

Culex (ku′leks) a genus of mosquitoes, species of which transmit various disease-producing agents, e.g. microfilariae, sporozoa and viruses.

culicide (ku′lĭ-sīd) an agent which destroys mosquitoes.

culicifuge (ku-lis′ĭ-fūj) an agent which repels mosquitoes.

Culicinae (ku-lĭ-si′ne) a tribe of mosquitoes, including the genera Aedes, Culex, Mansonia, Psorophora and others.

culling (kul′ing) a process of selective separation or removal.

culmen (kul′men), pl. *cul′mina* [L.] the anterior and upper part of the monticulus.

cultivation (kul″tĭ-va′shun) the propagation of living organisms, applied especially to the growth of microorganisms or other cells in artificial media.

culture (kul′tūr) 1. propagation of an organism. 2. a medium for propagating microorganisms. 3. the social heritage. adj., **cul′tural. fractional c.,** obtaining of a single species of microorganism from a culture containing more than one. **gelatin c.,** a bacterial culture on gelatin. **hanging-drop c.,** a culture in which the bacterium is inoculated into a drop of fluid on a coverglass. **plate c.,** a bacterial culture in agar or gelatin on a glass plate. **pure c.,** a culture of a single microorganism. **smear c.,** a culture prepared by smearing the infective material across the surface of the culture medium. **stab c.,** a bacterial culture into which the organisms are introduced by thrusting a needle deep into the medium. **streak c.,** a bacterial culture in which the infectious material is implanted in streaks. **type c.,** a culture that is generally agreed to represent a particular species of microorganisms.

cu. mm. cubic millimeter.

cumulus (ku′mu-lus), pl. *cu′muli* [L.] a small elevation. **c. ooph′orus,** the hillock of cells where the young ovum is buried in the graafian follicle.

cuneate (ku′ne-āt) wedge-shaped.

cuneiform (ku-ne′ĭ-form) wedge-shaped. **c. of carpus,** triquetral.

cuneocuboid (ku″ne-o-ku′boid) pertaining to cuneiform and cuboid bones.

cuneus (ku′ne-us), pl. *cu′nei* [L.] a wedge-shaped lobule on the medial aspect of the occipital lobe of the cerebrum.

cuniculus (ku-nik′u-lus), pl. *cunic′uli* [L.] burrow in the skin made by the itch mite.

cup (kup) a depression or hollow. **glaucomatous c.,** a depression of the optic disk due to persistently increased intraocular pressure, broader and deeper than a physiologic cup, and occurring first at the temporal side of the disk. **physiologic c.,** a slight depression sometimes observed in the optic disk.

cupola (ku'pŏ-lah) cupula.

cupping (kup'ing) 1. formation of a depression in the normally flat optic disk. 2. use or application of a cupping glass to the body surface. **dry c.,** application of a cupping glass to the intact skin to stimulate circulation in the region. **pathologic c.,** depression of the optic disk due to disease. **wet c.,** application of a cupping glass over incised or scarified skin, resulting in withdrawal of blood.

cupric (ku'prik) pertaining to or containing divalent copper. **c. sulfate,** blue crystalline powder, $CuSO_4.5H_2O$; used as an astringent and emetic.

cuprous (ku'prus) pertaining to or containing monovalent copper.

cupruresis (ku"proo-re'sis) the urinary excretion of copper.

cupruretic (-ret'ik) pertaining to or promoting the urinary excretion of copper.

cupula (ku'pu-lah), pl. *cu'pulae* [L.] a small, inverted cup or dome-shaped cap over a structure.

curare (koo-rah're) a South American arrow poison; used to produce muscle relaxation in shock therapy and surgical procedures.

curaremimetic (koo-rah"re-mi-met'ik) producing effects similar to those of curare.

curb (kerb) a thickening of the plantar tarsal ligament, producing an enlargement on the fibular tarsal bone and causing lameness in horses.

cure (kūr) 1. a system of treatment. 2. eradication of disease. **Banting c.,** treatment of corpulence by diet. **grape c.,** treatment by a diet consisting of grapes. **hunger c.,** treatment of disease by severe fasting. **Karell c.,** rest in bed and restricted milk diet; for cardiac weakness, renal insufficiency and high blood pressure. **mind c.,** supposed cure of disease by psychic processes. **starvation c.,** hunger cure. **water c.,** hydrotherapy.

curet (ku-ret') a spoon-shaped instrument for cleansing a diseased surface.

curettage (ku"rĕ-tahzh') [Fr.] the cleansing of a diseased surface with a curet. **medical c.,** induction of regression of and flow from the endometrium by administration and withdrawal of a progestational agent. **periapical c.,** removal with a curet of diseased periapical tissue without excision of the root tip.

curette (ku-ret') curet.

curettement (ku-ret'ment) curettage. **physiologic c.,** enzymatic debridement.

curie (ku're) a unit of radioactivity, defined as the quantity of any radioactive nuclide in which the number of disintegrations per second is 3.700×10^{10}.

curiegram (ku'ri-gram) a photographic print made by radium emanation.

curie-hour (ku're-our") a unit of dose equivalent to that obtained by exposure for one hour to radioactive material disintegrating at the rate of 3.7×10^{10} atoms per second.

curietherapy (ku"re-ther'ah-pe) radium therapy.

curioscopy (ku"re-os'ko-pe) the detection and mapping of objects by means of the nuclear radiations coming from them.

curium (ku're-um) a chemical element (*see table*), at. no. 96, symbol Cm.

current (kur'ent) that which flows; electric transmission in a circuit. **action c.,** an electric current aroused in a muscle by its action. **alternating c.,** a current which flows in opposite directions. **ascending c.,** an electric current passing toward a nerve center. **axial c.,** the central colored part of the blood stream. **centrifugal c.,** descending current. **centripetal c.,** ascending current. **constant c.,** **continuous c.,** an uninterrupted electric current. **d'Arsonval c.,** a high-frequency low-voltage current. **descending c.,** a current passed through a nerve from its origin toward its termination. **direct c.,** a current whose direction is always the same. **faradic c.,** a current of induced electricity. **galvanic c.,** a current of galvanic electricity. **high-frequency c.,** an extremely rapid alternating current. **induced c.,** secondary current. **interrupted c.,** a current that is alternately opened and closed. **labile c.,** a current applied to the body with electrodes moving over the surface. **Leduc's c.,** an interrupted direct electric current. **Oudin c.,** a high-frequency current of higher voltage than the ordinary diathermy current. **reversed c.,** a current produced by changing the poles. **secondary c.,** a current of induced electricity. **sinusoidal c.,** an alternating faradic current whose potential repeatedly rises from zero to maximum and returns to zero again. **stabile c.,** a current applied to the body with both electrodes stationary. **Tesla's c.,** d'Arsonval current.

curse (kers) an affliction thought to be invoked by a malevolent spirit. **Ondine's c.,** impairment of autonomic control of respiration, sometimes due to encephalitis, voluntary control remaining intact.

curtometer (ker-tom'ĕ-ter) instrument for measuring curved surfaces.

curvatura (ker"vah-tu'rah), pl. *curvatu'rae* [L.] curvature.

curvature (ker'vah-tūr) a nonangular deviation from a normally straight course. **Pott's c.,** curvature of the vertebral column after Pott's disease. **spinal c.,** abnormal deviation of the vertebral column.

curve (kerv) a line which is not straight, or which describes part of a circle, especially a line representing varying values in a graph. **Barnes' c.,** the segment of a circle the center of which is the sacral promontory, its concavity being directed dorsally. **c. of Carus,** the normal axis of the pelvic outlet. **dental c.,** the curve of the dental arch as viewed from the occlusal aspect. **frequency c.,** a curve representing graphically the probabilities of different numbers of recurrences of an event.

growth c., the curve obtained by plotting increase in size or numbers against the elapsed time. **isodose c's,** lines delimiting body areas receiving the same quantity of radiation in radiotherapy. **muscle c.,** myogram. **Price-Jones c.,** a graphic curve representing the variation in the size of the red blood corpuscles. **probability c.,** frequency curve. **Spee's c.,** the line described by the tops of the buccal cusps of the teeth from the first premolar to the third molar, viewed from the side. **temperature c.,** a graphic tracing showing the variations in temperature at different times. **tension c's,** lines observed in cancellous tissue of bones, determined by the exertion of stress during development. **Traube's c's,** long curves in a sphygmogram produced by holding the breath. **Wunderlich's c.,** the typical temperature curve of typhoid fever.

cushion (koosh'un) a soft or padlike part. **digital c.,** a wedge-shaped mass of white and elastic fibers, containing fat and cartilage, and overlying the frog of a horse's foot. **endocardial c's,** elevations on the atrioventricular canal of the embryonic heart which later help form the interatrial septum.

cusp (kusp) a pointed projection, such as on the crown of a tooth, or a segment of a cardiac valve.

cuspid (kus'pid) a canine tooth.

cuspidate (kus'pĭ-dāt) provided with cusps.

cuspis (kus'pis), pl. *cus'pides* [L.] a cusp.

cutaneous (ku-ta'ne-us) pertaining to the skin.

cutdown (kut'down) creation of a small incised opening, especially in a vein (*venous cut down*), to permit the passage of tubing to facilitate withdrawal of blood or transfusion of fluids.

cuticle (ku'tĭ-kl) 1. the outermost layer of the skin. 2. the flattened, elastic, keratinous rim of the posterior nail fold. **dental c.,** a membrane covering the surface of the crown of a tooth at the time of eruption. **enamel c.,** dental cuticle; Nasmyth's membrane.

cuticula (ku tik'u lah), pl. *cutic'ulae* [L.] cuticle.

cuticularization (ku-tik"u-ler-i-za'shun) epithelialization.

cutireaction (ku"tĭ-re-ak'shun) a response of the skin to application or introduction of an antigen. **von Pirquet's c.,** Pirquet reaction.

cutis (ku'tis) the outer protective covering of the body; the skin. **c. anseri'na,** erection of the papillae of the skin, as from cold or shock. **c. elas'tica, c. hyperelas'tica,** a hereditary condition with hyperelasticity of the skin, hyperlaxity of the joints, and other abnormalities. **c. lax'a,** a lax condition of the skin, with loss of elasticity and no tendency to return to normal when stretched. **c. marmora'ta,** transitory mottled discoloration of skin sometimes due to exposure to cold. **c. pen'dula,** cutis laxa. **c. rhomboida'lis nu'chae,** thickening of the skin of the neck with striking accentuation of its markings, giving an appearance of diamond-shaped plaques. **c. testa'cea,** a general seborrhea. **c. unctuo'sa,** seborrhea. **c.**

ve'ra, corium. **c. ver'ticis gyra'ta,** deep furrowing of the skin of the entire scalp or invading only a limited area, suggestive of the gyri of the cerebral hemispheres.

cutitis (ku-ti'tis) dermatitis.

cutization (ku"tĭ-za'shun) conversion into skin.

cuvette (ku-vet') [Fr.] a glass container generally having well defined characteristics (dimensions, optical properties), to contain solutions or suspensions for study.

cwt. hundredweight.

Cy. cyanogen.

cyan(o)- (si'ah-no) word element [Gr.], *blue.*

cyanemia (si"ah-ne'me-ah) blueness of the blood.

cyanephidrosis (si"an-ef"ĭ-dro'sis) the excretion of bluish sweat.

cyanhemoglobin (-he"mo-glo'bin) a compound formed by action of hydrocyanic acid on hemoglobin, which gives the bright red color to blood.

cyanhidrosis (-hī-dro'sis) cyanephidrosis.

cyanide (si'ah-nīd) a binary compound of cyanogen.

cyanmetmyoglobin (si"an-met-mi"o-glo'bin) a compound formed from metmyoglobin by addition of the cyanide ion to yield reduction to the ferrous state.

cyanochroia (si"ah-no-kroi'ah) cyanosis.

cyanocobalamin (si"ah-no-ko-bal'ah-min) a substance having hematopoietic activity apparently identical with that of the antianemia factor of liver; called also vitamin B_{12}. **radioactive c.,** cyanocobalamin containing radioactive cobalt of mass number 57 or 60, used in diagnosis of pernicious anemia.

cyanoderma (-der'mah) blueness of the skin.

cyanogen (si-an'o-jen) a poisonous gas, CN.CN.

cyanogenesis (si"ah-no-jen'ē-sis) the formation of cyanogen or hydrocyanic acid.

cyanogenetic (-jĕ-net'ik) pertaining to or characterized by the formation of hydrocyanic acid.

cyanomycosis (-mi-ko'sis) development of *Micrococcus pyocyaneus* in pus.

cyanopathy (si"ah-nop'ah the) cyanosis.

cyanophil (si-an'o-fil) a cell staining easily with blue dyes. adj., **cyanoph'ilous.**

cyanopia (si"ah-no'pe-ah) cyanopsia.

cyanopsia (si"ah-nop'se-ah) defect of vision in which objects appear tinged with blue.

cyanosed (si'ah-nōsd) affected with cyanosis.

cyanosis (si"ah-no'sis) a bluish discoloration of skin and mucous membranes due to excessive concentration of reduced hemoglobin in the blood. adj., **cyanot'ic. central c.,** severe generalized cyanosis with reduced oxygen saturation of arterial blood. **peripheral c.,** that due to an excessive amount of reduced hemoglobin in the venous blood as a result of extensive oxygen extraction at the capillary level. **pulmonary c.,** central cyanosis due to poor oxygenation of the blood in the lungs. **c. ret'inae,** cyanosis of the retina, observable in certain congenital cardiac defects. **shunt c.,** central cyanosis due to the mixing of unoxygenated blood with arterial blood in the heart or great vessels.

cyasma (si-az′mah) pigmentation of the skin of pregnant women.

cybernetics (si″ber-net′iks) the science of communication and control in the animal and in the machine.

cycl(o)- (si′klo) word element [Gr.], *round; recurring ciliary body of the eye.*

Cyclaine (si′klān) trademark for preparations of hexylcaine hydrochloride.

Cyclamycin (si′klah-mi″sin) trademark for preparations of triacetyloleandomycin.

cyclandelate (si-klan′dē-lāt) a vasodilator for peripheral vascular disease.

cyclarthrosis (si″klar-thro′sis) a rotary joint.

cycle (si′kl) a succession or recurring series of events. **carbon c.**, the steps by which carbon is extracted from the atmosphere, incorporated in the body of living organisms, and ultimately returned to the air. **cardiac c.**, a complete cardiac movement, or heart beat, including systole, diastole and intervening pause. **citric acid c.**, tricarboxylic acid cycle. **estrous c.**, the sequence of changes in the reproductive tract of female mammals other than primates, culminating in the interval of heightened intensity of the sex urge known as estrus. **glycolytic c.**, the successive steps by which glucose is broken down in living tissues. **hair c.**, the successive phases of hair growth, from initiation to loss from the follicle. **Krebs c.**, tricarboxylic acid cycle. **menstrual c.**, the correlated phenomena recurring in the reproductive system of female primates during the period of reproductive life, culminating in menstruation. **mosquito c.**, that period in the life of a malarial parasite that is spent in the body of the mosquito host. **nitrogen c.**, the steps by which nitrogen is extracted from the nitrates of soil and water, incorporated as amino acids and proteins in the body of living organisms, and ultimately reconverted to nitrates. **ornithine c.**, reactions in metabolism of proteins in the liver, involving sequential formation of ornithine and arginine, which splits into urea and a molecule of ornithine, which again begins the cycle. **ovarian c.**, the sequence of physiologic changes in the ovary involved in ovulation. **reproductive c.**, the cycle of physiologic changes in the reproductive organs, from the time of fertilization of the ovum through gestation and parturition. **sex c.**, **sexual c.**, 1. the physiologic changes recurring regularly in the genital organs of female mammals when pregnancy does not supervene. 2. the period of sexual reproduction in an organism which also reproduces asexually. **tricarboxylic acid c.**, the cyclic metabolic mechanism by which the complete oxidation of the acetyl moiety of acetyl-coenzyme A is effected. **uterine c.**, the phenomena occurring in the uterus coincident with the estrous or menstrual cycle. **vaginal c.**, the phenomena occurring in the vagina coincident with the estrous or menstrual cycle.

cyclectomy (si-klek′to-me) excision of a piece of the ciliary body.

cyclencephalus (si″klen-sef′ah-lus) a monster with one eye at the median line.

cyclicotomy (si″klī-kot′o-me) division of the ciliary body.

cyclitis (si-kli′tis) inflammation of the ciliary body.

cyclizine (si′klī-zēn) an antihistaminic and antinauseant to prevent motion sickness.

cyclobarbital (si″klo-bar′bī-tal) a short- to intermediate-acting barbiturate, $C_{24}H_{30}CaN_4$-O_6.

cyclocephalus (-sef′ah-lus) cyclencephalus.

cycloceratitis (-ser″ah-ti′tis) cyclokeratitis.

cyclochoroiditis (-ko″roi-di′tis) inflammation of ciliary body and choroid.

cyclodamia (-da″me-ah) suppression of visual accommodation, used in refraction of the eyes.

cyclodialysis (-di-al′ī-sis) creation of a communication between the anterior chamber of the eye and the suprachoroidal space, in glaucoma.

cyclodiathermy (-di″ah-ther′me) destruction of the ciliary body by diathermy.

cycloduction (-duk′shun) movement of the eyeball produced by the oblique muscle.

cycloelectrolysis (-e″lek-trol′ī-sis) destruction of the ciliary body by passage of electric current.

cyclogram (si′klo-gram) a tracing of the visual field made with a cycloscope.

Cyclogyl (si′klo-jil) trademark for a preparation of cyclopentolate.

cycloid (si′kloid) characterized by variations of mood from happiness to depression.

cyclokeratitis (si″klo-ker″ah-ti′tis) inflammation of cornea and ciliary body.

cyclomethycaine (-meth′ī-kān) a cyclohexyl-oxybenzoate derivative used as a surface anesthetic.

cyclopentamine (-pen′tah-mēn) a sympathomimetic nasal decongestant and hypertensive.

cyclopentolate (-pen′to-lāt) a drug used to produce parasympathetic blockade and topically to the conjunctiva to dilate the pupil and paralyze accommodation.

cyclophoria (-fo′re-ah) tendency of the eyeball to rotate on its anteroposterior axis. **negative c.**, tendency of the upper segment of the eye to rotate toward the median line. **positive c.**, tendency of the upper segment of the eye to rotate toward the temporal side.

cyclophosphamide (-fos′fah-mīd) a white, crystalline powder used as an antineoplastic agent.

cyclophrenia (-fre′ne-ah) cyclothymia.

cyclopia (si-klo′pe-ah) a developmental anomaly characterized by a single orbital fossa, with the globe absent or rudimentary, apparently normal or duplicated.

cycloplegia (si″klo-ple′je-ah) paralysis of the ciliary structure of the eye.

cycloplegic (-ple′jik) 1. causing cycloplegia. 2. an agent which produces cycloplegia.

cyclopropane (-pro′pān) a colorless, highly inflammable gas, C_3H_6, used in general anesthesia.

cyclops (si'klops) a fetal monster exhibiting cyclopia.

cycloscope (si'klo-skōp) a form of perimeter for mapping the visual fields.

cycloserine (si"klo-ser'ēn) an antibiotic substance elaborated by *Streptomyces orchidaceus* or *S. garyphalus*, used in treatment of urinary tract infections.

cyclosis (si-klo'sis) displacement of components in the protoplasm of a cell, without external deformation of the cell wall.

Cyclospasmol (si"klo-spaz'mol) trademark for preparations of cyclandelate.

cyclothymia (-th'mē-ah) a condition characterized by alternating moods of elation and dejection. adj., **cyclothy'mic.**

cyclotomy (si-klot'o-me) incision of the ciliary muscle.

cyclotron (si'klo-tron) an apparatus for accelerating protons or deutrons to high energies by means of a constant magnet and an oscillating electric field.

cyclotropia (si"klo-tro'pe-ah) rotation of the eyeball on its anteroposterior axis. **negative c.**, rotation of the upper segment of the eye toward the median line. **positive c.**, rotation of the upper segment of the eye toward the temporal side.

cycrimine (si'kri-min) an agent used to produce parasympathetic blockade and in treatment of parkinsonism.

cyesiognosis (si-e"se-og-no'sis) the diagnosis of pregnancy.

cyesiology (si-e"se-ol'o-je) scientific study of the phenomena of pregnancy.

cyesis (si-e'sis) pregnancy. adj., **cyet'ic.**

cyl. cylinder; cylindric (lens).

cylicotomy (sil"ĭ-kot'o-me) cyclotomy.

cylindroadenoma (sil"in-dro-ad"ē-no'mah) a degenerated adenoma containing cylindrical masses.

cylindrodendrite (-den'drīt) paraxon.

Cylindrogloea (-gle'ah) a genus of Schizomycetes (order Pseudomonadales, suborder Rhodobacterinieae, family Chlorobacteriaceae).

cylindroid (sil'in-droid) 1. shaped like a cylinder. 2. a mucous or spurious cast in urine.

cylindroma (sil"in-dro'mah) malignant tumor, especially about the face. adj., **cylindrom'-atous.**

cylindrosarcoma (sil"in-dro-sar-ko'mah) a tumor containing elements of cylindroma and sarcoma.

cylindruria (sil"in-droo're-ah) presence of cylindroids in the urine.

cyllosis (sĭ-lo'sis) clubfoot or other deformity of the foot.

cymbocephalic (sim"bo-sē-fal'ik) scaphocephalic.

cynanche (sĭ-nan'ke) severe sore throat with threatened suffocation. **c. malig'na**, putrid sore throat. **c. tonsilla'ris**, quinsy.

cynanthropy (sin-an'thro-pe) delusion in which the patient believes himself a dog.

cyniatrics (sin"e-at'riks) the study of the diseases of dogs.

cynobex (sin'o-beks) dry cough of early youth.

cynophobia (sin"o-fo'be-ah) morbid fear of dogs.

cyogenic (si"o-jen'ik) producing pregnancy.

cyotrophy (si-ot'ro-fe) nutrition of the fetus.

cypridopathy (sip"rĭ-dop'ah-the) any venereal disease.

cypridophobia (sip"rĭ-do-fo'be-ah) morbid fear of acquiring venereal disease.

cyprinin (sip'rĭ-nin) a toxic substance derived from the milt of the carp.

cyproheptadine (si"pro-hep'tah-dēn) a piperidine derivative used as an antihistaminic and antiserotonin.

cyrtometer (sir-tom'e-ter) an instrument for determining the dimensions of curved surfaces.

cyrtosis (sir-to'sis) backward curvature of the spine.

cyst (sist) a pathologic, epithelium-lined cavity usually containing fluid or semisolid material. **adventitious c.**, one formed about a foreign body. **Baker's c.**, a swelling about the knee due to escape of synovial fluid in popliteal bursitis. **Blessig's c's**, cystic spaces formed at the periphery of the retina. **blood c.**, hematoma. **blue dome c.**, a benign retention cyst of the breast which shows a blue color. **bone c., aneurysmal,** a solitary lesion of bone which causes a bulging of the overlying cortex, resembling somewhat the saccular protrusion of the aortic wall in aortic aneurysm. **Boyer's c.**, cyst of the subhyoid bursa. **branchial c., branchial cleft c., branchiogenetic c., branchiogenous c.**, one formed from an incompletely closed branchial cleft. **chocolate c.**, one with dark, syrupy contents, resulting from a collection of brownish serum, as may occur in the ovary in ovarian endometriosis. **colloid c.**, one with jelly-like contents. **daughter c.**, a small cyst developed from the walls of a large cyst. **dentigerous c.**, a common type of odontogenic cyst, nearly always involving or associated with the crown of a normal permanent tooth. **dermoid c.**, one containing bone, hair, teeth, etc. **echinococcus c.**, hydatid cyst. **fissural c.**, one occurring along the line separating adjoining processes or structures that normally fuse in embryonic development. **follicular c.**, dentigerous cyst. **globulo-maxillary c**, a bony cyst of the maxilla at the junction of the globular portion of the medial nasal process and the maxillary process. **hydatid c.**, echinococcus cyst; the cyst stage of an embryonic tapeworm, the cyst containing daughter cysts with many scolices. **incisive canal c.**, median anterior maxillary cyst. **keratinous c.**, a slow-growing globular tumor in the skin, distinguishable from a sebaceous cyst by its solid, crumbly content. **median anterior maxillary c.**, one in or near the incisive canal, arising from proliferation of epithelial remnants of the nasopalatine duct or from remnants of the dental lamina anterior to the incisive canal. **median palatal c.**, one in the midline of the hard palate, between the lateral palatal processes. **meibomian c.**, chalazion. **mother c.**, an echinococcus cyst containing smaller cysts. **nabothian**

c., a cystic dilatation caused by inflammatory stenosis of the glands of the uterine cervix. **nasoalveolar c.,** a fissural cyst arising at the junction of the globular portion of the medial nasal process, the lateral nasal process and the maxillary process. **nasolabial c.,** nasoalveolar cyst. **nasopalatine duct c.,** median anterior maxillary cyst. **odontogenic c.,** one derived from epithelium associated with development of the dental structures. **periodontal c., apical,** radicular cyst. **pilonidal c.,** a congenital lesion in the midline of the sacral region, overlying the junction of sacrum and coccyx, lined with epithelium and producing hair, sebum and keratin. **preauricular c.,** congenital, one due to imperfect fusion of the first and second branchial arches in formation of the auricle, communicating with a pitlike depression in front of the helix and above the tragus (ear pit). **primordial c.,** a rare type of odontogenic cyst developing before calcified enamel or dentin is formed, and found in place of a tooth. **radicular c.,** a lesion formed by proliferation of epithelial cells within an apical granuloma. **retention c.,** a tumor-like accumulation of secretion whose natural outlet is obstructed. **sebaceous c.,** a slow-growing, globular tumor in the skin, containing a milky or viscous cheeselike material. **seminal c.,** one containing semen. **sublingual c.,** ranula. **tarry c.,** one resulting from hemorrhage into a corpus luteum. **tarsal c.,** chalazion. **theca-lutein c.,** a cyst of the ovary in which the cystic cavity is lined with theca interna cells. **unilocular c.,** one with a single cavity. **wolffian c.,** a cyst of the broad ligament developed from vestiges of the wolffian body, or mesonephros.

cyst(o)- (sis'to) word element [Gr.], *cyst; bladder.*

cystadenoma (sis-tad″ē-no'mah) cystoma blended with adenoma. **mucinous c.,** a multilocular tumor of the ovary, filled with a stringy mucoid material. **serous c.,** a cystic tumor of the ovary containing thin, clear yellow serum and some solid tissue.

cystalgia (sis-tal'je-ah) pain in the bladder.

cystathionine (sis″tah-thi'o-nēn) a thio-ether of cysteine and methionine which occurs as an intermediate in cystine synthesis.

cystathioninuria (-thi″o-nin-u're-ah) the excretion of cystathionine in the urine.

cystatrophia (-tro'fe-ah) atrophy of the bladder.

cystduodenostomy (sist″du-od″ē-nos'to-me) internal drainage of a pseudocyst of the pancreas into the duodenum.

cystectasia (sis″tek-ta'ze-ah) incision of the urethra and dilatation of the neck of the bladder for extraction of stone.

cystectomy (sis-tek'to-me) 1. excision of a cyst. 2. excision of the urinary bladder.

cysteine (sis'te-in) an amino acid produced by acid hydrolysis of proteins, readily interconvertible with cystine.

cystencephalus (sis″ten-sef'ah-lus) a fetal monster with a brain like a membranous bag.

cysterethism (sis-ter'ē-thizm) irritability of the bladder.

cystgastrostomy (sist″gas-tros'to-me) internal drainage of a pseudocyst of the pancreas into the stomach.

cystic (sis'tik) 1. pertaining to cysts. 2. relating to a bladder, especially the urinary bladder.

cysticercosis (sis″tĭ-ser-ko'sis) infection with cysticerci.

cysticercus (-ser'kus), pl. *cysticer'ci* [Gr.], a larval form of tapeworm.

cystiform (sis'tĭ-form) resembling a cyst.

cystigerous (sis-tij'er-us) containing cysts.

cystine (sis'tēn, sis'tĭn) a naturally occurring amino acid, the chief sulfur-containing component of the protein molecule.

cystinemia (sis″tĭ-ne'me-ah) cystine in the blood.

cystinosis (-no'sis) a congenital metabolic disturbance characterized by deposition of cystine throughout the reticuloendothelial system and in various organs, notably the kidneys.

cystinuria (-nu're-ah) excretion in the urine of excessive cystine as a result of a genetically determined error of renal transport.

cystistaxis (-stak'sis) oozing of blood into the bladder.

cystitis (sis-ti'tis) inflammation of the urinary bladder. **allergic c.,** that due to some unusual hypersensitivity. **bacterial c.,** that occurring as a complication of bacterial infection elsewhere in the body. **catarrhal c., acute,** cystitis resulting from injury, irritation of foreign bodies, gonorrhea, etc., and by burning in the bladder, pain in the urethra and painful micturition. **croupous c.,** diphtheritic cystitis. **cystic c., c. cys'tica,** cystitis with the formation of submucosal cysts in the bladder neck. **diphtheritic c.,** that due to infection by *Corynebacterium diphtheriae,* with formation of a false membrane. **c. emphysemato'sa,** cystitis with gas-filled vesicles and cysts in the bladder mucosa and musculature. **eosinophilic c.,** a form with large numbers of eosinophils in the urinary sediment. **exfoliative c.,** cystitis with sloughing of the mucous membrane of the bladder. **c. follicula'ris,** cystitis in which the bladder mucosa is studded with nodules containing lymph follicles. **c. glandula'ris,** that in which the mucosa contains mucin-secreting glands. **interstitial c., chronic,** a bladder condition with an inflammatory lesion, usually in the vertex, and involving the entire thickness of the wall. **mechanical c.,** that due to irritation by a vesical calculus or a foreign body in the bladder. **panmural c.,** interstitial cystitis, chronic. **c. papillomato'sa,** inflammation of the trigone of the bladder. **c. seni'lis femina'rum,** chronic cystitis occurring in old women, marked by frequency of micturition, with tenesmus and burning. **submucous c.,** interstitial cystitis, chronic.

cystitome (sis'tĭ-tōm) an instrument for incising the capsule of the crystalline lens.

cystitomy (sis-tit'o-me) incision of the capsule of the crystalline lens.

cystjejunostomy (sist"je-ju-nos'to-me) internal drainage of a pseudocyst of the pancreas into the jejunum.

cystoadenoma (sis"to-ad"ĕ-no'mah) cystadenoma.

cystocarcinoma (-kar"sĭ-no'mah) cystoma blended with carcinoma.

cystocele (sis'to-sēl) herniation of the urinary bladder into the vagina.

cystodynia (sis"to-din'e-ah) pain in the bladder.

cystoelytroplasty (-el'ĭ-tro-plas"te) surgical repair of a vesicovaginal fistula.

cystoepithelioma (-ep"ĭ-the"le-o'mah) cystoma blended with epithelioma.

cystofibroma (-fi-bro'mah) fibroma blended with cystoma.

cystogastrostomy (-gas-tros'to-me) surgical anastomosis of a pancreatic cyst to the stomach.

cystogram (sis'to-gram) the film obtained by cystography. **voiding c.**, a radiograph of the urinary tract made while the patient is urinating.

cystography (sis-tog'rah-fe) radiography of the urinary bladder. **voiding c.**, radiography of the bladder while the patient is urinating.

cystoid (sis'toid) resembling a cyst.

cystojejunostomy (sis"to-je-ju-nos'to-me) surgical anastomosis of a pancreatic cyst to the jejunum.

cystolith (sis'to-lith) a vesical calculus.

cystolithectomy (sis"to-li-thek'to-me) removal of a vesical calculus.

cystolithiasis (-li-thi'ah-sis) formation of vesical calculi.

cystolithic (-lith'ik) pertaining to a vesical calculus.

cystolithotomy (-li-thot'o-me) incision of the urinary bladder with removal of calculus.

cystolutein (-lu'te-in) yellow pigment from ovarian cysts.

cystoma (sis-to'mah) a cystic tumor.

cystometer (sis-tom'ĕ-ter) an apparatus for measuring the capacity of the bladder and the pressure reactions caused by injecting fluid into it.

cystometrogram (sis"to-met'ro-gram) the record obtained by cystometrography.

cystometrography (-mĕ-trog'rah-fe) the graphic recording of intravesical volumes and pressures.

cystomorphous (-mor'fus) resembling a cyst or bladder.

cystomyxo-adenoma (-mik"so-ad"ĕ-no'mah) cystomyxoma blended with adenoma.

cystomyxoma (-mik-so'mah) myxoma with cystic degeneration.

cystonephrosis (-ne-fro'sis) cystiform dilatation of the kidney.

cystoneuralgia (-nu-ral'je-ah) neuralgia of the bladder.

cystoparalysis (-pah-ral'ĭ-sis) paralysis of the bladder.

cystopexy (sis'to-pek"se) fixation of bladder to abdominal wall.

cystoplasty (sis'to-plas"te) plastic repair of the bladder.

cystoplegia (sis"to-ple'je-ah) paralysis of the bladder.

cystoproctostomy (-prok-tos'to-me) surgical creation of a communication between the urinary bladder and the rectum.

cystoptosis (sis"top-to'sis) prolapse of the bladder into the urethra.

cystopyelitis (sis"to-pi"ĕ-li'tis) inflammation of bladder and renal pelvis.

cystopyelonephritis (-pi"ĕ-lo-ne-fri'tis) inflammation of bladder, renal pelvis and kidney.

cystorrhaphy (sis-tor'ah-fe) suture of the bladder.

cystorrhea (sis"to-re'ah) mucous discharge from the bladder.

cystosarcoma (-sar-ko'mah) sarcoma with contained cysts.

cystoschisis (sis-tos'kĭ-sis) fissure of the bladder.

cystoscirrhus (sis"to-skir'us) hard cancer of the bladder.

cystosclerosis (-skle-ro'sis) a cyst that has undergone sclerosis.

cystoscope (sis'to-skōp) an endoscope especially designed for passing through the urethra into the bladder to permit inspection of the interior of that organ.

cystoscopy (sis-tos'ko-pe) visual examination of the urinary tract with a cystoscope.

cystospermitis (sis"to-sper-mi'tis) inflammation of the seminal vesicles.

cystostomy (sis-tos'to-me) incision of the bladder, with drainage.

cystotomy (sis-tot'o-me) incision of the bladder.

cystoureteritis (sis"to-u-re"ter-i'tis) inflammation of the urinary bladder and ureters.

cystoureterogram (-u-re'ter-o-gram") a roentgenogram of bladder and ureter.

cystourethroscope (-u-re'thro-skōp") an instrument for examining the posterior urethra and bladder.

cyt(o)- (si'to) word element [Gr.], *cell.*

cytase (si'tās) an enzyme contained in phagocytes.

-cyte (sīt) word element [Gr.], *mature cell.*

cytoarchitectonic (si"to-ar"kĭ-tek-ton'ik) pertaining to the structural arrangement of cells.

cytobiology (-bi-ol'o-je) the biology of cells.

cytobiotaxis (-bi"o-tak'sis) cytoclesis.

cytoblast (si'to-blast) the cell nucleus.

cytoblastema (si"to-blas-te'mah) supposed mother liquid from which cells were held to form.

cytocannibalism (-kan'ĭ-bal-izm") destruction of one cell by another.

cytocentrum (-sen'trum) the attraction sphere.

cytocerastic (-sĕ-ras'tik) cytokerastic.

cytochemism (-kem'izm) reaction of body cells to injections of antitoxin, producing in the organism specific antitoxic substances.

cytochemistry (-kem'is-tre) the chemistry of cells.

cytochrome (si'to-krōm) a pigment universally present in aerobic cells; more than 20 such compounds, distinguishable by their spectra of absorption, have been studied.

cytochylema (si"to-ki-le'mah) hyaloplasm (1).

cytocide (si'to-sīd) an agent which destroys cells. adj., **cytoci'dal.**

cytocinesia (si"to-si-ne'ze-ah) cytokinesis.

cytoclasis (si-tok'lah-sis) the destruction of cells. adj., **cytoclas'tic.**

cytoclesis (si"to-kle'sis) a form of energy, totally unrelated to electricity, light, heat or sound, that is generated by living tissues. adj., **cytoclet'ic.**

cytocyst (si'to-sist) a cyst enclosing a mass of merozoites.

cytode (si'tōd) a non-nucleated cell or cell element.

cytodendrite (si"to dcn'drīt) a dendrite given off from the cell itself.

cytodiagnosis (-di"ag-no'sis) diagnosis by examination of cells in body fluids.

cytodieresis (-di-er'ē-sis) cytokinesis.

cytodistal (-dis'tal) remote from the cell of origin.

cytogene (si'to-jēn) a self-perpetuating cytoplasmic particle that traces origin to the genes of the nucleus.

cytogenesis (si"to-jen'ē-sis) development of the cell.

cytogenetic (-jē-net'ik) pertaining to the cellular constituents concerned in heredity, i.e. chromosomes and genes.

cytogeneticist (-jē-net'ĭ-sist) a specialist in cytogenetics.

cytogenetics (-jē-net'iks) the science concerned with cellular and molecular bases of heredity, variation, mutation, morphogenesis and evolution of organisms. adj., **cytogenet'- ical. clinical c.,** the branch of cytogenetics concerned with relations between chromosomal abnormalities and pathologic conditions.

cytogenic (-jen'ik) forming or producing cells.

cytogenous (si-toj'ē-nus) producing cells.

cytoglobin (si"to-glo'bin) a proteid from white blood corpuscles.

cytoglycopenia (-gli"ko-pe'ne-ah) deficient glucose content of blood cells.

cytogony (si-tog'o-ne) cytogenic reproduction.

cytohistogenesis (si"to-his"to-jen'ē-sis) development of the structure of cells.

cytoid (si'toid) resembling a cell.

cytokalipenia (si"to-kal"ĭ-pe'ne-ah) a deficiency of potassium in the cells of the body.

cytokerastic (-kē-ras'tik) pertaining to development of cells from a lower to a higher order.

cytokinesis (-ki-ne'sis) division of the cytoplasm of a cell in the formation of daughter cells.

cytology (si-tol'o-je) the scientific study of cells. **exfoliative c.,** microscopic examination of cells desquamated from a body surface as a means of detecting malignant change.

cytolymph (si'to-limf) hyaloplasm (1).

cytolysin (si-tol'ĭ-sin) a lysin or antibody which produces disintegration of cells.

cytolysis (si-tol'ĭ-sis) the dissolution of cells.

cytomegaloviruria (si"to-meg"ah-lo-vi-roo're-ah) presence in the urine of cytomegaloviruses.

cytomegalovirus (si"to-meg"ah-lo-vi'rus) one of a group of highly host-specific viruses infecting man, monkeys or rodents, producing unique large cells with intranuclear inclusions.

Cytomel (si'to-mel) trademark for a preparation of the sodium salt of liothyronine.

cytometaplasia (si"to-met"ah-pla'ze-ah) change in function or form of cells.

cytometer (si-tom'ē-ter) device for counting cells.

cytometry (si-tom'ē-tre) the counting of blood cells.

cytomitome (si"to-mi'tōm) a fibril, or fibrillar network, of spongioplasm.

cytomorphology (-mor-fol'o-je) the morphology of body cells.

cytomorphosis (-mor-fo'sis) the changes through which cells pass in development.

cytomycosis (-mi-ko'sis) histoplasmosis.

cyton (si'ton) the cell body of a neuron.

cytopathic (si"to-path'ik) pertaining to or characterized by pathologic changes in cells.

cytopathogenesis (-path"o-jen'ē-sis) production of pathologic changes in cells. adj., **cytopathogenet'ic.**

cytopathogenic (-path"o-jen'ik) capable of producing pathologic changes in cells.

cytopathogenicity (-path"o-je-nis'ĭ-te) the ability to cause pathologic changes in cells.

cytopathology (-pah-thol'o-je) the study of cells in disease.

cytopenia (-pe'ne-ah) deficiency in the cells of the blood.

Cytophaga (si-tof'ah-gah) a genus of Schizomycetes (order Myxobacterales, family Cytophagaceae) which dissolve vegetable fiber and hydrolyze cellulose.

Cytophagaceae (si"to-fah-ga'se-e) a family of Schizomycetes (order Myxobacterales) which are saprophytic soil microorganisms.

cytophagocytosis (-fag"o-si-to'sis) cytophagy.

cytophagous (si-tof'ah-gus) devouring or consuming cells.

cytophagy (si-tof'ah-je) absorption of cells by other cells.

cytophilic (si"to-fil'ik) having an affinity for cells.

cytophylaxis (-fi-lak'sis) the protection of cells against cytolysis.

cytophyletic (-fi-let'ik) pertaining to the genealogy of cells.

cytophysics (-fiz'iks) the physics of cell activity.

cytophysiology (-fiz"e-ol'o-je) the physiology of cells.

cytoplasm (si'to-plazm) the protoplasm of a cell surrounding the nucleus.

cytoplastin (si'to-plas"tin) the plastin of cytoplasm.

cytoproximal (si"to-prok'sĭ-mal) nearest the cell of origin.

cytoscopy (si-tos'ko-pe) examination of cells.

cytosine (si'to-sēn) a base, oxyaminopyrimidine, $C_4H_5N_3O$, one of the disintegration products of nucleic acid.

cytosome (si'to-sōm) the specific body of protoplasm in a particular cell.

cytospongium (si"to-spun'je-um) the spongioplasm of a cell.

cytost (si'tost) a specific toxin given off from a cell as a result of injury to it.

cytostatic (si"to-stat'ik) 1. checking the growth and multiplication of cells. 2. an agent that suppresses the growth and multiplication of cells.

cytostome (si'to-stōm) the oral aperture of protozoa.

cytostromatic (si"to-stro-mat'ik) pertaining to the stroma of a cell.

cytotaxis (-tak'sis) the movement of a cell in response to stimulation by another cell. adj., **cytotac'tic**.

cytotherapy (-ther'ah-pe) treatment by use of animal cells.

cytothesis (si-toth'ē-sis) restitution of cells to their normal condition.

cytotoxic (si"to-tok'sik) having a deleterious effect upon cells.

cytotoxicosis (si"to-tok"sī-ko'sis) a toxic state of the cells.

cytotoxin (-tok'sin) a toxin having a specific destructive effect on cells.

cytotrophoblast (-trof'o-blast) a relatively thin layer of the trophoblast located next to the cavity of the blastocyst and composed of distinct cells.

cytotropic (-trop'ik) having an affinity for cells.

Cytoxan (si-tok'san) trademark for preparations of cyclophosphamide.

cytozoic (si"to-zo'ik) 1. living within or attached to cells. 2. pertaining to a cytozoon.

cytozoon (-zo'on) a protozoan parasite inhabiting a cell.

cytozyme (si'to-zīm) thrombokinase.

cytula (sit'u-lah) the impregnated ovum.

cyturia (sī-tu're-ah) presence of cells in the urine.

D

D chemical symbol, *deuterium*.

D. 1. deciduous; density; [L.] *dex'ter* (right); diopter; dose; duration. 2. symbol, *closed circuit*.

dacry(o)- (dak're-o) word element [Gr.], *tears* (lacrimal apparatus of the eye).

dacryagogic (dak"re-ah-goj'ik) 1. inducing a flow of tears. 2. serving as a channel for discharge of secretion of the lacrimal glands.

dacryagogue (dak're-ah-gog) 1. causing a flow of tears. 2. an agent which provokes a flow of tears.

dacryelcosis (dak"re-el-ko'sis) ulceration of the lacrimal apparatus.

dacryoadenalgia (dak"re-o-ad"ē-nal'-je-ah) pain in a lacrimal gland.

dacryoadenectomy (-ad"ē-nek'to-me) excision of a lacrimal gland.

dacryoadenitis (-ad"ē-ni'tis) inflammation of a lacrimal gland.

dacryoblennorrhea (-blen"o-re'ah) mucous flow from the lacrimal apparatus.

dacryocele (dak're-o-sēl") hernia of the lacrimal sac.

dacryocyst (dak're-o-sist") the lacrimal sac.

dacryocystalgia (dak"re-o-sis-tal'je-ah) pain in the lacrimal sac.

dacryocystectasia (-sis"tek-ta'ze-ah) dilatation of the lacrimal sac.

dacryocystectomy (-sis-tek'to-me) excision of the lacrimal sac.

dacryocystitis (-sis-ti'tis) inflammation of the lacrimal sac.

dacryocystoblennorrhea (-sis"to-blen"o-re'ah) mucous flow from the lacrimal sac.

dacryocystocele (-sis'to-sēl) protrusion of the lacrimal sac.

dacryocystoptosis (-sis"top-to'sis) prolapse of the lacrimal sac.

dacryocystorhinostenosis (-sis"to-ri"no-ste-no'sis) narrowing of the passage through which the tears enter the nose.

dacryocystorhinostomy (dak"re-o-sis"to-ri-nos'to-me) formation of an opening between lacrimal sac and nasal cavity.

dacryocystorhinotomy (-ri-not'o-me) passage of a probe through the lacrimal sac into the nasal cavity.

dacryocystostenosis (-ste-no'sis) narrowing of the lacrimal sac.

dacryocystostomy (dak"re-o-sis-tos'to-me) incision of the lacrimal sac with drainage.

dacryocystotomy (-sis-tot'o-me) incision of the lacrimal sac.

dacryohemorrhea (-he"mo-re'ah) occurrence of a bloody discharge from the lacrimal glands.

dacryolith (dak're-o-lith") a lacrimal calculus.

dacryoma (dak"re-o'mah) a tumor-like swelling due to obstruction of the lacrimal duct.

dacryon (dak're-on) the point where the lacrimal, frontal and upper maxillary bones meet.

dacryops (dak're-ops) cystic distention of the lacrimal gland.

dacryopyorrhea (dak"re-o-pi"o-re'ah) the discharge of tears mixed with pus.

dacryopyosis (-pi-o'sis) suppuration of the lacrimal apparatus.

dacryorrhea (-re'ah) excessive flow of tears.

dacryostenosis (-ste-no'sis) narrowing of a lacrimal passage or duct.

dacryosyrinx (-sir'inks) lacrimal fistula.

Dactil (dak'til) trademark for preparations of piperidolate hydrochloride.

dactyl (dak'til) a digit.

dactyl(o)- (dak'tī-lo) word element [Gr.], *digit* (finger or toe).

dactylion (dak-til'e-on) webbing of the fingers or toes.

dactylitis (dak"tī-li'tis) inflammation of a finger or toe.

dactylography (-log'rah-fe) the study of fingerprints.

dactylogryposis (dak″tĭ-lo-grĭ-po′sis) permanent flexion of the fingers.

dactylology (dak″tĭ-lol′o-je) communication by signs made with the fingers.

dactylolysis (-lol′ĭ-sis) 1. surgical correction of syndactylia. 2. separation or loss of a finger or toe. **d. sponta′nea,** ainhum.

dactylomegaly (dak″tĭ-lo-meg′ah-le) large size of fingers and toes.

dactyloscopy (dak″tĭ-los′ko-pe) examination of fingerprints for identification.

dactylosymphysis (dak″tĭ-lo-sim′fĭ-sis) syndactyly.

dactylus (dak′tĭ lus), pl. *dac′tyli* [L.] a dactyl, or digit.

dahlin (dah′lin) a purple stain used in histology.

daltonism (dawl′ton-izm) red-green blindness.

damp (damp) a noxious gas in a mine. **after-d.,** a gaseous mixture of nitrogen, carbon dioxide and usually carbon monoxide, formed in a mine by explosion of fire damp or dust. **black d., choke d.,** a gaseous mixture formed in a mine by the gradual absorption of the oxygen and the giving off of carbon dioxide by the coal. **cold d.,** foggy vapor charged with carbon dioxide. **fire d.,** light explosive hydrocarbon gases, chiefly methane, CH_4, found in coal mines. **stink d.,** hydrogen sulfide. **white d.,** carbon monoxide.

damping (damp′ing) steady diminution of the amplitude of successive vibrations of an electric wave or current.

D. and C. dilation and curettement.

dandruff (dan′druf) scaly material shed from the scalp.

Danilone (dan′ĭ-lōn) trademark for a preparation of phenindione.

danthron (dan′thron) a drug used as a laxative.

daphnin (daf′nin) a bitter glycoside, $C_{15}H_{16}O_9$-H_2O, from bark of species of Daphne.

dapsone (dap′sōn) an antibacterial compound, $C_{12}H_{12}N_2O_2S$, used in leprosy and tuberculosis.

Daranide (dar′ah-nīd) trademark for a preparation of dichlorphenamide.

Daraprim (dar′ah-prim) trademark for a preparation of pyrimethamine.

Darbid (dar′bid) trademark for a preparation of isopropamide iodide.

Daricon (dar′ĭ-kon) trademark for a preparation of oxyphencyclimine hydrochloride.

Dartal (dar′tal) trademark for a preparation of thiopropazate dihydrochloride.

dartoid (dar′toid) resembling the dartos.

dartos (dar′tos) the contractile tissue under the skin of the scrotum.

Darvon (dar′von) trademark for a preparation of dextro propoxyphene hydrochloride.

darwinism (dar′wĭ-nizm) the theory of evolution propounded by Darwin.

dasymeter (dah-sim′ĕ-ter) an instrument for measuring density of gases.

daturine (da-tu′rin) hyoscyamine.

db. decibel.

DBI trademark for preparations of phenformin hydrochloride.

D.C. Dental Corps; direct current; Doctor of Chiropractic.

D.D.S. Doctor of Dental Surgery.

DDT dichloro-diphenyl-trichloro-ethane, a powerful insect poison; used in dilution as a powder or in an oily solution as a spray.

deacidification (de″ah-sid″ĭ-fĭ-ka′shun) neutralization of acidity.

deactivation (de-ak″tĭ-va′shun) the process of rendering inactive.

deaf-mute (def′mūt) a person unable to hear or speak.

deaf-mutism (def-mu′tizm) inability to hear or speak.

deafness (def′nes) impairment of hearing. **apoplectiform d.,** Meniere's syndrome. **bass d.,** deafness to certain low tones. **boilermakers' d.,** inability to hear ordinary conversation, with hearing perception increased amid loud noise. **cerebral d.,** that due to a brain lesion. **clang d.,** inability to perceive the more delicate qualities of tone. **conduction d.,** inability to hear due to defect of the impulse-conducting apparatus. **cortical d.,** that due to disease of the cortical centers. **functional d.,** that due to defective functioning of the auditory apparatus without organic lesions. **hysterical d.,** that which may appear or disappear in a hysterical patient without discoverable cause. **labyrinthine d.,** that due to disease of the labyrinth. **mind d.,** failure of perception of auditory stimuli caused by a brain lesion. **nerve d.,** inability to hear due to a lesion of the cochlear portion of the eighth cranial nerve. **perceptive d.,** that due to dysfunction of the end-organ of Corti or of the ganglion cells of the spiral ganglion of the auditory division of the eighth cranial nerve. **psychic d.,** mind deafness. **tone d.,** sensory amusia. **transmission d.,** conduction deafness. **word d.,** auditory aphasia.

dealcoholization (de-al″ko-hol-i-za′shun) removal of alcohol from an object.

deamidation (de-am″ĭ-da′shun) deamidization.

deamidization (-ĭ-za′shun) liberation of the ammonia from an amide.

deaminase (de-am′ĭ-nās) an enzyme that promotes the removal of an amino group from a compound.

deamination (de-am″ĭ-na′shun) removal of the amino group, $-NH_2$, from a compound.

Deaner (de′ner) trademark for a preparation of deanol.

deanol acetaminobenzoate (de′ah-nol as″et-am″ĭ-no-ben′zo-āt) a drug used as a cerebral stimulant.

dearterialization (de″ar-te″re-al-i-za′shun) 1. conversion of arterial blood into venous blood. 2. interruption of the supply of arterial (oxygenated) blood to an organ or part.

death (deth) the apparent extinction of life, as manifested by absence of heart beat and respiration. **apparent d.,** a state of complete interruption of bodily processes from which the patient can be resuscitated. **black d.,** plague. **brain d.,** absence of electrical activity in the brain as revealed by absence of deflection in the tracings obtained by electroencephalography. **cell d.,** complete degeneration or necrosis of cells. **cot d., crib d.,** the death, in its sleeping quarters, of an infant who had previously been apparently normal and well. **fetal d.,** death of the infant in utero, classified as *early* (in the first 20 weeks of gestation), *intermediate* (between 20 and 28 weeks) and *late* (after 28 weeks of gestation). **liver d.,** sudden death following surgical procedures on the gallbladder and bile tracts. **molecular d.,** death of cellular elements, as by ulceration. **neonatal d.,** death of an infant within 28 days after birth. **somatic d.,** death of the whole body.

debilitant (de-bil′ĭ-tant) 1. inducing weakness. 2. an agent which allays excitement.

debility (de-bil′ĭ-te) weakness. **nervous d.,** neurasthenia.

débride (da-brēd′) [Fr.] to subject to removal of foreign matter and devitalized tissue.

débridement (da-brēd-maw′) [Fr.] removal of all foreign material and aseptic excision (removal) of all contaminated and devitalized tissues. **enzymatic d.,** débridement of traumatized or diseased areas by use of proteolytic and fibrinolytic enzymes, such as streptodornase and streptokinase. **surgical d.,** removal of foreign material and devitalized tissue by mechanical methods.

deca- (dek′ah) 1. word element [Gr.], *ten.* See also *deka-.* 2. used in naming units of measurement to indicate a quantity 10 times the unit designated by the root with which it is combined.

decacurie (dek″ah-ku′re) a unit of radioactivity, being 10 curies.

Decadron (dek′ah-dron) trademark for preparations of dexamethasone.

decagram (dek′ah-gram) ten grams; 154.32 grains Troy.

decalcification (de-kal″sĭ-fĭ-ka′shun) removal of calcareous matter from tissues.

decalcify (de-kal′sĭ-fi) to deprive of calcium or its salts.

decaliter (dek′ah-le″ter) ten liters; 2.64 gallons.

decameter (dek′ah-me″ter) ten meters; 32.8 feet.

decannulation (de-kan″u-la′shun) the removal of a cannula.

decanormal (dek″ah-nor′mal) of ten times normal strength.

decantation (de″kan-ta′shun) the pouring of a clear supernatant liquid from a sediment.

decapeptide (dek″ah-pep′tĭd) a peptide containing 10 amino acids.

decapitation (de-kap″ĭ-ta′shun) removal of the head, as of the fetus in utero, or of a bone.

decapsulation (de-kap″su-la′shun) removal of a capsule.

decarboxylation (de″kar-bok″sĭ-la′shun) removal of the carboxyl group from a compound.

decay (de-ka′) 1. the gradual decomposition of dead organic matter. 2. the process or stage of decline; old age and its effects on mind and body. **beta d.,** disintegration of the nucleus

of an unstable radionuclide in which the mass number is unchanged, but atomic number is increased or decreased by 1, as a result of emission of a negatively or positively charged (beta) particle.

decerebrate (de-ser′ĕ-brāt) functionally or anatomically deprived of influence of the brain (cerebrum).

decerebration (de-ser″ĕ-bra′shun) excision of the brain or interruption of its influence by transection of the spinal cord.

decholesterolization (de-ko-les″ter-ol-i-za′-shun) extraction of cholesterol from the system.

Decholin (de′ko-lin) trademark for preparations of dehydrocholic acid.

deci- (des′ĭ) word element [L.], *one-tenth;* used in naming units of measurement to indicate one-tenth of the unit designated by the root with which it is combined (10^{-1}); symbol d.

decibel (des′ĭ-bel) the unit of loudness of sound.

decidua (de-sid′u-ah) the membranous lining of the uterus shed after childbirth or at menstruation. adj., **decid′ual. basal d., d. basa′lis,** that directly underlying the implanting ovum. **capsular d., d. capsula′ris,** that directly overlying the implanting ovum. **menstrual d., d. menstrua′lis,** that which is shed at menstruation. **parietal d., d. parieta′lis,** that lining the uterus elsewhere than at the site of the implanting ovum. **d. reflex′a,** capsular decidua. **d. seroti′na,** basal decidua. **true d., d. ve′ra,** parietal decidua.

decidualitis (de-sid″u-al-i′tis) a bacterial disease leading to changes in the decidua.

deciduate (de-sid′u-āt) characterized by shedding.

deciduation (de-sid″u-a′shun) the shedding of the decidua.

deciduitis (de-sid″u-i′tis) decidual endometritis.

deciduoma (de-sid″u-o′mah) intrauterine tumor derived from a retained decidua. **d. malig′num,** choriocarcinoma.

deciduomatosis (de-sid″u-o″mah-to′sis) excessive proliferation of decidual tissue in the nonpregnant state.

deciduosarcoma (-sar-ko′mah) chorioadenoma.

deciduous (de-sid′u-us) falling off; subject to being shed, as deciduous teeth.

decigram (des′ĭ-gram) one tenth of a gram; 1.54 grains.

deciliter (des′ĭ-le″ter) one tenth of a liter; 3.38 fluidounces.

decimeter (des′ĭ-me″ter) one tenth of a meter; 3.9 inches.

decinormal (des″ĭ-nor′mal) of one tenth normal strength.

decipara (des′ĭ-pah′rah) a woman who has had ten pregnancies which resulted in viable offspring; para X.

declination (dek″lĭ-na′shun) cyclophoria.

declivis (de-kli′vis) [L.] a slope or slanting surface. **d. cerebel′li,** sloping posterior surface of the superior vermis of the cerebellum.

Declomycin (dek'lo-mi"sin) trademark for preparations of demethylchlortetracycline.

decoction (de-kok'shun) 1. the process of boiling. 2. a preparation made by boiling.

décollement (da-kol-maw') [Fr.] separation of an organ from adjoining tissue to which it normally adheres.

decoloration (de-kul"er-a'shun) removal of color.

decompensation (de"kom-pen-sa'shun) failure of compensation, as in heart disease.

decomposition (de-kom"po-zish'un) dissolution, or chemical separation into component elements or simpler compounds. **emotional d.,** breakdown of an emotional adjustment previously stable, or of a defensive system seemingly adequate.

decompression (de"kom-presh'un) return to normal environmental pressure after exposure to greatly increased pressure. **cerebral d.,** removal of a flap of the skull and incision of the dura mater for the purpose of relieving intracranial pressure. **d. of heart,** incision of the pericardium with evacuation of a hematoma. **d. of pericardium,** decompression of heart. **d. of rectum,** proctotomy for imperforate anus. **d. of spinal cord,** incision of spinal cord with removal of hematoma, bone fragments, etc.

decongestant (de"kon-jes'tant) 1. tending to reduce congestion or swelling. 2. an agent that reduces congestion or swelling.

decongestive (-jes'tiv) reducing congestion.

decortication (de-kor"ti-ka'shun) removal of a cortex or of superficial substance. **chemical d., enzymatic d.,** decortication by means of chemical compounds or enzymes.

decrepitation (de-krep"i-ta'shun) crepitation.

decubitus (de-ku'bi-tus) 1. posture in bed. 2. act of lying down. 3. a decubitus ulcer. adj., **decu'bital. Andral's d.,** lying on the unaffected side in the early stages of pleurisy. **dorsal d.,** lying on the back. **lateral d.,** lying on one side, designated *right lateral decubitus* when the subject lies on the right side and *left lateral decubitus* when he lies on the left side. **ventral d.,** lying on the ventral surface, or belly.

decussate (de-kus'āt) 1. to cross in the form of an X. 2. crossed like the letter X.

decussatio (de"kus-sa'she-o), pl. *decussatio'-nes* [L.] decussation.

decussation (de"kus-sa'shun) 1. the position of one part crossing another, similar part. 2. the point of crossing; chiasma. **Forel's d.,** the ventral tegmental decussation of the rubrospinal and rubroreticular tracts in the mesencephalon. **fountain d. of Meynert,** the dorsal tegmental decussation of the tectospinal tract in the mesencephalon. **d. of the pyramids,** the crossing of the fibers of the pyramids of the oblongata from one pyramid to the other. **sensory d.,** the superior pyramidal decussation in the medulla oblongata.

dedifferentiation (de-dif"er-en"she-a'shun) re-

gression from a more specialized or complex form to a simpler state.

deerfly (dēr'fli) a member of the genus Chrysops.

defatted (de-fat'ed) deprived of fat.

defecation (def"ē-ka'shun) 1. elimination of wastes and undigested food, as feces, from the rectum. 2. a chemical process in which impurities are removed by heating, which causes their separation as a heavy scum and precipitate.

defect (de'fekt) a flaw or imperfection. **ectodermal d., congenital,** a rare hereditary condition marked by a smooth, glossy skin, diminished or absent sweat glands, abnormality of the teeth, and defective formation of hair and nails. **filling d.,** an interruption in the contour of the inner surface of stomach or intestine revealed by roentgenography. **retention d.,** a defect in the mental power of attention and remembrance. **septal d.,** a defect in the cardiac septum resulting in an abnormal communication between opposite chambers of the heart.

defective (de-fek'tiv) 1. imperfect. 2. a person lacking in some physical, mental or moral quality.

defeminization (de-fem"i-ni-za'shun) loss of normal secondary sex characters in the female.

defense (de-fens') resistance to or protection from attack. **d. mechanism,** a psychologic reaction or technique for protection against a stressful environmental situation or against anxiety.

deferens (def'er-ens) [L.] deferent.

deferent (def'er-ent) conducting or progressing away from a center or specific site of reference.

deferentectomy (def"er-en-tek'to-me) excision of a ductus deferens.

deferential (-en'shal) pertaining to the ductus deferens.

deferentitis (-en-ti'tis) inflammation of the ductus deferens.

defervescence (def"er-ves'ens) the decline of high temperature (fever) to normal.

defibrillator (de-fi'bri-la"tor) an apparatus to counteract fibrillation.

defibrination (de-fi"bri-na'shun) the destruction or removal of fibrin, as from the blood.

deficiency (de-fish'en-se) a lack or shortage; a condition characterized by presence of less than normal or necessary supply or competence. **oxygen d.,** anoxemia.

deformation (de"for-ma'shun) 1. deformity. 2. the process of deforming.

deformity (de-for'mi-te) distortion or malformation. **Akerlund d.,** indentation of the duodenal cap occurring in duodenal ulcer and revealed in roentgenograms. **Arnold-Chiari d.,** caudal displacement of brain stem, cerebellum and spinal cord. **gunstock d.,** deformity in which the forearm makes an angle with the arm, due to fracture near the elbow. **Madelung's d.,** distortion of the radius at the lower end, with ulnar displacement backward. **reduction d.**, congenital absence of a portion or all of a body part, especially of the limbs. **silver-fork d.**, the peculiar deformity seen in Colles' fracture. **Sprengel's d.**, congenital upward displacement of the scapula. **Volkmann's d.**, congenital tibiotarsal dislocation.

defunctionalization (de-funk"shun-al-i-za'-shun) destruction of a function.

defundation (de"fun-da'shun) excision of the fundus of the uterus.

defurfuration (de-fer"fer-a'shun) the shedding of branlike scales from the skin.

Deg. degeneration; degree.

deganglionate (de-gang'gle-o-nāt") to deprive of ganglia.

degenerate (de-jen'er-āt) 1. to change from a higher to a lower form. (de-jen'er-it). 2. characterized by degeneration. 3. a person whose moral or physical state is below the normal.

degeneration (de-jen"er-a'shun) alteration to a lower or to a less healthy or desirable state. adj., **degen'erative. Abercrombie's d.**, amyloid degeneration. **adipose d.**, fatty degeneration. **albuminoid d., albuminous d.**, cloudy swelling. **amyloid d.**, degeneration with deposit of lardacein in the tissues. **ascending d.**, degeneration of nerve fibers progressing from the site of the original lesion toward the spinal cord and brain. **atheromatous d**, atheroma. **bacony d.**, amyloid degeneration. **calcareous d.**, degeneration of tissue with deposit of calcareous material. **caseous d.**, caseation. **cellulose d.**, amyloid degeneration. **colloid d.**, degeneration with conversion into a gelatinous material. **congenital macular d.**, the infantile type of retinal atrophy. **cystic d.**, degeneration with formation of cysts. **descending d.**, degeneration of nerve fibers extending from the original lesion toward the periphery. **fatty d.**, degeneration of tissue with abnormal accumulation of fat. **fibrinous d.**, necrosis with deposit of fibrin within the cells of the tissue. **fibroid d.**, degeneration into fibrous tissue. **fibrous d.**, fibrosis. **gray d.**, degeneration of the white substance of the spinal cord. **hepatolenticular d.**, a group of diseases characterized by degeneration of the liver cells and of the lenticular nucleus. **hyaline d.**, a regressive change in cells in which the cytoplasm takes on a homogeneous, glassy appearance. **hyaloid d.**, amyloid degeneration. **hydropic d.**, appearance of vacuoles in cytoplasm of cells in certain tissues in relatively mild infections and other conditions. **lardaceous d.**, amyloid degeneration. **mucoid d.**, degeneration with deposit of myelin and lecithin in the cells. **mucous d.**, degeneration with accumulation of mucus in epithelial tissues. **myxomatous d.**, degeneration with accumulation of mucus in connective tissues. **parenchymatous d.**, cloudy swelling. **polypoid d.**, development of polypoid growths on a mucous membrane. **secondary d.**, wallerian degeneration. **vitreous d.**, hyaline degeneration. **wallerian d.**, degeneration of nerve

fibers after separation from their nutritive centers. **waxy d.**, amyloid degeneration. **Zenker's d.**, hyaline degeneration and necrosis of striated muscle.

deglutition (deg"loo-tish'un) the process of taking substance through the mouth and pharynx, past the cricopharyngeal constriction into the esophagus.

degradation (deg"rah-da'shun) conversion of a chemical compound to one less complex by splitting off one or more groups of atoms.

dehiscence (de-his'ens) separation of edges previously joined; the formation of a fissure.

dehumidifier (de"hu-mid'i-fi"er) an apparatus for reducing the content of moisture in the atmosphere.

dehydrase (de-hi'drās) an enzyme which catalyzes the transference of water from a compound.

dehydration (de"hi-dra'shun) the removal of water from a substance.

dehydroandrosterone (de-hi"dro-an-dros'ter-ōn) an androgenic compound derived from male urine.

dehydrocholesterol (-ko-les'ter-ol) calciferol. **activated 7-d.**, cholecalciferol.

dehydrocorticosterone (-kor"tĭ-ko'stēr-ōn) a steroid from the adrenal cortex.

dehydrogenase (de-hi'dro-jen-ās") an enzyme which catalyzes the transference of hydrogen ions. **lactic d.**, an enzyme that catalyzes the oxidation of alpha hydroxy acids to alpha keto acids.

dehydrogenate (de-hi'dro-jen-āt") 1. to remove hydrogen from. 2. a compound from which hydrogen has been removed.

dehypnotize (de-hip'no-tīz) to free from the hypnotic state.

deinsectization (de"in-sek"tĭ-za'shun) elimination of infesting insects.

de-iodination (de-i"o-din-a'shun) the loss or removal of iodine from a compound.

de-ionization (de-i"on-i-za'shun) the removal of ions from a compound.

déjà vu (da'zhah voo') [Fr.] an illusion that a new situation is a repetition of a previous experience.

dejecta (de-jek'tah) excrement.

dejection (de-jek'shun) 1. discharge of feces. 2. depression of spirits.

delacrimation (de-lak"rĭ ma'shun) excessive flow of tears.

delactation (de"lak-ta'shun) 1. weaning. 2. cessation of lactation.

Delalutin (del"ah-lu'tin) trademark for a preparation of hydroxyprogesterone caproate.

delamination (de-lam"ĭ-na'shun) the division of a blastoderm into layers.

Delatestryl (del"ah-tes'tril) trademark for a preparation of testosterone enanthate.

deletion (de-le'shun) in genetics, loss from a chromosome of genetic material.

deligation (de"li-ga'shun) 1. ligation. 2. bandaging.

delinquent (de-lin'kwent) 1. lacking in some respect; characterized by antisocial, illegal or criminal behavior. 2. a person whose conduct is antisocial, illegal or criminal; applied to a minor exhibiting such conduct (*juvenile delinquent*).

deliquescence (del"ĭ-kwes'ens) the process of becoming liquid by absorption of water from the air. adj., **deliques'cent.**

delirium (dĕ-lēr'e-um) a confused and excited state of organic origin marked by incoherence, illusions, hallucinations and disorientation. **chronic alcoholic d.**, Korsakoff's psychosis. **d. tre'mens,** a state of agitation, extreme restlessness, tremulousness, volubility, confusion of thought and speech, disorientation and distractibility, sometimes occurring as a withdrawal symptom in alcoholics.

deliver (de-lĭv'er) 1. to aid in childbirth. 2. to remove, as a fetus, placenta, or lens of the eye.

delivery (de-lĭv'er-e) 1. expulsion or extraction of the child at birth. 2. removal of a part, as the placenta or lens. **abdominal d.**, delivery of an infant through an incision made into the uterus through the abdominal wall. **postmortem d.**, delivery of a child after death of the mother. **spontaneous d.**, birth of an infant without any aid from an attendant. **vaginal d.**, delivery of an infant through the normal openings of the uterus and vagina.

delle (del'e) the clear area in the center of a stained erythrocyte.

delta (del'tah) 1. the fourth letter of the Greek alphabet, Δ or δ; used in chemical names to denote the fourth of a series of isomeric compounds or the carbon atom fourth from the carboxyl group, or to denote the fourth of any series. 2. a triangular area. **d. for'nicis,** a triangular striated depression on the lower side of the fornix.

Delta-cortef (del'tah kor"tef) trademark for a preparation of prednisolone.

deltacortisone (del"tah-kor'tĭ-sōn) prednisone.

Deltalin (del'tah-lin) trademark for a preparation of synthetic vitamin D_2.

Deltasone (del'tah-sōn) trademark for a preparation of prednisone.

deltoid (del'toid) triangular.

deltoiditis (del"toi-di'tis) inflammation of the deltoid muscle.

Deltra (del'trah) trademark for a tablet containing prednisone.

delusion (de-lu'zhun) a false belief inconsistent with an individual's own knowledge and experience. adj., **delu'sional. depressive d.,** a delusion of unworthiness or futility. **expansive d.,** abnormal belief in one's own greatness, goodness or power. **d. of grandeur,** abnormal belief in one's own importance, power, wealth, etc. **d. of negation,** a morbid belief that some part of the body is missing or that the world has ceased to exist. **nihilistic d.,** belief that the self and external reality no longer exist. **d. of persecution,** a morbid belief on the part of a patient that he is being persecuted, slandered and injured. **systematized d.,** a delusion which is organized by the patient in an orderly pattern. **unsystematized d.,** a delusion made up of disconnected parts.

Delvinal (del'vĭ-nal) trademark for preparations of vinbarbital.

demecarium (dem"e-ka're-um) a triethyl-ammonium compound used as a parasympathomimetic and to reduce intraocular pressure in glaucoma.

dementia (de-men'she-ah) progressive mental deterioration due to organic disease of the brain. **paralytic d., d. paralyt'ica,** a chronic disease of the brain characterized by degeneration of the cortical neurons and by progressive loss of mental and physical power, and resulting from antecedent syphilitic infection. **d. prae'cox,** a name formerly given a disorder beginning or exacerbating at puberty, and thought to lead inevitably to progressive mental deterioration (see *schizophrenia*). **secondary d.,** that following another kind of insanity. **senile d.,** a chronic brain disorder due to generalized atrophy of the brain characterized by deterioration in intellectual functions. **terminal d.,** that occurring near the end of another kind of insanity.

Demerol (dem'er-ol) trademark for meperidine.

demethylchlortetracycline (de-meth"il-klor"-tet-rah-si'klēn) a broad-spectrum antibiotic produced by a mutant strain of *Streptomyces aureofaciens;* closely related to the other tetracyclines.

demilune (dem'ĭ-lūn) a crescent-shaped structure or cell. **Heidenhain's d's,** Giannuzzi's crescents.

demineralization (de-min"er-al-i-za'shun) removal of mineral salts.

Demodex (dem'o-deks) a genus of mites parasitic within the hair follicles of the host, including the species *D. folliculo'rum* in man, and several other species in domestic and other animals. **D. ca'nis,** a species of mites that cause mange in dogs.

demogram (de'mo-gram) a graphic representation of the population of a given area according to the time period and the age and sex of the individuals composing it.

demography (de-mog'rah-fe) the science dealing with social statistics, including questions of health, disease, births and mortality.

demorphinization (de-mor"fĭ-nĭ-za'shun) gradual withdrawal of morphine from one addicted to its use.

demucosation (de"mu-ko-za'shun) removal of mucous membrane.

demulcent (de-mul'sent) 1. soothing; bland. 2. a soothing mucilaginous medicine.

denarcotize (de-nar'ko-tīz) to deprive of narcotics or of narcotic properties.

denatured (de-na'tūrd) having its chemical and physical properties changed from the native state, usually irreversibly.

dendraxon (den-drak'son) a nerve cell whose axon splits up into terminal filaments immediately after leaving the cell.

dendriform (den'drĭ-form) tree-shaped.

dendrite (den'drīt) a long, branching protoplasmic process, such as the branches conducting impulses toward the body of a nerve cell. adj., **den'dric.**

dendritic (den-drit'ik) treelike in appearance or form.

dendroid (den'droid) branching like a tree.

dendron (den'dron) dendrite.

dendrophagocytosis (den"dro-fag"o-si-to'sis) the absorption by microglia cells of broken portions of astrocytes.

denervation (de"ner-va'shun) interruption of the nerve connection to an organ or part.

dengue (den'ge) an infectious, eruptive, febrile disease of tropical countries marked by pains in the head, eyes, muscles and joints, and sore throat; caused by a filterable virus and transmitted by mosquitoes of the genus Aedes.

denidation (de"ni-da'shun) the disintegration and removal, during menstruation, of certain epithelial elements, potentially the nidus of an embryo.

dens (dens), pl. *den'tes* [L.] a tooth or toothlike structure. **d. in den'te,** a malformed tooth caused by invagination of the crown before it is calcified, giving the appearance of a "tooth within a tooth."

densimeter (den-sim'ĕ-ter) apparatus for determining density or specific gravity.

densitometer (den"si-tom'ĕ-ter) an instrument for determining the density of a liquid.

densitometry (-tom'ĕ-tre) determination of variations in density by comparison with that of another material or with a certain standard.

density (den'si-te) 1. the quality of being compact; the compactness of a substance. 2. the quantity of electricity in a given area or time.

densography (den-sog'rah-fe) the measurement of the contrast densities in a roentgen negative.

dent(o)- (den'to) word element [L.], *tooth; toothlike.*

dentagra (den-tag'rah) 1. toothache. 2. a forceps or key for pulling teeth.

dental (den'tal) pertaining to the teeth.

dentalgia (den-tal'je-ah) toothache.

dentate (den'tāt) notched; tooth-shaped.

dentia (den'she-ah) 1. dentition. 2. a condition relating to development or eruption of the teeth. **d. pre'cox,** premature eruption of the teeth; presence of teeth in the mouth at birth. **d. tar'da,** delayed eruption of the teeth, beyond the usual time for their appearance.

dentibuccal (den"ti-buk'al) pertaining to cheek and teeth.

denticle (den'ti-kl) 1. a small toothlike process. 2. a distinct calcified mass within the pulp chamber or in the dentin of a tooth.

dentification (den"ti-fi-ka'shun) formation of dentin or tooth substance.

dentifrice (den'ti-fris) a preparation for cleansing and polishing the teeth.

dentigerous (den-tij'er-us) containing or producing teeth.

dentilabial (den"ti-la'be-al) pertaining to teeth and lips.

dentilingual (-ling'gwal) pertaining to teeth and tongue.

dentimeter (den-tim'ĕ-ter) an instrument for measuring teeth.

dentin (den'tin) the chief substance of the teeth, forming the body, neck and roots, being covered by enamel on the exposed parts of the teeth and by cementum on the parts implanted in the jaws. adj., **den'tinal. adherent d., attached d.,** a calcified formation in a pulp chamber partially fused with the dentin. **adventitious d.,** secondary dentin. **circumpulpar d.,** the inner portion of dentin, adjacent to the pulp, consisting of thinner fibrils. **cover d.,** the peripheral portion of dentin, adjacent to the enamel or cementum, consisting of coarser fibers than the circumpulpar dentin. **interglobular d.,** imperfectly calcified dentinal matrix surrounded by calcified globules situated near the periphery of the dentin. **intermediate d.,** the soft matrix of the predentin. **irregular d.,** secondary dentin. **mantle d.,** cover dentin. **opalescent d.,** dentin giving an unusual translucent or opalescent appearance to the teeth, as occurs in dentinogenesis imperfecta. **primary d.,** dentin formed before the eruption of a tooth. **sclerotic d.,** transparent dentin. **secondary d.,** dentin formed after tooth eruption as a result of irritation from caries, abrasion, injury, etc. **transparent d.,** dentin in which Tomes's fibers are calcified.

dentinalgia (den"ti-nal'je-ah) pain in the dentin.

dentinification (den-tin"i-fi-ka'shun) the formation of dentin.

dentinoblast (den-tin'o-blast) a cell that forms dentin.

dentinoblastoma (den"ti-no-blas-to'mah) a tumor of odontogenic origin, composed of round or spindle-shaped connective tissue cells, among which are islands of irregularly shaped masses of dentin.

dentinogenesis (-jen'ĕ-sis) the formation of dentin. **d. imperfec'ta,** imperfect formation of dentin, resulting in an unusual translucent or opalescent hue to the teeth.

dentinogenic (-jen'ik) forming or producing dentin.

dentinoid (den'ti-noid) 1. resembling dentin. 2. predentin. 3. dentinoma.

dentinoma (den"ti-no'mah) an encapsulated tumor of the jaw, containing connective tissue and masses of dentin, with evidence of new dentin formation.

dentinum (den-ti'num) dentin.

dentist (den'tist) a person licensed to practice dentistry. **surgeon d.,** a practitioner of dentistry who has been authorized to excise or remove tooth tissue surgically.

dentistry (den'tis-tre) 1. that branch of the healing arts concerned with the teeth and associated structures of the oral cavity. 2. the work done by dentists, e.g. the creation of restorations, crowns and bridges, and surgical procedures performed in and about the oral cavity. 3. the practice of the dental profession collectively. **cosmetic d., esthetic d.,** dentistry concerned with the repair and restoration of carious, broken or defective teeth in such manner as to improve on their original appearance. **geriatric d.,** gerodontics. **operative d.,** dentistry concerned with restoration of parts of the teeth that are defective as a result of disease, trauma or abnormal development to a state of normal function, health and esthetics. **pediatric d.**, pedodontics. **preventive d.**, dentistry concerned with maintenance of a normal masticating mechanism by fortifying the structures of the oral cavity against damage and disease. **prosthetic d.**, prosthodontics.

dentition (den-tish'un) 1. appearance of the teeth exterior to the surface of the gingivae. 2. the entire array of teeth in a jaw, consisting of natural teeth in position in the alveoli. **deciduous d.**, the complement of teeth which erupt first and are later succeeded by the permanent teeth. **delayed d.**, retarded dentition. **mixed d.**, the complement of teeth in the jaws after eruption of some of the permanent teeth, but before all the deciduous teeth are shed. **permanent d.**, the complement of teeth that erupt after the deciduous teeth have been shed. **postpermanent d.**, teeth that sometimes erupt after extraction of the permanent teeth. **precocious d.**, abnormally accelerated appearance of the deciduous teeth. **predeciduous d.**, cornified epithelial structures resembling erupted teeth, found in the mouth before eruption of the true deciduous teeth. **primary d.**, deciduous dentition. **retarded d.**, abnormally delayed appearance of the deciduous teeth. **secondary d.**, permanent dentition. **transitional d.**, mixed dentition.

dentoalveolar (den″to-al-ve′o-ler) pertaining to a tooth alveolus.

dentoalveolitis (-al″ve-o-li′tis) periodontitis simplex.

dentotropic (-trop′ik) turning toward or having an affinity for tissues composing the teeth.

dentulous (den′tu-lus) having natural teeth.

denture (den′chur) a complement of teeth, either natural or artificial; ordinarily used to designate an artificial replacement for the natural teeth and adjacent tissues. **artificial d.**, an appliance worn in the mouth to replace missing natural teeth and associated structures. **clasp d.**, a partial denture retained with clasps. **complete d.**, an artificial denture replacing all the teeth of one jaw. **continuous gum d.**, an artificial denture consisting of teeth fused to a base covering the gum. **full d.**, complete denture. **immediate d.**, an artificial denture inserted immediately after extraction of the teeth. **implant d.**, one constructed with a metal substructure embedded within the underlying soft structures of the jaws. **partial d.**, a removable or permanently attached appliance replacing one or more missing teeth in one jaw and receiving support and retention from underlying tissues and some or all of the remaining teeth. **permanent d.**, an artificial denture inserted after the tissue layer becomes completely hardened. **trial d.**, an artificial denture made for verification of its esthetic qualities, the making of records or other procedures before the final denture is completed.

denucleated (de-nu″kle-āt″ed) deprived of the nucleus.

denudation (de″nu-da′shun) the stripping or laying bare of any part.

denutrition (de″nu-trish′un) lack or failure of nutrition.

deobstruent (de-ob′stroo-ent) 1. removing obstructions. 2. a medicine which removes obstructions.

deodorant (de-o′dor-ant) 1. destroying odors. 2. a deodorizing agent.

deodorize (de-o′dor-īz) to deprive of odor.

deodorizer (de-o′dor-īz″er) a deodorizing agent.

deontology (de″on-tol′o-je) medical ethics.

deorsum (de-or′sum) [L.] downward.

deorsumduction (de-or″sum-duk′shun) deorsumversion.

deorsumvergence (-ver′jens) deorsumversion.

deorsumversion (-ver′zhun) the turning downward of a part, especially of the eyes.

deossification (de-os″ĭ-fĭ-ka′shun) removal of the mineral elements of bone.

deoxidation (de-ok″sĭ-da′shun) deoxygenation.

deoxycorticosterone (de-ok″sĭ-kor″tĭ-ko-stēr′-ōn) desoxycorticosterone.

deoxygenation (-jĕ-na′shun) removal of oxygen.

deoxyribonuclease (-ri″bo-nu′kle-ās) an enzyme that catalyzes the depolymerization of deoxyribonucleic acid (DNA).

deoxyribonucleoprotein (-ri″bo-nu′kle-o-pro″-te-in) a nucleoprotein in which the sugar is D-2-deoxyribose.

deoxyribose (-ri′bōs) an aldopentose, $CH_2.OH.-(CHOH)_2.CH_2.CHO$, found in thymus nucleic acid.

depersonalization (de-per″sun-al-i-za′shun) a feeling of unreality or strangeness, related to one's self or to the external environment.

dephosphorylation (de-fos″for-ĭ-la′shun) removal of the trivalent PO group from organic molecules.

depilate (dep′ĭ-lāt) to remove hair.

depilation (dep″ĭ-la′shun) removal of hair.

depilatory (de-pil′ah-tor″e) 1. removing hair. 2. an agent which removes the hair.

deplasmolysis (de″plaz-mol′ĭ-sis) return to initial volume, after plasmolysis, of the protoplasm of a cell in hypertonic solution.

depolarization (de-po″lar-i-za′shun) the abolition or disappearance of a difference in electrical charge.

depolymerization (de-pol″ĭ-mer-i-za′shun) the conversion of a compound into one of smaller molecular weight and different physical properties without changing the percentage relations of the elements composing it.

depolymerize (de-pol′ĭ-mē-rīz″) to undergo depolymerization.

deposit (de-poz′it) 1. sediment or dregs. 2. extraneous inorganic matter collected in the tissues or in an organ of the body.

Depo-testosterone (de″po-tes-tos′ter-ōn) trademark for a sustained-action preparation of testosterone.

depressant (de-pres′ant) 1. depressing or retarding. 2. an agent which retards any function. **cardiac d.**, an agent that depresses excitability, conduction velocity and contractility of the myocardium.

depressed (de-prest') pressed down; retarded or lessened.

depression (de-presh'un) 1. reduction of vital or functional activity; in psychiatry, a feeling of morbid sadness or melancholy. 2. a hollow or fossa. **agitated d.,** depression with anxiety, as seen in involutional melancholy. **anaclitic d.,** impairment of an infant's physical, social and intellectual development which sometimes follows a sudden separation from the mothering person. **congenital chondrosternal d.,** congenital deformity with a deep, funnel-shaped depression in the anterior chest wall. **emotional d.,** undue sadness or melancholy, due to no recognizable cause. **involutional d.,** depression sometimes accompanying menopause in women or decline in sexual or vocational activity in men. **pacchionian d's,** depressions in the skull which lodge the pacchionian bodies. **reactive d.,** neurotic or psychotic depression due to environmental loss or stress. **situational d.,** reactive depression.

depressomotor (de-pres"o-mo'tor) diminishing motor action.

depressor (de-pres'or) that which depresses. **tongue d.,** an instrument for pressing down the tongue.

depth (depth) distance measured perpendicularly downward from a surface. **focal d.,** focal length.

deradelphus (der"ah-del'fus) a twin monster with one neck and head.

deradenitis (der"ad-ē-ni'tis) inflammation of the glands of the neck.

deradenoncus (-nong'kus) swelling of a gland of the neck.

derangement (de-rānj'ment) disorder.

dereistic (de"re-is'tik) giving the imagination free play.

derencephalus (der"en-sef'ah-lus) a monster with no cranium, the cervical vertebrae containing the relics of a brain.

derepression (de"re-presh'un) 1. in genetics, elevation of the level of an enzyme above the normal, either by lowering of the corepressor concentration or by a mutation that decreases the formation of aporepressor or the response to the complete repressor. 2. in psychiatry, the coming back of ideas or impulses into conscious awareness which were earlier pushed from such awareness into the unconscious because they were personally intolerable.

deric (der'ik) pertaining to ectoderm.

derma (der'mah) corium.

Dermacentor (der"mah-sen'tor) a genus of arthropods (family Ixodidae) parasitic on various animals, and vectors of disease-producing microorganisms. **D. albipic'tus,** a species of ticks found in Canada, and northern and western United States, parasitic on cattle, horses, moose and elk. **D. anderso'ni,** a species of tick common in the western United States, parasitic on numerous wild mammals,

most domestic animals, and man, and a vector of Rocky Mountain spotted fever, tularemia, Colorado tick fever and American Q fever. **D. varia'bilis,** a tick parasitic on dogs and man, as well as many wild animals and most other domestic animals; a vector of spotted fever and tularemia. **D. venus'tus,** *Dermacentor andersoni.*

dermad (der'mad) toward the skin.

dermadrome (der'mah-drōm) a complex of cutanous symptoms commonly associated with an internal disorder.

dermagraph (der'mah-graf) dermatograph.

dermagraphy (der-mag'rah-fe) dermographia.

dermal (der'mal) pertaining to the true skin.

dermalgia (der-mal'je-ah) neuralgia of the skin.

Dermanyssus (der"mah-nis'us) a genus of mites parasitic on birds. **D. galli'nae,** a species of mites parasitic on chickens; known also as the roost mite or red chicken mite; a vector of encephalomyelitis virus.

dermapostasis (-pos'tah-sis) a skin disease with abscess formation.

dermatalgia (-tal'je-ah) dermalgia.

dermatic (der-mat'ik) pertaining to the skin.

dermatitides (der"mah-ti'ti-dēz) inflammatory conditions of the skin considered collectively.

dermatitis (-ti'tis), pl. *dermatit'ides.* inflammation of the skin. **actinic d., d. actin'ica,** dermatitis produced by exposure to rays of the sun or to ultraviolet radiation. **d. artefac'ta,** factitial dermatitis. **atopic d.,** a skin condition occurring as a reaction to a substance to which the patient is sensitive. **berlock d.,** dermatitis about the neck, due to application of a liquid toilet preparation, e.g. perfume or eau de cologne. **d. congelatio'nis,** inflammation of the skin due to exposure to cold. **contact d.,** dermatitis due to contact with a vegetable, animal or mineral allergen, usually accompanied by severe itching. **d. dysmenorrhe'ica,** a rosacea-like eruption on the cheeks of women during the menstrual period. **d. exfoliati'va, exfoliative d.,** a cutaneous disorder marked by scaly desquamation of the skin. **d. exfoliati'va neonato'rum,** a rare, severe exfoliative skin inflammation in young infants. **d. facti'tia, factitial d.,** a condition of the skin characterized by lesions produced by the patient, who denies knowledge of their cause. **d. gangreno'sa,** gangrenous inflammation of the skin. **d. gestatio'nis,** a generalized pruritic skin eruption occurring during pregnancy. **d. herpetifor'mis,** dermatitis with grouped erythematous papular, vesicular, pustular or bulbous lesions, accompanied by burning and itching. **hypostatic d., d. hypostat'ica,** a pigmented purpuric eruption of the ankles and legs due to failure of venous return from the lower extremity. **industrial d.,** a dermatitis caused by material used in the patient's occupation. **d. infectio'sa eczematoi'des, infectious eczematoid d.,** secondary infection of the skin due to a bacterial infection elsewhere, as in the nose or ear. **d. medi-camento'sa,** a skin eruption due to sensitivity to a drug that was ingested, inhaled or injected. **d. multifor'mis,** dermatitis herpetiformis. **d. papilla'ris capillit'ii,** folliculitis keloidalis. **d. pediculoi'des ventrico'sus,** straw itch. **radiation d.,** radiodermatitis. **rat-mite d.,** inflammation of the skin due to a bite of the rat-mite, *Liponyssus bacoti.* **d. re'pens,** a recurrent inflammation of the skin of the hands and feet, with vesicles, pustules and crust formation. **roentgen-ray d.,** radiodermatitis due to exposure to x (roentgen) rays. **schistosome d.,** an itching dermatitis caused by penetration into the skin of larval forms of schistosomes. **seborrheic d., d. seborrhe'ica,** an inflammatory skin disease with yellowish, greasy scaling and usually itching. **uncinarial d.,** irritation of the skin due to larvae of the hookworm. **d. venena'ta,** contact dermatitis. **x-ray d.,** skin inflammation due to exposure to x-rays.

dermatoautoplasty (der″mah-to-aw′to-plas″te) grafting of the patient's own skin.

Dermatobia (der″mah-to′be-ah) a genus of flies whose larvae are parasitic in various animals and sometimes in man.

dermatocele (der′mah-to-sēl″) dermatolysis. **d. lipomato'sus,** a pedunculated lipoma showing cystic degeneration.

dermatocellulitis (der″mah-to-sel″u-li′tis) inflammation of the skin and subcutaneous cellular tissue.

dermatoconiosis (-ko″ne-o′sis) dermatitis caused by the irritation of dust.

dermatocyst (der′mah-to-sist″) a cyst of the skin.

dermatodynia (der″mah-to-din′e-ah) neuralgia of the skin.

dermatofibroma (-fi-bro′mah) a fibroma of the skin.

dermatofibrosarcoma (-fi″bro-sar-ko′mah) a fibrosarcoma of the skin.

dermatogen (der-mat′o-jen) an antigen of any skin disease.

dermatogenic (der″mah-to-jen′ik) producing skin.

dermatogenous (der″mah-toj′ĕ-nus) producing skin.

dermatoglyphics (der″mah-to-glif′iks) the study of the patterns of ridges of the skin of the fingers, palms, toes and soles, frequently found to be significant in genetic investigations.

dermatograph (der-mat′o-graf) 1. an instrument for marking the boundaries of the body. 2. a wheal made on the skin in dermographia.

dermatographia (der″mah-to-graf′e-ah) a condition in which persistent linear markings may be elicited by drawing a blunt instrument across the skin.

dermatographism (der″mah-tog′rah-fizm) dermographia.

dermatography (-tog′rah-fe) 1. a description or account of the skin. 2. dermographia.

dermatoheteroplasty (der″mah-to-het′er-o-plas″te) grafting of skin taken from the body of another.

dermatoid (der′mah-toid) skinlike.

dermatologist (der″mah-tol′o-jist) an expert in dermatology.

dermatology (-tol′o-je) that branch of medicine dealing with diseases of the skin.

dermatolysis (-tol′ĭ-sis) hypertrophy of the skin and subcutaneous tissues, with a tendency to hang in folds.

dermatoma (-to′mah) an abnormal growth of skin tissue.

dermatome (der′mah-tōm) 1. the ventrolateral portion of an embryonic somite, which develops into the fibrous layer of the integument. 2. the cutaneous area developed from a single embryonic somite and receiving the greater part of its innervation from a single spinal nerve. 3. an instrument for excising areas of skin to be used for grafting.

dermatomegaly (der″mah-to-meg′ah-le) a condition in which the skin is larger than necessary to cover the body, so that it hangs in folds.

dermatomere (der′mah-to-mēr″) any segment of the embryonic integument.

dermatomucosomyositis (der″mah-to-mu-ko″-so-mi″o-si′tis) inflammation of skin, mucous membrane and muscles.

dermatomycosis (-mi-ko′sis) a skin disease due to parasitic fungi.

dermatomyoma (-mi-o′mah) myoma involving the skin.

dermatomyositis (-mi″o-si′tis) an acute, subacute or chronic disease involving skin and skeletal muscles, usually symmetrically.

dermatoneurosis (-nu-ro′sis) a neurogenic skin disorder.

dermatopathology (-pah-thol′o-je) pathology which is especially concerned with lesions of the skin.

dermatopathy (der″mah-top′ah-the) disease of the skin.

dermatophobia (der″mah-to-fo′be-ah) morbid dread of skin disease.

dermatophylaxis (-fi-lak′sis) dermophylaxis.

dermatophyte (der′mah-to-fīt″) any one of a group of fungi which cause superficial infections of the skin, including Microsporum, Epidermophyton and Trichophyton.

dermatophytid (der″mah-tof′ĭ-tid) a secondary rash or eruption occurring in dermatomycosis.

dermatophytosis (der″mah-to-fi-to′sis) a superficial infection of the skin caused by a fungus. **d. furfura'cea,** tinea versicolor.

dermatoplasty (der′mah-to-plas″te) plastic repair of the skin. adj., **der'matoplastic.**

dermatopolyneuritis (der″mah-to-pol″ĭ-nu-ri′-tis) acrodynia.

dermatorrhea (-re′ah) morbid excess of sweat.

dermatosclerosis (-skle-ro′sis) scleroderma.

dermatoscopy (der″mah-tos′ko-pe) examination of the skin, especially microscopic examination of the capillaries of the skin.

dermatosiophobe (der″mah-to′se-o-fōb) a person with a morbid fear of skin disease.

dermatosis (der″mah-to′sis) any disorder of the skin. **angioneurotic d.,** a condition due to vasomotor disturbance of the cutaneous vessels. **Bowen's precancerous d.,** Bowen's disease. **chick nutritional d.**, a disease of chicks marked by eruptions on head and feet and due to lack of pantothenic acid. **industrial d.**, occupational dermatitis. **d. kapo'si,** xeroderma pigmentosum. **d. papulo'sa ni'gra,** a skin disease chiefly affecting Negroes, with hyperpigmented papules occurring over the cheek bones and increasing in number and size. **precancerous d.**, any skin condition in which the lesions—warts, moles or other excrescences—are likely to undergo malignant degeneration. **progressive pigmentary d.**, a slowly progressive disease of the skin affecting chiefly the shins, ankles, and dorsa of the feet. **Schamberg's d.**, progressive pigmentary dermatosis. **stasis d.**, skin disease marked by disturbances of the circulation and of lymphatic absorption. **subcorneal pustular d.**, a bullous dermatosis resembling dermatitis herpetiformis, with single and grouped vesicles and pustules beneath the horny layer of the skin. **Unna's d.,** seborrheic eczema.

dermatosome (der'mah-to-sōm") portion of the equatorial plate formed in mitosis.

dermatostomatitis (der"mah-to-sto"mah-ti'tis) ectodermosis erosiva pluriorificialis.

dermatotherapy (-ther'ah-pe) treatment of skin diseases.

dermatotropic (-trop'ik) having a specific affinity for the skin.

dermatoxerasia (-ze-ra'ze-ah) xeroderma.

dermatozoon (-zo'on) any animal parasite on the skin.

dermatrophia (der"mah-tro'fe-ah) atrophy of the skin.

dermiatrics (der"me-at'riks) the science of healing skin diseases.

dermis (der'mis) the true skin, or corium. adj., **der'mic.**

dermitis (der-mi'tis) inflammation of the skin.

dermoblast (der'mo-blast) part of mesoblast, developing into the true skin.

dermographia (der"mo-graf'e-ah) elicitation of a transient mark on the skin by stroking with a blunt-pointed instrument.

dermographism (der mog'rah-fizm) dermographia.

dermoid (der'moid) 1. skinlike. 2. a congenital cyst containing hair, skin, teeth, etc.

dermoidectomy (der"moi-dek'to-me) excision of a dermoid.

dermolysin (der-mol'ĭ-sin) a substance capable of dissolving the skin.

dermolysis (der-mol'ĭ-sis) destruction of the skin.

dermomycosis (der"mo-mi-ko'sis) a skin disease produced by a fungus.

dermomyotome (-mi'o-tōm) all but the sclerotome of a mesodermal somite; the primordium of skeletal muscle and, perhaps, of corium.

dermoneurosis (-nu-ro'sis) dermatoneurosis.

dermonosology (-no-sol'o-je) the pathology of skin diseases.

dermopathy (der-mop'ah-the) any skin disease.

dermophlebitis (der"mo-fle-bi'tis) inflammation of the veins of the skin.

dermophylaxis (der"mo-fi-lak'sis) the protective action of the skin against infections.

dermophyte (der'mo-fīt) a vegetable skin parasite.

dermoplasty (der'mo-plas"te) dermatoplasty.

dermoskeleton (der"mo-skel'ĕ-ton) the external and visible investments of the body: skin, teeth, hair and nails.

dermostenosis (-ste-no'sis) contraction of the skin.

dermosynovitis (-sin"o-vi'tis) malignant inflammation of the sole of the foot, with involvement of synovial sheaths.

dermosyphilopathy (-sif"ĭ-lop'ah-the) a syphilitic skin disease.

dermotropic (-trop'ik) having a special affinity for epithelial surfaces of the body.

dermovascular (-vas'ku-ler) pertaining to skin and blood vessels.

derodidymus (der"o-did'ĭ-mus) a fetal monster with one body, two necks and two heads.

Deronil (der'o-nil) trademark for a preparation of dexamethasone.

descemetitis (des"ē-mē-ti'tis) inflammation of Descemet's membrane.

descemetocele (des"ē-met'o-sēl) hernia of Descemet's membrane.

descensus (de-sen'sus), pl. *descen'sus* [L.] downward displacement or prolapse. **d. tes'tis,** normal migration of the testis from its fetal position in the abdominal cavity to its location within the scrotum, usually during the last three months of gestation. **d. u'teri,** prolapse of the uterus.

desensitization (de-sen"sĭ-tĭ-za'shun) the abolition of sensitivity to a particular antigen.

desensitize (de-sen'sĭ-tīz) to render less sensitive.

desequestration (de"se-kwes-tra'shun) the release of sequestered material, e.g. release into the general circulation of blood previously withheld from it by physiologic or mechanical means.

deserpidine (de-ser'pĭ-dēn) a reserpine derivative used as a tranquilizer.

desexualize (de-seks'u-al-īz) to deprive of sexual powers.

desiccant (des'ĭ-kant) promoting dryness.

desiccate (des'ĭ-kāt) to render thoroughly dry.

desiccation (des"ĭ-ka'shun) the act of drying.

desiccative (des'ĭ-ka"tiv) drying or lessening moisture.

deslanoside (des-lan'o sīd) a poisonous, white crystalline compound used as a cardiotonic.

desmalgia (des-mal'je-ah) pain in a ligament.

desmectasia (des"mek-ta'ze-ah) the stretching of a ligament.

desmepithelium (des"mep-ĭ-the'le-um) the epithelium of the blood vessels, lymphatics and synovial ligaments.

desmitis (des-mi'tis) inflammation of a ligament.

desmocranium (des"mo-kra'ne-um) the mass of dense mesenchyme enveloping the cranial end of the notochord at the fifth and sixth weeks, which is the earliest indication of the skull in the developing embryo.

desmocyte (des'mo-sīt) any supporting tissue cell.

desmodynia (des″mo-din'e-ah) pain in a ligament or ligaments.

desmoenzyme (-en'zīm) an enzyme which is bound to the protoplasm of a cell and which cannot be extracted by available methods.

desmogenous (des-moj'ĕ-nus) arising in connective tissue.

desmography (des-mog'rah-fe) a description of ligaments.

desmoid (des'moid) 1. fibrous. 2. a hard or tough fibroma.

desmolase (des'mo-lās) an enzyme that catalyzes the addition or removal of some chemical group, in the free state, to or from a substrate.

desmology (des-mol'o-je) science of ligaments.

desmoma (des-mo'mah) fibroma.

desmoneoplasm (des″mo-ne'o-plazm) a connective tissue neoplasm.

desmopathy (des-mop'ah-the) any disease of the ligaments.

desmoplastic (des″mo-plas″tik) producing adhesions.

desmorrhexis (des″mo-rek'sis) rupture of a ligament.

desmosis (des-mo'sis) a disease of the connective tissue.

desmosome (des'mo-sōm) a small thickening at the middle of an intercellular bridge.

desmosterol (des-mos'ter-ol) the immediate precursor of cholesterol in the biosynthetic pathway.

desmotomy (des-mot'o-me) incision or division of a ligament.

desoxy- (des-ok'se) for words beginning thus, see also those beginning *deoxy*-.

desoxycorticosterone (des-ok″sĭ-kor″tĭ-ko-stēr'ōn) a synthetic mineralocorticoid concerned in water and electrolyte metabolism, but having no effect on carbohydrate metabolism.

desoxyephedrine (des-ok″se-ĕ-fed'rin) methamphetamine.

Desoxyn (des-ok'sin) trademark for preparations of methamphetamine hydrochloride.

desoxyphenobarbital (des-ok″sĭ-fe″no-bar'bĭ-tal) primidone.

desoxyribonuclease (-ri″bo-nu'kle-ās) deoxyribonuclease.

desoxyribose (-ri'bōs) deoxyribose.

desquamation (des″kwah-ma'shun) shedding of material from a surface, as the shedding of cells from the skin or a mucous membrane. adj., **desquam'ative. siliquose d.,** the shedding of dried vesicles from the skin.

dest. [L.] *destilla'ta* (distilled).

Desulfovibrio (de-sul″fo-vib're-o) a genus of Schizomycetes (order Pseudomonadales, suborder Pseudomonadineae, family Spirillaceae).

detachment (de-tach'ment) the condition of being separated or set apart. **d. of retina, retinal d.,** separation of the inner layers of the retina from the pigment layer.

detector (de-tek'tor) an instrument or apparatus for revealing the presence of something. **lie d.,** polygraph.

detergent (de-ter'jent) 1. cleansing. 2. a substance that combines the properties of wetting and emulsifying agents, facilitating removal of oil and dirt.

deterioration (de-tēr″e-o-ra'shun) the act, process or state of growing worse. **emotional d.,** a condition in which the emotional response is not appropriate to or commensurate with the stimuli which arouse it. **mental d.,** a condition of progressive impairment of the mental faculties.

determinant (de-ter'mĭ-nant) a factor that establishes the nature of an entity or event. **antigenic d.,** haptene.

determination (de-ter″mĭ-na'shun) the establishment, during embryonic development, of the ultimate destiny of a particular region. **sex d.,** the process by which the sex of an organism is fixed, associated, in man, with the presence or absence of the Y chromosome.

determinism (de-ter'mĭ-nizm) the theory that all phenomena are the result of antecedent conditions and that nothing occurs by chance. **psychic d.,** the motivation of mental processes by factors in the unconscious.

dethyroidism (de-thi'roi-dizm) symptoms due to removal of the thyroid.

detoxicate (de-tok'sĭ-kāt) to deprive of toxic qualities.

detoxication (de-tok″sĭ-ka'shun) detoxification.

detoxification (-fī-ka'shun) the destruction of toxic properties of a substance, a major function of the liver. **metabolic d.,** reduction of the toxic properties of a substance by chemical changes induced in the body, producing a compound which is less poisonous or more readily eliminated.

detrition (de-trish'un) the wearing away, as of teeth, by friction.

detritivorous (de″trī-tiv'o-rus) consuming or subsisting on particulate matter (detritus), a mode of existence important in certain – e.g. aquatic – ecosystems.

detritus (de-tri'tus) particulate matter produced by or remaining after the wearing away or disintegration of a substance or tissue.

detruncation (de″trung-ka'shun) decollation; decapitation.

detubation (de″tu-ba'shun) the removal of a tube.

detumescence (de″tu-mes'ens) the subsidence of congestion and swelling.

deutan (du'tan) a person with anomalous color vision, marked by derangement or loss of the red-green sensory mechanism.

deuteranomalopia (du″ter-ah-nom″ah-lo'pe-ah) a variant of normal color vision with imperfect perception of the green hues.

deuteranomalopsia (-lop'se-ah) deuteranomalopia.

deuteranomaly (du″ter-ah-nom'ah-le) deuteranomalopia. adj., **deuteranom'alous.**

deuteranope (du″ter-ah-nōp″) a person exhibiting deuteranopia.

deuteranopia (du″ter-ah-no'pe-ah) defective color vision, with retention of the sensory mechanism for two hues only – blue and yellow. adj., **deuteranop'ic.**

deuteranopsia (du″ter-ah-nop′se-ah) deuteranopia.

deuterate (du′ter-āt) to treat (combine) with deuterium (H²).

deuterium (du-te′re-um) the mass two isotope of hydrogen, symbol H² or D. **d. oxide,** heavy water.

deutero-albumose (du″ter-o-al′bu-mōs) an albumose soluble in water and in saline solutions.

deutero-elastose (-e-las′tōs) a material formed in the digestion of elastin.

deuterohemophilia (-he″mo-fil′e-ah) a condition resembling classic hemophilia.

deuteromyosinose (-mi-os′i-nōs) a substance formed in digestion of myosin.

deuteron (du′ter-on) the nucleus of the deuterium atom, considered to consist of one proton and one neutron.

deuteropathy (du″ter-op′ah-the) a secondary or sympathetic affection.

deutoplasm (du′to-plazm) material in a cell which is elaborated by the protoplasm.

devasation (de″vas-a′shun) devascularization.

devascularization (de-vas″ku-ler-ĭ-za′shun) interruption of circulation of blood to a part due to obstruction or destruction of blood vessels supplying it.

Devegan (dev′e-gan) trademark for a preparation of acetarsone.

development (de-vel′up-ment) gradual change from lower to a higher state. **mosaic d.,** embryonic development in which the blastomeres just equal the fates which they achieve. **psychosexual d.,** development of the personality through the infantile and pregenital stages to sexual maturity. **regulative d.,** embryonic development in which the potencies of the blastomeres are greater than is indicated by their normal performance.

deviant (de′ve-ant) 1. varying from a determinable standard. 2. a person with characteristics varying from what is considered standard or normal. **color d.,** a person whose color perception varies from the norm. **sex d.,** a person whose sexual behavior varies from that normally considered biologically or socially accepted.

deviation (de″ve-a′shun) variation from the normal position or condition. **conjugate d.,** deviation of both eyes to the same side. **minimum d.,** the smallest deviation of a ray that a given prism can produce.

device (de-vīs′) something contrived for a specific purpose. **contraceptive d.,** one used to prevent conception, as a diaphragm or condom to prevent entrance of spermatozoa into the uterine cervix, or one inserted into the uterus (*intrauterine contraceptive device*) to prevent implantation of a fertilized ovum.

deviometer (de″ve-om′ě-ter) an instrument for measuring the deviation in strabismus.

devisceration (de-vis″er-a′shun) removal of viscera.

devitalization (de-vi′tal-i-za′shun) deprivation of vitality or life. **pulp d.,** destruction of vitality of the pulp of a tooth.

devolution (dev″o-lu′shun) the reverse of evolution; catabolic change.

dewlap (dū′lap) a heavy fold of skin on the ventral aspect of the neck in animals.

dexamethasone (dek″sah-meth′ah-sōn) an adrenocortical steroid of the glucogenic type, used as an anti-inflammatory steroid with little salt-retaining action.

dexbrompheniramine (deks″brōm-fen-i′rah-mēn) a pyridine derivative used as an antihistaminic.

dexchlorpheniramine (deks″klōr-fen-i′rah-mēn) a pyridine derivative used as an antihistaminic.

Dexedrine (dek′sě-drēn) trademark for preparations of dextroemphetamine.

dexiocardia (dek″se o kar′de ah) dextrocardia.

Dexoval (dek′so-val) trademark for a preparation of methamphetamine.

dexter (dek′ster) [L.] right; on the right side.

dextr(o)- (dek′stro) word element [L.], *right*.

dextrad (dek′strad) to or toward the right side.

dextral (dek′stral) pertaining to the right side.

dextrality (dek-stral′ĭ-te) dominance of the right member of paired organs.

dextran (dek′stran) a water-soluble, high-glucose polymer produced by the action of *Leuconostoc mesenteroides* on sucrose; used as a plasma substitute.

dextrase (dek′strās) an enzyme which changes dextrose into lactic acid.

dextraural (dek-straw′ral) hearing better with the right ear.

dextrin (dek′strin) a carbohydrate formed during the hydrolysis of starch to sugar.

dextrinosis (dek″stri-no′sis) a condition characterized by accumulation in the tissues of an abnormal polysaccharide. **limit d.,** a form of hepatic and muscle glycogen disease due to deficiency of debranching enzyme.

dextrinuria (dek″strin-u′re-ah) presence of dextrin in the urine.

dextroamphetamine (dek″stro-am-fet′ah-mēn) dextrorotatory isomer of amphetamine, having a more conspicuous stimulant effect on the central nervous system than racemic amphetamine in the same dosage.

dextrocardia (-kar′de-ah) location of the heart in the right side of the thorax, the apex pointing to the right. **mirror-image d.,** dextrocardia in which the right-to-left relation of the heart is reversed, venous blood passing through the chambers at the left, and arterial blood through the chambers at the right.

dextroclination (-kli′na′shun) rotation of the upper poles of the vertical meridians of the eyes to the right.

dextrocularity (dek″strok-u-lar′ĭ-te) dominance of the right eye.

dextroduction (dek″stro-duk′shun) movement of an eye to the right.

dextrogastria (-gas′tre-ah) displacement of the stomach to the right.

dextrogram (dek′stro-gram) an electrocardiographic tracing showing right axis deviation, indicative of right ventricular hypertrophy.

dextrogyration (dek″stro-ji-ra′shun) rotation to the right.

dextromanual (dek″stro-man′u-al) right-handed.

dextromethorphan (-meth′or-fan) a drug used as an antitussive.

dextropedal (dek-strop′ĕ-dal) right-footed.

dextrophobia (dek″stro-fo′be-ah) fear of objects on the right side of the body.

dextropropoxyphene (-pro-pok′sĭ-fēn) a drug used as an analgesic.

dextrorotatory (-ro′tah-tor″e) turning the plane of polarization to the right.

dextrose (dek′strōs) a white crystalline or granular powder, $C_6H_{12}O_6.H_2O$, usually obtained by hydrolysis of starch, used intravenously as a nutrient replenisher.

dextrosinistral (dek″stro-sin′is-tral) extending from right to left.

dextrosuria (-su′re-ah) dextrose in the urine.

dextrotorsion (-tor′shun) a twisting to the right.

dextrotropic (-trop′ik) turning to the right.

dextroversion (-ver′zhun) location to the right; especially location of the heart to the right side of the chest, the apex pointing to the right, without change in relation of the chambers.

dezymotize (de-zi′mo-tīz) to deprive of ferments or germs.

DFP diisopropyl fluorophosphate, a compound with anticholesterinase activity; a radioactive form containing P^{32} has been used in studies of the various formed elements of the blood.

D.G. distogingival.

dg. decigram.

dhurrin (du′rin) a cyanogenetic glucoside from sorghum, capable of causing poisoning in animals.

D.Hy. Doctor of Hygiene.

di- word element [Gr., L.], *two*.

diabetes (di″ah-be′tēz) inordinate and persistent increase in urinary secretions. **achrestic d.,** a condition characterized by inability of the tissues to utilize sugar despite the availability of biologically active insulin. **alimentary d.,** diabetes due to defective metabolism of the carbohydrates of the food. **biliary d.,** Hanot's disease. **bronze d.,** hemochromatosis. **d. insip′idus,** a condition characterized by excessive ingestion of water and urination without elevation of sugar in the urine. **d. insip′idus, nephrogenic,** diabetes insipidus due to congenital failure of renal tubules to reabsorb water, and characterized by failure to respond to administration of antidiuretic hormone. **latent d.,** the state following derangement of glucose tolerance, when the glucose tolerance test result is normal. **d. melli′tus,** a condition characterized by an elevated level of sugar in blood and urine, increased urination and increased intake of both fluid and food, with an absolute or relative insulin deficiency. **phlorizin d.,** that produced by administration of phlorizin. **phosphatic d.,** a variety in which there is excess of phosphates in urine. **puncture d.,** diabetes produced by puncture of the medulla oblongata. **renal d.,** renal glycosuria. **subclinical d.,** a state characterized by an abnormal glucose tolerance test result, but without any clinical signs of diabetes.

diabetic (di″ah-bet′ik) 1. pertaining to or characterized by diabetes. 2. a person exhibiting diabetes. **brittle d.,** a patient with diabetes who spontaneously shows considerable oscillation between high and low levels of sugar in the blood.

diabetid (di″ah-be′tid) a cutaneous manifestation of diabetes.

diabetogenic (-bet″o-jen′ik) producing diabetes.

diabetogenous (-be-toj′ĕ-nus) caused by diabetes.

diabetometer (-be-tom′ĕ-ter) a polariscope for use in estimating the percentage of sugar in urine.

diabetophobia (-be″to-fo′be-ah) morbid fear of diabetes.

diabetotherapy (-ther′ah-pe) the treatment of diabetes.

Diabinese (di-ab′ĭ-nēs) trademark for chlorpropamide.

diabrotic (di″ah-brot′ik) 1. ulcerative; caustic. 2. a corrosive or escharotic substance.

diacele (di′ah-sēl) diacoele.

diacetate (di-as′ĕ-tāt) a salt of diacetic acid.

diacetemia (di-as″ĕ-te′me-ah) diacetic acid in the blood.

diaceturia (-tu′re-ah) diacetic acid in the urine.

diacid (di-as′id) a compound containing two hydroxyl groups.

diaclasia (di″ah-kla′ze-ah) a fracture.

diaclast (di′ah-klast) an instrument used in fracturing the fetal head.

diacoele (di′ah-sēl) the third ventricle of the brain.

diacrisis (di-ak′rĭ-sis) 1. a disease characterized by change in the secretions. 2. a secretion or excretion. 3. diagnosis.

diacritical (di″ah-krit′ĭ-kal) diagnostic; pathognomonic.

diad (di′ad) a bivalent element or radical.

diaderm (di′ah-derm) the two-layered embryo, consisting of ectoderm and entoderm.

diadochokinesia (di″ah-do″ko-ki-ne′ze-ah) the function of arresting one motor impulse and substituting one that is diametrically opposite.

diadochokinesis (-ki-ne′sis) diadochokinesia.

Diadol (di′ah-dol) trademark for a preparation of diallyl barbituric acid.

Diafen (di′ah-fen) trademark for a preparation of diphenylpyraline hydrochloride.

diagnose (di′ag-nōs) to identify or recognize a disease.

diagnosis (di″ag-no′sis) determination of the disease producing the symptoms in a patient. adj., **diagnos′tic. clinical d.,** diagnosis based upon the symptoms shown by the patient. **differential d.,** the determination of which one of several diseases may be producing the symptoms. **d. by exclusion,** the determination of a disease by excluding all other conditions. **physical d.,** diagnosis based on information obtained by inspection, palpation, percussion and auscultation. **serum d.,**

diagnosis by means of serums and their reactions.

diagnostician (di″ag-nos-tish'an) an expert in diagnosis.

diagnostics (-nos'tiks) the science and practice of diagnosis of disease.

diagram (di'ah-gram) a graphic representation, in simplest form, of an object or concept, made up of lines and lacking pictorial elements. **vector d.**, a diagram representing the direction and magnitude of electromotive forces of the heart for one entire cycle, based on analysis of the scalar electrocardiogram.

diagraph (di'ah-graf) an instrument for recording outlines, as in craniometry.

Dialister (di″ah-lis'ter) a genus of Schizomycetes (order Eubacteriales, family Bacteroidaceae) found in the respiratory tract.

dialysance (di″ah-li'sans) the minute rate of net exchange of solute molecules passing through a membrane in dialysis.

dialysate (di al′ĭ-sāt) material obtained by dialysis (1).

dialysis (di-al'ĭ-sis) the diffusion of solute molecules through a semipermeable membrane, passing from the side of higher concentration to that of the lower; a method sometimes used, in patients with defective renal function, to remove from the blood elements that are normally excreted in the urine. **cross d.**, dialytic parabiosis. **lymph d.**, removal of urea and other elements from lymph collected from the thoracic duct, treated outside the body, and later reinfused. **peritoneal d.**, dialysis through the peritoneum, the dialyzing solution being introduced into and removed from the peritoneal cavity, as either a continuous or an intermittent procedure.

dialyzer (di'ah-līz″er) an apparatus for performing dialysis.

diamagnetic (di″ah-mag-net'ik) repelled by the magnet.

diameter (di-am'ē-ter) a straight line joining opposite points of a circle or other figure. **Baudelocque's d.**, external conjugate diameter. **conjugate d., true,** the anteroposterior diameter of the superior aperture of the minor pelvis, measured from the superior margin of the symphysis pubis to the sacrovertebral angle. **craniometric d's,** imaginary lines connecting points on opposite surfaces of the cranium; the most important are: *biparietal,* that joining the parietal eminences; *bitemporal,* that joining the extremities of the coronal suture; *occipitofrontal,* that joining the root of the nose and the most prominent point of the occiput; *occipitomental,* that joining the external occipital protuberance and the chin; *trachelobregmatic,* that joining the anterior fontanel and the junction of the neck with the floor of the mouth. **extracanthic d.,** the distance between the lateral points of junction of the upper and lower eyelids. **frontomental d.,** the distance from the forehead to the chin. **intercanthic d.,** the distance between the medial points of junction of the upper and lower eyelids. **d's of the pelvis,** imaginary lines connecting opposite points of the pelvis; the most important are: *anteroposterior* (of inlet), that joining the sacrovertebral angle and the pubic symphysis; *anteroposterior* (of outlet), that joining the tip of the coccyx and the subpubic ligament; *conjugate,* the anteroposterior diameter of the inlet; *diagonal conjugate,* that joining the sacrovertebral angle and the subpubic ligament; *external conjugate,* that joining the depression above the spine of the first sacral vertebra and the middle of the upper border of the pubic symphysis; *internal conjugate,* that joining the sacral promontory and the upper edge of the pubic symphysis; *true conjugate,* that joining the sacrovertebral angle and the most prominent portion of the posterior aspect of pubic symphysis; *transverse* (of inlet), that joining the two most widely separated points of inlet of pelvis; *transverse* (of outlet), that joining the ischial tuberosities. **pubosacral d.,** true conjugate diameter. **vertebromammary d.,** the anteroposterior diameter of the chest.

diamide (di-am'id) a double amide.

diamine (di-am'in, di'ah-min) a double amine.

diaminuria (di-am″ĭ-nu're-ah) diamines in the urine.

Diamox (di'ah-moks) trademark for preparations of acetazolamide.

diamthazole (di-am'thah-zōl) a drug used as an antifungal agent.

Dianabol (di-an'ah-bol) trademark for methandrostenolone.

Diaparene (di-ap'ah-rēn) trademark for preparations of methylbenzothonium chloride.

diapedesis (di″ah-pē-de'sis) the passage of blood corpuscles through intact vessel walls.

diaphane (di'ah-fān) the investing membrane of a cell.

diaphanometry (di″ah-fah-nom'ē-tre) measurement of the transparency of a liquid.

diaphanoscope (-fan'o-skōp) a device for examining closed cavities by means of transmitted light.

diaphanoscopy (-fah-nos'ko-pe) examination by the diaphanoscope.

diaphemetric (-fē-met'rik) pertaining to measurement of tactile sensibility.

diaphoresis (-fo-re'sis) profuse perspiration.

diaphoretic (-fo-ret'ik) 1. pertaining to, characterized by or promoting diaphoresis. 2. an agent that promotes diaphoresis.

diaphragm (di'ah-fram) 1. the strong, dome-shaped sheet of skeletal muscle separating the thoracic and abdominal cavities of the body. 2. a thin septum dividing a cavity. **Bucky d., Bucky-Potter d.,** a device used in radiography to prevent scattered radiation from reaching the plate, thereby securing better contrast and definition. **contraceptive d.,** a device of molded rubber or other soft plastic material, fitted over the cervix uteri to prevent entrance of spermatozoa. **pelvic d.,** the portion of the floor of the pelvis formed by the coccygeus muscles and the levator muscles of the anus, and their fascia. **poly-arcuate d.,** one showing abnormal scalloping of the margins on radiographic visualization. **urogenital d.,** the musculomembranous layer superficial to the pelvic diaphragm, extending between the ischiopubic rami and surrounding the urogenital ducts.

diaphragma (di″ah-frag′mah), pl. *diaphragmata* [Gr.] diaphragm.

diaphragmalgia (di″ah-frag-mal′je-ah) pain in the diaphragm.

diaphragmatocele (-mat′o-sēl) diaphragmatic hernia.

diaphragmitis (-mi′tis) inflammation of the diaphragm.

diaphragmodynia (di″ah-frag″mo-din′e-ah) pain in the diaphragm.

diaphysectomy (di″ah-fi-zek′to-me) excision of part of a diaphysis.

diaphyseal (di″ah-fiz′e-al) pertaining to or affecting the shaft of a long bone (diaphysis).

diaphysial (di″ah-fiz′e-al) diaphyseal.

diaphysis (di-af′ĭ-sis), pl. *diaph′yses* [Gr.] the shaft of a long bone, between the epiphyses.

diaphysitis (di″ah-fi-zi′tis) inflammation of a diaphysis.

diaplasis (di-ap′lah-sis) the setting of a fracture or reduction of a dislocation.

diaplexus (di″ah-plek′sus) the choroid plexus of third ventricle. adj., **diaplex′al.**

diapnoic (di″ap-no′ik) causing mild perspiration.

diapophysis (di″ah-pof′ĭ-sis) an upper transverse process of a vertebra.

diapyesis (di″ah-pi-e′sis) suppuration. adj., **diapyet′ic.**

diarrhea (di″ah-re′ah) frequent evacuation of watery feces. **choleraic d.,** severe, acute diarrhea with serous stools, accompanied by vomiting and collapse. **critical d.,** diarrhea occurring at the crisis of a disease or producing a crisis. **infantile d.,** summer diarrhea. **lienteric d.,** diarrhea marked by stools containing undigested food. **mucous d.,** diarrhea with mucus in the stools. **parenteral d.,** diarrhea due to infections outside the gastrointestinal tract. **summer d.,** acute diarrhea in children during the intense heat of summer. **tropical d.,** sprue (2).

diarthric (di-ar′thrik) pertaining to or affecting two different joints; biarticular.

diarthrosis (di″ar-thro′sis), pl. *diarthro′ses* [Gr.] a diarthrodial joint. **d. rotato′ria,** a joint characterized by mobility in a rotary direction.

diarticular (-tik′u-ler) pertaining to two joints.

diaschisis (di-as′kĭ-sis) loss of functional connection between various centers forming one of the cerebral mechanisms.

diascope (di′ah-skōp) a glass plate pressed against the skin for observing the changes other than those of congestion.

diascopy (di-as′ko-pe) 1. examination by means of a diascope. 2. transillumination.

Diasone (di′ah-sōn) trademark for a preparation of sulfoxone.

diastalsis (di″ah-stal′sis) the forward movement of the bowel contents.

diastaltic (-stal′tik) 1. pertaining to diastalsis. 2. performed reflexly.

diastase (di′ah-stās) an enzyme that catalyzes the decomposition of cooked or uncooked starches to maltose. **d. ve′ra,** pancreatin.

diastasis (di-as′tah-sis) a separation; an interval in time or space, e.g. a short period of the heart cycle *(dias′tasis cor′dis)* just before contraction, or a separation between normally contiguous structures, as bones or muscles.

diastema (di″ah-ste′mah) a space or cleft.

diastematocrania (-stem″ah-to-kra′ne-ah) longitudinal congenital fissure of the cranium.

diastematomyelia (-mi-e′le-ah) abnormal division of the spinal cord by a bony spicule protruding from a vertebra or two, each of the halves surrounded by a dural sac.

diastematopyelia (-pi-e′le-ah) congenital median fissure of the pelvis.

diaster (di-as′ter) the double star figure in karyokinesis.

diastole (di-as′to-le) the dilatation stage of the cardiac cycle. adj., **diastol′ic.**

diataxia (di″ah-tak′se-ah) ataxia affecting both sides of the body. **cerebral infantile d., d. cerebra′lis infanti′lis,** the ataxic form of birth palsy.

diatela (-te′lah) the roof of the third ventricle.

diaterma (-ter′mah) part of the floor of the third ventricle.

diathermal (-ther′mal) permeable by heat.

diathermia (-ther′me-ah) diathermy.

diathermy (-ther′me) generation of heat in body tissues due to resistance offered by the tissues to high-frequency electric currents passed through them. **short-wave d.,** diathermy with high-frequency current of wavelength less than 30 meters.

diathesis (di-ath′ĕ-sis) an unusual constitutional susceptibility or predisposition to a particular disease. adj., **diathet′ic. aneurysmal d.,** constitutional predisposition to aneurysms. **furuncular d.,** furunculosis. **gouty d.,** predisposition to gout. **hemorrhagic d.,** hemophilia. **rheumatic d.,** constitutional predisposition to rheumatism.

diatom (di′ah-tom) a unicellular microscopic plant.

diatomic (di″ah-tom′ik) 1. containing two atoms. 2. bivalent.

diauxie (di-awk′se) a phenomenon of bacterial growth in which two distinct periods of growth occur, separated by a perceptible lag. adj., **diaux′ic.**

diaxon (di-ak′son) a nerve cell with two axons.

diazo- (di-az′o) the group, $-N_2-$.

diazone (di′ah-zōn) one of the dark bands seen in cross section of a tooth.

dibasic (di-ba′sik) containing two replaceable hydrogen atoms, or furnishing two hydrogen ions.

dibenzothiazine (di-ben″zo-thi′ah-zēn) phenothiazine.

Dibenzyline (di-ben′zĭ-lēn) trademark for a

preparation of phenoxybenzamine hydrochloride.

dibothriocephaliasis (di-both″re-o-sef″ah-li′-ah-sis) diphyllobothriasis.

dibothriocephalus (-sef′ah-lus) diphyllobothrium.

dibucaine (di-bu′kān) a compound used as either a local or spinal anesthetic.

Dibuline (di′bu-lēn) trademark for a preparation of dibutoline sulfate.

dibutoline (di-bu′to-lēn) a compound used in parasympathetic blockade and as an antispasmodic.

dicentric (di-sen′trik) 1. pertaining to, developing from or having two centers. 2. having two centromeres.

dicephalous (di-sef′ah-lus) having two heads.

dicephalus (di-sef′ah-lus) a fetal monster with two heads.

dicephaly (di-sef′ah-le) a developmental anomaly characterized by the presence of two heads.

dichlorisone (di-klor′ĭ-sōn) a steroid used for topical anti-inflammatory action.

dichlorphenamide (di″klor-fen′ah-mīd) a compound used as a carbonic anhydrase inhibitor and to reduce intraocular pressure in glaucoma.

dichorial (di-ko′re al) pertaining to or characterized by the presence of two chorions.

dichorionic (di-ko″re-on′ik) dichorial.

dichotomization (di-kot″ŏ-mi-za′shun) the process of dividing, or the state of being divided, into two parts.

dichotomy (di-kot′o-me) division into two parts.

dichroic (di-kro′ik) characterized by dichroism.

dichroism (di′kro-izm) the showing of one color by reflected and of another by transmitted light.

dichromasy (di-kro′mah-se) dichromatism.

dichromat (di′kro-mat) a person exhibiting dichromatopsia.

dichromate (di kro′māt) a salt containing the bivalent Cr_2O_7 radical.

dichromatic (di″kro-mat′ik) pertaining to or characterized by dichromatism.

dichromatism (di-kro′mah-tizm) 1. the quality of existing in or exhibiting two different colors. 2. dichromatopsia.

dichromatopsia (di″kro-mah-top′se-ah) a condition characterized by ability to perceive only two of the 160 colors discriminated by the normal eye.

dichromic (di-kro′mik) 1. showing only two colors. 2. containing two atoms of chromium.

dichromophilic (di″kro-mo-fil′ik) staining with both acid and basic dyes.

dichromophilism (di″kro-mof′ĭ-lizm) the quality of being dichromophilic.

dicliditis (dik″lĭ-di′tis) inflammation of a valve, especially a heart valve.

diclidotomy (dik″lĭ-dot′o-me) incision of a valve.

Dicodid (di-ko′did) trademark for preparations of dihydrocodeinone.

dicoelous (di-se′lus) 1. hollowed on each of two sides. 2. having two cavities.

dicophane (di′ko-fān) chlorophenothane.

dicoria (di-ko′re-ah) double pupil.

dicoumarin (di-koo′mah-rin) dicumarol.

Dicrocoelium (dik″ro-se′le-um) a genus of flukes. **D. dentriticum,** a species of liver flukes that infest domestic animals and have been reported in man.

dicrotism (di′krŏ-tizm) the occurrence of two sphygmographic waves or elevations to one beat of the pulse. adj., **dicrot′ic.**

Dictyocaulus (dik″te-o-kaw′lus) a genus of worms parasitic in the lungs of domestic animals.

dictyoma (dik″te-o′mah) diktyoma.

dicumarol (di koo′mah-rol) registered name of a coumarin derivative originally isolated from spoiled sweet clover and later made synthetically; used as an anticoagulant in thrombotic states.

Dicurin (di-kur′in) trademark for a preparation of merethoxylline.

dicyclic (di-si′klik) pertaining to or having two cycles; in chemistry, having two rings in the atomic structure.

dicyclomine (di-si′klo-mēn) a compound used in parasympathetic blockade and as an antispasmodic.

didactylism (di-dak′tĭ-lizm) the presence of only two digits on a hand or foot.

didactylous (di-dak′tĭ-lus) having only two digits on a hand or foot.

didelphia (di del′fe-ah) the condition characterized by the presence of a double uterus.

didymalgia (did″ĭ-mal′je-ah) pain in a testis.

didymitis (did″ĭ-mi′tis) inflammation of a testis.

didymodynia (did″ĭ-mo-din′e-ah) pain in a testis.

didymous (did′ĭ-mus) occurring in pairs.

-didymus (did′ĭ-mus) word element [Gr.], *twin monster.*

die (di) a form used in the construction of something, as a positive reproduction of the form of a prepared tooth in a suitable hard substance.

diecious (di-e′shus) sexually distinct; having two sexes in separate individuals.

dielectric (di″e-lek′trik) transmitting electricity by induction, but not by conduction; the term is applied to an insulating substance through or across which electrice force is acting or may act by induction without conduction.

dielectrography (di″e-lek-trog′rah-fe) rheocardiography.

dielectrolysis (-trol′ĭ-sis) ionization and introduction of a drug into body tissues by passage of an electric current.

diembryony (di-em′bre-on″e) the production of two embryos from a single egg.

diencephalon (di″en-sef′ah-lon) the posterior part of the forebrain, consisting of the hypothalamus, thalamus, metathalamus and epithalamus.

dienestrol (-es′trol) a compound used as an estrogenic substance.

Dientamoeba (di-en″tah-me′bah) a genus of amebas commonly found in man. **D. frag′ilis,** a species frequently found in the appendix.

dieresis (di-er'ĕ-sis) 1. the division or separation of parts normally united. 2. mechanical separation of parts.

diet (di'et) 1. the total food consumed by an individual. 2. a prescription of food required or permitted to be eaten by a patient. 3. the regulation of food to the requirements of the body. adj., **dietet'ic. absolute d.,** fasting. **acid-ash d.,** one of meat, fish, eggs and cereals with little fruit or vegetables and no cheese or milk. **alkali-ash d.,** one of fruit, vegetables and milk with as little as possible of meat, fish, eggs and cereals. **balanced d.,** one containing foods which furnish all the nutritive factors in proper proportion for adequate nutrition. **Banting d.,** one designed to reduce obesity. **bland d.,** one that is free of irritating or stimulating foods. **Chittenden's d.,** one containing 47–55 gm. of protein. **Coleman-Shaffer d.,** a typhoid fever diet composed of eggs, cream, cocoa, milk sugar, and bread and butter, administered in small quantities, and frequently. **Dennett's d.,** a diet of fat-free buttermilk, baked potatoes, and large quantities of arrowroot; used in diarrheal conditions in infants. **diabetic d.,** one in which ordinary sugar, starchy food, fruits and ordinary bread are prohibited. **Ebstein's d.,** an obesity diet containing very little carbohydrate, a moderate amount of albumin and large quantities of fat. **elimination d.,** one for diagnosis of food allergy, based on omission of foods that might cause symptoms in the patient. **Gerson d., Gerson-Herrmannsdorfer d.,** one for lupus vulgaris and tuberculosis, low in sodium chloride and carbohydrate and rich in fats, proteins and vitamins. **Goldberger's d.,** one containing brewer's yeast for use in pellagra. **gouty d.,** one for mitigation of gout, restricting nitrogenous foods and prohibiting sweet wines and fermented liquors. **high calorie d.,** one which furnishes 4000 or more calories per day. **high fat d.,** ketogenic diet. **high protein d.,** one containing large amounts of protein, consisting largely of meats and vegetables. **Karell d.,** a milk diet for nephritis and heart disease. **ketogenic d.,** one containing large amounts of fat, with minimal amounts of protein and carbohydrate. **Lenhartz d.,** one rich in protein; for gastric ulcer. **low calorie d.,** one containing 1200 or less calories per day. **low fat d.,** one containing limited amounts of fat. **Minot-Murphy d.,** one containing large amounts of liver; given for pernicious anemia. **Prochownick d.,** one for the last weeks of pregnancy, designed to restrict the size and weight of the child, while strengthening the mother. **protective d.,** an extremely light diet for relieving the work of the digestive system. **purine-free d.,** one omitting meat, fowl and fish, but using milk, eggs, cheese and vegetables. **Sippy d.,** a graduated diet for gastric ulcer. **smooth d.,** one which avoids the use of roughage foods. **subsistence d.,** one that provides the minimal requirements for life. **Taylor's d.,** a preparation of white of egg, olive oil and sugar given when the urine is to be tested for chlorides. **Tufnell's d.,** a rich diet (with small allowance of liquids) prescribed in treatment of aneurysm.

dietary (di'ĕ-ter"e) 1. pertaining to diet. 2. a course or system of diet.

dietetics (di"ĕ-tet'iks) the science of diet and nutrition.

diethylcarbamazine (di-eth"il-kar-bam'ah-zēn) a compound used as an antifilarial agent.

diethylpropion (-pro'pe-on) a compound used as an anorectic.

diethylstilbestrol (-stil-bes'trol) white crystalline powder, $C_{18}H_{20}O_2$, an estrogenic compound.

diethyltoluamide (-tol-u'ah-mīd) a compound used as an insect repellant.

dietitian (di"ĕ-tish'an) one skilled in the use of diet in health and disease.

dietotherapy (di"ĕ-to-ther'ah-pe) the scientific regulation of food in treating disease, especially important in patients with inborn errors of metabolism and various other metabolic diseases.

differential (dif"er-en'shal) pertaining to differences; distinguishing separate elements.

differentiation (dif"er-en"she-a'shun) development into a more specialized or complex form.

diffract (di-frakt') to break up a ray of light into its component parts.

diffractometer (dif"frak-tom'ĕ-ter) erythrocytometer.

diffusate (di-fu'zāt) dialysate.

diffuse 1. (di-fūs') not definitely limited or localized. 2. (di-fūz') to pass through or to spread widely through a tissue or substance.

diffusible (di-fu'zī-bl) capable of rapid diffusion.

diffusion (di-fu'zhun) 1. the state or process of being widely spread. 2. the movement of a substance (molecules) from a region of high concentration to one of lower concentration.

digastric (di-gas'trik) having two bellies.

digenetic (di"jĕ-net'ik) having two stages of multiplication, one sexual in the mature forms, the other asexual in the larval stages.

digestant (di-jes'tant) 1. aiding digestion. 2. an agent capable of aiding digestion.

digestion (di-jes'chun) the conversion of material into simpler compounds, physically or chemically, especially conversion in the body of ingested nutrients into material that can be absorbed and utilized by the cells. adj., **diges'tive. artificial d.,** digestion carried on outside the body. **gastric d.,** digestion by the action of gastric juice. **intestinal d.,** digestion by the action of intestinal juices. **lipolytic d.,** the splitting of fat into fatty acid and glycerol. **pancreatic d.,** digestion by the action of pancreatic juice. **peptic d.,** gastric digestion. **primary d.,** digestion occurring in the gastrointestinal tract. **salivary d.,** digestion by the action of saliva. **secondary d.,** assimilation by body cells of nutritious material.

digit (dij'it) a finger or toe. adj., **dig'ital.**

Digitalin nativelle (dij"ĭ-tal'ēn na"tĭ-vel') trademark for preparations of the crystalline pure glycoside of *Digitalis purpurea.*

Digitalis (dij″i-tal′is)   a genus of herbs. **D. lana′ta,** a Balkan species which yields digoxin and lanatoside. **D. purpu′rea,** the foxglove whose leaves furnish digitalis.

digitalis (-tal′is)   dried leaf of *Digitalis purpurea;* used as a cardiotonic agent.

digitalism (dij′i-tal-izm)   the effect produced on the body by digitalis.

digitalization (dij″i-tal-i-za′shun)   production of the physiologic effect of digitalis on the body.

digitate (dij′i-tāt)   having digit-like branches.

digitation (dij″i-ta′shun)   1. a finger-like process.   2. surgical creation of a functioning digit by making a cleft between two adjacent metacarpal bones, after amputation of the fingers.

digitigrade (dij′i-ti-grād″)   characterized by walking or running on the toes; applied to animals whose digits only touch the ground, the posterior part of the foot being more or less raised, as horses and cattle.

digitonin (dij″i-to′nin)   a saponin from *Digitalis purpurea.*

digitoxin (dij″i-tok′sin)   a cardiotonic glycoside obtained from *Digitalis purpurea* and other species of the same genus; used in the treatment of congestive heart failure.

digitus (dij′i-tus), pl. *dig′iti* [L.]   a digit (finger or toe).

diglossia (di-glos′e-ah)   bifid tongue.

diglyceride (di-glis′er-īd)   a glyceride containing two fatty acid molecules.

dignathus (dig-na′thus)   a fetal monster with two lower jaws.

digoxin (di-jok′sin)   a cardiotonic glycoside obtained from the leaves of *Digitalis lanata;* used in the treatment of congestive heart failure.

dihydroergotamine (di-hi″dro-er-got′ah-mēn)   a product of the catalytic hydrogenation of ergotamine; used in the treatment of migraine.

dihydroestrin (-es′trin)   estradiol.

dihydrofolliculin (-fol-lik′u-lin)   estradiol.

dihydromorphinone hydrochloride (-mor′fi-nōn hi″dro-klo′rīd)   hydromorphone hydrochloride.

dihydrostreptomycin (-strep″to-mi′sin)   a substance produced by the hydrogenation of streptomycin; used as an antibiotic.

dihydrotachysterol (-tah-kis′ter-ol)   a compound derived from ergosterol by irradiation; used to increase the blood calcium level.

dihydroxyaluminum aminoacetate (di″hi-drok″se-ah-lu′mi-num am″i-no-as′ē-tāt)   an antacid compound.

dihydroxyfluorane (-floo′o-rān)   fluorescein.

dihydroxyphenylalanine (-fen″il-al′ah-nēn)   an amino acid produced by oxidation of tyrosine, and an intermediate product in the synthesis of both epinephrine and melanin.

dihyprylone (di-hi′pri-lōn)   a compound used as an antitussive.

diiodohydroxyquin (di″i-o″do-hi-drok′se-kwin)   an antiamebic and antitrichomonal.

diiodothyronine (-thi′ro-nēn)   an organic iodine-containing compound found in the thyroid gland, formed by conjugation of two molecules of monoiodothyronine.

diiodotyrosine (di″i-o″do-ti′ro-sēn)   an organic iodine-containing compound found in the thyroid gland, liberated from thyroglobulin by hydrolysis.

diktyoma (dik″te-o′mah)   a tumor of the ciliary epithelium.

dilaceration (di-las″er-a′shun)   the rending asunder of a part or organ.

Dilantin (di-lan′tin)   trademark for diphenylhydantoin.

dilatation (dil″ah-ta′shun)   an expanded area, or the state of being expanded. **d. of heart,** increase in size of one or more of the heart cavities from weakness or relaxation. **idiopathic d.,** dilatation of a vessel or other channel, especially of the pulmonary artery, not associated with any causative abnormality. **poststenotic d.,** dilatation of a vessel distal to a stenosed segment, often seen in the pulmonary artery.

dilatator (-ta′tor)   dilator.

dilation (di-la′shun)   the process of expanding or enlarging.

dilator (di-la′tor)   an instrument or agent, e.g. a muscle, that effects dilation. **Bailey d.,** an instrument designed especially for use in dilating the aortic valve in cardiac surgery.

Dilaudid (di-law′did)   trademark for preparations of hydromorphone.

Diloderm (di′lo-derm)   trademark for preparations of dichlorisone acetate.

diluent (dil′u-ent)   1. diluting.   2. an agent that dilutes or renders fluid.

dilution (di-lu′shun)   1. attenuation by admixture of a neutral agent.   2. an attenuated substance. **serial d.,** a method of obtaining a pure bacterial culture by rapid transfer of an exceedingly small amount of material from one nutrient medium to a succeeding one of the same volume.

dimenhydrinate (di″men-hi′dri-nāt)   an antihistaminic compound effective in relieving motion sickness and dizziness and nausea from other causes.

dimer (di′mer)   a compound formed by combination of two identical molecules.

dimercaprol (di″mer-kap′rol)   a compound used as an antidote against poisoning with arsenic, gold and mercury.

Dimetane (di′mē-tān)   trademark for preparations of brompheniramine.

dimethisoquin (di″mē-thi′so-kwin)   a compound used as a local anesthetic.

dimethoxanate (-thok′si-nāt)   a compound used as an antitussive.

dimethylamine (di-meth″il-am′in)   a nontoxic base, $(CH_3)_2NH$.

dimethylaminoazobenzene (-am″i-no-az″o-ben′zēn)   a carcinogenic compound formerly used to color oils, oleomargarine and other vegetable fat substitutes for butter.

Dimethylane (di-meth′i-lān)   trademark for a preparation of promoxolane.

dimethyl phthalate (di-meth′il thal′āt)   colorless oily liquid, $C_{10}H_{10}O_4$; insect repellent.

dimetria (di-me'tre-ah) a condition characterized by double uterus.

dimorphism (di-mor'fizm) the quality of existing in two distinct forms. adj., **dimor'phous. sexual d.,** the quality of sexual distinction based on characteristic differences.

dineuric (di-nu'rik) having two nerve cells.

dinitrobenzene (di-ni″tro-ben'zēn) a poisonous substance, $C_6H_4(NO_2)_2$, whose fumes may cause breathlessness and final asphyxia.

dinophobia (di″no-fo'be-ah) morbid fear of becoming dizzy.

diocoele (di'o-sēl) the cavity of the diencephalon; the third ventricle.

Dioctophyma (di-ok″to-ti'mah) a genus of nematode parasites. **D. rena'le,** a species found in the kidney in various carnivorous animals, and sometimes in man.

dioctyl calcium sulfosuccinate (di-ok'til kal'se-um sul″fo-suk'sī-nāt) a compound used as a fecal softener.

dioctyl sodium sulfosuccinate (so'de-um sul″fo-suk'sī-nāt) a compound used as a fecal softener and as a wetting agent.

Diodoquin (di″o-do'kwin) trademark for a preparation of diiodohydroxyquin.

Diodrast (di'o-drast) trademark for a preparation of iodopyracet for injection.

dioecious (di-e'shus) 1. having reproductive organs typical of only one sex in a single individual. 2. requiring two different hosts for completion of the life cycle.

Dioloxol (di″o-lok'sol) trademark for a preparation of mephenesin.

diopter (di-op'ter) a unit adopted for calibration of lenses, being the reciprocal of the focal length when expressed in meters; symbol D. **prism d.,** a unit of prismatic deviation, being the deflection of 1 cm. at a distance of one meter; symbol Δ.

dioptometer (di″op-tom'ĕ-ter) an instrument for testing ocular refraction.

dioptometry (-tom'ĕ-tre) the measurement of ocular accommodation and refraction.

dioptric (di-op'trik) 1. pertaining to refracted light. 2. pertaining to a diopter.

dioptrics (di-op'triks) the science of refracted light.

dioptry (di'op-tre) diopter.

diospyrobezoar (di″os-pi″ro-be'zōr) a bezoar made up of persimmon fibers.

diovulatory (di-ov'u-lah-to″re) ordinarily discharging two ova in one ovarian cycle.

dioxide (di-ok'sīd) oxide with two oxygen atoms.

dioxyline (di-ok'sī-lēn) a compound used as a vasodilator.

Dipaxin (di-pak'sin) trademark for a preparation of diphenadione.

dipeptidase (di-pep'ti-dās) an enzyme which attacks a dipeptide.

dipeptide (di-pep'tid) a compound of two amino acids, containing a peptide group.

diperodon (di-per'o-don) a compound used as a surface anesthetic.

Dipetalonema (di-pet″ah-lo-ne'mah) a genus of nematode parasites of the superfamily Filarioidea. **D. per'stans, D. streptocer'ca,** species primarily parasitic in man, other primates serving as reservoir hosts.

diphallus (di-fal'lus) a developmental anomaly characterized by duplication of the penis.

diphasic (di-fa'zik) having two phases.

diphebuzol (di-feb'u-zol) phenylbutazone.

diphemanil (di-fe'mah-nil) a compound used to produce parasympathetic blockade and as a relaxant for gastrointestinal spasm.

diphenadione (di-fen″ah-di'ōn) a yellow crystalline compound, $C_{23}H_{16}O_3$, used as an anticoagulant.

diphenhydramine hydrochloride (di″fen-hi'drah-min hi″dro-klo'rīd) white crystalline powder, $C_{17}H_{21}NO.HCl$; used in treatment of allergic disorders.

diphenoxylate (-ok'sī-lāt) a compound used to reduce intestinal motility.

diphenylhydantoin (di-fen″il-hi-dan'to-in) an anticonvulsant compound, $C_{15}H_{12}N_2O_2$. **sodium d.,** a compound of diphenylhydantoin and sodium, $C_{15}H_{11}N_2NaO_2$.

diphenylpyraline (-pi'rah-lēn) a compound used as an antihistaminic.

diphonia (di-fo'ne-ah) the production of two different voice tones in speaking.

diphtheria (dif-the're-ah) an infectious disease caused by *Corynebacterium diphtheriae,* characterized by formation of false membranes, especially in the throat and nose, by pain and by toxemia. adj., **diphthe'rial, diphther'ic, diphtherit'ic. Bretonneau's d.,** true diphtheria of the pharynx. **surgical d., wound d.,** formation of diphtheritic membrane on wounds.

diphtheritis (dif″the-ri'tis) diphtheria.

diphtheroid (dif'thĕ-roid) 1. resembling diphtheria. 2. pseudodiphtheria.

diphthongia (dif-thon'je-ah) the utterance at the same time of two vocal sounds of the same pitch.

diphyllobothriasis (di-fil″o-both-ri'ah-sis) infestation with Diphyllobothrium.

Diphyllobothrium (-both're-um) a genus of tapeworms. **D. la'tum,** a species of tapeworm found in man, dogs, cats and other fish-eating carnivores.

diphyodont (dif'e-o-dont″) having two sets of teeth.

diplacusis (dip″lah-koo'sis) the perception of a single auditory stimulus as two separate sounds. **binaural d.,** different perception by the two ears of a single auditory stimulus. **disharmonic d.,** a form of binaural diplacusis in which a pure tone is heard differently in the two ears. **echo d.,** a form of binaural diplacusis in which a sound of brief duration is heard at different times in the two ears. **monaural d.,** a form of diplacusis in which a pure tone is heard in the same ear as a split tone of two frequencies.

diplegia (di-ple'je-ah) paralysis of like parts on either side of the body. adj., **diple'gic.**

diplobacillus (dip″lo-bah-sil'us) a double bacillus.

diplobacterium (-bak-te're-um) a double bacterium.

diploblastic (-blas'tik) having two germ layers.

diplocardia (dip″lo-kar′de-ah) separation of the two halves of the heart.

diplococcemia (-kok-se′me-ah) diplococci in the blood.

Diplococcus (-kok′us) a genus of Schizomycetes (order Eubacteriales, family Lactobacillaceae, tribe Streptococceae). **D. pneumo′niae,** the commonest cause of lobar pneumonia, including some 80 serotypes distinguishable by the polysaccharide haptene of the capsular substance.

diplococcus (-kok′us), pl. *diplococ′ci.* 1. an individual of the genus Diplococcus. 2. an organism consisting of a pair of cells.

diplocoria (-ko′re-ah) double pupil.

diploë (dip′lo-e) the spongy layer between the inner and outer compact layers of the bones covering the brain. adj., **diploet′ic, diplo′ic.**

diplogenesis (dip″lo-jen′ĕ-sis) duplication of a part.

diploid (dip′loid) having a pair of each chromosome characteristic of a species (2 n or, in man, 46).

diploidy (dip′loi-de) the state of having two full sets of homologous chromosomes.

diplomyelia (dip″lo-mi-e′le-ah) lengthwise fissure of the spinal cord.

diploneural (-nu′ral) having a double nerve supply.

diplopia (di-plo′pe-ah) the perception of two images of a single object. **binocular d.,** perception of a separate image of a single object by each of the two eyes. **crossed d.,** horizontal diplopia in which the image perceived by the squinting eye is displaced to the opposite side of that perceived by the fixing eye. **direct d.,** horizontal diplopia in which the images bear the same lateral relation as the eyes to which they pertain. **heteronymous d.,** crossed diplopia. **homonymous d.,** direct diplopia. **horizontal d.,** diplopia in which the two images appear one beside the other. **monocular d.,** perception by one eye of two images of a single object. **paradoxical d.,** crossed diplopia. **torsional d.,** horizontal diplopia in which the upper pole of the vertical axis of one image is inclined toward or away from that of the other. **vertical d.,** diplopia in which one image appears above the other in the same vertical plane.

diplopiometer (di-plo″pe-om′e-ter) an instrument for measuring diplopia.

diploscope (dip′lo-skōp) an instrument for studying double vision.

diplosomatia (dip″lo-so-ma′she-ah) diplosomia.

diplosome (dip′lo-sōm) a figure seen by light microscopy, consisting of the two centrioles of a cell.

diplosomia (dip″lo-so′me-ah) doubling of the body of a fetus.

diprosopus (di-pros′o-pus) a fetal monster with a double face.

diprotrizoate (di″pro-tri′zo-āt) a compound used as a contrast medium in roentgenography of the urinary tract.

dipsesis (dip-se′sis) morbid thirst. adj., **dipset′ic.**

dipsia (dip′se-ah) thirst.

dipsogen (dip′so-jen) an agent or measure that induces thirst and promotes ingestion of fluids.

dipsomania (dip″so-ma′ne-ah) an uncontrollable craving for alcoholic drink.

dipsosis (dip-so′sis) morbid thirst.

dipsotherapy (dip″so-ther′ah-pe) limitation of amount of fluids ingested.

dipygus (di-pi′gus) a fetal monster with a double pelvis.

dipylidiasis (dip″ĭ-lĭ-di′ah-sis) infestation with Dipylidium.

Dipylidium (dip″ĭ-lid′e-um) a genus of tapeworms. **D. cani′num,** the dog tapeworm, parasitic in dogs and cats and occasionally found in man.

dipyridamole (di″pi-rid′ah-mōl) a compound used to improve coronary circulation.

dipyrone (di′pi-rōn) a compound used as an analgesic and antipyretic.

director (di-rek′tor) a grooved instrument for guiding a bistoury or other surgical instrument.

Dirofilaria (di″ro-fĭ-la′re-ah) a genus of nematode parasites of the super family Filarioidea. **D. immit′is,** a species found in domestic and wild animals, usually in the myocardium; the heartworm.

dirofilariasis (-fil″ah-ri′ah-sis) infection with organisms of the genus Dirofilaria.

dis- (dis) word element [L.], *reversal* or *separation;* [Gr.], *duplication.*

disaccharidase (di-sak′ah-rĭ-dās″) an enzyme that catalyzes the hydrolysis of disaccharides.

disaccharide (di-sak′ah-rid, di-sak′ah-rīd) a sugar each molecule of which yields two molecules of monosaccharide on hydrolysis.

disacchariduria (di-sak″ah-ri-du′re-ah) presence of a disaccharide (lactose or sucrose) in the urine.

disaccharose (di-sak′ah-rōs) disaccharide.

disarticulation (dis″ar-tik″u-la′shun) the separation of connecting bones at their site of articulation, as in amputation of an arm or leg.

disassimilation (dis″ah-sim″ĭ-la′shun) catabolic change.

disc (disk) disk.

discharge (dis-charj′) 1. a setting free, or liberation. 2. material or force set free, as electric energy, or an excretion or substance evacuated.

discharger (dis-char′jer) an instrument for liberating electricity.

discission (di-sizh′un) needling of lens capsule in operation for cataract.

discitis (dis-ki′tis) inflammation of a disk, especially of an interarticular cartilage.

disclination (dis″kli-na′shun) extorsion of both eyes.

discoblastula (dis″ko-blas′tu-lah) the specialized blastula formed by cleavage of a fertilized telolecithal ovum, consisting of a cellular cap separated by the blastocele from a floor of uncleaved yolk.

discogenic (-jen′ik) caused by derangement of an intervertebral disk.

discogram (dis′ko-gram) diskogram.

discography (dis-kog′rah-fe) diskography.

discoid (dis′koid) 1. shaped like or resembling

a disk. 2. a dental instrument with a disklike or circular blade.

discophorous (dis-kof'ŏ-rus) having a disklike organ or part.

discoplacenta (dis″ko-plah-sen'tah) a discoid placenta.

discordance (dis-kor'dans) failure of occurrence of a given trait in one member of a twin pair.

discus (dis'kus), pl. *dis'ci* [L.] disk. **d. ooph'-orus, d. ovig'erus, d. prolig'erus**, cumulus oophorus.

discutient (dis-ku'shent) 1. scattering or dispersing. 2. a scattering or dispersing remedy.

disdiaclast (dis-di'ah-klast) a small, doubly refracting element found in the contractile substance of muscle.

disease (dĭ-zēz′) a definite morbid process, often with a characteristic train of symptoms. **Abrami's d.**, acquired hemolytic icterus. **Acosta's d.**, mountain sickness. **Adams's d., Adams-Stokes d.**, see under *syndrome*. **Addison's d.**, a condition due to hypofunction of the adrenal cortex, and characterized by weakness, weight loss and pigmentation of the skin and mucous membranes. **akamushi d.**, scrub typhus. **Albers-Schönberg d.**, osteopetrosis. **Albright's d.**, osteitis fibrosa cystica. **alligator-skin d.**, ichthyosis. **Almeida's d.**, South American blastomycosis. **Alzheimer's d.**, presenile dementia. **Aran-Duchenne d.**, myelopathic muscular atrophy. **arc-welder's d.**, pulmonary siderosis. **Aujeszky's d.**, pseudorabies. **Australian X d.**, see under *encephalitis*. **autoimmune d.**, disease due to immunologic action of one's own cells or antibodies on components of the body. **Ayerza's d.**, a form of erythremia marked by chronic cyanosis, chronic dyspnea, chronic bronchitis, bronchiectasis, hepatosplenomegaly, hyperplasia of bone marrow, and associated with sclerosis of the pulmonary artery. **Bamberger-Marie d.**, hypertrophic pulmonary osteoarthropathy. **Bang's d.**, brucellosis of cattle, due to *Brucella abortus*. **Banti's d.**, a disease of the spleen with splenomegaly and pancytopenia, now considered secondary to portal hypertension. **Barlow's d.**, scurvy. **Barraquer-Simons d.**, progressive lipodystrophy. **Basedow's d.**, toxic diffuse goiter. **Bayle's d.**, progressive general paresis. **Bazin's d.**, tuberculosis indurativa (erythema induratum). **Bechterew's d.**, rheumatoid arthritis of spine. **Benson's d.**, a condition of unknown origin, sometimes occurring with age, characterized by small, dustlike, glistening particles in the vitreous. **Bernhardt's d.**, meralgia paresthetica. **Besnier-Boeck d.**, sarcoid of Boeck. **Best's d.**, congenital macular degeneration. **Beurmann's d.**, sporotrichosis. **Bielschowsky's d.**, late infantile amaurotic familial idiocy. **Bielschowsky-Jansky d.**, amaurotic familial idiocy. **Biermer's d.**, pernicious anemia. **bleeder's d.**, hemophilia. **Blocq's d.**, astasia-abasia. **Bloodgood's d.**, cystic disease of breast. **Blount's d.**, aseptic necrosis of the medial condyle of the tibia, sometimes causing lateral bowing of the

legs. **Boeck's d.**, multiple benign sarcoid. **Borna d.**, a fatal enzootic encephalitis of horses, cattle and sheep caused by a filterable virus. **Bornholm d.**, epidemic pleurodynia. **Bourneville's d.**, tuberous sclerosis. **Bowen's d.**, a precancerous condition characterized by scaly skin lesions resembling psoriasis and showing microscopic changes in the epidermal cells. **Breda's d.**, yaws. **Bright's d.**, any one of a group of kidney diseases attended with albuminuria and edema; glomerulonephritis. **Brill's d.**, recurrent typhus. **Brill-Symmers d.**, giant follicular lymphoma. **Brill-Zinnser d.**, recrudescent typhus. **Brocq's d.**, disseminated neurodermatitis. **Brown-Séquard d.**, see under *syndrome*. **Buerger's d.**, thromboangiitis obliterans. **Buerger-Grütz d.**, idiopathic hyperlipemia. **Busse-Buschke d.**, cryptococcosis. **Caffey's d.**, infantile cortical hyperostosis. **caisson d.**, decompression sickness. **California d.**, coccidioidomycosis. **caloric d.**, any disease due to exposure to high temperature. **Calvé-Perthes d.**, osteochondrosis of capitular epiphysis of femur. **Camurati-Engelmann d.**, progressive diaphyseal dysplasia. **Carrión's d.**, an infectious disease of South America due to *Bartonella bacilliformis*, and transmitted by sandflies, lice and ticks; an acute febrile anemia *(Oroya fever)* is followed by appearance of a nodular cutaneous eruption *(verruga peruana)*. **cat-scratch d.**, see under *fever*. **celiac d.**, a diarrheal condition, possibly hereditary or metabolic, with failure to thrive. **celiac d., adult**, nontropical sprue. **Chagas d.**, trypanosomiasis due to *Trypanosoma cruzi*. **Chagas-Cruz d.**, Chagas disease. **Charcot's d.**, neurogenic arthropathy. **Charcot-Marie-Tooth d.**, progressive neuropathic (peroneal) muscular atrophy. **Christian-Weber d.**, nodular nonsuppurative panniculitis. **Christmas d.**, a congenital hemorrhagic diathesis clinically similar to classic hemophilia, but due to deficiency of plasma thromboplastin component. **Civatte's d.**, see under *poikiloderma*. **Coats's d.**, exudative retinopathy. **collagen d's**, a group of diseases characterized by biochemical and structural alterations in the mesenchymal tissues, including rheumatoid arthritis, dermatomyositis, systemic lupus erythematosus, anaphylactoid purpura, periarteritis and scleroderma. **communicable d.**, a disease the causative agents of which may pass or be carried from one person to another directly or indirectly. **complicating d.**, one which occurs in the course of some other disease as a complication. **compressed-air d.**, decompression sickness. **Concato's d.**, polyserositis. **constitutional d.**, one in which the whole body or an entire system of organs is affected. **contagious d.**, communicable disease. **Coxsackie virus A d.**, herpangina. **Crigler-Najjar d.**, congenital familial jaundice. **Crocq's d.**, acrocyanosis. **Crohn's d.**, regional enteritis. **Crouzon's d.**, craniofacial dysostosis. **Cruveilhier's d.**, 1. simple ulcer of the stomach 2. progressive myelopathic muscular atrophy.

Cushing's d., 1. pituitary basophilism. 2. adrenal cortical hyperfunction. **cystic d. of breast,** a chronic condition characterized by pain and tenderness of the breast, accentuated, in the premenstrual period, with large, multiple brown to blue cysts apparent on section. **cystine storage d.,** Fanconi syndrome. **cytomegalic inclusion d.,** a disease, especially of newborns, due to infection with a cytomegalic virus, and characterized by hepatosplenomegaly and often by microcephaly and mental or motor retardation. **Darier's d.,** keratosis follicularis. **Darling's d.,** histoplasmosis. **deficiency d.,** a condition due to lack of some nutrient or other substance essential to well-being of the body. **Dejerine's d.,** hypertrophic interstitial neuritis in infants. **Dejerine-Sottas d.,** hypertrophic interstitial neuropathy. **demyelinating d.,** a condition characterized by destruction of myelin. **Dercum's d.,** adiposis dolorosa. **Devic's d.,** optic neuromyelitis. **Down's d.,** see under *syndrome.* **Duchenne's d.,** 1. myelopathic muscular atrophy. 2. bulbar paralysis. 3. tabes dorsalis. **Duchenne-Aran d.,** myelopathic muscular atrophy. **Duhring's d.,** dermatitis herpetiformis. **Duke's d.,** a mild contagious disease characterized by pharyngitis, lymphadenopathy and a generalized macular erythematous eruption. **Duplay's d.,** subacromial bursitis. **Durand-Nicolas-Favre d.,** lymphogranuloma venereum. **Duroziez's d.,** congenital stenosis of the mitral valve. **Ebstein's d.,** see under *anomaly.* **echinococcus d.,** unilocular hydatid disease. **Economo's d.,** encephalitis lethargica. **Engelmann's d.,** progressive diaphyseal dysplasia. **Engman's d.,** infectious eczematoid dermatitis. **epizootic d.,** a disease which affects a large number of animals in some particular region within a short period of time. **Erb's d.,** idiopathic muscular atrophy. **Erb-Goldflam d.,** myasthenia gravis. **Eulenburg's d.,** paramyotonia congenita. **Fabry's d.,** angiokeratoma corporis diffusum. **Fahr-Volhard d.,** malignant nephrosclerosis. **Fanconi's d.,** congenital aplastic anemia of childhood with musculoskeletal defects. **Feer's d.,** acrodynia. **fibrocystic d. of pancreas,** cystic fibrosis. **fifth d.,** erythema infectiosum. **fifth venereal d.,** lymphogranuloma venereum. **fish-skin d.,** ichthyosis. **fish-slime d.,** septicemia from puncture wound by a fish spine. **Flajani's d.,** exophthalmic goiter. **flint d.,** chalicosis. **focal d.,** a localized disease. **foot-and-mouth d.,** an acute and highly contagious viral disease primarily and almost exclusively limited to domestic and wild cloven-footed animals. **Fordyce d.,** congenital condition characterized by minute yellowish white papules on the oral mucosa. **Fothergill's d.,** trigeminal neuralgia. **fourth d.,** Duke's disease. **fourth venereal d.,** gangrenous balanitis. **Fox's d., Fox-Fordyce d.,** a condition of unknown causation characterized by plugging of the pores of the apocrine sweat glands and vesiculation of the epidermis. **Francis's d.,** tularemia. **Frei's d.,** lymphogranuloma venereum. **Freiberg's d.,**

osteochondritis of a metatarsal head, usually of the head of the second or third metatarsal bone. **Friedländer's d.,** endarteritis obliterans. **Friedreich's d.,** paramyoclonus multiplex. **functional d.,** any disease that alters body functions, but is not associated with any apparent organic lesion or change. **Gaisböck's d.,** polycythemia hypertonica. **Gamna's d.,** splenomegaly with thickening of the splenic capsule and the presence of small brownish areas (Gamna nodules), ferruginous pigment being deposited in the splenic pulp. **Garré's d.,** sclerotic nonsuppurative osteitis. **Gaucher's d.,** a familial disorder characterized by splenomegaly, skin pigmentation, scleral pingueculae, and presence of distinctive cells in the liver, spleen and bone marrow. **Gee's d., Gee-Herter d., Gee-Herter-Heubner d., Gee-Thaysen d.,** celiac disease. **genetotrophic d.,** a metabolic disease due to a genetically transmitted enzyme defect; called also *inborn error of metabolism.* **Gierke's d.,** glycogenosis. **Gilbert's d.,** constitutional hyperbilirubinemia. **Gilford-Hutchinson d.,** progeria. **Gilles de la Tourette's d.,** motor incoordination with echolalia and coprolalia. **Glanzmann's d.,** thrombasthenia. **glass-blowers' d.,** an infection with enlargement of the parotid gland occurring in glass-blowers. **Glénard's d.,** splanchnoptosis. **Glisson's d.,** rickets. **glycogen storage d.,** glycogenosis. **Goldflam's d., Goldflam-Erb d.,** myasthenia gravis. **Goldschieder's d.,** epidermolysis bullosa. **Graves's d.,** exophthalmic goiter. **Greenfield's d.,** late infantile metachromatic leukoencephalopathy. **Gull's d.,** atrophy of the thyroid gland with myxedema. **Gull-Sutton d.,** generalized arteriosclerosis. **Hartnup disease. Hailey-Hailey d.,** benign chronic familial pemphigus. **Hallervorden-Spatz d.,** see under *syndrome.* **Hallopeau's d.,** lichen sclerosus et atrophicus. **Hamman's d.,** spontaneous interstitial emphysema of the lungs. **Hand's d.,** Hand-Schüller-Christian disease. **hand-foot-and-mouth d.,** mild, highly infectious virus disease of children, with vesicular lesions in the mouth and on the hands and feet. **Hand-Schüller-Christian d.,** see under *syndrome.* **Hanot's d.,** biliary cirrhosis. **Hansen's d., benign,** the tuberculoid type of leprosy. **Hansen's d., malignant,** the lepromatous type of leprosy. **hardware d.,** gastritis in cattle due to ingestion of small metal objects. **Hartnup's d.,** a genetically determined disorder of tryptophan transport, with pellagra-like skin lesions, transient cerebellar ataxia, constant renal amino-aciduria and other biochemical abnormalities. **Hashimoto's d.,** chronic lymphocytic thyroiditis. **Heberden's d.,** rheumatic arthritis. **Hebra's d.,** erythema multiforme exudativum. **Heerfordt's d.,** uveoparotid fever. **Heine-Medin d.,** acute anterior poliomyelitis. **hemoglobin C d.,** a hereditary condition in Negroes characterized by a third type of adult hemoglobin, distinguishable from hemoglobin A and hemoglobin S. **hemolytic d. of newborn,** a condition in newborn infants marked by excessive blood destruction; caused, in the human patient, by transplacental transfer of antibodies produced by the mother in response to passage of incompatible blood from the fetal to the maternal circulation and usually the result of incompatibility of the Rh factor. **hemorrhagic d.**, any one of a group of diseases marked by a tendency to hemorrhages from the membranes and into the tissues. **hemorrhagic d. of newborn**, a self-limited hemorrhagic disorder of the first few days of life, due to deficiency of certain coagulation factors in the blood. **Hippel's d.**, angiomatosis of the retina. **Hirschsprung's d.**, aganglionic megacolon. **His's d.**, **His-Werner d.**, trench fever. **Hodgkin's d.**, a painless, progressive and fatal condition characterized by pruritus and enlargement of the lymph nodes, spleen and lymphoid tissues generally, which often begins in the neck and spreads through the body. **hoof-and-mouth d.**, foot-and-mouth disease. **Huebner-Herter d.**, celiac disease. **Hurler's d.**, a disorder of mucopolysaccharide metabolism, characterized by abnormal elimination of mucopolysaccharides and by typical craniofacial changes (gargoylism). **Hutchinson's d.**, progeria. **hyaline membrane d.**, idiopathic respiratory distress of newborn. **hydatid d.**, an infection due to larval forms of certain tapeworms (Echinococcus) and characterized by development of expanding cysts. **Hyde's d.**, prurigo nodularis. **hydrocephaloid d.**, a condition resembling hydrocephalus, but with depressed fontanels, following severe diarrhea. **Iceland d.**, benign myalgic encephalomyelitis. **idiopathic d.**, one that exists without any connection with any known cause. **infectious d.**, one caused by some parasitic organism and transmitted from one person to another by transfer of the organism. **intercurrent d.**, a disease occurring during the course of another disease with which it has no connection. **iron-storage d.**, hemochromatosis. **von Jaksch's d.**, infantile pseudoleukemia. **Janet's d.**, psychasthenia. **Jensen's d.**, retinochoroiditis juxtapapillaris. **Johne's d.**, paratuberculosis. **Kahler's d.**, multiple myeloma. **Kaposi's d.**, 1. xeroderma pigmentosum. 2. Kaposi's varicelliform eruption. 3. idiopathic hemorrhagic sarcoma (Kaposi). **Katayama d.**, schistosomiasis japonica. **Kedani d.**, scrub typhus. **Kienböck's d.**, chronic osteitis of the lunate bone. **Kimmelstiel's d.**, intercapillary nephrosclerosis. **Klippel-Feil d.**, arthritic general pseudoparalysis. **Köbner's d.**, epidermolysis bullosa. **Köhler's d.**, osteochondrosis of navicular bone. **Köhler's second d.**, osteochondritis of a metatarsal head, usually of the head of the second or third metatarsal bone. **Korsakoff's d.**, Korsakoff's psychosis. **Krabbe's d.**, diffuse infantile familial cerebral sclerosis. **Kümmel's d.**, see under *spondylitis*. **Kufs' d.**, late juvenile form of amaurotic familial idiocy. **Kussmaul's d.**, periarteritis nodosa. **Kyasanur Forest d.**, a highly fatal virus disease of monkeys in the Kyasanur Forest of India, communicable to man. **leaf-curl d.**, a virus disease of plants characterized by curling or crinkling of the leaves. **Leber's d.**, see under *atrophy*. **Legg's d.**, **Legg-Calvé d.**, **Legg-Calvé-Waldenström d.**, osteochondrosis of capitular epiphysis. **Legg-Calvé-Perthes d.**, osteochondrosis of epiphysis of the head of the femur. **Leiner's d.**, desquamative erythroderma in infants. **Leriche's d.**, Sudeck's atrophy. **Letterer-Siwe d.**, a rapidly fatal nonfamilial, nonlipoid reticuloendotheliosis of early childhood. **Lewandowsky's d.**, rosacea-like tuberculid. **Libman-Sacks d.**, nonbacterial verrucous endocarditis. **Lignac-Fanconi d.**, cystinosis. **Lindau's d.**, combined hemangioma of the cerebellum and of the retina occuring as a familial disease. **Lindau-von Hippel d.**, a hereditary condition of unknown origin, with hemangioblastomas of the cerebellum associated with hemangiomas of the skin. **Little's d.**, cerebral spastic infantile paralysis. **Lobstein's d.**, fragilitas ossium. **Lowe's d.**, oculocerebrorenal syndrome. **Lutembacher's d.**, mitral stenosis associated with an atrial septal defect. **Lutz-Splendore-Almeida d.**, South American blastomycosis. **Madelung's d.**, diffuse symmetrical lipomatosis. **Majocchi's d.**, annular telangiectatic purpura. **maple bark d.**, a granulomatous interstitial pneumonitis due to a rare mold found beneath the bark of maple logs. **maple syrup urine d.**, a genetotrophic disease involving deficiency of an enzyme necessary in the metabolism of branched-chain amino acids and named from the characteristic odor of the urine. **Marchiafava-Micheli d.**, see under *syndrome*. **Marfan's d.**, progressive spastic paraplegia in children with hereditary syphilis. **Marie's d.**, acromegaly. **Marie-Bamberger d.**, hypertrophic osteoarthropathy. **Marie-Strümpell d.**, rheumatoid spondylitis. **Marie-Tooth d.**, progressive neuropathic (peroneal) muscular atrophy. **Mediterranean d.**, thalassemia. **Menetrier's d.**, excessive proliferation of the gastric mucosa, producing diffuse thickening of the stomach wall. **Meniere's d.**, deafness, tinnitus, and dizziness, in association with nonsuppurative disease of the labyrinth. **Merzbacher-Pelizaeus d.**, aplasia axialis extracorticalis congenita. **Meyer's d.**, adenoids of the pharynx. **microdrepanocytic d.**, a disorder of the blood hemoglobin in which thalassemia is associated with the sickling trait. **Mikulicz's d.**, chronic lymphocytic infiltration and enlargement of the lacrimal and salivary glands of unknown origin. **Milroy's d.**, a hereditary condition with chronic lymphatic obstruction causing permanent edema of one or both legs. **Minamata d.**, a severe neurologic disorder due to poisoning by organic mercury and leading to severe permanent disability or death. **Mitchell's d.**, erythromelalgia. **Moebius' d.**, periodic migraine with paralysis of the oculomotor muscles. **Mondor's d.**, inflammation of a large subcutaneous vein crossing the lateral chest region and breast, the vessel appearing as a tender cord.

Morquio's d., familial osteochondrodystrophy. **Morton's d.**, tenderness or pain in the metatarsophalangeal joint of the third or fourth toe. **Morvan's d.**, syringomyelia. **mosaic d.**, a disease of plants, usually characterized by persistent chlorotic or necrotic spotting or mottling. **Murray Valley d.**, Australian X encephalitis. **Neumann's d.**, pemphigus vegetans. **Newcastle d.**, a viral disease of birds, including domestic fowl, characterized by respiratory and gastrointestinal or pneumonic and encephalitic symptoms; also transmissible to man. **Nicolas-Favre d.**, lymphogranuloma venereum. **Niemann's d., Niemann-Pick d.**, a heredofamilial disease with massive hepatosplenomegaly, brownish yellow discoloration of skin, nervous system involvement, and presence in the liver, spleen, lungs, lymph nodes and bone marrow of foamy reticular cells containing phospholipids. **occupational d.**, a disease arising from causes connected with the patient's occupation. **Oguchi's d.**, a form of hereditary night blindness common in Japan. **Ollier's d.**, dyschondroplasia. **Oppenheim's d.**, amyotonia congenita. **Oppenheim-Urbach d.**, necrobiosis lipoidica diabeticorum. **organic d.**, one due to structural changes. **Osgood-Schlatter d.**, osteochondritis of the tibial tubercle. **Osler's d.**, 1. polycythemia vera. 2. hereditary hemorrhagic telangiectasia. **Osler-Vaquez d.**, polycythemia vera. **Owren's d.**, parahemophilia. **Paget's d.**, 1. (of bone) osteitis deformans. 2. (of breast) an inflammatory cancerous affection of the areola and nipple. **parasitic d.**, one due to parasites. **Parkinson's d.**, parkinsonism. **parrot d.**, psittacosis. **Parrot's d.**, syphilitic pseudoparalysis. **Parry's d.**, exophthalmic goiter. **pearl d.**, tuberculosis of lower animals. **Pel-Ebstein d.**, Hodgkin's disease. **Pelizaeus-Merzbacher d.**, familial centrolobar sclerosis. **Pellegrini's d., Pellegrini-Stieda d.**, calcification of medial collateral ligament of knee due to trauma. **periodic d.**, a condition characterized by regularly recurring intermittent episodes of fever, edema, arthralgia or gastric pain and vomiting, continuing for years in otherwise healthy persons. **periodontal d.**, a disease process affecting the tissues about a tooth. **Perthes's d.**, osteochondrosis of the epiphysis of the head of the femur. **Peyronie's d.**, induration of the corpora cavernosa of the penis, with proliferation of connective tissue and possible presence of cartilage or bone. **Pfeiffer's d.**, infectious mononucleosis. **Pic's d.**, constrictive pericarditis. **Pick's d.**, circumscribed cerebral atrophy. **pink d.**, acrodynia. **Plaut-Vincent d.**, Vincent's angina. **Pompe's d.**, generalized glycogenosis. **Poncet's d.**, tuberculous arthritis. **porcupine d.**, ichthyosis. **Pott's d.**, tuberculosis of a vertebra, producing acute curvature of the spine, with convexity directed backward, and causing compression of the cord. **pulseless d.**, absence of the pulse and of perceptible blood pressure in the arms, with changes in the fundus of the eye and hypertension in the lower extremities. **de Quervain's d.**, inflammation of the long abductor, short extensor tendons of the thumb, with swelling and tenderness. **Quincke's d.**, angioneurotic edema. **Quinquaud's d.**, folliculitis decalvans. **Raynaud's d.**, intermittent pallor, cyanosis or redness of the fingers, brought on by exposure to cold; occurring chiefly in young females and sometimes leading to gangrene. **von Recklinghausen's d.**, 1. neurofibromatosis. 2. osteitis fibrosa cystica generalisata. **Reiter's d.**, a disease of males marked by initial diarrhea followed by urethritis, conjunctivitis and migratory polyarthritis and frequently accompanied by keratotic lesions of the skin. **Rendu-Weber-Osler d.**, hereditary hemorrhagic telangiectasia. **rheumatic heart d.**, the most important and constant manifestation of rheumatic fever, consisting of inflammatory changes with valvular deformations and other residua. **Rigg's d.**, periodontitis. **Ritter's d.**, dermatitis exfoliativa of infants. **Roger's d.**, an abnormal congenital communication between the ventricles of the heart. **Rokitansky's d.**, acute yellow atrophy of the liver. **runt d.**, a syndrome produced by immunologically competent cells in a foreign host that is unable to reject them, resulting in gross retardation of host development and in death. **sacroiliac d.**, chronic tuberculosis of the sacroiliac joint. **salivary gland inclusion d.**, cytomegalic inclusion disease. **San Joaquin Valley d.**, coccidioidal granuloma. **Sander's d.**, epidemic keratoconjunctivitis. **sartian d.**, an infectious disease of Turkestan, resembling cutaneous leishmaniasis. **Schamberg's d.**, progressive pigmentary dermatosis. **Schenck's d.**, sporotrichosis. **Scheuermann's d.**, osteochondritis deformans juvenilis dorsi. **Schilder's d.**, progressive subcortical encephalopathy. **Schimmelbusch's d.**, cystic disease of breast. **Schlatter-Osgood d.**, osteochondrosis of the tuberosity of the tibia. **Schmorl's d.**, herniation of nucleus pulposus. **Schönlein's d.**, nonthrombopenic purpura. **Schüller's d.**, 1. Hand-Schüller-Christian disease. 2. osteoporosis circumscripta cranii. **Schüller-Christian d.**, Hand-Schüller-Christian disease. **secondary d.**, 1. a morbid condition subsequent to or a consequence of another disease. 2. a condition due to introduction of mature, immunologically competent cells into a host rendered capable of accepting them by heavy exposure to ionizing radiation. **self-limited d.**, one which by its very nature runs a limited and definite course. **Senear-Usher d.**, pemphigus erythematosus. **septic d.**, one caused by putrefactive organisms within the body. **serum d.**, see under *sickness*. **silo-filler's d.**, a chronic inflammatory reaction, principally in interstitial tissues of the lung, due to exposure to dusty, moldy plant materials or to organic fertilizers. **Simmonds's d.**, a condition due to pituitary insufficiency and characterized by slowly progressive weakness, weight loss and mental deterioration. **sixth d.**, exanthem subitum. **sixth venereal**

d., lymphogranuloma venereum. **sleeping d.,** narcolepsy. **specific d.,** one caused by a specific virus or poison. **Spielmeyer-Vogt d.,** juvenile amaurotic familial idiocy. **Stanton's d.,** melioidosis. **Steinert's d.,** myotonia atrophica. **stiff lamb d.,** white muscle disease. **Still's d.,** juvenile rheumatoid arthritis. **Stokes's d.,** Graves's disease. **Stokes-Adams d.,** Adams-Stokes disease. **storage d.,** thesaurismosis. **structural d.,** one accompanied by anatomic or histologic change in the tissues. **Strümpell's d.,** 1. hereditary spastic spinal paralysis. 2. polioencephalomyelitis. **Strümpell-Leichtenstein d.,** hemorrhagic encephalitis. **Strümpell-Marie d.,** rheumatoid arthritis of spine. **Sturge-Weber d.,** telangiectases of the nervous system, with mental defect, focal epilepsy, buphthalmos, intracranial calcification and facial nevi, chiefly within the distribution of the ophthalmic nerve. **Stuttgart d.,** a disease of dogs due to *Leptospira canicola* or *Leptospira icterohaemorrhagiae*. **Sudeck's d.,** acute atrophy of a carpal or tarsal bone, resulting from trauma. **Sutton's d.,** 1. leukoderma acquisitum centrifugum. 2. granuloma fissuratum. **sweet clover d.,** a hemorrhagic disease of cattle due to ingestion of spoiled sweet clover. **Swift's d.,** acrodynia. **Symmers's d.,** giant follicular lymphoma. **systemic d.,** one affecting a number of tissues which perform a common function. **Tangier d.,** a familial disorder characterized by a deficiency of high-density lipoproteins in the blood serum, with storage of cholesterol esters in the tonsils and other tissues. **Tay-Sachs d.,** infantile amaurotic familial idiocy. **Teschen d.,** a viral encephalomyelitis in swine. **third d.,** an infectious disease characterized by fever, lymphadenitis, conjunctivitis and a macular erythematous eruption of the trunk. **Thomsen's d.,** myotonia congenita. **tsutsugamushi d.,** scrub typhus. **tunnel d.,** decompression sickness. **Urbach-Oppenheim d.,** necrobiosis lipoidica diabeticorum. **vagabonds' d.,** discoloration of the skin from lice. **Vaquez's d.,** polycythemia vera. **venereal d.,** one acquired in sexual contact or coitus. **vibration d.,** blanching and diminished flexion of the fingers, with loss of perception of cold, heat and pain, and osteoarthritic changes in joints of the arm, due to continued use of vibrating tools. **Vincent's d.,** ulceromembranous stomatitis. **Waldenström d.,** 1. (of blood) macroglobulinemia. 2. (of bone) osteochondrosis involving the hip joint. **Weber-Christian d.,** modular nonsuppurative panniculitis. **Weil's d.,** icterohemorrhagic leptospirosis. **Werlhof's d.,** idiopathic thrombocytopenia purpura. **Wernicke's d.,** hemorrhagic polioencephalitis. **Westphal-Strümpell d.,** hepatolenticular degeneration. **Whipple's d.,** intestinal lipodystrophy. **White-Darier d.,** keratosis follicularis. **white muscle d.,** a condition characterized by degeneration of muscles in young animals, chiefly in lambs and calves, whose dams have fed on legume hay. **Whitmore's d.,** melioidosis. **Willebrand's d.,** a hereditary familial

disease due to a deficiency of antihemophilic globulin and capillary defect, marked by severe epistaxis and bleeding from gums and genitalia. **Wilson's d.,** hepatolenticular degeneration. **woolsorter's d.,** pneumonia due to inhalation of spores of *Bacillus anthracis*, the organism causing anthrax. **x d.,** 1. hyperkeratosis in cattle. 2. a condition in fowl characterized by cyanosis of the head. **yellows d.,** a disease of flowering plants, with diffuse or stripelike yellowish discoloration of the foliage. **zymotic d.,** any disease produced by a living germ within the body.

disengagement (dis″en-gāj′ment) liberation of the fetus, or part thereof, from the vaginal canal.

disequilibrium (dis″e-kwī-lib′re-um) unstable equilibrium.

disgerminoma (dis-jer″mĭ-no′mah) dysgerminoma.

dish (dish) a vessel, usually of glass or porcelain, used for various laboratory purposes. **evaporating d.,** a laboratory vessel, usually wide and shallow, in which material is evaporated by exposure to heat. **Petri d.,** a round, shallow flat dish, usually of glass and of 100 mm. outside diameter, used in bacteriologic or biological laboratories. **Stender d.,** a glass vessel for biological preparations, staining, etc., with straight sides and ground plate glass covers of 50 to 130 mm. outside diameter, and 33 to 100 mm. high.

disimmunity (dis″ī-mu′nī-te) absence of immunity.

disimmunize (dis-im′u-nīz) to cause an organism to lose its immunity.

disimpaction (dis″im-pak′shun) relief of the impacted portion of a fracture.

disinfect (dis″in-fekt′) to free from infection.

disinfectant (-fek′tant) 1. destroying infection. 2. an agent which destroys infection-producing organisms.

disinfection (-fek′shun) destruction of pathogenic germs or agents. **concurrent d.,** disinfection of discharges and all infective matter all through the course of a disease. **terminal d.,** disinfection of a sick room and its contents at the termination of a disease.

disinfestation (-fes-ta′shun) the destruction of infesting insects, as lice.

disinsectization (-sek″tī-za′shun) removal of infesting insects.

disintegrator (dis-in″tē-gra′tor) an agent or device that produces disintegration of material, such as an apparatus that converts plant or animal tissues or other solid material into a homogeneous pulplike or semiliquid mass.

Disipal (dis′ĭ-pal) trademark for a preparation of orphenadrine hydrochloride.

disjunction (dis-junk′shun) the moving apart of chromosomes at anaphase of meiosis.

disk (disk) a flat, round structure or organ; often spelled with a *c* in names of anatomic structures. **articular d.,** a pad of fibrocartilage or dense fibrous tissue present in some synovial joints. **blood d.,** a blood platelet. **Bowman's d.,** one of the segments making up a striated muscle fiber. **choked d.,** an edematous optic disk, caused primarily by interference with circulation in the optic nerve, producing edema and hyperemia of the disk (papilledema). **cupped d.,** a pathologically depressed optic disk. **dental d.,** a thin, round piece of paper or other material for carrying polishing powders or specially treated for use in various procedures on the teeth. **embryonic d.,** the mass of cells of the developing fertilized ovum that gives rise to the new individual. **gelatin d.,** one prepared from gelatin, as those placed under an eyelid for introduction of substances acting on the eye. **germ d., germinal d.,** embryonic disk. **Hensen's d.,** pale line running transversely through a sarcous element. **intervertebral d.,** the layer of fibrocartilage between the bodies of adjoining vertebrae. **intra-articular d.,** fibrous structures within the capsules of diarthrodial joints. **optic d.,** circular area in the retina representing the termination of the optic nerve. **Placido's d.,** a keratoscopic disk marked with circles.

diskectomy (dis-kek'to-me)   excision of an intervertebral disk.

diskiform (dis'kī-form)   in the shape of a disk.

diskitis (dis-ki'tis)   inflammation of a disk, especially of an intervertebral disk.

diskogram (dis'ko-gram)   a film produced by diskography.

diskography (dis-kog'rah fe)   radiography of the vertebral column after injection of radiopaque material into an intervertebral disk.

dislocation (dis"lo-ka'shun)   displacement of a part. **complete d.,** one in which the surfaces are entirely separated. **compound d.,** one in which the joint communicates with the air through a wound. **consecutive d.,** one in which the displaced bone is not in the same position as when dislocated. **incomplete d.,** partial dislocation. **old d.,** one in which inflammatory changes have occurred. **partial d.,** one in which the surfaces remain in partial contact. **pathologic d.,** one due to disease of the joint or to paralysis of the muscles. **primitive d.,** one in which the bones remain as originally displaced. **recent d.,** one in which no inflammatory changes have occurred. **simple d.,** one in which there is no communication with the air through a wound. **sub spinous d.,** dislocation of the head of the humerus into the space below the spine of the scapula.

dismemberment (dis-mem'ber-ment)   amputation of an extremity, usually designating separation other than through a joint.

disobliteration (dis"ob-lit"er-a'shun)   the restoration of the lumen of a stenosed vessel or of other anatomic space which had previously been obliterated.

disocclude (dis"ō-klood')   to grind a tooth so that it does not touch its antagonist in the other jaw.

Disomer (di'so-mer)   trademark for preparations of dexbrompheniramine maleate.

disomus (di-so'mus)   a double-bodied monster.

disorder (dis-or'der)   an abnormality or derangement. **functional d.,** a disorder not associated with clearly defined physical cause or structural change.

disorientation (dis-o"re-en-ta'shun)   loss of recognition of time, place or persons.

dispensary (dis-pen'ser-e)   a place for dispensation of free or low-cost medical treatment.

dispensatory (dis-pen'sah-tor"e)   a book which describes medicines and their preparation and uses. **D. of the United States of America,** a collection of monographs on unofficial drugs and drugs recognized by the Pharmacopoeia of the United States, the Pharmacopoeia of Great Britain, and the National Formulary, also on general tests, processes, reagents and solutions of the U.S.P. and N.F., as well as drugs used in veterinary medicine.

dispersate (dis'per-sāt)   a suspension of finely divided particles of a substance.

disperse (dis-pers')   1. to scatter. 2. the particles suspended in a colloid solution.

dispersidology (dis-per"si-dol'o-je)   colloid chemistry.

dispersion (dis-per'zhun)   a preparation in which particles of one material are incorporated throughout the substance of another.

dispersoid (dis-per'soid)   a finely divided substance.

dispireme (di-spi'rēm)   the mitotic figure which follows the diaster.

displacement (dis-plās'ment)   removal to an abnormal location or position; in psychology, unconscious transference of an emotion from its original object onto a more acceptable substitute.

disproportion (dis"pro-por'shun)   abnormality of relation between two values or structures that are usually proportional. **cephalopelvic d.,** abnormally large size of fetal skull in relation to the maternal pelvis, leading to difficulties in delivery.

disruption (dis-rup'shun)   the act of separating forcibly, or the state of being abnormally separated.

dissect (dī-sekt', di-sekt')   to perform dissection.

dissection (dī-sek'shun)   1. cutting up of an organism for study. 2. the separation of tissues in surgical procedures. **blunt d.,** separation of tissues along natural lines of cleavage, by means of a blunt instrument or finger. **sharp d.,** separation of tissues by means of the sharp edge of a knife or scalpel, or with scissors.

dissector (dī-sek'tor)   1. one who dissects. 2. a handbook used as a guide for the act of dissecting.

dissimilation (dī-sim"ī-la'shun)   disassimilation.

dissociation (dī-so"se-a'shun)   1. separation into parts or elements. 2. a mental disorder in which ideas are split off from the personality and are buried in the unconscious.

dissogeny (dī-soj'e-ne)   the state of having sexual maturity in both a larval and an adult stage.

dissolution (dis"o-lu'shun)   1. death. 2. resolution into component elements.

dissolve (dī-zolv')   to liquefy by means of a solvent.

dissolvent (dĭ-zol′vent)   a solvent medium.

distad (dis′tad)   toward the distal part.

distal (dis′tal)   farthest from a point of reference, as from a center, a median line, the trunk, or the point of attachment or origin.

distalis (dis-ta′lis) [L.]   distal.

distance (dis′tans)   expression of the linear measurement of space separating two specified points. **focal d.,** focal length. **hearing d.,** the maximum distance at which sound-producing stimuli can be perceived by the ear. **infinite d.,** in optics, any distance over 20 feet (6 meters), from which rays of light striking the eye are practically parallel. **interarch d.,** the vertical distance between the maxillary and mandibular arches under specified conditions. **interocclusal d.,** the distance between the occluding surfaces of the maxillary and mandibular teeth with the mandible in physiologic rest position. **interocular d.,** the distance between the eyes, usually used in reference to the interpupillary distance. **target-skin d.,** the distance between the anode from which roentgen rays are reflected and the skin of the body surface interposed in their path. **working d.,** 1. the distance of the objective of a microscope from the specimen being examined. 2. the distance between the eye of a workman and the object on which he is working.

distemper (dis-tem′per)   an acute, highly infectious viral disease in animals.

distichia (dis-tik′e-ah)   presence of a double row of eyelashes, causing irritation of the cornea.

distichiasis (dis″tĭ-ki′ah-sis)   distichia.

distillate (dis′tĭ-lāt)   a product of distillation.

distillation (dis″tĭ-la′shun)   conversion of a liquid into vapors which are reconverted to liquid form, as a means of eliminating contaminants from the original solution. **destructive d.,** distillation at a high temperature in the absence of air, as in the preparation of coal tar from coal. **fractional d.,** separation of a mixture into a number of fractions, based on their different boiling points. **vacuum d.,** distillation under reduced pressure to avoid decomposition which might occur at atmospheric pressure.

distinctometer (dis″tink-tom′ĕ-ter)   an instrument for palpating the borders of the abdominal organs.

distobuccal (dis″to-buk′al)   pertaining to or formed by the distal and buccal surfaces of a tooth, or by the distal and buccal walls of a tooth cavity.

distobucco-occlusal (-buk″o-ŏ-kloo′zal)   pertaining to or formed by the distal, buccal and occlusal surfaces of a tooth.

distobuccopulpal (-pul′pal)   pertaining to or formed by the distal, buccal and pulpal walls of a tooth cavity.

distocervical (dis″to-ser′vĭ-kal)   1. pertaining to the distal surface of the neck of a tooth. 2. distogingival.

distoclusion (-kloo′zhun)   malrelation of the dental arches with the lower jaw in a distal or posterior position in relation to the upper.

distogingival (dis″to-jin-ji′val)   pertaining to or formed by the distal and gingival walls of a tooth cavity.

distomia (di-sto′me-ah)   the presence of two mouths.

distomiasis (dis″to-mi′ah-sis)   infection due to trematodes or flukes.

distomolar (-mo′lar)   a supernumerary molar.

distortion (dĭ-stor′shun)   the state of being twisted out of normal shape or position; in psychiatry, the conversion of material offensive to the superego into acceptable form. **parataxic d.,** distortions in judgment and perception, particularly in interpersonal relations, based upon the need to perceive objects and relationships in accord with a pattern from earlier experience.

distraction (di-strak′shun)   1. diversion of attention. 2. separation of joint surfaces without rupture of their binding ligaments and without displacement.

distress (dĭ-stres′)   physical or mental anguish or suffering. **idiopathic respiratory d. of newborn,** difficulty in breathing occurring in premature infants, infants of diabetic mothers and infants delivered by cesarean section.

distrix (dis′triks)   the splitting of the hairs at the end.

disulfiram (di-sul′fĭ-ram)   a disulfide compound used to treat chronic alcoholism.

dithiazanine (di″thi-az′ah-nēn)   a compound used as an anthelmintic.

diuresis (di″u-re′sis)   secretion of urine; often used to indicate increased function of the kidney.

diuretic (-ret′ik)   1. causing diuresis.   2. a medicine which stimulates the flow of urine.

Diuril (di′u-ril)   trademark for preparations of chlorothiazide.

diurnal (di-er′nal)   pertaining to or occurring during the daytime, or period of light.

divagation (di″vah-ga′shun)   incoherent or wandering speech.

divergence (di-ver′jens)   a moving part, or inclination away from a common point. adj., **diver′gent.**

diverticulectomy (di″ver-tik″u-lek′to-me)   excision of a diverticulum.

diverticulitis (-li′tis)   inflammation of a diverticulum.

diverticulogram (di″ver-tik′u-lo-gram)   an x-ray picture of a diverticulum.

diverticulosis (di″ver-tik″u-lo′sis)   the presence of diverticula.

diverticulum (di″ver-tik′u-lum), pl. *divertic′-ula* [L.]   a blind pouch. **false d.,** an intestinal diverticulum due to the protrusion of the mucous membrane through a tear in the muscular coat. **intestinal d.,** a pouch or sac formed by hernial protrusion of the mucous membrane through a defect in the muscular coat of the intestine. **Meckel's d.,** an occasional appendage of the ileum near the cecum; a relic of the vitelline duct. **Nuck's d.,** canal of Nuck. **pituitary d.,** Rathke's pouch. **pressure d., pulsion d.,** a sac or pouch formed by hernial protrusion of the mucous membrane through the muscular coat of the esophagus as a result of pressure from within. **Rokitansky's d.**, a traction diverticulum of the esophagus. **traction d.**, a localized distortion, angulation or funnel-shaped bulging of the esophageal wall, due to adhesions resulting from external lesion. **Zenker's d.**, a pulsion diverticulum of the esophagus.

division (dĭ-vizh'un) separation into parts. **cell d.**, the process by which cells reproduce. **indirect cell d.**, mitosis. **maturation d.**, meiosis.

divulsion (dĭ-vul'shun) forcible separation of parts.

divulsor (dĭ-vul'ser) instrument for forcible dilatation or separation of body parts.

dixenic (di-zen'ik) associated with two species of microorganisms.

dizygotic (di"zi-got'ik) pertaining to or derived from two separate zygotes (fertilized ova).

D.M.D. Doctor of Dental Medicine

D.M.F. decayed, missing, filled (teeth): an index used in dental surveys.

D.M.R.D. Diploma in Medical Radio-Diagnosis (Brit.)

D.M.R.E. Diploma in Medical Radiology and Electrology (Brit.)

D.M.R.T. Diploma in Medical Radio-Therapy (Brit.)

DMSO dimethyl sulfoxide, a chemical solvent with exceptional solvent properties, which has been used experimentally in a variety of clinical conditions.

DNA deoxyribonucleic acid.

D.N.B. dinitrobenzene.

D.O. Doctor of Osteopathy.

D.O.A. dead on admission (arrival).

DOCA (do'kah) trademark for desoxycorticosterone.

Docibin (do'si-bin) trademark for a crystalline preparation of vitamin B₁₂.

docimasia (do"si-ma'ze-ah) assay or examination; official test. adj., **docimas'tic.**

dodecadactylitis (do"dek-ah-dak"tĭ-li'tis) duodenitis.

dodecadactylon (dak'tĭ-lon) the duodenum.

dolich(o)- (dol'ĭ-ko) word element [Gr.], long.

dolichocephalic (dol'ĭ-ko-se fal'ik) having a cephalic index below 75.

dolichoderus (-der'us) an individual with a long neck.

dolichohieric (-hi-er'ik) having a sacral index below 100.

dolichomorphic (-mor'fik) a long, thin, asthenic body type.

dolichopellic (-pel'ik) having a pelvic index above 95.

dolichosigmoid (-sig'moid) an abnormally long sigmoid flexure.

dolichostenomelia (-ste"no-me'le-ah) extreme length and slenderness of the extremities, as in Marfan's syndrome.

Dolophine (do'lo-fēn) trademark for preparations of methadone.

dolor (do'lor) [L.] pain. **d. cap'itis,** headache.

dolorific (do"lor-if'ik) producing pain.

dolorogenic (do-lor"o-jen'ik) dolorific.

domatophobia (dom"ah-to-fo'be-ah) fear of being in a house.

dominance (dom'ĭ-nans) the greater strength of one of a pair or more of similar or contrasting factors or organs, so that the one appears to the exclusion of the other, or is used with greater ease or frequency; in genetics, the appearance, in a heterozygote, of one of two mutually antagonistic parental characters. **incomplete d.**, failure of one gene to be completely dominant, heterozygotes showing a phenotype intermediate between the two parents.

donor (do'ner) the person who furnishes blood or other body tissue to be transfused or grafted into the body of another. **hydrogen d.**, the molecule giving up hydrogen in an oxidation-reduction reaction. **universal d.**, a donor whose blood cells are not agglutinated by the blood of any patient.

donovanosis (don"o-van-o'sis) granuloma inguinale.

dopa (do'pah) 3,4-dihydroxyphenylalanine, produced by oxidation of tyrosine by tyrosinase, an intermediate product in the synthesis of both epinephrine and melanin.

dopamine (do'pah-mēn) a compound, hydroxytyramine, produced by the decarboxylation of dopa, an intermediate product in the synthesis of norepinephrine.

doraphobia (dor"ah-fo'be-ah) morbid dread of fur.

Dorbane (dor'bān) trademark for a preparation of danthron.

Doriden (dor'ĭ-den) trademark for preparations of glutethimide.

dormifacient (dor"mĭ-fa'shent) conducive to sleep.

Dormison (dor'mĭ-son) trademark for a preparation of methylparafynol.

dornase (dor'nās) deoxyribonuclease. **pancreatic d.**, a stabilized preparation of deoxyribonuclease, prepared from beef pancreas; used as an aerosol to reduce tenacity of pulmonary secretions.

Dornavac (dor'nah-vak) trademark for a preparation of pancreatic dornase.

dors(o)- (dor'so) word element [L.], the back; the dorsal aspect.

Dorsacaine (dor'sah-kān) trademark for a preparation of benoxinate hydrochloride.

dorsad (dor'sad) toward the back

dorsal (dor'sal) directed toward or situated on the back surface; opposite of ventral.

dorsalgia (dor-sal'je-ah) pain in the back.

dorsalis (dor-sa'lis) [L.] dorsal.

dorsiduct (dor'sĭ-dukt) to draw toward the back.

dorsiflexion (dor"sĭ-flek'shun) the act of bending a part backward.

dorsimesad (-mes'ad) traveling or directed toward the dorsimeson.

dorsimeson (-mes'on) the median lengthwise line of the back.

dorsocephalad (dor"so-sef'ah-lad) toward the back of the head.

dorsodynia (-din'e-ah) pain in the back.

dorsolateral (-lat'er-al) pertaining to the back and side.

dorsoventral (-ven'tral) 1. pertaining to the

back and belly surfaces of a body. 2. passing from the back to the belly surface.

dorsum (dor'sum), pl. *dor'sa* [L.] the back; the posterior or superior surface of a body or body part, as of the foot or hand.

dosage (do'sij) the determination and regulation of doses.

dose (dōs) a portion of any therapeutic agent (drug or radiation) to be administered at one time. **air d.,** the intensity of a roentgen-ray or gamma-ray beam in air. **curative d.,** that which is sufficient to restore normal health. **divided d.,** a relatively small dose repeated at short intervals. **effective d.,** that quantity of an agent sufficient to produce its characteristic effect. **effective d., median,** that which produces its effect in 50 per cent of the test subjects. **erythema d.,** that amount of roentgen rays which will cause a slight reddening of the skin. **lethal d.,** that quantity of an agent which is sufficient to cause death. **lethal d., median,** that which causes death of 50 per cent of the test subjects in 24 hours. **maximum d.,** the largest dose consistent with safety. **median curative d.,** one that abolishes symptoms in 50 per cent of test subjects. **minimum d.,** the smallest dose that will produce an effect. **organ tolerance d.,** that amount of radiation which can be administered without damage to the tissues of a normal organ. **permissible d.,** the largest amount of x-ray that a person may receive without harm. **skin d.,** the amount of radiation received on the surface of the skin, being the sum of primary radiation and the backscatter.

dosimeter (do-sim'ĕ-ter) instrument for measuring radiation dose.

dosimetry (do-sim'ĕ-tre) measurement of doses.

dossier (dos'e-a) the file containing the case history of a patient.

doublet (dub'let) a combination of two similar or complementary entities.

douche (dōōsh) [Fr.] a stream of water directed against a part or into a cavity. **air d.,** a current of air blown into a cavity, particularly into the tympanum to open the eustachian tube.

douglasitis (dug"lah-si'tis) inflammation of the cul-de-sac of Douglas.

dourine (doo-rēn') a contagious venereal disease of equine species, due to *Trypanosoma equiperdum.*

dowel (dow'el) a peg or pin for fastening an artificial crown or core to a natural tooth root, or affixing a die to a working model for construction of a crown, inlay or partial denture.

Doxinate (dok'sĭ-nāt) trademark for a preparation of dioctyl sodium sulfosuccinate.

doxogenic (dok'so-jen''ik) caused by one's own mental conceptions.

doxylamine (dok"sil-am'ēn) a pyridine compound used as an antihistaminic.

D.P. Doctor of Pharmacy.

D.P.H. Department of Public Health; Diplomate in Public Health; Doctor of Public Health.

D.R. reaction of degeneration.

Dr. Doctor.

dr. dram.

drachm (dram) dram.

dracunculiasis (drah-kung"ku-li'ah-sis) infection by nematodes of the genus Dracunculus.

dracunculosis (-lo'sis) dracunculiasis.

Dracunculus (drah-kung'ku-lus) a genus of nematode parasites. **D. medinen'sis,** a species widely distributed in North America, Africa, the Near East, East Indies and India; frequently found in man.

draft (draft) a copious liquid potion or dose.

drain (drān) an appliance or substance that affords a channel of exit for discharge from a wound. **cigaret d.,** a drain made by surrounding a small strip of gauze with a protective covering of rubber, gutta-percha, etc. **controlled d.,** a square of gauze, filled with gauze strips, pressed into a wound, the corners of the square and ends of the strips left protruding. **Mikulicz's d.,** a single layer of gauze, packed with several thick wicks of gauze, pushed into a wound cavity. **Penrose d.,** a piece of small rubber tubing through which gauze has been pulled. **quarantine d.,** a drain left in place after laparotomy to drain the peritoneal cavity and prevent external infection. **stab wound d.,** a drain brought out through a small puncture wound at some distance from the operative incision, to prevent infection of the operation wound. **Wylie d.,** a stem pessary of hard rubber with a groove along the stem, for draining the uterine cavity.

drainage (drān'ij) systematic withdrawal of fluids and discharges from a wound, sore or cavity. **basal d.,** withdrawal of the cerebrospinal fluid from the basal subarachnoid space for relief of increased intracranial pressure. **capillary d.,** drainage effected by strands of hair, catgut, spun glass or other material which acts by capillary attraction. **funnel d.,** drainage by glass funnels inserted into edematous tissues. **Monaldi's d.,** suction drainage of tuberculous cavities of the lungs. **postural d.,** therapeutic drainage in bronchiectasis and lung abscess by placing the patient head downward so that the trachea will be inclined downward and below the affected area. **through d.,** drainage effected by passing a perforated tube through the cavity, so that irrigation may be effected by injecting fluid into one aperture and letting it escape out of another. **tidal d.,** drainage of the urinary bladder by an apparatus which alternately fills the bladder to a predetermined pressure and empties it by a combination of siphonage and gravity flow.

dram (dram) a unit of weight in the avoirdupois (27.344 grains, 1.77 grams) or apothecaries' (60 grains, 3.89 grams) system. **fluid d.,** a unit of liquid measure of the apothecaries' system, containing 60 minims, and equivalent to 3.697 ml.

Dramamine (dram'ah-mēn) trademark for preparations of dimenhydrinate.

dramatism (dram'ah-tizm) dramatic behavior and speech.

drapetomania (drap"ĕ-to-ma'ne-ah) a morbid desire to run away.

drastic (dras'tik) 1. too effective. 2. a cathartic that produces watery stools and great irritation to the intestines.

Drepanidium (drep"ah-nid'e-um) a genus of parasitic protozoan animals.

drepanocyte (drep'ah-no-sīt") a sickle-shaped red blood corpuscle. adj., **drepanocyt'ic.**

drepanocytosis (drep"ah-no-si-to'sis) occurrence of drepanocytes in the blood.

dressing (dres'ing) a bandage or other application for an external wound. **antiseptic d.,** a dressing impregnated with an antiseptic solution. **occlusive d.,** one which completely closes a wound. **pressure d.,** one for maintaining constant pressure. **protective d.,** one which shields a part from injury or septic infection. **stent d.,** a dressing incorporating a mold of stent, such as is used to maintain position of a graft.

Drinalfa (drin-al'fah) trademark for preparations of methamphetamine hydrochloride.

drip (drip) a slow, drop-by-drop instillation of a solution. **Murphy d.,** slow instillation of fluid by rectum.

Drisdol (driz'dol) trademark for preparations of crystalline vitamin D.

drocarbil (dro-kar'bil) a compound used as an anthelmintic in veterinary medicine.

Drolban (drol'ban) trademark for a preparation of dromostanolone propionate.

dromograph (drom'o-graf) a recording hemodromometer.

dromomania (drom"o ma'ne-ah) a mania for traveling.

dromostanolone (dro"mo-stan'o-lōn) a steroid compound used as a palliative in advanced or metastatic carcinoma of the breast.

dromotropic (-trop'ik) affecting conductivity of a nerve fiber.

dromotropism (dro-mot'ro-pizm) the quality or property of affecting the conductivity of a nerve fiber

drop (drop) 1. a small spherical portion of liquid, which falls from the small opening in a pipet or medicine dropper; the quantity varies with the viscosity and specific gravity of the liquid, making use of this unit undesirable for medications requiring accurate measurement. 2. a descent or falling below the usual position. **ear d's,** medicated solution to be dropped into the external canal of the ear. **wrist d.,** paralysis of the extensor muscles of the hands and fingers, mainly due to metallic poisoning.

dropper (drop'er) a pipet or tube for dispensing liquid in drops.

dropsical (drop'si-kal) affected with dropsy.

dropsy (drop'se) accumulation of serous fluid in a cavity or in the tissues. **d. of belly,** ascites. **cardiac d.,** that due to heart disease. **d. of chest,** hydrothorax. **ovarian d.,** ovarian cyst.

drowning (drown'ing) suffocation and death resulting from filling of the lungs with water or other substance or fluid.

Dr.P.H. Doctor of Public Health.

drug (drug) any medicinal substance.

drum (drum) the cavity of the middle ear, closed by the tympanic membrane, to which the term "ear drum" is commonly applied.

drumstick (drum'stik) a nuclear lobule attached by a slender strand to the nucleus of a neutrophilic leukocyte; occurring in 2–3 per cent of neutrophils of normal females, but lacking in those of normal males.

drusen (droo'sen) 1. hyaline excrescences in the inner layer of the choroid of the eye. 2. rosettes of granules occurring in the lesions of actinomycosis.

D.T. distance test.

D.T.N. diphtheria toxin normal.

D.U. dog units.

dualism (du'al-izm) 1. the theory that there are two distinct stem cells for blood corpuscle formation: one for the lymphatic cells and the other for the myeloid cells. 2. the doctrine that body and mind are independent units.

Ducobee (doo'ko-be) trademark for preparations of vitamin B₁₂.

duct (dukt) a canal or passage for fluids. **aberrant d.,** any duct that is not usually present or that takes an unusual course or direction. **adipose d.,** an elongated sac in the cellular tissue filled with fat. **alimentary d.,** thoracic duct. **allantoic d.,** allantoic stalk. **auditory d.,** a space in the cochlea, between the tentorial and cochlear membranes. **d. of Bartholin,** the larger and longer of the sublingual ducts. **Bellini's d's,** large, short tubes emptying into the pelvis of the kidney. **biliary d's, biliferous d's,** the passages for the conveyance of bile in and from the liver. **Botallo's d.,** ductus arteriosus. **cochlear d.,** a spiral membranous tube in the bony canal of the cochlea. **common bile d.,** a duct formed by the union of the cystic and hepatic ducts. **d's of Cuvier,** two short venous trunks in the fetus opening into the atrium of the heart; the right one becomes the superior vena cava. **cystic d.,** the excretory duct of the gallbladder. **deferent d.,** vas deferens. **efferent d.,** the duct which gives outlet to a glandular secretion. **ejaculatory d.,** channel formed by union of the excretory ducts of testis and seminal vesicles, by which semen enters the urethra. **endolymphatic d.,** a tubular process of the membranous labyrinth of the ear. **excretory d.,** one through which the secretion is conveyed from a gland. **galactophorous d.,** one of the milk ducts of the mammary gland. **gall d's,** biliary ducts. **Gartner's d.,** a persistent relic of the wolffian duct. **genital d.,** genital canal. **hepatic d.,** the excretory duct of the liver, or one of its branches in the lobes of the liver. **interlobular d's,** channels between different lobules of a glandular organ. **lacrimal d.,** the excretory duct of the lacrimal gland. **lacrimonasal d.,** nasal duct. **lingual d.,** a depression on the dorsum of the tongue at the apex of the terminal sulcus. **Luschka's d's,** tubular structures in the wall of the gallbladder; some are connected with bile ducts, but none with the lumen of the gallbladder. **lymphatic d's,** channels for conducting lymph. **mesonephric d.,** an embryonic duct of the mesonephros, which in the male becomes the ductus deferens and in the female is largely obliterated. **metanephric d.,** ureter. **d. of Müller,** a duct in the embryo, developing into the oviducts, uterus and vagina. **nasal d., nasolacrimal d.,** the downward continuation of the lacrimal sac, opening on the lateral wall of the inferior meatus of the nose. **nephric d.,** ureter. **omphalomesenteric d.,** umbilical duct. **parotid d.,** duct by which the parotid gland empties into the mouth. **pronephric d.,** the duct of the pronephros, which later serves as the mesonephric duct (ductus mesonephricus). **prostatic d.,** any of the ducts conveying the prostatic secretion into the urethra. **renal d.,** ureter. **d. of Rivinus,** one of the ducts of the sublingual gland. **salivary d's,** the ducts of the salivary glands. **Santorini's d.,** the accessory duct of the pancreas. **secretory d.,** any one of the smaller ducts that are tributary to the excretory ducts of a gland and also have a secretory function. **segmental d.,** a tube, on either side of the body of the embryo, opening anteriorly into the body cavity, and posteriorly into the cloaca. **semicircular d's,** the long ducts of the membranous labyrinth of the ear. **seminal d's,** the passages for conveyance of spermatozoa and semen. **spermatic d.,** vas deferens. **d. of Steno, d. of Stensen,** parotid duct. **sublingual d's,** the ducts of the sublingual salivary glands. **tear d's,** lacrimal ducts. **thoracic d.,** a duct beginning in the receptaculum chyli and emptying into the left subclavian vein. **thyroglossal d.,** a channel in the fetus between the thyroid gland and tongue. **umbilical d.,** duct between umbilical vesicle and intestinal cavity of embryo. **urogenital d's,** the duct of Müller and the mesonephric duct. **vitelline d.,** umbilical duct. **d. of Wharton,** the duct of the submaxillary salivary gland. **d. of Wirsung,** the excretory duct of the pancreas. **wolffian d.,** mesonephric duct.

ductless (dukt'les) having no efferent duct.

ductule (duk'tūl) a minute duct.

ductulus (duk'tu-lus), pl. *duc'tuli* [L.] ductule.

ductus (duk'tus), pl. *duc'tus* [L.] duct. **d. arterio'sus,** fetal blood vessel which joins the aorta and pulmonary artery. **d. arterio'sus, patent,** persistence of the fetal channel between left pulmonary artery and aorta just distal to left subclavian artery. **d. choledo'chus commu'nis,** common bile duct. **d. def'erens,** the excretory duct of the testis which joins the excretory duct of the seminal vesicle to form the ejaculatory duct. **d. veno'sus,** a fetal vessel which connects the umbilical vein and the inferior vena cava.

duipara (du-ip'ah-rah) secundipara.

Dulcolax (dul'ko-laks) trademark for preparations of bisacodyl.

dull (dul) not resonant on percussion.

dullness (dul'nes) a quality of sound elicited by percussion, being short and high-pitched with little resonance.

dumb (dum) unable to speak.

dumbness (dum'nes) inability to speak.

duodenal (du″o-de'nal) pertaining to the duodenum.

duodenectomy (du″o-dě-nek'to-me) excision of the duodenum.

duodenitis (du″o-dě-ni'tis) inflammation of the duodenum.

duodenocholedochotomy (du″o-de″no-ko-led″-o-kot'o-me) incision of duodenum and common bile duct.

duodenoduodenostomy (-du″o-dě-nos'to-me) anastomosis of two previously remote portions of the duodenum.

duodenoenterostomy (-en″ter-os'to-me) anastomosis of the duodenum to some other part of the small intestine.

duodenohepatic (-hē-pat'ik) pertaining to duodenum and liver.

duodenoileostomy (-il″e-os'to-me) anastomosis of the duodenum to the ileum.

duodenojejunostomy (-je″ju-nos'to-me) anastomosis of the duodenum to the jejunum.

duodenorrhaphy (du″o-dě-nor'ah-fe) suture of the duodenum.

duodenoscopy (-nos'ko-pe) examination of the duodenum by an endoscope.

duodenostomy (-nos'to-me) fistulization of the duodenum.

duodenotomy (-not'o-me) incision of the duodenum.

duodenum (du″o-de'num) the first or proximal portion of the small intestine, being approximately twelve fingerbreadths in length.

Duphaston (du-fas'ton) trademark for a preparation of isopregnenone.

duplication (du-pli-ka'shun) in genetics, presence of an extra portion of a gene or chromosome.

Durabolin (du-rab'o-lin) trademark for a preparation of nandrolone phenpropionate.

Duracillin (du″rah-sil-in) trademark for preparations of crystalline procaine penicillin G.

dura mater (du'rah ma'ter) the outermost membrane of the brain and spinal cord.

dural (du'ral) pertaining to the dura mater.

duramatral (du″rah-ma'tral) dural.

duritis (du-ri'tis) inflammation of the dura mater.

duro-arachnitis (du″ro-ar″ak-ni'tis) inflammation of the dura mater and arachnoid.

dust (dust) a finely powdered substance. **blood d.,** hemoconia. **ear d.,** otoconia.

D.V.M. Doctor of Veterinary Medicine.

D.V.S. Doctor of Veterinary Science; Doctor of Veterinary Surgery.

dwale (dwāl) belladonna leaf.

dwarf (dwarf) an abnormally undersized person. **achondroplastic d.,** the commonest type of dwarf, showing relatively large head with saddle nose and brachycephaly, short extremities and usually lordosis. **aortic d.,** a person showing distinct underdevelopment as a result of severe aortic stenosis. **asexual d.,** an adult dwarf with deficient sexual development. **ateliotic d.,** a dwarf with infantile skeleton, with persistent nonunion between epiphyses and diaphyses. **infantile d.,** a person with retardation of mental and physical development. **micromelic d.,** a dwarf with very small limbs. **phocomelic d.,** a dwarf in whom the diaphyses of the long bones are abnormally short. **pituitary d.,** a dwarf

dysmyotonia (dis″mi-o-to′ne-ah) abnormal tonicity of muscle.

dysneuria (dis-nu′re-ah) impairment of the nervous power.

dysnomia (dis-no′me-ah) aphasia characterized by inability to correctly name certain things.

dysodontiasis (dis″o-don-ti′ah-sis) defective dentition.

dysontogenesis (dis″on-to-jen′ĕ-sis) defective development of the organism. adj., **dysontogenet′ic.**

dysopia (dis-o′pe-ah) defective vision.

dysorexia (dis″o-rek′se-ah) impairment of the appetite.

dysosmia (dis-oz′me-ah) impairment of the sense of smell.

dysostosis (dis″os-to′sis) a condition due to defective ossification of fetal cartilages. **cleidocranial d.,** a congenital condition in which there are defective ossification of the cranial bones and complete or partial absence of the clavicles **craniofacial d.,** deformity of the bones of the face and skull, attributed to premature fusion of the bones of the skull, a condition often having familial incidence. **mandibulofacial d.,** a congenital condition with hypoplasia of facial bones, antimongoloid slant of palpebral fissures, deformity of ears, macrostomia and other abnormalities of face and jaw. **metaphyseal d.,** a skeletal abnormality in which the epiphyses are normal or nearly so, and the metaphyseal tissues are replaced by masses of cartilage, producing interference with enchondral bone formation and expansion and thinning of the metaphyseal cortices. **d. mul′tiplex,** lipochondrodystrophy. **orodigitofacial d.,** anomalous development of the mouth and tongue, fingers, and frequently of the face, associated with a chromosomal abnormality.

dysoxidizable (dis-ok′sĭ-dīz″ah-bl) not easily oxidizable.

dyspancreatism (dis-pan′kre-ah-tizm″) disorder of the pancreas.

dyspareunia (dis″pah-ru′ne-ah) painful coitus.

dyspepsia (dis-pep′se-ah) indigestion; difficulty of digestion. adj., **dyspep′tic. acid d.,** dyspepsia with excessive formation of acid. **atonic d.,** that due to deficient quantity or quality of the gastric juice, or to defective action of the gastric muscles. **catarrhal d.,** that due to inflammation of the stomach. **intestinal d.,** that due to imperfect action of the intestinal juices. **nervous d.,** dyspepsia with gastric pains and various reflex nervous phenomena.

dyspeptone (dis-pep′tōn) an insoluble peptone.

dysphagia (dis-fa′je-ah) difficulty in swallowing.

dysphasia (dis-fa′ze-ah) impairment of ability to understand and use the symbols of language, both spoken and written.

dysphemia (dis-fe′me-ah) speech disorder due to psychoneurosis.

dysphonia (dis-fo′ne-ah) difficulty in speaking. adj., **dysphon′ic.**

dysphoria (dis-fo′re-ah) a feeling of misery.

dysphoriant (dis-fo′re-ant) 1. producing dysphoria. 2. an agent that produces dysphoria.

dysphrasia (dis-fra′ze-ah) difficulty in speaking due to mental defect.

dysphrenia (dis-fre′ne-ah) a functional psychosis.

dyspigmentation (dis″pig-men-ta′shun) any abnormality of pigmentation.

dyspinealism (dis-pin′e-al-izm) disordered activity of the pineal gland.

dyspituitarism (dis″pĭ-tu′ĭ-tar-izm″) disordered activity of the pituitary gland.

dysplasia (dis-pla′ze-ah) an abnormality of development. adj., **dysplas′tic. anteroposterior facial d.,** defective development resulting in abnormal anteroposterior relations of the maxilla and mandible to each other or to the cranial base. **cardiovascular d., hereditary,** a condition characterized by hypertrophy of the cephalic portion of the interventricular septum, disorganization of the myocardium and hypoplasia of the large arteries. **chondroectodermal d.,** achondroplasia with defective development of skin, hair and teeth, polydactyly, and defect of cardiac septum. **congenital alveolar d.,** idiopathic respiratory distress of newborn. **cretinoid d.,** developmental abnormality characteristic of cretinism, consisting of retarded ossification, smallness of internal and sexual organs. **dental d.,** developmental abnormality producing abnormal relationship of a varying number of teeth with their opposing members. **diaphyseal d.,** thickening of the cortex of the midshaft area of the long bones, progressing toward the epiphyses, and sometimes also in the flat bones. **epiphyseal d.,** faulty growth and ossification of the epiphyses with roentgenographically apparent stippling. **fibrous d.,** localized overgrowth of fibrous tissue in bone, causing destructive resorption of cancellous and adjacent cortical bone, and sometimes distention and distortion of the contours of the affected bones; it may affect a single bone (*monostotic fibrous dysplasia*) or many bones (*polyostotic fibrous dysplasia*). **hereditary ectodermal d.,** congenital ectodermal defect. **metaphyseal d.,** a disturbance in enchondral bone growth, failure of modeling causing the ends of the shafts to remain larger than normal in circumference.

dyspnea (disp-ne′ah) labored or difficult breathing. adj., **dyspne′ic. cardiac d.,** difficult breathing due to heart disease. **exertional d.,** dyspnea due to physical effort or exertion. **expiratory d.,** difficulty in breathing due to hindrance to the free egress of air from the lungs. **inspiratory d.,** difficulty in breathing due to hindrance to the free ingress of air into the lungs. **nonexpansional d.,** difficulty in breathing due to failure of expansion of the chest. **orthostatic d.,** difficulty in breathing when in the erect position. **paroxysmal d.,** respiratory distress occurring in attacks without apparent cause, usually during sleep at night. **renal d.,** a form ascribable to some renal disease. **sighing d.,** a syndrome characterized by abnormally deep inspiration without significant alteration in the respiratory rate and without wheezing.

dyspoiesis (dis″poi-e′sis) a disorder of formation, as of blood cells.

dysponderal (dis-pon′der-al) pertaining to disorder of weight, either obesity or underweight.

dyspragia (dis-pra′je-ah) the difficult performance of some function.

dyspraxia (dis-prak′se-ah) partial loss of previously acquired ability to perform skilled movements.

dysprosium (dis-pro′ze-um) chemical element (*see table*), at. no. 66, symbol Dy.

dysproteinemia (dis-pro″te-in-e′me-ah) disorder of the protein content of the blood.

dysraphia (dis-ra′fe-ah) malformation resulting from defective or delayed closure of the embryonic neural tube.

dysrhythmia (dis-rith′me-ah) disturbance of rhythm. **cerebral** (**electroencephalographic**) **d.**, disturbance or irregularity in the rhythm of the brain waves.

dyssomnia (dis-som′ne-ah) a disorder of sleep.

dysspermia (dis-sper′me-ah) impairment of the semen.

dysstasia (dis-sta′ze-ah) difficulty in standing. adj., **dysstat′ic.**

dyssymbolia (dis″sim-bo′le-ah) inability to express thoughts in intelligent language.

dyssynergia (dis″sin-er′je-ah) muscular incoordination.

dyssystole (dis-sis′to-le) asystole; incomplete systole.

dystaxia (dis-tak′se-ah) incomplete ataxia.

dystectia (dis-tek′she-ah) defective closure of the neural tube.

dysteleology (dis″te-le-ol′o-je) the science of rudimentary organs.

dysthermosia (dis″ther-mo′ze-ah) disturbance of heat production.

dysthymia (dis-thi′me-ah) mental distress.

dysthyroidism (dis-thi′roi-dizm) imperfect function of the thyroid gland.

dystimbria (dis-tim′bre-ah) defective resonance of the voice.

dystocia (dis-to′se-ah) difficult parturition. **fetal d.**, that due to malformation, abnormal position or size of fetus. **maternal d.**, that due to small or malformed pelvis of mother. **placental d.**, difficult delivery of the placenta.

dystonia (dis-to′ne-ah) impairment of muscular tonus. adj., **dyston′ic. d. musculo′rum defor′mans,** a disorder marked by muscular contractions which produce peculiar distortions of the spine and hip.

dystopia (dis-to′pe-ah) malposition; displacement. adj., **dystop′ic.**

dystrophia (dis-tro′fe-ah) [Gr.] dystrophy. **d. adiposogenita′lis,** adiposogenital dystrophy. **d. epithelia′lis cor′neae,** dystrophy of the corneal epithelium, with erosions. **d. hypophysopri′va chron′ica,** a condition caused by partial removal of the hypophysis cerebri, marked by obesity, increased carbohydrate tolerance, hypothermia, hypoplasia of the sex glands, retardation of skeletal growth and mental dullness. **d. myoton′ica,** a rare disease characterized by stiffness and progressive atrophy of the muscles. **d. un′guium,** alteration in texture and color of the nails, due to systemic or other disease. **d. un′guium media′na canalifor′mis,** solenonychia.

dystrophoneurosis (dis-trof″o-nu-ro′sis) nervous disease due to malnutrition.

dystrophy (dis′tro-fe) faulty nutrition. adj., **dystroph′ic. adiposogenital d.,** a condition associated with lesions of the hypophysis and hypothalamus, marked by prepuberal obesity and retarded sexual development. **elastic d.,** a disorder of the elastic components of the skin. **hypophyseal d.,** hypopituitarism. **median canaliform d. of the nail,** solenonychia. **papillary and pigmentary d.,** acanthosis nigricans. **progressive muscular d.,** progressive atrophy of the muscles with no discoverable lesion of the spinal cord. **pseudohypertrophic muscular d.,** a dystrophy of the muscles of the shoulder girdle and sometimes of the pelvic girdle, beginning in childhood with hypertrophy and followed later by atrophy. **Salzmann's nodular corneal d.,** a progressive hypertrophic degeneration of the epithelial layer, Bowman's membrane and the outer portion of the corneal stroma. **thyroneural d.,** a condition marked by chorea, athetosis, rigidity, ataxia and other indications of disturbed function of the vegetative nervous system with mental and thyroid defects.

dystropic (dis-tro′pik) abnormally concerned mentally toward either one's self or others.

dystrypsia (dis-trip′se-ah) intestinal dyspepsia.

dysuria (dis-u′re-ah) painful urination. adj., **dysu′ric.**

dysvitaminosis (dis″vi-tah-mĭ-no′sis) any disorder due to vitamin deficiency or excess.

dyszooamylia (dis-zo″o-ah-mi′le-ah) failure of the liver to store up glycogen.

dyszoospermia (dis″zo-o-sper′me-ah) a disorder of spermatozoa formation.

E

E. electromotive force; emmetropia; eye.

e. electron.

EACA epsilon-aminocaproic acid.

ear (ēr) the organ of hearing, especially the pinna or auricle. **Blainville's e.,** congenital difference in size or shape of the ears. **Cagot e.,** one without a lower lobe. **cauliflower e.,** deformity caused by trauma to the ear. **diabetic e.,** otitis media associated with diabetes. **external e.,** the auricle and external auditory meatus. **internal e.**, includes the vestibule, cochlea and semicircular canals. **middle e.**, the tympanum and ossicles.

earache (ēr'āk) pain in the ear; otalgia.

earwax (ēr'waks) cerumen.

ebonation (e″bo-na'shun) removal of loose pieces of bone from a wound.

ebullition (eb″u-lish'un) the state of boiling.

eburnation (e″ber-na'shun) conversion of bone into a hard, ivory-like mass.

eburneous (e-ber'ne-us) ivory-like.

ecaudate (e-kaw'dāt) tail-less.

ecbolic (ek-bol'ik) 1. stimulating the casting out of a material, as the secretion of a gland or the contents of the uterus. 2. an ecbolic agent.

eccentric (ek-sen'trik) away from a center; peripheral.

eccentrochondroplasia (ek-sen″tro-kon″dro-pla'ze-ah) excessive development of cartilage at the epiphysis of a bone.

eccentro-osteochondrodysplasia (-os″te-o-kon″dro-dis-pla'ze-ah) a condition in which ossification occurs from several centers instead of a single center, marked by dwarfing and bodily deformities.

eccentropiesis (-pi-e'sis) pressure from within outward.

ecchondroma (ek″kon-dro'mah) a hyperplastic growth of cartilaginous tissue on the surface of a cartilage or projecting under the periosteum of a bone.

ecchondrosis (-dro'sis) an outgrowth of cartilaginous tissue.

ecchymoma (ek″ĭ-mo'mah) swelling due to blood extravasation.

ecchymosis (ek″ĭ-mo'sis), pl. *ecchymoses* [Gr.] escape of blood into the tissues, producing a large and blotchy area of superficial discoloration (bruise). adj., **ecchymot'ic.**

eccrinology (ek″ri-nol'o-je) study of secreting glands and secretions.

eccrisis (ek'rĭ-sis) excretion of waste products.

eccritic (ek-krit'ik) 1. promoting excretion. 2. an agent which promotes excretion.

eccyesis (ek″si-e'sis) extrauterine pregnancy.

ecdemic (ek-dem'ik) brought into a region from without.

ecdemomania (ek″de-mo-ma'ne-ah) a morbid desire to go abroad.

ecderon (ek'der-on) epidermis.

ecdysis (ek'dĭ-sis) the shedding of an external covering, as the molting of larvae of certain animals.

ECG electrocardiogram.

echinococcosis (e-ki″no-kok-o'sis) infection with the larval form of *Echinococcus granulosus.*

Echinococcus (-kok'us) a genus of tapeworms. **E. granulo'sus,** a small tapeworm of dogs and wolves whose larvae may develop in mammals, forming hydatid tumors or cysts. **E. multilocula'ris,** a species resembling *E. granulosus,* but producing a multilocular or alveolar rather than a unilocular cyst.

echinulate (e-kin'u-lāt) having small prickles or spines.

echo (ek'o) a repeated sound, produced by reflection of the waves producing the original sound. **amphoric e.**, a resonant repetition of a sound heard on auscultation of the chest, occurring at an appreciable interval after the vocal sound. **metallic e.**, a ringing repetition of the heart sounds sometimes heard in patients with pneumopericardium and pneumothorax.

echo-acousia (ek″o-ah-koo'ze-ah) subjective hearing of repetition of a sound after stimuli producing it have ceased.

echocardiogram (-kar'de-o-gram″) the record produced by echocardiography.

echocardiography (-kar″de-og'rah fe) recording of the position and motion of the heart borders and valves by reflected echoes of ultrasonic waves transmitted through the chest wall.

echoencephalogram (-en-sef'ah-lo-gram″) the record produced by echoencephalography.

echoencephalography (-en-sef″ah-log'rah-fe) the mapping of intracranial structures by means of reflected echoes of ultrasound transmitted through the skull.

echolalia (-la'le-ah) automatic repetition by a patient of what is said to him.

echomimia (-mim'e-ah) purposeless repetition of the words of others.

echomotism (-mo'tizm) purposeless repetition of the movements of others.

echopathy (ek-op'ah-the) automatic repetition by a patient of words or movements of others.

echopraxia (ek″o-prak'se-ah) automatic repetition by a patient of movements noted in others.

echothiophate (-thi'o-fāt) a compound used as a cholinesterase inhibitor and to reduce intraocular pressure in glaucoma.

eclabium (ek-la'be-um) eversion of a lip.

eclampsia (e-klamp'se-ah) convulsive attack of peripheral origin; especially a toxemia of pregnancy (*e. of pregnancy*), marked by high blood pressure, albuminuria, convulsions, and coma. adj., **eclamp'tic. infantile e.**, reflex convulsions in children. **puerperal e.**, that occurring after or during childbirth. **uremic e.**, eclampsia due to uremia.

eclampsism (e klamp'sizm) puerperal eclampsia without convulsive seizures.

eclamptogenic (e-klamp″to-jen'ik) causing eclampsia.

eclecticism (e-klek'tĭ-sizm) a school of medicine treating diseases by application of single remedies to known pathologic conditions, special attention being given to indigenous plant remedies. adj., **eclec'tic.**

ecmnesia (ek-ne'ze-ah) forgetfulness of recent events with remembrance of more remote ones.

ecoid (e'koid) the colorless framework of a red blood corpuscle.

Ecolid (e'ko-lid) trademark for a preparation of chlorisondamine.

ecologist (e-kol'o-jist) a person skilled in ecology.

ecology (e-kol'o-je) the scientific study of the interrelations of living organisms and the nonliving elements of their environment. adj., **ecolog'ic. human e.**, application of the ecologic approach to the study of human societies.

ecomania (e″ko-ma′ne-ah) morbid bad temper of a patient in his domestic relations.

ecosystem (-sis′tem) the fundamental unit in ecology, comprising the living organisms and the nonliving elements interacting in a certain defined area.

ecphylaxis (ek″fi-lak′sis) impotency of the antibodies or phylactic agents in the blood. adj., **ecphylac′tic.**

ecphyma (ek-fi′mah) an outgrowth or protuberance.

écrasement (a″krahz-maw′) [Fr.] removal by means of an ecraseur.

écraseur (a″krah-zer′) [Fr.] instrument with a loop of chain or wire for removing parts.

ecstrophy (ek′stro-fe) exstrophy.

E.C.T. electroconvulsive therapy.

ect(o)- (ek′to) word element [Gr.], *external; outside.*

ectad (ek′tad) directed outward.

ectal (ek′tal) external.

ectasia (ek-ta′ze-ah) expansion; dilatation. adj., **ectat′ic. mammary duct e.,** dilatation of the collecting ducts of the mammary gland, with inspissation of gland secretion and inflammatory changes in the tissues.

ectental (ek-ten′tal) pertaining to ectoderm and the entoderm.

ectethmoid (ek-teth′moid) one of the lateral masses of the ethmoid bone.

ecthyma (ek-thi′mah) eruption of pustules with hard bases and areolae. **e. syphilit′icum,** an eruption of pustules in tertiary syphilis.

ectiris (ek-ti′ris) the retinal or external portion of the iris.

ecto-antigen (ek″to-an′tĭ-jen) an antigen loosely attached to the outside of bacteria.

ectoblast (ek′to-blast) the ectoderm.

ectocardia (ek″to-kar′de-ah) displacement of the heart.

ectochoroidea (-ko-roi′de-ah) outer layer of the choroid coat.

ectocinerea (-sĭ-ne′re-ah) the cortical gray matter of the brain.

ectocolon (-ko′lon) dilatation of the colon.

ectocommensal (-kom-men′sal) a commensal organism that lives outside the body of its symbiotic companion, but cannot be separated from it. adj., **ectocommensalis′tic.**

ectocondyle (-kon′dĭl) the external condyle of the bone.

ectocornea (-kor′ne-ah) outer layer of the cornea.

ectocuneiform (-ku-ne′ĭ-form) the lateral cuneiform bone.

ectocytic (-si′tik) outside the cell.

ectoderm (ek′to-derm) the outermost of the three primitive germ layers of the embryo; from it are derived the epidermis and epidermic tissues, such as the nails, hair, and glands of the skin, the nervous system, external sense organs (eye, ear, etc.) and mucous membrane of the mouth and anus. adj., **ectoder′mal, ectoder′mic. amniotic e.,** the inner layer of the amnion (and covering of the umbilical cord) that is continuous with body

ectoderm. **basal e.,** trophoblast covering the eroded uterine tissue that faces the placental sinuses. **extra-embryonic e.,** the epithelial covering of the chorion and lining of the amnion. **neural e.,** the region of the ectoderm destined to become the neural tube.

ectodermosis (ek″to-der-mo′sis) a disorder involving tissues developed from the ectoderm. **e. erosi′va pluriorificia′lis,** Stevens-Johnson syndrome.

ectoentad (-en′tad) from without inward.

ectoenzyme (-en′zim) an extracellular enzyme.

ectogenous (ek-toj′ĕ-nus) originating outside the organism.

ectoglia (ek-tog′le-ah) the external layer of the early embryonic medullary tube.

ectoglobular (ek″to-glob′u-lar) outside the blood corpuscles.

ectogony (ek-tog′o-ne) influence on the maternal organism by the developing zygote.

ectolecithal (ek″to-les′ĭ-thal) having the food yolk situated peripherally.

ectolysis (ek-tol′ĭ-sis) lysis or destruction of the ectoplasm.

ectomere (ek′to-mēr) one of the blastomeres taking part in formation of the ectoderm.

ectomesoblast (ek″to-mes′o-blast) the layer of cells not yet differentiated into ectoderm and mesoderm.

ectomorph (ek′to-morf) an individual exhibiting ectomorphy.

ectomorphy (ek′to-mor″fe) a type of body build in which tissues derived from the ectoderm predominate; a somatotype in which both visceral and body structures are relatively slightly developed, the body being linear and delicate. adj., **ectomor′phic.**

-ectomy (ek′to-me) word element [Gr.], *excision; surgical removal.*

ectonuclear (ek″to-nu′kle-ar) outside the nucleus of a cell.

ectopagus (ek-top′ah-gus) a twin monstrosity united at the thorax.

ectoparasite (ek″to-par′ah-sīt) a parasite attached to the outer surface or situated beneath the skin of the host. adj., **ectoparasit′ic.**

ectophyte (ek′to-fīt) an external vegetable parasite.

ectopia (ek-to′pe-ah) [Gr.] ectopy. **e. cor′dis,** location of the heart in an abnormal place, e.g. outside the chest wall or in the abdominal cavity. **e. i′ridis,** displacement of the iris, with abnormal smallness of the pupil. **e. len′tis,** abnormal position of the lens of the eye. **e. pupil′lae,** corectopia.

ectopic (ek-top′ik) situated elsewhere than in the normal place.

ectoplasm (ek′to-plazm) the more peripheral layer of cytoplasm of a cell.

ectoplastic (ek′to-plas″tik) having formative power on the exterior.

ectopterygoid (ek″to-ter′ĭ-goid) the external pterygoid muscle.

ectopy (ek′to-pe) displacement; abnormal situation.

ectoretina (ek″to-ret′ĭ-nah) the outermost layer of the retina.

ectoscopy (ek-tos′ko-pe) external inspection of an organ.

ectosite (ek′to-sīt) ectoparasite.

ectoskeleton (ek″to-skel′ĕ-ton) the dermoskeleton.

ectosphenoid (-sfe′noid) the third cuneiform bone.

ectosteal (ek-tos′te-al) situated outside of a bone.

ectostosis (ek″to-sto′sis) ossification beginning underneath the perichondrium.

ectosymbiont (-sim′be-ont) a symbiont that lives outside the body of the organism with which it is biologically related. adj., **ectosymbiot′ic.**

ectothrix (ek′to-thriks) a fungus which grows inside the shaft of a hair, but produces a conspicuous external sheath of spores.

ectozoon (ek″to-zo′on) an external animal parasite.

ectrodactyly (ek″tro-dak′tĭ-le) congenital absence of all or part of a digit *(partial ectrodactyly).*

ectromelia (-me′le-ah) gross hypoplasia or aplasia of one or more long bones of one or more limbs.

ectromelus (ek-trom′ĕ-lus) a fetus with rudimentary arms and legs.

ectrometacarpia (ek″tro-met″ah-kar′pe-ah) gross hypoplasia or aplasia of a metacarpal bone.

ectrometatarsia (-met″ah-tar′se-ah) gross hypoplasia or aplasia of a metatarsal bone.

ectrophalangia (-fah-lan′je-ah) gross hypoplasia or aplasia of one or more phalanges of a finger or toe.

ectropion (ek-tro′pe-on) eversion or turning outward, as of the margin of an eyelid. **e. u′veae,** eversion of the margin of the pupil.

ectropionize (ek-tro′pe-ŏ-nīz″) to put into a state of eversion.

ectrosyndactyly (ek″tro-sin-dak′tĭ-le) absence of some of the digits with fusion of the existing ones.

ectylurea (ek″til-u-re′ah) a urea compound used to produce mild depression of the central nervous system.

ecuresis (ek″u-re′sis) production of absolute dehydration of the body by excessive urinary excretion in relation to the intake of water.

eczema (ek′ze-mah) a skin disease, with itching, redness and infiltration. **atopic e.,** eczema resulting from ingestion of or contact with a substance to which the individual is sensitive. **e. bar′bae,** eczema affecting the beard area of the face and neck. **e. erythemato′sum,** a mild form with reddened skin. **e. herpet′icum,** a vesiculopustular eruption due to herpes simplex virus superimposed on areas of pre-existing eczema. **e. hypertroph′icum,** a form with permanent enlargement of the skin papillae. **linear e.,** eczema with lesions occurring in lines. **e. margina′tum,** tinea cruris. **e. papulo′sum,** a variety with itching papules of a deep red color. **e. parasit′icum,** eczema due to the presence of a parasitic microorganism. **e. pustulo′sum,** eczema marked by pustular eruption. **e. scrofuloder′ma,**

mycosis fungoides. **solar e.,** an eczematous eruption on exposed areas of the body due to the burn-producing wavelengths of sunlight. **e. squamo′sum,** eczema with adherent scales of epithelium. **stasis e.,** eczema of the legs, due to impeded circulation, with edema, pigmentation and ulceration. **e. vaccina′tum,** a vesiculopapular eruption due to vaccinia virus, superimposed on preexisting eczema. **e. verruco′sum,** eczema with wartlike excrescences. **vesicular e., e. vesiculo′sum,** eczema marked by presence of vesicles.

eczematous (ek-zem′ah-tus) of the nature of eczema.

E.D. effective dose; erythema dose.

E.D.₅₀. median effective dose.

edema (ĕ-de′mah) an abnormal accumulation of fluid in intercellular spaces of the body. adj., **edem′atous. angioneurotic e.,** temporary edema suddenly appearing in areas of skin or mucous membrane, of allergic, neurotic or unknown origin. **dependent e.,** edema affecting most severely the lowermost or dependent parts of the body. **malignant e.,** edema marked by rapid extension, quick destruction of tissue and the formation of gas. **e. neonato′rum,** a disease of newborn infants, with spreading edema and cold, livid skin. **nonpitting e.,** edema in which the tissues cannot be pitted by pressure. **pitting e.,** edema in which pressure of 30 seconds or so leaves a persistent depression in the tissues. **purulent e.,** edema with purulent effusion.

edematogenic (e-dem″ah-to-jen′ik) tending to produce or cause edema.

edentia (e-den′she-ah) absence of the teeth.

edentulate (e-den′tu-lāt) edentulous.

edentulous (e-den′tu-lus) without teeth.

edrophonium (ed″ro-fo′ne-um) an ammonium compound used as a curare antagonist and as a diagnostic agent in myasthenia gravis.

E.E.E. eastern equine encephalomvelitis.

EEG electroencephalogram.

E.E.N.T. eye-ear-nose-throat.

effacement (ĕ-fās′ment) the obliteration of form or features; applied to the cervix during labor when it is so changed that only the external os remains.

effect (ĕ-fekt′) a condition or alteration produced by some agent or force. **additive e.,** an enhanced effect produced by the combined action of two agents, being greater than the sum of their separate effects. **anachoretic e.,** anachoresis. **cumulative e.,** a sudden marked effect after administration of a number of ineffective doses of a medication. **photechic e.,** Russell effect. **position e.,** in genetics, the changed effect produced by alteration of the relative positions of various genes on the chromosomes. **pressure e.,** the sum of changes in any tissue due to abnormal pressure. **Russell e.,** making a photographic plate developable by substances other than light.

effectiveness (ĕ-fek′tiv-nes) the ability to produce a specific result or to exert a specific measurable influence. **relative biological**

e., an expression of the effectiveness of other types of radiation in comparison with that of 1 r of gamma or roentgen rays.

effector (ĕ-fek'tor) the organ which effects an organism's response to a stimulus.

effemination (ĕ-fem″ĭ-na'shun) development of feminine qualities in a man.

efferent (ef'er-ent) conducting or progressing away from a center or specific site of reference.

effleurage (ef″lu-rahzh') [Fr.] centripetal stroking movement in massage.

efflorescence (ef″lo-res'ens) quality of being efflorescent.

efflorescent (-res'ent) becoming powdery by losing the water of crystallization.

effluvium (ĕ-floo've-um), pl. *efflu'via* [L.] 1. an outflowing or shedding, as of the hair. 2. an exhalation or emanation, especially one of noxious nature.

effortil (ef'for-til) an alcoholic compound used as a sympathomimetic and as a pressor agent.

effusion (ĕ-fu'zhun) 1. escape of a fluid into a part. 2. effused material.

egesta (e-jes'tah) the excretions or discharges from the body.

egestion (e-jes'chun) elimination from the body of waste products and residue of ingested nutrients.

egg (eg) an ovum, especially the oval reproductive body of birds and many reptiles, in which the embryo of the new individual develops, the eggs of birds characteristically containing a yellow mass of nutritive material for the developing embryo, the yolk.

ego (e'go) that part of the psyche that has consciousness, maintains its identity and recognizes and tests reality.

egobronchophony (e″go-brong-kof'o-ne) peculiar bleating sound heard in pleuropneumonia.

egocentric (-sen'trik) overly self-centered; having one's interest largely centered in or directed toward one's self.

egoism (e'go-izm) a self-seeking for advantage at the expense of others; overevaluation of the self.

egomania (e″go-ma'ne-ah) pathologic self-centeredness and selfishness.

egophony (e-gof'o-ne) auscultation sound like the bleat of a goat.

egotism (e'go-tizm) overevaluation of one's self.

egotropic (e″go-trop'ik) egocentric.

Ehrlichia (ār-li'ke-ah) a genus of Microtatobiotes (order Rickettsiales, family Rickettsiaceae, tribe Ehrlichieae) causing disease in dogs, cattle and sheep, but nonpathogenic for man.

Ehrlichieae (ār″li-ki'e-e) a tribe of Microtatobiotes (order Rickettsiales, family Rickettsiaceae) pathogenic for certain vertebrates, but not for man.

eiconometer (i″ko-nom'ĕ-ter) eikonometer.

eidetic (i-det'ik) pertaining to or characterized by exact visualization of events or objects previously seen; a person having such an ability.

eidogen (i'do-jen) a substance elaborated by a second-grade inductor, which is capable of modifying the form of an organ already induced.

eidoptometry (i″dop-tom'ĕ-tre) measurement of the acuteness of visual perception.

eikonometer (i″ko-nom'ĕ-ter) an apparatus for measuring the difference in size of the retinal images in aniseikonia.

Eimeria (i-me're-ah) a multi-species genus of sporozoan parasites, including several economically important species, among them *E. bo'vis, E. stie'da* and *E. tenel'la.*

einsteinium (īn-sti'ne-um) chemical element (*see table*), at no. 99, symbol Es.

eisodic (i-sod'ik) afferent; centripetal.

ejaculatio (e-jak″u-la'she-o) [L.] ejaculation. **e. pre'cox,** premature ejaculation of semen in coitus.

ejaculation (-la'shun) forcible, sudden expulsion; especially expulsion of semen from the male urethra. adj., **ejac'ulatory.**

ejecta (e-jek'tah) refuse cast off from the body.

ejector (e-jek'tor) an apparatus for effecting the forcible expulsion or removal of a material or body. **saliva e.,** an apparatus for removal of saliva from the mouth of the patient during operations on the teeth.

EK, EKG electrocardiogram.

EKY electrokymogram.

elaboration (e-lab″o-ra'shun) a psychologic principle of expansion and greater detail.

elastase (e-las'tās) a factor or enzyme capable of catalyzing the digestion of elastic tissue.

elastic (e-las'tik) capable of resuming normal shape after distortion.

elasticin (e-las'tĭ-sin) elastin.

elasticity (e″las-tis'ĭ-te) the ability of a material to undergo distortion and resume its original size and shape.

elastin (e-las'tin) a scleroprotein present in fibers of connective tissues, digestible by pepsin and trypsin, but not converted to gelatin in boiling water.

elastinase (e-las'tĭ-nās) an enzyme which dissolves elastic tissue.

elastofibroma (e-las″to-fi-bro'mah) a tumor consisting of both elastin and fibrous elements. **e. dor'si,** a tumor of subscapular tissue occurring in old age.

elastolysis (e″las-tol'ĭ-sis) the digestion of elastic substance or tissue. adj., **elastolyt'ic.**

elastoma (-to'mah) pseudoxanthoma elasticum.

elastometer (-tom'ĕ-ter) an instrument for measuring elasticity of tissues.

elastometry (-tom'ĕ-tre) the measurement of elasticity.

elastomucin (e-las″to-mu'sin) a polysaccharide component of elastic tissue.

elastorrhexis (-rek'sis) rupture of fibers composing elastic tissue.

elastose (e-las'tōs) an albumose formed by treating elastin with ferments, acids or alkalis.

elastosis (e″las-to'sis) degeneration of elastic tissue. adj., **elastot'ic.**

elation (e-la'shun) emotional excitement

marked by acceleration of mental and bodily activity.

elbow (el'bo) the point of articulation of the humerus with the radius and ulna, or the corresponding joint in the foreleg of an animal. **capped e.,** a hard mass or swelling on the point of the elbow in horses and cattle. **miner's e.,** olecranon bursitis in miners. **tennis e.,** olecranon bursitis in tennis players.

elcosis (el-ko'sis) fetid ulceration.

eldrin (el'drin) rutin.

electric (e-lek'trik) having the properties of electricity.

electricity (e″lek-tris'ĭ-te) a form of energy generated by friction, induction or chemical means, which produces magnetic, chemical, thermal and radiant effects. adj., **elec'trical. faradic e.,** 1. electricity produced by induction. 2. electricity in intermittent currents. **franklinic e., frictional e.,** static electricity. **galvanic e.,** electricity generated by chemical action. **induced e.,** electricity produced in a body by proximity to an electrified body. **magnetic e.,** electricity developed by means of a magnet. **static e.,** electricity generated by friction, or which does not move in currents. **voltaic e.,** galvanic electricity.

electrization (e-lek″trĭ-za'shun) the act of charging with electricity.

electro-affinity (e-lek″tro-ah-fin'ĭ-te) the tenacity with which the ions of an element hold their charges.

electro-analysis (-ah-nal'ĭ-sis) chemical analysis by means of the electric current.

electro-anesthosia (-an″es-the'ze-ah) anesthesia produced by electricity.

electrobiology (-bi-ol'o-je) science of relations of electricity to living organisms.

electrobioscopy (-bi-os'ko-pe) electric test applied to determine whether life is extinct or not.

electrocardiogram (-kar'de-o-gram″) the record produced by electrocardiography. **scalar e.,** the conventional tracing showing only changes in magnitude of voltage and polarity (positive or negative) with time.

electrocardiograph (-kar'de-o-graf″) the apparatus used in electrocardiography.

electrocardiography (-kar″de-o'rah-fe) the graphic recording from the body surface of variation in electrical potential produced by the heart.

electrocardiophonograph (-kar″de-o-fo'no-graf) an instrument for simultaneously recording the electric potentials and sounds produced by contraction of the heart.

electrocatalysis (-kah-tal'ĭ-sis) catalysis produced by electricity.

electrocautery (-kaw'ter-e) galvanocautery.

electrochemistry (-kem'is-tre) scientific study of electricity in relation to chemical reactions.

electrochromatography (-kro″mah-tog'rah-fe) chromatography performed under the influence of an electric field.

electrocision (-sizh'un) excision by electric current.

electrocoagulation (-ko-ag″u-la'shun) coagulation of tissue by means of an electric current.

electrocontractility (e-lek″tro-kon″trak-til'ĭ-te) contractility to electric stimulation.

electrocorticogram (-kor'tĭ-ko-gram″) the record produced by electrocorticography.

electrocorticography (-kor″tĭ-kog'rah-fe) electroencephalography with the electrodes applied directly to the cerebral cortex.

electrocortin (-kor'tin) aldosterone.

electrode (e-lek'trōd) an electric conductor through which current enters or leaves a cell, apparatus or body. **active e.,** therapeutic electrode. **brush e.,** a wire brush connected with one of the poles of an electric battery; used for applying electricity to the body. **calomel e.,** an electrode consisting of metallic mercury in contact with calomel and hydrochloric acid, used as a standard in the determination of hydrogen ion concentration because it develops a constant potential. **depolarizing e.,** an electrode which has a resistance greater than that of the portion of the body enclosed in the circuit. **exciting e.,** therapeutic electrode. **hydrogen e.,** an electrode made by depositing platinum black on platinum and then allowing it to absorb hydrogen gas to saturation; used in determination of hydrogen ion concentration. **impregnated e.,** therapeutic electrode. **indifferent e.,** silent electrode. **negative e.,** cathode. **point e.,** an insulating handle having on one end a metallic point; used in applying sparks. **positive e.,** anode. **prescription e.,** an electrode impregnated with medicaments according to a physician's prescription. **silent e.,** the electrode which is not therapeutically active. **spark ball e.,** an insulating handle having on one end a metallic ball; used in applying static sparks. **therapeutic e.,** an electrode of carbon cored or filled with materials for medication.

electrodermography (e-lek″tro-der-mog'rah-fe) recording of the electrical resistance of the skin.

electrodesiccation (-des″ĭ-ka'shun) dehydration of tissue by use of a monopolar current through a needle electrode.

electrodiagnosis (-di″ag-no'sis) diagnosis by means of electricity.

electrodiagnostics (-di″ag-nos'tiks) the science and practice of electrodiagnosis.

electrodynamometer (-di″nah-mom'ĕ-ter) instrument to measure the faradic current.

electroencephalogram (-en-sef'ah-lo-gram″) the record produced by electroencephalography.

electroencephalograph (-en-sef'ah-lo-graf″) the instrument used in electroencephalography. adj., **electroencephalograph'ic.**

electroencephalography (-en-sef″ah-log'rah-fe) the recording of changes in electric potential in various areas of the brain by means of electrodes placed on the scalp or on or in the brain itself.

electrogastrography (-gas-trog'rah-fe) the synchronous recording of the electrical and mechanical activity of the stomach.

electrogenesis (-jen'ĕ-sis) the generation of electricity.

electrohemostasis (e-lek″tro-he″mo-sta′sis) arrest of hemorrhage by electrocautery.

electrohysterography (-his″ter-og′rah-fe) recording of changes in electric potential associated with contractions of the uterine muscle.

electrokymogram (-ki′mo-gram) the record produced by electrokymography.

electrokymograph (-ki′mo-graf) the instrument used in electrokymography.

electrokymography (-ki-mog′rah-fe) the graphic recording of the movements of an organ as they appear on a fluoroscopic screen, by means of a photoelectric device.

electrology (e″lek-trol′o jc) scientific study of the nature, effects and uses of electricity. **medical e.,** the scientific study of the use of electricity in diagnosis and treatment.

electrolysis (-trol′i-sis) 1. decomposition of a compound by means of electricity. 2. destruction of body tissue, as of hair roots, telangiectases, etc., by electricity.

electrolyte (e-lek′tro-lit) a compound which, dissolved in water, separates into charged particles (ions) capable of conducting an electric current.

electrolytic (e-lek″tro-lit′ik) pertaining to electrolysis or to an electrolyte.

electromagnet (-mag′net) a piece of metal rendered temporarily magnetic by passage of electricity through a coil surrounding it.

electromagnetism (-mag′nĕ-tizm) magnetism developed by an electric current.

electromassage (-mah-sahzh′) massage combined with electrization.

electrometer (e″lek-trom′ĕ-ter) an instrument for measuring electricity.

electromyogram (e-lek″tro-mi′o-gram) the record obtained by electromyography.

electromyography (-mi-og′rah-fe) the recording of the electric potentials developed in muscle.

electron (e-lek′tron) an elementary particle that is a constituent of every neutral atom; commonly used to designate the negative particle, also called negatron.

electronarcosis (e-lek″tro-nar-ko′sis) narcosis produced by passage of an electric current through electrodes placed on the temples.

electronegative (-neg′ah-tiv) 1. having a negative charge or an excess of electrons. 2. able to capture electrons.

electronic (e″lek-tron′ik) pertaining to or carrying electrons.

electrophoresis (e-lek″tro-fo-re′sis) the movement of charged particles suspended in a liquid on various media (e.g. paper, starch, agar), under the influence of an applied electric field. adj., **electrophoret′ic.**

electrophorus (e″lek-trof′o-rus) a device for obtaining static electricity by means of friction.

electrophysiology (e-lek″tro-fiz″e-ol′o-je) observation of the effects of electricity upon the body in health.

electroplexy (-plek′se) electric shock.

electropneumatotherapy (-nu″mah-to-ther′-ah-pe) treatment of voice weakness by air forced electrically into the larynx.

electropositive (e-lek″tro-poz′i-tiv) 1. having a positive charge or a deficiency of electrons. 2. able to give up electrons.

electroprognosis (-prog-no′sis) prognosis by means of an electric test.

electropuncture (e-lek′tro-punk″tūr) puncture of tissues by electric needles.

electropyrexia (e-lek″tro-pi-rek′se-ah) production of high body temperature by electric means.

electroradiometer (-ra″de-om′ĕ-ter) an electroscope for measuring radiant energy.

electroresection (-re-sek′shun) resection by electric cautery.

electroscission (-sish′un) excision by electricity.

electroscope (e-lek′tro-skōp) an instrument for detecting static electricity.

electroshock (e-lek′tro-shok) shock produced by applying electric current to the brain.

electrosleep (e-lek′tro-slēp) sleep induced by electrical stimulation of the brain.

electrostatics (e-lek″tro-stat′iks) the science of static or frictional electricity.

electrostimulation (-stim-u-la′shun) a form of electroshock treatment.

electrostriatogram (-stri-a′to-gram) an electroencephalogram showing differences in electric potential recorded at various levels of the corpus striatum.

electrosurgery (-ser′jer-e) the use of electricity in surgery.

electrosynthesis (-sin′thĕ-sis) the formation of a compound under the influence of electricity.

electrotaxis (-tak′sis) taxis in response to electric stimuli.

electrotherapy (-ther′ah-pe) treatment of disease by electricity.

electrotonus (e″lek-trot′o-nus) the change effected in a nerve or muscle by passage of an electric current.

electrotropism (e″lek-trot′ro-pizm) tropism in response to electric stimuli.

electuary (e-lek′tu-er″e) a soft medicated confection.

eleidin (el-e′ĭ-din) a principle in the granular layer of the skin.

element (el′ĕ-ment) 1. a substance composed of atoms all of which have the same number of protons in their nuclei and therefore the same number of electrons circling in their orbits. 2. an integral part of an entity. **formed e's of the blood,** the erythrocytes, leukocytes and thrombocytes. **radioactive e.,** a chemical element which spontaneously transmutes into another element, with emission of corpuscular or electromagnetic radiations. **sarcous e.,** one of the minute parts into which a sarcostyle may be divided. **stable e.,** one that does not change readily, such as a chemical element that does not spontaneously transmute into another with emission of corpuscular or electromagnetic radiations. **trace e.,** a chemical element present or needed in extremely small amount by plants and animals, such as manganese, copper, cobalt, zinc, iron. **transcalifornium e's,** chemical elements with atomic numbers higher than 98. **transuranium e's,** chemical elements with atomic numbers higher than 92, all of which have been produced artificially on earth by nuclear reactions and synthesis.

ele(o)- (el′e-o) word element [Gr.], *oil.*

eleoma (el″e-o′mah) a tumor caused by injection of oil into the tissues.

eleometer (el″e-om′ĕ ter) an instrument for measuring the oil in a mixture.

eleopten (-op′ten) the liquid part of a volatile oil.

eleotherapy (el″e-o-ther′ah-pe) therapeutic use of oil.

eleothorax (-tho′raks) injection of oil into the pleural cavity.

elephantiasis (el″ĕ-fan-ti′ah-sis) massive subcutaneous edema, with accompanying thickening of the skin, the result of lymphatic obstruction. **e. filarien′sis,** elephantiasis caused by filariasis of the lymphatic channels. **e. graeco′rum,** leprosy. **e. neuromato′sa,** hypertrophy caused by Schwann cell proliferation. **e. nos′tras,** that due to recurrent streptococcal cellulitis. **e. nos′tras verruco′sa,** persistent swelling of the lower leg, with crowded, wartlike growths on the skin of the foot and ankle.

elevator (el′ĕ-va″tor) an instrument for raising a part.

elimination (e-lim″ĭ na′shun) discharge from the body of indigestible materials and of waste products of body metabolism.

Elipten (e-lip′ten) trademark for a preparation of amino glutethimide.

elix. elixir.

elixir (e-lik′ser) a clear, sweetened, hydroalcoholic liquid for oral use. **aromatic e.,** a preparation containing compound orange spirit, sugar, talc and alcohol; used as a vehicle for various drugs. **aromatic e., red,** aromatic elixir colored by addition of amaranth solution. **benzaldehyde e., compound,** a preparation of benzaldehyde, vanillin, orange, flower water, alcohol, simple syrup and water. **high-alcoholic e.,** a preparation of compound orange spirit, saccharin and glycerin in water. **iso-alcoholic e.,** one prepared by combining calculated volumes of the high- and low-alcoholic elixirs. **lowalcoholic e.,** a preparation of compound orange spirit, alcohol, glycerin, sucrose and purified water, containing only 10 per cent alcohol by volume. **terpin hydrate e.,** a preparation of terpin hydrate, sweet orange peel tincture, benzaldehyde, glycerin, alcohol and syrup in purified water; used as an expectorant. **three bromides e.,** a mixture of ammonium, potassium and sodium bromides, amaranth solution and compound benzaldehyde elixir.

elkoplasty (el′ko-plas″te) helcoplasty.

Elkosin (el′ko-sin) trademark for preparations of sulfisomidine.

elliptocyte (e-lip′to-sīt) an elliptical red blood corpuscle.

elliptocytosis (e-lip″to-si-to′sis) a hereditary disorder in which the erythrocytes are largely elliptical and which is characterized by increased red cell destruction and anemia.

Elorine (el′o-rēn) trademark for a preparation of tricyclamol.

elution (e-loo′shun) separation of substances by extraction with a solvent.

elutriation (e-loo″tre-a′shun) purification of a substance by dissolving it in a solvent and pouring off the solution, thus separating it from the undissolved foreign material.

Em. emmetropia.

emaciation (e-ma″se-a′shun) a wasted, lean habit of body.

emailloblast (e-ma′lo-blast) adamantinoblast.

emailloid (e-ma′loid) a tumor developing from tooth enamel.

emanation (em″ah-na′shun) 1. an effluvium. 2. a product given off from radioactive substances. **actinium e.,** actinon. **radium e.,** radon. **thorium e.,** thoron.

emanotherapy (em″ah-no-ther′ah-pe) treatment by means of emanations, such as radium emanation.

emasculation (e-mas″ku-la′shun) removal of the penis or testes.

embalming (em-bahm′ing) treatment of a dead body to retard decomposition.

embedding (em-bed′ing) fixation of tissue in a firm medium before cutting microscopic sections.

embolalia (em″bo la′le-ah) interpolation of meaningless words in a spoken sentence.

embole (em′bo-le) emboly.

embolectomy (em″bo-lek′to-me) removal of an embolus through an incision in the blood vessel wall.

embolic (em-bol′ik) pertaining to embolism or an embolus.

embolism (em′bo-lizm) impaction in a blood vessel of any undissolved material conveyed to the site in the blood stream. **air e.,** obstruction by an air bubble. **cerebral e.,** embolism of a cerebral artery. **coronary e.,** embolism of a coronary artery, leading to myocardial infarction. **fat e.,** obstruction by fat globules. **infective e.,** obstruction by an embolus containing bacteria or septic poison. **miliary e.,** embolism affecting many small blood vessels. **paradoxical e.,** blockage of an artery by a thrombus carried from a systemic vein that has passed through a defect in the interatrial or interventricular septum. **pulmonary e.,** obstruction of the pulmonary artery or one of its branches by an embolus.

embolophrasia (em″bo-lo-fra′ze-ah) interpolation of meaningless phrases in a spoken sentence.

embolus (em′bo-lus) a mass of undissolved material, usually part or all of a thrombus, carried in the blood stream and frequently obstructing a vessel. **saddle e.,** one situated astride the bifurcation of a large artery, sometimes blocking both branches.

TABLE OF CHEMICAL ELEMENTS

ELEMENT (DATE OF DISCOVERY)	SYMBOL	ATOMIC NUMBER	ATOMIC WEIGHT[a]	VALENCE	SP. GR. OR DENSITY (GRAMS/LITER)	DESCRIPTIVE COMMENT
Actinium (1899)	Ac	89	[227]	....	10.07	radioactive element associated with uranium
Aluminum (1827)	Al	13	26.9815	3	2.6989	silvery-white metal, abundant in earth's crust, but not in free form
Americium (1944)	Am	95	[243]	3, 4, 5, 6	11.7	fourth transuranium element discovered
Antimony (prehistoric)	Sb	51	121.75	3, 5	6.691	exists in 4 allotropic forms
Argon (1894)	Ar	18	39.948	0?	1.7837 g./l.	colorless, odorless gas
Arsenic (1250)	As	33	74.9216	3, 5	5.73 / 4.73 / 1.97	(gray) semimetallic solid / (black) / (yellow)
Astatine (1940)	At	85	[210]	1, 3, 5, 7		radioactive halogen
Barium (1808)	Ba	56	137.34	2	3.5	silvery-white, alkaline earth metal
Berkelium (1949)	Bk	97	[247]	3, 4		fifth transuranium element discovered
Beryllium (1798)	Be	4	9.0122	2	1.848	light, steel-gray metal
Bismuth (1753)	Bi	83	208.980	3, 5	9.747	pinkish-white, crystalline, brittle metal
Boron (1808)	B	5	10.811	3	2.34, 2.37	crystalline or amorphous element, not occurring free in nature
Bromine (1826)	Br	35	79.909	1, 3, 5, 7	3.12	mobile, reddish-brown liquid, volatilizing readily red vapor with disagreeable odor
Cadmium (1817)	Cd	48	112.40	2	8.65	soft, bluish-white metal
Calcium (1808)	Ca	20	40.08	2	1.55	metallic element, forming more than 3 per cent of earth's crust
Californium (1950)	Cf	98	[249]	....	1.8-2.1	sixth transuranium element discovered
Carbon (prehistoric)	C	6	12.01115	2, 3, 4	1.9-2.3 / 3.15-3.53	(amorphous) element widely distributed in nature / (graphite) / (diamond)
Cerium (1803)	Ce	58	140.12	3, 4	6.67-8.23	most abundant rare earth metal
Cesium (1860)	Cs	55	132.905	1	1.873	silvery-white, soft, alkaline metal
Chlorine (1774)	Cl	17	35.453	1, 3, 5, 7	3.214 g./l.	greenish-yellow gas of the halogen group
Chromium (1797)	Cr	24	51.996	2, 3, 6	7.18-7.20	steel-gray, lustrous, hard metal
Cobalt (1735)	Co	27	58.9332	2, 3	8.9	brittle, hard metal
Copper (prehistoric)	Cu	29	63.54	1, 2	8.96	reddish, lustrous, malleable metal
Curium (1944)	Cm	96	[247]	3	7	third transuranium element discovered
Dysprosium (1886)	Dy	66	162.50	3	8.536	rare earth metal with metallic bright silver luster
Einsteinium (1952)	Es	99	[254]	....		seventh transuranium element discovered

Element (year)	Symbol	At. No.	At. Weight	Valence	Density	Description
Erbium (1843)	Er	68	167.26	3	9.051	soft, malleable rare earth metal
Europium (1896)	Eu	63	151.96	2, 3	5.259	lustrous, silvery-white rare earth metal
Fermium (1953)	Fm	100	[253]	. . . .		eighth transuranium element discovered
Fluorine (1771)	F	9	18.9984	1	1.696 g./l.	pale yellow, corrosive gas of the halogen group
Francium (1939)	Fr	87	[223]	1		product of alpha disintegration of actinium
Gadolinium (1880)	Gd	64	157.25	3	7.8, 7.895	lustrous, silvery-white rare earth metal
Gallium (1875)	Ga	31	69.72	2, 3	5.907	beautiful, silvery-appearing metal
Germanium (1886)	Ge	32	72.59	2, 4	5.323	grayish-white, brittle metal
Gold (prehistoric)	Au	79	196.957	1, 3	19.32	malleable yellow metal
Hafnium (1923)	Hf	72	178.49	4	13.29	gray metal associated with zirconium
Helium (1895)	He	2	4.0026	0	0.177 g./l.	inert gas
Holmium (1879)	Ho	67	164.930	3	8.803	relatively soft and malleable rare earth metal
Hydrogen (1766)	H	1	1.00797	1	0.08988 g./l. 0.070	(gas) most abundant element in the universe (liquid)
Indium (1863)	In	49	114.82	1, 2?, 3	7.31	soft, silvery-white metal
Iodine (1811)	I	53	126.9004	1, 3, 5, 7	4.93 11.27 g./l.	grayish-black, lustrous solid or violet-blue gas
Iridium (1803)	Ir	77	192.2	3, 4	22.42	white, brittle metal of platinum family
Iron (prehistoric)	Fe	26	55.847	2, 3, 4, 6	7.874	fourth most abundant element in earth's crust
Krypton (1898)	Kr	36	83.80	0	3.733 g./l.	inert gas
Lanthanum (1839)	La	57	138.91	3	5.98–6.186	silvery-white, ductile, rare earth metal
Lawrencium (1961)	Lw	103	[257]	. . . .		last of transuranium elements discovered
Lead (prehistoric)	Pb	82	207.19	2, 4	11.35	bluish-white, lustrous, malleable metal
Lithium (1817)	Li	3	6.939	1	0.534	lightest of all metals
Lutetium (1907)	Lu	71	174.97	3	9.872	rare earth metal
Magnesium (1808)	Mg	12	24.312	2	1.738	silvery-white metallic element, eighth in abundance in earth's crust
Manganese (1774)	Mn	25	54.938)	1, 2, 3, 4, 6, 7	7.21–7.44	exists in 4 allotropic forms
Mendelevium (1955)	Md	101	[256]	. . . .		ninth transuranium element discovered
Mercury (prehistoric)	Hg	80	200.59	1, 2	13.546	heavy, silvery-white metal, liquid at ordinary temperatures
Molybdenum (1782)	Mo	42	95.94	2, 3, 4?, 5?, 6	10.22	silvery-white, very hard metal
Neodymium (1885)	Nd	60	144.24	3	6.80, 7.004	exists in 2 allotropic forms
Neon (1898)	Ne	10	20.183	0?	0.89990 g./l.	inert gas
Neptunium (1940)	Np	93	[237]	3, 4, 5, 6	18.0–20.45	first transuranium element discovered
Nickel (1751)	Ni	28	58.71	0, 1, 2, 3	8.902	silvery-white, malleable metal
Niobium (1801)	Nb	41	92.906	2, 3, 4?, 5	8.57	shiny white, soft, ductile metal
Nitrogen (1772)	N	7	14.0067	3, 5	1.2506 g./l.	colorless, odorless, inert element, making up 78 per cent of the air
Nobelium (?) (1958)	No	102	[253]	. . . .		acceptance of this element considered premature
Osmium (1803)	Os	76	190.2	2, 3, 4, 8	22.57	bluish-white, hard metal of platinum family
Oxygen (1774)	O	8	15.9994	2	1.429 g./l.	colorless, odorless gas, third most abundant element in the universe

TABLE OF CHEMICAL ELEMENTS (*Continued*)

ELEMENT (DATE OF DISCOVERY)	SYMBOL	ATOMIC NUMBER	ATOMIC WEIGHT*	VALENCE	SP. GR. OR DENSITY (GRAMS/LITER)	DESCRIPTIVE COMMENT
Palladium (1803)	Pd	46	106.4	2, 3, 4	12.02	steel-white metal of the platinum family
Phosphorus (1669)	P	15	30.9738	3, 5	1.82	(white) waxy solid, transparent when pure
					2.20	(red)
					2.25–2.69	(black)
Platinum (1735)	Pt	78	195.09	1?, 2, 3, 4	21.45	silvery-white, malleable metal
Plutonium (1940)	Pu	94	[242]	3, 4, 5, 6	19.84	second transuranium element discovered
Polonium (1898)	Po	84	[210]	2, 4, 6	9.32	very rare natural element
Potassium (1807)	K	19	39.102	1	0.862	soft, silvery, alkali metal, seventh in abundance in earth's crust
Praseodymium (1885)	Pr	59	140.907	3, 4	6.782, 6.64	soft, silvery rare earth metal
Promethium (1941)	Pm	61	[147]	3		produced by irradiation of neodymium and praseodymium; identity established in 1945
Protactinium (1917)	Pa	91	[231]	4 or 5	15.37	bright lustrous metal
Radium (1898)	Ra	88	[226]	2	5(?)	brilliant white, radioactive metal
Radon (1900)	Rn	86	[222]	0	9.73 g./l.	heaviest known gas
Rhenium (1925)	Re	75	186.2	– 1, 2, 3, 4, 5, 6, 7	21.02	silvery-white lustrous metal
Rhodium (1803)	Rh	45	102.905	– 2, 3, 4, 5, 6, 7	12.41	silvery-white metal of platinum family
Rubidium (1861)	Rb	37	85.47	1, 2, 3, 4	1.532	soft, silvery-white, alkali metal
Ruthenium (1844)	Ru	44	101.07	0, 1, 2, 3, 4, 5, 6, 7, 8	12.41	hard white metal of platinum family
Samarium (1879)	Sm	62	150.35	2, 3	7.536–7.40	bright silver lustrous metal
Scandium (1879)	Sc	21	44.956	3	2.992	soft, silvery-white metal
Selenium (1817)	Se	34	78.96	2, 4, 6	4.79, 4.28	exists in several allotropic forms
Silicon (1823)	Si	14	28.086	4	2.33	a relatively inert element, second in abundance in earth's crust
Silver (prehistoric)	Ag	47	107.870	1, 2	10.50	malleable, ductile metal with brilliant white luster
Sodium (1807)	Na	11	22.9898	1	0.971	most abundant of alkali metals, sixth in abundance in earth's crust
Strontium (1808)	Sr	38	87.62	2	2.54	exists in 3 allotropic forms
Sulfur (prehistoric)	S	16	32.064	2, 4, 6	1.957, 2.07	exists in several isotopic and many allotropic forms
Tantalum (1802)	Ta	73	180.948	2?, 3, 4?, 5	16.6	gray, heavy, very hard metal
Technetium (1937)	Tc	43	[99]	3?, 4, 6, 7	11.50	first element produced artificially
Tellurium (1782)	Te	52	127.60	2, 4, 6	6.24	silvery-white, lustrous element

Element (year)	Symbol	At. No.	Mass	Oxidation states	Density	Description
Terbium (1843)	Tb	65	158.924	3, 4	8.272	silvery-gray, malleable, ductile rare earth metal
Thallium (1861)	Tl	81	204.37	1, 3	11.85	very soft, malleable metal
Thorium (1828)	Th	90	232.038	4	11.66	silvery-white, lustrous metal
Thulium (1879)	Tm	69	168.934	2, 3		least abundant rare earth metal
Tin (prehistoric)	Sn	50	118.69	2, 4	5.75	(gray) malleable metal existing in 2 or 3 allotropic forms, changing from white to gray on cooling and back to white on warming
					7.31	(white)
Titanium (1791)	Ti	22	47.90	2, 3, 4	4.54	lustrous white metal
Tungsten (1783)	W	74	183.85	2, 3, 4, 5, 6	19.3	steel-gray to tin-white metal
Uranium (1789)	U	92	238.03	3, 4, 5, 6	18.95	heavy, silvery-white metal
Vanadium (1801)	V	23	50.942	2, 3, 4, 5	6.11	bright, white metal
Xenon (1898)	Xe	54	131.30	0?	5.887 g/l.	one of the so-called rare or inert gases
Ytterbium (1878)	Yb	70	173.04	2, 3	6.977, 6.54	exists in 2 allotropic forms
Yttrium (1794)	Y	39	88.905	3	4.45	rare earth metal with silvery metallic luster
Zinc (1746)	Zn	30	65.37	2	7.133	bluish-white, lustrous metal, malleable at 100–150° C.
Zirconium (1789)	Zr	40	91.22	4	6.4	grayish-white, lustrous metal

*Figures in brackets represent mass number of most stable isotope.

Table of Elements by Atomic Numbers

1 hydrogen
2 helium
3 lithium
4 beryllium
5 boron
6 carbon
7 nitrogen
8 oxygen
9 fluorine
10 neon
11 sodium
12 magnesium
13 aluminum
14 silicon
15 phosphorus
16 sulfur
17 chlorine
18 argon
19 potassium
20 calcium
21 scandium
22 titanium
23 vanadium
24 chromium
25 manganese
26 iron
27 cobalt
28 nickel
29 copper
30 zinc
31 gallium
32 germanium
33 arsenic
34 selenium
35 bromine
36 krypton
37 rubidium
38 strontium
39 yttrium
40 zirconium
41 niobium
42 molybdenum
43 technetium
44 ruthenium
45 rhodium
46 palladium
47 silver
48 cadmium
49 indium
50 tin
51 antimony
52 tellurium
53 iodine
54 xenon
55 cesium
56 barium
57 lanthanum
58 cerium
59 praseodymium
60 neodymium
61 promethium
62 samarium
63 europium
64 gadolinium
65 terbium
66 dysprosium
67 holmium
68 erbium
69 thulium
70 ytterbium
71 lutetium
72 hafnium
73 tantalum
74 tungsten
75 rhenium
76 osmium
77 iridium
78 platinum
79 gold
80 mercury
81 thallium
82 lead
83 bismuth
84 polonium
85 astatine
86 radon
87 francium
88 radium
89 actinium
90 thorium
91 protactinium
92 uranium
93 neptunium
94 plutonium
95 americium
96 curium
97 berkelium
98 californium
99 einsteinium
100 fermium
101 mendelevium
102 [see nobelium]
103 lawrencium

emboly (em'bo-le) invagination of the blastula to form the gastrula.

embrasure (em-bra'zhur) the interproximal space occlusal to the area of contact of adjacent teeth in the same dental arch.

embrocation (em"bro-ka'shun) a liniment or medicine for external application.

embryectomy (em"bre-ek'to-me) excision of an extrauterine embryo or fetus.

embryo (em'bre-o) an early formative stage; the earliest stage of development of an organism; applied to human young from the time the longitudinal axis is identifiable until all organs and major structures have been formed, seven to nine weeks after fertilization of the ovum. adj., **embry'onal, embryon'ic. presomite e.,** the embryo at any stage before the appearance of the first somite. **previllous e.,** the embryo at any stage before the appearance of the chorionic villi. **somite e.,** the embryo at any stage between the appearance of the first and the last somites.

embryocardia (em"bre-o-kar'de-ah) a fetal state of the heart or its pulsation.

embryoctony (em"bre-ok'to-ne) destruction of the fetus in utero.

embryogeny (-oj'ĕ-ne) development of the embryo. adj., **embryogenet'ic, embryogen'ic.**

embryography (-og'rah-fe) description of the embryo.

embryology (-ol'o-je) the science of the development of embryos. adj., **embryolog'ic.**

embryoma (em"bre-o'mah) a tumor containing embryonic elements.

embryonization (em-bre"o-ni-za'shun) return of a tissue to embryonic form.

embryonoid (em'bre-ŏ-noid") resembling an embryo.

embryopathia (em"bre-o-path'e-ah) embryopathy. **e. rubeola'ris,** developmental anomalies in infants of mothers who had rubeola during pregnancy.

embryopathy (em"bre-op'ah-the) disordered embryonic development with consequent congenital anomalies. **rubella e.,** congenital deformities in an infant due to rubella in the mother during early pregnancy.

embryoplastic (em"bre-o-plas"tik) pertaining to formation of an embryo.

embryotocia (em"bre-o-to'se-ah) abortion.

embryotomy (em"bre-ot'o-me) dissection of the fetus in difficult labor.

embryotoxon (em"bre-o-tok'son) congenital opacity of the margin of the cornea.

embryotroph (em'bre-o-trŏf") the nutritive material utilized by the early embryo.

embryotrophy (em"bre-ot'ro-fe) nourishment of the early embryo.

embryulcus (-ul'kus) a hooked instrument for extracting a dead fetus from the uterus.

emedullate (e-med'u-lāt) to deprive of marrow.

emergent (e-mer'jent) 1. coming out from a cavity or other part. 2. coming on suddenly.

emery (em'er-e) an abrasive substance consisting of corundum and various impurities, such as iron oxide.

emesis (em'ĕ-sis) the act of vomiting.

emetic (e-met'ik) 1. causing vomiting. 2. an agent that causes vomiting.

emetine (em'ĕ-tēn) an alkaloid derived from ipecac or produced synthetically. **e. hydrochloride,** a white or slightly yellowish crystalline compound, $C_{29}H_{40}N_2O_4 \cdot 2HCl \cdot xH_2O$, used in treatment of amebiasis.

emetism (em'ĕ-tizm) poisoning by ipecac.

emetocathartic (em"ĕ-to-kah-thar'tik) both emetic and cathartic.

emetology (em"ĕ-tol'o-je) sum of knowledge regarding emetics.

E.M.F. electromotive force.

-emia (e'me-ah) word element [Gr.], *condition of the blood.*

eminence (em'ĭ-nens) a projection or boss.

eminentia (em"ĭ-nen'she-ah), pl. *eminen'tiae* [L.] eminence.

emissary (em'ĭ-sār"e) affording an outlet, as the veins exiting from the skull to drain blood from the dural sinuses.

emission (e-mish'un) discharge, especially of semen. **nocturnal e.,** involuntary discharge of semen during sleep.

Emivan (em'i-van) trademark for preparations of ethamivan.

emmenagogue (ĕ-men'ah-gog) 1. promoting menstruation. 2. a drug that promotes the menstrual flow.

emmenia (ĕ-me'ne-ah) the menses. adj., **emmen'ic.**

emmenology (em"ĕ-nol'o-je) sum of what is known about menstruation.

emmetrope (em'ĕ-trōp) a person with normal vision.

emmetropia (em"ĕ-tro'pe-ah) the ideal optical condition, parallel rays coming to a focus on the retina. adj., **emmetrop'ic.**

emollient (e-mol'yent) 1. soothing and softening. 2. a soothing medicine.

emotion (e-mo'shun) a state of mental excitement characterized by alteration of feeling tone.

emotivity (e"mo-tiv'ĭ-te) capacity for emotion.

empathize (em'pah-thīz) to comprehend intellectually the feelings of another.

empathy (em'pah-the) intellectual understanding of something in another person which is foreign to one's self. adj., **empath'ic.**

emphlysis (em'fli-sis) a vesicular eruption.

emphractic (em-frak'tik) clogging or obstructive.

emphysema (em"fĭ-se'mah) abnormal presence of air or gas in body tissue. **atrophic e.,** emphysema with wasting of lung substance. **bullous e.,** emphysema characterized by the development of bullae which may be single or multiple, and varying in size from 1 or 2 cm. up to the volume of the entire hemithorax. **centrilobular e.,** emphysema in which the destructive lesions occur in the region of the respiratory bronchioles, which tend to become confluent and form enlarged spaces toward the center of the lobules; called also *bronchostenotic* or *bronchiolostenotic obstructive emphysema.* **cutaneous e.,** air or gas in the connective tissues under the skin. **familial e.,** emphysema occurring in different encephalitis

members of a family and considered to be due to a familial predisposition to the disease. **interlobular e.**, air between the lobes of the lung. **interstitial e.**, pulmonary emphysema due to destruction of the walls of the alveoli. **interstitial e., spontaneous,** presence of air in the interstitial tissues of the lungs after spontaneous rupture of the alveoli. **intestinal e.**, a condition marked by accumulation of gas under the serous tunic of the intestine. **lobar e.**, emphysema involving less than all the lobes of the affected lung. **lobar e., infantile,** a condition characterized by overinflation, commonly affecting one of the upper lobes and causing respiratory distress in early life, usually necessitating lobectomy; called also *congenital lobar emphysema*. **e. of lungs,** pulmonary emphysema. **mediastinal e.**, pneumomediastinum. **panlobular e.**, emphysema in which the destructive lesions unselectively involve an entire lobule of the lung; called also *panacinar emphysema, destructive panacinar emphysema, diffuse* or *generalized emphysema,* and *atrophic senile emphysema*. **pulmonary e.**, increase beyond normal in the size of the air space in the lungs distal to the terminal bronchioles. **surgical e.**, subcutaneous emphysema following operation. **unilateral e.**, a condition in which an entire lung is overinflated and does not empty on expiration. **vesicular e.**, pulmonary emphysema due to dilatation of the alveoli.

empiricism (em-pir'ĭ-sizm) skill or knowledge from mere experience. adj., **empir'ic.**

Empirin (em'pĭ-rin) trademark for tablets containing acetylsalicylic acid, acetophenetidin and caffeine.

emporiatrics (em-po"re-at'riks) that branch of medicine particularly concerned with health problems of travelers about the world.

emprosthotonos (em"pros-thot'o-nos) tetanic forward flexure of the body.

emptysis (emp-ti'sis) pulmonary hemorrhage.

empyema (em"pi-e'mah) the presence of a frank purulent exudate within the pleural cavity.

empyesis (-e'sis) a pustular eruption.

empyocele (em-pi'o-sēl) a purulent tumor of the scrotum.

emul. emulsion.

emulgent (e-mul'jent) draining out.

emulsifier (em-ul"si-fi'er) a substance used to make an emulsion.

emulsion (e-mul'shun) 1. a mixture of two immiscible liquids, one being dispersed throughout the other in small droplets; a colloid system in which both the dispersed phase and the dispersion medium are liquids. 2. a pharmaceutical preparation with acacia or gelatin, tragacanth, agar or mixtures of these.

emulsoid (e-mul'soid) a colloid system in which there is a mutual attraction between the two phases.

emulsum (e-mul'sum) [L.] emulsion.

emunctory (e-mungk'to-re) 1. excretory or cleansing. 2. an excretory organ.

emylcamate (e-mil'kah-māt) a compound used as a tranquilizer.

enamel (e-nam'el) calcified tissue of ectodermal origin covering the crown of a tooth. **brown e., hereditary,** amelogenesis imperfecta. **curled e.**, enamel in which the columns are bent. **dwarfed e.**, enamel which is less thick than normal. **mottled e.**, defective enamel, with a chalky white appearance or brownish stain, caused by excessive amounts of fluorine in drinking water during period of enamel calcification. **nanoid e.**, dwarfed enamel.

enameloma (en-am"el-o'mah) a small spherical nodule of enamel attached to a tooth at the cervical line or on the root.

enamelum (e-nam'el-um) [L.] enamel.

enanthem (en-an'them) an eruption upon a mucous surface. adj., **enanthem'atous.**

enanthesis (en-an"the'sis) a skin eruption from an internal disease.

enanthrope (en'an-thrōp) a source of disease within the body.

enantiobiosis (en-an"te-o-bi-o'sis) commensalism in which the associated organisms are mutually antagonistic.

enantiomorph (en-an'te-o-morf") one of a pair of isomeric substances, the structures of which are mirror opposites of each other.

enantiopathy (en-an"te-op'ah-the) 1. any disease antagonistic to another. 2. the curing of one disease by inducing an antagonistic disease.

enarthritis (en"ar-thri'tis) inflammation of an enarthrosis.

enarthrosis (-thro'sis) a joint in which the rounded head of one bone fits in a cuplike depression in another, permitting motion in any direction.

encapsulation (en-kap"su-la'shun) enclosure within a capsule.

encarditis (en"kar-di'tis) endocarditis.

encelialgia (en"se le-al'je-ah) pain in an abdominal organ.

encephal(o)- (en-sef'ah-lo) word element [Gr.], *brain.*

encephalalgia (en"sef-ah-lal'je-ah) cephalalgia.

encephalasthenia (en"sef-al-as-the'ne-ah) lack of brain power.

encephalatrophy (en"sef-ah-lat'ro-fe) atrophy of the brain.

encephalic (en"se-fal'ik) pertaining to the brain.

encephalin (en-sef'ah-lin) a nitrogenous glycoside said to be obtained from the brain.

encephalitis (en"sef-ah-li'tis) inflammation of the brain. **e. A,** lethargic encephalitis. **acute disseminated e.**, postinfection encephalitis. **Australian X e.**, an acute encephalitis of viral origin observed in Australia during the summer months between 1917 and 1926. **e. B,** Japanese B encephalitis. **e. C,** St. Louis encephalitis. **cortical e.**, inflammation involving only the cortex of the brain. **Economo's e., epidemic e.**, a viral disease of obscure pathology, occurring epidemically. **equine e.**, equine encephalomyelitis. **hemorrhagic e., e. hemorrha'-gica**, inflammation of the brain with hemorrhagic exudate. **herpes e.**, a viral disease resembling equine encephalomyelitis. **e. hyperplas'tica**, acute nonsuppurating encephalitis. **infantile e.**, inflammation of the brain in children following infections, injury, etc., and causing the cerebral palsies of children. **influenzal e.**, epidemic encephalitis. **Japanese B e.**, a form of epidemic encephalitis of varying severity occurring in Japan and other Pacific islands, China, Manchuria, U.S.S.R. and probably much of the Far East. **lead e.**, encephalitis with cerebral edema due to lead poisoning. **lethargic e.**, a form of epidemic encephalitis characterized by increasing languor, apathy and drowsiness. **Murray Valley e.**, a disease endemic in Murray Valley in 1951, believed to be identical to Australian X encephalitis. **e. neonato'rum**, encephalitis of the newborn. **e. periaxia'lis**, massive inflammation of the white matter of the cerebral hemispheres, beginning in the occipital lobes and characterized by early disappearance of the myelin; the disease occurs mostly in children and young subjects and begins with occipital blindness. **postinfection e.**, an acute disease of the central nervous system seen in patients convalescing from infectious diseases. **postvaccinal e.**, encephalitis following vaccination against virus diseases. **purulent e., pyogenic e.**, suppurative encephalitis. **Russian autumnal e.**, Japanese B encephalitis. **Russian endemic e., Russian forest-spring e., Russian spring-summer e.**, a form of epidemic encephalitis acquired in forests from infected ticks and transmitted in other ways. **Russian tick-borne e., Russian vernal e.**, Russian spring-summer encephalitis. **St. Louis e.**, a viral disease first observed in Illinois in 1932, closely resembling western equine encephalomyelitis. **Schilder's e.**, progressive subcortical encephalopathy. **e. subcortica'lis chron'ica**, sclerotic changes in the vessels of the subcortical white matter of the brain. **suppurative e.**, encephalitis accompanied by suppuration and abscess formation. **vaccinal e.**, postvaccinal encephalitis. **vernal e.**, Russian spring-summer encephalitis.

encephalitogenic (en″sef-ah-lĭ-to-jen′ik) causing encephalitis.

encephalocele (en-sef′ah-lo-sēl″) local herniation of neural tissue through a defect in the skull.

encephalocystocele (en-sef″ah-lo-sis′to-sēl) hernial protrusion of the brain distended by fluid.

encephalodialysis (-di-al′ĭ-sis) softening of the brain.

encephalogram (en-sef′ah-lo-gram″) the film obtained by encephalography.

encephalography (en-sef″ah-log′rah-fe) radiography of the brain.

encephaloid (en-sef′ah-loid) 1. like the brain. 2. encephaloma.

encephalolith (en-sef′ah-lo-lith″) a brain calculus.

encephalology (en-sef″ah-lol′o-je) scientific study of the encephalon.

encephaloma (en-sef″ah-lo′mah) encephaloid cancer.

encephalomalacia (en-sef″ah-lo-mah-la′she-ah) abnormal softening of the brain.

encephalomeningitis (-men″in-ji′tis) meningoencephalitis.

encephalomeningocele (-mĕ-ning′go-sēl) protrusion of the brain and meninges through the skull.

encephalomeningopathy (-men″in-gop′ah-the) disease involving brain and meninges.

encephalomere (en-sef′ah-lo-mēr″) one of the segments making up the embryonic brain.

encephalometer (en″sef-ah-lom′ē-ter) an instrument for measuring the skull.

encephalomyelitis (en-sef″ah-lo-mi″ĕ-li′tis) inflammation of the brain and spinal cord. **acute disseminated e.**, postinfection encephalitis. **benign myalgic e.**, a disease, usually occurring in epidemics, characterized by headache, fever, myalgia, muscular weakness and emotional lability. **disseminated e.**, a disease in which disseminated focal lesions of a demyelinated type are scattered through the central nervous system. **equine e.**, a viral disease of horses and mules, occurring as epizootics in the western hemisphere. **equine e., eastern**, a viral disease similar to western equine encephalomyelitis, but occurring principally in the Atlantic and Gulf states. **equine e., Venezuelan**, a viral disease of horses and mules; the infection in man resembles influenza, with little or no indication of nervous system involvement. **equine e., western**, a viral disease of horses and mules, communicable to man, occurring chiefly as a meningoencephalitis, with little involvement of the medulla or spinal cord; observed in the United States chiefly west of the Mississippi River. **granulomatous e.**, a disease marked by granulomas and necrosis of the walls of the cerebral and spinal ventricles. **postvaccinal e.**, inflammation of the brain and spinal cord following vaccination or infection with vaccinia virus.

encephalomyeloneuropathy (-mi″ĕ-lo-nu-rop′-ah-the) disease involving brain, spinal cord and nerves.

encephalomyelopathy (-mi″ĕ-lop′ah-the) disease involving brain and spinal cord.

encephalomyeloradiculitis (mi″ĕ-lo-rah-dik″-u-li′tis) inflammation of brain, spinal cord and spinal nerve roots.

encephalomyeloradiculopathy (-mi″ĕ-lo-rah-dik″u-lop′ah-the) disease involving brain, spinal cord and spinal nerve roots.

encephalomyocarditis (-mi″o-kar-di′tis) a disease of virus origin, characterized by lesions in the central nervous system and by degenerative and inflammatory changes in skeletal and cardiac muscle.

encephalon (en-sef′ah-lon) the brain; with the spinal cord (medulla spinalis) constituting the central nervous system.

encephalopathy (en-sef″ah-lop′ah-the) any disorder of the brain. **boxer's e.,** a syndrome of prize fighters due to cumulative punishment absorbed in the boxing ring, characterized by slowing of mental functions, bouts of confusion and scattered memory loss. **lead e.,** brain disease caused by lead poisoning. **progressive subcortical e.,** a familial lesion of unknown origin, characterized by headache, dysphasia, weakness of the arms and legs, and visual failure progressing to blindness. **Wernicke's e.,** see under *syndrome.*

encephalopuncture (en-sef″ah lo-punk′tūr) puncture into the brain substance.

encephalopyosis (-pi-o′sis) a purulent condition in the brain.

encephalorachidian (-rah-kid′e-an) cerebrospinal.

encephalorrhagia (-ra′je-an) cerebral hemorrhage.

encephalosclerosis (-skle-ro′sis) hardening of the brain.

encephalosis (en″sef-ah-lo′sis) any organic brain disease.

encephalotomy (-lot′o-me) incision of the fetal head in difficult labor.

enchondroma (en″kon-dro′mah) a hyperplastic growth of cartilaginous tissue remaining in the interior of a cartilage or bone.

enchondromatosis (en-kon″dro-mah-to′sis) a condition characterized by hamartomatous proliferation of cartilage cells within the metaphysis of several bones, causing thinning of the overlying cortex and distortion of the growth in length.

enchondrosarcoma (-sar-ko′mah) sarcoma containing cartilaginous tissue.

enchondrosis (en″kon-dro′sis) hyperplastic growth within a cartilage or bone.

enchylema (en″ki-le′mah) hyaloplasm (1).

enclave (en′klāv) tissue detached from its normal connection and enclosed within another organ.

enclitic (en-klit′ik) having the planes of the fetal head inclined to those of the maternal pelvis.

encopresis (en″ko-pre′sis) incontinence of feces not due to organic defect or illness.

encranial (en-kra′ne-al) situated within the cranium.

encyesis (en″si-e′sis) normal uterine pregnancy.

encyst (en-sist′) to enclose in a sac or cyst.

end(o)- (en′do) word element [Gr.], *within; inward.*

endadelphos (end″ah-del′fos) a fetal monster in which a parasitic twin is enclosed within the body of another.

Endamoeba (en″dah-me′bah) a genus of amebas parasitic in the intestines of invertebrates, distinguishable from Entamoeba by the characteristics of the nucleus.

endangium (en-dan′je-um) membrane which lines blood vessels.

endaortitis (en″da-or-ti′tis) inflammation of the membrane lining the aorta. **bacterial e.,** the presence of bacterial vegetations on the endothelial surface of the aorta.

endarterectomize (en″dar-ter-ek′to-mīz) to subject to endarterectomy.

endarterectomy (-ek′to-me) excision of thickened areas of the innermost coat of an artery.

endarteritis (-i′tis) inflammation of the innermost coat of an artery. **e. oblit′erans,** a form in which the lumen of the vessel becomes obliterated.

endarteropathy (-op′ah-the) noninflammatory disorder of the innermost coat of an artery.

end-artery (end-ar′ter-e) one which does not anastomose with other arteries.

end-body (-bod′e) complement.

end-brain (end′brān) telencephalon.

end-bud (end′bud) 1. the ovoid termination of sensory nerves in mucous membrane. 2. tail bud.

end-bulb (end′bulb) end-bud (1).

endeictic (en-dīk′tik) symptomatic.

endemic (en-dem′ik) 1. present in a community at all times, but occurring in only small numbers of cases. 2. a disease of low morbidity that is constantly present in a human community.

endemiology (en-de″me-ol′o-je) the science dealing with all the factors relating to occurrence of endemic disease.

endemo-epidemic (en″de-mo-ep″ĭ-dem′ik) endemic, but occasionally becoming epidemic.

endorgonic (en″der-gon′ik) characterized or accompanied by the absorption of energy; requiring the input of free energy.

endermic (en-der′mik) administered through the skin.

endermosis (en″der-mo′sis) 1. administration of medicines by absorption through the skin. 2. herpetic affection of mucous membranes.

enderon (en′der-on) the deeper part of the skin or mucous membrane.

endoaneurysmorrhaphy (en″do-an″u-riz-mor′ah-fe) opening of an aneurysmal sac and suture of the orifices.

endoangiitis (-an″je-i′tis) inflammation of the intima of blood vessels.

endoantitoxin (-an″tĭ-tok′sin) an antitoxin contained within a cell.

endoappendicitis (-ah-pen″dĭ-si′tis) inflammation of mucous membrane of the appendix vermiformis.

endoarteritis (-ar″ter-i′tis) endarteritis.

endoblast (en′do-blast) the cell nucleus.

endobronchitis (en″do-brong-ki′tis) inflammation of the lining membrane of the bronchia.

endocarditis (-kar-di′tis) inflammation of the endocardium. adj., **endocar′dial. bacterial e.,** an acute or subacute, febrile, systemic disease characterized by focal bacterial infection of the heart valves, with formation of bacteria-laden vegetations. **Libman-Sacks e.,** nonbacterial verrucous endocarditis. **mural e.,** parietal endocarditis. **nonbacterial verrucous e.,** involvement of the heart in disseminated lupus erythematosus, with formation of small warty excrescences on the valve leaflets and collagenous fibrosis of underlying tissue. **parietal e.,** endocarditis involving the inner lining of the cardiac chambers. **rheumatic e.**, cardiac involvement in rheumatic fever. **syphilitic e.**, endocarditis resulting from extension of syphilitic infection from the aorta. **tuberculous e.**, endocarditis resulting from extension of a tuberculous infection from the pericardium and myocardium. **vegetative e.**, bacterial endocarditis.

endocardium (en″do-kar′de-um) the membrane lining the chambers of the heart and covering the cusps of the various valves.

endocervicitis (-ser″vĭ-si′tis) inflammation of the endocervix.

endocervix (-ser′viks) 1. the mucous membrane lining the canal of the cervix uteri. 2. the region of the opening of the uterine cervix into the uterine cavity.

endochondral (-kon′dral) developed within cartilage.

endochorion (-ko′re-on) the inner chorion.

endochrome (en′do-krōm) the coloring matter within a cell.

endocolitis (en″do-ko-li′tis) inflammation of the mucous membrane of the colon.

endocolpitis (-kol-pi′tis) inflammation of vaginal mucous membrane.

endocommensal (-kom-men′sal) a commensal organism which lives inside the body of its symbiotic companion. adj., **endocommensalis′tic.**

endocomplement (-kom′ple-ment) a complement contained within the erythrocyte.

endocorpuscular (-kor-pus′ku-ler) contained within a corpuscle.

endocranial (-kra′ne-al) within the cranium.

endocranitis (-kra-ni′tis) inflammation of endocranium.

endocranium (-kra′ne-um) the dura mater lining the cranium.

endocrinasthenia (-krin″es-the′ne-ah) endocrine exhaustion.

endocrine (en′do-krin) secreting internally.

endocrinism (en-dok′rĭ-nizm) endocrinopathy.

endocrinology (en″do-krĭ-nol′o-je) study of the glands of internal secretion.

endocrinopathy (-nop′ah-the) a disorder of the internal secretions. adj., **endocrinopath′ic.**

endocrinosis (en″do-krĭ-no′sis) dysfunction of an endocrine gland.

endocrinotherapy (-kri″no-ther′ah-pe) treatment of disease by the administration of endocrine preparations.

endocrinotropic (-trop′ik) having an affinity for the endocrine glands.

endocrinous (en-dok′rĭ-nus) pertaining to internal secretions.

endocritic (en″do-krit′ik) endocrinous.

endocystitis (-sis-ti′tis) inflammation of the bladder mucosa.

endoderm (en′do-derm) entoderm.

Endodermophyton (en″do-der-mof′ĭ-ton) a genus of fungi causing skin infections.

endodontia (-don′she-ah) endodontics.

endodontics (-don′tiks) the branch of dentistry concerned with the etiology, prevention, diagnosis and treatment of conditions that affect the tooth pulp and apical periodontal tissues.

endodontist (en″do-don′tist) a dentist who practices endodontics.

endodontitis (-don-ti′tis) inflammation of the dentinal pulp.

endodontium (-don′she-um) dental pulp.

endoenteritis (-en″ter-i′tis) inflammation of the intestinal mucosa.

endoenzyme (-en′zīm) an enzyme which is apparently adsorbed or bound to the plasma membrane and which can be extracted only when the membrane is mechanically or chemically destroyed.

endogain (en′do-gān) the primary gain of emotional illness, which operates on a deeply unconscious level in its initiation.

endogamy (en-dog′ah-me) 1. fertilization by union of separate cells having the same chromatin ancestry. 2. restriction of marriage to persons within the same community. adj., **endog′amous.**

endogastrectomy (en″do-gas-trek′to-me) excision of gastric mucosa.

endogastritis (-gas-tri′tis) inflammation of the gastric mucosa.

endogenic (-jen′ik) endogenous.

endogenous (en-doj′ĕ-nus) produced within or caused by factors within the organism.

endoglobular (en″do-glob′u-lar) within the blood corpuscles.

endo-intoxication (-in-tok″sĭ-ka′shun) poisoning by an endogenous toxin.

endolabyrinthitis (-lab″ĭ-rin-thi′tis) inflammation of the membranous labyrinth.

endolaryngeal (-lah-rin′je-al) in the larynx.

Endolimax (-li′maks) a genus of amebas found in the colon of man, other mammals, birds, amphibians and cockroaches.

endolumbar (-lum′bar) within the lumbar portion of the spinal cord.

endolymph (en′do-limf) fluid within the membranous labyrinth. adj., **endolymphat′ic.**

endolympha (en″do-lim′fah) endolymph.

endolysin (en-dol′ĭ-sin) a lysin existing in a leukocyte and acting directly on bacteria.

endolysis (en-dol′ĭ-sis) dissolution of the cytoplasm of a cell.

endomastoiditis (en″do-mas″toi-di′tis) inflammation of interior of mastoid cavity and cells.

endomesoderm (-mes′o-derm) mesoderm originating from the entoderm of the two-layered blastodisk.

endometrectomy (-me-trek′to-me) excision of uterine mucosa.

endometrial (-me′tre-al) pertaining to the endometrium.

endometrioid (-me′tre-oid) resembling endometrium.

endometrioma (-me″tre-o′mah) a tumor containing endometrium.

endometriosis (-me″tre-o′sis) the presence of endometrial tissue in abnormal locations. adj., **endometriot′ic. external e.**, presence of endometrial glands or stroma outside the uterus. **internal e.**, adenomyosis.

endometritis (-me-tri′tis) inflammation of the endometrium. **puerperal e.**, endometritis following childbirth.

endometrium (en"do-me'tre-um) the mucous membrane lining the uterus.

endomitosis (-mi-to'sis) mitosis taking place without dissolution of the nuclear membrane, resulting in doubling of the number of chromosomes within the nucleus (endoreduplication). adj., **endomitot'ic.**

endomixis (-mik'sis) mingling of nuclear and cytoplasmic substance of a cell.

endomorph (en'do-morf) an individual exhibiting endomorphy.

endomorphy (en'do-mor"fe) a type of body build in which tissues derived from the endoderm predominate; a somatotype in which the digestive viscera are massive and highly developed, and the body structure is relatively weak and undeveloped. adj., **endomor'phic.**

endomyocarditis (en"do-mi"o-kar-di'tis) inflammation of endocardium and myocardium.

endomysium (-mis'e-um) delicate connective tissue stroma covering the individual muscle cells in a fasciculus of striated muscle.

endoneuritis (-nu-ri'tis) inflammation of the endoneurium.

endoneurium (-nu're-um) connective tissue between the fibers of a fasciculus of a nerve.

endoparasite (-par'ah-sīt) a parasite that lives within the body of the host. adj., **endoparasit'ic.**

endopelvic (-pel'vik) within the pelvis.

endopeptidase (-pep'tĭ-dās) a peptidase capable of acting on any peptide linkage in a peptide chain.

endopericarditis (-per"ĭ-kar-di'tis) inflammation of endocardium and pericardium.

endoperimyocarditis (-per"ĭ-mi"o-kar-di'tis) inflammation of endocardium, pericardium and myocardium.

endoperitonitis (-per"ĭ-to-ni'tis) inflammation of serous lining of peritoneal cavity.

endophlebitis (-fle-bi'tis) inflammation of the intima of a vein.

endophthalmitis (en"dof-thal-mi'tis) inflammation of internal structures of the eye.

endophyte (en'do fīt) entophyte.

endophytic (en"do-fit'ik) growing inward; proliferating internally.

endoplasm (en'do-plazm) the more centrally located cytoplasm of a cell.

endoplast (en'do-plast) nucleus of a cell.

endopolyploid (en"do-pol'ĭ-ploid) having reduplicated chromatin within an intact nucleus, with or without an increase in the number of chromosomes (applied only to cells and tissues).

endopolyploidy (-pol"ĭ-ploi'de) 1. endomitosis. 2. polysomaty. 3. autopolyploidy due to a previous endomitotic cycle.

endopredator (-pred'ah-tor) an individual or species that lives within the body of an organism of another species, which it feeds upon and destroys.

endoreduplication (-re-du"plĭ-ka'shun) reproduction of elements within the nucleus of a cell not followed by chromosome movements and cytoplasmic division (endomitosis).

end-organ (end"or'gan) any terminal structure of a nerve.

endorhinitis (en"do-ri-ni'tis) inflammation of the mucous membrane of the nasal passages.

endosalpingitis (-sal"pin-ji'tis) inflammation of the lining membrane of the oviduct.

endosalpingoma (-sal"ping-go'mah) an epithelial tumor of the oviduct.

endosalpingosis (-sal"ping-go'sis) adenomyosis of an oviduct.

endosalpinx (-sal'pinks) the mucous membrane lining the oviduct.

endoscope (en'do-skōp) a tubular instrument, usually carrying an illumination source, inserted into a hollow organ or body cavity to permit direct visual inspection of its interior.

endoscopy (en-dos'ko-pe) visual examination of interior structures of the body with an endoscope. adj., **endoscop'ic. peroral e.,** endoscopic examination of organs accessible to observation through an endoscope passed through the mouth.

endosepsis (en"do-sep'sis) septicemia originating from causes inside the body.

endosite (en'do-sīt) an internal parasite.

endoskeleton (en"do-skel'ĕ-ton) the framework of hard structures, imbedded in and supporting the soft tissues of the body of higher animals, derived principally from the mesoderm.

endosmometer (en"dos-mom'ĕ-ter) instrument for measurement of endosmosis.

endosmosis (-mo'sis) inward osmosis; inward passage of liquid through a membrane.

endosome (en'do-sōm) a body thought to consist of deoxyribonucleic acid, observed in the vesicular nucleus of certain cells.

endospore (en'do-spōr) a spore formed within a parent cell.

endosteal (en-dos'te-al) occurring inside a bone.

endosteitis (en-dos"te-i'tis) inflammation of the endosteum.

endosteoma (en-dos"te-o'mah) a tumor in the medullary cavity of a bone.

endosteum (en dos'te-um) lining membrane of a hollow bone.

endostoma (en"dos-to'mah) a bony tumor within a bone.

endosymbiont (en"do sim'be-ont) a symbiont that lives within the cells of its partner. adj., **endosymbiot'ic.**

endothelial (-the'le-al) pertaining to endothelium.

endothelialization (-the"le-al-ĭ-za'shun) the complete coverage of an exposed area by endothelial cells growing out from the margin.

endothelioangiitis (-the"le-o-an"je-i'tis) a condition resembling lupus erythematosus, attended by fever, arthritis, pericarditis and angiitis.

endotheliochorial (-the"le-o-ko're-al) denoting a type of placenta in which syncytial trophoblast embeds maternal vessels bared to their endothelial lining.

endotheliocyte (-the'le-o-sīt") a large mononuclear phagocytic cell of the blood and tissues.

endotheliocytosis (en″do-the″le-o-si-to′sis) abnormal increase of endotheliocytes.

endothelio-inoma (-ĭ-no′mah) fibrous tumor arising from endothelium.

endotheliolysin (en″do-the″le-ol′ĭ-sin) an antibody which causes the dissolution of endothelial cells. adj., **endotheliolyt′ic.**

endothelioma (-the″le-o′mah) an endothelial tumor.

endotheliomatosis (-the″le-o″mah-to′sis) formation of multiple, diffuse endotheliomas.

endotheliomyoma (-the″le-o-mi-o′mah) myoma arising from endothelium.

endotheliomyxoma (mik-so′mah) myxoma arising from endothelium.

endotheliosis (-the″le-o′sis) proliferation of endothelial elements.

endotheliotoxin (-the″le-o-tok′sin) a toxin which destroys endothelium.

endothelium (-the′le-um), pl. *endothe′lia* [Gr.] the layer of epithelial cells that lines the cavities of the heart and of the blood and lymph vessels, and the serous cavities of the body.

endothermal (-ther′mal) endothermic.

endothermic (-ther′mik) 1. characterized by the absorption of heat. 2. pertaining to endothermy.

endothermy (en′do-ther″me) production of heat in the tissues by the resistance they offer to the passage of the high frequency current.

endothoracic (en″do-tho-ras′ik) within the thorax; situated internal to the ribs.

endothrix (en′do-thriks) a fungus whose growth is confined chiefly within the shaft of a hair, without formation of conspicuous external spores.

endotoscope (en-do′to-skōp) otoscope.

endotoxic (en″do-tok′sik) retaining its toxin within itself; said of certain bacteria.

endotoxicosis (-tok″sĭ-ko′sis) poisoning by an endotoxin.

endotoxin (-tok′sin) a toxin present in the bacterial cell, but not in cell-free filtrate of intact bacteria.

endotoxoid (-tok′soid) a toxoid prepared from an endotoxin.

endotracheal (-tra′ke-al) within the trachea.

endotracheitis (-tra″ke-i′tis) inflammation of the mucous membrane of the trachea.

endotrachelitis (-tra″kel-i′tis) endocervicitis.

endovasculitis (-vas″ku-li′tis) inflammation of the endangium.

endovenous (-ve′nus) within a vein.

endoxan (en-dok′san) cyclophosphamide.

end-plate (end′plāt) the discoid terminal expansion of motor nerve branches.

enem. enema.

enema (en′ĕ-mah) 1. introduction of fluid into the rectum. 2. a solution introduced into the rectum to promote evacuation of feces or as a means of introducing nutrient or medicinal substances, or opaque material in roentgen examination of the lower intestinal tract. **double contrast e.,** injection and evacuation of a barium suspension, followed by inflation of the intestines with air, to facilitate roentgen visualization of the intestinal mucosa.

enepidermic (en″ep-ĭ-der′mik) applied to or injected into the skin.

energometer (en″er-gom′ĕ-ter) an instrument for studying the pulse.

energy (en′er-je) power which may be translated into motion, overcoming resistance or effecting physical change; the ability to do work. **kinetic e.,** that which produces motion. **potential e.,** that which may be translated into an effect.

enervation (en″er-va′shun) 1. lack of nervous energy. 2. removal of a nerve or a section of a nerve.

enflagellation (en-flaj″ĕ-la′shun) the formation of flagella; flagellation.

engagement (en-gāj′ment) the entrance of the fetal head or presenting part into the superior pelvic strait.

engastrius (en-gas′tre-us) a double fetal monster in which one fetus is contained within the abdomen of the other.

engine (en′jin) a mechanical apparatus by which energy is converted from one form to another. **dental e.,** a machine operated by footpower or electricity to activate instruments used by dentists in procedures on the teeth; such machines are capable of producing 10,000 *(high speed)* to more than 100,000 *(ultra-speed)* revolutions a minute. **surgical e.,** a machine similar to the dental engine, used in surgery.

engorgement (en-gorj′ment) excessive fulness of any organ or passage.

engram (en′gram) the traces allegedly left in the nervous system by any experience.

engraphia (en-gra′fe-ah) the production by stimuli of definite traces (engrams) on the protoplasm, which, with repetition, induce a habit that persists after the stimuli have ceased.

enhematospore (en-hem′ah-to-spōr″) a spore of the malarial parasite found in the blood.

enhexymal (en-hek′sĭ-mal) hexobarbital.

enkatarrhaphy (en″kah-tar′ah-fe) suturing together of the sides of tissues alongside a structure, burying it.

enomania (e″no-ma′ne-ah) 1. periodic craving for strong drink. 2. delirium tremens.

enophthalmos (en″of-thal′mos) abnormal recession of the eyeballs in the orbit.

enostosis (en″os-to′sis) bony growth in the hollow of a bone.

ensiform (en′sĭ-form) sword-shaped.

ensomphalus (en-som′fah-lus) a double monster with bodies partially united.

enstrophe (en′stro-fe) inversion; a turning inward.

entad (en′tad) toward a center; inwardly.

ental (en′tal) inner; central.

entamebiasis (en″tah-me-bi′ah-sis) infection by Entamoeba.

Entamoeba (en″tah-me′bah) a genus of amebas parasitic in the intestines of vertebrates. **E. bucca′lis,** *Entamoeba gingivalis.* **E. co′li,** a nonpathogenic form found in the intestinal tract of man. **E. gingiva′lis,** a species found in the mouth, about the gums and in the tartar of the teeth. **e. histolyt′ica,** a species causing amebic or tropical dysentery and tropical abscess of the liver. **E. tropica'lis,** *Entamoeba histolytica.*

entasia (en-ta'ze-ah)   a constrictive spasm.

entelechy (en-tel'ĕ-ke)   completion of anything; attainment of an end.

enter(o)- (en'ter-o)   word element [Gr.], *intestines.*

enteradenitis (en"ter-ad"ĕ-ni'tis)   inflammation of the intestinal glands.

enteral (en'ter-al)   within the intestine.

enteralgia (en"ter-al'je-ah)   pain in the intestine.

enteramine (-am'ēn)   serotonin.

enterectomy (-ek'to-me)   excision of a portion of the intestine.

enterelcosis (-el-ko'sis)   ulceration of the intestine.

enterepiplocele (-e-pip'lo-sēl)   hernia of bowel and omentum.

enteric (en-ter'ik)   pertaining to the intestine.

enteric-coated (en-ter"ik-kōt'ed)   coated with a substance that is disintegrated only by the intestinal enzymes.

entericoid (en-ter'ĭ-koid)   resembling typhoid fever.

enteritis (en"ter-i'tis)   inflammation of the intestine. **choleriform e.,** an acute choleralike diarrheal disease with a high fatality rate prevalent in epidemic and endemic forms in the Western Pacific area since 1938. **e. cys'tica chron'ica,** a form marked by cystic dilatations of the intestinal glands, due to closure of their openings. **diphtheritic e.,** diphtheria of the intestines. **e. gra'vis,** an often fatal disease characterized by severe abdominal pain, nausea, vomiting and bloody diarrhea, with mucosal necrosis and hemorrhage and edema of the submucosa, most prominent in the jejunum and proximal ileum. **e. membrana'cea, membranous e., muco-membraneous e., mucous e., myxomembranous e.,** mucous colitis. **e. necrot'icans,** an inflammation of the intestines due to *Clostridium perfringens* and characterized by necrosis. **e. nodula'ris,** enteritis with enlargement of the lymph nodes. **pellicular e.,** mucous enteritis. **phlegmonous e.,** a condition with symptoms resembling those of peritonitis, and secondary to other intestinal diseases, e.g. chronic obstruction, strangulated hernia, carcinoma. **e. polypo'sa,** enteritis marked by polypoid growths in the intestine, due to proliferation of the connective tissue. **protozoan e.,** enteritis in which the intestine is infested with protozoan organisms of various species. **pseudomembranous e.,** enteritis without fever and with profuse exudate of mucin. **regional e.,** inflammation involving a segment of the small intestine. **streptococcal e.,** primary phlegmonous enteritis due to *Streptococcus pyogenes.* **terminal e.,** regional enteritis.

enteroanastomosis (en"ter-o-ah-nas"to-mo'sis)   enteroenterostomy.

enteroantigen (-an'tĭ-jen)   an antigen derived from feces.

Enterobacteriaceae (-bak-te"re-a'se-e)   a family of Schizomycetes (order Eubacteriales) occurring as plant or animal parasites.

enterobiasis (en"ter-o-bi'ah-sis)   infection by *Enterobius vermicularis.*

enterobiliary (-bil'i-er"e)   pertaining to the intestines and the bile passages.

Enterobius (en"ter-o'be-us)   a genus of nematode worms. **E. vermicula'ris,** the seatworm or pinworm, a small white worm parasitic in the upper part of the large intestine.

enterocele (en'ter-o-sēl")   intestinal hernia.

enterocentesis (en"ter-o-sen-te'sis)   surgical puncture of the intestine.

enterochirurgia (-ki-rur'je-ah)   intestinal surgery.

enterocholecystostomy (-ko"le-sis-tos'to-me)   surgical creation of an opening from the gallbladder to the small intestine.

enterocholecystotomy (-ko"le-sis-tot'o-me)   incision of the gallbladder and intestine.

enterocinesia (-si-ne'se-ah)   peristalsis. adj., **enterocinet'ic.**

enteroclysis (en"ter-ok'lĭ-sis)   the injection of liquids into the intestine.

enterococcus (en"ter-o-kok'kus)   a streptococcus of the human intestine.

enterocoele (en'ter-o-sēl")   the abdominal or body cavity, formed by outpouchings from the archenteron.

enterocolectomy (en"ter-o-ko-lek'to-me)   resection of part of the small intestine and colon

enterocolitis (-ko-li'tis)   inflammation of small intestine and colon. **hemorrhagic e.,** inflammation of the small intestine and colon, characterized by hemorrhagic breakdown of the intestinal mucosa, with inflammatory cell infiltration. **necrotizing e., pseudomembranous e.,** an acute, superficial necrosis of the mucosa of the small intestine and colon, characterized by passage of shreds or casts of the bowel wall.

enterocolostomy (-ko-los'to-me)   anastomosis of the small intestine to the colon.

enterocrinin (en"ter-ok'rĭ-nin)   a hormone from animal intestines which stimulates the glands of the small intestine.

enterocutaneous (en"ter-o-ku-ta'ne-us)   pertaining to or communicating with the intestine and the skin, or surface of the body.

enterocyst (en'ter-o-sist")   a cyst proceeding from subperitoneal tissue.

enterocystocele (en"ter-o-sis'to-sēl)   hernia of bladder and intestine.

enterocystoma (-sis-to'mah)   cystic tumor of the intestine.

enterodynia (-din'e-ah)   pain in the intestine.

enteroenterostomy (-en"ter-os'to-me)   anastomosis between two formerly remote parts of the intestine.

entero-epiplocele (en"ter-o-e-pip'lo-sēl)   hernia of intestine and omentum.

enterogastritis (-gas-tri'tis)   combination of enteritis and gastritis.

enterogastrone (-gas'trōn)   a hormone of the duodenum which mediates the humoral inhibition of gastric secretion and motility produced by ingestion of fat.

enterogenous (en″ter-oj′ĕ-nus) arising within the intestine.

enterogram (en′ter-o-gram″) an instrumental tracing of the movements of the intestine.

enterography (en″ter-og′rah-fe) a description of the intestines.

enterohepatitis (en″ter-o-hep″ah-ti′tis) 1. inflammation of the intestine and liver. 2. an infectious disease of turkeys.

enterohepatocele (-hep′ah-to-sēl″) an umbilical hernia containing intestine and liver.

enterohepatopexy (-hep″ah-to-pek′se) fixation to the liver of a seromuscular flap of a defunctionalized loop of the proximal small intestine.

enterohydrocele (-hi′dro-sēl) hernia with hydrocele.

enterokinase (-ki′nās) an enzyme present in intestinal juice that catalyzes conversion of trypsinogen to trypsin.

enterolith (en′ter-o-lith″) a calculus in the intestine.

enterolithiasis (en″ter-o-li-thi′ah-sis) the formation of enteroliths.

enterology (en″ter-ol′o-je) scientific study of the intestines.

enterolysis (-ol′ĭ-sis) surgical separation of intestinal adhesions.

enteromegaly (en″ter-o-meg′ah-le) enlargement of the intestines.

enteromycosis (-mi-ko′sis) bacterial disease of the intestine.

enteron (en′ter-on) the intestine.

enteroneuritis (en″ter-o-nu-ri′tis) inflammation of the nerves of the intestine.

enteronitis (-ni′tis) inflammation of the small intestine.

enteroparesis (-par′ĕ-sis) relaxation and dilatation of the intestine.

enteropathogen (-path′o-jen) a microorganism which causes a disease of the intestines. adj., **enteropathogen′ic.**

enteropathogenesis (-path″o-jen′ĕ-sis) the production of disease or disorder of the intestines.

enteropathy (en″ter-op′ah-the) a disease of the intestine.

enteropexy (en′ter-o-pek″se) surgical fixation of the intestine.

enteroplasty (en′ter-o-plas″te) plastic repair of the intestine.

enteroplegia (en″ter-o-ple′je-ah) paralysis of the intestine.

enteroptosis (en″ter-op-to′sis) abnormal downward displacement of the intestines.

enterorrhagia (en″ter-o-ra′je-ah) intestinal hemorrhage.

enterorrhaphy (en″ter-or′ah-fe) suture of the intestine.

enterorrhexis (en″ter-o-rek′sis) rupture of the intestine.

enteroscope (en′ter-o-skōp″) instrument for inspecting the inside of the intestine.

enterosepsis (en″ter-o-sep′sis) sepsis developed from the intestinal contents.

enterosorption (-sorp′shun) accumulation of a substance in the bowel by virtue of its passage from the circulating blood.

enterospasm (en′ter-o-spazm″) intestinal colic.

enterostasis (en″ter-o-sta′sis) intestinal stasis.

enterostenosis (-ste-no′sis) narrowing or stricture of the intestine.

enterostomy (en″ter-os′to-me) fistulization of the intestine.

enterotomy (-ot′o-me) incision of the intestine.

enterotoxigenic (en″ter-o-tok″sĭ-jen′ik) producing, produced by or pertaining to production of enterotoxin.

enterotoxin (-tok′sin) 1. a toxin specific for the cells of the intestinal mucosa. 2. a toxin arising in the intestine. 3. an exotoxin that is protein in nature and relatively heat-stable, produced by staphylococci.

enterotoxism (-tok′sizm) absorption of toxins from the intestine.

enterotropic (-trop′ik) affecting the intestines.

enterovaginal (-vaj′ĭ-nal) pertaining to or communicating with the intestine and the vagina.

enterovesical (-ves′ĭ-kal) pertaining to or communicating with the intestine and urinary bladder.

Entero-vioform (en″ter-o-vi′o-form) trademark for a preparation of iodochlorhydroxyquin.

enterovirus (-vi′rus) one of a group of morphologically similar viruses infecting the gastrointestinal tract and discharged in the excreta, including the poliovirus and Coxsackie and ECHO viruses.

enterozoon (-zo′on) an animal parasite in the intestines. adj., **enterozo′ic.**

enthalpy (en′thal-pe) the heat content of a physical system.

enthesis (en′the-sis) the use of nonliving material in the repair of a defect or deformity of the body.

enthetic (en-thet′ik) 1. pertaining to enthesis. 2. brought in from outside.

entoblast (en′to-blast) the entoderm.

entocele (en′to-sēl) internal hernia.

entochondrostosis (en″to-kon″dros-to′sis) the development of bone within cartilage.

entochoroidea (-ko-roi′de-ah) the inner layer of the choroid.

entocineria (-sĭ-ne′re-ah) the internal gray matter of the brain or cord.

entocone (en′to-kōn) the inner posterior cusp of an upper molar tooth.

entocornea (en″to-kor′ne-ah) Descemet's membrane.

entocyte (en′to-sīt) the cell contents.

entoderm (en′to-derm) the innermost of the three primitive germ layers of the embryo; from it are derived the epithelium of the pharynx, respiratory tract (except the nose), digestive tract, bladder and urethra. adj., **entoder′mal, entoder′mic.**

entoectad (en″to-ek′tad) from within outward.

entomere (en′to-mēr) a blastomere normally destined to become entoderm.

entomesoderm (en″to-mes′o-derm) endomesoderm.

entomion (en-to′me-on) tip of mastoid angle of parietal bone.

entomology (en″to-mol′o-je) that branch of biology concerned with the study of insects.

economic e., that concerned with insects that affect the production of economically important plants and animals. **medical e.**, that concerned with insects which cause disease or serve as vectors of microorganisms that cause disease in man. **veterinary e.**, that concerned with insects which cause disease or serve as vectors of microorganisms that cause disease in animals.

entomophilous (en″to-mof′ĭ-lus) fertilized by insect-borne pollen; said of certain flowers.

entomophobia (en″to-mo-fo′be-ah) morbid dread of insects, mites, ticks, etc.

entophyte (en′to-fīt) an internal plant parasite.

entopic (en-top′ik) occurring in the proper place.

entoptic (en-top′tik) originating within the eye.

ontoptoscopy (en″top-tos′ko-pe) inspection of the interior of the eye.

entoretina (en″to-ret′ĭ-nah) the nervous or inner layer of the retina.

entotic (en-tot′ik) originating within the ear.

entozoon (en″to-zo′on) an internal animal parasite. adj., **entozo′ic.**

entropion (en-tro′pe-on) inversion, or the turning inward, as of the margin of an eyelid. **e. u′veae**, inversion of the margin of the pupil.

entropionize (en-tro′pe-ŏ-nīz″) to put into a state of inversion.

entypy (en′tĭ-pe) a method of gastrulation in which the entoderm lies external to the amniotic ectoderm.

enucleation (e-nu″kle-a′shun) removal of an organ or other mass intact from its supporting tissues, as of the eyeball from the orbit.

enuresis (en″u-re′sis) incontinence of urine not due to organic defect or illness; usually referring to the involuntary passage of urine at night in persons past the age of three years. adj., **enuret′ic.**

Enzactin (en-zak′tin) trademark for preparations of triacetin.

enzootic (en″zo-ot′ik) 1. present in an animal community at all times, but occurring in only small numbers of cases. 2. a disease of low morbidity which is constantly present in an animal community.

enzygotic (en″zi-got′ik) developed from one zygote.

enzyme (en′zim) a complex organic compound secreted by living cells, which is capable of causing or accelerating some change in a substrate for which it is often specific. **activating e.**, one which activates a given amino acid by attaching it to the corresponding transfer ribonucleic acid. **adaptive e.**, induced enzyme. **amylolytic e.**, one that catalyzes the conversion of starch into sugar. **autolytic e.**, one which produces autolysis. **branch-point e.**, the enzyme of a reaction that branches off a common pathway to initiate a specific biosynthetic pathway. **catheptic e.**, a proteolytic enzyme that has the property of being activated by hydrocyanic acid, hydrogen sulfide and other substances. **clotting e.**, one that catalyzes the conversion of soluble into insoluble proteins. **coagulating e.**, clotting enzyme. **constitutive e.**, one produced by a

microorganism regardless of the presence or absence of the specific substrate acted upon. **curdling e.**, clotting enzyme. **deamidizing e.**, one which splits up the amino acids into ammonia compounds. **decarbolizing e.**, one that splits carbon dioxide from organic acids. **digestive e.**, a substance that catalyzes the process of digestion. **extracellular e.**, one secreted outside the cell. **glycolytic e.**, one which catalyzes the oxidation of sugar. **induced e.**, one whose production requires or is stimulated by a specific small molecule, the inducer, which is the substrate of the enzyme or a compound structurally related to it.

inhibitory e., antienzyme. **inorganic e.**, a colloidal solution of a metal which has an action similar to that of enzymes. **intracellular e.**, one retained within the cell. **inverting e.**, one which splits up sugar, as invertin. **lipolytic e.**, one that catalyzes the decomposition of fat. **mucolytic e.**, one that catalyzes the depolymerization of mucopolysaccharides. **oxidation e.**, oxidase. **peptolytic e.**, one that catalyzes the decomposition of peptone. **proteolytic e.**, one that catalyzes the hydrolysis of proteins and protein split products to peptone. **redox e.**, one that catalyzes oxidation-reduction reactions. **reducing e.**, reductase. **steatolytic e.**, one which splits up fat, as steapsin. **sucroclastic e.**, one which decomposes sugar. **transferring e.**, one which catalyzes the transference of various radicals between molecules. **uricolytic e.**, one which metabolizes uric acid into urea. **Warburg's respiratory e.**, a protein existing in many tissues and serving as an important factor in tissue respiration.

enzymolysis (en″zi-mol′ĭ-sis) disintegration induced by an enzyme.

enzymosis (-mo′sis) fermentation induced by an enzyme.

enzymuria (-mu′re-ah) presence of enzymes in the urine.

eonism (e′o-nizm) the wearing of feminine clothing or the adoption of feminine habits and sexual behavior by a male.

eosin (e′o-sin) a coloring matter used as a dye in preparing various specimens for microscopic study.

eosinopenia (e″o-sin″o-pe′ne-ah) deficiency of eosinophil cells in the blood.

eosinophil (e″o-sin′o-fil) 1. an element readily stainable by eosin. 2. a medium-sized leukocyte, with a two- or three-lobed nucleus and cytoplasm containing large granules which stain bright red, normally constituting 1–2 per cent of the leukocytes in the blood.

eosinophilia (e″o-sin″o-fil′e-ah) 1. affinity for eosin. 2. an excess in the number of eosinophils. **tropical e.**, a disease characterized by anorexia, malaise, cough, leukocytosis and an increase in eosinophils.

eosinophilic (-fil′ik) staining readily with eosin.

eosinophilous (e″o-sĭ-nof′ĭ-lus) eosinophilic.

eosinotactic (e″o-sin″o-tak′tik) attracting or repelling eosinophilic cells.

epactal (e-pak′tal) 1. supernumerary. 2. any wormian bone.

epaxial (ep-ak'se-al) situated above the axis.

epencephalon (ep″en-sef'ah-lon) embryonic structure from which arise the pons and cerebellum.

ependyma (ĕ-pen'dĭ-mah) the membrane lining the cerebral ventricles and the central canal of the spine. adj., **epen'dymal.**

ependymitis (ep″en-dĭ-mi'tis) inflammation of the ependyma.

ependymoblast (ep″en-di'mo-blast) an embryonic ependymal cell.

ependymocyte (ĕ-pen'dĭ-mo-sīt″) an ependymal cell.

ependymoma (ĕ-pen″dĭ-mo'mah) a tumor containing ependymal elements.

ependymopathy (-mop'ah-the) disease of the ependyma.

Eperythrozoon (ep″ĕ-rith″ro-zo'on) a genus of Microtatobiotes (order Rickettsiales, family Bartonellaceae).

ephebiatrics (e-fe″be-at'riks) the branch of medicine which deals especially with the diagnosis and treatment of diseases and problems peculiar to youth.

ephebic (ĕ-fe'bik) pertaining to puberty.

ephebogenesis (ef″e-bo-jen'ĕ-sis) the bodily changes occurring at puberty. adj., **ephebogenet'ic.**

ephebogenic (-jen'ik) leading to the changes associated with puberty.

ephebology (ef″e-bol'o-je) the study of puberty.

Ephedra (ef'ĕ-drah) a genus of low, branching shrubs found in various parts of the world.

ephedrine (ĕ-fed'rin, ef'ĕ-drin) a sympathomimetic compound, $C_{10}H_{15}NO$, used as **e. hydrochloride** ($C_{10}H_{15}NO.HCl$) or **e. sulfate** ($[C_{10}H_{15}NO]_2.H_2SO_4$).

ephelis (ĕ-fe'lis), pl. *ephel'ides* [Gr.] a freckle.

ephidrosis (ef″ĭ-dro'sis) profuse perspiration. **e. cruen'ta,** bloody sweat.

Ephynal (ef'ĭ-nal) trademark for a preparation of vitamin E.

epi- (ep'ĭ) word element [Gr.], *upon.*

epiblast (ep'ĭ-blast) ectoderm. adj., **epiblas'tic.**

epiblepharon (ep″ĭ-blef'ah-ron) congenital anomaly, with horizontal fold of the lower eyelid, covering the lid margin and part of the eyelashes when the patient looks down.

epiboly (e-pib'o-le) the rapid segmentation of certain embryonic cells, enclosing another, less rapidly segmenting tissue.

epibulbar (ep″ĭ-bul'bar) situated upon the eyeball.

epicanthus (-kan'thus) a vertical fold of skin on either side of the nose, sometimes covering the inner canthus; a normal characteristic in persons of certain races, but anomalous in others. adj., **epican'thal.**

epicardia (-kar'de-ah) the portion of esophagus below the diaphragm.

epicardiectomy (-kar″de-ek'to-me) an operation by which the heart is supplied with a collateral circulation from the pericardium.

epicardium (-kar'de-um) the layer of the pericardium which is in contact with the heart.

epicele (ep'ĭ-sēl) the fourth ventricle of the brain.

epichorion (ep″ĭ-ko're-on) the portion of uterine mucosa enclosing the fertilized ovum.

epicomus (-ko'mus) a fetal monster with double head joined at summit.

epicondylalgia (-kon″dĭ-lal'je-ah) pain in the muscles attached to the epicondyle of the humerus.

epicondyle (-kon'dīl) an eminence or projection above the condyle of a bone.

epicondylus (-kon'dĭ-lus), pl. *epicon'dyli* [L.] epicondyle.

epicranium (-kra'ne-um) structures collectively which cover the skull.

epicrisis (-kri'sis) a secondary crisis.

epicritic (-krit'ik) determining accurately; said of cutaneous nerve fibers which are sensitive to fine variations of touch or temperature.

epicystitis (-sis-ti'tis) inflammation above the bladder.

epicystotomy (-sis-tot'o-me) cystotomy by the suprapubic method.

epicyte (ep'ĭ-sīt) the wall or envelope of a cell.

epidemic (ep″ĭ-dem'ik) 1. occurring in a great number of cases in a community at the same time. 2. the simultaneous occurrence in a human community of a great many cases of a specific disease.

epidemicity (-dĕ-mis'ĭ-te) the quality of being widely diffused and rapidly spreading throughout a community.

epidemiogenesis (-de″me-o-jen'ĕ-sis) the spread of a communicable disease to epidemic proportions.

epidemiography (-de″me-og'rah-fe) literature of epidemic diseases.

epidemiology (-ol'o-je) the scientific study of factors that influence the frequency and distribution of infectious diseases in man.

epidermal (-der'mal) 1. any material originating from animal epidermis (hairs, scales, feathers) which may cause allergy in hypersensitive persons. 2. epidermic.

epidermidization (-der″mid-ĭ-za'shun) development of stratified squamous epithelium from mucous cells, especially the downgrowth of such epithelium encircling the glands of the uterine cervix.

epidermidolysis (-der″mĭ-dol'ĭ-sis) epidermolysis.

epidermidosis (-der″mĭ-do'sis) disease of the epidermis.

epidermis (-der'mis) the outermost, nonvascular layer of the skin, derived from the embryonic ectoderm, varying in thickness from $^{1}/_{200}$ to $^{1}/_{20}$ inch, and composed of four layers: the desquamating horny layer, replaced by growth from below; the clear layer; the granular layer; a transition state between the innermost, the malpighian, layer and the outer two. adj., **epider'mic.**

epidermitis (-der-mi'tis) inflammation of the epidermis.

epidermodysplasia (-der″mo-dis-pla'ze-ah) faulty development of the epidermis. **e. verrucifor'mis,** an inherited dysplasia of the upper layers of the epidermis.

epidermoid (-der'moid) 1. resembling the

epidermis. 2. a brain tumor formed by inclusion of epidermal cells.

epidermoidoma (ep″ĭ-der″moi-do′mah) a usually benign tumor developing in the scalp, in the diploic space or between the dura and inner table of the skull.

epidermolysis (-der-mol′ĭ-sis) looseness of the skin. **e. bullo′sa,** a variety with formation of deep-seated bullae which appear after irritation.

epidermoma (-der-mo′mah) an outgrowth on the skin.

epidermomycosis (-der″mo-mi-ko′sis) any dermatitis caused by fungi or yeasts.

epidermophytid (-der-mof′ĭ-tid) a skin eruption occurring as an allergic response to Epidermophyton.

epidermophytin (-der-mof′ĭ-tin) a vaccine for epidermophytosis prepared from cultures of Epidermophyton.

Epidermophyton (-der-mof′ĭ-ton) a genus of fungi.

epidermophytosis (-der″mo-fi-to′sis) infection by the fungus Epidermophyton.

epidermosis (-der-mo′sis) disease of the epidermis.

epidiascope (-di′ah-skōp) an instrument for projecting the images of opaque bodies upon a screen.

epididymectomy (-did″ĭ-mek′to-me) excision of the epididymis.

epididymis (-did′ĭ-mis) an elongated, cordlike structure along the posterior border of the testis. adj., **epidid′ymal.**

epididymitis (-did″ĭ-mi′tis) inflammation of the epididymis.

epididymodeferentectomy (-did″-ĭ-mo-def″er-en-tek′to-me) excision of epididymis and vas deferens.

epididymodeferential (-def″er-en′shal) pertaining to epididymis and vas deferens.

epididymo-orchitis (-or-ki′tis) inflammation of epididymis and testis.

epididymotomy (ep″ĭ-did″ĭ-mot′o-me) incision of the epididymis.

epididymovasostomy (ep″ĭ-did″ĭ-mo-vas-os′to-me) anastomosis of the epididymis to the vas deferens.

epidural (ep″ĭ-du′ral) external to the dura mater.

epifolliculitis (-fo-lik″u-li′tis) inflammation of the hair follicles.

epigain (ep′ĭ-gān) the unconscious portion of the secondary external advantage to be derived from an emotional illness.

epigaster (ep″ĭ-gas′ter) hindgut.

epigastralgia (-gas-tral′je-ah) pain in the epigastrium.

epigastrium (-gas′tre-um) the upper abdominal region, overlying the stomach. adj., **epigas′tric.**

epigastrius (-gas′tre-us) a double fetal monster in which the parasite forms a tumor on the epigastrium of the autosite.

epigastrocele (-gas′tro-sēl) epigastric hernia.

epigenesis (-jen′ĕ-sis) development from simpler to more complex forms through division and progressive differentiation of the component cells.

epigenetics (ep″ĭ-jĕ-net′iks) the science concerned with the causal analysis of development.

epiglottectomy (-glŏ-tek′to-me) epiglottidectomy.

epiglottidean (-glŏ-tid′e-an) pertaining to the epiglottis.

epiglottidectomy (-glot″ĭ-dek′to-me) excision of the epiglottis.

epiglottiditis (-glot″ĭ-di′tis) epiglottitis.

epiglottis (-glot′is) cartilaginous lid of the larynx.

epiglottitis (-glŏ-ti′tis) inflammation of the epiglottis.

epilation (-la′shun) removal of hair.

epilatory (e-pil′ah-tor″e) 1. pertaining to removal of hair. 2. an agent for removing hair.

epilemma (ep″ĭ-lem′ah) the sheath of a terminal nerve fiber.

epilepsy (ep′ĭ-lep″se) a disorder characterized by convulsive seizures or disturbances of consciousness, or both, and associated with disturbance of electrical activity of the brain. **abdominal e.,** paroxysmal abdominal pain as an expression of neuronal discharge from the brain. **cardiac e.,** epilepsy with profound disturbance of heart's action, probably due to disease of the heart or of its nerves. **cortical e., focal e.,** localized epileptiform spasm on one side without loss of consciousness. **idiopathic e.,** true or typical epilepsy. **jacksonian e.,** a progression of involuntary clonic movement or sensation, with retention of consciousness. **myoclonus e.,** a condition characterized by intermittent or continuous clonus of muscle groups with mental deterioration, often interspersed with convulsive seizures. **nocturnal e.,** that in which the attack comes on during sleep. **procursive e.,** that in which at the beginning of the attack the patient runs swiftly. **psychomotor e.,** a condition characterized by purposeful motor or psychic activity which is irrelevant for the time and place, the patient being amnesic afterward for events that occurred during the seizure. **reflex e.,** a form due to peripheral irritation. **sensory e.,** epilepsy in which convulsions are replaced by delusions of sense and by hallucinations. **sleep e.,** narcolepsy. **spinal e.,** succession of clonic and tonic spasms in spastic paraplegia. **thalamic e.,** sensory epilepsy ascribed to disease of the thalamus. **tonic e.,** a seizure characterized by involuntary movements marked by rigidity. **toxemic e.,** that due to a toxic influence.

epileptic (ep″ĭ-lep′tik) 1. pertaining to epilepsy. 2. a person subject to attacks of epilepsy.

epileptiform (-lep′tĭ-form) epileptoid.

epileptogenic (-lep″to-jen′ik) causing an epileptic seizure.

epileptoid (-lep′toid) 1. resembling epilepsy or its manifestations. 2. occurring in severe or sudden paroxysms.

epileptology (-lep-tol′o-je) the study of epilepsy.

epiloia (ep″ĭ-loi′ah) tuberous sclerosis.

epimandibular (-man-dib′u-lar) situated on the lower jaw.

epimenorrhagia (-men″o-ra′je-ah) abnormally profuse menstruation.

epimenorrhea (-men″o-re′ah) abnormally frequent menstruation.

epimer (ep′ĭ-měr) one of two or more optical isomers which differ only in the position of one carbon atom.

epimere (ep′ĭ-měr) one of the dorsal portions of the fusing myotomes in embryonic development, forming muscles innervated by the dorsal rami of the spinal nerves.

epimerite (ep″ĭ-mer′ĭt) an organ of protozoa by which they attach themselves to epithelial cells.

epimicroscope (-mi′kro-skōp) a microscope in which the specimen is illuminated by light passing through a condenser built around the objective.

epimorphosis (-mor-fo′sis) the regeneration of a piece of an organism by proliferation at the cut surface. adj., **epimor′phic.**

epimysium (-mis′e-um) the outer investment of a striated muscle.

epinephrectomy (-ne-frek′to-me) adrenalectomy.

epinephrine (-nef′rin) a hormone secreted by the adrenal medulla and released in response to hypoglycemia, or produced synthetically, used as a sympathomimetic, a cardiac stimulant, a pressor substance and to relax bronchial smooth muscle.

epinephrinemia (-nef″rĭ-ne′me-ah) epinephrine in the blood.

epinephritis (-ne-fri′tis) inflammation of an adrenal gland.

epinephroma (-ne-fro′mah) hypernephroma.

epinephros (-nef′ros) an adrenal gland.

epineural (-nu′ral) situated upon a neural arch.

epineurium (-nu′re-um) the sheath of a nerve.

epinosis (-no′sis) a psychic or imaginary state of illness secondary to an original illness.

epionychium (ep″e-o-nik′e-um) situated on or above the ear.

epipharynx (ep″ĭ-far′inks) nasopharynx. adj., **epipharyn′geal.**

epiphenomenon (-fē-nom′ē-non) an exceptional phenomenon not necessarily associated with the circumstances it accompanied.

epiphora (e-pif′o-rah) overflow of tears from obstruction of lacrimal duct.

epiphylaxis (ep″ĭ-fĭ-lak′sis) increase of normal phylaxis. adj., **epiphylac′tic.**

epiphysiolysis (-fiz″e-ol′ĭ-sis) separation of the epiphysis from the diaphysis of a bone.

epiphysis (e-pif′ĭ-sis), pl. *epiph′yses* [Gr.] 1. portion of a bone which in early life is distinct from the shaft. 2. the pineal gland (*e. cer′ebri*). adj., **epiphys′eal. slipped e.**, dislocation of the epiphysis of a bone, as of the epiphysis of the head of the femur. **stippled e′s**, chondrodystrophia fetalis calcificans.

epiphysitis (e-pif″ĭ-si′tis) inflammation of the cartilage joining the epiphysis to a shaft.

epiphyte (ep′ĭ-fīt) an external plant parasite.

epiphytic (ep″ĭ-fit′ik) 1. growing or proliferating externally. 2. pertaining to an external vegetable parasite.

epipial (-pi′al) situated upon the pia mater.

epiplocele (e-pip′lo-sēl) omental hernia.

epiploectomy (ep″ĭ-plo-ek′to-me) omentectomy.

epiploenterocele (-en′ter-o-sēl″) hernia containing intestine and omentum.

epiploitis (-i′tis) inflammation of the epiploon.

epiplomerocele (-me′ro-sēl) femoral hernia containing omentum.

epiplomphalocele (ep″ĭ-plom-fal′o-sēl) umbilical hernia containing omentum.

epiploon (e-pip′lo-on), pl. *epip′loa* [Gr.] the greater omentum. adj., **epiplo′ic.**

epiplopexy (e-pip′lo-pek″se) omentopexy.

epiplorrhaphy (e″pip-lor′ah-fe) omentorrhaphy.

epiplosarcomphalocele (e-pip″lo-sar″kom-fal′-o-sēl) umbilical hernia with a local fleshy excrescence.

epiploscheocele (e″pip-los′ke-o-sēl″) scrotal hernia containing omentum.

epipygus (ep″ĭ-pi′gus) pygomelus.

episcleral (-skle′ral) over the sclera of the eye.

episcleritis (-skle-ri′tis) inflammation of the outer layers of the sclera.

episcope (ep′ĭ-skōp) epidiascope.

episioclisia (e-piz″e-o-kli′se-ah) surgical closure of the vulva.

episioperineoplasty (-per″ĭ-ne′o-plas″te) plastic repair of vulva and perineum.

episioperineorrhaphy (-per″ĭ-ne-or′ah-fe) suture of vulva and perineum.

episioplasty (ep-iz′e-o-plas″te) plastic repair of the vulva.

episiorrhaphy (e-piz″e-or′ah-fe) suture of the vulva.

episiostenosis (e-piz″e-o-ste-no′sis) narrowing of the vulva.

episiotomy (e-piz″e-ot′o-me) incision of the vulva.

episome (ep′ĭ-sōm) a block of genetic material capable of existing in the cell in two alternate forms, one replicating autonomously in the cytoplasm and the other replicating as part of the chromosome.

epispadias (ep″ĭ-spa′de-as) a congenital malformation with absence of the upper wall of the urethra, occurring in both sexes, but more commonly in the male, the urethral opening being located anywhere on the dorsum of the penis. adj., **epispa′diac.**

epispastic (-spas′tik) vesicant; blistering.

episplenitis (-sple-ni′tis) inflammation of the capsule of the spleen.

epistaxis (-stak′sis) hemorrhage from the nose, usually due to rupture of small vessels overlying the anterior part of the cartilaginous nasal septum.

episternal (-ster′nal) situated upon the sternum.

episternum (-ster′num) the manubrium, or upper piece of the sternum.

epistropheus (ep″ĭ-stro′fe-us) axis.

epitendineum (-ten-din′e-um) the fibrous sheath covering a tendon.

epithalamus (-thal′ah-mus) the pineal body and adjacent structures of the forebrain.

epithalaxia (-thah-lak′se-ah) desquamation of the epithelium, especially of the intestine.

epithelialization (-the″le-al-i-za′shun) the covering of a denuded area with epithelium; conversion into epithelium.

epithelialize (-the′le-al-īz″) to cover with or change into epithelium.

epitheliitis (-the″le-i′tis) inflammation of epithelium.

epithelioblastoma (-the″le-o-blas-to′mah) a tumor made up of cells of epithelial origin.

epitheliochorial (-ko′re-al) denoting a type of placenta in which the uterine lining is not eroded, but merely lies in apposition.

epitheliofibril (-fi′bril) a fibril running through the protoplasm of epithelial cells.

epitheliogenetic (-jĕ-net′ik) due to epithelial proliferation.

epithelioid (ep″ĭ-the′le-oid) resembling epithelium.

epitheliolysin (ep″ĭ-the″le-ol′ĭ-sin) an antibody which causes dissolution of epithelial cells.

epitheliolysis (-ol′ĭ-sis) destruction of epithelial tissue.

epithelioma (ep″ĭ-the″le-o′mah) cancer composed largely of epithelial cells. adj., **epithelio′matous. e. adenoi′des cys′ticum,** a rare form of basal cell carcinoma, appearing as heaped-up lesions on the skin, especially of the face.

epitheliosis (-o′sis) proliferation of conjunctival epithelium, forming trachoma-like granules.

epitheliotropic (-o-trop′ik) having a special affinity for epithelial cells.

epithelium (ep″ĭ-the′le-um), pl. *epithe′lia* [Gr.] cellular substance of skin and mucous membrane. adj., **epithe′lial. ciliated e.,** epithelium having motile, hairlike processes on its free surface. **columnar e.,** epithelium whose cells are of much greater height than width. **cuboidal e.,** epithelium whose cells are of approximately the same height and width, and appear square in transverse section. **germinal e.,** a layer of cells between the primitive mesentery and each mesonephros which becomes the epithelial covering of the gonad and perhaps gives rise to the germ cells. **glandular e.,** that composed of secreting cells. **laminated e.,** stratified epithelium. **pavement e.,** a variety composed of flattened cells in layers. **pigmented e.,** that made up of cells containing melanin or other pigment. **pseudostratified e.,** epithelium whose cells appear to be arranged in layers because of location of the nuclei at different levels and loss by some of the cells of their connection with the free surface. **pyramidal e.,** columnar epithelium whose cells have been modified by pressure into truncated pyramids. **rod e.,** peculiarly striated epithelium of certain glands. **sense e.,** epithelium containing end-organs receiving stimuli of sensation. **squamous e.,** epithelium whose cells are thin and platelike. **stratified e.,** epithelium made up of cells arranged in two or more layers. **tessellated e.,** pavement epithelium. **transitional e.,** a type characteristically found lining hollow organs that are subject to great mechanical change due to contraction and distention, originally thought to represent a transition between stratified squamous and columnar epithelium.

epithelization (ep″ĭ-the″li-za′shun) the formation of skin over a denuded area or wound.

epitonic (ep″ĭ-ton′ik) abnormally tense and tonic.

epitrichium (-trik′e-um) superficial layer of the epidermis of the embryo and fetus.

epitrochlea (-trok′le-ah) inner condyle of the humerus.

epituberculosis (-tu-ber″ku-lo′sis) a condition resembling tuberculosis, but not caused by tubercle bacilli.

epiturbinate (-ter′bi-nāt) the soft tissue covering the turbinate bone.

epitympanum (-tim′pah-num) the upper part of the tympanum.

epizoicide (-zo′ĭ-sīd) an agent which destroys epizoa.

epizoon (-zo′on), pl. *epizo′a* [Gr.] an external animal parasite. adj., **epizo′ic.**

epizoonosis (-zo-o-no′sis), pl. *epizoono′ses*, a morbid condition due to external animal parasites.

epizootic (-zo-ot′ik) 1. occurring in a great number of cases in an animal community at the same time. 2. the simultaneous occurrence in an animal community of a great many cases of a specific disease. 3. a disease of high morbidity which is only occasionally present in an animal community.

epizootiology (-zo-ot″e-ol′o-je) the scientific study of factors in the frequency and distribution of infectious diseases among animals.

eponychium (ep″o-nik′e-um) 1. an extension of the horny layers of the skin over the nail. 2. the horny embryonic membrane from which the nail is developed.

eponym (ep′o-nim) name of a person used to designate a disease, organ or other entity, e.g. Hodgkin's disease, Cowper's gland, Schick test. adj., **eponym′ic.**

epoophorectomy (ep″o-of″o-rek′to-me) excision of the epoophoron.

epoophoron (-of′o-ron) a vestigial structure associated with the ovary.

epornithology (ep″or-ni-thol′o-je) the scientific study of epidemic diseases of birds.

epoxytropine tropate (e-pok″se-tro′pēn tro′-pāt) methscopolamine.

EPR electrophrenic respiration.

Eprolin (ep′ro-lin) trademark for a preparation of vitamin E.

epulis (ep-u′lis), pl. *epu′lides* [Gr.] a fibrous tumor of the gum.

epulosis (ep″u-lo′sis) cicatrization. adj., **epulot′ic.**

Equanil (ek′wah-nil) trademark for preparations of meprobamate.

equation 230

equation (e-kwa'zhun) an expression of equality. **Henderson-Hasselbalch e.,** a formula for calculating the pH of a buffer solution such as blood plasma, pH = pK′ + log $\frac{(BA)}{(HA)}$; (HA) is the concentration of a weak acid; (BA) the concentration of a weak salt of this acid; pK′ the buffer system. **personal e.,** the variation introduced into any study or relationship because of the differences in individuals.

equator (e-kwa'tor) an imaginary line encircling the globe midway between its poles. adj., **equato′rial.**

equiaxial (e″kwe-ak'se-al) having axes of the same length.

equilibration (e″kwī-li-bra'shun) the achievement of a balance between opposing elements or forces. **occlusal e.,** modification of the occlusal forms of teeth to equalize occlusal stress or achieve harmonious occlusion.

equilibrium (e″kwī-lib're-um) a state of balance between opposing forces or influences.

equine (e'kwīn) pertaining to, characteristic of or derived from the horse.

equinophobia (e-kwi″no-fo'be-ah) morbid fear of horses.

equinovarus (-va'rus) talipes equinovarus.

equipotential (e″kwī-po-ten'shal) having similar and equal power or capability.

equipotentiality (-po-ten″she-al'ī-te) the quality or state of having similar and equal power; the capacity for developing in the same way and to the same extent.

equivalent (e-kwiv'ah-lent) 1. of equal force, power or value. 2. the unvarying quantity of one body necessary to replace a fixed weight of another body. **epilepsy e.,** any disturbance, mental or physical, which may take the place of an epileptic seizure. **Joule's e.,** energy expended in raising the temperature of one unit weight of water 1 degree. **neutralization e.,** the equivalent weight of an acid as determined by neutralization with a standard base.

E.R. external resistance.

Er chemical symbol, *erbium.*

E.R.A. Electroshock Research Association.

erasion (e-ra'zhun) abrasion or scraping.

erbium (er'be-um) chemical element *(see table),* at. no. 68, symbol Er.

erection (e-rek'shun) process of becoming upright and turgid.

erector (e-rek'tor) [L.] that which erects.

eredosome (e-red'o-sōm) amorphous hemoglobin filling the meshes of the stroma of erythrocytes.

eremacausis (er″ĕ-mah-kaw'sis) slow oxidation and decay of organic matter.

eremophobia (-mo-fo'be-ah) morbid fear of being alone.

erepsin (e-rep'sīn) an enzyme of the intestinal juice.

erethin (er'ĕ-thin) poisonous principle of tuberculin.

erethism (er'ĕ-thizm) morbid excitability. adj., **erethis′mic, erethis′tic.**

erethisophrenia (er″ĕ-thiz″o-fre'ne-ah) exaggerated mental excitability.

erg (erg) a unit of work or energy, equivalent to 2.4 × 10⁻⁸ gram calories, or to 0.624 × 10¹² electron volts.

ergasia (er-ga'ze-ah) 1. a hypothetical substance which stimulates the activity of body cells. 2. the total of an individual's functions and behavior.

ergasiology (er-ga″se-ol'o-je) objective psychobiology.

ergasiomania (er-ga″se-o-ma'ne-ah) a morbid desire to be continually at work.

ergasiophobia (-fo'be-ah) morbid fear of overexertion.

ergasthenia (er″gas-the'ne-ah) debility from overwork.

ergastic (er-gas'tik) having potential energy.

ergastoplasm (er-gas'to-plazm) granular endoplasmic reticulum, so called because of the activity of the ribosomes studding its surface.

ergocalciferol (er″go-kal-sif'er-ol) calciferol.

ergocardiogram (-kar'de-o-gram) the graphic record obtained by ergocardiography.

ergocardiography (-kar″de-og'rah-fe) the recording of moment-to-moment electromotive forces of the heart while the subject is engaging in muscular activity.

ergograph (er'go-graf) instrument for measuring work done in muscular action.

ergonomics (er″go-nom'iks) the science relating to man and his work, including the factors affecting the efficient use of human energy.

ergonovine (-no'vin) an ergot alkaloid used as an oxytocic and to relieve migraine headache.

ergophobia (-fo'be-ah) morbid dread of work.

ergophore (er'go-fōr) the group of atoms in a molecule that brings about the specific activity of the substance.

ergoplasm (er'go-plazm) kinoplasm.

ergosome (er'go-sōm) polyribosome.

ergostat (er'go-stat) a machine to be worked for muscular exercise.

ergosterol (er-gos'ter-ol) a sterol occurring in animal and plant tissues which on ultraviolet irradiation becomes a potent antirachitic substance.

ergot (er'got) the dried sclerotium of *Claviceps purpurea;* smooth muscle stimulant, oxytocic; fatal epidemics have been caused by use of bread made from rye contaminated with the fungus.

ergotamine (er-got'ah-min) an alkaloid derived from ergot, used as an oxytocic and in treatment of migraine.

ergotherapy (er″go-ther'ah-pe) treatment by physical exertion.

ergotism (er'go-tizm) chronic poisoning produced by ingestion of ergot.

Ergotrate (er'go-trāt) trademark for preparations of ergonovine.

eriodictyon (er″e-o-dik'te-on) the dried leaf of *Eriodictyon californicum,* used in pharmaceutical preparations.

erogenous (ĕ-roj'ĕ-nus) causing sexual excitement.

erosio (e-ro'ze-o) [L.] erosion. **e. intergita′-**

lis blastomycet'ica, a fungus infection causing maceration between the fingers.

erosion (e-ro'zhun) an eating or gnawing away; a kind of ulceration; in dentistry, the wasting away or loss of substance of a tooth by a chemical process that does not involve known bacterial action. adj., **ero'sive. cervical e.,** ulceration of the endocervix and of the vaginal portion of the cervix, due to chemical irritation. **dental e.,** the disintegration of tooth substance on surfaces free from attrition by mastication. **Dieulafoy's e.,** ulcerative gastroenteritis occurring as a complication of pneumonia.

erotic (ē-rot'ik) pertaining to love or to sexual energy.

erotism (er'o-tizm) the expression of one's instinctual energy or drive, often used in special reference to the sex drive. **anal e.,** fixation of libido at (or regression to) anal phase of infantile development, producing egotistic, dogmatic, stubborn, miserly character. **genital e.,** achievement and maintenance of libido at genital phase of psychosexual development, permitting acceptance of normal adult relationships and responsibilities. **oral e.,** fixation of libido at (or regression to) oral phase of infantile development, producing passive, insecure, sensitive character.

erotize (er'o-tīz) to endow with erotic meaning or significance.

erotogenic (ē-ro″to-jen'ik) arousing sexual desire.

erotology (er″o-tol'o-je) the study of love.

erotomania (ē-ro″to-ma'ne-ah) morbidly exaggerated sexual behavior.

erotophobia (-fo'be-ah) morbid dread of sexual love.

errhine (er'īn) causing sneezing and secretion from the nose.

Ertron (er'tron) trademark for preparations of vitamin D_2.

eructation (e″ruk-ta'shun) the oral ejection of gas or air from the stomach.

eruption (e-rup'shun) emergence from beneath a surface, as of teeth through the gingivae or of lesions on the skin; applied also to various skin lesions not due to external injury. **bullous e.,** an eruption of large blebs or blisters. **creeping e.,** larva migrans. **drug e.,** dermatitis medicamentosa. **fixed e.,** circumscribed lesions that persist or persistently recur at the same site on the body over a period of months or years. **Kaposi's varicelliform e.,** a vesiculopustular eruption of viral origin, superimposed upon a pre-existing eczema.

eruptive (e-rup'tiv) attended with a breaking out or rash.

ERV expiratory reserve volume.

Erwinia (er-win'e-ah) a genus of Schizomycetes (order Eubacteriales, family Enterobacteriaceae, tribe Erwinieae).

Erwinieae (er″wi-ni'e-e) a tribe of Schizomycetes (order Eubacteriales, family Enterobacteriaceae).

erysipelas (er″ĭ-sip'ĕ-las) a febrile disease characterized by inflammation and redness of skin, mucous membranes, etc., and due to *Streptococcus pyogenes.*

erysipelatous (er″ĭ-sĭ-pel'ah-tus) of the nature of erysipelas.

erysipeloid (er″ĭ-sip'ĕ-loid) a disease similar to erysipelas, caused by *Erysipelothrix insidiosa.*

Erysipelothrix (er″ĭ-sip'ĕ-lo-thriks″) a genus of Schizomycetes (order Eubacteriales, family Corynebacteriaceae).

erysiphake (er-is'ĭ-fāk) an instrument for removing the lens in cataract by suction.

erythema (er″ĭ-the'mah) redness of the skin due to congestion of the capillaries. **e. ab ig'ne,** persistent erythema and pigmentation from long-continued exposure to excessive heat without burning. **e. annula're,** an erythema with circinate lesions 1–2 cm. in diameter, thought by some to be pathognomonic of rheumatic fever. **e. annula're centrif'ugum,** a rare disease with erythematous ringed lesions on the trunk that tend to grow eccentrically, break up and disappear, to be replaced by new lesions that follow a similar course. **e. bullo'sum,** a type of erythema multiforme characterized by eruption of vesicles or bullae. **epidemic arthritic e., e. arthrit'icum epidem'icum,** Haverhill fever. **e. indura'tum,** tuberculosis indurativa. **e. infectio'sum,** an afebrile exanthem occurring in epidemics or endemics, with an erythematous, edematous plaque on the face and a maculopapular eruption on the trunk. **e. i'ris,** a type of erythema multiforme in which the lesions form concentric rings, producing a target-like appearance. **e. margina'tum,** a type of erythema multiforme in which the reddened areas are disk-shaped, with elevated edges. **e. mi'grans,** geographic tongue. **e. multifor'me,** a disease state with highly polymorphic skin lesions, including macular papules, vesicles and bullae. **e. multifor'me exudati'vum,** Stevens-Johnson syndrome. **e. nodo'sum,** a form marked by tender, light red, round or oval raised nodules, chiefly on the legs. **e. puncta'tum, e. scarlatinifor'me,** redness of the skin resembling the appearance of scarlet fever. **toxic e., e. tox'icum,** a generalized erythematous or erythematomacular eruption due to administration of a drug or to bacterial toxins or other toxic substances. **e. tox'icum neonato'rum,** a self-limited urticarial condition affecting infants in the first few days of life. **e. venena'tum,** toxic erythema.

erythematous (er″ĭ-them'ah-tus) of the nature of erythema.

erythemogenic (er″ĭ-the″mo-jen'ik) producing erythema.

erythr(o)- (ē-rith'ro) word element [Gr.], *red.*

erythralgia (er″ĭ-thral'je-ah) erythromelalgia.

erythrasma (-thraz'mah) skin disease marked by patches in groin or axilla, and due to fungus infection.

erythredema polyneuropathy (ē-rith″rĕ-de'-mah pol″ĭ-nu-rop'ah-the) acrodynia.

erythremia (er″ĭ-thre'me-ah) polycythemia vera.

erythrin (er'ĭ-thrin) an antibacterial peptide isolated from red blood corpuscles.

erythrism (ĕ-rith'rizm) redness of the hair and beard. adj., **erythris'tic.**

erythrityl (ĕ-rith'rĭ-til) the univalent radical, C_4H_9, from erythritol. **e. tetranitrate,** a compound, $C_4H_6(NO_3)_4$; vasodilator.

erythroblast (ĕ-rith'ro-blast) an immature cell from which a red blood corpuscle develops. **basophilic e.,** a cell with a slightly clumped nuclear chromatin and basophilic cytoplasm without hemoglobin, which follows the pronormoblast developmentally. **early e.,** basophilic erythroblast. **late e., polychromatophilic e.,** a cell of the stage following the basophilic erythroblast, in which there is increased chromatin clumping and the earliest appearance of pink cytoplasmic hemoglobin.

erythroblastemia (ĕ-rith″ro-blas-te′me-ah) presence in the peripheral blood of abnormally large numbers of nucleated red cells.

erythroblastoma (-blas-to′mah) a tumor arising from erythroblasts.

erythroblastomatosis (-blas″to-mah-to′sis) a condition marked by the formation of erythroblastomas.

erythroblastopenia (-blas″to-pe′ne-ah) abnormal deficiency of erythroblasts.

erythroblastosis (-blas-to′sis) the presence of erythroblasts in the circulating blood. adj., **erythroblastot′ic. e. feta′lis, e. neonato′rum,** a hemolytic anemia of the fetus or newborn infant, due to transplacental transmission of maternally formed antibody.

erythrochloropia (-klo-ro′pe-ah) visual recognition of only red and green.

erythrochromia (-kro′me-ah) hemorrhagic, red pigmentation of the spinal fluid.

erythroclasis (er″ĭ-throk′lah-sis) fragmentation of the red blood corpuscles. adj., **erythroclas′tic.**

erythrocuprein (ĕ-rith″ro-koo′prin) a copperprotein compound contained in erythrocytes.

erythrocyanosis (-si″ah-no′sis) bluish or red discoloration of skin, with swelling, burning and itching.

erythrocyte (ĕ-rith′ro-sīt) one of the formed elements in peripheral blood, containing hemoglobin and transporting oxygen. **achromic e.,** a colorless erythrocyte. **basophilic e.,** one that takes the basic stain. **"Mexican hat" e.,** leptocyte. **orthochromatic e.,** one that takes only the acid stain. **polychromatic e., polychromatophilic e.,** one that, on staining, shows shades of blue combined with tinges of pink. **target e.,** leptocyte.

erythrocythemia (ĕ-rith″ro-si-the′me-ah) erythremia.

erythrocytin (-si′tin) a substance in red cells thought to function in the first stage of blood coagulation.

erythrocytolysis (-si-tol′ĭ-sis) dissolution of erythrocytes.

erythrocytometer (-si-tom′ĕ-ter) a laboratory instrument utilizing the principle of light diffraction in measuring the diameter of red blood cells or other microscopic particles in a thin film.

erythrocyto-opsonin (ĕ-rith″ro-si″to-op-so′nin) an opsonin that acts on erythrocytes.

erythrocytophagy (-si-tof′ah-je) the engulfment of erythrocytes by other cells. adj., **erythrocytoph′agous.**

erythrocytorrhexis (-si″to-rek′sis) the breaking up of erythrocytes.

erythrocytoschisis (-si-tos′kĭ-sis) degeneration of erythrocytes into disklike bodies.

erythrocytosis (-si to′sis) increase in number of red cells as a result of a known stimulus. **leukemic e., e. megalosplen′ica,** polycythemia vera. **stress e.,** a relative polycythemia observed in anxiety-prone persons.

erythrocytotropic (-si″to-trop′ik) having a special affinity for erythrocytes.

erythrodegenerative (-de-jen′er-a″tiv) characterized by degeneration of erythrocytes.

erythroderma (-der′mah) abnormal redness of the skin over widespread areas of the body. **atopic e.,** a chronic diffuse dermatitis occurring in allergic infants. **congenital ichthyosiform e.,** a generalized hereditary dermatitis with scaling. **e. desquamati′vum,** severe seborrheic dermatitis, leading to desquamation of skin and exposure of corium. **e. ichthyosifor′me congen′itum,** congenital ichthyosiform erythroderma. **lymphoblastic e.,** a condition marked by chronic redness of the skin, associated with absolute leukocytosis, with relative increase in the lymphocytes. **lymphomatous e.,** widespread redness of the skin associated with lymphoma. **maculopapular e.,** a reddish eruption composed of macules and papules. **psoriatic e., e. psorat′icum,** a generalized psoriasis vulgaris, showing the chemical characteristics of exfoliative dermatitis. **squamous e., e. squamo′sum,** an eruption of scaly groups of papules.

erythrodermatitis (-der″mah-ti′tis) inflammation of the skin, with redness.

erythrodermia (-der′me-ah) abnormal redness in the skin.

erythrodextrin (-dek′strin) a dextrin stained red by iodine.

erythrogenesis (-jen′ĕ-sis) the production of erythrocytes. **e. imperfec′ta,** congenital hypoplastic anemia.

erythrogonium (-go′ne-um) a very immature erythroblast.

erythrogranulose (-gran′u-lōs) a form of granulose stained red by iodine.

erythroid (er′ĭ-throid) of a red color.

erythrokatalysis (ĕ-rith″ro-kah-tal′ĭ-sis) phagocytosis of red blood corpuscles.

erythrokinetics (-ki-net′iks) the quantitative, dynamic study of in-vivo production and destruction of erythrocytes.

erythroleukemia (-lu-ke′me-ah) a malignant blood dyscrasia with atypical erythroblasts and myeloblasts in the peripheral blood.

erythroleukosis (-lu-ko′sis) excessive formation of both erythrocytes and leukocytes in the blood.

erythrolysin (er″ĭ-throl′ĭ-sin) a substance capable of causing erythrocytolysis.

erythrolysis (er″ĭ-throl′ĭ-sis) erythrocytolysis.

erythromania (ĕ-rith″ro-ma′ne-ah) uncontrollable blushing.

erythromelalgia (-mel-al′je-ah) neuritis marked by burning pain and redness of the extremities.

erythromelia (-me′le-ah) progressive redness of the skin on the extensor surfaces of the legs and arms.

erythrometer (er″ĭ-throm′ĕ-ter) an instrument for measuring redness.

erythromycin (ĕ-rith″ro-mi′sin) an antibiotic compound for oral or intravenous use.

erythron (er′ĭ-thron) the circulating erythrocytes and the erythrocyte-forming tissues of the body.

erythroneocytosis (ĕ-rith″ro-ne″o-si-to′sis) presence of immature erythrocytes in the blood.

erythronoclastic (er″ĭ-thron′o-klas″tik) destroying erythron.

erythroparasite (ĕ-rith″ro-par′ah-sīt) a parasite of the erythrocytes.

erythropathy (er″ĭ-throp′ah-the) any disorder of the erythrocytes.

erythropenia (ĕ-rith″ro-pe′ne-ah) deficiency in the number of erythrocytes.

erythrophage (ĕ-rith′ro-fāj) a phagocyte which absorbs blood pigments and destroys erythrocytes.

erythrophagia (ĕ-rith″ro-fa′je-ah) destruction of blood pigments and erythrocytes by phagocytes.

erythrophagocytosis (-fag″o-si-to′sis) phagocytosis of erythrocytes.

erythrophil (ĕ-rith′ro-fil) an element which stains easily with red.

erythrophilic (ĕ-rith″ro-fil′ik) having a special affinity for red dye (acid fuchsin).

erythrophilous (er″ĭ-throf′ĭ-lus) easily staining red.

erythrophobia (ĕ-rith″ro-fo′be-ah) 1. morbid flushing. 2. morbid aversion to red.

erythrophobic (-fo′bik) having no affinity for red dye (acid fuchsin).

erythrophose (ĕ-rith′ro-fōz) any red phose.

erythrophthisis (ĕ-rith″ro-thi′sis) a condition characterized by severe impairment of the restorative power of the erythrocyte-forming tissues.

erythroplasia (-pla′ze-ah) a condition of mucous membrane characterized by erythematous papular lesions. **e. of Queyrat,** a condition characterized by an erythematous papular lesion on the glans penis, coronal sulcus or prepuce.

erythroplastid (-plas′tid) erythrocyte.

erythropoiesis (-poi-e′sis) the formation of erythrocytes. adj., **erythropoiet′ic.**

erythropoietin (-poi′ĕ-tin) a factor in the plasma that stimulates the production of red cells.

erythroprecipitin (-pre-sip′ĭ-tin) a precipitin specific for erythrocytes.

erythroprosopalgia (-pros″o-pal′je-ah) a nervous disorder marked by redness and pain in the face.

erythropsia (er″ĭ-throp′se-ah) a defect of

vision in which objects appear tinged with red.

erythropsin (er″ĭ-throp′sin) rhodopsin.

erythrorrhexis (ĕ-rith″ro-rek′sis) erythrocytorrhexis.

erythrosedimentation (-sed″ĭ-men-ta′shun) the sedimentation of erythrocytes.

erythrosis (er″ĭ-thro′sis) reddish discoloration of skin and mucous membranes.

erythrotoxin (ĕ-rith″ro-tok′sin) a toxin acting on erythrocytes.

erythruria (er″ĭ-throo′re-ah) excretion of red urine.

E.S. The Endocrine Society.

Es chemical symbol, *einsteinium.*

eschar (es′kar) a lesion such as that due to a bite of the infected mite, resulting in scrub typhus, or by application of a caustic or corrosive agent, a necrotic mass ultimately separating from healthy tissue and being cast off. adj., **escharot′ic.**

Escherichia (esh″ĕ-rik′e-ah) a genus of Schizomycetes (order Eubacteriales, family Enterobacteriaceae, tribe Escherichieae) occasionally pathogenic for man.

Escherichieae (esh″er-ĭ-ki′e-e) a tribe of Schizomycetes (order Eubacteriales, family Enterobacteriaceae) that comprises the coliform bacteria.

eschrolalia (es″kro-la′le-ah) coprolalia.

eserine (es′er-ēn) physostigmine.

E.S.F. erythropoietic-stimulating factor.

Esidrix (es′ĭ-driks) trademark for a preparation of hydrochlorothiazide.

-esis (e′sis) word element, *state; condition.*

Eskabarb (es′kah-barb) trademark for a preparation of phenobarbital.

Eskadiazine (es″kah-di′ah-zēn) trademark for a preparation of sulfadiazine.

esmarch (es′mark) an Esmarch bandage.

eso- (es′o) prefix [Gr.], *within.*

esodic (e-sod′ik) afferent, centripetal.

eso-ethmoiditis (es″o-eth″moid-i′tis) inflammation of the ethmoid sinuses.

esogastritis (-gas-tri′tis) inflammation of the gastric mucosa.

esophageal (e-sof″ah-je′al) pertaining to the esophagus.

esophagectasia (e-sof″ah-jek-ta′se-ah) dilatation of the esophagus.

esophagectomy (e-sof″ah-jek′to-me) excision of the esophagus.

esophagism (e-sof″ah-jizm) spasm of the esophagus.

esophagitis (e-sof″ah-ji′tis) inflammation of the esophagus. **peptic e.,** inflammation of the esophagus due to a reflux of acid and pepsin from the stomach.

esophagobronchial (e-sof″ah-go-brong′ke-al) pertaining to or communicating with esophagus and a bronchus.

esophagocele (e-sof′ah-go-sēl″) esophageal hernia.

esophagoduodenostomy (e-sof″ah-go-du″o-de-nos′to-me) anastomosis of the esophagus to the duodenum.

esophagodynia (-din′e-ah) pain in the esophagus.

esophagoenterostomy (e-sof″ah-go-en″ter-os′-to-me) creation of an opening between the esophagus and a part of the intestine.

esophagoesophagostomy (-e-sof″ah-gos′to-me) anastomosis between two formerly remote parts of the esophagus.

esophagogastrectomy (-gas-trek′to-me) excision of esophagus and stomach.

esophagogastroanastomosis (-gas″tro-ah-nas″to-mo′sis) esophagogastrostomy.

esophagogastroplasty (-gas′tro-plas″te) plastic repair of esophagus and stomach.

esophagogastroscopy (-gas-tros′ko-pe) endoscopic inspection of esophagus and stomach.

esophagogastrostomy (-gas-tros′to-me) anastomosis of esophagus to the stomach.

esophagography (e-sof″ah-gog′rah-fe) roentgenography of the esophagus.

esophagojejunoplasty (e-sof″ah-go-je-joo′no-plas″te) restoration of the esophagus with a segment of jejunum.

esophagojejunostomy (-je″ju-nos′to-me) anastomosis of the esophagus to the jejunum.

esophagolaryngectomy (-lar″in-jek′to-me) excision of the upper cervical esophagus and larynx.

esophagology (e-sof″ah-gol′o-je) scientific study of the esophagus and its diseases.

esophagomalacia (e-sof″ah-go-mah-la′she-ah) softening of the walls of the esophagus.

esophagometer (e-sof″ah-gom′ĕ-ter) an instrument for measuring the esophagus.

esophagomyotomy (e-sof″ah-go-mi-ot′o-me) incision through the muscular coat of the esophagus.

esophagoplasty (e-sof′ah-go-plas″te) plastic repair of the esophagus.

esophagoplication (e-sof″ah-go-pli-ka′shun) infolding of the wall of an esophageal pouch.

esophagoptosis (e-sof″ah-gop-to′sis) prolapse of the esophagus.

esophagorespiratory (e-sof″ah-go-re-spir′ah-to″re) pertaining to or communicating with the esophagus and respiratory tract (trachea or a bronchus).

esophagoscope (e-sof′ah-go-skōp″) an endoscope for examination of the esophagus.

esophagospasm (e-sof′ah-go-spazm″) spasm of the esophagus.

esophagospasm (e-sof′ah-go-spazm) spasm of the esophagus.

esophagostenosis (e-sof″ah-go-ste-no′sis) stricture of the esophagus.

esophagostomy (e-sof″ah-gos′to-me) fistulization of the esophagus.

esophagotomy (-got′o-me) incision of the esophagus.

esophagotracheal (e-sof″ah-go-tra′ke-al) pertaining to or communicating with esophagus and trachea.

esophagus (e-sof′ah-gus) the muscular tube extending from the pharynx to the stomach, consisting of an outer fibrous, a muscular, a submucous and an inner mucous coat.

esophoria (es″o-fo′re-ah) deviation of the visual axis toward that of the other eye when fusion is prevented.

esosphenoiditis (es″o-sfe″noid-i′tis) osteomyelitis of the sphenoid bone.

esotropia (-tro′pe-ah) deviation of a visual axis toward that of the other eye when fusion is a possibility.

E.S.P. extrasensory perception.

E.S.R. erythrocyte sedimentation rate.

essence (es′ens) 1. the distinctive or individual principle of anything. 2. mixture of alcohol with a volatile oil. **e. of peppermint,** peppermint spirit (U.S.P.). **pepsin e.,** pepsin and rennin elixir (N.F.).

E.S.T. electric shock therapy.

ester (es′ter) a compound formed from an alcohol and an acid by removal of water. **Cori e.,** a compound which is an important intermediate in the alcoholic fermentation of sugars, glucose-1-dihydrogen phosphate. **Robison e.,** a compound which is an important intermediate in the alcoholic fermentation of sugars, glucose-6-dihydrogen phosphate.

esterase (es′ter-ās) an enzyme which catalyzes the hydrolysis of esters.

esterification (es-ter″ĭ-fi-ka′shun) conversion of an acid into an ester by combination with an alcohol and removal of a molecule of water.

esterify (es-ter′ĭ-fi) to combine with an alcohol with elimination of a molecule of water, forming an ester.

esterolysis (es″ter-ol′ĭ-sis) the hydrolysis of an ester into its alcohol and acid. adj., **esterolyt′ic.**

esthematology (es″them-ah-tol′o-je) esthesiology.

esthesioblast (es-the′ze-o-blast″) ganglioblast.

esthesiology (es-the″ze-ol′o-je) the scientific study or description of the sense organs and sensations.

esthesiomania (es-the″ze-o-ma′ne-ah) mental disorder with perverted moral sense.

esthesiometer (es-the″ze-om′ĕ-ter) an instrument for measuring tactile sensibility.

esthesioneurosis (es-the″ze-o-nu-ro′sis) disease of the sensory nerves.

esthesiophysiology (-fiz″e-ol′o-je) the physiology of sensation and sense organs.

esthesioscopy (es-the″ze-os′ko-pe) marking on the skin of areas in which pain is felt.

esthesodic (es″the-zod′ik) conveying sense impressions.

estheticokinetic (es-thet″ĭ-ko-ki-net′ik) both sensory and motor.

esthetics (es-thet′iks) the branch of philosophy dealing with beauty; in dentistry, a philosophy concerned especially with the appearance of a dental restoration, as achieved through its color or form.

Estinyl (es′tĭ-nil) trademark for a preparation of ethinyl estradiol.

estival (es′tĭ-val, ĕ-sti′val) pertaining to or occurring in summer.

estivation (es″tĭ-va′shun) the dormant state in which certain animals pass the summer.

estivo-autumnal (es″tĭ-vo-aw-tum′nal) occurring in summer and autumn.

estradiol (es″trah-di′ol, es-tra′de-ol) an estrogenic compound available as **e. benzoate** ($C_{25}H_{28}O_3$), **e. cyprionate** ($C_{26}H_{36}O_3$), **e. dipropionate** ($C_{24}H_{32}O_4$) or **e. valerate** ($C_{23}H_{32}O_3$).

estrin (es'trin) estrogen.

estrinization (es''trin-ī-za'shun) production of the cellular changes in the vaginal epithelium characteristic of estrus.

estrogen (es'tro-jen) an estrus-producing substance.

estrogenic (es''tro-jen'ik) producing estrus.

estrogenicity (es''tro jē-nis'ĭ-te) the quality of exerting or the ability to exert an estrus-producing effect.

estrone (es'trōn) an estrogenic steroid, $C_{18}H_{22}O_2$.

estrous (es'trus) having the characteristics of estrus.

estruation (es''troo-a'shun) the state of being in estrus.

Estrugenone (es''troo-jen'ōn) trademark for a preparation of estrone.

estrum (es'trum) estrus.

estrus (es'trus) 1. the recurrent period of sexual excitement in adult female mammals. 2. the cycle of changes in the genital tract produced as a result of ovarian hormonal activity. adj., **es'trual**.

e.s.u. electrostatic unit.

Etamon (et'ah-mon) trademark for a solution of tetraethylammonium (chloride).

ethal (eth'al) cetyl alcohol.

ethamivan (ē-tham'ĭ-van) a compound used as a respiratory stimulant and to hasten recovery from general anesthesia.

ethaverine (eth''ah-ver'ēn) a compound used as a relaxant for vascular smooth muscle.

ethchlorvynol (eth-klor'vī-nol) a hypnotic and sedative compound.

ethene (eth'ēn) ethylene.

ether (e'ther) 1. the subtle fluid believed to fill all space. 2. a colorless, transparent, volatile liquid, $C_4H_{10}O$, used by inhalation to produce general anesthesia. adj., **ethe'real. acetic e.**, ethyl acetate. **chloric e.**, a mixture of chloroform and ether. **formic e.**, ethyl formate. **hydriodic e.**, ethyl iodide. **hydrobromic e.**, ethyl bromide. **hydrochloric e.**, ethyl chloride. **nitrofurfuryl methyl e.**, a compound used as a topical fungicide and sporicide for skin infections. **nitrous e.**, ethyl nitrite. **vinyl e.**, an anesthetic compound, $CH_2{:}CH.O.CH{:}CH_2$, a clear liquid used by inhalation to produce general anesthesia.

etherism (e'ther-izm) more or less complete anesthesia produced by ether.

etherization (e''ther-i-za'shun) induction of anesthesia by means of ether.

ethinamate (ē-thin'ah-māt) a central nervous system depressant, $C_9H_{13}NO_2$.

ethinyl trichloride (eth'ĭ-nil tri-klo'rīd) trichloroethylene.

ethisterone (ē-this'ter-ōn) a progestational steroid.

ethmocarditis (eth''mo-kar-di'tis) inflammation of the connective tissue of the heart.

ethmocephalus (-sef'ah-lus) a monster with defective nose, and eye orbits partly fused.

ethmoid (eth'moid) sievelike; cribriform.

ethmoidal (eth-moi'dal) pertaining to the ethmoid bone.

ethmoidectomy (eth''moi-dek'to-me) excision of the ethmoid bone.

ethmoiditis (eth''moi-di'tis) inflammation of the ethmoid bone.

ethmoidotomy (eth''moi-dot'o-me) incision of the ethmoid bone.

ethmoturbinal (eth''mo-tur'bī-nal) the superior and middle nasal conchae.

ethnic (eth'nik) pertaining to the races of mankind.

ethnobiology (eth''no-bi-ol'o-je) the scientific study of physical characteristics of different races of mankind.

ethnology (eth-nol'o-je) the science dealing with comparison and analytical study of the human races.

ethoheptazine (eth''o-hep'tah-zēn) a compound used as an analgesic.

ethohexadiol (-heks-a'de-ol) a compound used as an insect repellant.

ethologist (e-thol'o-jist) a person skilled in ethology.

ethology (e-thol'o-je) the scientific study of animal behavior.

ethopropazine (eth''o-pro'pah-zēn) a phenothiazine compound used to produce parasympathetic blockade and to reduce tremors in parkinsonism.

ethosuximide (-suk'sī-mīd) a succinimide compound used as an anticonvulsant in treatment of petit mal epilepsy.

ethotoin (e-tho'to-in) a phenylhydantoin compound used as an anticonvulsant in grand mal epilepsy.

ethoxazene (eth-ok'sah-zēn) a compound used to relieve pain associated with chronic urinary tract infections.

ethoxzolamide (eth''ok-zol'ah-mīd) a diuretic of the carbonic anhydrase inhibitor type.

ethyl (eth'il) the monovalent radical, C_2H_5. **e. acetate**, a transparent, colorless liquid used as a flavoring agent. **o. aminobenzoate**, a white, crystalline substance used as a local anesthetic. **e. biscoumacetate**, a white, odorless, bitter, crystalline solid used as an anticoagulant. **e. bromide**, a colorless, volatile liquid having anesthetic properties. **e. carbamate**, urethane. **e. chloride**, a colorless, volatile liquid used as a general and a topical anesthetic. **e. oxide**, a transparent, colorless liquid used as a solvent. **e. phenylephrine**, effortil. **e. vanillin**, fine white or slightly yellowish crystals used as a flavoring agent.

ethylcellulose (eth''il-sel'u-lōs) an ethyl ether of cellulose used in preparing pharmaceuticals.

ethylene (eth'ĭ-lēn) a colorless, highly flammable gas with a slightly sweet taste and odor, used for inducing general anesthesia.

ethylmorphine hydrochloride (eth''il-mor'fēn hi''dro-klo'rīd) white or faintly yellow microcrystalline powder; used as a narcotic and antitussive.

ethylnoradrenaline (-nor-ah-dren'ah-lin) ethylnorepinephrine.

ethylnorepinephrine (-nor-ep''ī-nef'rin) a

compound used as a sympathomimetic and in treatment of bronchial asthma.

ethylnorsuprarenin (eth″il-nor-su″prah-ren′-in) ethylnorepinephrine.

etiolation (e″te-o-la′shun) blanching of a plant grown in the dark due to lack of chlorophyll.

etiology (e″te-ol′o-je) the science dealing with causes of disease. adj., **etiolog′ic.**

etioporphyrin (e″te-o-por′fir-in) a porphyrin obtained from hematoporphyrin.

etryptamine (e-trip′tah-min) a compound formerly used as a psychomotor stimulant.

Eu chemical symbol, *europium.*

eu- (u) word element [Gr.], *normal; good; well; easy.*

euangiotic (u″an-je-ot′ik) well supplied with blood vessels.

Eubacteriales (u″bak-te″re-a′lēz) an order of Schizomycetes comprising the true bacteria.

Eubacterium (u″bak-te′re-um) a genus of Schizomycetes (order Eubacteriales, family Lactobacillaceae, tribe Lactobacilleae) found in the intestinal tract as parasites and as saprophytes in soil and water.

eubiotics (u″bi-ot′iks) the science of healthy living.

eubolism (u′bo-lizm) a condition of normal metabolism.

eucalyptol (u″kah-lip′tol) a colorless liquid obtained from eucalyptus oil and other sources; used as an expectorant and flavoring agent.

eucatropine (u-kat′ro-pēn) white granular, odorless powder, $C_{17}H_{25}O_3N.HCl$; mydriatic.

euchlorhydria (u″klor-hi′dre-ah) normal amount of acid in the gastric juice.

eucholia (u-ko′le-ah) normal condition of the bile.

euchromatin (u-kro′mah-tin) material of the chromosomes that is dispersed and lightly staining during interphase, considered the genetically active form.

euchromatopsy (u-kro′mah-top″se) normal color vision.

euchylia (u-ki′le-ah) normal condition of the chyle.

eucrasia (u-kra′ze-ah) the proper balance of different factors constituting a healthy state.

eudiemorrhysis (u″di-ē-mor′ĭ-sis) the normal flow of blood through the capillaries.

eudiometer (u″de-om′ē-ter) an instrument for measuring and analyzing gases.

eudipsia (u-dip′se-ah) ordinary, normal thirst.

euergasia (u″er-ga′ze-ah) normal mental functioning.

euesthesia (u″es-the′ze-ah) a normal state of the senses.

eugamy (u′gah-me) the union of gametes each of which contains the proper complement of chromosomes.

eugenics (u-jen′iks) the scientific study and practice of principles that will improve the hereditary qualities of future generations. **negative e.,** that concerned with prevention of reproduction by individuals having inferior or undesirable traits. **positive e.,** that concerned with promotion of optimal mating and

reproduction by individuals having desirable or superior traits.

eugenol (u′jĕ-nol) a phenol from clove oil and other sources, used as a dental analgesic.

euglycemia (u″gli-se′me-ah) a normal level of glucose in the blood. adj., **euglyce′mic.**

eugnathic (u-nath′ik) pertaining to or characterized by a normal state of the maxilla and mandible.

eugonic (u-gon′ik) growing luxuriantly; said of bacteria.

eukaryosis (u″kar-e-o′sis) the state of having a true nucleus. adj., **eukaryot′ic.**

eukinesia (u″ki-ne′ze-ah) normal or proper motor function or activity. adj., **eukinet′ic.**

eumetria (u-me′tre-ah) a normal condition of nerve impulse, so that a voluntary movement just reaches the intended goal; the proper range of movement.

eunuch (u′nuk) a castrated male.

eunuchoid (u′nŭ-koid) 1. resembling a eunuch. 2. a person who resembles a eunuch.

eunuchoidism (u′nŭ-koi-dizm″) hypogonadism.

eupancreatism (u-pan′kre-ah-tizm″) normal functioning of the pancreas.

eupepsia (u-pep′se-ah) good digestion. adj., **eupep′tic.**

euphoretic (u″fo-ret′ik) 1. pertaining to or characterized by euphoria. 2. an agent that produces euphoria.

euphoria (u-fo′re-ah) a subjectively pleasant feeling of well-being, marked by confidence and assurance. adj., **euphor′ic.**

euphoriant (u-for′e-ant) 1. conducive to a feeling of well-being. 2. an agent that is conducive to a feeling of well-being.

eupiesis (u″pi-e′sis) normal pressure. adj., **eupiet′ic.**

euplastic (u-plas′tik) forming sound tissues.

euploid (u′ploid) 1. having a balanced set or sets of chromosomes, in any number. 2. an individual or cell having a balanced set or sets of chromosomes, in any number.

euploidy (u′ploi-de) the state of having a balanced set or sets of chromosomes, in any number.

eupnea (ūp-ne′ah) normal respiration. adj., **eupne′ic.**

eupraxia (u-prak′se-ah) intactness of reproduction of coordinated movements. adj., **euprac′tic.**

eupyrexia (u″pi-rek′se-ah) a slight fever in the early stage of an infection.

Eurax (u′raks) trademark for preparations of crotamiton.

eurhythmia (u-rith′me-ah) regularity of the pulse.

europium (u-ro′pe-um) chemical element *(see table),* at. no. 63, symbol Eu.

Eurotium (u-ro′she-um) a genus of fungi or molds.

eury- (u′re) word element [Gr.], *wide; broad.*

eurycephalic (u″rĭ-sĕ-fal′ik) having a wide head.

euryon (u′re-on) a point on either parietal bone marking either end of the greatest transverse diameter of the skull.

euryphotic (u″rĭ-fo′tik) able to see in a wide range of light intensity.

euscope (u′skōp) a device for projecting the image of a microscopic field upon a screen.

eusitia (u-sit′e-ah) normal appetite.

eusplanchnia (u-splangk′ne-ah) a normal state of the internal organs.

eusplenia (u-sple′ne-ah) normal functioning of the spleen.

eusthenuria (u″sthen-u′re-ah) a normal state of the urine as to osmolality.

eusystole (u-sĭs′to-le) a normal state of systole of the heart.

euthanasia (u″thah-na′zhe-ah) 1. an easy death. 2. the painless induction of death in a patient with an incurable disease or condition.

euthenics (u-then′iks) the science of race improvement by regulation of environment.

euthermy (u ther′me) the state of being tolerant of a wide range of temperature. adj., **euther′mic.**

euthyroid (u-thi′roid) characterized by normal activity (secretion) of the thyroid gland.

eutocia (u-to′she-ah) natural or normal parturition.

Eutrombicula (u″trom-bik′u-lah) a genus of mites.

eutrophia (u-tro′fe-ah) a state of normal (good) nutrition. adj., **eutroph′ic.**

evacuant (e-vak′u-ant) 1. promoting evacuation. 2. an agent which promotes evacuation.

evacuation (e-vak″u-a′shun) 1. removal, especially the removal of any material from the body by discharge through a natural or artificial passage. 2. material discharged from the body, especially the discharge from the bowels.

evagination (e-vaj″ĭ-na′shun) protrusion of a part or organ.

eventration (e″ven-tra′shun) 1. protrusion of abdominal viscera. 2. removal of abdominal viscera. **e. of the diaphragm,** elevation of the diaphragm into the thoracic cavity.

eversion (e-ver′zhun) a turning outward.

Evipal (ev′ĭ-pal) trademark for a preparation of hexobarbital.

evisceration (e-vis″er-a′shun) removal of the viscera or the internal contents of a body, as removal of the contents of the eyeball.

evocation (ev″o-ka′shun) the calling forth of morphogenetic potentialities through contact with organizer material, living or dead.

evocator (ev′o-ka″tor) a chemical substance emitted by an organizer, by which its effect is mediated in the developing embryo.

evolution (ev″o-lu′shun) a gradual, orderly transition from one condition to another. **convergent e.,** the development, in animals that are only distantly related, of similar structures in adaptation to similar environment. **inorganic e.,** evolution occurring in inorganic or inanimate elements of the universe. **organic e.,** the evolution of living things; the theory that organisms now living have developed by gradual modifications from simpler organisms.

evulsion (e-vul′shun) forcible tearing away of a part.

ex (eks) preposition [L.], *out; away from.*

exacerbation (eg-zas″er-ba′shun) increase in severity.

exacrinous (eks-ak′rĭ-nus) pertaining to external secretion of a gland.

examination (eg-zam″ĭ-na′shun) inspection and investigation of a patient as a means of diagnosing disease. **physical e.,** examination of the bodily state of a patient by ordinary physical means, as inspection, palpation, percussion and auscultation.

exangia (eks-an′je-ah) dilatation of a blood vessel.

exanthem (eg-zan′them) an eruption or rash on the skin. **e. sub′itum,** an acute viral disease of infants, with fever and a macular or maculopapular eruption.

exanthema (eg″zan-the′mah), pl. *exanthem′-ata* [Gr.] exanthem.

exanthematous (-them′ah-tus) characterized by an eruption or rash.

exanthrope (ek′zan-thrōp) a source of disease outside the body.

exarteritis (eks″ar-ter-i′tis) inflammation of the outer arterial coat

exarticulation (eks″ar-tik-u-la′shun) amputation at a joint.

excalation (eks″kah-la′shun) absence or exclusion of one member of a normal series, such as a vertebra.

excavatio (eks″kah-va′she-o), pl. *excavatio′nes* [L.] excavation.

excavation (-va′shun) 1. the act of hollowing out. 2. a hollowed-out space, or pouchlike cavity. **atrophic e.,** cupping of the optic disk, due to atrophy of the optic nerve fibers. **dental e.,** removal of carious material from a tooth in preparation for filling.

excavator (eks′kah-va″tor) a scoop or gouge for surgeons' use. **dental e.,** an instrument for removing carious material from a tooth and shaping the internal walls of a cavity.

excementosis (ek″se-men-to′sis) hypertrophy of the cementum of the root of a tooth.

excentric (ek-sen′trik) out of, or away from, a center.

excerebration (ek″ser-ĕ-bra′shun) removal of the brain.

excernant (ek-ser′nant) causing an evacuation or discharge.

exchanger (eks-chānj′er) an apparatus by which something may be exchanged. **heat e.,** a device placed in the circuit of extracorporeal circulation to induce rapid cooling and rewarming of blood.

excipient (ek-sip′e-ent) a gummy or syrupy material in which an active ingredient (powder) is incorporated to be made into pills.

excise (ek-sīz′) to remove by cutting.

excision (ek-sizh′un) removal by cutting out or off, often applied to surgical removal of an entire organ or body structure.

excitant (ek-sīt′ant) a medicine which arouses functional activity.

excitation (ek″si-ta′shun) stimulation or irritation. **direct e.,** stimulation of a muscle by means of an electrode on the muscle substance. **indirect e.**, stimulation of a muscle through stimulation of its nerve.

excitomotor (ek-si″to-mo′tor) arousing muscular activity.

excitonutrient (-nu′tre-ent) stimulating nutrition.

excitor (ek-si′tor) a nerve which stimulates a part to greater activity.

excitosecretory (ek-si″to-se-kre′to-re) producing increased secretion.

excitovascular (-vas′ku-ler) causing vascular changes.

exclave (eks′klāv) a detached part of an organ.

exclusion (ek-skloo′zhun) 1. a shutting out or elimination. 2. surgical isolation of a part, as of a segment of intestine, without removal from the body.

excochleation (eks″kok-le-a′shun) curettement of a cavity.

excoriation (ek-sko″re-a′shun) removal of an area of skin.

excrement (ek′skrĕ-ment) excreted or fecal matter.

excrementitious (ek″skrĕ-men-tish′us) pertaining to excrement.

excrescence (ek-skres′ens) an abnormal outgrowth.

excreta (ek-skre′tah) substances excreted.

excrete (ek-skrēt′) to separate and eliminate useless matter.

excretion (ek-skre′shun) 1. the expulsion of nonmodified substances along favorable concentration gradients, without the expenditure of energy by the cell. 2. any substance excreted. adj., **ex′cretory.**

excursion (ek-sker′zhun) a range of movement regularly repeated in performance of a function, e.g. excursion of the jaws in mastication. adj., **excur′sive.**

excyclophoria (ek″si-klo-fo′re-ah) tendency of the upper segment of the eye to rotate toward the temporal side.

excyclotropia (-tro′pe-ah) rotation of the upper segment of the eye toward the temporal side.

excystation (ek″sis-ta′shun) escape or removal from a cyst.

exemia (ek-se′me-ah) loss of blood from circulation, though not from the body.

exencephalus (eks″en-sef′ah-lus) monster with brain outside, or partly outside, the cranium.

exenteration (ek-sen″ter-a′shun) surgical removal of the inner organs; evisceration. **pelvic e.**, excision of the organs and adjacent structures of the pelvis.

exercise (ek′ser-sīz) performance of physical exertion for improvement of health or correction of physical deformity. **active e.**, motion imparted to a part by voluntary contraction and relaxation of its controlling muscles. **active resistive e.**, motion voluntarily imparted to a part against resistance. **passive e.**, motion imparted to a part by another person or outside force, without voluntary participation by the patient.

exeresis (ek-ser′ĕ-sis) removal of a nerve, vessel or other part or organ.

exergonic (ek″ser-gon′ik) accompanied by the release of free energy.

exfetation (eks″fe-ta′shun) extrauterine pregnancy.

exflagellation (eks-flaj″ē-la′shun) the formation of flagella by a protozoan.

exfoliation (eks-fo″le-a′shun) separation of fragments of dead bone or of skin in scales.

exhalation (eks″hah-la′shun) 1. the expulsion of air or other vapor from the lungs. 2. escape in form of vapor. 3. vapor escaping from a body or substance.

exhaustion (eg-zos′chun) loss of ability to react or to function because of continued stimulation or activity. **heat e.**, heat stroke or shock; called also *heat prostration*. **heat e., anhidrotic**, tropical anhidrotic asthenia.

exhibit (eg-zib′it) to administer as a remedy.

exhibitionism (ek″sī-bish′ĕ-nizm) an abnormal tendency to make a display of one's self, in its severest form leading to exposure of the genitals.

exhibitionist (ek″sī-bish′ĕ-nist) a person who indulges in exhibitionism.

exo- (ek′so) prefix [Gr.], *outside of; outward.*

exobiology (ek″so-bi-ol′o-je) the science concerned with study of life on planets other than the earth.

exocardia (-kar′de-ah) abnormal position of the heart.

exocardial (-kar′de-al) 1. situated outside the heart. 2. pertaining to exocardia.

exocoelom (-se′lum) the portion of the coelom external to the embryo.

exocolitis (-ko-li′tis) inflammation of the outer coat of the colon.

exocrine (ek′so-krin) secreting externally.

exocrinology (ek″so-krī-nol′o-je) the study of substances secreted externally by individuals which effect integration of a group of organisms.

exodeviation (-de″ve-a′shun) a turning outward.

exodic (ek-sod′ik) efferent; centrifugal.

exodontia (ek″so-don′she-ah) exodontics.

exodontics (-don′tiks) that branch of dentistry dealing with extraction of teeth.

exodontist (-don′tist) a dentist who practices exodontics.

exodontology (-don-tol′o-je) the department of dentistry dealing with extraction of teeth.

exo-enzyme (-en′zīm) an enzyme which acts outside the cell which secretes it.

exoerythrocytic (-ē-rith″ro-sit′ik) occurring or situated outside red blood cells (erythrocytes).

exogamy (ek-sog′ah-me) 1. fertilization by union of elements derived from different cells. 2. heterosexuality.

exogastritis (ek″so-gas-tri′tis) inflammation of the external coat of the stomach.

exogenous (ek-soj′ĕ-nus) originating outside or caused by factors outside the organism.

exometritis (ek″so-me-tri′tis) inflammation of the outer surface of the uterus.

exomphalos (ek-som′fah-lus) undue prominence of the navel.

exopathic (ek″so-path′ik) originating outside the body.

exopeptidase (ek″so-pep″tĭ-dās) a proteolytic enzyme whose action is limited to terminal peptide linkages.

exophoria (-fo′re-ah) deviation of a visual axis away from that of the other eye when fusion is prevented.

exophthalmia (ek″sof-thal′me-ah) exophthalmos.

exophthalmogenic (-thal″mo-jen′ik) causing or producing exophthalmos.

exophthalmometry (-thal-mom′ĕ-tre) measurement of the extent of protrusion of the eyeball in exophthalmos. adj., **exophthalmomet′ric.**

exophthalmos (-thal′mus) abnormal protrusion of the eye. adj., **exophthal′mic.**

exophylaxis (ek″so-fi-lak′sis) protective against disease from the outside. adj., **exophylac′tic.**

exophytic (-fit′ik) growing outward; proliferating externally or on the surface of an organ or other structure.

exoplasm (ek′so-plazm) the peripheral part of the protoplasm of a cell.

exorbitism (ek-sor′bĭ-tizm) protrusion of the eyeball.

exormia (ek-sor′me-ah) a papular skin eruption.

exosepsis (ek″so-sop′sis) septic poison originating outside the body.

exoserosis (-se-ro′sis) an oozing of serum or exudate.

exoskeleton (-skel′ĕ-ton) an external hard framework which supports and protects the soft tissues of lower animals, derived from the ectoderm.

exosmosis (ek″sos-mo′sis) osmosis or diffusion from within outward.

exostosis (ek″sos-to′sis), pl. *exosto′ses* [Gr.] a benign new growth protruding from the outer contour of bones and characteristically capped by growing cartilage. **e. mul′tiplex cartilagin′ea,** dyschondroplasia.

exothermal (ek″so-ther′mal) exothermic.

exothermic (-ther′mik) marked by evolution of heat; liberating heat.

exotoxin (-tok′sin) a toxin exuded from the bacterial cell and found in the culture medium. adj., **exotox′ic.**

exotropia (-tro′pe-ah) deviation of a visual axis away from that of the other eye when fusion is a possibility. adj., **exotro′pic.**

expander (ek-span′der) an agent which increases volume or bulk. **plasma volume e.,** a solution given instead of blood transfusion, to increase the volume of fluid circulating in the blood vessels.

expectancy (ek-spek′tan-se) the probability of occurrence of a specific event. **life e.,** the number of years, based on statistical averages, that a given person of a specific age or class may expect to continue living.

expectation (ek″spek-ta′shun) that which may reasonably be anticipated. **e. of life,** life expectancy.

expectorant (ek-spek′to-rant) 1. promoting expectoration. 2. an agent that promotes expectoration. **liquefying e.,** an expectorant that promotes the ejection of mucus from the respiratory tract by decreasing the viscosity of that already present.

expectoration (ek-spek″to-ra′shun) the ejection of sputum from the air passages.

experiment (ek-sper′ĭ-ment) an operation undertaken under controlled conditions, to determine its outcome or effects. adj., **experimen′tal. check e.,** crucial experiment. **control e.,** one made under standard conditions, to test the correctness of other observations. **crucial e.,** one so designed and prepared for by previous work that it will settle some point. **Cyon's e.,** stimulus to an intact anterior spinal nerve root induces stronger contraction of muscle than the same stimulus to the peripheral end of a divided nerve root. **Valsalva's e.,** see under *maneuver.*

expiration (ek″spi-ra′shun) the expulsion of air or other vapor from the lungs. adj., **expi′ratory.**

expire (ek-spīr′) 1. to breathe out. 2. to die.

explant 1. (eks-plant′) to take from the body and place in an artificial medium for growth. 2. (eks′plant) material taken from the body and grown in an artificial medium.

expression (-presh′un) 1. the act of squeezing out. 2. the process of making manifest, especially the revelation of emotions by facial lineaments.

expressivity (eks″pres-siv′ĭ-te) the extent to which a heritable trait is manifested by an individual carrying the principal gene or genes conditioning it.

expulsive (ek-spul′siv) tending to expel or extrude.

exsanguination (-sang″gwĭ-na′shun) 1. forcible expulsion of blood from a part. 2. the state of being deprived of blood.

exsection (ek-sek′shun) an excision or cutting out.

exsiccation (ek″sĭ-ka′shun) a thorough drying by heat.

exsiccosis (ek″sĭ-ko′sis) the bodily state produced by low intake of water.

exsorption (ek-sorp′shun) outward movement of material through a membrane.

exstrophy (ek′stro-fe) the turning inside out of an organ, as the bladder.

exsufflation (ek″suf-fla′shun) the act of exhausting the air content of a cavity by artificial or mechanical means.

exsufflator (ek″suf-fla′tor) an apparatus which, by the sudden production of negative pressure, can reproduce in the bronchial tree the effects of a natural, vigorous cough.

ext. external; extract.

extender (ek-sten′der) something that increases dimension in space or duration in time. **plasma volume e.,** plasma volume expander.

extension (-sten′shun) 1. an increase in measurement or duration. 2. the straightening of a flexed limb. **Buck's e.,** extension of fractured leg by weights, the foot of the bed being raised so that the body makes counterextension. **Codivilla's e.,** extension for fractures made by a weight pulling on a nail passed through the lower end of the bone. **Steinmann e.**, see under *pin*.

extensor (ek-sten'sor) [L.] that which extends.

exteriorization (ek-stēr″e-or-i-za'shun) the process of bringing an interior body structure temporarily outside the body; in psychiatry, the turning of interests and drives outwardly into work, recreation and social pursuits.

extern (ek'stern) 1. a physician belonging to the staff of a hospital, but attending only during the day. 2. one of the hospital staff who attends to the outpatient department.

externalization (ek-ster″nah-li-za'shun) a mental mechanism operating outside of and beyond conscious awareness in which the emotion of an internal conflict is directed outwardly.

externe (ek'stern) extern.

externus (ek-ster'nus) external; in official anatomic nomenclature, designating a structure farther from the center of an organ or cavity.

exteroception (ek″ster-o-sep'shun) the perception of stimuli originating outside or at a distance from the body.

exteroceptive (-sep'tiv) receiving impulses from the ectodermal covering or exterior of the body.

exteroceptor (-sep'tor) a receptor organ which responds to stimuli arising outside the body.

exterofective (-fek'tiv) responding to external stimuli; a term applied to the cerebrospinal nervous system.

exterogestate (-jes'tāt) 1. developing outside the uterus, but still requiring complete care to meet all physical needs. 2. an infant during the period of exterior gestation.

extima (ek'stī-mah) the outermost coat of a blood vessel.

extirpation (ek″ster-pa'shun) complete removal; eradication.

extra- (ek'strah) prefix [L.], *outside; beyond the scope of; in addition.*

extra-articular (ek″strah-ar-tik'u-ler) outside a joint.

extracapsular (-kap'su-ler) outside a capsule.

extracerebral (-ser'ĕ-bral) outside the cerebrum.

extracorporeal (-kor-po're-al) outside the body.

extract (ek'strakt) a concentrated preparation of a vegetable or animal drug. **allergenic e.**, an extract of the protein of any substance to which a person may be sensitive. **beef e.**, a concentrate from beef broth. **dry e.**, one prepared in a dry form. **Goulard's e.**, lead subacetate solution. **liver e.**, a brownish, somewhat hygroscopic powder prepared from mammalian livers; used as a hematopoietic. **malt e.**, a product containing dextrin, maltose, a small amount of glucose and amylolytic enzymes; used as a nutritive and emulsifying agent. **ox bile e.**, a brown or brownish or greenish yellow powder with a characteristic odor and bitter taste; used as a choleretic. **parathyroid e.**, a preparation of the active principles of parathyroid glands. **pilular e.**, one whose solvent has been partially evaporated, leaving a plastic mass. **powdered e.**, one whose solvent has been entirely evaporated, leaving a fine, dry powder. **semiliquid e.**, one evaporated to a syrupy consistency. **solid e.**, pilular extract. **trichinella e.**, an aqueous extract of specially treated larvae of *Trichinella spiralis*, usually obtained from inoculated rodents; used as a skin test for trichinella infection.

extraction (ek-strak'shun) 1. the act of removing or pulling out. 2. the separation of a constituent from a compound or mixture by use of a suitable volatile solvent. **breech e.**, extraction of an infant from the uterus in cases of breech presentation. **flap e.**, removal of a cataractous lens by making a flap in the cornea.

extractive (ek-strak'tiv) a substance separated by extraction.

extractor (ek-strak'tor) an instrument for removing bullets, etc.

extractum (ek-strak'tum) [L.] extract.

extracystic (ek″strah-sis'tik) outside a bladder or cyst.

extradural (-du'ral) outside the dura mater.

extragenital (-jen'ĭ-tal) unconnected with the genital organs.

extrahepatic (-hĕ-pat'ik) unconnected with the liver.

extraligamentous (-lig″ah-men'tus) outside a ligament.

extramalleolus (-mal-e'o-lus) the external malleolus.

extramarginal (-mar'jĭ-nal) below the limit of consciousness.

extramastoiditis (-mas″toi-di'tis) inflammation of tissues adjoining the mastoid process.

extramedullary (-med'u-ler″e) 1. outside the medulla oblongata. 2. outside a bone marrow cavity.

extranuclear (-nu'kle-ar) outside a nucleus.

extraocular (-ok'u-lar) situated outside the eyeball.

extraperitoneal (-per″ĭ-to-ne'al) outside the peritoneum.

extrapleural (-ploo'ral) outside the pleura.

extrapolar (-po'lar) outside or beyond the poles.

extrasystole (-sis'to-le) a cardiac contraction caused by an impulse arising outside the sinoatrial node and occurring earlier than expected in the dominant or usual rhythm. **atrial e.**, an extrasystole in which the stimulus is thought to arise in the remains of the cardiac tube incorporated in the atrium elsewhere than at the sinus. **atrioventricular e.**, one in which the stimulus is supposed to arise in the atrioventricular node. **infranodal e.**, ventricular extrasystole. **interpolated e.**, a contraction taking place between two normal heart beats. **nodal e.**, atrioventricular extrasystole. **retrograde e.**, a premature ventricular contraction, followed by a premature atrial contraction, due to transmission of the stimulus backward over the bundle of His. **ventricular e.**, one in which the stimulus is thought to arise in the ventricular portion of the atrioventricular bundle.

extrauterine (-u'ter-īn) outside the uterus.

extravaginal (ek″strah-vag′ĭ-nal) outside the vagina.

extravasation (ek-strav″ah-za′shun) escape of fluid from its proper vessel into the tissues.

extravascular (ek″strah-vas′ku-ler) outside a vessel.

extraventricular (-ven-trik′u-ler) outside a ventricle.

extraversion (-ver′zhun) extroversion.

extravert (ek′strah-vert) extrovert.

extremitas (ek′strem′ĭ-tas), pl. *extremita′tes* [L.] extremity.

extremity (ek-strem′ĭ-te) 1. a termination of an elongated or pointed structure. 2. a limb of the body.

extrinsic (ek-strin′sik) of external origin.

extroversion (ek″stro-ver′zhun) direction of one's energy and interests toward external environmental and social phenomena.

extrovert (ek′stro-vert) a person whose interest is turned outward.

extrudoclusion (ek-stroo″do-kloo′zhun) extrusion (2).

extrusion (ek-stroo′zhun) 1. a pushing out. 2. in dentistry, the condition of a tooth pushed too far forward from the line of occlusion.

extubation (eks″tu-ba′shun) removal of a tube.

exudate (eks′u-dāt) material which has escaped from blood vessels and been deposited in tissues or on tissue surfaces, usually as a result of inflammation.

exudation (eks″u-da′shun) 1. the escape of fluid, cells or cellular debris from blood vessels and deposition in or on the tissue. 2. exudate.

exudative (ek-soo′dah-tiv) of the nature of exudation.

exumbilication (eks″um-bil″ĭ-ka′shun) protrusion of the umbilicus.

exuvia (ek-su′ve-ah), pl. *exu′viae* [L.] something that is shed; the exoskeleton shed by an animal in molting.

eye (i) the organ of vision. **crab's e's**, concretions from the stomach of crawfish. **Klieg e.**, severe inflammation of the eyes caused by exposure to the intense (Klieg) lights used in motion picture studios. **pink e.**, acute contagious conjunctivitis. **schematic e.**, a diagram or model of the eye for anatomic study. **shipyard e.**, epidemic keratoconjunctivitis. **wall e.**, 1. leukoma of the cornea. 2. exophoria.

eyeball (i′bawl) the ball or globe of the eye.

eyebrow (i′brow) hairy ridge above the eye; supercilium.

eyecup (i′kup) 1. a small vessel for application of cleansing or medicated solution to the exposed area of the eyeball. 2. optic cup.

eyeglass (i′glas) a lens for aiding the sight.

eyeground (i′grownd) the fundus of the eye.

eyelash (i′lash) one of the hairs growing on the edge of an eyelid.

eyelid (i′lid) either of two movable folds (upper and lower) protecting the anterior surface of the eyeball.

eyepiece (i′pēs) the lens or system of lenses of a microscope nearest the eye of the observer when the instrument is in use.

F

F chemical symbol, *fluorine*.

F. Fahrenheit; Fellow; field of vision, formula; French; Fusiformis.

F₁ first filial generation.

F₂ second filial generation.

fabella (fah-bel′ah), pl. *fabel′lae* [L.] a sesamoid fibrocartilage in the gastrocnemius.

fabism (fa′bizm) favism.

F.A.C.D. Fellow of American College of Dentists.

face (fās) the anterior aspect of the head. **frog f.**, flatness of the face due to intranasal disease. **hippocratic f.**, facies hippocratica. **moon f.**, the peculiar rounded face resulting from excess of adrenocortical hormones or adrenal corticoids.

face-bow (fās′bo) a device used in dentistry to record the positional relations of the maxillary ridge to the temporomandibular joints, and to transfer these relations to the articulator.

facet (fas′et) a small, nearly plane area on a bone or other hard surface.

facetectomy (fas″ĕ-tek′to-me) excision of a facet of a bone.

faci(o)- (fa′she-o) word element [L.], *face*.

facial (fa′shal) pertaining to the face.

facies (fa′she-ēz), pl. *fa′cies* [L.] 1. a specific surface, e.g. the anterior aspect of the head, or face. 2. the expression or appearance of the face. **adenoid f.**, the stupid expression, with open mouth, in children with adenoid growths. **f. hepat′ica**, a thin face with sunken eyeballs, sallow complexion and yellow conjunctivae, characteristic of certain chronic liver disorders. **f. hippocrat′ica**, a drawn, pinched and livid appearance indicative of approaching death. **f. leonti′na**, a lion-like appearance seen in certain cases of leprosy. **f. ovari′na**, anxious look indicative of ovarian disease.

facilitation (fah-sil″ĭ-ta′shun) hastening or assistance of a natural process.

facing (fās′ing) a piece of porcelain cut to represent the outer surface of a tooth.

faciobrachial (fa″she-o-bra′ke-al) pertaining to face and arm.

faciocephalalgia (-sef″ah-lal′je-ah) neuralgia of the face and head.

faciocervical (-ser′vĭ-kal) pertaining to face and neck.

faciolingual (-ling′gwal) pertaining to face and tongue.

facioplasty (fa′she-o-plas″te) plastic surgery of the face.

facioplegia (fa"she-o-ple'je-ah) facial paralysis.

facioscapulohumeral (-skap"u-lo-hu'-mer-al) pertaining to face, scapula and arm.

F.A.C.O.G. Fellow of the American College of Obstetricians and Gynecologists.

F.A.C.P. Fellow of American College of Physicians.

F.A.C.S. Fellow of American College of Surgeons.

F.A.C.S.M. Fellow of the American College of Sports Medicine.

factitious (fak-tish'us) artificial.

factor (fak'tor) an agent or element that contributes to the production of a result. **animal protein f.**, a substance found in animal protein essential to the growth of certain organisms. **antianemia f.**, an element essential for the maturation of erythrocytes and the prevention of anemia. **antihemorrhagic f.**, vitamin K. **antipernicious anemia f.**, cyanocobalamin. **antirachitic f.**, vitamin D. **antiscorbutic f.**, ascorbic acid. **antisterility f.**, vitamin E. **Bittner milk f.**, mouse mammary tumor agent. **Castle's intrinsic f.**, an element in gastric juice which combines with the extrinsic factor to produce blood formation and which is absent in pernicious anemia. **citrovorum f.**, folinic acid, a factor necessary for the growth of *Leuconostoc citrovorum*. **coagulation f.**, a factor essential to normal blood clotting, whose absence, diminution or excess may lead to abnormality of the clotting; 12 factors, commonly designated by Roman numerals, have been described. **Curling f.**, griseofulvin. **Duran Reynals' permeability f.**, hyaluronidase. **extrinsic f.**, a constituent of food which combines with Castle's intrinsic factor to produce blood formation. **intrinsic f.**, Castle's intrinsic factor. **modifying f's**, multiple factors which affect the degree of expressivity of another gene. **multiple f's**, two or more independent pairs of genes which affect the same character in the same way and in an additive fashion. **platelet f's**, factors important in hemostasis which are contained in or attached to the platelets. **Rh f.**, **Rhesus f.**, an antigen found in some 25 different serologically distinct types in about 85 per cent of the Caucasian population. **rheumatoid f.**, a protein of high molecular weight in the serum of most patients with rheumatoid arthritis, detectable by serologic tests. **spreading f.**, hyaluronidase.

facultative (fak'ul-ta"tiv) capable of adaptation to different conditions.

faculty (fak'ul-te) 1. a normal power or function, especially of the mind. 2. the teaching staff of an institution of learning.

fae- for words beginning thus, see those beginning *fe-*.

Fahr. Fahrenheit.

failure (fāl'yer) inability to perform or to function properly. **left ventricular f.**, inadequate output of blood by the left ventricle, leading to pulmonary edema. **right ventricular f.**, inability of right ventricle to expel adequate amount of blood, usually due to enlargement consequent to left ventricular failure.

faint (fānt) syncope.

falcate (fal'kāt) sickle-shaped.

falcial (fal'shal) pertaining to a falx.

falciform (fal'si-form) sickle-shaped.

falcula (fal'ku-lah) the falx cerebelli.

falcular (fal'ku-ler) sickle-shaped.

fallout (fawl'owt) the settling of radioactive fission products from the atmosphere after explosion of an atomic or thermonuclear bomb.

falx (falks), pl. *fal'ces* [L.] a sickle-shaped structure. **f. cerebel'li**, a fold of dura mater separating the cerebral hemispheres.

F.A.M.A. Fellow of American Medical Association.

familial (fah-mil'e-al) tending to occur in families, but without the mechanism of its occurrence being known.

family (fam'i-le) 1. a group descended from a common ancestor. 2. a taxonomic category subordinate to an order (or suborder) and superior to a tribe (or subfamily); names of families end typically in *-aceae* (plants) or *-idae* (animals).

fang (fang) the root of a tooth.

Fannia (fan'e-ah) a genus of flies whose larvae have caused both intestinal and urinary myiasis in man.

fantasy (fan'tah-se) an imagined series of events.

far. faradic.

farad (far'ad) the unit of electric capacity; capacity to hold 1 coulomb with a potential of 1 volt.

faradism (far'ah-dizm) 1. faradization. 2. faradic electricity.

faradization (far"ah-di-za'shun) therapeutic use of faradic electricity.

farcinoma (far"si-no'mah) a glandulous tumor.

farcy (far'se) glanders; applied especially to the cutaneous form of the disease.

fardel-bound (far'del-bownd) having an inflamed abomasum and a distended omasum, making chewing of the cud impossible.

farinaceous (far"i-na'shus) prepared from flour; starchy.

fasc. fasciculus.

fascia (fash'e-ah), pl. *fas'ciae* [L.] a band or sheet of tissue investing and connecting muscles. adj., **fas'cial. aponeurotic f.**, **deep f.**, a dense, firm, fibrous membrane investing the trunk and limbs and giving off sheaths to the various muscles. **extrapleural f.**, a prolongation of the endothoracic fascia, important as possibly modifying the auscultatory sounds at the apex of the lung. **Scarpa's f.**, part of deep layer of superficial abdominal fascia crossing Poupart's ligament. **superficial f.**, the thin tough membrane covering the muscles and lying immediately under the skin. **Tenon's f.**, see under *capsule*. **thyrolaryngeal f.**, the fascia covering the thyroid body and attached to the cricoid cartilage. **f. transversa'lis**, **transverse f.**, that fascia between the transversalis muscle and the peritoneum **Tyrrell's f.**, the fascia between the bladder and rectum.

fascicle (fas'ĭ-kl) a small bundle or cluster, especially of nerve or muscle fibers.

fascicular (fah-sik'u-lar) clustered together; pertaining to or arranged in bundles or clusters.

fasciculation (fah-sik″u-la'shun) spontaneous contractions of a number of muscle fibers supplied by a single motor nerve filament.

fasciculus (fah-sik'u-lus), pl. *fascic'uli* [L.] fascicle.

fasciectomy (fas″e-ek'to-me) excision of fascia.

fasciitis (fas″e-i'tis) inflammation of a fascia. **nodular f., proliferative f.**, a benign, reactive proliferation of fibroblasts in the subcutaneous tissues and commonly associated with the deep fascia. **pseudosarcomatous f.**, a benign soft tissue tumor occurring subcutaneously and sometimes arising from deep muscle and fascia.

fasciodesis (-od'ĕ-sis) suture of a fascia to skeletal attachment.

Fasciola (fah-si'o-lah) a genus of flukes. **F. hepat'ica**, a species parasitic in the liver and bile ducts of herbivorous mammals; found also in man.

fasciola (fah-si'o-lah), pl. *fasci'olae* [L.] 1. a small band or striplike structure as a small bandage. 2. a fluke of the genus Fasciola.

fasciolar (fah-si'o-lar) pertaining to the fascia dentata.

fascioliasis (fas″e-o-li'ah-sis) infection of the body with Fasciola.

fasciolopsiasis (-lop-si'ah-sis) infection with Fasciolopsis.

Fasciolopsis (fas″e-o-lop'sis) a genus of trematodes, or flukes. **F. bus'ki**, a species of flukes parasitic in the intestines.

fascioplasty (fas″e-o-plas″te) plastic repair of a fascia.

fasciorrhaphy (fas″e-or'ah-fe) suture of a fascia.

fasciotomy (-ot'o-me) incision of a fascia.

fast (fast) 1. resistant to treatment by. 2. abstention from food.

fastigatum (fas″tǐ-ga'tum) the red nucleus.

fastigium (fas-tij'e-um) the highest point.

fat (fat) 1. adipose tissue. 2. an organic salt consisting of the glycerol radical, C_3H_5, combined with a fatty acid. **wool f.**, anhydrous fat. **wool f., hydrous**, lanolin. **wool f., refined**, wool fat.

fatigue (fah-tēg') a state of diminished capacity to respond effectively to a stimulus.

fauces (faw'sēz) the passage between throat and pharynx. adj., **fau'cial.**

faucitis (faw-si'tis) inflammation of the fauces.

fauna (faw'nah) the collective animal organisms of a given locality.

faveolate (fah-ve'o-lāt) honeycombed; alveolate.

faveolus (fah-ve'o-lus) a small pit or depression.

favid (fa'vid) the general eruption occurring in favus.

favism (fa'vizm) an acute hemolytic anemia precipitated by fava beans (ingestion, or in-

halation of pollen), but caused by deficiency of glucose-6-phosphate dehydrogenase in the erythrocytes.

favus (fa'vus) a type of tinea capitis, with formation of prominent honeycomb-like masses, due to *Trichophyton schoenleini.*

F-Cortef (ef-kor'tef) trademark for a preparation of fludrocortisone.

F.D. fatal dose; focal distance.

F.D.₅₀ median fatal (lethal) dose.

F.D.I. Fédération Dentaire Internationale (International Dental Association).

Fe chemical symbol, *iron* (L. *ferrum*).

febricide (feb'rĭ-sīd) 1. destroying fever. 2. an agent which destroys fever.

febrifacient (feb″rĭ-fa'shent) producing fever.

febrific (fĕ-brif'ik) producing fever.

febrifugal (fĕ-brif'u-gal) dispelling fever.

febrifuge (feb'rĭ-fūj) a remedy that dispels fever.

febrile (feb'ril) pertaining to fever; feverish.

febriphobia (feb″rĭ-fo'be-ah) morbid fear of fever.

febris (feb'ris) [L.] fever. **f. enter'ica**, typhoid fever. **f. meliten'sis, f. un'dulans**, brucellosis.

fecalith (fe'kah-lith) an intestinal concretion composed of fecal material.

fecaloid (fe'kal-oid) resembling feces.

fecaloma (fe″kal-o'mah) a tumor-like accumulation of feces in the rectum.

fecaluria (-u'rc-ah) presence of fecal matter in the urine.

feces (fe'sēz), pl. of *faex* [L.] excrement discharged from the bowels. adj., **fe'cal.**

fecula (fek'u-lah) 1. lees or sediment. 2. starch.

feculent (fek'u-lent) having sediment.

fecundation (fe″kun-da'shun) fertilization; impregnation. **artificial f.**, fertilization by mechanical introduction of semen.

fecundity (fe-kun'dĭ-te) the ability to produce offspring frequently and in large numbers.

feeblemindedness (fe″bl-mīnd'ed-nes) mental deficiency with I.Q. 50–69.

feedback (fēd'bak) the return of some of the output of a system as input.

feeding (fēd'ing) the taking or giving of food. **artificial f.**, feeding of a baby with food other than mother's milk. **extrabuccal f.**, administration of food other than through the mouth. **Finkelstein's f.**, feeding of infants based upon decrease in the milk sugar of the food. **forced f.**, administration of food by force to those who cannot or will not receive it.

felon (fel'on) a purulent infection involving the pulp of the distal phalanx of a finger.

feltwork (felt'werk) a complex of closely interwoven fibers, as of nerve fibers.

female (fe'māl) an individual of the sex that produces ova or bears young.

feminism (fem'ĭ-nizm) the possession of female characteristics, usually referring to the presence of such characteristics in the male.

feminization (fem″ĭ-ni-za'shun) the development of female characteristics. **testicular f.**, a condition in which the subject is phenotypically female, but lacks nuclear sex chromatin and is of XY chromosomal sex.

feminonucleus (fem″ĭ-no-nu′kle-us) the female pronucleus.

femoral (fem′o-ral) pertaining to the femur or to the thigh.

femorocele (fem′o-ro-sēl″) femoral hernia.

femorotibial (fem″o-ro-tib′e-al) pertaining to femur and tibia.

femur (fe′mur), pl. *fem′ora* [L.] the bone that extends from the pelvis to the knee; called also *thigh bone.* 2. the proximal portion of the lower member of the body – the thigh.

fenestra (fĕ-nes′trah), pl. *fenes′trae* [L.] a small opening or window. **f. coch′leae,** a small, round, membrane-filled opening between the middle ear and internal ear. **f. ova′lis,** fenestra vestibuli. **f. rotun′da,** fenestra cochleae. **f. vestib′uli,** a small, oval opening between the middle ear and internal ear into which the foot of the stapes fits.

fenestrate (fen′es-trāt) to pierce with one or more openings.

fenestration (fen″es-tra′shun) the act of perforating or condition of being perforated. **aortopulmonary f.,** a congenital anomaly consisting of a communication between the aorta and the pulmonary artery just above the semilunar valves.

fennel (fen′el) the dried ripe fruit of cultivated varieties of *Foeniculum vulgare;* aromatic, carminative.

Feosol (fe′o-sol) trademark for preparations of ferrous sulfate.

Fergon (fer′gon) trademark for preparations of ferrous gluconate.

ferment (fer′ment) a substance which causes fermentation.

fermentation (fer″men-ta′shun) the decomposition of an organic substance into simpler compounds through the agency of an enzyme. **acetic f.,** conversion of alcoholic solution into acetic acid or vinegar. **alcoholic f.,** formation of alcohol from carbohydrates. **ammoniacal f.,** formation of ammonia and carbon dioxide from urea. **butyric f.,** change of carbohydrates, milk, etc., into butyric acid. **caseous f.,** the coagulation of soluble casein. **diastatic f.,** the change of starch into glucose. **lactic f.,** the souring of milk. **viscous f.,** production of gummy substances, as in wine, milk or urine, under the influence of various bacilli.

fermentogen (fer-men′to-jen) a substance which may be converted into a ferment.

fermentum (fer-men′tum) [L.] yeast.

fermium (fer′me-um) chemical element (*see table*), at. no. 100, symbol Fm.

Ferribacterium (fer″rĭ-bak-te′re-um) a genus of Schizomycetes (order Pseudomonadales, suborder Pseudomonadineae, family Siderocapsaceae).

ferric (fer′ik) containing iron in its trivalent form and yielding trivalent ions in aqueous solution. **f. ammonium citrate,** an iron preparation sometimes used in anemia. **f. ammonium tartrate,** a compound used orally in iron deficiency anemia. **f. chloride,** $FeCl_3$, sometimes used as an astringent for skin disorders and as a styptic. **f. glycerophosphate,** orange to greenish yellow transparent scales, $C_9H_{21}Fe_2O_{18}P_3$. **f. hypophosphite,** grayish white powder, $Fe(PH_2O_2)_3$. **f. oxide, red,** reddish brown powder, containing 90 per cent of ferric oxide. **f. oxide, yellow,** yellowish orange powder containing at least 97.5 per cent of ferric oxide. **f. phosphate, soluble,** bright green, transparent scales, yielding 12–15 per cent of iron. **f. subsulfate,** an iron-containing compound used in solution as a styptic.

ferricyanide (fer″ĭ-si′ah-nīd) a compound containing the trivalent $Fe(CN)_6$ radical.

ferritin (fer′ĭ-tin) the iron-apoferritin complex, which is one of the forms in which iron is stored in the body.

Ferrobacillus (fer″o-bah-sil′lus) a genus of Schizomycetes (order Pseudomonadales, suborder Pseudomonadineae, family Siderocepsaceae) which oxidize ferrous iron in the ferric state.

ferrocholinate (-ko′lin-āt) a compound of ferric chloride and choline dihydrogen citrate, used as a hematinic.

ferrocyanide (-si′ah-nīd) a compound containing the tetravalent $Fe(CN)_6$ radical.

ferrokinetics (-ki-net′iks) the scientific study of the turnover or rate of change of iron in the body.

Ferrolip (fer′o-lip) trademark for preparations of ferrocholinate.

ferrometer (fer-om′ĕ-ter) instrument for estimating the amount of iron in the blood.

ferropectic (fer″o-pek′tik) fixing iron.

ferrotherapy (-ther′ah-pe) therapeutic use of iron and iron compounds.

ferrous (fer′us) pertaining to iron in its lower valency; containing divalent iron. **f. carbonate** ($FeCO_3$), **f. fumarate** ($C_4H_2FeO_4$), **f. gluconate** ($C_{12}H_{22}FeO_{14}.2H_2O$) and **f. sulfate** ($FeSO_4.7H_2O$) have been used in iron deficiency anemia.

ferruginous (fĕ-roo′jĭ-nus) containing iron.

ferrule (fer′ōol) a band of metal applied to a tooth to strengthen it.

ferrum (fer′um) [L.] iron (symbol Fe).

fertility (fer-til′ĭ-te) the ability to produce offspring. adj., **fer′tile.**

fertilization (fer″tĭ-lĭ-za′shun) union of male and female elements, leading to development of a new individual. **external f.,** union of the gametes outside the bodies of the originating organisms, as in aquatic animals. **internal f.,** union of the gametes inside the body of the female, the sperm having been transferred from the body of the male by an accessory sex organ or other means.

fertilizin (fer″tĭ-li′zin) a substance of the plasma membrane and gelatinous coat of the ovum; thought to bind the spermatozoon to the ovum and also to be concerned with its engulfment by the ovum.

fervescence (fer-ves′ens) increase of fever or body temperature.

festinant (fes′tĭ-nant) hastening; rapidly accelerating.

festination (fes″tĭ-na′shun) a gait in which quicker and quicker steps are taken.

festoon (fes-toon') the curving margin of gum around the neck of a tooth.

fetalization (fe″tal-i-za'shun) retention in the adult of characters that at an earlier stage of evolution were only infantile and were rapidly lost as the organism attained maturity.

fetation (fe-ta'shun) 1. development of the fetus. 2. pregnancy.

feticide (fēt'ĭ-sid) the killing of a fetus in utero.

fetid (fet'id) having a rank, disagreeable smell.

fetish (fet'ish, fe'tish) an object or act to which special significance is attributed, e.g. an object, body part or maneuver charged with special erotic interest.

fetography (fe-tog'rah-fe) radiography of the fetus in utero.

fetometry (fe-tom'ē-tre) measurement of the fetus or of the fetal head.

fetoplacental (fe″to-plah-sen'tal) pertaining to fetus and placenta.

fotor (fe'tor) stench or offensive odors. **f. o'ris,** halitosis.

fetus (fe'tus) [L.] the developing young in the uterus; applied especially to the human young from the seventh to ninth week of gestation until birth. adj., **fe'tal. f. acardi'acus,** acardius. **calcified f.,** lithopedion. **f. compres'sus,** fetus papyraceus. **f. in fe'tu,** a teratoma within the body of an infant produced by separate growth of cells split off from the developing embryo. **harlequin f.,** an infant born with ichthyosis. **mummified f.,** a dried up and shriveled fetus. **f. papyra'ceus,** a fetus flattened by being pressed against the uterine wall by a living twin. **parasitic f.,** an incomplete minor fetus attached to a larger, more completely developed fetus, or autosite.

fever (fe'ver) 1. elevation of body temperature above the normal value (98.6° F. or 37° C.). 2. a morbid condition characterized by elevation of body temperature. **African tick f.,** tick-borne relapsing fever. **American mountain f.,** Colorado tick fever. **aphthous f.,** foot-and-mouth disease. **Assam f.,** kala-azar. **biliary f. of dogs,** a condition in dogs due to *Piroplasma canis;* called also malignant jaundice of dogs. **boutonneuse f.,** a fever of southern Europe and northern Africa, caused by *Rickettsia conorii,* transmitted by bite of ticks. **breakbone f.,** dengue. **carbuncular f.,** a kind of anthrax in horses and cattle, with gangrenous swellings in the skin. **cat-scratch f.,** a condition marked by headache, fever and malaise following a scratch or bite by a cat, and thought to be of viral origin. **Chagres f.,** a malignant type of malarial fever. **child-bed f.,** puerperal septicemia. **Colorado tick f.,** a nonexanthematous febrile disease occurring in the Rocky Mountain regions of the United States. **continuous f.,** persistently elevated body temperature, showing no or little variation and never falling to normal during any 24-hour period. **dandy f.,** dengue. **deer fly f.,** tularemia. **desert f.,** coccidioidomycosis. **elephantoid f.,** a recurrent acute febrile condition occurring with filariasis; it may be associated with elephantiasis or lymphangitis or may occur without inflammatory phenomena.

enteric f., typhoid. **epidemic hemorrhagic f.,** an acute infectious disease characterized by fever, purpura, peripheral vascular collapse and acute renal failure, caused by a filterable agent thought to be transmitted to man by mites or chiggers. **eruptive f., exanthematous f.,** any fever accompanied by eruption on the skin. **exanthematous f. of Marseille,** boutonneuse fever. **famine f.,** relapsing fever; typhus. **Far East hemorrhagic f.,** epidemic hemorrhagic fever. **Gibraltar f.,** brucellosis. **glandular f.,** infectious mononucleosis. **harvest f.,** spirochetosis affecting harvest workers. **Hasami f.,** a disease of Japan caused by *Leptospira autumnalis.* **Haverhill f.,** a spirochetal infection due to a bite by an infected rat. **hay f.,** annually recurring acute conjunctivitis and coryza, followed by bronchitis and asthma, usually due to sensitivity to the pollen of ragweed. **hectic f.,** a fever recurring daily. **hemoglobinurie f.,** malarial hemoglobinuria. **hospital f.,** epidemic typhus. **icterohemorrhagic f.,** leptospiral jaundice. **Ikwa f.,** trench fever. **induced f.,** fever brought on artificially, as by diathermy or by the injection of malarial organisms. **intermittent f.,** elevated body temperature showing fluctation each day, with periods when it falls to normal or below normal values. **jail f.,** epidemic typhus. **Japanese river f.,** scrub typhus. **jungle f.,** a severe form of tropical remittent fever. **Kagami f.,** infectious mononucleosis. **Kedani f.,** scrub typhus. **Kenya f.,** Kenya typhus. **Kew Gardens spotted f.,** rickettsialpox. **lung f.,** pneumonia. **Malta f.,** brucellosis. **march f.,** leptospiral jaundice; malaria. **Mediterranean f.,** brucellosis. **metal fume f.,** zinc poisoning. **miliary f.,** an epidemic fever marked by sweating and the formation of papules followed by pustules. **milk f.,** 1. mild puerperal septicemia. 2. fever said to attend the establishment of lactation after delivery. 3. endemic fever said to be caused by the use of unwholesome cow's milk. **mountain f.,** 1. Colorado tick fever. 2. Rocky Mountain spotted fever. 3. brucellosis. **mountain tick f.,** Colorado tick fever. **mouse f.,** mouse septicemia. **mud f.,** leptospiral jaundice. **Murchison-Pel-Ebstein f.,** a type observed in some patients with Hodgkin's disease, characterized by irregular episodes of pyrexia of several days' duration, with intervening periods in which the temperature is normal. **Neapolitan f.,** brucellosis. **nodal f.,** erythema nodosum. **nonexanthematous tick f.,** Colorado tick fever. **Oroya f.,** an anemic condition caused by *Bartonella bacilliformis.* **paludal f.,** malaria. **Panama f.,** Chagres fever. **pappataci f.,** phlebotomus fever. **paratyphoid f.,** a continued fever with symptoms of true typhoid, but without the Widal reaction, and caused by paratyphoid bacillus, Salmonella. **paraundulant f.,** a fever resembling brucellosis. **parenteric f.,** a fever resembling typhoid fever, but due to other bacteria than those of typhoid and paratyphoid fever. **parrot f.,** psittacosis. **periodic f.,** a hereditary condition characterized by repetitive febrile episodes and anatomic disturbances, occurring in precise or irregular cycles of days, weeks or months. **petechial f.**, cerebrospinal meningitis. **pharyngoconjunctival f.**, a febrile disease of viral origin occurring in epidemic form and characterized by fever, pharyngitis, rhinitis, conjunctivitis and enlarged cervical lymph nodes. **Philippine hemorrhagic f.**, dengue. **phlebotomus f.**, a febrile viral disease resembling dengue, occurring in Mediterranean countries. **pinta f.**, a disease observed in northern Mexico, identical with Rocky Mountain spotted fever. **pretibial f.**, a disease marked by rash on the front of the tibial region, by pain in the lumbar region and by fever and coryza. **puerperal f.**, see under *septicemia*. **Q f.**, a febrile rickettsial infection, usually respiratory, first described in Australia, caused by *Coxiella burnetii*. **quartan f.**, a form of malarial fever caused by *Plasmodium vivax*, in which the paroxysm recurs every three days. **quintan f.**, trench fever. **rabbit f.**, tularemia. **rat-bite f.**, an infectious fever following the bite of a rat, caused by *Spirillum minus*. **recurrent f.**, **relapsing f.**, elevated body temperature for one or several days, alternating with similar periods of normal or subnormal temperature; an acute infectious disease due to a species of Borrelia. **remittent f.**, elevated body temperature showing fluctuation each day, but never falling to normal. **rheumatic f.**, acute rheumatic arthritis. **Rift Valley f.**, a febrile disease of viral origin; its symptoms resemble those of dengue, and it is rarely fatal. **rock f.**, brucellosis. **Rocky Mountain spotted f.**, an infectious disease caused by *Rickettsia rickettsii*, marked by high fever, a spotted red eruption which later turns blue, and by mental symptoms. **sandfly f.**, phlebotomus fever. **scarlet f.**, an acute contagious disease caused by a group A hemolytic streptococcus and characterized by fever and a rash of thickly set red spots, followed by desquamation of the skin in scales or flakes. **septic f.**, remittent fever. **seven-day f.**, 1. a fever attacking Europeans in India and having symptoms like those of dengue. 2. nanukayami. **shin bone f.**, trench fever. **ship f.**, epidemic typhus. **slime f.**, leptospiral jaundice. **slow f.**, brucellosis. **solar f.**, dengue. **Songo f.**, epidemic hemorrhagic fever. **South African tick-bite fever**, a rickettsial infection similar to boutonneuse fever. **spirillum f.**, relapsing fever. **splenic f.**, anthrax. **spotted f.**, a febrile disease characterized by a skin eruption, such as Rocky Mountain spotted fever, boutonneuse fever and other infections due to tick-borne rickettsiae, and typhus fever and epidemic cerebrospinal meningitis. **sun f.**, dengue. **swamp f.**, 1. leptospiral jaundice. 2. equine infectious anemia. 3. malaria. **sweating f.**, miliary fever. **tertian f.**, a form of malarial fever caused by *Plasmodium malariae*, in which the paroxysms recur every two days. **thermic f.**, sunstroke. **three-day f.**, phlebotomus fever. **tick f.**, Rocky Mountain spotted fever. **trench**

f., a louse-borne disease marked by sudden fever with pain and soreness in muscles, bones and joints and by a tendency to relapse. **tsutsugamushi f.**, scrub typhus. **typhoid f.**, a specific eruptive communicable fever with lesions of the spleen and Peyer's patches and caused by the bacterium *Eberthella typhosa*. **typhomalarial f.**, malarial fever with typhoidal symptoms. **typhus f.**, typhus. **undulant f.**, brucellosis. **uveoparotid f.**, an infectious fever marked by inflammation of the parotid gland and uvea. **valley f.**, coccidioidomycosis. **Van der Scheer's f.**, a disease resembling dengue with sudden fever, headache, backache and eruption; it usually lasts for five days. **vesicular f.**, 1. pemphigus. 2. a fever of Ceylon marked by pain and a vesicular eruption. **Volhynia f.**, trench fever. **yellow f.**, an acute, infectious viral disease transmitted by infected mosquitoes or through human serum, and characterized by high fever, hemorrhagic diathesis and damage to kidneys and liver.

FFA free fatty acids.

fiber (fi'ber) an elongated threadlike structure of organic tissue. **A f's**, myelinated somatic afferent and efferent nerve fibers conducting at speeds of 5–120 meters per second. **adrenergic f's**, nerve fibers that liberate epinephrine-like substances at the time of passage of nerve impulses across a synapse. **alveolar f's**, fibers of the periodontal membrane extending from the cementum of the tooth root to the walls of the alveolus. **apical f's**, fibers of the periodontal membrane extending from the cementum of the tooth to the deepest portion of the alveolus. **arciform f.**, **arcuate f.**, bow-shaped fiber crossing the anterior aspect of the medulla. **axial f.**, the axis-cylinder of a nerve fiber. **B f's**, myelinated efferent preganglionic fibers of autonomic nerves, conducting at 3–15 meters per second. **basilar f's**, those that form the middle layer of the zona arcuata and the zona pectinata of the organ of Corti. **Beale's f.**, a spiral nerve fiber **C f's**, unmyelinated fibers of the autonomic nervous system, conducting at a velocity of 0.6–2.3 meters per second. **chromosomal f.**, traction fiber. **collagenous f.**, a soft, flexible white fiber which is the most characteristic constituent of all types of connective tissues. **Corti's f's**, rods of Corti. **dark f's**, muscle fibers rich in sarcoplasm and having a dark appearance. **dendritic f's**, those which pass in a treelike form from the cortex to the white substance of Schwann. **Gerdy's f's**, fibers of the superficial ligament bridging the cleft between the fingers on the palm of the hand. **Gottstein's f's**, nerve fibers of auditory nerve in the cochlea. **gray f's**, nonmedullated nerve fibers found largely in the sympathetic nerves. **Herxheimer's f's**, spiral fibers in the stratum mucosum of the skin. **internuncial f's**, fibers connecting nerve cells. **lattice f's**, reticular fibers. **light f's**, muscle fibers poor in sarcoplasm and more transparent than dark fibers. **motor f's**, nerve fibers transmitting motor impulses only. **Müller's f's,** supporting fibers of neuroglia in the retina. **muscle f.,** a unit of structure of muscle, made up of the coalesced protoplasm of a varying number of cells, and containing contractile fibrils. **nerve f.,** a slender process of a neuron, especially the prolonged axon which conducts nerve impulses. **nonmedullated f's,** nerve fibers which lack the myelin sheath. **osteogenetic f's, osteogenic f's,** precollagenous fibers formed by osteoclasts and becoming the fibrous component of bone matrix. **oxytalan f.,** a distinctive type of connective tissue fiber found typically in periodontal membrane of man and certain other animals, including monkeys. **perforating f's,** Sharpey's fibers. **postganglionic f's,** nerve fibers passing to involuntary muscle and gland cells, the cell bodies of which lie in the autonomic ganglia. **precollagenous f.,** a reticular fiber, so called on the supposition that it is an immature collagenous fiber. **preganglionic f's,** nerve fibers passing to the autonomic ganglia, the cell bodies of which lie in the brain or spinal cord. **projection f's,** bundles of axon fibers which connect the cerebral cortex with the brain stem. **Purkinje's f's,** moniliform fibers in the subendocardial tissue of the heart. **radicular f's,** fibers in the roots of the spinal nerves. **f's of Remak,** gray fibers. **reticular f.,** one of the connective tissue fibers, staining with silver, forming the reticular framework of lymphoid and myeloid tissue, and occurring in interstitial tissue of glandular organs, papillary layer of the skin, and elsewhere. **Rolando's f's,** the external arcuate fibers of the medulla oblongata. **Sharpey's f's,** those that pass from the periosteum and embed in the periosteal lamellae. **spindle f's,** achromatic filaments extending between the poles of a dividing cell and making a spindle-shaped configuration. **T f.,** a fiber given off at right angles from the axon of a unipolar ganglion cell. **Tomes's f's,** branched processes of odontoblasts filling the dentinal tubules. **traction f's,** those of the spindle in mitosis along which the daughter chromosomes move apart. **white f's,** collagenous fibers.

fiberscope (fi'ber-skōp) a flexible instrument for direct visual examination of the interior of hollow organs or body cavities, constructed of fibers having special optical properties.

fibr(o)- (fi'bro) word element [L.] *fiber; fibrous.*

fibra (fi'brah), pl. *fi'brae* [L.] fiber.

fibralbumin (fi"bral-bu'min) globulin.

fibremia (fi-bre'me-ah) presence of fibrin in the blood.

fibril (fi'bril) a minute fiber or filament. adj., **fibril'lar, fib'rillary. dentinal f's,** component fibrils of the dentinal matrix.

fibrilla (fi-bril'ah), pl. *fibril'lae* [L.] a fibril.

fibrillation (fi"bri-la'shun) 1. a transitory muscular contraction resulting from spontaneous activation of single muscle cells or muscle fibers. 2. the quality of being made up of fibrils. **atrial f., auricular f.,** a cardiac arrhythmia characterized by extremely rapid, irregular atrial impulses, ineffectual vermicular atrial contractions and irregular, rapid ventricular beats. **ventricular f.,** a cardiac arrhythmia characterized by rapid, irregular and ineffective twitchings of the ventricles.

fibrilloblast (fi-bril'o-blast) odontoblast.

fibrilloceptor (fi-bril'o-sep"tor) a receptor at the terminal of a neurofibril which receives the stimuli.

fibrillolysis (fi"bril-ol'i-sis) the dissolution of fibrils. adj., **fibrillolyt'ic.**

fibrin (fi'brin) an insoluble protein that is essential to clotting of blood, formed from fibrinogen by action of thrombin.

fibrination (fi"bri-na'shun) excess of fibrin in the blood.

fibrinemia (-ne'me-ah) presence of fibrin in the blood.

fibrinocellular (-no-sel'u-ler) made up of fibrin and cells.

fibrinogen (fi-brin'o-jen) a plasma protein of high molecular weight that is converted to fibrin through the action of thrombin; a sterile preparation is used to promote clotting of blood.

fibrinogenesis (fi"bri-no-jen'e-sis) the production of fibrin.

fibrinogenic (fi-brin"o-jen'ik) giving origin to fibrin.

fibrinogenolysis (-je-nol'i-sis) dissolution or inactivation of fibrinogen in the blood. adj., **fibrinogenolyt'ic.**

fibrinogenopenia (-jen"o-pe'ne-ah) decreased fibrinogen in the blood. adj., **fibrinogenope'-nic.**

fibrinoid (fi'bri-noid) a homogeneous, eosinophilic, relatively acellular refractile substance with some of the staining properties of fibrin.

fibrinokinase (fi"bri-no-ki'nās) a nonwater-soluble plasminogen activator derived from animal tissues.

fibrinolysin (fi"bri-nol'i-sin) any enzyme that catalyzes the digestion of fibrin.

fibrinolysis (-nol'i-sis) the splitting up or dissolution of fibrin. adj., **fibrinolyt'ic.**

fibrinopenia (fi"bri-no-pe'ne-ah) deficiency of fibrin in the blood.

fibrinopeptide (-pep'tīd) a substance split off from fibrinogen, during coagulation, by the action of thrombin.

fibrinoplastic (-plas'tik) of the nature of paraglobulin.

fibrinoplastin (-plas'tin) paraglobulin.

fibrinopurulent (-pu'roo-lent) characterized by precipitation of fibrin and production of pus.

fibrinorrhea (-re'ah) a profuse discharge containing fibrin. **f. plas'tica,** membranous dysmenorrhea.

fibrinoscopy (fi"bri-nos'ko-pe) the diagnosis of disease by artificial digestion and examination of the fibers or fibrinous matter of the sputum, blood, effusions, etc.

fibrinosis (fi"bri-no'sis) excess of fibrin in the blood.

fibrinous (fi'bri-nus) of the nature of fibrin.

fibrinuria (fi"bri-nu're-ah) discharge of fibrin in the urine.

fibroadamantoblastoma (fi"bro-ad"ah-man"-to-blas-to'mah) ameloblastic fibroma.

fibroadenia (fi″bro-ah-de′ne-ah) fibroid degeneration of gland tissue.

fibroadenoma (-ad″ĕ-no′mah) adenoma containing fibrous elements.

fibroadipose (-ad′ĭ-pōs) both fibrous and fatty.

fibroangioma (-an″je-o′mah) an angioma containing fibrous elements.

fibroareolar (-ah-re′o-lar) both fibrous and areolar.

fibroblast (fi′bro-blast) an immature fiber-producing cell capable of differentiating into chondroblast, collagenoblast or osteoblast.

fibroblastoma (fi″bro-blas-to′mah) a tumor arising from connective tissue cells. **arachnoid f., meningeal f.**, meningioma.

fibrobronchitis (-brong-ki′tis) plastic bronchitis.

fibrocalcific (-kal-sif′ik) pertaining to or characterized by partially calcified fibrous tissue.

fibrocarcinoma (-kar″sĭ-no′mah) carcinoma containing fibrous elements.

fibrocartilage (-kar′tĭ-lĭj) cartilage made up of parallel, thick, compact collagenous bundles, separated by narrow clefts containing the typical cartilage cells. **elastic f.**, that containing elastic fibers. **interarticular f.**, any articular disk.

fibrocartilago (-kar″tĭ-lah′go), pl. *fibrocartilag′ines* [L.] fibrocartilage.

fibrocellular (-sel′u-ler) both fibrous and cellular.

fibrochondritis (-kon-dri′tis) inflammation of fibrocartilage.

fibrochondroma (-kon-dro′mah) chondroma containing fibrous elements.

fibrocyst (fi′bro-sist) fibroma that has undergone cystic degeneration.

fibrocystic (fi″bro-sis′tik) characterized by an overgrowth of fibrous tissue and the development of cystic spaces.

fibrocystoma (-sis-to′mah) cystoma containing fibrous elements.

fibrocyte (fi′bro-sīt) a cell which produces fibrous tissue.

fibrocytogenesis (fi″bro-si″to-jen′ĕ-sis) development of connective tissue fibrils.

fibroelastic (-e-las′tik) both fibrous and elastic.

fibroelastosis (-e″las-to′sis) overgrowth of fibroelastic elements. **endocardial f.**, a condition characterized by left ventricular hypertrophy, conversion of the endocardium into a thick fibroelastic coat, and reduction in ventricular capacity.

fibroenchondroma (-en″kon-dro′mah) enchondroma containing fibrous elements.

fibrofascitis (-fah-si′tis) fibrositis.

fibrogen (fi′bro-jen) fibrinogen.

fibrogenic (fi″bro-jen′ik) conducive to the development of fibers.

fibroglia (fi-brog′le-ah) a fibrillar substance produced by connective tissue cells.

fibroglioma (fi″bro-gli-o′mah) glioma containing fibrous elements.

fibroid (fi′broid) 1. resembling fiber or a fibrous structure. 2. fibroma.

fibroidectomy (fi″broid-ek′to-me) excision of a uterine fibroma.

fibrolipoma (fi″bro-lĭ-po′mah) a lipoma containing fibrous elements.

fibroma (fi-bro′mah) a tumor composed mainly of fibrous or fully developed connective tissue. **ameloblastic f.**, an odontogenic tumor. **chondromyxoid f. of bone**, a benign neoplasm apparently derived from cartilage-forming connective tissue. **nonosteogenic f.**, a degenerative and proliferative lesion of the medullary and cortical tissues of bone. **odontogenic f.**, a benign tumor of the jaw arising from the embryonic portion of the tooth germ, the dental papilla or dental follicle, or later from the periodontal membrane.

fibromatogenic (fi-bro″mah-to-jen′ik) producing or causing fibroma.

fibromatosis (fi″bro-mah-to′sis) a condition characterized by presence of numerous fibromas. **f. gingi′vae**, a diffuse fibroma of the gingivae and palate, manifested as a dense, smooth or nodular overgrowth of the tissues.

fibromatous (fi-bro′mah-tus) of the nature of fibroma.

fibromembranous (fi″bro-mem′brah-nus) both fibrous and membranous.

fibromuscular (-mus″ku-ler) both fibrous and muscular.

fibromyectomy (-mi-ek′to-me) excision of a fibromyoma.

fibromyitis (-mi-i′tis) inflammation of muscle with fibrous degeneration.

fibromyoma (-mi-o′mah) a myoma containing fibrous elements.

fibromyomectomy (-mi″o-mek′to-me) excision of a fibromyoma.

fibromyositis (-mi″o-si′tis) inflammation of fibromuscular tissue.

fibromyotomy (-mi-ot′o-me) the excision of a fibroma.

fibromyxoma (-mik-so′mah) a myxoma containing fibrous elements.

fibromyxosarcoma (-mik″so-sar-ko′mah) a sarcoma containing fibrous and mucous elements.

fibroneuroma (-nu-ro′mah) a neuroma containing fibrous elements.

fibropapilloma (-pap″ĭ-lo′mah) a papilloma containing fibrous tissue.

fibropericarditis (-per″ĭ-kar-di′tis) fibrous pericarditis.

fibroplasia (-pla′ze-ah) the formation of fibrous tissue. adj., **fibroplas′tic. retrolental f.**, a condition characterized by the presence of opaque tissue behind the lens, leading to detachment of the retina and arrest of growth of the eye, generally attributed to use of high concentrations of oxygen in the care of premature infants.

fibroplastin (-plas′tin) paraglobulin.

fibropsammoma (-sam-o′mah) a tumor containing fibromatous and psammomatous elements.

fibropurulent (-pu′roo-lent) containing both fibers and pus.

fibrosarcoma (-sar-ko′mah) sarcoma blended with fibroma. **odontogenic f.**, a malignant tumor of the jaws, originating from one of the mesenchymal components of the tooth or tooth germ.

fibrosis (fi-bro'sis) formation of fibrous tissue; fibroid degeneration. adj., **fibrot'ic. arteriocapillary f.,** fibrous obstruction of capillaries and minute arteries. **cystic f.,** overgrowth of fibrous tissue in an organ, with development of cystic spaces. **cystic f. of pancreas,** a generalized hereditary disorder with widespread dysfunction of exocrine glands, chronic pulmonary disease, pancreatic deficiency, high levels of electrolytes in sweat and sometimes biliary cirrhosis. **mediastinal f.,** development of whitish, hard fibrous tissue in the upper portion of the mediastinum, sometimes obstructing the air passages and large blood vessels. **neoplastic f.,** proliferative fibrosis. **panmural f. of the bladder,** chronic interstitial cystitis. **periureteric f.,** progressive development of fibrous tissue spreading from the great midline vessels and causing strangulation of one or both ureters. **postfibrinous f.,** that occurring in tissues in which fibrin has been deposited. **proliferative f.,** that in which the fibrous elements continue to proliferate after the original causative factor has ceased to operate. **pulmonary f., interstitial, diffuse,** progressive fibrosis of the walls of pulmonary alveoli, leading to deficient aeration of the blood, dyspnea, cyanosis and cor pulmonale. **f. u'teri,** a morbid condition characterized by overgrowth of the smooth muscle and increase in the collagenous fibrous tissue, producing a thickened, coarse, tough myometrium.

fibrositis (fi″bro-si'tis) inflammatory hyperplasia of the white fibrous tissue, especially of the muscle sheaths and fascial layers of the locomotor system.

fibrous (fi'brus) composed of fibers.

fibulocalcaneal (fib″u-lo″kal-ka'ne-al) pertaining to fibula and calcaneus.

F.I.C.D. Fellow of the International College of Dentists.

F.I.C.S Fellow of the International College of Surgeons.

fiction (fik'shun) an untrue or invented story. **directive f.,** fantasy conceived by the patient to compensate for a feeling of inferiority.

field (feld) a limited area, such as the area of a slide visible through the lens system of a microscope. **auditory f.,** the area within which stimuli will produce the sensation of sound. **high-power f.,** the area of a slide visible under the high magnification system of a microscope. **individuation f.,** a region in which an organizer influences adjacent tissue to become a part of a total embryo. **Krönig's f.,** see under *area*. **low-power f.,** the area of a slide visible under the low magnification system of a microscope. **morphogenetic f.,** an embryonic region out of which definite structures normally develop. **visual f.,** the area within which stimuli will produce the sensation of sight with the eye in a straight-ahead position.

FIGLU formiminoglutamic acid.

figure (fig'ūr) a body or object having shape or form. **mitotic f's,** stages exhibiting a pattern characteristic of mitosis.

filaceous (fi-la'shus) composed of filaments.

filament (fil'ah-ment) a delicate fiber or thread.

filamentum (fil″ah-men'tum), pl. *filamen'ta* [L.] filament.

Filaria (fi-la're-ah) a name formerly given a genus of nematode parasitic worms. **F. bancrof'ti,** *Wuchereria bancrofti.* **F. medinen'sis,** *Dracunculus medinensis.* **F. san'-guinis-hom'inis,** *Wuchereria bancrofti.*

filaria (fi-la're-ah), pl. *fila'riae* [L.] a slender, threadlike worm, especially one of a species formerly included in the genus Filaria. adj., **fila'rial.**

filariasis (fil″ah-ri'ah-sis) infection by nematodes of the superfamily Filarioidea.

filaricide (fi-lār'i-sid) an agent which destroys filariae. adj., **filaricid'al.**

Filarioidea (fi-la″re-oi'de-ah) a superfamily of nematode parasites, the adults of which are long, threadlike worms found in lymph nodes, other tissues and body cavities, and the larvae of which (microfilariae) are found in the blood.

filiform (fil'iform, fi'li-form) threadlike.

filipuncture (fil'i-punk″tūr) insertion of wire or thread in an aneurysm.

fillet (fil'et) 1. a loop, as of cord or tape, for making traction. 2. a loop-shaped structure, such as a band of nerve fibers in the brain. **olivary f.,** nerve fasciculus surrounding the olivary body.

filling (fil'ing) 1. material inserted in a prepared tooth cavity. 2. restoration of the crown with appropriate material after removal of carious tissue from a tooth. **combination f.,** a filling made up of two or more materials, usually one on top of the other. **complex f.,** one for a complex cavity. **composite f.,** combination filling. **compound f.,** one for a cavity that involves two surfaces of a tooth. **contour f.,** one that is shaped to restore the anatomic form of a tooth. **nonleaking f.,** a filling so well fitted to the cavity as to prevent the penetration of moisture between the filling and the tooth. **permanent f.,** a filling intended to be left in place permanently. **provisional f.,** temporary filling. **submarine f.,** a filling inserted while the tooth of the cavity is covered with the fluids of the mouth. **temporary f.,** a filling designed to be removed after a short period of insertion.

film (film) 1. a thin layer or coating. 2. a thin sheet of material (e.g. gelatin, cellulose acetate) specially treated for use in photography or radiography; used also to designate the sheet after exposure to the energy to which it is sensitive. **bite-wing f.,** an x-ray film for radiography of oral structures, with a protruding tab to be held between the upper and lower teeth. **gelatin f., absorbable,** sterile, nonantigenic, absorbable, water-insoluble film used as an aid in surgical closure and repair of defects in dura and pleura. **spot f.,** a radiograph of a small anatomic area obtained (*a*) by rapid exposure during fluoroscopy to provide a permanent record of a transiently observed abnormality, or (*b*) by limitation of radiation passing through the area to improve definition and detail of the image produced. **x-ray f.**, film sensitized to roentgen (x-) rays, either before or after exposure.

filopod (fĭl′o-pod) filopodium.

filopodium (fĭ″lo-po′de-um), pl. *filopo′dia* [L.] a filamentous pseudopodium composed of ectoplasm.

filopressure (-presh′ūr) compression of a blood vessel by a thread.

filter (fĭl′ter) a device for eliminating certain elements, as (1) particles of certain size from a solution, or (2) rays of certain wavelength from a stream of radiant energy. **Berkefeld's f.**, one composed of diatomaceous earth, impermeable to ordinary bacteria. **Kitasato's f.**, an unglazed porcelain bougie through which liquids are drawn by suction. **Pasteur-Chamberland's f.**, a hollow column of unglazed porcelain through which liquids are forced by pressure. **Wood's f.**, a screen permitting passage of ultraviolet rays and absorbing rays of visible light.

filterable (fĭl′ter-ah-bl) capable of passing through the pores of a filter.

filtrable (fĭl′trah-bl) filterable.

filtrate (fĭl′trāt) a liquor which has passed through a filter.

filtration (fĭl-tra′shun) passage through a filter or through a material that prevents passage of certain molecules.

filtratometer (fĭl″trah-tom′ē-ter) an instrument for measuring gastric filtrates.

filum (fĭ′lum), pl. *fi′la* [L.] a threadlike structure. **f. termina′le**, the slender fibrous strand anchoring the spinal cord to the coccyx.

fimbria (fĭm′bre-ah), pl. *fim′briae* [L.] an elongated process such as one of the components making up a fringe.

fimbriate (fĭm′bre-āt) fringed.

fimbriatum (fĭm″bre-a′tum) corpus fimbriatum.

fimbriocele (fĭm′bre-o-sēl″) hernia containing the fimbria of the oviduct.

finger (fĭng′ger) one of the five digits of the hand. **Brodie's f.**, herpes zoster infection of the finger. **clubbed f.**, enlargement of the distal phalanx of a finger. **hammer f.**, mallet finger. **index f.**, the second digit of the hand; the forefinger. **mallet f.**, permanent flexion of the distal phalanx of a finger. **ring f.**, the fourth digit of the hand. **webbed f's**, fingers abnormally joined by strands of tissue at their base.

fingerprint (fĭng′ger-print) an impression of the cutaneous ridges of the fleshy distal portion of a finger.

fire (fīr) burning heat, or inflammation. **grass f.**, stalk disease of cattle. **St. Anthony's f.**, 1. ergotism. 2. erysipelas. 3. contagious anthrax.

first aid (ferst ād) emergency care and treatment of an injured person before complete medical and surgical treatment can be secured.

fission (fish′un) division into parts; segmentation. **binary f.**, the halving of the nucleus and then the cytoplasm of the cell, as in protozoa. **nuclear f.**, disintegration of a heavy atomic nucleus into smaller nuclei.

fissiparous (fĭ-sip′ah-rus) propagated by fission.

fissula (fis′u-lah), pl. *fis′sulae* [L.] a small cleft.

fissura (fis-su′rah), pl. *fissu′rae* [L.] fissure. **f. in a′no**, anal fissure.

fissure (fish′er) a narrow slit or cleft, especially one of the deeper or more constant furrows separating the gyri of the brain. **abdominal f.**, a congenital cleft in the abdominal wall. **anal f.**, painful lineal ulcer at the margin of the anus. **anterior median f.**, a longitudinal furrow along the midline of the ventral surface of the spinal cord, extending nearly one third of the anteroposterior diameter. **ape f.**, any fissure in the human brain that is found also in apes, especially the sulcus lunatus. **auricular f.**, one in the petrous bone. **basirhinal f.**, a cerebral fissure at the base of the olfactory lobe. **basisylvian f.**, the transverse basilar portion of the fissure of Sylvius. **f. of Bichat**, transverse fissure between the fornix and upper surface of the cerebellum. **branchial f.**, branchial cleft. **Broca's f.**, one which surrounds the third left frontal convolution. **Burdach's f.**, one between lateral surface of insula and inner surface of operculum. **calcarine f.**, one between the cuneate lobe and the lingual lobule on the mesial aspect of the cerebrum. **callosomarginal f.**, one on the median surface of each cerebral hemisphere midway between the callosum and the margin of the surface. **central f.**, Rolando's fissure. **craniofacial f.**, a vertical fissure separating the mesethmoid into two parts. **enamel f.**, a fault in the enamel surface of a tooth. **exoccipital f.**, Wernicke's fissure. **glaserian f.**, a fissure between the tympanic and squamous parts of the temporal bone. **Henle's f's**, spaces filled with connective tissue between the muscular fibers of the heart. **hippocampal f.**, one from the splenium to the tip of the temporal lobe. **interparietal f.**, one between the parietal convolutions of the brain. **longitudinal f.**, the deep fissure between the cerebral hemispheres. **maxillary f.**, a groove on the maxilla for the maxillary process of the palatal bone. **occipital f.**, a deep fissure between the parietal and occipital lobes of the cerebrum. **palpebral f.**, the slit or opening between the eyelids. **portal f.**, the transverse fissure of the liver. **precentral f.**, one parallel to the fissure of Rolando and anterior to it. **presylvian f.**, the anterior branch of the fissure of Sylvius. **Rolando's f.**, one between the parietal and frontal lobes. **Santorini's f's**, clefts in the fibrocartilage of the pinna. **sphenoid f.**, a cleft in the wings and body of sphenoid and orbital plate of frontal bone for various nerves and vessels. **f. of Sylvius**, one which separates the anterior and middle lobes of the cerebrum. **transverse f.,** 1. fissure crossing transversely the under surface of the right lobe of the liver. 2. horseshoe-shaped fissure from the descending cornu of the cerebrum on one side to that on the other. **umbilical f.,** the anterior part of the longitudinal fissure of the liver. **Wernicke's f.,** one separating the parietal and temporal lobe from the occipital lobe. **zygal f.,** a cerebral fissure consisting of two branches connected by a stem.

fistula (fis'tu-lah) a deep sinuous passage or tract, often leading to an internal hollow organ. **anal f.,** a fistula near the anus which may or may not communicate with the rectum. **arteriovenous f.,** a fistula between an artery and a vein. **blind f.,** one open at one end only, opening on the skin. (*external blind fistula*) or on a mucous surface (*internal blind fistula*). **branchial f.,** an unclosed branchial cleft. **complete f.,** one extending from the skin to an internal body cavity. **craniosinus f.,** one between the cerebral space and one of the sinuses, permitting escape of cerebrospinal fluid into the nose. **Eck's f.,** an artificial communication made between the portal vein and the vena cava. **fecal f.,** one which communicates with the intestine. **horseshoe f.,** a semicircular fistulous tract about the anus. **incomplete f.,** blind fistula. **pulmonary arteriovenous f., congenital,** a congenital anomalous communication between the pulmonary arterial and venous systems, allowing unoxygenated blood to enter the systemic circulation. **Thiry's f.,** an opening created into the intestine to obtain specimens of intestinal juice. **umbilical f.,** an abnormal passage communicating with the gut or the urachus at the umbilicus. **vesicovaginal f.,** an opening from the bladder to the vagina.

fistulatome (fis'tu-lah-tōm") a knife for cutting a fistula.

fistulectomy (fis"tu-lek'to-me) excision of a fistula.

fistulization (-li-za'shun) surgical creation of an opening from the body surface to an internal organ or passage.

fistulotomy (-lot'o-me) incision of a fistula.

fistulous (fis'tu-lus) of the nature of a fistula.

fit (fit) a convulsion, paroxysm or sudden attack. **running f's,** an episode of uncontrolled running in an animal.

fixation (fik-sa'shun) 1. process of making or the state of being immovable. 2. in psychiatry, the cessation of the development of personality at a stage short of complete maturity. 3. in microscopy, the hardening and preserving for microscopic examination of fresh tissue or microorganisms by heating or by immersion in a hardening solution. 4. in chemistry, the rendering of a compound nonvolatile or solid. **f. of complement,** addition of another serum containing an antibody and the corresponding antigen to a hemolytic serum, making the complement incapable of producing hemolysis. **parent f.,** pathologic devotion of an offspring to one of the parents. **skeletal f.,** immobilization of the ends of a

fractured bone by metal wires or plates applied directly to the bone (*internal skeletal fixation*) or on the body surface (*external skeletal fixation*).

fixative (fik'sah-tiv) an agent for hardening and preserving specimens for histologic study.

flabellum (flah-bel'um) a set of radiating white fibers in the corpus striatum.

flagellate (flaj'ē-lāt) an organism of the subphylum Mastigophora, having one or more flagella.

flagelliform (flah-jel'ī-form) shaped like a flagellum or lash.

flagellosis (flaj"ē-lo'sis) infestation with a flagellate protozoan.

flagellospore (flah-jel'o-spōr) a spore having one or more flagella.

flagellum (flah-jel'um), pl. *flagel'la* [L.] a filamentous, cytoplasmic projection from a cell, such as the specific organelle characteristic of protozoa of the subphylum Mastigophora.

flange (flanj) a projecting border or edge; in dentistry, applied to that part of the denture base which extends from around the embedded teeth to the border of the denture.

flank (flank) the side of the body between ribs and ilium.

flap (flap) a portion of superficial tissue (skin with subcutaneous tissue, cornea, etc.) detached from underlying tissue, except at one side, permitting it to be restored easily to the same site. **cellulocutaneous f.,** a flap cut from skin and subcutaneous tissue. **circular f.,** a flap of somewhat circular outline. **island f.,** a segment of skin and subcutaneous tissue, with a pedicle made up of only the nutrient vessels. **liver f.,** asterixis. **musculocutaneous f.,** a flap containing skin and muscle. **skin f.,** a thin flap containing little subcutaneous tissue. **sliding f.,** a flap carried to its new position by sliding.

flare (flār) an area of redness on the skin around an infective lesion or around the point of application of an irritant.

flask (flask) 1. a laboratory vessel, usually of glass and with a constricted neck. 2. a case in which materials used in making artificial dentures are placed for processing. **Erlenmeyer f.,** one of a conical shape, with a broad, flat bottom and a short, narrow neck. **volumetric f.,** a narrow-necked vessel of glass calibrated to contain or deliver an exact volume at a given temperature.

flatfoot (flat'foot) absence of the normal arch of the sole of the foot.

flatness (flat'nes) a quality of sound elicited by percussion, being short and high-pitched.

flatulence (flat'u-lens) excessive formation of gases in stomach or intestine.

flatulent (flat'u-lent) characterized by flatulence.

flatus (fla'tus) gas or air in stomach or intestine.

flatworm (flat'werm) an individual organism of the phylum Platyhelminthes.

flav(o)- (fla'vo) word element [L.], *yellow.*

flavanone (fla'vah-nōn) a compound formed

by reduction of the 2:3 double bond of a flavone.

flavedo (flah-ve'do) yellowness, as of the skin.

flavism (fla'vizm) yellowness of the hair.

Flavobacterium (fla"vo-bak-te're-um) a genus of Schizomycetes (order Eubacteriales, family Achromobacteraceae) found in soil and water.

flavone (fla'vōn) a substance, $C_{15}H_{10}O_2$, the basis of several yellow dyes.

flavonoid (fla'vo-noid) one of a group of substances resembling vitamin P and having antihemorrhagic properties.

flavonol (fla'vo-nol) a yellow, crystalline substance, a hydroxyl derivative of flavone.

flavoprotein (fla"vo-pro'te-in) an enzyme containing riboflavin.

flaxseed (flak'sēd) linseed.

fl.dr. fluid dram.

flea (fle) a small, wingless insect with mouthparts of the piercing-sucking type, ectoparasitic on birds and mammals.

fleece (flēs) a mass of interlacing fibrils. **f. of Stilling,** the lacework of white fibers surrounding the dentate nucleus.

flesh (flesh) soft tissue of plant or animal organisms; muscular tissue of animals. **goose f.,** cutis anserina. **proud f.,** soft, edematous, unhealthy-looking granulation tissue.

fletcherism (flech'er-izm) thorough mastication of food.

flex (fleks) to bend or put in a state of flexion.

flexibilitas (flek"sī-bil'ī-tas) [L.] flexibility. **f. ce'rea,** passive retention by the body or limbs of any position in which they are placed.

flexibility (-bil'ī-te) the state of being unusually pliant. **waxy f.,** flexibilitas cerea.

flexion (flek'shun) the act of bending; decreasing of the angle at the joint between two bones.

flexor (flek'ser) that which flexes.

flexura (flek-shu'rah), pl. *flexu'rae* [L.] flexure.

flexure (flek'sher) a bend or fold; a curvation. **caudal f.,** bend at the aboral end of the embryo. **cephalic f.,** a sharp bend at the level of the midbrain of an early vertebrate embryo. **cervical f.,** a gentle curvature in the early vertebrate embryo, in the region of the future neck. **colic f., left,** the angular junction of the transverse and descending colon. **colic f., right,** the angular junction of the ascending and transverse colon. **cranial f.,** cephalic flexure. **dorsal f.,** a flexure in the mid-dorsal region of the embryo. **duodenojejunal f.,** the bend at the junction of duodenum and jejunum. **hemal f.,** a curvature of the cerebral vesicles toward the hemal or ventral aspect. **hepatic f.,** the bend at the junction of the ascending and transverse colon. **lumbar f.,** the ventral curvature in the lumbar region of the back. **mesencephalic f.,** a bend in the neural tube of the embryo at the level of the mesencephalon. **nuchal f.,** cervical flexure. **pontine f.,** a flexure of the hindbrain in the embryo. **sacral f.,** caudal flexure. **sigmoid f.,** the bend at the junction of descending colon and rectum.

floccillation (flok"sī-la'shun) carphology.

floccose (flok'ōs) resembling wool.

flocculent (flok'u-lent) containing downy or flaky shreds.

flocculoreaction (flok"u-lo-re-ak'shun) a serum reaction characterized by flocculation.

flocculus (flok'u-lus), pl. *floc'culi.* [L.] a small tuft or mass, as of wool or other fibrous material. adj., **floc'cular.**

flora (flo'rah) the collective plant organisms of a given locality. **intestinal f.,** the bacteria normally residing within the lumen of the intestine.

florantyrone (flo-ran'ti-rōn) a butyric acid compound used as a hydrocholeretic.

Floraquin (flor'ah-kwin) trademark for a preparation of diiodohydroxyquin.

Florinef (flor'ī-nef) trademark for preparations of fludrocortisone.

Floropryl (flor'o-pril) trademark for preparations of isoflurophate.

fl.oz. fluid ounce.

flucticuli (fluk-tik'u-li) [L.] wavelike markings on lateral wall of third ventricle.

fluctuation (fluk"tu-a'shun) a wavelike motion or alteration of condition or position.

fludrocortisone (floo"dro-kor'tī-sōn) a synthetic adrenal corticoid with effects similar to those of hydrocortisone and desoxycorticosterone.

fluid (floo'id) 1. one of the four ultimate states of matter, being composed of molecules that can move about within limits, permitting change in the shape of the mass without disruption of the substance. 2. composed of elements that yield to pressure without disruption of the mass. 3. a material that flows readily in the natural state; a liquid. **allantoic f.,** the fluid contained in the allantois. **amniotic f.,** the fluid within the amnion that bathes the developing fetus. **cerebrospinal f.,** the fluid contained within the ventricles of the brain, the subarachnoid space and the central canal of the spinal cord. **Dakin's f.,** see under *solution.* **interstitial f.,** that portion of the body water outside the cells and the plasma volume; the extracellular water minus the plasma volume. **labyrinthine f.,** the perilymph. **Müller's f.,** a fluid for preserving anatomic specimens. **Scarpa's f.,** the endolymph of the ear. **serous f.,** normal lymph of a serous cavity. **spinal f., subarachnoid f.,** cerebrospinal fluid. **synovial f.,** synovia.

fluidextract (floo"id-ek'strakt) a liquid preparation of a vegetable drug, containing alcohol as a solvent or preservative, or both, each milliliter of which contains the therapeutic constituents of 1 gm. of the standard drug it represents.

fluidrachm (floo'ī-dram) fluid dram.

fluke (flook) an organism of the class Trematoda (phylum Platyhelminthes), characterized by a body that is usually flat and often leaflike.

flumen (floo'men), pl. *flu'mina* [L.] a stream. **flu'mina pilo'rum,** the lines along which the hairs of the body are arranged.

flumethiazide (floo"mē-thi'ah-zīd) a sulfonamide compound used as a diuretic and antihypertensive.

fluocinolone acetonide (floo-o-sin'o-lōn ah-set'-o-nīd) a steroid compound with anti-inflammatory action used for topical application to skin lesions.

fluohydrisone (-hi'drī-sōn) fludrocortisone.

fluohydrocortisone (-hi"dro-kor'tĭ-sōn) fludrocortisone.

fluorescein (-res'e-in) an orange-red powder, $C_{20}H_{12}O_4$, used in manufacture of various dyes. **sodium f.**, a compound, $C_{20}H_{10}Na_2O_5$, used in solution applied topically to the eye to detect injury to the cornea.

fluorescence (-res'ens) the emission of radiation as a result of exposure to and absorption of radiation from another source.

fluoridation (floo"or-ĭ-da'shun) treatment with fluorides; the addition of fluorides to a public water supply as a public health measure to reduce the incidence of dental caries.

fluoride (floo'o-rīd) any binary compound of fluorine.

fluoridization (floo"or-ĭ-di-za'shun) fluoridation.

fluorimetry (floo"or-im'ē-tre) determination of the spectral range of fluorescence of a substance in solution.

fluorination (floo"or-ĭ-na'shun) 1. treatment with fluorine. 2. fluoridation.

fluorine (floo'or-ēn) chemical element (see table), at no. 9, symbol F.

fluorography (floo"or-og'rah-fe) photography of the image revealed on a fluorescent screen.

fluorometholone (floor"o-meth'o-lōn) a compound used as a glucocorticoid with anti-inflammatory effects on the skin.

fluorophosphate (floo"or-o-fos'fāt) an organic compound containing fluorine and phosphorus.

fluoroscope (floo'or-o-skōp) an instrument for visual observation of the deep structures of the body by means of roentgen rays. **biplane f.**, a fluoroscope permitting simultaneous examination in both horizontal and vertical planes.

fluoroscopy (floo"or-os'ko-pe) examination by means of the fluoroscope.

fluorosis (floo"o-ro'sis) a condition due to ingestion of excessive amounts of fluorine. **dental f.**, a mottled discoloration of the enamel of the teeth occurring in chronic endemic fluorosis. **endemic f., chronic,** a condition due to long-continued ingestion of excessive amounts of fluorine.

Fluothane (floo'o-thān) trademark for a preparation of halothane.

fluoxymesterone (floo-ok"se-mes'ter-ōn) a compound used as an anabolic androgen in palliative treatment of certain cancers.

fluphenazine (floo-fen'ah-zēn) a compound used as a tranquilizer and antiemetic.

fluprednisolone (floo"pred-nis'o-lōn) a compound used as an anti-inflammatory corticosteroid in treatment of joint disease and allergic disturbances.

flurandrenolone (floor"an-dren'o-lōn) a corticosteroid applied locally to skin lesions.

flush (flush) redness of the face and neck. **hectic f.**, the peculiar flush of the face in wasting disease. **malar f.**, hectic flush at the malar eminence in pulmonary tuberculosis.

flutter (flut'er) a tremulous, generally ineffective movement. **atrial f.**, rapid heart action with the atria contracting regularly at a rate of 250–350 per minute. **impure f.**, a form in which the atrial rhythm is irregular. **mediastinal f.**, mobility of the mediastinum, each inspiration of the healthy lung drawing the mediastinum toward itself. **pure f.**, a form in which the atrial rhythm is regular. **ventricular f.**, a possible transition stage between ventricular tachycardia and ventricular fibrillation, the electrocardiogram showing rapid, uniform and virtually regular oscillations, 250 or more per minute.

flux (fluks) 1. an excessive discharge. 2. matter discharged. **alvine f.**, diarrhea. **bilious f.**, tropical dysentery with a copious discharge of bile. **bloody f.**, dysentery. **hepatic f.**, bilious flux.

fly (fli) a two-winged insect which is often the vector of organisms causing disease. **deer f.**, Chrysops. **tsetse f.**, Glossina.

Fm chemical symbol, *fermium.*

FMD foot-and-mouth disease.

F.N.I.F. Florence Nightingale International Foundation.

focus (fo'kus) pl. *fo'ci* [L.] 1. the point of convergence of light rays or sound waves. 2. chief center of a morbid process. adj., **fo'cal. epileptogenic f.**, the area of the cortex responsible for causing epileptic seizures, as revealed in the encephalogram. **Simon's foci,** hematogenous areas in the apices of the lungs of children, regarded as precursors of apical tuberculosis.

foe- for words beginning thus, see those beginning *fe-*.

fog (fog) a colloid system in which the dispersion medium is a gas and the disperse particles are liquid.

fogging (fog'ing) dimming of the vision by use of appropriate lenses before the eyes, as a means of relaxing accommodation.

foil (foil) metal in the form of an extremely thin, pliable sheet.

fold (fold) a doubling or reflection of a body structure. **aryepiglottic f's, aryepiglottidean f's,** folds of mucous membrane extending between arytenoid cartilage and epiglottis. **costocolic f.**, a fold of peritoneum from the diaphragm to the splenic flexure of the colon. **Douglas's semilunar f.**, the lower part of the posterior wall of the sheath of the rectus abdominis muscle. **gluteal f.**, the crease separating the buttocks from the thigh. **head f.**, a fold of blastoderm at the cephalic end of the developing embryo. **Kohlrausch's f.**, fold of mucous membrane projecting into the lumen of the rectum. **Marshall's f.**, vestigial fold. **medullary f.**, neural fold. **mesonephric f.**, mesonephric ridge. **nail f.**, the fold of connective tissue embracing the base and sides of the nail of a finger or toe. **neural f.**, one of the paired folds lying on either side of the neural plate that form the neural tube. **tail f.**, a fold in the early embryo, ensheathing the hindgut. **urogenital f.**, urogenital ridge. **vestigial f.**, a pericardial fold over the root of the left lung.

folie (fo-le′) [Fr.] psychosis. **f. à deux** (ah duh′) occurrence of psychosis simultaneously in two closely associated persons. **f. circulaire** (ser-ku-lair′) the circular form of manic-depressive psychosis. **f. du doute** (du doot) persistent obsessive doubting, vacillation and indecision. **f. du pourquoi** (du poor-kwah′) psychopathologic constant questioning. **f. gémellaire** (zha-mĕ-lair′) psychosis occurring simultaneously in twins. **f. musculaire** (mus″ku-lār′) severe chorea. **f. raisonnante** (rez-un-nahnt′) the delusional form of any psychosis.

folium (fo′le-um), pl. **fo′lia** [L.] a leaflike structure, especially one of the leaflike subdivisions of the cerebellar cortex.

follicle (fol′lĭ-kl) a sac or pouchlike depression or cavity. adj., **follic′ular. atretic f.**, a graafian follicle which has involuted. **dental f.**, the structure within the substance of the jaws enclosing a tooth before its eruption; the dental sac and its contents. **Fleischmann's f.**, one in the mucosa of the floor of the mouth. **gastric f's**, lymphoid masses in the gastric mucosa. **graafian f.**, an ovarian follicle in which an ovum matures, before its rupture containing an eccentric cavity filled with fluid. **hair f.**, a pouchlike depression in the skin in which a hair develops from the matrix at its base and grows to emerge from its opening on the body surface. **intestinal f's**, intestinal glands. **f's of Lieberkühn**, little tubular pits on the mucous membrane of the small intestine. **lingual f's**, nodular masses of lymphoid tissue at the root of the tongue, constituting the lingual tonsil. **lymph f.**, an aggregation of adenoid substance; chiefly found on mucous surfaces. **lymphatic f.**, 1. a small collection of actively proliferating lymphocytes in the cortex of a lymph node. 2. a small collection of lymphoid tissue in the mucous membrane of the gastrointestinal tract, where they occur singly (*solitary lymphatic follicle*) or closely packed together (*aggregated lymphatic follicles*). **Montgomery's f's, Naboth's f's, nabothian f's**, cystlike formations due to occlusion of the lumina of glands in the mucosa of the uterine cervix, causing them to be distended with retained secretion. **ovarian f.**, one of the crypts in the cortex of the ovary in which the ova develop. **primordial f.**, an ovarian follicle consisting of an egg enclosed by a single layer of cells. **sebaceous f.**, a sebaceous gland of the skin. **solitary f.**, any discrete lymph follicle on the mucous membrane of the intestine. **thyroid f's**, discrete cystlike units filled with a colloid substance, constituting the lobules of the thyroid gland. **vesicular f.**, a graafian follicle before rupture and discharge of the ovum.

folliclis (fol′ĭ-klis) papulonecrotic tuberculid with lesions on the hands.

folliculin (fŏ-lik′u-lin) estrone.

folliculitis (fŏ-lik″u-li′tis) inflammation of a follicle. **f. bar′bae**, inflammation of the hair follicles of the beard. **f. decal′vans**, a spreading folliculitis, with inflammation and loss of hair from the beard area and eyebrows. **keloid f., f. keloida′lis**, infection of hair follicles of back of neck and scalp, occurring chiefly in men, producing large, irregular keloidal plaques and scarring. **f. ulerythemato′sa reticula′ta**, inflammatory condition with reddened cheeks and symmetrical eruption with honeycomb appearance. **f. variolifor′mis**, acne varioliformis.

folliculoma (-lo′mah) an ovarian tumor derived from epithelium of the graafian follicles.

folliculosis (-lo′sis) excessive development of lymph follicles.

folliculus (fŏ-lik′u-lus), pl. **follic′uli** [L.] follicle.

Follutein (fol-lu′te-in) trademark for a preparation of chorionic gonadotropin.

Folvite (fōl′vīt) trademark for preparations of folic acid.

fomentation (fo″men-ta′shun) a warm, moist application.

fomes (fo′mēz), pl. **fo′mites** [L.] an inanimate object or material on which disease-producing agents may be conveyed.

fontanel (fon′tah-nel) one of the membrane-covered spaces remaining at the junction of the sutures in an incompletely ossified skull.

fontanelle (fon′tah-nel) fontanel.

fonticulus (fon-tik′u-lus), pl. **fontic′uli** [L.] a fontanel.

food (food) anything that serves to nourish, or supplies building material or energy for the body. **isodynamic f's**, foods which generate equal amounts of force in heat units.

foodstuff (food′stuf) any nutrient material taken in by a living organism for production of energy or building of tissue.

foot (foot) the terminal part of the leg or lower (posterior) extremity of a primate. **athlete's f.**, tinea pedis. **drop f.**, paraplegia of the anterior tibial muscles. **fungus f.**, mycetoma. **immersion f.**, a morbid condition occurring in persons in water for considerable periods. **Madura f.**, mycetoma. **march f.**, painful swelling of the foot, usually with fracture of a metatarsal bone. **sucker f.**, an expansion of a process of an astrocyte, by which it is attached to a small blood vessel. **trench f.**, a morbid condition resulting from inaction and prolonged exposure to cold and moisture.

foot-candle (foot-kan′dl) a unit of illumination, the amount of light at 1 foot from a standard candle; it is 1 lumen per foot.

footdrop (foot′drop) dropping of the foot from paralysis of the anterior muscles of the leg.

foot-pound (foot′pownd) the amount of energy necessary to raise 1 pound of mass a distance of 1 foot.

foramen (fo-ra′men), pl. *foram′ina* [L.] an opening; applied to numerous apertures in various tissues of the body for passage of other structures, as blood and other vessels, spinal cord and nerves. **aortic f.**, the hindmost of the openings of the diaphragm. **apical f.**, the foramen at the end of the root of a tooth. **arachnoid f.**, foramen of Magendie. **auditory f., external**, the external meatus of auditory canal. **auditory f., internal**, passage for auditory and facial nerves in petrous bone. **Bichat's f.**, a canal from subarachnoid space to third ventricle. **Botallo's f.**, foramen ovale (1). **f. cae'cum, cecal f.**, 1. foramen between the frontal bone and crista galli. 2. a canal over the root and dorsum of the tongue. 3. one in the mucous membrane of the posterior wall of the pharynx. **condyloid f., anterior**, passage in occipital bone for hypoglossal nerve. **condyloid f., posterior**, a fossa behind either occipital condyle. **cotyloid f.**, passage between the margin of acetabulum and transverse ligament. **dental f., inferior**, the outer aperture of the inferior dental canal in the ramus of the lower jaw. **epiploic f.**, foramen of Winslow. **esophageal f.**, passage for esophagus through the diaphragm. **ethmoid f., anterior**, a canal formed by the ethmoid and frontal bones. **frontal f.**, the supraorbital notch. **great f.**, foramen magnum. **incisor f.**, the aperture for anterior palatine artery in the alveolar margin. **infraorbital f.**, passage for infraorbital nerve and artery. **intervertebral f., anterior**, passage for spinal nerves and vessels between laminae of adjacent vertebrae. **intervertebral f., posterior**, space between the articular processes of adjacent vertebrae. **jugular f.**, foramen lacerum posterius. **Key-Retzius foramina**, two passages from cisterna magna to the fourth ventricle. **f. la'cerum ante'rius**, sphenoidal fissure. **f. la'cerum me'dium**, a cleft in petrous bone and great wing of sphenoid for carotid artery, etc. **f. la'cerum poste'rius**, space made by jugular notches of the temporal and occipital bones. **f. of Magendie, Magendie's f.**, orifice in the pia of the roof of fourth ventricle. **f. mag'num**, large opening in anterior inferior part of occipital bone, between the cranial cavity and vertebral canal. **mastoid f.**, small hole behind mastoid process. **medullary f.**, passage which admits the nutrient vessels to the medullary cavity of a bone. **mental f.**, foramen of lower jaw for mental nerve and vessels. **f. of Monro**, passage from third to lateral ventricle of brain. **nutrient f.**, medullary foramen. **obturator f.**, the large opening between os pubis and ischium. **olfactory foramina**, many openings of the cribriform plate of ethmoid bone. **optic f.**, passage for optic nerve and ophthalmic artery at apex of orbit. **f. ova'le**, 1. fetal opening between the heart's atria. 2. aperture in great wing of sphenoid for vessels and nerves. **palatine f., anterior**, an orifice in anterior part of roof of mouth for a nerve and artery. **palatine f., posterior**, orifice in hard palate for descending palatine canal. **parietal f.**, passage in parietal bone for vessels. **pterygopalatine f.**, passage for pterygopalatine vessels and nerve. **quadrate f.**, passage for postcava in the diaphragm. **f. rotun'dum**, a round opening in great wing of sphenoid for the superior maxillary nerve. **sacral foramina, anterior**, eight passages for anterior branches of sacral nerves. **sacral foramina, posterior**, eight passages for posterior branches of sacral nerves. **sacrosciatic f., great**, oval space between the innominate bone and lesser sacrosciatic ligament. **sacrosciatic f., smaller**, space between the greater and lesser sacrosciatic ligaments and innominate bone. **Scarpa's f.**, aperture in maxilla for nasopalatine nerve. **Sömmering's f.**, fovea centralis. **sphenopalatine f.**, space between the orbital and sphenoidal processes of palate bone. **f. spino'sum**, hole in great wing of sphenoid for middle meningeal artery. **Stensen's foramina**, two incisive foramina of the maxilla. **stylomastoid f.**, a foramen between the styloid and mastoid processes of the temporal bone. **supraorbital f.**, notch of frontal bone for supraorbital vessels and nerve. **Thebesius' foramina**, the orifices of the thebesian veins in the right atrium. **thyroid f.**, obturator foramen. **vertebral f.**, space between body and arch of a vertebra and the spinal cord and its meninges. **vertebro-arterial f.**, foramen in transverse process of a cervical vertebra for vertebral vessels. **f. of Vesalius**, opening at inner side of the foramen ovale of the sphenoid. **Weitbrecht's f.**, a foramen in the capsule of the shoulder joint. **f. of Winslow**, aperture between greater and lesser peritoneal cavities. **zygomatico-temporal f.**, opening on temporal surface of zygomatic bone.

force (fōrs) energy or power; that which originates or arrests motion or other activity. **catabolic f.**, energy derived from the metabolism of food. **coriolian f., Coriolis' f.**, the force produced by rotation of the earth on its axis. **electromotive f.**, that which gives rise to an electric current. **nerve f., nervous f.**, 1. the ability of nerve tissue to conduct stimuli. 2. in psychiatry, the amount of nervous capital or stamina a person possesses. **occlusal f.**, the force exerted on opposing teeth when the jaws are brought into approximation. **vital f.**, that which characterizes a living organism.

forceps (fōr'seps), pl. *for'cipes* [L.] 1. a two-pronged instrument for grasping or seizing. 2. any organ or part shaped like a forceps. **f. ante'rior**, forceps minor. **artery f.**, a forceps for grasping and compressing an artery. **aural f.**, a forceps for operations on the ear. **axis-traction f.**, an obstetrical forceps. **bayonet f.**, a forceps whose blades are offset from the axis of the handles. **capsule f.**, a forceps for removing the lens capsule in cataract. **Chamberlen f.**, the original form of obstetrical forceps. **clamp f.**, a forceps-like clamp with an automatic lock, for compressing arteries. **dental f.**, one for the extraction of teeth. **dressing f.**, a forceps for handling wound dressings. **epilating f.**, a forceps for pulling out hairs. **extracting f.**, dental forceps. **fixation f.**, forceps for holding a part steady during operation. **Hodge's f.**, a form of obstetrical forceps. **Knapp's f.**, a forceps with roller blades for expressing trachomatous granules. **Kocher's f.**, a strong forceps for holding tissues during operation or for compressing bleeding tissue. **Laborde's f.**, a flat forceps for making traction on the tongue. **Laplace's f.**, a forceps for holding portions of the intestines together in enterostomy. **Levret's f.**, an obstetrical forceps, curved to correspond with the curve of the parturient canal. **ligature f.**, forceps for holding delicate parts. **Liston's f.**, a bone-cutting forceps. **lithotomy f.**, a forceps for removing stone from the bladder. **Löwenberg's f.**, a forceps for removing adenoid growth. **f. ma'jor**, the terminal fibers of the callosum that pass into the occipital lobe. **f. mi'nor**, the terminal fibers of the callosum that pass from the splenium into the anterior region of each cerebral hemisphere. **mouse-tooth f.**, a forceps with two or more fine teeth at the tip of each blade. **obstetrical f.**, forceps for making traction on the fetus in difficult labor. **Péan's f.**, a clamp for hemostasis. **f. poste'rior**, forceps major. **roller f.**, a forceps with a roller at the end of each blade for expressing trachomatous granules. **sequestrum f.**, a forceps with small but strong serrated jaws. **Simpson's f.**, a form of obstetrical forceps. **speculum f.**, a long, slender forceps for use through a speculum. **Tarnier's f.**, axis-traction forceps. **tenaculum f.**, a forceps having a sharp hook at the end of each jaw. **torsion f.**, a forceps for making torsion on an artery to arrest hemorrhage. **tracheal f.**, a long, slender forceps for removing foreign bodies from the trachea. **trachoma f.**, roller forceps. **tubular f.**, a slender forceps for use through a tubular instrument. **volsella f., vulsellum f.**, vulsella. **Willett f.**, an obstetrical forceps for scalp traction.

forcipate (fôr'sĭ-pāt) shaped like a forceps.

forcipressure (fôr'sĭ-presh″ŭr) pressure by a forceps to check hemorrhage.

forearm (fôr'arm) the part of the arm between elbow and wrist.

forebrain (fôr'brān) the portion of the brain developed from the rostral of the three primary brain vesicles in the early embryo, and comprising the diencephalon and telencephalon.

forefinger (fôr'fing-ger) the first, or index finger.

foreconscious (fōr'kon-shus) preconscious; material not ordinarily in consciousness, but subject to voluntary recall.

forefoot (fōr'fut) the front part of the foot, comprising the toes and metatarsal region.

foregut (fōr'gut) the embryonic organ from which pharynx, esophagus, stomach and part of the small intestine are derived.

forehead (fōr'ed) part of the head above the eyes; the anterior portion of the cranium. **bony f.**, the skeleton of the forehead, formed by the anterior part of the skull (frontal bone).

foreskin (fōr'skin) the prepuce.

formaldehyde (fōr-mal'dĕ-hīd) a gaseous compound, CH_2O, with strongly disinfectant properties.

formaldehydogenic (fōr-mal″dĕ-hi″do-jen'ik) producing formaldehyde.

formalin (fōr'mah-lin) a 40 per cent solution of gaseous formaldehyde.

formate (fôr'māt) a salt of formic acid.

formatio (fôr-ma'she-o), pl. *formatio'nes* [L.] formation.

formation (fôr-ma'shun) 1. the giving or taking of form. 2. something given form or shape. **reaction f.**, development of attributes which hold in check and repress the components of infantile sexuality. **reticular f.**, a network of fibers in the medulla oblongata, passing to the pons. **rut f.**, the limitation of affective interest to a narrow track or rut.

forme (fôrm), pl. *formes* [Fr.] form. **f. fruste** (fôrm froost) (pl. *formes frustes*) an atypical form of a disease. **f. tardive** (fôrm tahr-dēv') a late-occurring form of a disease that usually appears at an earlier age.

formication (fôr″mĭ-ka'shun) sensation as if ants were creeping on the body.

formiciasis (-sĭ'ah-sis) morbid condition caused by ant bites.

formilase (fôr'mĭ-lās) an enzyme which changes acetic acid into formic acid.

formol (fôr'mol) formaldehyde solution.

formula (fôr'mu-lah), pl. *for'mulae, for'mulas* [L.] an expression, using numbers or symbols, of the composition of, or directions for preparing, a compound, such as a medicine, or of a procedure to follow to obtain a desired result, or of a single concept. **chemical f.**, a combination of chemical symbols representing the elements and the number of their atoms in a molecule of a chemical compound. **configurational f.**, spatial formula. **constitutional f.**, structural formula. **dental f.**, an expression of the number of each kind of teeth normally present in the jaw; the human dental formula is, for deciduous teeth, i. $\frac{2-2}{2-2}$ c. $\frac{1-1}{1-1}$ m. $\frac{2-2}{2-2} = 20$; for permanent teeth, i. $\frac{2-2}{2-2}$ c. $\frac{1-1}{1-1}$ pm. $\frac{2-2}{2-2}$ m. $\frac{3-3}{3-3} = 32$. **digital f.**, one that expresses the relative lengths of the digits, usually $3 > 4 > 2 > 5 > 1$, or $3 > 2 > 4 > 5 > 1$ for the fingers, and $1 > 2 > 3 > 4 > 5$ or $2 > 1 > 3 > 4 > 5$ for the toes. **empirical f.**, a chemical formula which expresses the proportions of the elements composing the molecule. **graphic f.**, structural formula. **molecular f.**, a chemical formula expressing the number of atoms of each element of which the molecule is composed. **official f.**, one officially established by a pharmacopeia or other recognized authority. **rational f.**, structural formula. **spatial f.**, a chemical formula giving the numbers of atoms of each element present in a molecule of a substance, which atom is linked to which, the types of linkages involved and the relative positions of the atoms in space. **stereochemical f.**, spatial formula. **structural f.**, a chemical formula showing the spatial arrangement of the atoms and the linkage of every atom. **vertebral f.**, an expression of the number of vertebrae in each region of the spinal column; the human vertebral formula is $C_7T_{12}L_5S_5Cd_4 = 33$.

formulary (fôr'mu-ler″e) a collection of formulae. **National F.**, a book published at regular intervals under supervision of the

Council of the American Pharmaceutical Association, establishing official standards for certain drugs.

fornix (fôr′niks), pl. *for′nices* [L.] an archlike structure or the vaultlike space created by such a structure.

Foroblique (fôr-o-blēk′) trademark for a system of lenses for cystoscope and urethroscope, giving both forward and deflected vision.

Forthane (fôr′thān) trademark for a preparation of methylhexaneamine.

fossa (fos′ah), pl. *fos′sae* [L.] a pit or depression; applied to numerous depressions in various tissues of the body where they come in contact with or articulate with other structures. **acetabular f.**, acetabulum. **adipose fossae**, spaces in the female breast which contain fat. **amygdaloid f.**, the depression in which the tonsil is lodged. **canine f.**, depression on external surface of superior maxilla. **cerebral f.**, any of the depressions on the floor of the cranial cavity. **coronoid f.**, a depression in the humerus for the coronoid process of the ulna. **cranial f.**, any one of three hollows in base of cranium for lobes of the brain. **digastric f.**, groove on inner aspect of mastoid process. **digital f.**, a depression at base of inner surface of mastoid process. **duodenojejunal f.**, a pouch of peritoneum from the anterior wall of the duodenum. **glenoid f.**, fossa in the temporal bone for condyle of lower jaw. **f. hemiellip′tica,** the uppermost of two recesses in fore part of vestibule. **f. hemisphe′rica,** one of the recesses of the anterior part of vestibule. **hyaloid f.**, fossa patellaris. **hypogastric f.**, a depression on the interior surface of the anterior abdominal wall, between the hypogastric folds. **iliac f., external,** wide depression on outer surface of ilium. **iliac f., internal,** wide depression on inner surface of ilium. **interpeduncular f.**, a depression on the inferior surface of the mesencephalon, between the two cerebral peduncles, the floor of which is the posterior perforated substance. **ischiorectal f.**, triangular space between rectum and tuberosity of the ischium. **Jobert's f.**, a fossa in the popliteal region bounded by the adductor magnus and the gracilis and sartorius. **Jonnesco's f.**, duodenojejunal fossa. **jugular f.**, part of the jugular foramen for passage of the jugular vein. **lacerate f.**, an irregularly shaped opening in the orbit just above the disphenoid. **lacrimal f.**, in roof of orbit, lodges the lacrimal gland. **nasal f.**, the portion of the nasal cavity anterior to the middle meatus. **navicular f., f. navicula′ris,** 1. cavity behind the vaginal aperture. 2. expansion of urethra in the glans penis. 3. fossa between helix and antihelix. 4. depression on internal pterygoid process of sphenoid bone. **olfactory f.**, a depression on the inner surface of the cranium for the olfactory lobes. **oral f.**, stomodeum. **f. ova′lis,** fossa in right atrium of heart; remains of fetal foramen ovale. **ovarian f.**, a shallow pouch on the posterior surface of the broad ligament in which the ovary is located. **f.**

patella′ris, depression in front of vitreous body which lodges the lens. **pituitary f.**, depression in the sphenoid which lodges the pituitary gland. **rhomboid f.**, fourth ventricle. **f. of Rosenmüller,** cavity of Rosenmüller. **sigmoid f.**, the curved fossa on the mastoid process. **subarcuate f.**, a depression in the posterior inner surface of the petrous portion of the temporal bone. **sublingual f.**, space on inside of lower jaw which lodges the sublingual gland. **submaxillary f.**, depression on the inner surface of inferior maxillary bone for the submaxillary gland. **subpyramidal f.**, a depression on the internal wall of the middle ear. **subsigmoid f.**, a fossa between the mesentery of the sigmoid flexure and that of the descending colon. **supraspinous f.**, a depression above the spine of the scapula. **sylvian f.**, a depression of the cerebral hemispheres between the arms of the fissure of Sylvius. **tibiofemoral f.**, a space between the articular surfaces of the tibia and femur mesial or lateral to the inferior pole of the patella. **Treitz's f.**, the duodenojejunal fossa. **trochanteric f.**, digital fossa. **Waldeyer's f.**, the two duodenal fossae regarded as one. **zygomatic f.**, cavity below and within the zygoma.

fossette (fô-set′) 1. a small depression. 2. a small, deep corneal ulcer.

fossula (fos′u-lah), pl. *fos′sulae* [L.] a small fossa.

foulage (foo-lahzh′) [Fr.] kneading and pressing of the muscles in massage.

foul brood (fowl brōōd) a contagious disease of honey bees.

foundation (fown-da′shun) the structure or basis on which something is built. **denture f.**, the portion of the structures and tissues of the mouth available to support a denture.

fourchette (foor-shet′) [Fr.] the posterior junction of labia majora.

fovea (fo′ve-ah), pl. *fo′veae* [L.] a small pit or depression. **f. centra′lis,** a depression in the macula lutea, resulting from absence of most of the layers of the retina except the neuroepithelial layer.

foveate (fo′ve-āt) pitted.

foveation (fo″ve-a′shun) formation of pits on a surface as on the skin.

foveola (fo-ve′o-lah), pl. *fove′olae* [L.] a minute pit or depression.

foxglove (foks′gluv) digitalis.

F.P. freezing point.

F.R. flocculation reaction.

Fr chemical symbol, *francium.*

fracture (frak′tūr) a break in the continuity of a bone. **avulsion f.**, separation of a small fragment of bone cortex at the site of attachment of a ligament. **Barton's f.**, one involving only a small portion of the articular surface of the distal end of the radius. **Bennett's f.**, a longitudinal fracture of the first metacarpal bone, complicated by subluxation. **birth f.**, one in an infant, caused by trauma incident to a difficult delivery. **capillary f.**, one that appears on a radiogram as a fine, hairlike line, the segments of bone not being separated;

sometimes seen in fractures of the skull. **chip f.**, avulsion fracture. **closed f.**, one in which there is no wound on the body surface communicating with the break in the bone. **Colles f.**, a break in the lower end of the radius, the distal fragment being displaced backward. **Colles f., reversed**, one in the lower end of the radius, the distal fragment being displaced anteriorly. **comminuted f.**, one in which two or more communicating breaks divide the bone into more than two fragments. **complete f.**, one involving the entire cross section of the bone. **compound f.**, open fracture. **compression f.**, disruption of the normal continuity and structure of a bone resulting from unusual and excessive compressive force. **depressed f.**, one in which the fragment of bone is forced beneath the line of its normal contour. **double f.**, one in which the bone is divided by two noncommunicating lines of fracture. **Dupuytren's f.**, Pott's fracture. **Duverney's f.**, fracture of the ilium just below the anterior inferior spine. **fissure f.**, one extending longitudinally along the shaft of a long bone. **greenstick f.**, an incomplete fracture of a long bone, with a longitudinal split of the shaft. **gunshot f.**, a fracture produced by a bullet. **impacted f.**, fracture in which one fragment is firmly driven into the other. **incomplete f.**, one which does not involve the complete cross section of the bone. **interperiosteal f.**, greenstick fracture. **intrauterine f.**, fracture of a fetal bone incurred in utero. **lead pipe f.**, buckling of the cortex on one side of the shaft of a long bone. **Monteggia's f.**, one in the proximal half of the shaft of the ulna, with dislocation of the head of the radius. **open f.**, one in which a wound through the adjacent or overlying soft tissues communicates with the site of the break. **parry f.**, Monteggia's fracture. **pathologic f.**, one occurring in diseased bone with only slight or no trauma. **ping-pong f.**, fracture of the skull with the bone fragment depressed below the normal level of the surface. **Pott's f.**, fracture of lower part of fibula with serious injury of the lower tibial articulation. **silverfork f.**, see under *deformity.* **simple f.**, closed fracture. **Smith's f.**, Colles fracture, reversed. **spiral f.**, a fracture twisting around the shaft of a bone. **spontaneous f.**, pathologic fracture. **sprain f.**, avulsion fracture. **Stieda's f.**, a fracture of the internal condyle of the femur sometimes causing hypertrophy of the condyle. **transcervical f.**, one through the neck of the femur. **trophic f.**, one due to a trophic disturbance. **Wagstaffe's f.**, separation of the internal malleolus.

frae- for words beginning thus, see those beginning *fre-.*

fragilitas (frah-jil′ĭ-tas) [L.] fragility. **f. crin′ium**, fragility of the hair, with resultant longitudinal splitting of the shaft. **f. os′sium congen′ita**, osteogenesis imperfecta. **f. san′guinis**, fragility of the blood. **f. un′guium**, abnormal brittleness of the nails.

fragility (frah-jil′ĭ-te) susceptibility or lack of resistance to influences capable of causing disruption of continuity or integrity. **f. of blood**, erythrocyte fragility. **capillary f.**, abnormal susceptibility of capillary walls to rupture. **erythrocyte f.**, susceptibility of erythrocytes to hemolysis when exposed to increasingly hypotonic saline solutions *(osmotic fragility)* or when subjected to mechanical trauma *(mechanical fragility).*

fragilocyte (frah-jil′o-sīt) an erythrocyte abnormally sensitive to hypotonic salt solution.

fragilocytosis (frah-jil″o-si-to′sis) the presence of fragilocytes in the blood.

fragmentation (frag″men-ta′shun) division into small pieces.

frambesia (fram-be′ze-ah) yaws. **f. trop′ica**, yaws.

frambesioma (fram-be″ze-o′mah) mother yaw.

frame (frām) a rigid supporting structure. **Balkan f.**, an apparatus for continuous extension in treatment of fractures of the femur, consisting of an overhead bar, with pulleys attached, by which the leg is supported in a sling. **Bradford f.**, a rectangular structure of gas pipe across which are stretched two strips of canvas, used for patients with fractures or disease of the hip or spine. **quadriplegic standing f.**, a device for supporting in the upright position a patient whose four limbs are paralyzed. **spectacle f.**, a device for holding lenses before the eyes. **trial f.**, a spectacle frame designed to permit ready insertion and removal of different lenses used in testing vision.

francium (fran′se-um) chemical element *(see table)*, at. no. 87, symbol Fr.

franklinization (frank″li-ni-za′shun) therapeutic use of static electricity.

F.R.C.P. Fellow of the Royal College of Physicians.

F.R.C.S. Fellow of the Royal College of Surgeons.

freckle (frek′l) a pigmented spot on the skin due to accumulation of melanin resulting from exposure to sunlight. **cold f.**, lentigo.

freemartin (fre′mar-tin) a female calf born as a twin of a male calf; it is usually sterile and intersexual as a result of male hormone reaching it through anastomosed placental vessels.

fremitus (frem′ĭ-tus) a thrill, especially one perceptible on palpation or auscultation. **friction f.**, thrill caused by the rubbing together of two dry surfaces. **hydatid f.**, tremulous impulse felt in palpation over a hydatid cyst. **rhonchal f.**, vibration produced by passage of air through a large bronchial tube loaded with mucus. **tactile f.**, vibration or thrill of the chest wall in speaking, perceived on palpation. **tussive f.**, thrill felt on chest while patient coughs. **vocal f.**, vibration or thrill of the chest wall in speaking, perceived on auscultation.

frenectomy (fre-nek′to-me) excision of a frenum (frenulum).

frenosecretory (fre″no-se-kre′to-re) restraining secretion.

frenotomy (fre-not′o-me) the cutting of a frenum (frenulum).

frenulum (fren′u-lum), pl. *fren′ula* [L.] a small

fold of integument or mucous membrane that limits the movements of an organ or part. **f. of clitoris,** a fold on the urethral surface of the clitoris, formed by the anterior junction of the labia minora. **f. labio′rum,** a fold of mucous membrane on the midline of each lip, connecting lip and gum. **f. labio′rum puden′di,** fourchette. **f. lin′guae,** the midline fold connecting the under surface of the tongue and floor of the mouth. **f. of Morgagni,** a ridge formed by extension of the conjoined edges of the ileocecal valve, partially encircling the intestine. **f. of penis,** a fold of thin integument from inferior angle of exterior urethral orifice to the inner sheath of the prepuce. **f. val′vulae co′li,** frenulum of Morgagni. **f. ve′li,** a continuation of the white substance of the inferior quadrigeminal bodies in the roof of the fourth ventricle.

frenum (fre′num), pl. *fre′na* [L.] a restraining structure; frenulum. adj., **fre′nal.**

frequency (fre′kwen-se) the number of occurrences of a determinable entity per unit of population or of time, e.g. cases of a disease per 100,000 population. **audio f.,** a frequency corresponding to a normal audible sound wave. **infrasonic f.,** a frequency below the audio frequency range. **subsonic f.,** infrasonic frequency. **supersonic f., ultrasonic f.,** a frequency above the audio frequency range.

freudian (froi′de-an) pertaining to Sigmund Freud and his doctrines that certain nervous disorders are caused by the existence of unconscious sexual repressions, and that they can be cured by bringing these repressions into consciousness by psychoanalysis.

friable (fri′ah-bl) broken easily into small pieces.

friction (frik′shun) the act of rubbing.

frigidity (fri-jid′i-te) partial or complete inability of the female to be aroused sexually or to achieve orgasm.

frigolabile (frig″o-la′bil) easily affected by cold.

frigorific (-rif′ik) producing coldness.

frigostabile (-sta′bil) not easily affected by cold.

frigotherapy (-ther′ah-pe) treatment of disease by cold.

frit (frit) imperfectly fused material used as a basis for making glass and in formation of porcelain teeth.

frog (frog) the forked band of horny substance on the sole of a horse's foot.

frolement (frōl-maw′) [Fr.] 1. a rustling sound heard in pericardial disease. 2. a brushing movement in massage.

frondose (fron′dōs) bearing villi or fronds.

frons (fronz) [L.] the forehead.

frontad (frun′tad) toward a front, or frontal aspect.

frontal (frun′tal) pertaining to the upper, anterior part of the head, or forehead.

frontalis (fron-ta′lis) [L.] frontal.

frontomalar (frun″to-ma′lar) pertaining to frontal and malar bones.

frontomaxillary (-mak′si-ler″e) pertaining to frontal bone and maxilla.

frontoparietal (frun″to-pah-ri′e-tal) pertaining to frontal and parietal bones.

frontotemporal (-tem′po-ral) pertaining to frontal and temporal bones.

frost (frost) a deposit resembling frozen dew or vapor. **urea f.,** the appearance on the skin of salt crystals left by evaporation of the sweat in urhidrosis.

frostbite (frost′bīt) injury to tissues due to exposure to cold.

frottage (fro-tahzh′) [Fr.] rubbing movement in massage.

fructivorous (fruk-tiv′o-rus) subsisting on or eating fruit.

fructose (fruk′tōs) a colorless or white crystalline compound, $C_6H_{12}O_6$, used in solution as a fluid and nutrient replenisher.

fructosuria (fruk″to-su′re-ah) fructose in the urine.

fruit (frōot) the matured ovary of a flowering plant, containing the seeds.

frustration (frus-tra′shun) the feeling aroused by the blocking of sought gratifications and satisfactions, ordinarily by forces outside one's self.

FSH follicle-stimulating hormone.

Fuadin (fu′ah-din) trademark for a preparation of stibophen.

fuchsin (fook′sin) a dark red dye with germicidal properties. **acid f.,** a compound used in preparation of a staining solution. **basic f.,** a compound used in preparation of an antifungal solution.

fuchsinophilia (fook″sin-o-fil′e-ah) the property of staining readily with fuchsin dyes. adj., **fuchsinophil′ic.**

fugacity (fu-gas′i-te) tendency to escape, as of gas or liquids from material in which they are absorbed.

-fugal (fu′gal) word element [L.] *driving away; fleeing from; repelling.*

fugue (fūg) transitory abnormal behavior marked by aimless wandering and some alteration of consciousness, usually but not always followed by amnesia.

fulgurate (ful′gu-rāt) 1. to come and go like a flash of lightning. 2. to subject to treatment by electric sparks.

fulguration (ful″gu-ra′shun) treatment by electric sparks.

fulminate (ful′mī-nāt) to occur suddenly with great intensity. adj., **ful′minant.**

Fulvicin (ful′vi-sin) trademark for a preparation of griseofulvin.

fumagillin (fu″mah-jil′in) an antibiotic elaborated by strains of *Aspergillus fumigatus;* used as an amebicide.

fumarate (fu′mar-āt) a salt of fumaric acid. **ferrous f.,** the anhydrous salt of a combination of ferrous iron and fumaric acid; used as a hematinic.

fumigation (fu″mī-ga′shun) exposure to disinfecting fumes.

fuming (fūm′ing) emitting a visible vapor.

Fumiron (fum′i-ron) trademark for a preparation of ferrous fumarate.

functio (fungk′she-o) [L.] function. **f. lae′sa,** loss of function.

function (fungk'shun)   a special action or purpose.

functional (fungk'shun-al)   pertaining to or fulfilling a function.

fundament (fun'dah-ment) 1. a base or foundation upon which something rests. 2. the anus and parts adjacent to it.

fundectomy (fun-dek'to-me)   excision of the fundus of an organ, as of the stomach or uterus.

fundiform (fun'dĭ-form)   shaped like a loop or sling.

fundoplication (fun"do-pli-ka'shun)   mobilization of the lower end of the esophagus and plication of the fundus of the stomach up around it, in the treatment of reflux esophagitis.

fundus (fun'dus), pl. *fun'di* [L.]   a bottom or base; applied to the interior of the back of the eyeball, the part of the uterus between the orifices of the fallopian tubes, farthest from the opening of the cervix, and the base or posterior portion of the urinary bladder. adj., **fun'dal, fun'dic. f. of eye,** the back portion of the interior of the eyeball, visible through the pupil by use of the ophthalmoscope. **f. of gallbladder,** the rounded end of the gallbladder, remote from its opening into the cystic ducts. **f. of stomach,** the part of the stomach to the left and above the level of the opening between stomach and esophagus. **f. tym'pani,** the floor of the tympanic cavity. **f. of urinary bladder,** the posterior wall of the bladder. **f. of uterus,** the rounded end of the uterus, remote from its junction with the cervix.

fundusectomy (fun"du-sek'to-me)   excision of the fundus of the stomach.

fungate (fun'gāt)   to grow in fungus-like masses.

fungemia (fun-je'me-ah)   the presence of fungi in the blood stream.

fungicide (fun'jĭ-sīd)   an agent that destroys fungi. adj., **fungici'dal.**

fungicidin (fun"jĭ-si'din)   nystatin.

fungiform (fun'jĭ-form)   shaped like a fungus (puff ball).

fungistasis (fun"jĭ-sta'sis)   inhibition of the growth of fungi. adj., **fungistat'ic.**

fungistat (fun'jĭ-stat)   a substance that checks the growth of fungi.

fungitoxic (fun"jĭ-tok'sik)   exerting a toxic effect upon fungi.

Fungizone (fun'jĭ-zōn)   trademark for a preparation of amphotericin B.

fungoid (fun'goid)   resembling a fungus. **chignon f.,** a nodular growth on the hair.

fungosity (fun-gos'ĭ-te)   a fungoid growth or excrescence.

fungous (fun'gus)   of the nature of a fungus.

fungus (fun'gus), pl. *fun'gi* [L.] 1. any vegetable organism of the class to which mushrooms and molds belong, many genera being pathogenic for man.   2. a mushroom-like growth. **cerebral f.,** a mass of cerebral tissue protruding through a defect in the skull and overlying layers of the scalp. **foot f.,** the fungus that produces mycetoma. **f. hemato'-** **des,** a bleeding and vascular malignant tumor. **ray f.,** Actinomyces.

funicle (fu'nĭ-kl)   funiculus.

funiculitis (fu-nik"u-li'tis)   inflammation of the spermatic cord.

funiculus (fu-nik'u-lus), pl. *funic'uli* [L.]   a cordlike structure or part, especially one of the large bundles of nerve tracts making up the white substance of the spinal cord. adj., **funic'ular. anterior f., f. ante'rior,** the ventral mass of fibers on either side of the spinal cord, between the anterior median fissure and the anterolateral sulcus. **cuneate f., f. cunea'tus,** continuation of the fasciculus cuneatus on the dorsal aspect of the medulla oblongata. **f. gra'cilis,** continuation of the fasciculus gracilis on the dorsal aspect of the medulla oblongata. **lateral f., f. latera'lis,** the lateral mass of fibers on either side of the spinal cord, between the anterolateral and posterolateral sulci. **posterior f., f. poste'rior,** the posterior mass of fibers on either side of the spinal cord, between the posterolateral and posterior median sulci. **f. spermat'icus,** the spermatic cord.

funiform (fu'nĭ-form)   resembling a rope or cord.

funis (fu'nis)   a cord, especially the umbilical cord. adj., **fu'nic.**

Furacin (fu'rah-sin)   trademark for preparations of nitrofurazone.

Furadantin (fūr"ah-dan'tin)   trademark for preparations of nitrofurantoin.

furaltadone (fūr-al'tah-dōn)   a compound formerly used as an antibacterial.

Furaspor (fūr'ah-spōr)   trademark for a preparation of nitrofurfuryl methyl ether.

furazolidone (fu"rah-zol'ĭ-dōn)   a yellow, odorless, crystalline powder; used as a local antibacterial and antiprotozoal.

furca (fer'kah), pl. *fur'cae* [L.]   the area between and at the base of normally divided tooth roots.

furcal (fer'kal)   forked.

furfuraceous (fer"fu-ra'shus)   like dandruff or bran.

furibund (fu'rĭ-bund)   full of fury; raging; maniacal.

furmethonol (fer-meth'o-nol)   furaltadone.

furor (fu'ror)   fury; rage. **f. epilep'ticus,** an attack of intense anger occurring in epilepsy. **f. secan'di,** tomomania. **f. uteri'nus,** nymphomania.

Furoxone (fer-ok'sōn)   trademark for preparations of furazolidone.

furrow (fur'o)   a groove or trench. **atrioventricular f.,** the transverse groove marking off the atria of the heart from the ventricles. **digital f.,** any one of the transverse lines on the palmar surface of a finger. **genital f.,** a groove that appears on the genital tubercle of the fetus at the end of the second month. **gluteal f.,** the furrow which separates the buttocks. **interventricular f.,** see under *groove.* **Jadelot's f's,** see under *line.* **Liebermeister's f's,** depressions sometimes seen on the upper surface of the liver from pressure of the ribs, generally from tight lacing. **mentolabial f.**, the hollow just above the chin. **nympholabial f.**, a furrow between the labia majora and labia minora on each side. **primitive f.**, the primitive groove. **Schmorl's f.**, a depression over the apex of the lung, said to be indicative of a tendency to tuberculosis. **scleral f.**, scleral sulcus. **Sibson's f.**, the under border of the pectoralis major muscle.

furuncle (fu'rung-kl) a focal suppurative inflammation of the skin and subcutaneous tissues.

furunculoid (fu-rung'ku-loid) furunculous.

furunculosis (fu-rung″ku-lo'sis) the occurrence of a number of furuncles.

furunculus (fu-rung'ku-lus) [L.] furuncle. adj., **furun'culous. f. orienta'lis**, cutaneous leishmaniasis.

fuscin (fus'in) a brown pigment of the retinal epithelium.

fusible (fu'zĭ-bl) capable of being melted.

fusiform (fu'zĭ-form) spindle-shaped.

fusion (fu'zhun) the combining or blending of distinct bodies into one, as (*a*) the fusion into a single image of the separate impressions received by the two eyes, or (*b*) the surgical process of making a formerly movable structure (joint) immovable. **diaphyseal-epiphyseal f.**, operative establishment of bony union between epiphysis and diaphysis of a bone. **nerve f.**, nerve anastomosis done to induce regeneration for resupplying empty tracts of a nerve with new growth of fibers. **spinal f.**, spondylosyndesis.

fusional (fu'zhun-al) marked by fusion.

Fusobacterium (fu″zo-bak-te're-um) a genus of Schizomycetes (order Eubacteriales, family Bacteroidaceae) occurring in the mouth and large bowel. **F. plau'ti-vincen'ti**, a microorganism found in necrotizing ulcerative gingivitis.

fusocellular (-sel'u-ler) having spindle-shaped cells.

fusospirillosis (-spi″rĭ-lo'sis) Vincent's angina.

fusospirochetal (-spi″ro-ke'tal) caused by fusiform bacilli and spirochetes.

fusospirochetosis (-spi″ro-ke-to'sis) Vincent's angina.

fusus (fu'sus), pl. *fu'si* [L.] 1. a spindle-shaped structure. 2. a minute air vesicle in a hair shaft.

G

G. gram; gingival.

Ga chemical symbol, *gallium.*

gadolinium (gad″o-lin'e-um) chemical element (*see table*), at. no. 64, symbol Gd.

Gaffkya (gaf'ke-ah) a genus of Schizomycetes (order Eubacteriales, family Micrococcaceae).

gag (gag) a device to hold the mouth open.

gait (gāt) the manner of progression in walking. **antalgic g.**, a manner of walking adopted to minimize pain experienced when moving normally. **ataxic g.**, a gait in which the foot is raised high, the sole striking the ground at once and suddenly. **cerebellar g.**, a staggering walk indicative of cerebellar disease. **spastic g.**, a gait in which the legs are held together and move in a stiff manner, the toes seeming to drag and catch. **steppage g.**, one in which the toe is strongly lifted and the heel reaches the ground first. **tabetic g.**, ataxic gait. **waddling g.**, a ducklike gait seen in pseudohypertrophic paralysis.

galactacrasia (gah-lak″tah-kra'ze-ah) an abnormal state of mother's milk.

galactagogue (gah-lak'tah-gog) 1. increasing the flow of milk. 2. an agent which increases the flow of milk.

galactan (gah-lak'tan) a carbohydrate which yields galactose upon hydrolysis.

galactase (gah-lak'tās) an enzyme which ripens cheese.

galactemia (gal″ak-te'me-ah) presence of milk in the blood.

galactic (gah-lak'tik) pertaining to milk.

galactidrosis (gah-lak″tĭ-dro'sis) the sweating of a milky fluid.

galactin (gah-lak'tin) a basic principle found in milk.

galactoblast (gah-lak'to-blast) a colostrum corpuscle in the gland acini.

galactocele (gah-lak'to-sēl) 1. milk-containing tumor of the mammary gland. 2. hydrocele filled with milky fluid.

galactokinase (gah-lak″to-ki'nās) an enzyme that catalyzes transfer of a high-energy phosphate group from a donor to D-galactose, producing D-galactose-1-phosphate.

galactoma (gal″ak-to'mah) galactocele (1).

galactometer (-tom'ĕ-ter) lactometer.

galactopexy (gah-lak'to-pek″se) fixation of galactose by the liver. adj., **galactopec'tic.**

galactophagous (gal″ak-tof'ah-gus) subsisting upon milk.

galactophlysis (-tof'lĭ-sis) eruption of vesicles with milk contents.

galactophorous (-tof'o-rus) conveying milk.

galactophygous (-tof'ĭ-gus) arresting the flow of milk.

galactoplania (gah-lak″to-pla'ne-ah) secretion of milk in some abnormal part.

galactopoietic (-poi-et'ik) concerned in production of milk.

galactopyra (-pi'rah) milk fever.

galactorrhea (-re'ah) excessive secretion by the mammary gland.

galactoschesis (gal″ak-tos'kĕ-sis) suppression of milk secretion.

galactoscope (gah-lak″to-skōp) lactoscope.

galactose (gah-lak′tōs) a monosaccharide derived from lactose.

galactosemia (gah-lak″to-se′me-ah) 1. a hereditary disorder of carbohydrate metabolism, characterized by vomiting, diarrhea, jaundice, poor weight gain and malnutrition in early infancy. 2. the presence of galactose in the blood.

galactosis (gal″ak-to′sis) the formation of milk.

galactostasis (-tos′tah-sis) 1. cessation of milk secretion. 2. abnormal collection of milk.

galactosuria (gal-lak″to-su′re-ah) galactose in the urine.

galactotherapy (-ther′ah-pe) treatment of a nursing infant by medication given the mother.

galactotoxicon (-tok′sĭ-kon) a poisonous compound formed in decomposed milk.

galactotoxin (-tok′sin) a poison produced in milk by growth of a microorganism.

galactotoxism (-tok′sizm) poisoning by milk.

galactotrophy (gal″ak-tot′ro-fe) feeding with milk.

galactoxism (-tok′sizm) galactotoxism.

galactozymase (gah-lak″to-zi′mās) a starch-liquefying enzyme.

galacturia (gal″ak-tu′re-ah) chyluria.

galea (ga′le-ah), pl. *ga′leae* [L.] a helmet-shaped structure. **g. aponeurot′ica,** the aponeurosis connecting the two bellies of the epicranius muscle. **tendinous g.,** galea aponeurotica.

galeanthropy (ga″le-an′thro-pe) morbid belief that one has become a cat.

galenicals (gah-len′ĭ-kals) galenics.

galenics (gah-len′iks) medicines of vegetable origin.

galeophilia (ga″le-o-fil′e-ah) abnormal fondness for cats.

galeophobia (-fo′be-ah) morbid fear of cats.

gallamine triethiodide (gal′ah-min tri″eth-i′o-dĭd) a compound used to relax skeletal muscles.

gallate (gal′āt) a salt of gallic acid.

gallbladder (gawl′blad-er) the pear-shaped reservoir for bile on the posterior surface of the liver.

Gallionella (gal″le-o-nel′ah) a genus of Schizomycetes (order Pseudomonadales, suborder Pseudomonadineae, family Caulobacteraceae) growing only in iron-containing fresh or salt water.

gallium (gal′le-um) chemical element *(see table),* at. no. 31, symbol Ga.

gallon (gal′on) a unit of liquid measure (4 quarts, or 3.785 liters).

gallstone (gawl′stōn) a calculus formed in the gallbladder or bile duct.

galv. galvanic.

galvanism (gal′vah-nizm) uninterrupted electric current.

galvanization (gal″vah-ni-za′shun) treatment by galvanism.

galvanocautery (gal″vah-no-kaw′ter-e) cautery by a wire that is heated by galvanic electricity.

galvanocontractility (gal″vah-no-kon″trak-til′ĭ-te) contractility on stimulation by galvanic electricity.

galvanofaradization (-far″ah-dĭ-za′-shun) application of continuous and interrupted currents together.

galvanogustometer (-gus-tom′ĕ-ter) an apparatus for clinical determination of taste thresholds by use of a galvanic current.

galvanometer (gal″vah-nom′ĕ-ter) instrument for measuring galvanic electricity.

galvanomuscular (gal″vah-no-mus′ku-ler) produced by application of galvanic electricity to a muscle.

galvanonarcosis (-nar-ko′sis) electronarcosis.

galvanonervous (-ner′vus) produced by application of galvanic electricity to a nerve.

galvanopalpation (-pal-pa′shun) testing of nerves of the skin by means of galvanic electricity.

galvanopuncture (-punk′tūr) puncture and galvanism conjoined.

galvanoscope (gal-van′o-skōp) instrument which shows the presence of galvanic electricity.

galvanosurgery (-ser′jer-e) surgical application of galvanism.

galvanotaxis (-tak′sis) 1. taxis in response to the influence of an electric current. 2. arrangement of a living organism in a fluid medium in relation to the direction of flow of the medium.

galvanotherapy (-ther′ah-pe) treatment by means of uninterrupted electric current.

galvanothermy (-ther′me) heating by galvanic electricity.

galvanotonus (gal″vah-not′o-nus) tonic response to galvanism.

galvanotropism (gal″vah-not′ro-pizm) movements in organs of animals and plants under the influence of an electric current.

gamete (gam′ēt) 1. one of two cells, male and female, whose union is necessary in sexual reproduction to initiate the development of a new individual. 2. the complete sexual form of malarial plasmodium as found in the anopheles mosquito. adj., **gamet′ic.**

gametocide (gam′ē-to-sīd″) an agent which destroys malarial gametes. adj., **gametoci′-dal.**

gametocyte (gah-met′o-sīt) the sexual plasmodial cell in malarial blood which produces gametes in the insect host.

gametogenesis (gam″ē-to-jen′ē-sis) the formation or production of gametes.

gametologist (gam″ē-tol′o-jist) a scientist whose special study is gametology.

gametology (-tol′o-je) the study of gametes.

gamma (gam′ah) third letter of the Greek alphabet, γ; used in names of chemical compounds to distinguish one of three or more isomers or to indicate position of substituting atoms or groups.

gamma benzene hexachloride (gam′ah ben′-zēn hek″sah-klor′ĭd) lindane.

gammacism (gam′ah-sizm) imperfect utterance of *g* and *k* sounds.

gammaglobulinopathy (gam″ah-glob″u-lin-op'ah-the) abnormality of the gamma globulins in the blood.

gammagram (gam'ah-gram) 1. a graphic record of the gamma rays emitted by an object or substance. 2. a radiogram produced by use of gamma rays as the radiant energy.

gammagraph (gam'ah-graf) scintiscanner.

gammagraphic (gam"ah-graf'ik) pertaining to the recording of gamma rays in the study of organs after the administration of radioactive isotopes.

gamma-lactone (-lak'tōn) a compound having a five-membered ring structure formed by internal reaction of a carboxylic acid group with a hydroxyl group on the gamma carbon of a carbon chain.

gamma-pipradol (-pip'rah-dol) azacyclonol.

gammopathy (gam-mop'ah-the) gammaglobulinopathy.

gamogenesis (gam"o-jen'ē-sis) sexual reproduction. adj., **gamogenet'ic.**

gamogony (gam-og'o-ne) the development of merozoites into male and female gametes, which later fuse to form a zygote.

gamophobia (gam"o-fo'be-ah) morbid fear of marriage.

gampsodactylia (gamp"so-dak-til'e-ah) clawlike deformity of the toes.

gangli(o)- (gang'gle-o) word element [Gr.], *ganglion.*

gangliasthenia (gang"gle-as-the'ne-ah) asthenia due to disease of the ganglion.

gangliated (gang'gle-āt"ed) provided with ganglia.

gangliectomy (gang"gle-ek'to-me) excision of a ganglion.

gangliform (gang'glī-form) resembling a ganglion.

gangliitis (gang"gle-i'tis) inflammation of a ganglion.

ganglioblast (gang'gle-o-blast") an embryonic cell of the spinal ganglia.

gangliocyte (gang'gle-o-sīt") a ganglion cell.

gangliocytoma (gang"gle-o-si-to'mah) a tumor containing ganglion cells.

ganglioform (gang'gle-o-form") gangliform

ganglioglioma (gang"gle-o-gli-o'mah) a glioma containing ganglion cells.

ganglioglioneuroma (-gli"o-nu-ro'mah) a nerve tumor containing ganglion cells, glia cells and nerve fibers.

gangliolytic (-lit'ik) ganglioplegic.

ganglioma (gang"gle-o'mah) tumor of the lymphatic ganglia.

ganglion (gang'gle-on), pl. *gan'glia, ganglions* [Gr.] 1. a mass of gray substance in the nervous system, especially an aggregation of cell bodies of neurons occurring outside the central nervous system. 2. a form of cystic tumor on an aponeurosis or a tendon. adj., **gan'glial, ganglion'ic.** Acrel's **g.,** one on the extensor tendons of the wrist. **Andersch's g.,** petrous ganglion. **Arnold's g., auricular g.,** situated below the foramen ovale, sending nerves to the tympanic muscles and tensor palati. **Auerbach's g.,** any of the small ganglia of Auerbach's plexus. **autonomic ganglia,** aggregations of cell bodies of neu-

rons of the autonomic nervous system. **azygous g.,** coccygeal ganglion. **basal ganglia,** the thalami, corpora striata, corpora quadrigemina, tuber cinereum, and geniculate bodies. **Bidder's ganglia,** two ganglia of the auricular septum of a frog's heart. **Bochdalek's g.,** swelling at junction of anterior and middle dental nerves. **cardiac g.,** a ganglion of the superficial cardiac plexus under the aortic arch. **carotid g.,** one in the lower part of the cavernous sinus. **carotid g., inferior,** one in the lower part of the carotid canal. **carotid g., superior,** one in the upper part of the carotid canal. **casserian g.,** gasserian ganglion. **celiac ganglia,** two large masses, one on either side of the midline, near the adrenal glands, which with the nerve fibers uniting them form the celiac plexus. **cephalic ganglia,** the ciliary, Arnold's, Meckel's and submaxillary ganglia, all mainly of the trisplanchnic system. **cerebral g.,** thalamus. **cerebrospinal ganglia,** those associated with the cranial and spinal nerves. **cervical g., inferior,** between transverse process of lowest cervical vertebra and the neck of the first rib. **cervical g., middle,** adjacent to fifth cervical vertebra. **cervical g., superior,** opposite the second and third cervical vertebrae. **cervical g. of uterus,** near the cervix uteri. **ciliary g.,** in the posterior part of the orbit. **Cloquet's g.,** swelling of nasopalatine nerve in anterior palatine canal. **coccygeal g.,** glomus coccygeum. **Corti's g.,** spiral ganglion. **dorsal root g.,** spinal ganglion. **Ehrenritter's g.,** jugular ganglion. **false g.,** an enlargement on a nerve that does not have a true ganglionic structure. **Frankenhäuser's g.,** a ganglion near the cervix uteri. **gasserian g.,** on larger root of fifth cranial nerve. **geniculate g.,** on facial nerve in aqueduct of Fallopius. **hepatic g.,** around the hepatic artery. **g. im'par,** the ganglion commonly found in front of the coccyx, where the sympathetic trunks of the two sides unite. **inframaxillary g., anterior,** on inferior maxillary nerve near incisor teeth. **inframaxillary g., posterior,** near last molar teeth. **intercarotic g., intercarotid g.,** carotid gland. **jugular g.,** node on (1) root of vagus nerve or (2) on glossopharyngeal nerve, both in the jugular foramen. **Lee's g.,** cervical ganglion of the uterus. **lenticular g.,** ciliary ganglion. **lingual g.,** on an anterior branch from the superior cervical ganglion. **Ludwig's g.,** at right atrium of heart. **lumbar ganglia,** four or five pairs on either side behind abdominal aorta. **lymphatic g.,** any lymphatic node. **Meckel's g.,** in the sphenomaxillary fossa. **Meissner's g.,** see under *plexus.* **mesenteric g., inferior,** on the inferior mesenteric artery. **mesenteric g., lateral,** in the superior mesenteric plexus, left side. **mesenteric g., superior,** in the superior mesenteric plexus. **Müller's g.,** prostatic ganglion. **nasal g.,** Meckel's ganglion. **ophthalmic g., orbital g.,** ciliary ganglion. **otic g.,** Arnold's ganglion. **parasympathetic ganglia,** aggregations of cell bodies of neurons of the parasympathetic nervous system. **petrous g.**, on glossopharyngeal nerve at lower border of petrous bone. **pharyngeal g.**, on an anterior branch from the cavernous plexus. **phrenic g.**, beneath diaphragm at junction of right phrenic nerve and phrenic plexus. **prostatic g.**, on the prostate gland; connected with prostatic plexus. **pterygopalatine g.**, Meckel's ganglion. **Remak's g.**, in the wall of the right atrium. **renal g.**, around the renal artery. **Ribes's g.**, the alleged cephalic ending of the sympathetic nervous system. **sacral ganglia**, four or five pairs on ventral face of the sacrum. **Scarpa's g.**, vestibular ganglion. **Schacher's g.**, ciliary ganglion. **semilunar g.**, 1. celiac ganglion (ganglia). 2. gasserian ganglion. **sensory g.**, a name sometimes applied to the collective masses of nerve cell bodies in the brain subserving the function of sensation. **simple g.**, a cystic tumor in a tendon sheath. **solar ganglia**, celiac ganglia. **sphenopalatine g.**, Meckel's ganglion. **spinal ganglia**, on posterior root of each spinal nerve. **spiral g.**, between plates of the spiral lamina, sending filaments to the organ of Corti. **splanchnic ganglia**, celiac ganglia. **stellate g.**, the first dorsal sympathetic nerve ganglion. **submaxillary g.**, above the submaxillary gland. **suprarenal g.**, at the junction of the great splanchnic nerves. **sympathetic ganglia**, aggregations of cell bodies of neurons of the sympathetic nervous system. **synovial g.**, a synovial cyst. **thoracic ganglia**, 12 pairs between transverse processes of vertebrae and head of ribs. **thyroid g., inferior**, cervical ganglion, middle. **thyroid g., superior**, cervical ganglion, superior. **tympanic g.**, on the tympanic branch of the glossopharyngeal nerve. **vagal g., inferior**, near the jugular foramen. **Valentin's g.**, at junction of the posterior and middle dental nerves. **ventricular ganglia**, Bidder's ganglia. **vestibular g.**, a ganglion on the vestibular nerve near the external auditory meatus. **Walther's g.**, glomus coccygeum. **Wrisberg's g.**, cardiac ganglion.

ganglionated (gang'gle-o-nāt"ed) provided with ganglia.

ganglionectomy (gang"gle-o-nek'to-me) excision of a ganglion.

ganglionervous (-ner'vus) pertaining to the sympathetic nervous system.

ganglioneure (gang'gle-o-nūr") any cell of a nerve ganglion.

ganglioneuroma (gang"gle-o-nu-ro'mah) a tumor made up of ganglion cells.

ganglionitis (-ni'tis) inflammation of a ganglion.

ganglionostomy (-nos'to-me) surgical creation of an opening into a cystic tumor on a tendon sheath or aponeurosis.

ganglioplegic (-ple'jik) 1. blocking transmission of impulses through the sympathetic and parasympathetic ganglia. 2. an agent that blocks impulses through the sympathetic and parasympathetic ganglia.

gangosa (gang-go'sah) destructive ulceration of the pharynx, nose and face.

gangrene (gang'grēn) death of tissue in considerable mass, usually associated with loss of vascular (nutritive) supply and followed by bacterial invasion and putrefaction. **anemic g.**, gangrene due to obstruction of the blood supply. **angioneurotic g.**, a condition due to thrombosis of the arteries and veins. **diabetic g.**, moist gangrene associated with diabetes. **dry g.**, that occurring without subsequent bacterial decomposition, the tissues becoming dry and shriveled. **embolic g.**, a condition following cutting off of blood supply by embolism. **gas g.**, a rapidly spreading, necrotizing inflammation caused by various species of Clostridium. **moist g.**, that associated with proteolytic decomposition resulting from bacterial action. **primary g.**, a form which does not follow a local inflammation. **secondary g.**, a form which follows a local inflammation. **senile g.**, a form that attacks the extremities of the aged. **symmetric g.**, gangrene of corresponding parts on either side, due to vasomotor disturbances. **white g.**, gangrene from local anemia following complete lymphatic obstruction.

gangrenosis (gang"grē-no'sis) a general gangrenous condition.

gangrenous (gang'grē-nus) affected with gangrene.

ganoblast (gan'o-blast) ameloblast.

Gantrisin (gan'tri-sin) trademark for preparations of sulfisoxazole.

gap (gap) an unoccupied interval in time or an opening in space. **air-bone g.**, the variation between the audiographic curves for air- and bone-conducted stimuli, as an indication of loss of bone conduction of the ear. **auscultatory g.**, a period in which sound is not heard in the auscultatory method of sphygmomanometry. **chromatid g.**, a nonstaining region in a chromatid. **interocclusal g.**, interocclusal distance. **isochromatid g.**, a nonstaining region at the same level in two sister chromatids. **silent g.**, auscultatory gap. **spark g.**, the space between the terminals of a high-tension circuit across which the spark is to jump.

gargle (gar'gl) 1. a solution for rinsing mouth and throat. 2. to rinse the mouth and throat by holding a solution in the open mouth and agitating it by expulsion of air from the lungs.

gargoylism (gar'goil-izm) a hereditary condition with large head, grotesque facies, thickening of lips, nostrils and ears, deformed limbs and clawlike hands, associated with Hurler's syndrome.

gas (gas) 1. one of the four ultimate states of matter, being composed of widely scattered molecules that are freely movable. 2. an aeriform fluid without independent shape or volume. adj., **gas'eous. laughing g.**, nitrous oxide. **marsh g.**, methane. **olefiant g.**, ethylene. **tear g.**, one which produces severe lacrimation by irritating the conjunctivae.

gaskin (gas'kin) the thigh of a horse.

gasometry (gas-om'ĕ-tre) measurement of the amount of gas present in a mixture.

gaster (gas'ter) [Gr.] stomach.

gasterangiemphraxis (gas″ter-an″je-em-frak′sis) obstruction of blood vessels of the stomach.

Gasterophilus (-of′ĭ-lus) a genus of flies, the horse bot flies, the larvae of which develop in the gastrointestinal tract of horses and may sometimes infect man.

gastr(o)- (gas′tro) word element [Gr.], *stomach.*

gastradenitis (gas″trad-ĕ-ni′tis) inflammation of the stomach glands.

gastralgia (gas-tral′je-ah) pain in the stomach.

gastramine (gas′trah-min) betazole.

gastraneuria (gas″trah-nu′re-ah) defective nervous tone of the stomach.

gastrasthenia (gas″tras-the′ne-ah) a weak state of the stomach.

gastratrophia (gas″trah-tro′fe-ah) atrophy of the stomach.

gastrectasia (gas″trek-ta′ze-ah) dilatation of the stomach.

gastrectomy (gas-trek′to-me) excision of the stomach (*total gastrectomy*) or of a portion of it (*partial* or *subtotal gastrectomy.*)

gastrectosis (gas″trek-to′sis) gastrectasia.

gastric (gas′trik) pertaining to the stomach.

gastricsin (gas-trik′sin) a proteolytic enzyme isolated from gastric juices, differing from pepsin in molecular weight and amino acids at the N terminal.

gastricism (gas′trĭ-sizm) gastric disorder.

gastrin (gas′trin) a substance in extracts of pyloric mucosa which stimulates secretion by the gastric glands.

gastritis (gas-tri′tis) inflammation of the stomach. **atrophic g.,** a form with atrophy of mucous membrane and glands. **hypertrophic g.,** gastritis with infiltration and enlargement of the glands. **phlegmonous g.,** a variety with abscesses in the stomach walls. **polypous g.,** hypertrophic gastritis with polyp-like projections of the mucosa. **pseudomembranous g.,** a variety in which false membrane occurs in patches within the stomach.

gastroacephalus (gas″tro-a-sef′ah-lus) a twin monster, the autosite bearing a headless parasite on its abdomen.

gastroanastomosis (-ah-nas″to-mo′sis) gastrogastrostomy.

gastroblonorrhea (-blen″o-re′ah) excessive secretion of mucus in the stomach.

gastrobrosis (-bro′sis) perforation of the stomach.

gastrocele (gas′tro-sēl) hernia of the stomach.

gastrocolitis (gas″tro-ko-li′tis) inflammation of stomach and colon.

gastrocoloptosis (-ko″lop-to′sis) downward displacement of stomach and colon.

gastrocolostomy (-ko-los′to-me) anastomosis of the stomach to the colon.

gastrocolotomy (-ko-lot′o-me) incision of stomach and colon.

gastrocutaneous (-ku-ta′ne-us) pertaining to the stomach and skin, or communicating with stomach and the cutaneous surface of the body.

gastrodiaphane (-di′ah-fān) electric light for use in gastrodiaphanoscopy.

gastrodiaphanoscopy (-di-af″ah-nos′ko-pe)

examination of the stomach by transillumination of its walls.

gastrodidymus (gas″tro-did′ĭ-mus) symmetrical conjoined twins joined in the abdominal region.

Gastrodiscoides (-dis-koi′dēz) a genus of trematodes parasitic in the intestinal tract.

gastroduodenal (-du″o-de′nal) pertaining to stomach and duodenum.

gastroduodenectomy (-du″o-de-nek′to-me) excision of stomach and duodenum.

gastroduodenitis (-du-od″ĕ-ni′tis) inflammation of stomach and duodenum.

gastroduodenostomy (-du″o-dē-nos′to-me) anastomosis of the stomach to a formerly remote part of the duodenum.

gastrodynia (-din′e-ah) pain in the stomach.

gastroenteralgia (-en″ter-al′je-ah) pain in stomach and intestines.

gastroenteric (-en-ter′ik) pertaining to stomach and intestines.

gastroenteritis (-en″ter-i′tis) inflammation of stomach and intestines.

gastroenteroanastomosis (-en″ter-o-ah-nas″-to-mo′sis) anastomosis of the stomach to the intestine.

gastroenterocolitis (-en″ter-o-ko-li′tis) inflammation of stomach, small intestine and colon.

gastroenterologist (-en″ter-ol′o-jist) a specialist in gastroenterology.

gastroenterology (-en″ter-ol′o-je) study of diseases of stomach and intestine.

gastroenteropathy (-en″ter-op′ah-the) any disease of stomach and intestine.

gastroenteroptosis (-en″ter-op-to′sis) downward displacement of stomach and intestines.

gastroenterostomy (-en″ter-os′to-me) anastomosis of stomach to intestine.

gastroenterotomy (-en″ter-ot′o-me) incision of stomach and intestine.

gastroepiploic (-ep″ĭ-plo′ik) pertaining to stomach and epiploon.

gastroesophagitis (-e-sof″ah-ji′tis) inflammation of stomach and esophagus.

gastroesophagostomy (-e-sof″ah-gos′to-me) anastomosis between the stomach and esophagus.

gastrogastrostomy (-gas-tros′to-me) anastomosis of two previously remote portions of the stomach.

gastrogavage (-gah-vahzh′) artificial feeding through a tube passed into the stomach.

gastrogenic (-jen′ik) originating in the stomach.

gastrograph (gas′tro-graf) instrument for registering motions of stomach.

gastrohelcosis (gas″tro-hel-ko′sis) ulceration of the stomach.

gastrohepatic (-hĕ-pat′ik) pertaining to stomach and liver.

gastrohepatitis (-hep″ah-ti′tis) inflammation of stomach and liver.

gastrohydrorrhea (-hi″dro-re′ah) secretion of watery fluid by the stomach.

gastrohyperneuria (-hi″per-nu′re-ah) excessive activity of the stomach nerves.

gastrohyponeuria (gas″tro-hi″po-nu′re-ah) defective activity of the stomach nerves.

gastroileac (-il′e-ak) pertaining to stomach and ileum.

gastroileitis (-il″e-i′tis) inflammation of stomach and ileum.

gastroileostomy (-il″e-os′to-me) anastomosis of the stomach to the ileum.

gastrointestinal (-in-tes′tī-nal) pertaining to stomach and intestine.

gastrojejunocolic (-je-ju″no-kol′ik) pertaining to stomach, jejunum and colon.

gastrojejunostomy (-je-ju-nos′to-me) anastomosis of the stomach to the jejunum.

gastrolienal (-li′ē-nal) pertaining to stomach and spleen.

gastrolith (gas′tro-lith) a calculus in the stomach.

gastrolithiasis (gas″tro-lī-thi′ah-sis) formation of gastroliths.

gastrology (gas-trol′o-je) study of the stomach and its diseases.

gastrolysis (gas-trol′ī-sis) freeing of the stomach from adhesions.

gastromalacia (gas″tro-mah-la′she-ah) softening of the wall of the stomach.

gastromegaly (-meg′ah-le) enlargement of the stomach.

gastromelus (gas-trom′ē-lus) a fetal monster with a leg on the abdomen.

gastromycosis (gas″tro-mi-ko′sis) fungus infection of the stomach.

gastromyotomy (-mi-ot′o-me) pyloromyotomy.

gastromyxorrhea (-mik″so-re′ah) excessive secretion of mucus by the stomach.

gastronephritis (-ne-fri′tis) inflammation of stomach and kidney.

gastropancreatitis (-pan″kre-ah-ti′-tis) inflammation of stomach and pancreas.

gastroparalysis (-pah-ral′ī-sis) paralysis of the stomach.

gastroparesis (-par′ē-sis) gastroparalysis.

gastropathy (gas-trop′ah-the) any disease of the stomach.

gastrophrenic (gas″tro-fren′ik) pertaining to stomach and diaphragm.

Gastrophilus (gas-trof′ī-lus) Gasterophilus.

gastroplasty (gas′tro-plas″te) plastic repair of the stomach.

gastroplegia (gas″tro-ple′je-ah) gastroparalysis.

gastroplication (-pli-ka′shun) reefing and stitching of the stomach wall.

gastroptosis (gas″trop-to′sis) downward displacement of the stomach.

gastroptyxis (gas″tro-tik′sis) an operation for reducing a dilated stomach.

gastropulmonary (-pul′mo-ner″e) pertaining to the stomach and lungs.

gastropylorectomy (-pi″lo-rek′to-me) excision of pyloric part of the stomach.

gastropyloric (-pi-lor′ik) pertaining to the stomach and pylorus.

gastrorrhagia (-ra′je-ah) hemorrhage from the stomach.

gastrorrhaphy (gas-tror′ah-fe) suture of the stomach.

gastrorrhea (gas″tro-re′ah) excessive secretion by the glands of the stomach.

gastrorrhexis (-rek′sis) rupture of the stomach.

gastroschisis (gas-tros′kī-sis) developmental anomaly resulting from faulty closure of the body wall along the midventral line.

gastroscope (gas′tro-skōp) an endoscope especially designed for passage into the stomach to permit examination of its interior.

gastroscopy (gas-tros′ko-pe) inspection of the interior of the stomach with a gastroscope.

gastrosis (gas-tro′sis) any disease of the stomach.

gastrospasm (gas′tro-spazm) spasm of the stomach.

gastrospiry (gas′tro-spi″re) aerophagy.

gastrosplenic (gas″tro-splen′ik) pertaining to stomach and spleen.

gastrostaxis (-stak′sis) oozing of blood from the stomach.

gastrostenosis (-ste-no′sis) abnormal constriction of the stomach.

gastrogavage (gas-tros″to-gah-vahzh′) feeding through a gastric fistula.

gastrostolavage (-lah-vahzh′) washing of the stomach through a gastric fistula.

gastrostoma (gas-tros′to-mah) a gastric fistula.

gastrostomy (gas-tros′to-me) fistulization of the stomach.

gastrosuccorrhea (gas″tro-suk″ō-re′ah) continuous secretion of gastric juice.

gastrotherapy (-ther′ah-pe) 1. treatment of stomach diseases. 2. treatment of pernicious anemia with extract of gastric mucosa.

gastrothoracopagus (-thor″ah-kop′ah-gus) symmetrical conjoined twins joined at the abdomen and thorax.

gastrotomy (gas-trot′o-me) incision of the stomach.

gastrotonometer (gas″tro-to-nom′ē-ter) an instrument for measuring intragastric pressure.

gastrotrachelotomy (-tra″kel-ot′o-me) cesarean section with a transverse incision across the cervix.

gastrotropic (-trop′ik) having affinity for the stomach.

gastrotympanites (-tim″pah-ni′tēz) tympanitic distention of the stomach.

gastrula (gas′troo-lah) the developing product of conception when it consists of the three germ layers (ectoderm, mesoderm and entoderm), occupying their characteristic positions.

gastrulation (gas″troo-la′shun) the formation of a gastrula.

gatophilia (gat″o-fil′e-ah) abnormal fondness for cats.

gatophobia (-fo′be-ah) morbid dread of cats.

gauntlet (gawnt′let) a bandage covering hand and fingers like a glove.

gauss (gows) the unit of magnetic flux density.

gauze (gawz) white cotton cloth of plain weave of varying closeness. **absorbent g.,** white cotton cloth of various thread counts and weights, supplied in various lengths and widths and in different forms (rolls or folds).

petrolatum g., a sterile material produced by saturation of sterile absorbent gauze with sterile white petrolatum.

gavage (gah-vahzh′) [Fr.] feeding by a tube passed into the stomach.

g.cal. gram calorie (small calorie).

g-cm. gram-centimeter.

Gd chemical symbol, *gadolinium*.

Ge chemical symbol, *germanium*.

gel (jel) 1. a suspension in a water medium of an insoluble drug in hydrated form, the suspended particles approaching or attaining colloidal size. 2. a solid colloidal solution. **aluminum hydroxide g.**, a preparation of aluminum oxide in the form of hydrated oxide; used to reduce gastric acidity, as a demulcent and protective for gastric mucosa, as a vehicle to increase absorption of orally administered penicillin, and in conjunction with a low phosphorus diet in the treatment of renal disease. **aluminum phosphate g.**, a water suspension of aluminum phosphate and some flavoring agents; used as a gastric antacid, astringent and demulcent.

gelasmus (jē-las′mus) hysterical laughter.

gelatin (jel′ah-tin) a substance obtained by partial hydrolysis of collagen derived from skin, white connective tissue, and bones of animals; used as a vehicle for various drugs or in manufacture of capsules, and suggested for intravenous use as a plasma substitute. **zinc g.**, a preparation of zinc oxide, gelatin, glycerin and purified water, applied topically as a protective.

gelatinase (jē-lat′ĭ-nās) an enzyme which liquefies gelatin.

gelatiniferous (jel″ah-tin-if′er-us) producing gelatin.

gelatinize (jē-lat′ĭ-nīz) to convert into a jelly.

gelatinoid (jē-lat′ĭ-noid) resembling gelatin.

gelatinolytic (jē-lat″ĭ-no-lit′ik) splitting up gelatin.

gelatinosa (jel″ah-tĭ-no′sah) substantia gelatinosa.

gelatinous (jē-lat′ĭ-nus) like jelly or gelatin.

gelation (jē-la′shun) conversion of a sol into a gel.

Gelfilm (jel′film) trademark for absorbable gelatin film.

Gelfoam (jel′fōm) trademark for preparations of absorbable gelatin sponge.

gelose (jel′ōs) agar.

gelosis (je-lo′sis) a hard, swollen lump.

gemellology (jem″el-ol′o-je) the scientific study of twins and twinning.

geminate (jem′ĭ-nāt) paired; in twos.

geminus (jem′ĭ-nus), pl. *gem′ini* [L.] a twin. **gem′ini aequa′les,** monozygotic twins.

gemmangioma (jem″an-je-o′mah) a vascular tumor composed of embryonal cells.

gemmation (jē-ma′shun) development of a new organism from a protuberance on the body of the parent, a form of asexual reproduction.

gemmule (jem′ūl) early name for one of the submicroscopic particles in a cell which manifest specific functions.

Gemonil (jem′o-nil) trademark for a preparation of metharbital.

gen (jēn) gene.

-gen (jen) word element [Gr.], *an agent that produces.*

genal (je′nal) pertaining to the cheek.

gender (jen′der) the category (male, female or intersex) to which an individual is assigned on the basis of sex.

gene (jēn) one of the biologic units of heredity contained in the chromosome, each of which controls the inheritance of one or more characteristics. **allelic g's**, genes situated at corresponding loci in a pair of chromosomes **complementary g's**, two independent pairs of genes, neither of which will produce its effect in the absence of the other. **dominant g.**, an allele that produces an effect in the organism regardless of the state of the corresponding allele. **holandric g's**, genes located on the Y chromosome and appearing only in male offspring. **hologenic g's**, genes located on the X chromosome and appearing only in female offspring. **lethal g.**, one whose presence brings about the death of the organism or permits survival only under certain conditions. **mutant g.**, one that has undergone a detectable mutation. **nonstructural g.**, units of a chromosome that are not concerned with formation of templates, i.e. messenger RNA; the operator and regulator genes. **operator g.**, one that controls, through interaction with a repressor, the activity of adjacent structural genes. **recessive g.**, one that produces an effect in the organism only when it is transmitted by both parents. **regulator g.**, a segment of a chromosome that directs the synthesis of a repressor. **repressor g.**, one that controls formation of a repressor. **sex-linked g.**, one that is carried on or linked to a sex chromosome (X or Y). **structural g.**, one that forms templates (messenger RNA) and is thereby responsible for the amino acid sequence of specific polypeptides. **supplementary g's**, two independent pairs of genes which interact in such a way that one dominant will produce its effect even in the absence of the other, but the second requires the presence of the first to be effective.

generation (jen″ē-ra′shun) 1. the process of reproduction. 2. a class composed of all individuals removed by the same number of successive ancestors from a common predecessor, or occupying positions on the same level in a genealogical (pedigree) chart. **alternate g.**, the alternate generation by asexual and sexual means in an animal or plant species. **asexual g.**, production of a new organism not originating from union of gametes. **direct g.**, asexual generation. **filial g., first**, the offspring of the first mating in a particular genetic experiment. **filial g., second,** offspring resulting from mating of two individuals of the first filial generation in a particular genetic experiment. **nonsexual g.**, asexual generation. **parental g.**, the two individuals first mating in a particular genetic study. **sexual g.**, production of a new organism from the zygote formed by the union of gametes. **spontaneous g.**, the alleged development of living organisms from lifeless matter; abiogenesis.

generative (jen′ĕ-ra″tiv) pertaining to reproduction

generic (jĕ-ner′ik) 1. pertaining to a genus. 2. distinctive of a kind.

genesiology (jĕ-ne″ze-ol′o-je) the science of generation.

genesis (jen′ĕ-sis) creation; origination; used as a word termination joined to an element indicating the thing created, e.g. carcinogenesis.

-genesis (jen′ĕ-sis) word element [Gr.], *creation.* adj., **-genet′ic.**

genetic (jĕ-net′ik) pertaining to or carried by a gene or genes; hereditary.

geneticist (jĕ-net′ĭ-sist) a student of genetics.

genetics (jĕ-net′iks) the branch of biology dealing with the phenomena of heredity and the laws governing it. **biochemical g.**, the science concerned with the chemical and physical nature of genes and the mechanism by which they control the development and maintenance of the organism. **clinical g.**, the study of the possible genetic factors influencing the occurrence of a pathologic condition.

genetopathy (jen″ĕ-top′ah-the) any disease affecting the reproductive function.

genetous (jen′ĕ-tus) dating from fetal life.

Geneva Convention (jĕ-ne′vah) an international agreement of 1864, whereby the signatory nations pledged themselves to treat the wounded and the army medical and nursing staffs as neutrals on the field of battle.

genial (je′ne-al) pertaining to the chin.

genic (jen′ik) pertaining to genes.

-genic (jen′ik) word element [Gr.], *giving rise to; causing.*

genicular (jĕ-nik′u-lar) pertaining to the knee.

geniculate (jĕ-nik′u-lāt) bent like a knee.

geniculum (jĕ-nik′u-lum), pl. *genic′ula* [L.] a little knee; used in anatomic nomenclature to designate a sharp kneelike bend in a small structure or organ.

genion (je′ne-on) apex of lower genial tubercle.

genioplasty (je′ne-o-plas″te) plastic surgery of the chin.

genital (jen′ĭ-tal) pertaining to reproduction.

genitalia (jen″ĭ-ta′le-ah) the organs of the reproductive system. **external g.**, those organs of the reproductive system that are external to the body, including the penis and scrotum in the male and the pudendum and clitoris in the female. **indifferent g.**, the reproductive organs of the embryo prior to the establishment of definitive sex.

genitaloid (jen′ĭ-tal-oid″) pertaining to the primordial sex cells, before future sexuality is distinguishable.

genito- (jen′ĭ-to) word element [L.], relating to the organs of reproduction.

genitofemoral (jen″ĭ-to-fem′o-ral) pertaining to the genital organs and thigh.

genitoplasty (jen′ĭ-to-plas″te) plastic surgery on the genital organs.

genitourinary (jen″ĭ-to-u′rĭ-ner″e) pertaining to reproductive and urinary organs.

genoblast (jen′o-blast) 1. the nucleus of the impregnated ovum. 2. a mature germ cell.

genoceptor (jen′o-sep″ter) the reproductive element of a cell.

genocide (jen′o-sīd) the mass destruction of individuals because of their race.

genodermatosis (je″no-der″mah-to′sis), pl. *genodermato′ses*, a genetically determined disease or malformation which involves the skin.

genome (je′nōm) the complete set of hereditary factors contained in the haploid set of chromosomes. adj., **genom′ic.**

genoneme (jen′o-nēm) the axial thread of a chromosome in which lie the genes.

genotype (je′no-tīp) the hereditary constitution of an organism. adj., **genotyp′ic.**

-genous (jen′us) word element [Gr.], *arising or resulting from; produced by.*

gentian (jen′shan) the dried rhizome and roots of *Gentiana lutea;* used as a bitter tonic.

gentianophilous (jen″shan-of′ĭ-lus) staining readily with gentian violet.

gentianophobous (jen″shan-of′ŏ-bus) not staining with gentian violet.

gentiavern (jen′sha-vern) methylrosaniline.

genu (je′nu), pl. *gen′ua* [L.] the knee. **g. extror′sum,** bowleg. **g. intror′sum,** knock knee. **g. recurva′tum,** hyperextensibility of the knee joint. **g. val′gum,** knock knee. **g. va′rum,** bowleg.

genuclast (jen′u-klast) an instrument for breaking up adhesions of the knee joint.

genus (je′nus), pl. *gen′era* [L.] a taxonomic category (taxon) subordinate to a tribe (or subtribe) and superior to a species (or subgenus).

genyantralgia (jen″e-an-tral′je-ah) pain in the maxillary antrum.

genyantritis (-an-tri′tis) inflammation of maxillary antrum.

genyplasty (jen′ĭ-plas″te) plastic surgery of the cheek.

geobiology (je″o-bi-ol′o-je) the biology of terrestrial life.

geode (je′ōd) a dilated lymph space.

geomedicine (je″o-med′ĭ-sin) the branch of medicine dealing with the influence of climatic and environmental conditions on health.

geophagism (je-of′ah-jizm) geophagy.

geophagy (je-of′ah-je) the eating of earth (soil) or clay.

geotaxis (je″o-tak′sis) an orientation movement in response to the stimulation of gravity.

geotragia (-tra′je-ah) geophagy.

geotrichosis (-trĭ-ko′sis) infection with fungus of the genus Geotrichum.

Geotrichum (je-ot′rĭ-kum) a genus of fungi sometimes found in lesions in the lungs.

geotropism (je-ot′ro-pizm) a growth curvature occurring in response to the stimulation of gravity.

gephyrophobia (je-fi″ro-fo′be-ah) fear of walking on a bridge or other structure near the water.

geratic (jĕ-rat′ik) pertaining to old age.

geratology (jer″ah-tol′o-je) gereology.

gereology (jer″e-ol′o-je) the science dealing with old age.

geriatrics (-at′riks) the department of medicine dealing especially with the problems of aging and diseases of the elderly. **dental g.,** gerodontics.

geriodontics (-o-don′tiks) gerodontics.

germ (jerm) 1. a pathogenic microorganism. 2. a spore. 3. the primitive beginning of a developing embryo. **dental g.,** collective tissues from which a tooth is formed. **enamel g.,** the epithelial rudiment of the enamel organ. **wheat g.,** the embryo of wheat which contains tocopherol, thiamine, riboflavin and other vitamins.

germanin (jer′mah-nin) suramin sodium.

germanium (jer-ma′ne-um) chemical element *(see table),* at. no. 32, symbol Ge.

germicidal (jer″mǐ-si′dal) destructive to pathogenic microorganisms.

germicide (jer′mǐ-sīd) an agent that destroys pathogenic microorganisms.

germinal (jer′mǐ-nal) pertaining to a germ.

germination (jer″mǐ-na′shun) the beginning of development of a plant embryo.

germinative (jer′mǐ-na″tiv) germinal.

gerocomia (jer″o-ko′me-ah) the hygiene of old age.

geroderma (-der′mah) wrinkling and thickening of the skin, like that of old age.

gerodermia (-der′me-ah) geroderma.

gerodontics (-don′tiks) dentistry dealing with the dental problems of older people. adj., **gerodon′tic.**

gerodontist (-don′tist) a dentist specializing in gerodontics.

gerodontology (-don-tol′o-je) study of the dentition and dental problems in the aged and aging.

geromarasmus (-mah-raz′mus) the emaciation of old age.

geromorphism (-mor′fizm) premature old age.

gerontal (jě-ron′tal) pertaining to old age.

gerontologist (jer″on-tol′o-jist) a specialist in the problems of aging in all their aspects—clinical, biological, historical and sociological.

gerontology (-tol′o-je) the study of old age, its phenomena, diseases, etc.

gerontopia (-to′pe-ah) the improved sight of old age.

gerontotherapeutics (je-ron″to-ther″ah-pu′-tiks) the science of retarding and preventing the development of many of the aspects of senescence.

gerontoxon (jer″on-tok′son) arcus senilis.

gestagen (jes′tah-jen) a hormone with progestational activity.

gestaltism (gě-stawl′tizm) the theory in psychology that the objects of mind, as immediately presented to direct experience, come as complete unanalyzable wholes or forms (Gestalten) which cannot be split up into parts.

gestation (jes-ta′shun) the development of the new individual within the uterus, from conception to birth. **abdominal g.,** development of the fertilized ovum in the abdominal cavity. **ectopic g.,** development of the fertilized ovum

outside the uterine cavity; ectopic pregnancy. **exterior g.,** development of an infant after emergence from the uterus until the time of quadrupedal locomotion, when it might still be considered a fetus. **interior g.,** development of the human young up to the time of emergence from the uterus. **tubular g.,** tubal pregnancy.

gestosis (jes-to′sis) any toxemic manifestation in pregnancy.

geumaphobia (gu″mah-fo′be-ah) abnormal fear of tastes or flavors.

GFR glomerular filtration rate.

ghost (gōst) a faint or shadowy figure lacking the customary substance of reality. **blood g.,** phantom corpuscle.

G.I. gastrointestinal; globin (or) insulin.

giantism (ji′an-tizm) gigantism.

Giardia (je-ar′de-ah) a genus of flagellate protozoa parasitic in many species of vertebrates. **G. intestina′lis,** a species parasitic in the intestines of man. **G. lam′blia,** *Giardia intestinalis.*

giardiasis (je″ar-di′ah-sis) infection with Giardia.

gibbosity (gǐ-bos′ǐ-te) the condition of being humped.

gibbous (gib′us) humped; protuberant.

gid (gid) staggers.

giga- (gi′gah) word element [Gr.], *huge;* used in naming units of measurement to designate an amount 10^9 (one billion) times the size of the unit to which it is joined, e.g. gigameter (10^9 meters); symbol G.

gigantism (ji-gan′tizm) abnormal overgrowth of the body or of a part. **eunuchoid g.,** gigantism in which the body shows the proportions of a eunuch and sexual deficiency.

gigantocyte (ji-gan′to-sīt) a very large erythrocyte.

gigantosoma (ji-gan″to-so′mah) gigantism.

ginger (jin′jer) the dried rhizome of *Zingiber officinale,* with outer cortical layers partially or completely removed; used as a flavoring agent.

gingiva (jin-ji′vah), pl. *gingi′vae* [L.] the fleshy structure covering the tooth-bearing border of the jaw. adj., **gingi′val. alveolar g.,** the portion overlying the alveolar process and firmly attached to it. **areolar g.,** the portion attached to the alveolar process by loose areolar connective tissue. **cemental g.,** the portion attached to cementum of a tooth, but lying crownward of the alveolar process. **free g.,** the portion covering part of the crowns of the teeth, but not attached to them. **marginal g.,** free gingiva.

gingivalgia (jin″jǐ-val′je-ah) neuralgia of the gingiva.

gingivally (jin-ji′val-e) toward the gingiva.

gingivectomy (jin″jǐ-vek′to-me) surgical excision of all loose infected and diseased gingival tissue.

gingivitis (-vi′tis) inflammation of the gingiva. **atrophic g., senile,** a condition characterized by hyperkeratinization and areas of desquamation in the gingiva. **fusospirochetal g.,** ulcerative gingivitis, necrotizing.

herpetic g., infection of gingiva by the herpetic virus. **ulcerative g.**, **necrotizing**, an infection characterized by redness and swelling, necrosis, pain, hemorrhage, a necrotic odor and often a pseudomembrane. **ulceromembranous g.**, **Vincent's g.**, ulcerative gingivitis, necrotizing.

gingivo- (jin″ji-vo) word element [L.], *gingival*.

gingivoglossitis (jin″ji-vo-glos-si′tis) inflammation of the gingiva and tongue.

gingivolabial (-la′be-al) pertaining to the gingiva and lips.

gingivoplasty (jin″ji-vo-plas″te) surgical remodeling of the gingiva.

gingivosis (jin″ji-vo′sis) a chronic, diffuse inflammation of the gingivae, with desquamation of papillary epithelium and mucous membrane.

gingivostomatitis (jin″ji-vo-sto″mah-ti′tis) inflammation of the gingiva and oral mucosa. **herpetic g.**, an infection of the gingivae and oral mucosa by herpetic virus, characterized by fever, redness and swelling, without necrosis of the gingival papillae or gingival margins.

ginglymo-arthrodial (jing″gli-mo-ar-thro′de-al) partly ginglymoid and partly arthrodial.

ginglymoid (jing′gli-moid) resembling a hinge.

ginglymus (jing′gli-mus) a joint that allows movement in but one plane, forward and backward like a door hinge; called also *hinge joint*.

girdle (ger′dl) an encircling or confining structure. **pectoral g.**, shoulder girdle. **pelvic g.**, the encircling bony structure supporting the lower limbs. **shoulder g.**, the encircling bony structure supporting the upper limbs. **thoracic g.**, shoulder girdle.

Gitaligin (ji-tal′i-jin) trademark for a preparation of amorphous gitalin.

gitalin (jit′ah-lin) a glycoside of digitalis. **amorphous g.**, a glycosidal constituent of the leaves of *Digitalis purpurea*; used as a cardiotonic.

githagism (gith′ah-jizm) a condition caused by poisoning with corn-cockle, *Lychnis githago*.

gizzard (giz′ard) the muscular second stomach of a bird.

glabella (glah-bel′ah) space between the eyebrows.

glabrous (gla′brus) smooth.

gladiolus (glah-di′o-lus) the main portion of the sternum.

glairy (glār′e) resembling white of an egg.

gland (gland) an organ that produces a specific product or secretion. adj., **glan′dular. accessory g.**, a detached mass of glandular tissue near or at some distance from a gland of similar structure. **acinar g.**, **acinous g.**, one made up of several oval or spherical sacs (acini). **adrenal g.**, a triangular structure above either kidney, an endocrine gland consisting of cortex and medulla, the latter secreting epinephrine and the cortex secreting hormones affecting growth and the gonads of the individual. **aggregate g's**, **agminated g's**, Peyer's patches. **albuminous g's**, certain glands of the digestive tract secreting a watery fluid. **alveolar g.**, acinar gland. **anacrine g.**, exocrine gland. **anomalous g.**, endocrine gland. **aortic g.**, aortic body. **apocrine g.**, one whose discharged secretion contains part of the secreting cells. **axillary g's**, lymphatic nodes situated in the axilla. **g. of Bartholin**, vulvovaginal gland. **Blandin's g.**, Nuhn's gland. **Bowman's g's**, tubular glands in the olfactory mucosa. **bronchial g's**, lymph nodes at the root of a bronchus. **Bruch's g's**, lymph follicles in conjunctiva of lower lid. **Brunner's g's**, glands in the duodenum secreting intestinal juice. **bulbocavernous g.**, **bulbourethral g.**, one of two glands embedded in the substance of the sphincter of the urethra, posterior to the membranous part of the urethra. **cardiac g's**, those of the cardiac extremity of the stomach. **carotid g.**, see under *body*. **celiac g's**, lymph nodes anterior to the abdominal aorta. **ceruminous g's**, glands which secrete cerumen. **cervical g's**, lymph nodes of the neck. **choroid g.**, the choroid plexus, regarded as the secretor of the cerebrospinal fluid. **circumanal g's**, specialized sweat and sebaceous glands around the anus. **closed g.**, endocrine gland. **Cobelli's g's**, glands in the mucous membrane of the esophagus. **coccygeal g.**, a vascular body near tip of coccyx. **compound g.**, one with branching ducts. **conglobate g.**, a lymphatic node. **conglomerate g.**, compound gland. **Cowper's g's**, two glands near bulb of corpus spongiosum. **dental g.**, one of the white areas on the mucous membrane of the jaw over the point of emergence of the tooth. **ductless g.**, endocrine gland. **duodenal g's**, Brunner's glands. **Duverney's g.**, vulvovaginal gland. **Ebner's g's**, mucous glands of the tongue. **eccrine g.**, one which produces a simple fluid secretion without admixture of cell plasm or cell contents. **endocrine g.**, one whose secretion enters directly into the blood or lymph and is not discharged through a duct. **enterochromaffin g.**, a type found in the mucosa of the intestinal canal, characterized by the presence in the cell protoplasm of granules which stain with chromium salts and are impregnable with silver. **excretory g.**, one that excretes waste products from the system. **exocrine g.**, one whose secretion is discharged through a duct opening on an internal or external surface of the body. **Fränkel's g's**, minute glands that open below the edge of the vocal cord. **fundus g's**, delomorphous cells. **Galeati's g's**, the crypts of Lieberkühn. **gastric g's**, the secreting glands of the stomach, including the fundus, cardiac and pyloric glands. **Gay's g's**, highly developed sweat glands. **genal g's**, glands in the submucous tissue of the cheek. **glossopalatine g's**, mucous glands at the posterior end of the smaller sublingual glands. **gustatory g's**, Ebner's glands. **guttural g.**, one of the mucous glands of the pharynx. **hair g.**, the sebaceous gland of a hair follicle. **Harder's g's**, **harderian g's**, accessory lacrimal glands at the inner corner of the eye in animals that have nictitating membranes. **haversian g's**, folds on synovial surfaces regarded as se-cretors of synovial fluid. **hematopoietic g's,** glands which take part in formation of the blood elements. **hemolymph g's,** glands containing blood sinuses occurring along with the lymph nodes. **heterocrine g's,** those having a mixed (mucous and albuminous) secretion. **hibernating g.,** a collection of brown fatty tissue in various regions of the body in hibernating animals. **holocrine g.,** one whose discharged secretion contains the entire secreting cells. **Huguier's g's,** two minor vaginal glands. **incretory g's,** endocrine glands. **interscapular g.,** a mass of lymphoid tissue in the embryo. **intestinal g's,** straight tubular glands in the mucous membrane of the intestines, opening, in the small intestine, between the bases of the villi, and containing argentaffin cells. **jugular g.,** a lymph node behind the clavicular insertion of the sternomastoid muscle. **Krause's g's,** mucous glands in the middle portion of the conjunctiva. **lacrimal g's,** the glands which secrete tears. **g's of Lieberkühn,** intestinal glands. **Littre's g's,** racemose glands in spongy portion of urethra. **Luschka's g.,** coccygeal gland. **lymph g., lymphatic g.,** see under *node*. **mammary g.,** the milk-se-creting organ of female mammals, existing also in a rudimentary state in the male. **meibomian g's,** sebaceous follicles between the cartilage and conjunctiva of eyelids. **merocrine g.,** one whose discharged secretion contains no part of the secreting cells. **Méry's g's,** Cowper's glands. **mixed g's,** those that are both mucous and serous. **Moll's g's,** small glands at the edges of the eyelids. **monoptychic g.,** one in which the tubules or alveoli are lined with a single layer of secreting cells. **Montgomery's g's,** sebaceous glands in the mammary areola. **Morgagni's g's,** Littre's glands. **muciparous g's, mucous g's,** glands which secrete mucus. **nabothian g's,** see under *cyst*. **Nuhn's g.,** a mucous gland on either side of the frenulum linguae; a sebaceous gland. **open g.,** exocrine gland. **pacchionian g's,** see under *body*. **parathyroid g's,** small bodies in the region of the thyroid gland, developed from the entoderm of the branchial clefts, numbering one to four, commonly two; they are concerned with the metabolism of calcium and phosphorus. **parotid g.,** the large salivary gland in front of the ear. **peptic g's,** a set of mucous glands on the mucous membrane of the stomach, believed to secrete the gastric juice. **Peyer's g's,** see under *patch*. **pilous g.,** the sebaceous gland of a hair follicle. **pineal g.,** a small, conelike, glandular body between the two superior quadrigeminal bodies and connected with the thalami by the habenula. **pituitary g.,** an epithelial body of dual origin, resting on the sphenoid bone and connected to the brain by a stalk; it consists of two lobes, the *anterior lobe,* secreting several important hormones which regulate the proper functioning of the other endocrine glands, and the *posterior lobe,* whose cells are sites of storage

for a pressor and an oxytocic principle; called also *hypophysis*. **preen g.,** a large, compound alveolar structure on the back of birds, above the base of the tail, which secretes an oily "water-proofing" material that the bird applies to its feathers and skin by preening. **pregnancy g's,** those containing female genital hormone, i.e. the ovarian follicle, corpus luteum and placenta. **prostate g.,** see *prostate*. **pyloric g's,** the pepsin-secreting glands of the stomach situated near the pylorus. **racemose g.,** acinar gland. **Rivini's g.,** sublingual gland. **saccular g.,** one consisting of a sac or sacs, lined with glandular epithelium. **salivary g.,** any gland that secretes saliva, as the parotid, submaxillary or sublingual. **Schueller's g's,** urethral glands. **sebaceous g.,** one of the tiny glands of the skin that secrete an oily material into the hair follicles. **sentinel g.,** an enlarged lymph node, considered to be pathogenic of some pathologic condition elsewhere. **seromucous g.,** one that contains both serous and mucous secreting cells. **serous g's,** albuminous glands. **simple g.,** one with a nonbranching duct. **Skene's g's,** two glands just within the meatus of the female urethra. **solitary g's,** isolated lymphoid nodules in mucosa of the large and small intestines. **sublingual g.,** a salivary gland on either side under the tongue. **submandibular g., submaxillary g.,** a salivary gland on the inner side of each ramus of the lower jaw. **sudoriparous g's,** sweat glands. **suprarenal g.,** adrenal gland. **Susanne's g.,** a mucous gland of the mouth, beneath the alveolingual groove. **sweat g.,** one of the glands of the skin that secrete sweat. **sweat g., apocrine,** a vestigial structure in man, occurring only in certain areas of the body, whose excretory duct coincides with that of a sebaceous gland. **sweat g., eccrine,** one of the glands distributed over the entire body surface which promote cooling of the body by evaporation of their secretion. **target g.,** one specifically affected by a pituitary hormone. **thymus g.,** see *thymus*. **thyroid g.,** an endocrine gland concerned with metabolism, situated in the neck at the level of the fifth to seventh cervical vertebrae, and serving an important function in regulating body metabolism. **tubular g.,** one without an excretory duct, the terminal portion being a straight tubule that opens directly on an epithelial surface. **Tyson's g's,** small sebaceous glands of the corona of the penis and of the labia pudenti. **urethral g's,** Littre's glands. **vaginal g.,** any gland of the vaginal mucosa. **Virchow's g.,** signal node. **vulvovaginal g.,** a minute gland on either side of the vagina, the duct opening on the vulva. **Waldeyer's g's,** glands in the attached edge of the eyelid. **Weber's g's,** the tubular mucous glands of the tongue. **Willis's g's,** corpora albicantia. **Zeis's g's, zeisian g's,** sebaceous glands whose ducts open on the edge of the eyelid. **Zuckerkandl's g.,** small yellow mass sometimes seen between the geniohyoid muscles.

glanders (glan'derz) a contagious and chronic

disease of horses and mules due to infection by *Actinobacillus mallei.*

glandilemma (glan″dĭ-lem′ah) capsule or outer envelope of a gland.

glandula (glan′du-lah), pl. *glan′dulae* [L.] a small gland.

glandule (glan′dūl) a small gland.

glans (glanz), pl. *glan′des* [L.] a small, rounded mass or glandlike body. **g. clitor′idis,** distal end of clitoris. **g. pe′nis,** the cap-shaped expansion of the corpus spongiosum at the end of the penis.

glass (glas) 1. an amorphous, transparent or translucent substance, usually consisting of a mixture of silicates. 2. a container, usually round and straight-sided, made from glass. 3. a lens for aiding vision. **cupping g.,** a glass to be applied to the skin for drawing blood or for local stimulation. **soluble g.,** a potassium or sodium silicate sometimes used in preparing immovable bandages. **water g.,** soluble glass. **Wood's g.,** glass containing nickel oxide, for filtering light rays.

glasses (glas′ez) lenses arranged in a frame holding them in the proper position before the eyes, as an aid to vision. **bifocal g.,** those having two segments which give the proper correction for near and for far vision. **Franklin g., pantoscopic g.,** bifocal glasses.

glaucarubin (glaw″kah-ru′bin) a crystalline glycoside obtained from the fruit of *Simaruba glauca;* used as an amebicide.

glaucoma (glaw-ko′mah) a condition of the eye characterized by increased intraocular pressure. **Donders' g.,** glaucoma simplex. **primary g.,** increased intraocular pressure occurring in an eye without previous disease. **secondary g.,** increased intraocular pressure due to disease or injury to the eye. **g. sim′plex,** glaucoma without pronounced symptoms, but attended with progressive loss of vision.

glaucomatous (glaw-ko′-mah-tus) of the nature of glaucoma.

glaze (glāz) in dentistry, the vitreous coating fused onto porcelain of artificial teeth, to simulate enamel.

gleet (glēt) chronic gonorrheal urethritis.

glenoid (gle′noid) resembling a pit or socket.

glia (gli′ah) neuroglia.

gliacyte (gli′ah-sīt) a cell of the neuroglia.

gliadin (gli′ah-din) tough protein from wheat gluten.

glial (gli′al) pertaining to glia or neuroglia.

gliarase (gli′ah-rās) a mass of astrocytes whose cytoplasm has undergone fission.

gliobacteria (gli″o-bac-te′re-ah) rod-shaped Schizomycetes surrounded by a zooglea.

glioblastoma (-blas-to′mah) glioma.

gliococcus (-kok′us) micrococcus forming gelatinous matter.

gliocyte (gli′o-sīt) gliacyte.

gliocytoma (gli″o-si-to′mah) a tumor composed of neuroglia cells.

gliogenous (gli-oj′ĕ-nus) produced or formed by neuroglia.

glioma (gli-o′mah) a tumor composed of neuroglia in any of its stages of development. **g.**

ret′inae, a tumor of the retina resembling glioma.

gliomatosis (gli″o-mah-to′sis) overdevelopment of neuroglia in spinal cord.

gliomatous (gli-o′mah-tus) of the nature of glioma.

gliomyoma (gli″o-mi-o′mah) glioma combined with myxoma.

gliomyxoma (-mik-so′mah) a tumor containing gliomatous and myxomatous elements.

glioneuroma (-nu-ro′mah) glioma combined with neuroma.

gliopil (gli′o-pil) a dense feltwork of glial processes, as in the subependymal matrix of the ventricular system.

gliosarcoma (gli″o-sar-ko′mah) glioma combined with sarcoma.

gliosis (gli-o′sis) excessive development of neuroglia tissue.

gliosome (gli′o-sōm) a small granule seen in neuroglia cells.

glissonitis (glis″o-ni′tis) inflammation of Glisson's capsule.

globin (glo′bin) a protein from hemoglobin.

globinometer (glo″bĭ-nom′ĕ-ter) instrument for determining proportion of oxyhemoglobin in the blood.

globomyeloma (glo″bo-mi″ĕ-lo′mah) a round cell sarcoma.

globulariacitrin (glob″u-la″re-ah-sit′rin) rutin.

globule (glob′ūl) a small spherical mass, especially a red blood corpuscle. **polar g's,** polar bodies.

globulimeter (glob″u-lim′ĕ-ter) an instrument for estimating the number of red blood corpuscles in a given quantity of blood.

globulin (glob′u-lin) one of a class of simple proteins which are insoluble in water, soluble in dilute salt solution, and precipitated by half-saturation with ammonium sulfate; found in serum and tissue, and in seeds and nuts. **accelerator g.,** a substance present in plasma, but not in serum, which functions in the formation of intrinsic and extrinsic thromboplastin. **alpha g's,** globulins in plasma which, in neutral or alkaline solutions, have the greatest electrophoretic mobility, in this respect most nearly resembling the albumins. **antihemophilic g.,** a sterile preparation containing a fraction of normal human plasma of unknown composition which shortens the coagulation time of shed hemophilic blood. **beta g's,** globulins in plasma which, in neutral or alkaline solutions, have an electrophoretic mobility between that of the alpha and that of the gamma globulins. **gamma g's,** globulins in plasma which, in neutral or alkaline solutions, have the slowest electrophoretic mobility. **immune g.,** a serum globulin that has been modified in response to infection or to injection of certain materials and contains antibodies to the antigens eliciting their production; used as a passive immunizing agent against measles or tetanus and in prophylaxis or treatment of pertussis.

globulinemia (glob″u-lin-e′me-ah)   globulin in the blood.

globulinuria (-u′re-ah) globulin in the urine.

globulolysis (glob″u-lol′ĭ-sis) destruction of red blood corpuscles. adj., **globulolyt′ic.**

globulose (glob′u-lōs) a product of the digestion of globulins.

globus (glo′bus), pl. *glo′bi* [L.] 1. a sphere or ball; a large spherical mass. 2. a subjective sensation as of a lump or mass. **g. hyster′icus,** subjective sensation of a lump in the throat. **g. pal′lidus,** the smaller and more medial part of the lentiform nucleus.

glomangioma (glo-man″je-o′mah) an extremely painful, small, firm, rounded, redblue tumor, usually occurring in the distal portion of a finger or toe, in the skin or in deeper tissues.

glomectomy (glo-mek′to-me) excision of a glomus.

glomerulitis (glo-mer″u-li′tis) inflammation of glomeruli of kidney.

glomerulonephritis (glo-mer″u-lo-ne-fri′tis) nephritis with inflammation of the capillary loops in the glomeruli of the kidneys.

glomerulopathy (glo-mer″u-lop′ah-the) a noninflammatory disease of the kidney glomeruli. **diabetic g.,** intercapillary glomerulosclerosis.

glomerulosclerosis (glo mer″u-lo-skle-ro′sis) arteriolar nephrosclerosis. **intercapillary g.,** a degenerative complication of diabetes, manifested as albuminuria, nephrotic edema, hypertension, renal insufficiency and retinopathy.

glomerulus (glo-mer′u-lus), pl. *glomer′uli* [L.] a small tuft or cluster, as of blood vessels or nerve fibers; applied especially to the coils of blood vessels, one projecting into the expanded end or capsule of each of the uriniferous tubules of the kidney *(renal glomeruli).* adj., **glomer′ular. olfactory glomeruli,** coiling fibrillar structures in the olfactory bulb. **renal g.,** the small cluster of blood vessels projecting into the expanded end marking the beginning of a renal tubule.

glomoid (glo′moid) resembling a glomus.

glomus (glo′mus), pl. *glom′era* [L.] a small histologically recognizable body composed primarily of fine arterioles connecting directly with veins, and having a rich nerve supply. **g. carot′icum,** the carotid gland. **g. choroi′-deum,** an enlargement of the choroid plexus of the lateral ventricle.

glonoin (glon′o-in) glyceryl trinitrate.

glonoinism (glon′o-in-izm″) poisoning with glonoin.

gloss(o)- (glos′o) word element [Gr.], *tongue.*

glossal (glos′al) pertaining to the tongue.

glossalgia (glŏ-sal′je-ah) pain in the tongue.

glossectomy (glŏ-sek′to-me) excision of the tongue.

Glossina (glŏ-si′nah) a genus of biting flies, including the tsetse fly; important as vectors of trypanosomes. **G. palpa′lis,** the species which transmits the trypanosomes causing sleeping sickness.

glossitis (glŏ-si′tis) inflammation of the tongue. **rhomboid g., median,** a congenital

anomaly of the tongue, with a flat or slightly raised reddish patch or plaque on the dorsal surface.

glossocele (glos′o-sēl) swelling and protrusion of the tongue.

glossodynia (glos″o-din′e-ah) pain in the tongue.

glossoepiglottidean (-ep″ĭ-glŏ-tid′e-an) pertaining to tongue and epiglottis.

glossograph (glos′o-graf) apparatus for registering tongue movements in speech.

glossohyal (glos″o-hi′al) pertaining to tongue and hyoid bone.

glossolalia (-la′le-ah) unintelligible speech.

glossology (glŏ-sol′o-je) 1. sum of knowledge regarding the tongue. 2. treatise on nomenclature.

glossolysis (glŏ-sol′ĭ-sis) paralysis of tongue.

glossopathy (glŏ-sop′ah-the) disease of the tongue.

glossopharyngeal (glos″o-fah-rin′je-al) pertaining to tongue and pharynx.

glossoplasty (glos′o-plas″te) plastic surgery of the tongue.

glossoplegia (glos″o-ple′je-ah) paralysis of tongue.

glossorrhaphy (glŏ-sōr′ah-fe) suture of the tongue.

glossospasm (glos′o-spazm) spasm of the tongue.

glossotomy (glŏ-sot′o-me) incision of the tongue.

glossotrichia (glos″o-trik′e-ah) hairy tongue.

glottic (glot′ik) pertaining to glottis or tongue.

glottis (glot′tis), pl. *glot′tides* [Gr.] the vocal apparatus of the larynx, consisting of the true vocal cords (vocal folds) and the opening between them.

glottitis (glŏ-ti′tis) glossitis.

glottology (glŏ-tol′o-je) glossology.

glucagon (gloo′kah-gon) a secretion of the pancreas that increases concentration of sugar in the blood; a preparation from the pancreas of domestic mammals used for food by man is used parenterally as a hyperglycemic agent. **g. hydrochloride,** a pharmaceutical preparation used in treatment of hypoglycemia.

glucase (gloo′kās) an enzyme from plants changing starch into dextroglucose.

glucide (gloo′sīd) a simple reducing sugar.

glucinium (gloo-sin′e-um) beryllium.

glucocorticoid (gloo″ko-kor′ti-koid) a type of hormone secreted by the adrenal cortex which stimulates the conversion of proteins to carbohydrates.

Gluco-ferrum (-fer′rum) trademark for preparations of ferrous gluconate.

glucogenic (-jen′ik) producing sugar.

glucohemia (-he′me-ah) sugar in the blood.

glucokinase (-ki′nās) an enzyme which catalyzes the conversion of glucose to glucose phosphate.

glucokinetic (-ki-net′ik) activating sugar so as to maintain the sugar level of the body.

glucokinin (-kin′in) a substance obtained from vegetable tissues which produces hyperglycemia when injected into animals.

gluconate (gloo″ko-nāt) a salt of gluconic acid, containing the $HOCH_2(CHOH)_5COO—$ radical. **ferrous g.**, a compound used in the treatment of iron deficiency anemia.

gluconeogenesis (gloo″ko-ne″o-jen′ĕ-sis) the formation of sugar by the liver from non-carbohydrate molecules.

glucophore (gloo′ko-fōr) the group of atoms in a molecule which gives the compound a sweet taste.

glucoprotein (gloo″ko-pro′te-in) glycoprotein.

glucosamine (gloo″ko-sam′in) a derivative of glycoprotein, $C_6H_{11}O_5.NH_2$.

glucosan (gloo′ko-san) a polysaccharide of indefinite composition, yielding chiefly glucose on hydrolysis.

glucosazone (gloo″ko-sa′zōn) a crystalline principle found in urine after the phenyl-hydrazine test.

glucose (gloo′kōs) a sugar, $C_6H_{12}O_6$. **liquid g.**, a product obtained by incomplete hydrolysis of starch, consisting chiefly of dextrose with dextrins, maltose and water.

glucoside (gloo′ko-sīd) a vegetable principle decomposable into glucose and another substance.

glucosin (gloo′ko-sin) a base derived from glucose by action of ammonia.

glucosulfone (gloo″ko-sul′fōn) a compound derived from dapsone. **sodium g.**, $C_{24}H_{34}N_2$-$Na_2O_{18}S_3$, used in treatment of leprosy.

glucosuria (-su′re-ah) abnormally high sugar in the urine.

glucurolactone (gloo″ku-ro-lak′tōn) a compound used in treatment of arthritis, neuritis and fibrositis.

glucuronidase (gloo″ku-ron′ĭ-dās) an enzyme which splits compounds of glucuronic acid.

glucuronolactone (gloo″ku-ro″no-lak′tōn) glucurolactone.

glutamine (gloo′tah-min) a naturally occurring amino acid found in the juices of many plants.

Glutan H-C-L (gloo′tan) trademark for capsules containing glutamic acid hydrochloride.

glutaraldehyde (gloo″tahr-al′dĕ-hīd) a compound, $CHO.(CH_2)_3.CHO$, used as a tissue fixative for light and electron microscopy because of its preservation of fine structural detail and localization of enzyme activity.

glutathione (gloo″tah-thi′ōn) a compound in animal and plant tissues which acts as a carrier of oxygen. **oxidized g.**, the precursor of reduced glutathione. **reduced g.**, a tripeptide present in red cells, deficiency of which probably predisposes erythrocytes to the oxidant and hemolytic effects of certain drugs.

gluteal (gloo′te-al) pertaining to the buttocks.

glutelin (gloo′tĕ-lin) a simple protein from the seeds of cereals.

gluten (gloo′ten) a viscous, tenacious principle of various grains.

glutethimide (gloo-teth′ĭ-mīd) a compound used as a central nervous system depressant.

glutin (gloo′tin) a viscid constituent found in cereal proteins and collagen.

glutinous (gloo′tĭ-nus) adhesive; sticky.

glutitis (gloo-ti′tis) inflammation of glutei muscles.

glycase (gli′kās) an enzyme which converts maltose and maltodextrin into dextrose.

glycemia (gli-se′me-ah) sugar in the blood.

glyceride (glis′er-īd) an organic acid ester of glycerol, designated, according to the number of ester linkages, as a mono-, di- or triglyceride.

glycerin (glis′er-in) glycerol; the official (USP) name of the preparation used as an emollient and pharmaceutic aid (solvent).

glycerite (glis′er-īt) a preparation of a medicinal substance in glycerin.

glycerol (glis′er-ol) glycerin. **g. borogly-cerite,** boroglycerin glycerite.

glycerophosphate (glis″er-o-fos′fāt) a combination of a base with glycerin and phosphoric acid.

glyceryl (glis′er-il) the radical, C_3H_5, of glycerin. **g. monostearate,** a white, waxlike solid, used in cosmetic creams. **g. triacetate,** triacetin. **g. trinitrate,** a colorless or yellowish, oily liquid, $C_3H_5N_3O_9$; used principally in angina pectoris and asthma.

glycine (gli′sēn) aminoacetic acid.

glycobiarsol (gli″ko-bi-ar′sol) an odorless, slightly colored amorphous powder, used in amebiasis.

glycocholate (-ko′lāt) a salt of glycocholic acid.

glycoclastic (-klas′tik) breaking up sugars.

glycocoll (gli′ko-kol) aminoacetic acid.

glycogen (gli′ko-jen) the form in which carbohydrates are stored in animal tissue. adj., **glycogen′ic.**

glycogenase (gli′ko-jĕ-nās″) an enzyme which splits glycogen into dextrin and maltose.

glycogenesis (gli″ko-jen′ĕ-sis) production of sugar or glycogen. adj., **glycogenet′ic.**

glycogenolysis (-jĕ-nol′ĭ-sis) the splitting up of glycogen into dextrose. adj., **glycogenolyt′-ic.**

glycogenosis (-jĕ-no′sis) a disease due to abnormal storage of glycogen in children; marked by enlargement of the liver and hypoglycemia.

glycogenous (gli-koj′ĕ-nus) glycogenic.

glycogeusia (gli″ko-gu′se-ah) a sweet taste in the mouth.

glycohemia (-he′me-ah) sugar in the blood.

glycol (gli′kol) any diatomic alcohol.

glycolipid (gli″ko-lip′id) a compound of an alcohol, fatty acids and a carbohydrate.

glycolysis (gli-kol′ĭ-sis) the breaking down of sugars into simpler compounds. adj., **glycolyt′ic.**

glycometabolic (gli″ko-met″ah-bol′ik) pertaining to metabolism of sugar.

glyconeogenesis (-ne″o-jen′ĕ-sis) formation of carbohydrates from molecules which are not themselves carbohydrates.

glyconucleoprotein (-nu″kle-o-pro′te-in) a nucleoprotein having the carbohydrate group largely developed.

glycopenia (-pe′ne-ah) abnormally low blood sugar.

glycopexis (-pek′sis) fixation or storing of sugar. adj., **glycopec′tic.**

glycophilia (-fil′e-ah) a condition in which a small amount of glucose produces hyperglycemia.

glycopolyuria (gli"ko-pol"e-u're-ah) diabetes with moderate increase of sugar in urine, and great increase of uric acid in blood.

glycoprival (-pri'val) deprived of carbohydrates.

glycoprotein (-pro'te-in) a protein combined with a carbohydrate, but not containing phosphoric acid, purines or pyrimidines.

glycoptyalism (-ti'ah-lizm) glucose in the saliva.

glycopyrrolate (-pir'o-lāt) a compound used to produce parasympathetic blockade and to reduce gastric acid secretion and hypermotility.

glycorachia (-ra'ke-ah) sugar in the cerebrospinal fluid.

glycoregulation (-reg"u-la'shun) the control of sugar metabolism. adj., **glycoreg'ulatory.**

glycorrhea (-re'ah) any sugary discharge from the body.

glycosamine (-sam'in) a base, $C_6N_{13}NO_5$, from decomposition of chitin.

glycosecretory (-se-kre'to-re) concerned in secretion of glycogen.

glycosemia (-se'me-ah) glucose in the blood.

glycosialia (-si-a'le-ah) sugar in the saliva.

glycosialorrhea (-si"ah-lo-re'ah) excessive flow of saliva containing sugar.

glycoside (gli'ko-sīd) a compound containing a carbohydrate molecule, especially such a compound occurring in plants, convertible, by hydrolytic cleavage, into a sugar and a nonsugar component (aglycone), and named specifically for the sugar contained, as glucoside (glucose), pentoside (pentose), fructoside (fructose), etc.; used in various heart conditions (cardiac glycosides).

glycosine (gli-ko'sin) 1. a principle which sometimes unites with urea in the kidneys, forming uric acid. 2. an extract from the pancreas.

glycosomotor (gli"ko-som'ĕ-ter) instrument for determining proportion of sugar in urine

glycostatic (-stat'ik) tending to maintain a constant sugar level.

glycosuria (-su're-ah) abnormally high sugar content in the urine. **renal g.,** glycosuria due to an abnormally low threshold of the kidney for glucose.

glycotaxis (-tak'sis) metabolic distribution of glucose to body tissues.

glycotropic (-trop'ik) having an affinity for sugar; causing hyperglycemia.

glycuresis (gli"ku-re'sis) an abnormal amount of sugar in the urine.

glycylglycine (glis"il-glis'in) the simplest polypeptide.

glycyltryptophan (-trip'to-fan) a dipeptide used as a test for cancer of the stomach.

glycyrrhiza (glis"ĭ-ri'zah) dried rhizome and roots of *Glycyrrhiza glabra;* used in various pharmaceutical preparations.

glycyrrhizin (glis"ĭ-ri'zin) a principle, $C_{24}H_{36}$-O_9, from glycyrrhiza.

glyphylline (gli-fil'in) dyphilline.

Glytheonate (gli-the'o-nāt) trademark for a preparation of theophylline sodium glycinate.

Gm., gm. gram.

gnath(o)- (nath'o) word element [Gr.], *jaw.*

gnathion (na'the-on) lowest point of median line of lower jaw.

gnathitis (na-thi'tis) inflammation of the jaw.

gnathocephalus (na"tho-sef'ah-lus) headless fetal monster with jaws.

gnathodynamometer (-di"nah-mom'ĕ-ter) an instrument for measuring the force exerted in closing the jaws.

gnathology (nah-thol'o-je) a science dealing with the masticatory apparatus as a whole, including morphology, anatomy, histology, physiology, pathology and therapeutics.

gnathoplasty (na'tho-plas"te) plastic repair of the jaw.

gnathoschisis (nah-thos'kĭ-sis) congenital cleft of the upper jaw.

Gnathostoma (nah-thos'to-mah) a genus of nematode worms affecting cats, swine, cattle.

gnathostomiasis (nah-thos"to-mi'ah-sis) infestation with worms of the genus Gnathostoma.

G.N.C. General Nursing Council.

gnosia (no'se-ah) the faculty of perceiving and recognizing. adj., **gnos'tic.**

gnotobiota (no"to-bi-o'tah) the specifically and entirely known microfauna and microflora of a specially reared laboratory animal.

gnotobiote (-bi'ōt) a specially reared laboratory animal whose microflora and microfauna are specifically known in their entirety. adj., **gnotobiot'ic.**

gnotobiotics (-bi-ot'iks) the science of rearing laboratory animals whose microflora and microfauna are specifically known in their entirety.

goiter (goi'ter) enlargement of the thyroid, causing a swelling in the front part of the neck. **aberrant g.,** goiter of an accessory thyroid gland. **adenomatous g.,** enlargement caused by adenoma of the thyroid gland. **basedow g.,** a colloid goiter which has become hyperfunctioning after administration of iodine. **colloid g.,** a large, soft thyroid gland with distended spaces filled with colloid. **cystic g.,** one with cysts formed by mucoid or colloid degeneration. **diving g.,** a movable goiter, located sometimes above and sometimes below the sternal notch. **exophthalmic g.,** goiter characterized by exophthalmos. **fibrous g.,** goiter in which the capsule and the stroma of the thyroid gland are hyperplastic. **follicular g.,** parenchymatous goiter. **intrathoracic g.,** goiter which is situated in the thoracic cavity. **lingual g.,** enlargement of the upper end of the thyroglossal duct, forming a tumor at the posterior part of the dorsum of the tongue. **nodular g.,** thyroid enlargement with circumscribed nodules within the gland. **papillomatous g.,** adenomatous goiter. **parenchymatous g.,** goiter marked by increase in follicles and proliferation of epithelium. **perivascular g.,** goiter growing around a blood vessel. **plunging g.,** diving goiter. **retrovascular g.,** goiter with a process or processes behind an important blood vessel. **simple g.**, simple hyperplasia of the thyroid gland. **substernal g.**, goiter situated below the sternum. **suffocative g.**, one which causes dyspnea by pressure. **toxic g.**, exophthalmic goiter. **vascular g.**, enlargement of the thyroid due chiefly to dilatation of the blood vessels. **wandering g.**, diving goiter.

goitrin (goi'trin) a goitrogenic substance isolated from rutabagas and turnips.

goitrogen (goi'tro-jen) a goiter-producing agent.

goitrogenicity (goi″tro-jĕ-nis'ĭ-te) the tendency to produce goiter.

goitrogenous (goi-troj'ĕ-nus) producing goiter.

gold (gōld) chemical element (see table), at. no. 79, symbol Au; used in treatment of rheumatoid arthritis. **adhesive g.**, annealed gold with cohesive properties. **annealed g.**, gold which has been heated in a flame to increase its cohesive properties. **g. aurothiosulfate,** gold sodium thiosulfate. **cohesive g.**, chemically pure gold that forms a solid mass when properly condensed into a tooth cavity. **crystal g.**, **crystalline g.**, **fibrous g.**, **mat g.**, pure gold composed of flakelike crystals formed by electrodeposition. **g. sodium thiomalate,** an odorless, fine, white to yellowish powder with a metallic taste; used in treatment of rheumatoid arthritis and nondisseminated lupus erythematosus. **g. sodium thiosulfate,** $Na_3Au(S_2O_3)_2.2H_2O$; used in treatment of rheumatoid arthritis. **g. thioglucose,** aurothioglucose.

gomphiasis (gom-fi'ah-sis) looseness of the teeth.

gomphosis (gom-fo'sis) articulation in which a spike of bone fits into a bony socket.

gonad (go'nad, gon'ad) an ovary or testis. **indifferent g.**, the sexually undifferentiated gonad of the early embryo. **third g.**, the adrenal gland, so called because of its interrelations with the sex glands.

gonadal (go-nad'al) derived from or pertaining to a gonad.

gonadectomize (go″na-dek'to-mīz) to deprive of the gonads by surgical excision.

gonadectomy (-dek'to-me) removal of a gonad.

gonadial (go-nad'e-al) gonadal.

gonadogenesis (gon″ah-do-jen'ĕ-sis) development of the gonads in the embryo, especially the development of gonads typical of one or the other sex.

gonadokinetic (-ki-net'ik) stimulating activity of the gonads.

gonadopathy (gon″ah-dop'ah-the) disease of the gonads.

gonadotherapy (gon″ah-do-ther'ah-pe) treatment with gonadal hormones.

gonadotrophic (-trōf'ik) gonadotropic (2).

gonadotrophin (-trōf'in) gonadotropin.

gonadotropic (-trop'ik) 1. pertaining to gonadotropism. 2. having a stimulating effect upon the gonads.

gonadotropin (-trōp'in) a substance which has a stimulating effect upon the gonads, especially the hormone secreted by the anterior pituitary. **chorionic g.**, such a substance

found in human pregnancy urine; used in treatment of underdevelopment of sex glands.

gonadotropism (gon″ah-dot'ro-pizm) dominance of the gonads in the endocrine constitution.

gonaduct (gon'ah-dukt) a tubular channel for passage of ova or spermatozoa.

gonagra (go-nag'rah) gouty seizure of the knee.

gonalgia (go-nal'je-ah) pain in the knee.

gonangiectomy (go-nan″je-ek'to-me) excision of the vas deferens.

gonarthritis (gon″ar-thri'tis) inflammation of the knee joint.

gonarthrocace (-throk'ah-se) white swelling of knee.

gonarthrotomy (-throt'o-me) incision into the knee joint.

gonecystis (gon″e-sis'tis) a seminal vesicle.

gonecystitis (-sis-ti'tis) inflammation of a seminal vesicle.

gonecystolith (-sis'to-lith) a concretion in a seminal vesicle.

gonecystopyosis (-sis″to-pi-o'sis) suppuration of a seminal vesicle.

gonepoiesis (-poi-e'sis) formation of the semen.

gonidium (go-nid'e-um) pl. *gonid'ia* [Gr.] 1. a spore which is not born free, but is formed in a case or receptacle; an endospore. 2. one of the chlorophyll-bearing elements of lichens.

goniometer (go″ne-om'ĕ-ter) an instrument for measuring angles. **finger g.**, one for measuring the limits of flexion and extension of the interphalangeal joints of the fingers.

gonion (go'ne-on), pl. *go'nia* [Gr.] the most inferior, posterior and lateral point on the angle of the mandible.

goniopuncture (go″ne-o-punk'tūr) insertion of a knife blade through clear cornea, just within the limbus, across the anterior chamber of the eye and through the opposite corneoscleral wall, in treatment of glaucoma.

gonioscope (go'ne-o-skōp″) an instrument for examination of the angle of the anterior chamber of the eye.

gonioscopy (go″ne-os'ko-pe) examination of the angle of the anterior chamber of the eye.

goniotomy (-ot'o-me) an operation for glaucoma; it consists in opening Schlemm's canal under direct vision.

gonocele (gon'o-sēl) spermatocele.

gonococcemia (gon″o-kok-se'me-ah) gonococci in the blood.

gonococcide (-kok'sīd) an agent destructive to gonococci.

gonococcus (-kok'us), pl. *gonococ'ci* [L.] the causative organism of gonorrhea, *Neisseria gonorrhoeae.* adj., **gonococ'cal, gonococ'cic.**

gonocyte (gon'o-sit) the primitive reproductive cell of the embryo.

gonophore (gon'o-fōr) an accessory generative organ.

gonorrhea (gon″o-re'ah) inflammation of the genital mucous membrane caused by *Neisseria gonorrhoeae.* adj., **gonorrhe'al.**

gonotoxemia (-tok-se'me-ah) toxemia with gonorrheal pus.

gonycampsis (gon″ĭ-kamp′sis) curvature of the knee.

gonycrotesis (-kro-te′sis) knock-knee.

gonyocele (gon′e-o-sēl″) synovitis of the knee.

gonyoncus (gon″e-ong′kus) tumor of the knee.

gorget (gor′jet) wide-grooved lithotomy director.

Gossypium (gŏ-sip′e-um) a genus of tropical and subtropical plants found in both hemispheres, including 10 species, three of which yield most of the world's cotton: *G. barbadense, G. herbaceum* and *G. hirsutum.*

GOT glutamic-oxalacetic transaminase.

gouge (gowj) an instrument for cutting bone.

goundou (gōōn′doo) osteoplastic periostitis of the nose.

gout (gowt) painful constitutional disease with joint inflammation and chalky deposits, due to disturbance of the purine metabolism of the body. adj., **gout′y.** **latent g., masked g.,** lithemia without the typical features of gout. **misplaced g., retrocedent g.,** gout in which the arthritic symptoms have disappeared and are followed by severe constitutional disturbances. **rheumatic g.,** atrophic arthritis.

G.P. general paresis; general practitioner.

GPT glutamic-pyruvic transaminase.

gr. grain.

gracile (gras′il) slender; delicate.

gradatim (gra-da′tim) [L.] by degrees; gradually.

gradient (gra′de-ent) rate of increase or decrease of a variable value, or its representative curve.

graduate (grad′u-āt) 1. a cylindrical or tapered laboratory vessel, usually of glass, with a scale showing the capacity in milliliters or fluid ounces. 2. person who has received an academic or professional degree.

graduated (grad′u-āt″ed) marked by a succession of lines; progressing by regularly marked intervals or degrees.

graft (graft) a fragment of skin or other body tissue for transplantation. **accordion g.,** a full-thickness graft in which slits have been made so that the graft may be stretched to cover a large area. **animal g.,** a graft of tissue transferred from one of the lower animals to man. **autodermic g., auto-epidermic g.,** a skin graft taken from the patient's own body. **autologous g.,** autograft. **autoplastic g.,** a graft taken from another area of the patient's own body. **avascular g.,** a graft of tissue in which not even transient vascularization is achieved. **Blair-Brown g.,** a split-skin graft of intermediate thickness. **bone g.,** a piece of bone used to take the place of a removed bone or bony defect. **cable g.,** a nerve graft made up of several sections of nerve in the manner of a cable. **cutis g.,** skin from which epidermis and subcutaneous fat have been removed, used instead of fascia in various plastic procedures. **Davis g.,** a thick pinch graft. **dermic g.,** a graft composed of a bit of derma or corium. **Dragstedt g.,** accordion graft. **epidermic g.,** a piece of epidermis implanted on a raw surface. **Esser g.,**

a graft spread over a mold of Stent preparation and sutured in position along with the mold. **fascia g.,** a graft of tissue taken from the fascia lata. **fascicular g.,** a nerve graft in which bundles of nerve fibers are approximated and sutured separately. **full-thickness g.,** a skin graft consisting of the full thickness of the skin. **heterodermic g.,** a skin graft taken from a person other than the patient. **heteroplastic g.,** a graft of tissue derived from an individual of a different species, or of synthetic or nonorganic material. **homologous g.,** homograft. **homoplastic g.,** autoplastic g. **isologous g.,** isograft. **isoplastic g.,** one taken from another individual of the same species. **lamellar g.,** replacement of the superficial layers of an opaque cornea by a thin layer of clear cornea from a donor eye. **nerve g.,** replacement of an area of defective nerve with a segment from a sound one. **omental g's,** strips of omentum to cover the line of enterorrhaphy. **pedicle g.,** one consisting of the full thickness of the skin and the subcutaneous tissue. **penetrating g.,** a full-thickness corneal transplant. **periosteal g.,** a piece of periosteum to cover a denuded bone. **pinch g.,** a piece of skin graft about ¼ inch in diameter, obtained by elevating the skin with a needle and slicing it off with a knife. **post-mortem g.,** tissue taken from a body after death and stored under proper conditions, to be used later in a patient requiring a graft of such tissue (skin, cornea, etc.). **Reverdin g.,** epidermic graft. **rope g.,** one made by elevating a strip of tissue from its bed except at its two extremities, the cut edges of the tissue being then sutured together to form a rope or tube. **sieve g.,** one so taken that islands of attached skin are left behind to stimulate regeneration. **skin g.,** a bit of skin implanted to replace a lost part of the integument. **sponge g.,** a bit of sponge inserted into a wound to promote the formation of granulations. **Thiersch's g.,** a skin graft in which long, broad strips of skin are used, which include the epidermis, the rete and part of the cutis vera. **thyroid g.,** a piece of thyroid tissue implanted in the body as a remedy for myxedema. **tube g., tunnel g.,** rope graft. **white g.,** avascular graft. **Wolfe's g.,** a full-thickness skin graft. **zooplastic g.,** animal graft.

grafting (graf′ting) the replacement of injured or damaged body tissue with healthy tissue removed from another area of the body or from the body of another individual of the same or a different species. **skin g.,** implantation of patches of healthy skin on a denuded area to form centers of cicatrization.

Grahamella (gra″ah-mel′ah) a genus of Microtatobiotes (order Rickettsiales, family Bartonellaceae).

grain (grān) 1. seed of cereal plants. 2. a unit of weight in the avoirdupois or apothecaries' system, being the equivalent of 64.8 milligrams; abbreviated gr.

gram (gram) the basic unit of mass (weight)

of the metric system, being the equivalent of 15.432 grains; abbreviated G. or gm.

-gram (gram) word element [Gr.], *written; recorded.*

gram-equivalent (gram″e-kwiv'ah-lent) the equivalent weight of a substance in grams.

gramicidin (gram″ĭ-si'din) an antibacterial substance produced by the growth of *Bacillus brevis,* one of the two principal components of tyrothricin; called also *gramicidin D.*

graminivorous (-niv'o-rus) eating or subsisting on cereal grains.

gram-molecule (gram-mol'ĕ-kūl) a quantity in grams equal to the molecular weight of the substance.

gram-negative (-neg'ah-tiv) not staining by Gram's method.

gram-positive (-poz'ĭ-tiv) staining by Gram's method.

grand mal (grahn mal) [Fr.] a major epileptic attack attended by loss of consciousness.

granular (gran'u-lar) made up of granules or grains.

granulatio (gran″u-la'she-o), pl. *granulatio'-nes* [L.] a granular mass.

granulation (-la'shun) 1. a small rounded mass. 2. the production of small rounded masses, as in the healing of a wound of soft tissue. **exuberant g's,** excessive proliferation of granulation tissue in the healing of a wound.

granule (gran'ūl) 1. a small rounded body. 2. a medicinal pellet. **acidophil g's,** alpha granules. **agminated g's,** small proplasmic particles occurring in the blood, supposed to be disintegrated blood corpuscles. **albuminous g's,** granules seen in the cytoplasm of many normal cells, which disappear on the addition of acetic acid, but are not affected by ether or chloroform. **aleuronoid g's,** colorless myeloid colloidal bodies found in the base of pigment cells. **alpha g's,** coarse, highly refractive, eosinophil granules of leukocytes, composed of albuminous matter. **Altmann's g's,** mitochondria. **amphophil g's,** beta granules. **azur g's, azurophil g's,** granules that stain easily with azure dyes; they are coarse, reddish granules and are seen in many lymphocytes. **Babes-Ernst g's,** metachromatic granules. **Balfour's infective g.,** a small refractive granule seen in the erythrocytes in spirochetosis of fowls. **basal g.,** a minute granule in the cytoplasm of a protozoon, from which the flagellum arises. **basophil g's,** granules staining with basic dyes. **beta g's,** presecretion granules found in the hypophysis and pancreatic islands. **Bettelheim's g's,** small mobile granules seen in the blood. **Bütschli's g's,** swellings on the bipolar rays of the amphiaster in the ovum. **carbohydrate g's,** particles of carbohydrate matter in body fluids in course of being assimilated. **chromatic g's, chromophilic g's,** Nissl's bodies. **cone g's,** nuclei of visual cells in outer nuclear layer of the retina which are connected with the cones. **cytoplasmic g's,** albuminous granules. **delta g's,** fine basophilic granules in the lympho-

cytes. **elementary g's,** hemoconiae. **eosinophil g's,** those staining with eosin. **epsilon g's,** neutrophil granules from protoplasm of polymorphonuclear leukocytes. **Fauvel's g's,** peribronchitic abscesses. **fuchsinophil g's,** those staining with fuchsin. **gamma g's,** basophilic granules found in the blood, marrow and tissues. **Grawitz's g's,** minute granules seen in the red blood corpuscles in lead poisoning. **hyperchromatin g.,** azure granule. **infective g.,** a small granular body which carries the infection in trypanosomiasis. **iodophil g's,** granules staining brown with iodine, seen in polymorphonuclear leukocytes in various acute infectious diseases. **juxtaglomerular g's,** osmophilic secretory granules present in the juxtaglomerular cells, closely resembling zymogen granules. **kappa g.,** azur granule. **Kölliker's interstitial g's,** granules seen in the sarcoplasm of muscle fibers. **metachromatic g's,** deeply staining masses irregular in size and number seen in the protoplasm of various bacteria. **Much's g's,** granules and rods found in tuberculous sputum which do not stain by the usual processes for acid-fast bacilli, but do stain with Gram stain. **Neusser's g's,** basophil granules seen about the nuclei of leukocytes. **neutrophil g's,** epsilon granules. **Nissl's g's,** Nissl's bodies. **oxyphil g's,** alpha granules. **pigment g's,** small masses of coloring matter in pigment cells. **Plehn's g's,** basophil granules in the conjugating form of malarial parasite. **protein g's,** minute particles of various proteins, some anabolic and others catabolic. **rod g's,** nuclei of visual cells in outer nuclear layer of the retina which are connected with the rods. **Schridde's g's,** granules similar to Altmann's granules, but smaller, found in plasma cells and lymphocytes. **Schrön's g.,** a small body, of doubtful origin, seen in the germinal spot of the ovum. **Schrön-Much g's,** Much's granules. **Schüffner's g's,** coarse red granules in parasitized erythrocytes in tertian malarial fever staining with polychrome methylene blue. **Schüle's g's,** Plehn's granules. **seminal g's,** the small granular bodies in the spermatic fluid. **thread g's,** mitochondria. **yolk g's,** see under *cell.* **zymogen g's,** granules in the cells of the salivary gland.

granulitis (gran″u-li'tis) miliary tuberculosis.

granuloadipose (gran″u-lo-ad'ĭ-pōs) containing granules of fat.

granuloblast (gran″u-lo-blast″) an immature granulocyte.

granuloblastosis (gran″u-lo-blas-to'sis) a disease of fowl with increase in the immature blood cells of the granular series.

granulocyte (gran'u-lo-sīt″) any blood cell containing specific granules, including neutrophils, basophils and eosinophils. **band-form g.,** a stage in the development of the granulocytic leukocyte in which the nuclear indentation is more than half the width of the hypothetical round nucleus, and its opposite ends become approximately parallel for an appreciable distance.

granulocytemia (gran″u-lo-si-te′me-ah) an excess of granulocytes in the blood.

granulocytopenia (-si″to-pe′ne-ah) deficiency of granulocytes in the blood. **primary g.,** agranulocytosis.

granulocytopoiesis (-si″to-poi-e′sis) the production of granulocytes. adj., **granulocytopoiet′ic.**

granulocytosis (-si-to′sis) granulocytemia.

granulofilocyte (-fil′o-sit) a reticulocyte.

granuloma (gran″u-lo′mah) a circumscribed mass consisting mainly of histiocytes, occurring in reaction to the presence of a living agent (infective granuloma) or a foreign body, or sometimes idiopathically. **apical g.,** periodontal cyst. **benign g. of thyroid,** chronic inflammation of the thyroid gland, converting it into a bulky tumor which later becomes extremely hard. **coccidioidal g., g. coccidioida′le,** a disease due to infection with the fungus *Coccidioides immitis.* **dental g.,** a proliferating mass of chronic inflammatory tissue contained within an extension of the periodontal membrane of a tooth. **g. endem′icum,** cutaneous leishmaniasis. **g. fissura′tum,** a firm, whitish, fissured, fibrotic granuloma of the gum and buccal mucosa, occurring in the fold between the jaw and cheek. **foreign body g.,** a localized histiocytic reaction to a foreign body in the tissue. **g. fungoi′des,** mycosis fungoides. **Hodgkin's g.,** Hodgkin's disease. **infective g.,** one due to the presence in the tissues of living agents. **g. inguina′le,** ulcerating granuloma affecting genitals and neighboring parts, sometimes with inguinal adenitis. **g. ir′idis,** a nonmalignant and highly vascular growth of the iris. **lipoid g.,** a granuloma containing lipoid cells. **lipophagic g.,** a granuloma attended by the loss of subcutaneous fat. **Majocchi's g.,** a condition characterized by the development of nodules at the borders of indistinct scaling patches of the lower half of the lower leg, due to *Trichophyton rubrum* infection. **malignant g., g. malig′num,** Hodgkin's disease. **paracoccidioidal g.,** South American blastomycosis. **peripheral giant cell reparative g.,** a pedunculated or sessile lesion apparently arising from periodontal membrane or mucoperiosteum, and usually due to trauma. **g. pyogen′icum,** a fungating pedunculated growth in which the granulations consist of masses of pyogenic organisms. **g. sarcomato′des,** mycosis fungoides. **septic g.,** granuloma pyogenicum. **swimming pool g.,** a papular lesion at the site of a swimming pool injury, caused by an organism related to the tubercle bacillus, which tends to heal spontaneously in a few months or years. **g. telangiectat′icum,** a form characterized by numerous dilated blood vessels. **g. trop′icum,** yaws. **ulcerating g. of the pudenda, venereal g., g. vene′reum,** granuloma inguinale.

granulomatosis (gran″u-lo″mah-to′sis) the formation of multiple granulomas. **g. siderot′ica,** Gamna's disease. **Wegener's g.,** progressive disease, with granulomatous lesions of the respiratory tract, focal necrotizing arteriolitis and, finally, widespread inflammation of all organs of the body.

granulomere (gran′u-lo-mēr″) the center portion of a platelet in a dry, stained blood smear, apparently filled with fine, purplish red granules, thought possibly to be due to an artefact.

granulopenia (gran″u-lo-pe′ne-ah) decreased number of granulocytes in the blood.

granulopexis (-pek′sis) the fixation of granules.

granuloplastic (gran′u-lo-plas″tik) forming granules.

granulopoiesis (gran″u-lo-poi-e′sis) the formation and development of granulocytes. adj., **granulopoiet′ic.**

granulopotent (-po′tent) able to form granules.

granulosarcoma (-sar-ko′mah) mycosis fungoides.

granulose (gran′u-lōs) the more soluble portion of starch.

granulosis (gran″u-lo′sis) the formation of granules. **g. ru′bra na′si,** a red granular eruption of the skin of the nose.

granulotherapy (gran″u-lo-ther′ah-pe) treatment by stimulating production of leukocytes.

granum (gra′num) [L.] grain.

graph (graf) a diagram showing relationship between different variable factors.

graphorrhea (graf″o-re′ah) the writing of a meaningless flow of words.

graphospasm (graf′o-spazm) writers' cramp.

-graphy (graf′e) word element [Gr.], *making of a graphic record.* adj., **-graph′ic.**

grattage (grah-tahzh′) [Fr.] removal of granulations or follicles by scraping.

gravedo (grah-ve′do) coryza, or nasal catarrh.

gravel (grav′el) calculus occurring in small particles.

gravid (grav′id) pregnant.

gravida (grav′ĭ-dah) a pregnant woman. **g. I,** primigravida. **g. II,** secundigravida. **g. III,** tertigravida.

gravidocardiac (grav″ĭ-do-kar′de-ak) pertaining to heart disease in pregnancy.

gravidopuerperal (-pu-er′per-al) pertaining to or occurring during pregnancy and the puerperium.

gravimetric (grav″ĭ-met′rik) performed by weight and measure.

gravity (grav′ĭ-te) weight; tendency toward the center of the earth. **specific g.,** the weight of a substance compared with that of another taken as a standard.

grease (grēs) an inflammatory swelling in a horse's leg, with formation of cracks in the skin and excretion of oily matter.

green (grēn) 1. the color of grass or of an emerald. 2. a green dye. **benzaldehyde g.,** malachite green. **indocyanine g.,** a dye used in tests of cardiovascular function. **malachite g.,** a triphenyl methane dye used as a stain for bacteria and as an antiseptic for wounds. **Paris g.,** an emerald green powder, Cu-$(C_2H_3O_2)_2.3Cu(AsO_2)_2$, used as an insecticide on plants. **Schweinfurt g.,** Paris green.

Gregarina (greg″ah-ri′nah) a genus of protozoans, parasitic in invertebrates.

grid (grid) 1. a grating. 2. a chart with horizontal and vertical lines for plotting curves. **baby g.**, a direct-reading chart on infant growth. **Wetzel g.**, a direct-reading chart for evaluating physical fitness in terms of body build, developmental level and basal metabolism.

grip (grip) 1. influenza. 2. a grasping or clasping. **devil's g.**, epidemic pleurodynia.

griseofulvin (gris″e-o-ful′vin) a substance produced by growth of *Penicillium griseofulvum* or by other means; used in treatment of superficial fungus infections of the skin.

groin (groin) the junction of abdomen and thigh.

groove (groōv) a narrow, linear hollow or depression. **branchial g.**, an external furrow lined with ectoderm, occurring in the embryo between two branchial arches. **Harrison's g.**, one on the thorax, caused by contraction of the diaphragm. **labial g.**, one produced by degeneration of the central cells of the labial lamina, which later becomes the vestibule of the oral cavity. **medullary g.**, **neural g.**, that formed by beginning invagination of the neural plate to form the neural tube.

group (groōp) a collection of similar units or of closely related entities, such as a number of different atoms that act as a unit when entering or leaving chemical combination (a radical), or a particular combination of atoms in a molecule responsible for a characteristic (e.g. taste, odor) of the compound. **acetyl g.**, the radical, CH_3CO. **alcohol g.**, an organic radical consisting of one atom each of carbon and oxygen with three atoms of hydrogen (*primary alcohol group*), with two atoms of hydrogen (*secondary alcohol group*), or with only one atom of hydrogen (*tertiary alcohol group*). **alkyl g.**, an organic radical produced by loss of one hydrogen atom from an aliphatic hydrocarbon. **amino g.**, the radical, NH_2. **aryl g.**, an organic radical. **azo g.**, the divalent radical, $-N=N-$. **blood g.**, see *blood type*. **butyl g.**, an organic radical. **carbonyl g.**, a functional group consisting of carbon joined to oxygen with a double bond, two carbon electrons remaining unpaired (C:O). **carboxyl g.**, a carbonyl group united with a hydroxyl group, one electron of the carbon remaining unpaired (COOH). **coli-aerogenes g.**, a group of microorganisms including *Escherichia coli*, *Aerobacter aerogenes* and a variety of intermediate forms; called also *coliform bacilli* or *coliform bacteria*. **hydroxyl g.**, the univalent radical, OH. **methyl g.**, the organic radical, $-CH_3$. **nitro g.**, the monovalent radical, $-NO_2$. **nitroso g.**, the monovalent radical, $-N=O$. **peptide g.**, the bivalent radical, $-CO.NH-$, formed by reaction between the NH_2 and COOH groups of adjacent amino acids. **prosthetic g.**, the nonamino acid portion of a protein molecule. **saccharide g.**, a combination of carbon, hydrogen and oxygen atoms in a hypothetical molecule, $C_6H_{10}O_5$, the number of which in the compound determines the specific name of the polysaccharide. **zymotic g.**, zymophore.

grouping (groōp′ing) arrangement or classification in groups. **antigenic structural g.**, haptene. **g. of blood**, classification of blood according to the blood type to which it belongs. **haptenic g.**, haptene.

growth (groth) 1. increase in size, usually referring to a normal process resulting from accretion of tissue of a constitution similar to that originally present. 2. an abnormal formation of tissue, such as a tumor. **absolute g.**, an expression of the absolute increase in size of an organism or of a particular organ or part. **allometric g.**, the growth of different organs or parts of an organism at different rates. **appositional g.**, growth by structure or part. **interstitial g.**, that occurring in the interior of parts or structures already formed.

grumous (groo′mus) lumpy or clotted.

grutum (groo′tum) milium.

G.S. Gerontological Society.

GSH reduced glutathione.

G6PD glucose-6-phosphate dehydrogenase.

GSSG oxidized glutathione.

Gt. [L.] *gutta* (drop).

Gtt. [L.] *guttae* (drops).

G.U. genitourinary.

guanase (gwan′ās) an enzyme found in the thymus, adrenals and pancreas.

guanethidine (gwan-eth′ĭ-dēn) a compound used as an antihypertensive.

guanidine (gwan′ĭ-dēn) a base, $NH:C(NH_2)_2$, the amidine of aminocarbamic acid.

guaranine (gwah-rah′nin) caffeine.

gubernaculum (goo″ber-nak′u-lum), pl. *gubernac′ula* [L.] a guiding structure. **g. den′tis**, a connective tissue band joining the sac of an unerupted tooth with the gum. **g. tes′tis**, a cord in the fetus connecting the epididymis and bottom of the scrotum.

guide (gīd) 1. a grooved sound. 2. a filiform bougie over which a tunneled sound is passed.

guillotine (gil′o-tēn) a surgical instrument with a movable blade which slides in the grooves of a rigid frame, used for removing tonsils; a similar knife is used in surgery on the heart.

guilt (gilt) the subjective feeling of having committed an error, offense or sin.

gullet (gul′et) the passage to the stomach.

gum (gum) 1. mucilaginous excretion of various plants. 2. gingiva. **g. arabic**, acacia. **Bassora g.**, gum resembling gum arabic from Persia. **British g.**, dextrin. **g. camphor**, camphor. **g. karaya**, sterculia gum. **g. opium**, opium. **sterculia g.**, dried gummy exudation from species of Sterculia or Cochlospermum; used in forming viscous dispersions and as a bulk cathartic. **g. tragacanth**, tragacanth.

gumma (gum′ah) a soft, gummy tumor in tertiary syphilis.

gummatous (gum′ah-tus) of the nature of gumma.

gummy (gum′e) resembling gum or gumma.

gustation (gus-ta′shun) the sense of taste. adj., **gus′tatory**.

gustometer (gus-tom′ĕ-ter) an instrument used in the quantitative determination of taste thresholds.

gustometry (gus-tom″ĕ-tre) measurement of acuity of the sense of taste.

gut (gut) 1. the bowel or intestine. 2. catgut. **head g.**, foregut. **preoral g.**, Seessel's pouch. **primitive g.**, archenteron. **tail g.**, prolongation of the archenteron into the tail of the early embryo.

gutta (gut′ah), pl. *gut′tae* [L.] drop. **g. rosa′- cea,** acne rosacea. **g. sere′na,** amaurosis.

gutta-percha (gut″ah-per′chah) the coagulated latex of a number of tropical trees of the family Sapotaceae, resembling rubber and used in medicine and surgery for mechanical purposes.

guttat. [L.] *guttatim* (drop by drop).

guttate (gut′āt) resembling a drop.

guttatim (gū-ta′tim) drop by drop.

guttering (gut′er-ing) cutting of a gutter-like excision in bone.

guttural (gut′er-al) pertaining to the throat.

gymnastics (jim-nas′tiks) systematic muscular exercise. **Swedish g.**, a system of exercise following a rigid pattern of movement, utilizing little equipment and stressing correct body posture.

gymnobacterium (jim″no-bak-te′re-um) a microorganism which has no flagella.

gymnocyte (jim′no-sīt) a cell with no cell wall.

gymnophobia (jim″no-fo′be-ah) morbid fear of the naked body.

gymnospore (jim′no-spōr) a spore without an envelope.

Gymnothorax (jim″no-tho′raks) a genus of moray eels whose flesh is sometimes used as food.

gynaeco- for words beginning thus, see those beginning *gyneco-*.

gynandrism (jin-an′drizm) a mixture of female and male characteristics in the male.

gynandroblastoma (jī-nan″dro-blas-to′mah) a tumor containing elements of both male and female sex cells.

gynandroid (jī-nan′droid) a female with masculine characteristics.

gynandromorph (jī-nan′dro-morf) an organism exhibiting gynandromorphism.

gynandromorphism (jī-nan″dro-mor′fizm) the presence of chromosomes of both sexes in different tissues of the body, producing a mosaic of male and female sex characteristics.

gynecic (jī-ne′sik) pertaining to women.

gynecogenic (jin″ĕ-ko-jen′ik) producing female characteristics or reactions.

gynecography (jin″ĕ-kog′rah-fe) radiography of the female reproductive tract.

gynecoid (jin′ĕ-koid) woman-like.

gynecologist (jin″ĕ-kol′o-jist) a specialist in gynecology.

gynecology (-kol′o-je) the branch of medicine dealing with diseases of the genital tract in women. adj., **gynecolog′ic.**

gynecomania (jin″ĕ-ko-ma′ne-ah) satyriasis.

gynecomastia (-mas′te-ah) overdevelopment of mammary glands in the male.

gynecopathy (jin″ĕ-kop′ah-the) disease peculiar to women.

gyneduct (jin′ĕ-dukt) the primitive female duct; müllerian duct.

gynephobia (jin″ĕ-fo′be-ah) morbid aversion to women.

Gynergen (jin′er-jen) trademark for ergotamine tartrate.

gyniatrics (jin″e-at′riks) the treatment of diseases of women.

gynomerogon (jin″o-mer′o-gon) an organism produced by gynomerogony and containing only the maternal set of chromosomes.

gynomerogony (-mer-og′o-ne) development of a portion of a fertilized ovum containing only the female pronucleus.

gynopathic (-path′ik) pertaining to disease of women.

gynoplastics (jin′o-plas″tiks) plastic surgery of female genitalia.

gypsum (jip′sum) calcium sulfate.

gyration (ji-ra′shun) revolution about a fixed center.

gyre (jīr) gyrus.

gyrectomy (ji-rek′to-me) surgical ablation of a cerebral gyrus.

Gyrencephala (ji″ren-sef′ah-lah) a group of higher mammals having a brain marked by gyri.

gyrencephalic (ji″ren-sē-fal′ik) having a brain marked by gyri.

gyroma (ji-ro′mah) a tumor of the ovary, consisting of a convoluted, highly refracting mass.

gyrose (ji′rōs) marked by curved lines or circles.

gyrospasm (ji′ro-spazm) rotatory spasm of the head.

gyrotrope (ji′ro-trōp) rheotrope.

gyrous (ji′rus) gyrose.

gyrus (ji′rus), pl. *gy′ri* [L.] one of the many well developed folds in the white medullary layer of the cerebral cortex, separated by fissures or sulci. **angular g.**, one continuous anteriorly with the supramarginal gyrus. **annectant g.**, any one of four gyri connecting occipital and parietotemporal lobes. **gy′ri bre′ves in′sulae,** preinsular gyri. **Broca's g.**, inferior frontal gyrus. **callosal g.**, **g. callo′- sus,** gyrus cinguli. **central g., anterior,** one on the frontal lobe between the precentral and central sulci. **central g., posterior,** one on the parietal lobe between the central and postcentral sulci. **g. cin′guli,** one embracing the entire upper surface of the corpus callosum and continuous with the gyrus hippocampi. **dentate g.**, an imperfect gyrus within the dentate fissure. **g. forni′catus,** 1. the marginal portion of the cerebral cortex on the medial aspect of the hemisphere, including the gyrus cinguli, gyrus hippocampi and others. 2. gyrus cinguli. **frontal g.**, any of the three (inferior, middle and superior) gyri of the frontal lobe. **fusiform g.**, one connecting temporal and occipital lobes, under the collateral and over the subtemporal fissure. **g. genic′uli,** a vestigial gyrus at the anterior end of the corpus callosum. **Heschl's g.**, transverse temporal gyrus. **hippocampal g., g. hippocam′pi,** one between the hippocampal and collateral fissures. **infracalcarine g.**, one on the under surface of the temporal lobe.

lingual g., median occipitotemporal gyrus. **g. lon'gus in'sulae**, a long gyrus forming the postinsula. **marginal g.**, one in the frontal lobe bordering on the callosomarginal fissure. **occipital g.**, any of the three (superior, middle and inferior) gyri of the occipital lobe. **occipitotemporal g., lateral**, fusiform gyrus. **occipitotemporal g., median**, one on the tentorial surface of the temporal lobe, continuous anteriorly with the hippocampal gyrus and ending posteriorly in the occipital lobe. **g. olfacto'rius media'lis of Retzius**, Broca's area. **orbital g.**, irregular gyri on the orbital surface of the frontal lobe. **paracentral g.**, one on the mesial surface of a cerebral hemisphere, between the paracentral fissure and the precuneus. **parietal g., ascending**, one between the fissure of Rolando, the intraparietal fissure and the fissure of Sylvius. **parietal g., superior**, the superomedial border of the parietal lobe. **paroccipital g.**, the first, or superior occipital, gyrus of the cerebrum. **preinsular gyri**, radiating gyri forming the preinsula. **g. profun'di cer'ebri**, a deep cerebral gyrus. **quadrate g.**, an upward extension of the gyrus fornicatus on the median surface of the parietal lobe. **g. rec'tus**, a cerebral convolution on the orbital aspect of the frontal, between the olfactory fissure and the mesial margin. **Retzius' g., sagittal g.**, a large gyrus of the brain running parallel with the sagittal suture of the skull. **g. subcallo'sus**, a narrow fold of cortex below the rostrum of the corpus callosum. **subcollateral g.**, fusiform gyrus. **g. supracallo'sus**, a rudimentary gyrus on the upper surface of the corpus callosum. **supramarginal g.**, that part of the inferior parietal convolution which curves around the upper end of the sylvian fissure. **temporal g.**, any gyrus of the temporal lobe. **temporal g., inferior**, the gyrus of the temporal lobe, between the middle and inferior temporal sulci. **temporal g., middle**, that between the superior and middle temporal sulci. **temporal g., superior**, the gyrus of the temporal lobe, between the lateral fissure and the superior temporal sulcus. **temporal gyri, transverse**, horizontal convolutions marking the posterior extremity of the superior temporal gyrus; the more marked of these, the *anterior transverse temporal gyrus*, represents the cortical center for hearing. **g. transiti'vus**, annectant gyrus. **uncinate g., g. uncina'tus**, the hook-shaped forward continuation of the hippocampal gyrus.

H

H chemical symbol, *hydrogen.*
H. Holzknecht unit; L. *ho'ra* (hour); horizontal; hyperopia.
H⁺ symbol, *hydrogen ion.*
habena (hah-be'nah) habenula (def. 2). adj., **habe'nal, habe'nar.**
habenula (hah-ben'u-lah), pl. *haben'ulae* [L.] 1. any frenulum, especially one of a series of structures in the cochlea. 2. a triangular area in the dorsomedial aspect of the thalamus rostral to the pineal body. adj., **haben'ular.**
habit (hab'it) 1. an action which has become automatic or characteristic by repetition. 2. predisposition; bodily temperament. **drug h.**, see *addiction.* **full h.**, a plethoric bodily condition.
habituation (hah-bit″u-a'shun) acquired tolerance from repeated use or exposure to a specific stimulus or substance; applied to a condition due to repeated consumption of a drug, with a desire to continue its use, but with little or no tendency to increase the dose.
habitus (hab'ĭ-tus) [L.] habit; body conformation. **h. apoplec'ticus**, full habit. **h. enterop'toticus**, the body conformation seen in enteroptosis, marked by a long, narrow abdomen. **h. phthis'icus**, a body conformation predisposing to pulmonary tuberculosis, marked by pallor, emaciation, poor muscular development and small bones.
Habronema (hab″ro-ne'mah) a genus of nematode worms causing dermatitis in horses and other animals.
habronemiasis (hab″ro-ne-mi'ah-sis) infection with Habronema.
hachement (ahsh-maw') [Fr.] hacking or chopping stroke in massage.
hae- for words beginning thus, see also those beginning *he-.*
Haemadipsa (he″mah-dip'sah) a genus of leeches.
Haemaphysalis (hem″ah-fis'ah-lis) a genus of arthropods (family Ixodidae), several species of which are important as vectors of disease.
Haemobartonella (he″mo-bar″to-nel'ah) a genus of Microtatobiotes (order Rickettsiales, family Bartonellaceae).
Haemophilus (he-mof'ĭ-lus) a genus of Schizomycetes (order Eubacteriales, family Brucellaceae). **H. aegyp'tius**, an organism related to *H. influenzae*, and the cause of acute contagious conjunctivitis. **H. ducrey'i**, the causative agent of chancroid. **H. influen'zae**, a species which produces a serious form of meningitis, especially in infants. **H. vagina'lis**, a hemophilic bacterium associated, possibly causally, with human vaginitis.
hafnium (haf'ne-um) chemical element (*see table*), at. no. 72, symbol Hf.
hair (hār) a threadlike structure, especially the specialized epidermal structure developing from a papilla sunk in the corium, pro-

duced only by mammals and characteristic of that group of animals. **auditory h's,** epithelial hairs of the internal ear. **beaded h.,** hair marked with alternate swellings and constrictions; seen in monilethrix. **burrowing h.,** one which grows horizontally in the skin. **club h.,** a hair whose root is surrounded by a bulbous enlargement composed of keratinized cells, preliminary to normal loss of the hair from the follicle. **embedded h.,** burrowing hair. **Frey's h's,** stiff hairs mounted in a handle; used for testing the sensitiveness of pressure points of the skin. **ingrown h.,** one which has curved and re-entered the skin. **lanugo h.,** the fine hair on the body of the fetus, constituting the lanugo. **moniliform h.,** beaded hair. **resting h.,** one that has ceased growing, but has not yet been shed from the follicles. **ringed h.,** a condition in which a hair appears to be marked by alternating bands of white. **sensory h's,** hairlike projections on the surface of sensory epithelial cells. **stellate h.,** a hair split at the end in a starlike form. **tactile h's,** hairs sensitive to touch. **taste h's,** short hairlike processes projecting freely into the lumen of the pit of a taste bud from the peripheral ends of the taste cells. **terminal h.,** the coarse hair on various areas of the body during adult years. **twisted h.,** a hair which at spaced intervals is twisted through an axis of 180 degrees, being abnormally flattened at the site of twisting. **wooly h.,** lanugo.

hairball (hār'bawl) trichobezoar.

halation (hah-la'shun) indistinctness of the visual image by illumination from the wrong direction.

halazone (hal'ah-zōn) a white, crystalline powder used as a disinfectant for water supplies.

Haldrone (hal'drōn) trademark for a preparation of paramethasone acetate.

half-life (haf'līf) the time in which the radioactivity usually associated with a particular isotope is reduced by half through radioactive decay.

halide (hal'īd) a compound of a halogen with an element or radical.

halisteresis (hah-lis"ter-e'sis) deficiency of mineral salts in a part, as in bone. adj., **halisteret'ic.**

halitosis (hal'ī-to'sis) offensive odor of the breath.

halitous (hal'ī-tus) covered with vapor or moisture.

halitus (hal'ī-tus) an expired breath.

hallucination (hah-lu"sī-na'shun) a sensory impression (sight, touch, sound, smell or taste) that has no basis in external stimulation. **auditory h.,** a hallucination of hearing. **gustatory h.,** a hallucination of taste. **haptic h.,** tactile hallucination. **hypnagogic h.,** a hallucination occurring between sleeping and awakening. **olfactory h.,** a hallucination of smell. **tactile h.,** a hallucination of touch. **visual h.,** a hallucination of sight.

hallucinogen (hah-lu'sī-no-jen") an agent capable of producing hallucinations. adj., **hallucinogen'ic.**

hallucinogenesis (hah-lu"sī-no-jen'ē-sis) the production of hallucinations. adj., **hallucinogenet'ic.**

hallucinosis (hah-lu"sī-no'sis) the experiencing of hallucinations. **acute h., alcoholic h.,** alcoholic psychosis marked by auditory hallucinations and delusions of persecution.

hallux (hal'uks) the great toe. **h. doloro'sa,** a painful disease of the great toe, usually associated with flatfoot. **h. flex'us,** a bent great toe. **h. mal'leus,** hammer toe affecting the great toe. **h. rig'idus,** painful stiffness of the first metatarsophalangeal joint due to degenerative arthritis. **h. val'gus,** angulation of the great toe toward the other toes of the foot. **h. va'rus,** angulation of the great toe away from the other toes of the foot.

halmatogenesis (hal"mah-to-jen'ē-sis) a sudden alteration of type from one generation to another.

halo (ha'lo) a circular structure, such as a luminous circle seen surrounding an object or light. **Fick's h.,** a colored circle appearing around a light, due to the wearing of contact lenses. **h. glaucomato'sus, glaucomatous h.,** a narrow light zone surrounding the optic disk in glaucoma. **senile h.,** a zone of variable width around the optic papilla, due to exposure of various elements of the choroid as a result of senile atrophy of the pigmented epithelium.

Halobacterium (ha"lo-bak-tc're-um) a genus of Schizomycetes (order Pseudomonadales, suborder Pseudomonadineae, family Pseudomonadaceae).

haloduric (hal"o-du'rik) capable of existing in a medium containing a high concentration of salt.

halogen (hal'o-jen) a nonmetallic element of the seventh group of the periodic system: chlorine, iodine, bromine or fluorine.

halometer (hal-lom'ē-ter) erythrocytometer.

halophil (hal'o-fil) a microorganism that requires a high concentration of salt for optimal growth.

halophilic (hal"o-fil'ik) pertaining to or characterized by an affinity for salt; requiring a high concentration of salt for optimal growth.

Halotestin (-tes'tin) trademark for a preparation of fluoxymesterone.

haluthane (hal'o-thān) a colorless, mobile, nonflammable, heavy liquid used by inhalation to produce general anesthesia.

hamarthritis (ham"ar-thri'tis) arthritis of all the joints.

hamartia (ham-ar'she-ah) defect in tissue combination during development.

hamartoblastoma (ham-ar"to-blas-to'mah) a specific tumor of embryonic tissue.

hamartoma (ham"ar-to'mah) a mixture of tissue commonly present in an organ, but not existing in the usual arrangement. **vascular h.,** hemangioma.

hamartomatosis (-to"mah-to'sis) the presence of multiple hamartomas.

hamartoplasia (-to-pla'ze-ah) overdevelopment of tissue in response to trauma.

hammer (ham'er) the malleus. **Major's h.,** a

metal hammer intended to be heated in boiling water and applied to the skin as a counter-irritant.

hamster (ham'ster) a small rodent, used extensively in laboratory experiments.

hamstring (ham'string) a tendon which laterally bounds the popliteal space. **inner h's,** tendons of gracilis, sartorius and two other muscles of leg. **outer h.,** tendon of biceps flexor femoris.

hamulus (ham'u-lus), pl. *ham'uli* [L.] any hook-shaped process. adj., **ham'ular.**

hand (hand) the terminal part of an arm, or of the upper (anterior) extremity of a primate. **ape h.,** one with the thumb permanently extended. **drop h.,** wrist drop. **Krukenberg's h.,** a forklike stump created by separating the distal ends of the radius and ulna and covering them with skin, after amputation proximal to the carpus. **writing h.,** in paralysis agitans, assumption of the position by which a pen is commonly held.

H and E hematoxylin and eosin (stain).

handedness (hand'ed-nes) the preferential use of the hand of one side in all voluntary motor acts.

handpiece (hand'pēs) a device which engages the bur or working point used in procedures on the teeth while it is revolved by the dental engine.

hansenarium (han″sĕ-na're-um), pl. *hansena'-ria* [L.] a term suggested to replace leprosarium, as the name of an institution devoted to care of patients with leprosy (Hansen's disease).

hapalonychia (hap″ah-lo-nik'e-ah) abnormal softening of the nails.

haphalgesia (haf″al-je'ze-ah) pain on touching objects.

haphephobia (haf″e-fo'be-ah) morbid fear of contact.

haploid (hap'loid) having half the number of chromosomes characteristically found in the somatic cells of an organism; typical of the gametes of a species whose union restores the diploid number.

haploidy (hap'loi-de) the state of having only one member of each pair of homologous chromosomes.

haploscope (hap'lo-skōp) a form of stereoscope.

hapten (hap'ten) haptene.

haptene (hap'tēn) the portion of an antigenic molecule or complex that determines its immunologic specificity.

haptic (hap'tik) tactile.

haptics (hap'tiks) the science of the sense of touch.

haptoglobin (hap″to-glo'bin) a serum alpha-2 globulin glycoprotein that binds free hemoglobin; different types, genetically determined, are distinguished electrophoretically.

haptophore (hap'to-fōr) the specific group of atoms in a toxin molecule by which it attaches itself to another molecule; it is capable of neutralizing antitoxin and of acting as an antigen to stimulate specific antitoxin production by body cells. adj., **haptoph'orous.**

harelip (hār'lip) congenitally cleft lip.

harmony (har'mo-ne) the state of working together smoothly. **occlusal h.,** proper occlusion of the teeth in various positions of the mandible.

Harmonyl (har'mo-nil) trademark for preparations of deserpidine.

haustration (hos-tra'shun) 1. the formation of a haustrum. 2. a haustrum.

haustrum (hos'trum), pl. *haus'tra* [L.] one of the pouches of the colon, produced by collection of circular muscle fibers at 1- or 2-cm. distances, and responsible for the sacculated appearance. adj., **haus'tral.**

Hb hemoglobin.

H.C. Hospital Corps.

He chemical symbol, *helium.*

head (hed) the anterior or superior part of a structure or organism, in vertebrates containing the brain and the organs of special sense. **articular h.,** an eminence on a bone by which it articulates with another bone. **big h.,** swelled head. **hourglass h.,** one in which the coronal suture is depressed. **nerve h.,** the optic disk. **saddle h.,** a head with a sunken crown. **steeple h.,** oxycephaly. **swelled h.,** a condition in young rams due to infection by *Clostridium novyi,* and characterized by intense edematous swelling of the head, face and neck. **tower h.,** oxycephaly.

headache (hed'āk) pain in the head, conventionally designating that restricted to the forehead and regions covered by the scalp. **cough h.,** stabbing pain produced by traction on pain-sensitive structures on coughing or straining. **sick h.,** that accompanied by considerable malaise; migraine. **tension h.,** a type due to prolonged overwork, emotional strain, or both.

headgrit (hed'grit) cholera of sheep.

healing (hēl'ing) the restoration of structure and function of injured or diseased tissues. **h. by first intention,** union of accurately co-apted edges of a wound, with an irreducible minimum of granulation tissue. **h. by second intention,** union by adhesion of granulating surfaces. **h. by third intention,** union by filling of wound with granulations.

health (helth) a state of physical, mental and social well-being.

healthy (helth'e) pertaining to, characterized by or promoting health.

heart (hart) the muscular component of the cardiovascular system that maintains the circulation of the blood. **athlete's h.,** aortic incompetence due to strain in athletic exercise. **bovine h.,** cor bovinum. **cervical h.,** a heart situated high up in the neck. **chaotic h.,** a heart which exhibits frequent premature systoles. **fatty h.,** replacement of heart muscle by deposit of normal fat beneath the epicardium, chiefly in the anterior wall of the right ventricle. **fibroid h.,** heart affected with fibroid degeneration. **irritable h.,** neurocirculatory asthenia. **luxus h.,** dilatation with hypertrophy of the left ventricle. **Quain's fatty h.,** fatty degeneration of the myocardium. **soldier's h.,** neurocirculatory asthenia. **tobacco h.,** cardiac disturbance from excessive use of tobacco. **triatrial h.,** cor triatriatum.

heart block (hart′blok) interruption of muscular connection between atrium and ventricle so that they beat independently of each other. **arborization h. b.,** a form in which there is interference with the fine terminal subendocardial fibers of the Purkinje system. **atrioventricular h. b., auriculoventricular h. b.,** a form in which the blocking is at the atrioventricular junction. **bundle-branch h. b.,** a form of heart block in which the two ventricles contract independently of each other. **complete h. b.,** a condition in which the functional relation between the parts of the bundle of His is destroyed by a lesion, so that the atria and ventricles act independently of each other. **interventricular h. b.,** bundle-branch heart block. **sinoatrial h. b.,** a form in which the blocking is located between the atria and the mouths of the great veins and coronary sinus.

heartburn (hart′bern) burning sensation in the epigastrium.

heart failure (hart′fāl-ūr) inability of the heart to perform its proper function of expelling blood from the ventricles. **backward h. f.,** heart failure produced by passive engorgement of the venous system. **congestive h. f.,** a condition resulting from cardiac output inadequate for physiologic needs, with shortness of breath, edema and abnormal retention of sodium and water in body tissues. **forward h. f.,** diminution in amount of blood propelled in a forward direction by the heart. **left ventricular h. f.,** failure of the left ventricle to maintain a normal output of blood. **total h. f.,** a condition due to weakening of the myocardium as a whole, with engorgement of neck veins and liver, and edema of the legs. **unilateral h. f.,** inadequate output of blood involving only one side of the heart.

heartworm (hart′werm) an individual of the species *Dirofilaria immitis*.

HEAT human erythrocyte agglutination test.

heat (hēt) 1. a form of kinetic energy communicable from one body to another, and appreciable by the thermal sense. 2. estrus. **h. of combustion,** the amount of energy released per mole of a compound on oxidation or combustion. **latent h.,** the heat which a body may absorb without changing its temperature. **molecular h.,** the product of the molecular weight of a substance multiplied by its specific heat. **prickly h.,** miliaria. **sensible h.,** the heat which, when absorbed by a body, produces a rise in temperature. **specific h.,** the number of calories required to raise the temperature of 1 gm. of a particular substance 1 degree centigrade.

hebephrenia (he″bē-fre′ne-ah) hebetic schizophrenia. adj., **hebephren′ic.**

hebetic (hē-bet′ik) pertaining to puberty.

hebetude (heb′ē-tūd) mental dullness.

hebiatrics (he″be-at′riks) ephebiatrics.

heboidophrenia (hē-boi″do-fre′ne-ah) dementia praecox marked by simple dementia.

hebosteotomy (he-bos″te-ot′o-me) pubiotomy.

hebotomy (he-bot′o-me) pubiotomy.

hecatomeric (hek″ah-to-mer′ik) having processes which divide in two, one going to each side of the spinal cord, said of certain neurons.

hecto- (hek′to) word element [Fr.], *hundred,* used in naming units of measurements to designate an amount 100 times (10^2) the size of the unit to which it jointed, e.g. hectoliter (100 liters); symbol h.

hectogram (hek′to-gram) one hundred grams; 3.53 ounces.

hectoliter (hek′to-le″ter) one hundred liters; 26.42 gallons.

hectometer (hek′to-me″ter) one hundred meters; 109.36 yards.

hedonism (he′do-nizm) excessive devotion to pleasure.

Hedulin (hed′u-lin) trademark for a preparation of phenindione.

heel (hēl) the hindmost part of the foot; by extension, a part comparable to the heel of the foot, or the hindmost portion of an elongate structure. **Thomas h.,** a shoe correction consisting of a heel ½ inch longer and ⅙–⅛ inch higher on the inside; used to bring the heel of the foot into varus and to prevent depression in the region of the head of the talus.

height (hīt) distance measured perpendicularly upward from a surface. **h. of contour,** a line surrounding the crown of a tooth and marking the junction of the surfaces sloping occlusally and those sloping cervically.

helcoid (hel′koid) like an ulcer.

helcology (hel-kol′o-je) the science of ulcers.

helcoplasty (hel′ko-plas″te) plastic surgery of ulcers.

helcosis (hel-ko′sis) the formation of an ulcer.

Heleidae (hē-le′ī-de) a family of flies of the order Diptera, species of which suck the blood of man and may serve as vectors of disease.

heli(o)- (he′le-o) word element [Gr.], *sun.*

helianthin (he″le-an′thin) an orange-yellow aniline dye.

helicine (hel′ī-sin) spiral.

helicoid (hel′ī-koid) coiled; spiral.

helicopid (hel′ī-ko-pod″) having a peculiar dragging gait, seen in certain paralyses.

helicotrema (hel″ī-ko-tre′mah) a foramen between the scala tympani and scala vestibuli.

heliencephalitis (he″le-en-sef″ah-li′tis) encephalitis from exposure to the sun.

heliophobia (he″le-o-fo′be-ah) morbid fear of sunlight.

heliotaxis (-tak′sis) the motile response of an organism to the stimulus of light.

heliotherapy (-ther′ah-pe) the sun cure.

heliotropism (he″le-ot′ro-pizm) the tendency of an organism to orient itself in relation to the stimulus of light.

helium (he′le-um) chemical element (*see table*), at. no. 2, symbol He.

helix (he′liks) 1. a coiled structure. 2. the superior and posterior free margin of the pinna of the ear. **Watson-Crick h.,** a representation of the structure of DNA, consisting of two coiled chains, each of which contains information completely specifying the other chain.

helminth (hel'minth) a worm or wormlike parasitic organism.

helminthagogue (hel-min'thah-gog) vermifuge.

helminthemesis (hel″min-them'ĕ-sis) the vomiting of worms.

helminthiasis (-thi'ah-sis) morbid state due to infestation with worms.

helminthicide (hel-min'thĭ-sīd) vermicide.

helminthology (hel″min-thol'o-je) the scientific study of worms.

helminthoma (-tho'mah) a tumor caused by a parasitic worm.

heloma (he-lo'mah) a corn. **h. du′rum,** hard corn, the usual type occurring over joints of the toes. **h. mol′le,** a soft corn.

helotomy (he-lot'o-me) excision of a corn or callus.

hemabarometer (hem″ah-bah-rom'ĕ-ter) instrument for ascertaining specific gravity of blood.

hemachrome (he'mah-krōm, hem'ah-krōm) the red coloring matter of blood.

hemacyanine (he″mah-si'ah-nin) hematocyanine.

hemacyte (he'mah-sīt) hemocyte.

hemacytometer (he″mah-si-tom'ĕ-ter) an instrument used in counting blood cells, commonly applied to a combination of counting chambers with cover glasses and pipets for red and white cells, all meeting established specifications.

hemacytozoon (-si″to-zo'on) any cellular microparasite in the blood.

hemad (he'mad) toward the hemal or ventral side.

hemadynamometer (he″mah-di″nah-mom'ĕ-ter) instrument for measuring blood pressure.

hemadynamometry (-di″nah-mom'ĕ-tre) measurement of blood pressure.

hemafacient (-fa'shent) 1. producing blood. 2. an agent which induces the production of blood.

hemagglutination (-gloo″tĭ-na'shun) agglutination of blood erythrocytes.

hemagglutinin (-gloo'tĭ-nin) an antibody that causes agglutination of erythrocytes. **cold h.,** one which acts only at temperatures near 4°C. **warm h.,** one which acts only at temperatures near 37°C.

hemagogue (he'mah-gog) promoting the flow of blood.

hemal (he'mal) pertaining to blood or blood vessels.

hemanalysis (he″mah-nal'ĭ-sis) analysis of the blood.

hemangiectasis (he-man″je-ek'tah-sis) dilatation of blood vessels.

hemangioameloblastoma (he-man″je-o-ah-mel″o-blas-to'mah) ameloblastic hemangioma.

hemangioblast (he-man'je-o-blast) a mesodermal cell which gives rise to both vascular endothelium and hemocytoblasts.

hemangioblastoma (he-man″je-o-blas-to'mah)

a true mesodermal tumor presumably arising from the primitive mesenchymal vascular network.

hemangioendothelioblastoma (he-man″je-o-en″do-the″le-o-blas-to'mah) angiosarcoma.

hemangioendothelioma (-en″do-the″le-o'mah) a true neoplasm consisting predominantly of masses of endothelial cells growing in and about vascular channels.

hemangioendotheliosarcoma (-en″do-the″le-o-sar-ko'mah) a vascular tumor with masses of endothelial cells showing the atypia and anaplasia characteristic of all malignant growths.

hemangioma (he-man″je-o'mah) a benign tumor made up of newly formed blood vessels. **ameloblastic h.,** a tumor composed of an ameloblastoma and hemangioma occurring concomitantly. **cavernous h.,** a growth on skin or mucous membrane, sometimes found in brain and other organs, consisting of dilated vascular channels filled with blood. **h. congenita′le,** a vascular nevus seen at birth or shortly after. **sclerosing h.,** one which has been transformed into a solidly cellular lesion by proliferation of endothelial cells and connective tissue stroma. **h. sim′plex,** a vascular nevus made up of red elevations composed of aggregations of small blood vessels, present at or appearing soon after birth. **strawberry h.,** nevus vasculosus.

hemangiopericyte (he-man″je-o-per'ĭ-sīt) pericyte.

hemangiopericytoma (-per″ĭ-si-to'mah) a tumor composed of spindled cells with a rich vascular network, which apparently arises from pericytes.

hemangiosarcoma (-sar-ko'mah) a malignant tumor of vascular tissue.

hemaphein (hem″ah-fe'in) a brown coloring matter of the blood and urine. adj., **hemaphe′ic.**

hemapoiesis (hem″ah-poi-e'sis) hemopoiesis.

hemapoietic (-poi-et'ik) hemopoietic.

hemapophysis (-pof'ĭ-sis) a costal cartilage.

hemarthros (hem-ar'thros) hemarthrosis.

hemarthrosis (hem″ar-thro'sis) blood in a joint cavity.

hemase (he'mās) an enzyme found in the blood.

hemasthenosis (hem″as-the-no'sis) defective state or defective circulation of the blood.

hemat(o)- word element [Gr.], *blood.* See also words beginning *hem-* and *hemo-.*

hematachometer (hem″ah-tah-kom'ĕ-ter) instrument for measuring speed of blood currents.

hemataerometer (hem″at-a″er-om'ĕ-ter) an instrument for measuring gases in the blood.

hematein (hem″ah-te'in) a compound, $C_{16}H_{12}O_6$, occurring in reddish brown plates with a metallic luster; the coloring principle of hematoxylin.

hematemesis (-tem'e-sis) the vomiting of blood.

hematencephalon (hem″at-en-sef'ah-lon) effusion of blood in the brain.

hematherapy (hem″ah-ther'ah-pe) treatment of disease by administration of blood.

hemathermous (hem″ah-ther′mus) warm-blooded.

hematic (he-mat′ik) pertaining to the blood.

hematidrosis (hem″ah-tī-dro′sis) excretion of bloody sweat.

hematimeter (hem″ah-tim′ē-ter) device for counting blood corpuscles.

hematin (hem′ah-tin) heme.

hematinemia (hem″ah-tī-ne′me-ah) presence of hematin in the blood.

hematinic (hem″ah-tin′ik) 1. increasing the number of erythrocytes and the hemoglobin concentration. 2. an agent that improves the quality of the blood.

hematinometer (hem″ah-tī-nom′ē-ter) instrument for measuring hemoglobin of the blood.

hematinuria (hem″ah-tin-u′re-ah) hematin in the urine.

hematobilia (hem″ah-to-bil′ĭ-ah) bleeding into the biliary passages.

hematobium (hem″ah-to′be-um) an organism living in the blood.

hematoblast (hem′ah-to-blast″) cell which develops into a red blood corpuscle.

hematocele (hem′ah-to-sēl″) an effusion of blood into a cavity, especially into the tunica vaginalis testis. **retrouterine h.,** a tumor formed by effusion of blood into the pouch of Douglas.

hematocelia (hem″ah-to-se′le-ah) effusion of blood into the peritoneal cavity.

hematochezia (-ke′ze-ah) the passage of bloody stools.

hematochromatosis (-kro″mah-to′sis) staining of tissues with blood pigment.

hematochyluria (-ki-lu′re-ah) blood and chyle in the urine.

hematocolpometra (-kol″po-me′trah) progressive accumulation of menstrual blood in vagina and uterus.

hematocolpos (-kol′pos) accumulation of blood in vagina.

hematocrit (he-mat′o-krit) the volume percentage of erythrocytes in whole blood.

hematocryal (hcm″ah to kri′al) cold-blooded.

hematocrystallin (-kris′tah-lin) hemoglobin.

hematocyanin (-sī′ah-nin) hemocyanin.

hematocyst (hem′ah-to-sist″) effusion of blood in the bladder or in a cyst.

hematocytopenia (hem″ah-to-si″to-pe′ne-ah) decrease in cellular elements of the blood.

hematocytosis (-si-to′sis) increase in cellular elements of the blood.

hematocyturia (-si-tu′re-ah) blood corpuscles in urine.

hematodialysis (-di-al′ĭ-sis) hemodialysis.

hematogen (hem′ah-to-jen″) any blood-producing substance.

hematogenesis (hem″ah-to-jen′ē-sis) the formation of blood.

hematogenic (-jen′ik) 1. hematopoietic. 2. hematogenous.

hematogenous (hem″ah-toj′ē-nus) produced by or derived from the blood; disseminated through the blood stream.

hematoid (hem′ah-toid) like blood.

hematoidin (hem″ah-toi′din) a crystalline pigment lacking iron, generally found where blood has extravasated into the tissues.

hematologist (he″mah-tol′o-jist) a specialist in hematology.

hematology (-tol′o-je) the science dealing with study of the blood.

hematolymphangioma (hem″ah-to-lim-fan″-je-o′mah) a tumor composed of blood and lymph vessels.

hematolysis (hem″ah-tol′ĭ-sis) hemolysis. adj., **hematolyt′ic.**

hematoma (he″mah-to′mah) a tumor-like mass produced by coagulation of extravasated blood in a tissue or cavity. **subdural h.,** a massive blood clot beneath the dura mater that causes neurologic symptoms by pressure on the brain.

hematomediastinum (hem″ah-to-me″de-as-ti′num) effusion of blood in the mediastinum.

hematometra (-me′trah) progressive accumulation of menstrual blood in the uterus.

hematometry (he″mah-tom′ē-tre) measurement of hemoglobin and various cells of the blood.

hematomphalocele (hem″at-om-fal′o-sēl) umbilical hernia containing blood.

hematomphalus (hem″at-om′fah-lus) 1. hematomphalocele. 2. blue discoloration around the navel in ruptured ectopic pregnancy.

hematomycosis (hem″ah-to-mi-ko′sis) the presence of a fungus in the blood.

hematomyelia (-mi-e′le-ah) hemorrhage into the gray substance of the spinal cord.

hematomyelitis (-mi″ē-li′tis) acute myelitis with bloody effusion.

hematomyelopore (-mi″ĕ-lo-pōr″) formation of canals in spinal cord due to hemorrhage.

hematonephrosis (-ne-fro′sis) blood in the renal pelvis.

hematonosis (hem″ah-ton′o-sis) a disease of the blood.

hematopathology (hem″ah-to-pah-thol′o-je) the study of diseases of the blood.

hematophagous (hem″ah-tof′ah-gus) subsisting on blood.

hematophilia (hcm″ah-to-fil′e ah) hemophilia.

hematophyte (hem″ah-to-fīt″) any vegetative microorganism or species living in the blood. adj., **hematophyt′ic.**

hematopneic (hem″ah-top-ne′ik) pertaining to oxygenation of the blood.

hematopoiesis (hem″ah-to-poi-e′sis) production of blood or of its constituent elements. adj., **hematopoiet′ic.**

hematoporphyria (-por-fir′e-ah) a disorder with large quantities of hematoporphyrin in the urine.

hematoporphyrin (-por′fī-rin) an iron-free derivative of heme, a product of the decomposition of hemoglobin.

hematoporphyrinemia (-por″fī-rī-ne′me-ah) hematoporphyrin in the blood.

hematoporphyrinism (-por′fī-rin-izm″) a condition marked by hematoporphyrinemia and sensitiveness to sunlight.

hematoporphyrinuria (-por″fī-rī-nu′re-ah) hematoporphyrin in urine.

hematorrhachis (hem″at-o′rah-kis) hemorrhage into or beneath the meninges of the spinal cord.

hematorrhea (hem″ah-to-re′ah) copious hemorrhage.

hematosalpinx (-sal′pinks) an accumulation of blood in the uterine tube.

hematoscheocele (hem″ah-tos′ke-o-sēl″) hematoma of the scrotum.

hematoscope (hem″ah-to-skōp″) device used in examining thin layers of blood.

hematoscopy (hem″ah-tos′ko-pe) the inspection of blood.

hematosepsis (hem″ah-to-sep′sis) septicemia.

hematospectroscopy (-spek-tros′ko-pe) spectroscopic examination of blood.

hematospermatocele (-sper-mat′o-sēl) a spermatocele containing blood.

hematospermia (-sper′me-ah) blood in the semen.

hematosteon (hem″ah-tos′te-on) hemorrhage into the medullary cavity of a bone.

hematothermal (hem″ah-to-ther′mal) warm-blooded.

hematotoxic (-tok′sik) pertaining to blood poisoning.

hematotoxicosis (-tok″sĭ-ko′sis) toxic damage to the blood-forming organs.

hematotrachelos (-trah-ke′los) distention of the cervix uteri with blood.

hematotropic (-trop′ik) having a special affinity for the blood or red blood corpuscles.

hematoxylin (hem″ah-tok′sĭ-lin) an acid coloring matter obtained from the wood of a tree (*Haematoxylon campechianum*); used as a stain for histologic specimens.

hematozoon (hem″ah-to-zo′on) any animal microorganism or species living in the blood. adj., **hematozo′ic**.

hematuresis (hem″ah-tu-re′sis) hematuria.

hematuria (hem″ah-tu′re-ah) excretion of urine containing blood. **endemic h.**, urinary schistosomiasis. **enzootic bovine h.**, disease of cattle marked by blood in the urine, anemia and debilitation. **essential h.**, renal bleeding of undetermined cause. **false h.**, redness of the urine due to ingestion of food or drugs containing pigment. **renal h.**, hematuria in which the blood comes from the kidney. **urethral h.**, hematuria in which the blood comes from the urethra. **vesical h.**, hematuria in which the blood comes from the bladder.

heme (hēm) an iron compound of protoporphyrin which constitutes the pigment portion or protein-free part of the hemoglobin molecule.

hemeralopia (hem″er-ah-lo′pe-ah) day blindness.

hemi- (hem′i) word element [Gr.], *half*.

hemiacardius (hem″e-ah-kar′de-us) an unequal twin in which the heart is rudimentary.

hemiachromatopsia (-a″kro-mah-top′se-ah) loss of the normal perception of color in half of the visual field.

hemialbumin (-al-bu′min) antialbumin.

hemialbumose (-al′bu-mōs) a digestion product of certain proteids; normally found in bone marrow.

hemialbumosuria (hem″e-al″bu-mo-su′re-ah) hemialbumose in urine.

hemiamyosthenia (-ah-mi″os-the′ne-ah) lack of muscular power on one side of the body.

hemianacusia (-an″ah-ku′ze-ah) loss of hearing in one ear.

hemianalgesia (-an″al-je′ze-ah) analgesia on one side of the body.

hemianencephaly (-an″en-sef′ah-le) congenital absence of one side of the brain.

hemianesthesia (-an″es-the′ze-ah) anesthesia of one side of the body.

hemianopia (-ah-no′pe-ah) defective vision or blindness in half of the visual field; usually applied to bilateral defects caused by a single lesion. adj., **hemiano′pic. absolute h.**, blindness to light, color and form in half of the visual field. **altitudinal h.**, defective vision or blindness in a horizontal half of the visual field. **binasal h.**, crossed hemianopia in which the defect is in the nasal half of the visual field in each eye. **binocular h.**, true hemianopia. **bitemporal h.**, crossed hemianopia in which the defect is in the temporal half of the visual field in each eye. **complete h.**, that affecting an entire half of the visual field in each eye. **congruous h.**, that in which the defect is approximatedly the same in each eye. **crossed h.**, that in which the defect is in different vertical halves (one right and one left) of the visual field in the two eyes. **equilateral h.**, homonymous hemianopia. **heteronymous h.**, crossed hemianopia. **homonymous h.**, loss of vision in half the visual field on the same side (right or left) in both eyes. **horizontal h.**, altitudinal hemianopia. **lateral h.**, blindness for the right or left half of the field of vision. **lower h.**, defective vision in the lower half of the visual field. **nasal h.**, defective vision or blindness in the medial vertical half of the visual field, i.e. nearest the nose. **quadrant h., quadrantic h.**, quadrantanopia. **temporal h.**, defective vision or blindness in the lateral vertical half of the visual field, i.e. the half nearest the temple. **true h.**, defective vision or blindness in one vertical half of each eye, due to a single lesion of the optic tract, at or above the level of the chiasm. **unilateral h.**, defective vision or blindness in half of the visual field of one eye only. **uniocular h.**, unilateral hemianopia. **upper h.**, defective vision in the upper half of the visual field. **vertical h.**, lateral hemianopia.

hemianopsia (-ah-nop′se-ah) hemianopia.

hemianosmia (-an-oz′me-ah) absence of sense of smell in one nostril.

hemiapraxia (-ah-prak′se-ah) inability to perform coordinated movements on one side of the body.

hemiataxia (-ah-tak′se-ah) ataxia on one side of the body.

hemiathetosis (-ath″ĕ-to′sis) athetosis of one side of the body.

hemiatrophy (-at′ro-fe) atrophy of one side of the body.

hemiautotroph (-aw′to-trōf) an organism

which can build up protein from inorganic nitrogen, but requires organic carbon. adj., **hemiautotroph'ic.**

hemiballismus (hem″ĭ-ba-liz′mus) violent motor restlessness of half of the body, most marked in the upper extremity.

hemic (he′mik, hem′ik) pertaining to blood.

hemicardia (hem″ĭ-kar′de-ah) 1. the presence of only one side of a four-chambered heart. 2. one side of a four-chambered heart.

hemicellulose (-sel′u-lōs) a cellular plant material which is more soluble than cellulose.

hemicentrum (-sen′trum) either lateral half of a vertebral centrum.

hemicephalia (-sĕ-fa′le-ah) congenital absence of one side of the skull.

hemicephalus (-sef′ah-lus) a fetal monster with one cerebral hemisphere.

hemichorea (ko-re′ah) chorea affecting only one side of the body.

hemichromatopsia (-kro″mah-top′se-ah) defective perception of color in half of the visual field.

hemicolectomy (-ko-lek′to-me) excision of approximately half of the colon. **left h.,** excision of the entire left colon, from the middle of the transverse colon to the rectum. **right h.,** excision of the entire right colon, from the ileum to the middle of the transverse colon.

hemicorporectomy (-kor″po-rek′to-me) surgical removal of the lower part of the body, including the bony pelvis, external genitals and the lower part of the rectum and anus.

hemicrania (-kra′ne-ah) 1. headache on one side of the head. 2. developmental anomaly with absence of half of the cranium, or brain case.

hemicraniosis (-kra″ne-o′sis) hyperostosis of one side of the cranium and face.

hemidiaphoresis (-di″ah-fo-re′sis) sweating of one side of the body.

hemidysergia (-dis-er′je-ah) dysergia on one side of the body.

hemidysesthesia (-dis″es-the′ze-ah) disorder of sensation affecting only one side of the body.

hemidystrophy (-dis′tro-fe) unequal development of the two sides of the body.

hemiectromelia (-ek″tro-me′le-ah) developmental anomaly with imperfect limbs on one side of the body.

hemiepilepsy (hem″e-ep′ĭ-lep″se) epilepsy of one side of the body.

hemifacial (hem″ĭ-fa′shal) affecting one side of the face.

hemigastrectomy (-gas-trek′to-me) excision of half of the stomach.

hemigeusia (-gu′ze-ah) absence of sense of taste on one side of the tongue.

hemiglossectomy (-glŏ-sek′to-me) excision of part of the tongue.

hemiglossitis (-glŏ-si′tis) inflammation of half of the tongue.

hemignathia (-na′the-ah) a developmental anomaly characterized by partial or complete lack of the lower jaw on one side.

hemihidrosis (-hī-dro′sis) sweating on one side of the body.

hemihypalgesia (hem″ĭ-hīp″al-je′ze-ah) diminished sensitivity to pain on one side of the body.

hemihyperesthesia (-hi″per-es-the′ze-ah) increased sensitiveness of one side of the body.

hemihyperhidrosis (-hi″per-hī-dro′sis) excessive perspiration on one side of the body.

hemihyperplasia (-hi″per-pla′ze-ah) overdevelopment of one side of the body or of half of an organ or part.

hemihypertonia (-hi″per-to′ne-ah) increased tonicity of muscles on one side of the body.

hemihypertrophy (-hi-per′tro-fe) overgrowth of one side of the body.

hemihypesthesia (-hīp″es-the′ze-ah) diminished sensitiveness on one side of the body.

hemihypoplasia (-hi″po-pla′ze-ah) underdevelopment of one side of the body or of half of an organ or part.

hemihypotonia (-hi″po-to′ne-ah) diminished tonicity of one side of the body.

hemilaminectomy (-lam″ĭ-nek′to-me) excision of part of a vertebral lamina.

hemilaryngectomy (-lar″ĭn-jek′to-me) excision of part of the larynx.

hemilateral (-lat′er-al) affecting one side of the body only.

hemilesion (-le′zhun) a lesion on one side of the spinal cord.

hemimelia (-me′le-ah) developmental anomaly characterized by absence of all or part of the distal half of a limb.

hemimelus (hem-im′ĕ-lus) a fetus with defective limbs.

heminephrectomy (hem″ĭ-ne-frek′to-me) excision of part (half) of a kidney.

hemiopia (hem″e-o′pe-ah) hemianopia. adj., **hemiop′ic.**

hemipagus (hem-ip′ah-gus) twin fetuses joined at the thorax.

hemiparalysis (hem″ĭ-pah-ral′ĭ-sis) paralysis of one side of the body.

hemiparanesthesia (-par″an-es-the′ze-ah) anesthesia of the lower half of one side.

hemiparaplegia (-par″ah ple′je-ah) paralysis of the lower half of one side.

hemiparesis (-par′ĕ-sis) paralysis affecting one side of the body.

hemiparesthesia (-par″es-the′ze-ah) perverted sensation on one side.

hemipeptone (-pep′tōn) a form of peptone obtained from pepsin digestion.

hemiplacenta (-plah-sen′tah) an organ composed of the chorion, yolk sac and, usually, allantois which puts marsupial embryos into temporary relation with the maternal uterus.

hemiplegia (-ple′je-ah) paralysis of one side of the body. adj., **hemiple′gic. alternate h.,** paralysis of one side of the face and opposite side of the body. **cerebral h.,** hemiplegia due to brain lesion. **crossed h.,** alternate hemiplegia. **facial h.,** paralysis of one side of face. **flaccid h.,** hypotonia. **spastic h.,** hemiplegia with spasms and atrophy; usually infantile. **spinal h.,** hemiplegia due to lesion of spinal cord.

hemiprostatectomy (-pros″tah-tek′to-me) excision of half of the prostate.

hemiprotein (hem″ĭ-pro′te-in) antialbumin.

Hemiptera (hem-ip′ter-ah) an order of arthropods (class Insecta) characterized usually by the presence of two pairs of wings; including some 30,000 species, known as the true bugs.

hemipyocyanin (hem″ĭ-pi″o-si′ah-nin) an antibiotic produced by the growth of *Pseudomonas pyocyanea*, which is active against *Achorion schoenleini* and *Candida albicans*.

hemirachischisis (-rah-kis′kĭ-sis) fissure of the vertebral column without prolapse of the spinal cord.

hemisacralization (-sa″kral-i-za′shun) fusion of the fifth lumbar vertebra to the first segment of the sacrum on only one side.

hemisection (-sek′shun) bisection.

hemispasm (hem′ĭ-spazm) spasm affecting *sphe′ria* [L.] hemisphere.

hemisphere (hem′ĭ-sfēr) half of a spherical or roughly spherical structure or organ. **animal h.,** the half of the mass of cells formed by cleavage of a fertilized telolecithal ovum that is nearest the animal pole. **cerebral h.,** one of the paired structures constituting the largest part of the brain, consisting of the extensive cerebal cortex, corpus striatum and rhinencephalon, and containing the lateral ventricle. **dominant h.,** that cerebral hemisphere which is more concerned than the other in the integration of sensations and the control of many functions. **vegetal h.,** the half of the mass of cells formed by cleavage of a fertilized telolecithal ovum that is nearest the vegetal pole.

hemispherium (hem″ĭ-sfe′re-um), pl. *hemisphe′ria* [L.] hemisphere.

hemisystole (-sis′to-le) absence of contraction of left ventricle after every other contraction of the atrium.

hemithorax (-tho′raks) one side of the chest; the cavity lateral to the mediastinum.

hemithyroidectomy (-thi″roi-dek′to-me) excision of one lobe of the thyroid.

hemivagotony (-va-got′o-ne) irritability of the vagus nerve on one side.

hemivertebra (-ver′tĕ-brah) 1. either lateral half of a vertebra. 2. a developmental anomaly in which only half of a vertebra is present.

hemizygosity (-zi-gos′ĭ-te) the state of having only one of a pair of alleles transmitting a specific character. adj., **hemizy′gous.**

hemizygote (-zi′gōt) an individual exhibiting hemizygosity.

hemo- (he′mo) word element [Gr.], *blood.* See also words beginning *hem-* and *hemato-*.

hemo-alkalimeter (he″mo-al″kah-lim′ĕ-ter) an apparatus for estimating alkalinity of the blood.

hemobilia (-bil′e-ah) hematobilia.

hemobilinuria (-bil″ĭ-nu′re-ah) blood cells and bile pigments in the urine.

hemoblast (he′mo-blast) hemocytoblast. **lymphoid h. of Pappenheim,** proerythroblast.

hemocatheresis (he″mo-kah-ther′ĕ-sis) the destruction of red blood corpuscles. adj., **hemocatheret′ic.**

hemochorial (-ko′re-al) denoting a type of

placenta in which maternal blood comes in direct contact with the chorion.

hemochromatosis (he″mo-kro″mah-to′sis) a disorder of iron metabolism with excess deposition of iron in the tissues, skin pigmentation, hepatic cirrhosis and decreased carbohydrate tolerance. adj., **hemochromatot′ic.**

hemochrome (he′mo-krōm) an oxygen-carrying pigment of the blood.

hemochromogen (he″mo-kro′mo-jen) a compound formed by the combination of heme with a nitrogenous compound.

hemochromometer (-kro-mom′ĕ-ter) an instrument for making color tests of the blood.

hemochromoprotein (-kro″mo-pro′te-in) a colored, conjugated protein with respiratory functions, found in the blood of animals.

hemocidal (-si′dal) destroying blood cells.

hemoclasis (he-mok′lah-sis) destruction of red blood corpuscles. adj., **hemoclas′tic.**

hemoconcentration (he″mo-kon″sen-tra′shun) increase in the proportion of formed elements in the blood.

hemoconia (-ko′ne-ah), pl. *hemoco′niae* [L.] small, round or dumbbell-shaped bodies exhibiting active brownian movement, observed in darkfield microscopy of a wet film of blood.

hemoconiosis (-ko″ne-o′sis) presence in blood of excessive amounts of hemoconia.

hemocrystallin (-kris′tah-lin) hemoglobin.

hemoculture (-kul′tūr) a bacteriologic culture of the blood.

hemocuprein (-ku′pre-in) a copper and protein compound isolated from erythrocytes.

hemocyanin (-si′ah-nin) a blue-green blood pigment from crabs and lobsters, containing copper instead of iron.

hemocyte (he′mo-sīt) a blood corpuscle.

hemocytoblast (he″mo-si′to-blast) a primitive cell from which all blood corpuscles develop.

hemocytoblastoma (-si″to-blas-to′mah) a tumor containing undifferentiated blood cells.

hemocytocatheresis (-kah-ther′ĕ-sis) destruction of blood cells.

hemocytogenesis (-jen′ĕ-sis) formation of blood cells.

hemocytology (he″mo-si-tol′o-je) the study of blood cells.

hemocytolysis (-si-tol′ĭ-sis) disintegration of blood cells.

hemocytoma (-si-to′mah) a tumor containing undifferentiated blood cells.

hemocytometer (-si-tom′ĕ-ter) hematimeter. **Thomas-Zeiss h.,** an instrument for counting blood corpuscles.

hemocytophagy (-si-tof′ah-je) ingestion and destruction of blood cells by the histiocytes of the reticuloendothelial system. adj., **hemocytophag′ic.**

hemocytopoiesis (-si″to-poi-e′sis) formation of blood cells.

hemocytotripsis (-trip′sis) disintegration of blood cells by pressure.

hemocytozoon (-zo′on) an animal microparasite inhabiting blood cells.

hemodiagnosis (he″mo-di″ag-no′sis) diagnosis by examination of the blood.

hemodialysis (he″mo-di-al′ĭ-sis) removal of certain elements from the blood by virtue of difference in rates of their diffusion through a semipermeable membrane while being circulated outside the body.

hemodialyzer (-di′ah-līz″er) an apparatus for performing hemodialysis.

hemodiastase (-di′as-tās) an enzyme found in the blood.

hemodilution (-di-lu′shun) increase in fluid content of blood, resulting in diminution of proportion of formed elements.

hemodipsia (-dip′se-ah) a desire to drink blood to assuage thirst.

hemodromometer (-dro-mom′ĕ-ter) instrument for measuring speed of the blood current.

hemodynamics (-di-nam′iks) the study of the movements of the blood.

hemodynamometer (-di″nah-mom′ĕ-ter) hemadynamometer.

hemoendothelial (-en-do-the′le-al) denoting a type of placenta in which maternal blood comes in contact with the endothelium of chorionic vessels.

hemoferrum (-fer′um) oxyhemoglobin.

hemoflagellate (-flaj′ĕ-lāt) a flagellate protozoan parasitic in the blood.

hemofuscin (-fus′in) brown coloring matter of blood.

hemogenesis (jen′ĕ sis) hematogenesis.

hemogenic (-jen′ik) pertaining to production of blood.

hemoglobin (-glo′bin) the oxygen-carrying pigment of the blood, made up of four different globin polypeptide chains, each composed of several hundred amino acids. **fetal h.**, the hemoglobin found in erythrocytes of the fetus, capable of taking up and giving off oxygen at lower oxygen tensions than that in erythrocytes of the adult. **muscle h.**, myohemoglobin. **reduced h.**, the hemoglobin of venous blood, which has given up its oxygen in the tissues.

hemoglobinated (-glo′bin-āt″ed) filled with or containing hemoglobin.

hemoglobinemia (-glo″bī-ne′me-ah) abnormal presence of hemoglobin in the blood plasma.

hemoglobinolysis (-glo″bī-nol′ĭ-sis) the splitting up of hemoglobin.

hemoglobinometer (-nom′ĕ-ter) a laboratory instrument for colorimetric determination of the hemoglobin content of the blood.

hemoglobinophilia (he″mo-glo″bī-no-fil′e-ah) fondness for hemoglobin. adj., **hemoglobinophil′ic.**

hemoglobinorrhea (-glo″bī-no-re′ah) escape of hemoglobin from the red blood corpuscles.

hemoglobinous (-glo′bī-nus) containing hemoglobin.

hemoglobinuria (-glo″bī-nu′re-ah) presence of hemoglobin in the urine. adj., **hemoglobinu′ric. epidemic h.**, hemoglobinuria of young infants, with cyanosis, jaundice, etc. **intermittent h., paroxysmal h.**, that occurring episodically, after exertion (*march hemoglobinuria*) or idiopathically, with

hemolytic anemia, leukopenia and possible thrombocytopenia (*nocturnal paroxysmal hemoglobinuria*). **paroxysmal cold h.**, sudden passage of hemoglobin in the urine following exposure to cold. **toxic h.**, that which is consequent upon the ingestion of various poisons.

hemogram (he′mo-gram) a graphic representation of the differential blood count.

hemohistioblast (he″mo-his′te-o-blast″) promonocyte.

hemoid (he′moid) resembling blood.

hemokinesis (he″mo-ki-ne′sis) augmentation of the flow of blood in the body. adj., **hemokinet′ic.**

hemokonia (-ko′ne-ah) hemoconia.

hemokoniosis (-ko″ne-o′sis) hemoconiosis.

hemolith (he′mo-lith) a concretion in the walls of a blood vessel.

hemolymph (he′mo-limf) 1. blood and lymph. 2. nutrient fluid or blood of certain invertebrates.

hemolymphangioma (he″mo-lim-fan″je-o′-mah) hematolymphangioma.

hemolysate (he-mol′ĭ-sāt) the product resulting from hemolysis.

hemolysin (he-mol′ĭ-sin) a substance produced in the body of an animal which disintegrates red corpuscles.

hemolysis (he-mol′ĭ-sis) disintegration of elements in the blood. adj., **hemolyt′ic. immune h.**, lysis of erythrocytes by complement in the presence of antibody to the erythrocyte. **passive h.**, lysis of erythrocytes on which antigen has been adsorbed in the presence of complement and antiserums to that antigen.

hemolytopoietic (he″mo-lit″o-poi-et′ik) pertaining to destruction and formation of blood cells.

hemomediastinum (-me″de-as-ti′num) hematomediastinum.

hemometer (he-mom′ĕ-ter) hemoglobinometer.

hemometra (he″mo-me′trah) hematometra.

hemonephrosis (-ne-fro′sis) effused blood in the kidney pelvis.

hemopathology (-pah-thol′o-je) the study of diseases of the blood.

hemopathy (he-mop′ah-the) disease of the blood. adj., **hemopath′ic.**

hemoperfusion (he″mo-per-fu′zhun) continuous circulation of blood outside the body through a material, such as charcoal, for removal of injurious factors from the blood stream.

hemopericardium (-per″ĭ-kar′de-um) effused blood in the pericardial cavity.

hemoperitoneum (-per″ĭ-to-ne′um) effused blood in the peritoneal cavity.

hemopexin (-pek′sin) an enzyme which coagulates blood.

hemopexis (-pek′sis) coagulation of blood.

hemophagocyte (-fag′o-sīt) a cell which destroys blood corpuscles.

hemophil (he′mo-fil) 1. thriving on blood. 2. a microorganism which grows best in media containing hemoglobin.

hemophilia (he″mo-fil′e-ah) a hereditary hemorrhagic diathesis characterized by hemarthroses and deep tissue bleeding, due to deficient generation of intrinsic thromboplastin. **h. A,** a hereditary hemophilic state transmitted by the female to the male as a sex-linked recessive abnormality, and due to absence of a specific coagulation factor. **h. B,** a hereditary hemorrhagic diathesis due to lack of coagulation factor IX, transmitted by the female to the male as a sex-linked recessive abnormality; called also *Christmas disease*. **h. C,** a hemorrhagic diathesis transmitted as an autosomal dominant and due to a lack of coagulation factor XI. **h. calcipri′va,** a bleeding tendency due to deficiency of calcium in the blood. **classic h.,** hemophilia A. **hereditary h.,** a bleeding tendency due to a genetically determined deficiency of some factor in the blood. **vascular h.,** angiohemophilia.

hemophiliac (he″mo-fil′e-ak) 1. a person affected with hemophilia. 2. pertaining to hemophilia.

hemophilic (-fil′ik) 1. pertaining to hemophilia. 2. living or growing especially well in blood.

hemophilioid (-fil′e-oid) resembling classic hemophilia clinically, but not due to the same deficiency in the blood.

Hemophilus (he-mof′ĭ-lus) a genus name formerly given a taxon of microorganisms growing best (or only) in the presence of hemoglobin. **H. bronchisep′ticus,** *Bordetella bronchiseptica*. **H. parapertus′sis,** *Bordetella parapertussis*. **H. pertus′sis,** *Bordetella pertussis*.

hemophobia (he″mo-fo′be-ah) fear of blood.

hemophoric (-for′ik) conveying blood.

hemophthalmia (he″mof-thal′me-ah) extravasation of blood inside the eye.

hemoplastic (he′mo-plas″tik) concerned with elaboration of the blood.

hemopleura (he″mo-ploo′rah) hemothorax.

hemopneumopericardium (-nu″mo-per″ĭ-kar′-de-um) effused blood and air in the pericardium.

hemopneumothorax (-nu″mo-tho′raks) hemothorax and penumothorax together.

hemopoiesis (-poi-e′sis) hematopoiesis. adj., **hemopoiet′ic.**

hemoposia (-po′ze-ah) the drinking of blood.

hemoptysis (he-mop′tĭ-sis) spitting of blood. **parasitic h.,** a disease due to *Paragonimus westermanii* in the lungs.

hemorrhage (hem′ŏ-rij) the escape of blood from a ruptured vessel. adj., **hemorrhag′ic. accidental h.,** caused by premature detachment of placenta. **capillary h.,** oozing from minute vessels. **concealed h.,** internal hemorrhage. **critical h.,** that which occurs at a crisis. **fibrinolytic h.,** that due to abnormalities in the fibrinolytic system and not dependent on hypofibrinogenemia. **internal h.,** that in which the extravasated blood remains within the body. **nasal h.,** epistaxis. **petechial h.,** subcutaneous hemorrhage occurring in minute spots. **postpartum h.,** that which follows soon after labor. **primary h.,** that which soon follows an accident. **secondary h.,** that which follows an accident after a con-

siderable lapse of time. **unavoidable h.,** caused by detachment of a placenta previa.

hemorrhagenic (hem″o-rah-jen′ik) causing hemorrhage.

hemorrhea (-re′ah) hematorrhea.

hemorrheology (he″mo-re-ol′o-je) the scientific study of the deformation and flow properties of cellular and plasmatic components of blood in macroscopic, microscopic and submicroscopic dimensions, and the rheological properties of vessel structure with which the blood comes in direct contact.

hemorrhoid (hem′ŏ-roid) a varicose dilatation of a vein of the superior or inferior hemorrhoidal plexus. adj., **hemorrhoi′dal. external h.,** a varicose dilatation of a vein of the inferior hemorrhoidal plexus, distal to the pectinate line and covered with modified anal skin. **internal h.,** a varicose dilatation of a vein of the superior hemorrhoidal plexus, originating above the pectinate line and covered by mucous membrane. **lingual h.,** a varicose dilatation of a vein at the root of the tongue. **prolapsed h.,** an internal hemorrhoid which has descended below the pectinate line and protruded outside the anal sphincter. **strangulated h.,** an internal hemorrhoid which has been prolapsed sufficiently and for long enough time for its blood supply to become occluded by the constricting action of the anal sphincter. **thrombosed h.,** one containing clotted blood.

hemorrhoidectomy (hem″o-roi-dek′to-me) excision of hemorrhoids.

hemosiderin (he″mo-sid′er-in) an insoluble form of storage iron, visible microscopically both with and without the use of special stains.

hemosiderosis (-sid″ĕ-ro-sis) a focal or general increase in tissue iron stores without associated tissue damage.

hemosozic (-so′zik) preventing destruction of blood corpuscles.

hemospasia (-spa′ze-ah) withdrawal of blood.

hemospermia (-sper′me-ah) hematospermia.

hemostasis (-sta′sis) arrest of the escape of blood by either natural (clot formation or vessel spasm) or artificial (compression or ligation) means. adj., **hemostat′ic.**

hemostat (he′mo-stat) an agent (instrument or drug) used to check the escape of blood.

hemostyptic (he″mo-stip′tik) chemically hemostatic.

hemotachometer (-tah-kom′e-ter) instrument for measuring speed of the blood flow.

hemotherapy (-ther′ah-pe) the use of blood in treating disease.

hemothorax (-tho′raks) collection of blood in the pleural cavity.

hemotoxic (-tok′sik) pertaining to or producing toxic destruction of blood cells.

hemotoxin (-tok′sin) an exotoxin characterized by hemolytic activity.

hemotroph (he′mo-trof) nutritive material from the circulating blood of the maternal body, utilized by the early embryo. adj., **hemotro′phic.**

hemotympanum (he″mo-tim′pah-num) blood in the tympanic cavity.

henbane (hen′bān) hyoscyamus.

hepar (he′par) [L.] liver.

heparin (hep′ah-rin) a mucopolysaccharide acid occurring in tissues, but most abundantly in the liver, or a mixture of active principles from the livers or lungs of domestic animals, which renders the blood incoagulable; used in the prevention and treatment of thrombosis and bacterial endocarditis, postoperative pulmonary embolism, frostbite and in repair of vascular injury. **sodium h.,** a mixture of principles from liver, lungs, intestinal mucosa or other tissues of domestic animals, used as a food by man, given to prolong clotting time of blood.

heparinize (hep′ĕr-ĭ-nīz″) to render blood incoagulable with heparin.

hepat(o)- word element [Gr.], *liver.*

hepatalgia (hep″ah-tal′je-ah) pain in the liver.

hepatargia (-tar′je-ah) autointoxication from defective liver action.

hepatatrophia (hep″ah-tah-tro′fe-ah) atrophy of the liver.

hepatectomize (hep″ah-tek′to-mīz) to deprive of the liver by surgical removal.

hepatectomy (-tek′to-me) surgical excision of liver tissue.

hepatic (hē-pat′ik) pertaining to the liver.

hepatic(o)- (hē-pat′ĭ-ko) word element [Gr.], *hepatic duct.*

hepaticoduodenostomy (hē-pat″ĭ-ko-du″o-dē-nos′to-me) anastomosis of the hepatic duct to the duodenum.

hepaticoenterostomy (-en″ter-os′to-me) anastomosis of hepatic duct to intestine (duodenum or jejunum).

hepaticogastrostomy (-gas-tros′to-me) anastomosis of the hepatic duct to the stomach.

hepaticojejunostomy (-je″ju-nos′to-me) anastomosis of hepatic duct to jejunum.

hepaticolithotomy (-lĭ-thot′o-me) incision of the hepatic duct with removal of calculi.

hepaticolithotripsy (-lith′o-trip″se) crushing of a stone in the hepatic duct.

hepaticostomy (hē-pat″ĭ-kos′to-me) fistulization of the hepatic duct.

hepaticotomy (-kot′o-me) incision of the hepatic duct.

hepatin (hep′ah-tin) glycogen.

hepatitis (hep″ah-ti′tis) inflammation of the liver. **homologous serum h.,** serum hepatitis. **infectious h.,** a subacute disease due to a virus, with liver enlargement, fever, gastrointestinal distress, headache, anorexia and jaundice. **infectious necrotic h. of sheep,** black disease. **serum h.,** a virus infection transmitted by inadequately sterilized syringes and needles and by administration of infectious blood, plasma or blood products. **transfusion h.,** serum hepatitis. **viral h.,** a viral infection causing minimal to severe necrosis of hepatic cells.

hepatization (hep″ah-tĭ-za′shun) conversion of the air-containing lung into solid tissue, resembling that of the liver, occurring in lobar pneumonia. **gray h.,** a late stage, in which the fibrinosuppurative exudate produces a gray color. **red h.,** the early stage, when the tissue is red because of the extravasated erythrocytes.

hepatoblastoma (hep″ah-to-blas-to′mah) a hamartoma of the liver.

hepatocele (hep′ah-to-sēl″) hernia of the liver.

hepatocirrhosis (hep″ah-to-sĭ-ro′sis) cirrhosis of liver.

hepatocolic (-kol′ik) pertaining to liver and colon.

hepatocuprein (-ku′prin) a copper-containing compound present in liver tissue.

hepatocystic (-sis′tik) pertaining to liver and gallbladder.

hepatodynia (-din′e-ah) pain in the liver.

hepatoflavin (-fla′vin) a flavin occurring in the liver.

hepatogenic (-jen′ik) giving rise to or forming liver tissue.

hepatogenous (hep″ah-toj′ĕ-nus) originating in or caused by the liver.

hepatogram (hep′ah-to-gram″) 1. a tracing of the liver pulse in the sphygmogram. 2. a roentgenogram of the liver.

hepatography (hep″ah-tog′rah-fe) 1. a treatise on the liver. 2. radiography of the liver.

hepatoid (hep′ah-toid) resembling the liver.

hepatolienography (hep″ah-to-li″ĕ-nog′rah-fe) radiography of liver and spleen.

hepatolith (hep′ah-to-lith″) a calculus in the liver.

hepatolithectomy (hep″ah-to-lĭ-thek′to-me) excision of a calculus from the liver.

hepatolithiasis (-lĭ-thi′ah-sis) formation of calculi in liver or gallbladder.

hepatology (hep″ah-tol′o-je) the scientific study of the liver and its diseases.

hepatolysin (-tol′ĭ-sin) a substance destructive to liver cells.

hepatolysis (-tol′ĭ-sis) destruction of the liver cells. adj., **hepatolyt′ic.**

hepatoma (hep″ah-to′mah) a tumor of the liver.

hepatomalacia (hep″ah-to mah-la′she-ah) softening of the liver.

hepatomegaly (-meg′ah-le) enlargement of the liver.

hepatomelanosis (-mel″ah-no′sis) melanosis of the liver.

hepatometry (hep″ah-tom′ĕ-tre) determination of the size of the liver.

hepatomphalocele (hep″ah-tom′fah-lo-sel″) omphalocele with liver also in the membranous sac outside the abdomen.

hepatonephric (hep″ah-to-nef′rik) pertaining to the liver and kidney.

hepatopathy (hep″ah-top′ah-the) any disease of liver.

hepatopexy (hep′ah-to-pek″se) fixation of displaced liver to abdominal wall.

hepatopleural (hep″ah-to-ploo′ral) pertaining to liver and pleura.

hepatoptosis (-to′sis) downward displacement of the liver.

hepatopulmonary (-pul′mo-ner″e) pertaining to liver and lungs.

hepatorenal (-re′nal) pertaining to liver and kidneys.

hepatorrhaphy (hep″ah-tor′ah-fe)   suture of the liver.

hepatorrhexis (hep″ah-to-rek′sis)   rupture of the liver.

hepatoscopy (hep″ah-tos′ko-pe)   examination of the liver.

hepatosis (hep″ah-to′sis)   any functional disorder of the liver. **serous h.,** veno-occlusive disease of the liver.

hepatosolenotropic (hep″ah-to-so-le″no-trop′-ik)   having an affinity for or exerting a specific effect on the cholangioles and interlobular ducts of the liver.

hepatosplenography (-sple-nog′rah-fe)   roentgenography of the liver and spleen.

hepatosplenomegaly (-sple″no-meg′ah-le)   enlargement of liver and spleen.

hepatotherapy (-ther′ah-pe)   administration of liver or liver extract.

hepatotomy (hep″ah-tot′o-me)   incision of the liver.

hepatotoxemia (hep″ah-to-tok-se′me-ah)   blood poisoning originating in the liver.

hepatotoxicity (-tok-sis′i-te)   the property of exerting a deleterious effect upon the liver cells.

hepatotoxin (-tok′sin)   a toxin that destroys liver cells.

hepatotropic (-trop′ik)   having a special affinity for the liver.

hepta- (hep′tah)   word element [Gr.], *seven.*

heptabarbital (hep″tah-bar′bĭ-tal)   a short- to intermediate-acting barbiturate.

heptachromic (-kro′mik)   1. pertaining to or exhibiting seven colors.   2. having vision for all seven colors of the spectrum.

heptad (hep′tad)   an element with a valence of seven.

heptapeptide (hep″tah-pep′tīd)   a polypeptide containing seven amino acids.

heptaploid (hep′tah-ploid)   1. pertaining to or characterized by heptaploidy.   2. an individual or cell having seven sets of chromosomes.

heptaploidy (hep′tah-ploi″de)   the state of having seven sets of chromosomes.

heptose (hep′tōs)   a sugar whose molecule contains seven carbon atoms.

heptosuria (hep″to-su′re-ah)   heptose in the urine.

herb (herb, erb)   a plant whose stems are soft and perishable, and which are supported chiefly by turgor pressure. **death's h.,** belladonna leaf.

hereditary (hĕ-red′ĭ-tār″e)   transmissible or transmitted from parent to offspring; genetically determined.

heredity (hĕ-red′ĭ-te)   transmission of characters from parent or other ancestor to offspring; the resemblance of individual organisms to their progenitors. **autosomal h.,** transmission of a quality or trait by a gene located on an autosome. **sex-linked h.,** transmission of a quality or trait by a gene located on a sex chromosome.

heredopathia (her″ĕ-do-path′e-ah)   any inherited pathologic condition.

heredosyphilis (-sif′ĭ-lis)   congenital syphilis.

hermaphrodism (her-maf′ro-dizm)   hermaphroditism.

hermaphrodite (her-maf′ro-dīt)   an individual organism having gonads of both sexes.

hermaphroditism (her-maf′ro-di-tizm″)   presence of both ovarian and testicular tissue in the same individual. **bilateral h.,** that in which gonadal tissue typical of both sexes occurs on each side of the body. **false h.,** pseudohermaphroditism. **lateral h.,** presence of gonadal tissue typical of one sex on one side of the body and tissue typical of the other sex on the opposite side. **protandrous h.,** that in which the male organs develop first, and those typical of the female sex develop later. **protogynous h.,** that in which the female gonads function first, the sexual role later being reversed. **synchronous h.,** that in which the gonads of both sexes are functional at the same time. **true h.,** coexistence in the same person of both ovarian and testicular tissue, with somatic characters typical of both sexes.

hermetic (her-met′ik)   impervious to the air.

hernia (her′ne-ah)   abnormal protrusion of an organ or a part thereof through structures normally containing it. adj., **her′nial. h. adipo′sa,** fat hernia. **Béclard's h.,** femoral hernia at the saphenous opening. **h. cer′ebri,** protrusion of brain substance through the skull. **Cloquet's h.,** pectineal hernia. **crural h.,** femoral hernia. **cystic h.,** cystocele. **diaphragmatic h.,** hernia through the diaphragm. **extrasaccular h.,** sliding hernia. **fat h.,** hernial protrusion of peritoneal fat through the abdominal wall. **femoral h.,** protrusion of a loop of intestine into the femoral canal. **Hesselbach's h.,** femoral hernia with a pouch through the cribriform fascia. **hiatal h., hiatus h.,** protrusion of any structure through the esophageal hiatus of the diaphragm. **Holthouse's h.,** hernia that is both femoral and inguinal. **incarcerated h.,** one which cannot be readily reduced, but without obstruction or strangulation; sometimes applied to an irreducible hernia with intestinal obstruction but no strangulation. **inguinal h.,** hernia into the inguinal canal. **interparietal h.,** one in which the loop of intestine does not protrude outside the abdominal wall. **interstitial h.,** a hernia lying in one of the planes of the abdominal wall, between the transverse fascia and a muscle layer. **ischiatic h.,** hernia through sacrosciatic foramen. **Littre's h.,** protrusion of a congenital diverticulum of the gut. **lumbar h.,** hernia in the loin. **mesocolic h.,** hernia into a pouch of the mesocolon. **obturator h.,** protrusion through obturator foramen. **pectineal h.,** hernia beneath the pectineal fascia. **properitoneal h.,** a hernia lying between the peritoneum and transverse fascia. **Richter's h.,** hernia involving only part of the lumen or the gut. **scrotal h.,** inguinal hernia which has passed into the scrotum. **sliding h., slip h., slipped h.,** hernia of the colon in which a portion of the part is drawn into or slips into a hernial sac by the inclusion in the sac of the parietal peritoneum to which it is attached. **strangulated h.,** one which is tightly constricted, and may become gangrenous. **umbilical h.,** herniation of part of the umbilicus, the defect in the abdominal wall and protruding bowel being covered with skin and subcutaneous tissue. **vaginal h.,** hernia in the vagina. **ventral h.,** hernia through the abdominal wall.

herniation (her″ne-a′shun) abnormal protrusion of an organ or other body structure through a defect or natural opening in a covering membrane, muscle or bone. **h. of nucleus pulposus,** rupture or prolapse of the nucleus pulposus into the spinal cord.

hernioid (her′ne-oid) resembling hernia.

herniology (her″ne-ol′o-je) the study of hernia.

hernioplasty (her′ne-o-plas″te) surgical repair of hernia, with reconstruction of the abdominal wall.

herniorrhaphy (her″ne-or′ah-fe) surgical repair of hernia, with suture of abdominal wall.

herniotomy (-ot′o-me) surgical repair of hernia.

heroin (her′o-in) a white, bitterish, crystalline powder, the diacetic acid ester of morphine, used as an anodyne and sedative. Its importation into the United States is illegal.

heroinism (her′o-in-izm″) addiction to heroin.

herpangina (her″pan-ji′nah) a febrile disease of children marked by vesicular or ulcerated lesions on the fauces or soft palate.

herpes (her′pēz) an infectious disease characterized by sudden onset of fever of short duration and appearance of vesicular or ulcerated lesions in the faucial area or on the soft palate, due to a virus of the Coxsackie A group. adj., **herpet′ic. h. catarrha′lis,** herpes simplex. **h. circina′tus,** tinea circinata. **h. febri′lis,** herpes simplex. **h. gestatio′nis,** a herpes peculiar to pregnant women. **h. i′ris,** a form seen in rings on the hands and feet. **h. praeputia′lis,** herpes on the genitalia. **h. sim′plex,** an acute infectious virus disease characterized by groups of watery blisters on the skin and mucous membranes. **h. ton′surans,** tinea tonsurans. **h. veg′etans,** pemphigus vegetans. **h. zos′ter,** an acute virus disease characterized by inflammation of dorsal root ganglia and by a vesicular eruption along the area of distribution of a cutaneous nerve. **h. zos′ter auricula′ris, h. zos′ter o′ticus,** herpes zoster of the ear. **h. zos′ter ophthal′micus,** herpes zoster affecting structures of the eye.

herpesvirus (her″pēz-vi′rus) the viral agent causing herpes simplex.

herpetiform (her-pet′i-form) resembling herpes.

hertz (herts) a unit of frequency, equal to one cycle per second.

HES hydroxyethyl starch.

hesperidin (hes-per′i-din) a citrin factor which influences permeability of blood vessels.

heter(o)- word element [Gr.], *other; dissimilar.*

heteradelphus (het″er-ah-del′fus) a twin monster with one fetus more developed than the other.

heteradenia (-de′ne-ah) an abnormality of gland tissue. adj., **heteraden′ic.**

heterecious (het″er-e′shus) requiring different hosts in different stages of development; a characteristic of certain parasites.

heteresthesia (het″er-es-the′ze-ah) variation of cutaneous sensibility on adjoining areas.

heteroagglutination (het″er-o-ah-glu″ti-na′shun) heterohemagglutination.

heteroalbumose (-al′bu-mōs) hemialbumose insoluble in water.

heteroantibody (-an″ti-bod′e) an antibody combining with antigens originating from a species foreign to the antibody producer.

heteroantigen (-an″ti-jen) an antigen originating from a species foreign to the antibody producer.

heteroautoplasty (-aw′to-plas″te) transfer of tissue from one part of the body to another.

heteroblastic (-blas′tik) originating in a different kind of tissue.

heterocephalus (-sef′ah-lus) a fetal monster with two unequal heads.

heterochromatin (-kro′mah-tin) material of the chromosomes that remains condensed and deeply staining during interphase, considered metabolically inert.

heterochromatosis (-kro″mah-to′sis) abnormal staining.

heterochromia (-kro′me-ah) diversity of color in a part normally of one color. **h. i′ridis,** difference in color of the iris in the two eyes, or in different areas in the same iris.

heterochronia (-kro′ne-ah) irregularity in time; occurrence at abnormal times.

heterochronic (-kron′ik) 1. pertaining to or characterized by heterochronia. 2. existing for different periods of time; showing a difference in ages.

heterochthonous (het″er-ok′tho-nus) originating in an area other than that in which it is found.

heterocyclic (het″er-o-si′klik) having an abnormal chain structure.

heterodermic (-der′mik) performed with skin from another individual.

heterodont (het′er-o-dont″) having teeth of different shapes, as molars, incisors, etc.

heterodromous (het″er-od′ro-mus) moving or acting in other than the usual direction.

heterodymus (het″er-od′i-mus) a fetal monster with a second head on the abdomen.

heteroerotism (het″er-o-er′o-tizm) sexual feeling directed toward another person.

heterogamety (-gam′ĕ-te) production by an individual of one sex (as the human male) of unlike gametes with respect to the sex chromosomes. adj., **heterogamet′ic.**

heterogamy (het″er-og′ah-me) the conjugation of gametes differing in size and structure, to form the zygote from which the new organism develops. adj., **heterog′amous.**

heterogeneity (het″er-o-jĕ-ne′i-te) the state of being heterogeneous.

heterogeneous (-je′ne-us) not of uniform composition, quality or structure.

heterogenesis (-jen′ĕ-sis) 1. alternation of generation. 2. asexual generation. adj., **heterogenet′ic.**

heterogenote (het′er-o-je″nōt) a cell which has

an additional genetic fragment, different from its intact genotype; usually resulting from transduction.

heterogenous (het″er-oj′ĕ-nus) of other origin; not originating in the body.

heterogony (het″er-og′o-ne) heterogenesis.

heterograft (het′er-o-graft″) a graft of tissue obtained from an animal of a species other than that of the recipient.

heterography (het″er-og′rah-fe) writing of other than the intended words.

heterohemagglutination (het″er-o-hem″ah-glu″tī-na′shun) agglutination of erythrocytes by a hemagglutin derived from an individual of a different species.

heterohemoagglutinin (-hem″ah-glu′tī-nin) a hemagglutinin that agglutinates erythrocytes of organisms of other species.

heterohemolysin (het″er-o-he-mol′ĭ-sin) a hemolysin which destroys red blood corpuscles of animals of other species than that of the animal in which it is formed.

heteroinoculation (-ĭ-nok″u-la′shun) inoculation from another organism.

heterokaryon (-kar′e-on) a cell or hypha containing two or more nuclei of different genetic constitution.

heterokinesis (-ki-ne′sis) the differential distribution of the sex chromosomes in the developing gametes of a heterogametic organism.

heterolalia (-la′le-ah) utterance of inappropriate or meaningless words instead of those intended.

heterologous (het″er-ol′o-gus) 1. made up of tissue not normal to the part. 2. derived from an individual of a different species or one having a different genetic constitution.

heterolysin (-ol′ĭ-sin) heterohemolysin.

heterolysis (-ol′ĭ-sis) destruction of blood cells of an animal by serum from another species.

heteromeric (het″er-o-mer′ik) sending processes through one of the commissures to the white matter of the opposite side of the spinal cord.

heterometaplasia (-met″ah-pla′ze-ah) formation of tissue foreign to the part where it is formed.

heteromorphosis (-mor-fo′sis) the development, in regeneration, of an organ or structure different from the one that was lost.

heteromorphous (-mor′fus) of abnormal shape or structure.

heteronomous (het″er-on′ŏ-mus) subject to different laws; in biology, subject to different laws of growth or specialized along different lines.

heteronymous (-on′ĭ-mus) standing in opposite relations.

hetero-osteoplasty (het″er-o-os′te-o-plas″te) osteoplasty with bone taken from another individual.

heteropagus (het″er-op′ah-gus) a conjoined twin monster consisting of unequally developed components.

heteropathy (-op′ah-the) abnormal or morbid sensibility to stimuli.

heterophany (het″er-of′ah-ne) a difference in manifestations of the same condition.

heterophasia (het″er-o-fa′ze-ah) the utterance of words other than those intended by the speaker.

heterophemia (-fe′me-ah) utterance of other than the intended words.

heterophil (het′er-o-fil″) a finely granular polymorphonuclear leukocyte represented by neutrophils in man, but characterized in other mammals by granules which have variable sizes and staining characteristics. adj., **heterophil′ic.**

heterophonia (het″er-o-fo′ne-ah) any abnormality of the voice.

heterophoria (-fo′re-ah) deviation of the visual axis of one eye when the other eye is covered and fusion is prevented.

heterophthalmos (het″er-of-thal′mos) heterochromia iridis.

heteroplasia (het″er-o-pla′ze-ah) replacement of normal by abnormal tissues. adj., **heteroplas′tic.**

heteroplasty (het′er-o-plas″te) plastic repair with tissue derived from an individual of a different species or with synthetic or nonorganic material.

heteroploid (het′er-o-ploid″) 1. characterized by heteroploidy. 2. an individual or cell with an abnormal number of chromosomes.

heteroploidy (het′er-o-ploi″de) the state of having an abnormal number of chromosomes.

heteropsia (het″er-op′se-ah) unequal vision in the two eyes.

heteropyknosis (het″er-o-pik-no′sis) 1. the quality of showing variations in density throughout. 2. a state of differential condensation observed in different chromosomes, or in different regions of the same chromosome; it may be attenuated (*negative heteropyknosis*) or accentuated (*positive heteropyknosis*). adj., **heteropyknot′ic.**

heterosexual (-seks′u-al) 1. pertaining to or characteristic of the opposite sex. 2. a person with erotic interests directed toward one of the opposite sex.

heterosexuality (-seks″u-al′ĭ-te) attraction to persons of the opposite sex.

heterosis (het″er-o′sis) the existence, in the first generation of a hybrid, of greater vigor than is shown by either parent.

heterostimulation (het″er-o-stim″u-la′shun) stimulation of an animal with antigenic material originating from foreign species.

heterotaxia (-tak′se-ah) abnormal position of viscera.

heterotherm (het′er-o-therm″) an organism that exhibits different temperatures at different times or under different conditions.

heterothermy (het′er-o-ther″me) exhibition of widely different body temperatures at different times or under different conditions. adj., **heterother′mic.**

heterotonia (het″er-o-to′ne-ah) a state characterized by variations in tension or tone. adj., **heteroton′ic.**

heterotopia (-to′pe-ah) displacement or misplacement of parts. adj., **heterotop′ic.**

heterotoxin (het″er-o-tok′sin) a toxin derived from an external source.

heterotransplant (-trans′plant) tissue taken from one individual and transplanted into one of a different species.

heterotrichosis (-tri-ko′sis) growth of hairs of different colors on the body.

heterotroph (het′er-o-tröf″) a heterotrophic organism.

heterotrophic (het″er-o-tröf′ik) not self-sustaining; requiring complex organic substances (growth factors) for nutrition.

heterotropia (-tro′pe-ah) deviation of the visual axis of one eye when the other eye is fixing, with the result that single binocular vision is prevented. **comitant h., concomitant h.,** deviation of a visual axis in which the angular relation between the visual axes remains fairly constant, whatever the position of the fixing eye. **noncomitant h.,** deviation in which there is no maintenance of the angular relation between the visual axes. **paralytic h.,** heterotropia due to paralysis of one or more of the extraocular muscles.

heterotypic (-tip′ik) pertaining to, characteristic of or belonging to a different type. adj., **heterotyp′ical.**

heteroxenous (het″er-ok′sĕ-nus) requiring more than one host to complete the life cycle.

heterozygosity (het″er-o-zi-gos′ĭ-te) the state of having different alleles in regard to a given character. adj., **heterozy′gous.**

heterozygote (-zi′gōt) an individual exhibiting heterozygosity.

HETP hexaethyltetraphosphate.

Hetrazan (het′rah-zan) trademark for preparations of diethylcarbamazine.

heuristic (hu-ris′tik) encouraging or promoting investigation; conducive to discovery.

hex(a)- (hek′sah) word element [Gr.], *six.*

hexabasic (hek″sah-ba′sik) having six atoms replaceable by a base.

Hexa-betalin (-be′tah lin) trademark for preparations of pyridoxine hydrochloride.

hexachlorophene (-klo′ro-fēn) a crystalline compound, $C_{13}H_6Cl_6O_2$, used for its detergent and germicidal properties.

hexachromic (-kro′mik) 1. pertaining to or exhibiting six colors. 2. able to distinguish only six of the seven colors of the spectrum.

hexad (hek′sad) 1. a group or combination of six similar or related entities. 2. an element with a valence of six.

hexadimethrine (hek″sah-di-meth′rēn) a compound used to neutralize the anticoagulant action of heparin.

hexamethonium (-mĕ-tho′ne-um) an ammonium compound used in blockade of autonomic ganglia and to produce hypotension.

hexamine (hek′sah-min) methenamine.

hexaploid (hek′sah-ploid) 1. pertaining to or characterized by hexaploidy. 2. an individual or cell having six sets of chromosomes.

hexaploidy (hek′sah-ploi″de) the state of having six sets of chromosomes (6n).

hexatomic (hek″sah-tom′ik) containing six replaceable atoms.

hexavalent (-va′lent) having a valence of six.

Hexavibex (hek″sah-vi′beks) trademark for a preparation of pyridoxine hydrochloride.

hexavitamin (-vi′tah-min) a preparation of vitamin A, vitamin D, ascorbic acid, thiamine hydrochloride, riboflavin and nicotinamide.

hexestrol (hek-ses′trol) a compound used as an estrogenic substance.

hexethal (hek′se-thal) a short- to intermediate-acting barbiturate.

hexetidine (hek-set′ĭ-dēn) a compound used as an antibacterial, antifungal and antitrichomonal agent.

hexobarbital (hek″so-bar′bĭ-tal) an ultrashort-acting barbiturate. **sodium h.,** a white, crystalline powder, $C_{12}H_{15}N_2NaO_3$, used intravenously to produce general anesthesia.

hexobarbitone (-bar′bĭ-tōn) hexobarbital.

hexocyclium (-si′kle-um) a compound used in parasympathetic blockade and as an antispasmodic.

hexokinase (-ki′nās) an enzyme that catalyzes the transfer of a high-energy phosphate group of a donor to D-glucose, producing D-glucose-6-phosphate.

hexonic (hek-son′ik) pertaining to hexone bases.

hexose (hek′sōs) a monosaccharide containing six carbon atoms in a molecule.

hexosephosphate (hek″sōs-fos′fāt) a substance in muscle which, during contraction, splits into lactic acid and phosphoric acid.

hexylcaine (hek′sil-kān) a compound used as a local anesthetic.

hexylresorcinol (hek″sil-rĕ-zor′sĭ-nol) a compound, $C_{12}H_{18}O_2$, used as an anthelmintic.

Hf chemical symbol, *hafnium.*

HF Hageman factor.

Hg chemical symbol, *mercury* (L., *hydrargyrum*).

Hg. hectogram.

Hgb. hemoglobin.

HGF hyperglycemic-glycogenolytic factor (glucagon).

hiatus (hi-a′tus), pl. *hia′tus* [L.] a gap, cleft or opening. adj., **hia′tal. h. aor′ticus,** the aortic opening in the diaphragm. **esophageal h., h. esophage′us,** the opening in the diaphragm for the passage of the esophagus and the vagus nerves. **h. fallo′pii,** opening for vidian nerve in petrous bone. **h. semiluna′ris,** the groove in the nasal fossa into which open the antrum of Highmore and the middle ethmoid cells.

hibernation (hi″ber-na′shun) the dormant state in which certain animals pass the winter. **artificial h.,** a state of reduced metabolism, muscle relaxation and a twilight sleep resembling narcosis, produced by controlled inhibition of the sympathetic nervous system and causing attenuation of the homeostatic reactions of the organism.

hibernoma (-no′mah) a rare tumor made up of large polyhedral cells with a coarsely granular cytoplasm, occurring on the back or around the hips.

hiccough (hik′up) hiccup.

hiccup (hik'up) sharp inspiratory sound with spasm of glottis and diaphragm.

hidr(o)- (hid'ro) word element [Gr.], *sweat*.

hidradenitis (hi"drad-ĕ-ni'tis) inflammation of sweat glands. **h. suppurati'va,** a severe, chronic, recurrent suppurative infection of the apocrine sweat glands.

hidradenoma (-no'mah) adenoma of the sweat glands.

hidrocystoma (hi"dro-sis-to'mah) a sweat gland tumor.

hidropoiesis (-poi-e'sis) the formation of sweat. adj., **hidropoiet'ic.**

hidrorrhea (-re'ah) profuse perspiration.

hidroschesis (hi-dros'kĕ-sis) suppression of perspiration.

hidrosis (hi-dro'sis) 1. sweating. 2. disease of the sweat glands.

hieralgia (hi"er-al'je-ah) pain in the sacrum.

hierolisthesis (hi"er-o-lis-the'sis) displacement of the sacrum.

hilitis (hi-li'tis) inflammation of a hilus.

hilum (hi'lum) hilus.

hilus (hi'lus), pl. *hi'li* [L.] a depression or pit on an organ, giving entrance and exit to vessels and nerves. adj., **hi'lar.**

hindbrain (hīnd'brān) the portion of the brain developed from the most caudal of the three primary brain vesicles of the early embryo, comprising the metencephalon and myelencephalon.

hindfoot (hīnd'foot) the posterior portion of the foot, comprising the region of the talus and calcaneus.

hindgut (hīnd'gut) a pocket formed beneath the caudal portion of the developing embryo, which develops into the distal portion of the small intestine, the colon and rectum.

hip (hip) the region of the articulation of femur and innominate bone. **snapping h.,** slipping of the hip joint, sometimes with an audible snap, due to slipping of a tendinous band over the greater trochanter.

hippo (hip'o) ipecac.

hippocampus (hip"o-kam'pus), pl. *hippocam'-pi* [L.] a curved structure on the floor of the inferior horn of the lateral ventricle. **h. ma'jor,** hippocampus. **h. mi'nor,** a white elevation on the floor of the posterior cornu of the lateral ventricle.

hippuria (hĭ-pu're-ah) excess of hippuric acid in urine.

hippus (hip'us) abnormal exaggeration of the rhythmic contraction and dilation of the pupil, independent of changes in illumination or in fixation of the eyes.

hircus (her'kus), pl. *hir'ci* [L.] 1. the hair growing in the axilla. 2. tragus.

hirsute (her'sūt) shaggy; hairy.

hirsuties (her-su'she-ēz) hirsutism.

hirsutism (her'sūt-izm) abnormal growth of hair.

hirudicide (hĭ-roo'dĭ-sīd) an agent that is destructive to leeches. adj., **hirudici'dal.**

hirudin (hĭ-roo'din) the active principle of the buccal secretion of leeches.

Histadyl (his'tah-dil) trademark for preparations of methapyrilene.

Histalog (his'tah-log) trademark for a preparation of betazole.

histaminase (his-tam'ĭ-nās) an enzyme which inactivates histamine.

histamine (his'tah-min) a decomposition product of histidine, formed in the intestines and found in most body tissues, or produced synthetically; it causes dilatation and increased permeability of capillaries and stimulates gastric secretion and visceral muscle contraction. **h. phosphate,** $C_5H_9N_3.2H_3PO_4$; used in tests of gastric function and to reduce sensitivity to histamine.

histaminemia (his"tah-min-e'me-ah) histamine in the blood.

histaminia (his"tah-min'e-ah) shock produced by histamine.

histenzyme (his-ten'zīm) an enzyme from the kidney which catalyzes the splitting of hippuric acid into benzoic acid and glycocoll.

histidine (his'tĭ-din) a naturally occurring amino acid, first found as a decomposition product of protamine of sturgeon testes. **h. monohydrochloride,** small, colorless crystals, $C_6H_9N_3O_2.HCl.H_2O$; used in ulceration of the intestines.

histidinemia (his"tĭ-dĭ-ne'me-ah) excessive histidine in the blood.

histioblast (his'te-o-blast") an immature histiocyte.

histioblastoma (his"te-o-blas-to'mah) reticuloendothelioma.

histiocyte (his'te-o-sīt") a large phagocytic interstitial cell of the reticuloendothelial system.

histiocytoma (his"te-o-si-to'mah) a tumor containing histiocytes.

histiocytomatosis (-si-to"mah-to'sis) any general disorder of the reticuloendothelial system.

histiocytosis (-si-to'sis) a condition marked by an abnormal appearance of histiocytes in the blood. **lipid h.,** Niemann-Pick disease. **h. X,** a generic term embracing eosinophilic granuloma, Letterer-Siwe disease and Hand-Schüller-Christian disease.

histiogenic (-jen'ik) formed by the tissues.

histioid (his'te-oid) histoid.

histio-irritative (his"te-o-ir"ĭ-ta'tiv) irritative to tissue.

histoblast (his'to-blast) a tissue cell.

histochemistry (his"to-kem'is-tre) that branch of histology that deals with the disposition of chemical components in cells and in the intercellular materials of tissues.

histochromatosis (-kro"mah-to'sis) a general term for affections of the reticuloendothelial system.

histoclastic (-klas'tik) breaking down tissue.

histocompatibility (-kom-pat"ĭ-bil'ĭ-te) the quality of a cellular or tissue graft enabling it to be accepted and functional when transplanted to another organism. adj., **histocompat'ible.**

histodiagnosis (-di"ag-no'sis) diagnosis by microscopic examination of the tissues.

histodialysis (-di-al'ĭ-sis) disintegration or breaking down of tissue.

histogenesis (-jen'ĕ-sis) differentiation of

cells into the specialized tissues forming the various organs and parts of the body. adj., **histogenet'ic.**

histogram (his'to-gram) a graph in which values found in a statistical study are represented by lines or symbols placed horizontally or vertically.

histography (his-tog'rah-fe) description of the tissues.

histohematin (his"to-hem'ah-tin) one of a group of red tissue pigments.

histohematogenous (-hem"ah-toj'ĕ-nus) formed from tissues and blood.

histohypoxia (-hi-pok'se-ah) abnormally diminished concentration of oxygen in the tissues.

histoid (his'toid) developed from one tissue.

histoincompatibility (his"to-in"kom-pat"ĭ-bil'-ĭ-te) the quality of a cellular or tissue graft preventing its acceptance or functioning when transplanted to another organism. adj., **histoincompat'ible.**

histokinesis (-ki-ne'sis) movement in the tissues of the body.

histology (his-tol'o-je) microscopic study of the form and structure of the various tissues making up living organisms. **normal h.,** science of healthy tissues. **pathologic h.,** science of diseased tissues.

histolysis (his-tol'ĭ-sis) breaking down of tissues. adj., **histolyt'ic.**

histoma (his-to'mah) any tissue tumor.

histone (his'tōn) a simple protein, soluble in water and insoluble in dilute ammonia, found combined as salts with acidic substances, such as nucleic acids or heme, in animal tissues.

histonomy (his-ton'o-me) the scientific study of tissues based on the translation into biological terms of quantitative laws derived from histologic measurement.

histonuria (his"to-nu're-ah) histone in the urine.

histopathology (-pah-thol'o-je) pathologic histology.

histophysiology (-fiz"e-ol'o-je) physiology of the minute elements of tissues.

Histoplasma (-plaz'mah) a genus of fungi.

histoplasmin (-plaz'min) a preparation of growth products of *Histoplasma capsulatum,* injected intracutaneously as a test for histoplasmosis.

histoplasmosis (-plaz-mo'sis) infection with *Histoplasma capsulatum,* producing a variety of clinical pictures.

historrhexis (-rek'sis) the breaking up of tissue.

histoteliosis (-tēl"e-o'sis) the final differentiation of cells whose fate has already been determined irreversibly.

histotherapy (-ther'ah-pe) treatment by administration of animal tissues.

histothrombin (-throm'bin) thrombin derived from connective tissue.

histotome (his'to-tōm) a cutting instrument used in microtomy.

histotomy (his-tot'o-me) dissection of tissues; microtomy.

histotribe (his'to-trīb) an instrument for crushing tissues to secure hemostasis.

histotroph (his'to-trōf) amorphous nutritive material derived from maternal tissue, utilized by the early embryo.

histotrophic (his"to-trōf'ik) encouraging formation of tissue.

histotropic (-trop'ik) having affinity for tissue cells.

histozyme (his'to-zīm) an enzyme which causes fermentation in a tissue.

histrionism (his'tre-o-nizm") a morbid or hysterical adoption of an exaggerated manner and gestures. adj., **histrion'ic.**

hitch (hich) a knot. **clove h.,** a knot formed by a double loop: used in traction and forcible extension.

hives (hīvz) urticaria.

Hl. hectoliter; latent hyperopia.

Hm. hectometer; manifest hyperopia.

Ho chemical symbol, *holmium.*

hodoneuromere (ho"do-nu'ro-mēr) a segment of the embryonic trunk with its pair of nerves and their branches.

holandric (hol-an'drik) inherited exclusively through the male descent; transmitted through genes located on the Y chromosome.

holarthritis (hol"ar-thri'tis) inflammation of all the joints.

holergasia (hol"er-ga'ze-ah) a psychiatric disorder involving the entire personality. adj., **holergas'tic.**

holistic (ho-lis'tik) pertaining to totality, or to the whole.

holmium (hol'me-um) chemical element *(see table),* at. no. 67, symbol Ho.

holoacardius (hol"o-ah-kar'de-us) an unequal twin in which the heart is entirely absent. **h. aceph'alus,** one which has no head. **h. acor'mus,** one without a body, in which the head only is present. **h. amor'phus,** one which has no recognizable organs, being only a shapeless mass.

holoblastic (-blas'tik) undergoing cleavage in which the entire ovum participates; completely dividing.

Holocaine (ho'lo-kān) trademark for a preparation of phenacaine.

holocrine (hol'o-krēn) having the whole secretory cell, laden with its characteristic product passing off as secretion.

holodiastolic (hol"o-di"ah-stol'ik) pertaining to the entire diastole.

holoendemic (-en-dem'ik) affecting practically all the residents of a particular region.

holoenzyme (-en'zīm) an active substance formed by combination of a coenzyme and apoenzyme.

hologynic (-jin'ik) inherited exclusively through the female descent; transmitted through genes located on attached X chromosomes.

holophytic (-fit'ik) resembling a plant in every respect.

holorachischisis (-rah-kis'kĭ-sis) fissure of the entire vertebral column with prolapse of the spinal cord.

holoschisis (ho-los'kĭ-sis) amitosis.

holosystolic (hol″o-sis-tol′ik) pertaining to the entire systole.

holotetanus (-tet′ah-nus) general tetanus.

holothurin (-thu′rin) a hemotoxic substance derived from sea cucumbers.

holotonia (-to′ne-ah) muscular spasm of the whole body. adj., **holoton′ic.**

holozoic (-zo′ik) resembling an animal in every respect.

homaluria (hom″ah-lu′re-ah) production and excretion of urine at a normal, even rate.

homatropine (ho-mat′ro-pin) an alkaloid obtained by the condensation of tropine and mandelic acid; used to produce parasympathetic blockade and as a mydriatric. **h. hydrobromide,** a compound, $C_{16}H_{21}NO_3 \cdot HBr$, used topically in the eye as a cycloplegic and mydriatic. **h. methylbromide,** a compound, $C_{17}H_{24}BrNO_3$, parasympatholytic; used in treatment of gastrointestinal spasm and hyperchlorhydria.

homaxial (ho-mak′se-al) having all axes similar.

homeo- (ho′me-o) word element [Gr.], *similar, same; unchanging.*

homeochrome (ho′me-o-krōm″) staining with mucin stains after formol-bichromate fixation.

homeokinesis (ho″me-o-ki-ne′sis) the reception of identical amounts and kinds of chromation by the daughter cells in meiosis.

homeomorphous (-mor′fus) of like form and structure.

homeo-osmosis (-os-mo′sis) the maintenance by a cell, tissue, organ or organism of its fluid milieu at relatively constant and stable osmotic pressure (or tonicity), independent of the tonicity of the surrounding medium.

homeopathy (ho″me-op′ah-the) a system of medicine based on use of infinitesimal doses of medicines capable of producing symptoms like those of the disease treated.

homeoplasia (ho″me-o-pla′ze-ah) formation of new tissue like that adjacent to it. adj., **homeoplas′tic.**

homeostasis (-sta′sis) a tendency to uniformity or stability in the normal body states of the organism. adj., **homeostat′ic.**

homeotherapy (-ther′ah-pe) treatment with a substance similar to the causative agent of the disease.

homeothermal (-ther′mal) homothermal.

homeotransplant (-trans′plant) tissue taken from one individual and transplanted into another of the same species.

homeotransplantation (-trans″plan-ta′shun) transfer of tissue from one individual to another of the same species.

homeotypical (-tip′ĭ-kal) resembling the normal or usual type.

homergy (hom′er-je) normal metabolism.

homo- (ho′mo) word element [Gr.], *same; similar.*

homoarterenol (ho″mo-ar″tĕ-re′nol) nordefrin.

homocerebrin (-ser′ĕ-brin) principle obtainable from brain substance.

homochrome (ho′mo-krōm) taking the same color as the stain.

homodromous (ho-mod′ro-mus) moving or acting in the same or in the usual direction.

homogametic (ho″mo-gah-met′ik) having only one kind of gametes with respect to the sex chromosomes.

homogamy (ho-mog′-ah-me) inbreeding.

homogenate (ho-moj′ĕ-nāt) material obtained by homogenization.

homogeneity (ho″mo-jĕ-ne′ĭ-te) the state of being homogeneous.

homogeneous (-je′ne-us) of uniform quality, composition or structure.

homogenesis (-jen′ē-sis) reproduction by the same process in each generation. adj., **homogenet′ic.**

homogenic (-jen′ik) homozygous.

homogenicity (-je-nis′ĭ-te) homogeneity.

homogenize (ho-moj′ĕ-nīz) to convert into material that is of uniform quality or consistency throughout.

homoglandular (ho″mo-glan′du-lar) pertaining to the same gland.

homograft (ho′mo-graft) a graft of tissue from another animal of the same species, but having a different genotype.

homohemotherapy (ho″mo-he″mo-ther′ah-pe) treatment by injection of blood from another individual of the same species.

homoiopodal (ho″moi-op′ō-dal) having processes of one kind only.

homoiotherm (ho-moi′o-therm) an animal which exhibits homoiothermy; a so-called warm-blooded animal.

homoiothermy (ho-moi′o-ther″me) maintenance of a constant body temperature despite variation in environmental temperature. adj., **homoiother′mic.**

homolateral (ho″mo-lat′er-al) ipsilateral.

homologous (ho-mol′ŏ-gus) arising from common primordia and similar in basic plan and development, but having a different function.

homologue (hom′o-log) any homologous organ or part.

homology (ho-mol′o-je) the state of being homologous.

homolysin (ho-mol′ĭ-sin) isohemolysin.

homonomous (ho-mon′ŏ-mus) subject to the same laws; in biology, subject to the same laws of growth or developed along the same line.

homonymous (ho-mon′ĭ-mus) standing in the same relation.

homophil (ho′mo-fīl) acting only with a specific antigen.

homoplasty (ho′mo-plas″te) transplantation of tissue of the same sort as the tissue it replaces. adj., **homoplas′tic.**

homorganic (hom″or-gan′ik) produced by the same or by homologous organs.

homosexual (ho″mo-seks′u-al) 1. sexually attracted by persons of the same sex. 2. an individual sexually attracted by persons of the same sex.

homosexuality (-seks″u-al′ĭ-te) sexual attraction toward persons of the same sex.

homostimulant (-stim′u-lant) stimulating the organ from which it is derived.

homotherm (ho′mo-therm) homoiotherm.

homotonia (ho″mo-to′ne-ah) isotonia. adj., **homoton′ic.**

homotopic (-top′ik) occurring at the same place upon the body.

homotype (ho′mo-tīp) a part or object similar to another, but oppositely oriented. adj., **homotyp′ic.**

homozygosis (ho″mo-zi-go′sis) the formation of a zygote by the union of gametes of similar genetic constitution.

homozygosity (-zi-gos′ĭ-te) the state of having identical alleles in regard to a given character. adj., **homozy′gous.**

homozygote (-zi′gōt) an individual exhibiting homozygosity.

homunculus (ho-mung′ku-lus) a dwarf without deformity or disproportion of parts.

hoof-bound (hoof′bownd) dryness and contraction of a horse's hoof, causing lameness.

hook (hook) curved instrument for traction or holding. **Braun's h.,** an instrument used in fetal decapitation. **Malgaigne's h's,** adjustable double hooks for treating a fractured patella. **palate h.,** one for raising the palate in rhinoscopy. **Tyrrell's h.,** a blunt hook for drawing the iris through a hole in the cornea.

hookworm (hook′werm) an individual organism of the family Ancylostomidae. **American h., New World h.,** an individual of the species *Necator americanus.* **Old World h.,** an individual of the species *Ancylostoma duodenale.*

hordeolum (hōr-de′o-lum) inflammation of a gland of the eyelid. **h. exter′num,** suppuration of a gland of Zeis, near the edge of the eyelid. **h. inter′num,** suppuration of a meibomian gland, in the tarsus of the eyelid.

horismascope (ho-ris′mah-skōp) an instrument for examining the urine for albumin.

horismology (hor″iz-mol′o-je) the science dealing with the definition of terms.

horizocardia (ho-ri″zo-kar′de-ah) horizontal position of the heart.

horizon (ho-ri′zon) a specific anatomic stage of embryonic development, of which 23 have been defined, beginning with the unicellular fertilized egg and ending seven to nine weeks later, with beginning of the fetal stage.

hormesis (hōr-me′sis) stimulation by a subinhibitory concentration of a toxic substance.

hormion (hōr′me-on) point of union of sphenoid bone with posterior border of vomer.

hormonagogue (hōr-mōn′ah-gog) an agent which increases the production of hormones.

hormone (hōr′mōn) a chemical substance produced in the body which has a specific effect on the activity of a certain organ or organs. adj., **hormo′nal, hormon′ic. adaptive h.,** one which is secreted during adaptation to unusual circumstances. **adrenocortical h.,** one of the steroids produced by the adrenal cortex, of which there are four main types: (1) estrogen, (2) androgens, (3) progesterone, and (4) corticoids. **adrenocorticotropic h.,** a hormone elaborated by the anterior lobe of the pituitary gland, which influences the action of the adrenal cortex. **adrenomedullary h's,** substances secreted by the adrenal medulla, including epinephrine and norepinephrine. **androgenic h's,** the masculinizing hormones, androsterone and testosterone. **antidiuretic h.,** one which suppresses the secretion of urine; vasopressin. **A.P.L. h.,** chorionic gonadotropin. **chromaffin h.,** epinephrine. **corpus luteum h.,** progesterone. **cortical h.,** adrenocortical hormone. **estrogenic h.,** one which produces estrus in female mammals. **follicle-stimulating h.,** hormone of the anterior pituitary which stimulates follicular growth in the ovary and spermatogenesis in the testis. **gonadotropic h.,** one which has an influence on the gonads. **growth h.,** a substance that stimulates growth, especially a secretion of the anterior lobe of the pituitary gland, that directly influences protein, carbohydrate and lipid metabolism and controls rate of skeletal and visceral growth. **interstitial cell-stimulating h.,** luteinizing hormone. **lactation h., lactogenic h.,** a hormone of the anterior pituitary that regulates lactation. **luteinizing h.,** hormone of the anterior pituitary concerned in production of corpora lutea in the ovary and secretion of testosterone by the interstitial cells of the testis. **luteotropic h.,** lactogenic hormone. **melanin-stimulating h.,** a product of the anterior pituitary gland which influences the intracellular distribution of melanin. **ovarian h.,** estrin. **parathyroid h.,** a substance secreted by the parathyroid glands which influences calcium and phosphorus metabolism and bone formation. **placental h.,** an estrogenic hormone derived from the placenta. **sex h's,** hormones having estrogenic *(female sex hormones)* or androgenic *(male sex hormones)* activity. **somatotrophic h., somatotropic h.,** growth hormone.

hormonology (hōr″mo-nol′o-je) the science of hormones; clinical endocrinology.

hormonopexic (hōr-mo″no-pek′sik) fixing hormones.

hormonopoiesis (-poi-e′sis) the production of hormones. adj., **hormonopoiet′ic.**

hormonoprivia (-priv′e-ah) a morbid condition resulting from a lack of hormones; it may be the result of hyposecretion or of surgical removal of an endocrine gland. adj., **hormonopriv′ic.**

hormonotherapy (-ther′ah-pe) treatment by the use of hormones.

horn (hōrn) a pointed projection such as the paired processes on the head of various animals, or other structure resembling them in shape. **cicatricial h.,** a hard, dry outgrowth from a cicatrix, commonly scaly and rarely osseous. **h. of clitoris,** an occasional formation of a horny mass, resembling a talon, under the prepuce of the clitoris. **cutaneous h.,** cornu cutaneum. **h. of pulp,** an extension of the pulp into an accentuation of the roof of the pulp chamber directly under a cusp or a developmental lobe of the tooth. **sebaceous h.,** a hard outgrowth of the contents of a sebaceous cyst. **warty h.,** a hard, pointed outgrowth of a wart.

horopter (hōr-op′ter) sum of all points seen in binocular vision with the eyes fixed.

horror (hor′er) dread; terror. **h. autotox′icus,** a term coined by Ehrlich and Morgenroth in 1900 to express refusal of a normal animal to form autoantibodies. **h. fusio′nis,** antipathy to single binocular fusion, manifested in the tendency of one eye to move away from the fixation state in which the retinal image falls on the macula of each eye.

hortobezoar (hor″to-be′zor) phytobezoar.

hosp. hospital.

hospital (hos′pĭ-tl) an institution for the shelter and care of persons who require medical or surgical treatment. **lying-in h.,** an institution for the care of obstetric or gynecologic patients. **open h.,** one for care of psychiatric patients in which no restraints or locked doors are used to enforce confinement.

hospitalization (hos″pĭ-tal-i-za′shun) 1. the placing of a patient in a hospital for treatment. 2. the term of confinement in a hospital.

host (hōst) 1. an animal or plant which harbors and provides sustenance for another organism. 2. the recipient of an organ or other tissue derived from another organism. **accidental h.,** one that accidentally harbors an organism that is not ordinarily parasitic in the particular species. **alternate h.,** intermediary host. **definitive h., final h.,** the organism in which a parasite passes its adult and sexual existence. **intermediary h., intermediate h.,** the organism in which a parasite passes its larval or nonsexual existence. **h. of predilection,** the host preferred by a parasite. **primary h.,** definitive host. **reservoir h.,** one that becomes infected by a pathogenic parasite and may serve as the source from which the parasite is transmitted to other animals. **secondary h.,** intermediary host. **transfer h.,** one that is used until the appropriate definitive host is reached, but is not necessary to completion of the life cycle of the parasite.

H.P. House Physician.

Hp haptoglobin.

hr. hour.

H.S. House Surgeon.

HSA human serum albumin.

5-HT serotonin (5-hydroxytryptamine).

ht. height.

hum (hum) a low, steady, prolonged sound. **venous h.,** a continuous steady sound heard over the larger veins.

Humatin (hu′mah-tin) trademark for preparations of paromomycin sulfate.

humectant (hu-mek′tant) 1. moistening. 2. a diluent medicine.

humectation (hu″mek-ta′shun) the act of moistening.

humeral (hu′mer-al) of or pertaining to the humerus.

humeroradial (hu″mer-o-ra′de-al) pertaining to humerus and radius.

humidifier (hu-mid′ĭ-fi′er) an apparatus for controlling humidity by adding moisture to the air.

humidistat (hu-mid′ĭ-stat) a device interposed in a humidifying system for the automatic control of the humidity within a certain range.

humidity (hu-mid′ĭ-te) degree of moisture in the air.

humor (hu′mor), pl. *humo′res, humors* [L.] any fluid or semifluid of the body. **aqueous h.,** the fluid produced in the eye and filling the spaces (anterior and posterior chambers) in front of the lens and its attachments. **crystalline h.,** the crystalline lens. **ocular h.,** any one of the humors of the eye—aqueous, crystalline or vitreous. **vitreous h.,** the fluid portion of the vitreous body; often used to designate the entire gelatinous mass.

humoralism (hu′mor-al-izm″) obsolete doctrine that all diseases arise from some change of the humors.

Humorsol (hu′mor-sol) trademark for a solution of demecarium bromide.

hunchback (hunch′bak) 1. kyphosis. 2. a person with a rounded deformity of the back, or kyphosis.

hunger (hung′ger) a craving, as for food. **air h.,** dyspnea affecting both inspiration and expiration.

HVL half-value layer.

hyalin (hi′ah-lin) a principle obtainable from the products of amyloid degeneration.

hyaline (hi′ah-lĭn) glassy; pellucid.

hyalinosis (hi″ah-lĭ-no′sis) hyaline degeneration.

hyalinuria (-nu′re-ah) hyalin in the urine.

hyalitis (hi″ah-li′tis) inflammation of the vitreous body. **asteroid h.,** hyalitis marked by spherical or star-shaped bodies in the vitreous. **h. puncta′ta,** a form marked by small opacities. **h. suppurati′va,** purulent inflammation of the vitreous humor of the eye.

hyaloenchondroma (hi″ah-lo-en″kon-dro′mah) a chondroma of hyaline cartilage.

hyalogen (hi-al′o-jen) an albuminous substance occurring in cartilage, vitreous humor, etc., and convertible into hyalin.

hyaloid (hi′ah-loid) pellucid; like glass.

hyaloidin (hi″ah-loi′din) a carbohydrate radical from mucoproteins.

hyaloiditis (hi″ah-loi-di′tis) hyalitis.

hyaloma (-lo′mah) colloid milium.

hyalomere (hi′ah-lo-mēr″) the pale, homogeneous portion of a blood platelet.

hyalomitome (hi″ah-lo-mi′tōm) hyaloplasm (1).

Hyalomma (hi″ah-lom′ah) a genus of arthropods (family Ixodidae) occurring only in Africa, Asia and Europe; ectoparasites of animals and man, they may transmit disease and cause serious injury by their bite.

hyalomucoid (hi″ah-lo-mu′koid) the mucoid of the vitreous body.

hyalonyxis (-nik′sis) puncturing of the vitreous body.

hyalophagia (-fa′je-ah) the eating of glass.

hyalophobia (-fo′be-ah) fear of glass.

hyaloplasm (hi′ah-lo-plazm″) 1. the fluid portion of the cytoplasm of a cell, in which the other elements are dispersed. 2. the conducting medium of the axon. **nuclear h.,** karyolymph.

hyaloserositis (hi″ah-lo-se″ro-si′tis) inflammation of serous membranes marked by formation of a fibrohyaline investment.

progressive multiple h., polyorrhomenitis.

hyalosome (hi-al'o-sōm) a structure resembling the nucleolus of a cell, but staining only slightly.

hyaluronidase (hi″ah-lu-ron'ĭ-dās) an enzyme that catalyzes the hydrolysis of hyaluronic acid.

Hyazyme (hi'ah-zīm) trademark for a preparation of hyaluronidase for injection.

hybrid (hi'brid) an offspring of parents of different species.

hybridism (hi'brid-izm) the state of being a hybrid; the production of hybrids.

hybridization (hi″brid-ĭ-za'shun) the production of hybrids.

hydantoin (hi-dan'to-in) a crystalline base, glycolyl urea, derivable from allantoin.

hydatid (hi'dah-tid) a cystlike structure; applied especially to an individual of the species *Echinococcus granulosus*. **h. of Morgagni,** a cystlike remnant of the müllerian duct attached to a testis or to the oviduct. **sessile h.,** the hydatid of Morgagni connected with a testis. **stalked h.,** the hydatid of Morgagni connected with an oviduct.

hydatidiform (hi″dah-tid'ĭ-form) resembling a hydatid.

hydatidocele (-tid'o-sēl) tumor of the scrotum containing hydatids.

hydatidoma (-tī-do'mah) a tumor containing hydatids.

hydatidosis (-do'sis) infestation with hydatids.

hydatidostomy (-dos'to-me) incision and drainage of a hydatid cyst.

hydatiduria (-du're-ah) excretion of hydatid cysts in the urine.

Hydeltra (hi-del'trah) trademark for preparations of prednisolone.

hydr(o)- word element [Gr.], *hydrogen; water.*

hydracetin (hi-dras'ĕ-tin) acetylphenylhydrazine.

hydracid (hi-dras'id) any hydrogen acid containing no oxygen.

hydraeroperitoneum (hi-dra″er o-per″ĭ-to-ne'um) water and gas in the peritoneal cavity.

hydragogue (hi'drah-gog) 1. increasing the fluid content of the feces. 2. a purgative that causes evacuation of watery stools.

hydralazine (hi-dral'ah-zēn) a compound used as a hypotensive agent.

hydramnios (hi-dram'ne-os) polyhydramnios.

hydranencephaly (hi″dran-en-sef'ah-le) absence of the cerebral hemispheres, their normal site being occupied by fluid. adj., **hydranencephal'ic.**

hydrargyria (hi″drar-ji're-ah) mercurialism.

hydrarthrosis (-thro'sis) dropsical effusion into a joint.

hydrate (hi'drāt) 1. compound of hydroxyl with a radical. 2. a salt or other compound which contains water. 3. to combine with water.

hydraulics (hi-draw'liks) science of liquids in motion.

hydrazine (hi'drah-zin) 1. a gaseous diamine, H_4N_2. 2. any one of its substitution derivatives.

hydremia (hi-dre'me-ah) excess of water in the blood.

hydrencephalus (hi″dren-sef'ah-lus) hydrocephalus.

hydrencephaly (-sef'ah-le) hydrocephalus.

hydriatrist (hi″dre-at'rist) a specialist in hydrotherapy.

hydroa (hi-dro'ah) skin disease with vesicular patches.

hydroappendix (hi″dro-ah-pen'diks) distention of vermiform appendix with watery fluid.

hydrobilirubin (-bil″ĭ-roo'bin) a bile pigment.

hydrobromate (-bro'māt) a salt of hydrobromic acid.

Hydrocal (hi'dro-kal) trademark for an artificial stone used in dentistry.

hydrocalycosis (hi″dro-kal″ĭ-ko'sis) distention of a single calyx of the kidney with accumulated urine.

hydrocarbon (-kar'bon) an organic compound that contains carbon and hydrogen only. **alicyclic h.,** one that has cyclic structure and aliphatic properties. **aliphatic h.,** one in which no carbon atoms are joined to form a ring. **aromatic h.,** one that has cyclic structure and a closed conjugated system of double bonds. **cyclic h.,** one of a series of hydrocarbons having the general formula CnH_{2n}, the carbon atoms being thought of as having a closed ring structure. **saturated h.,** one that has the maximum number of hydrogen atoms for a given carbon structure. **unsaturated h.,** an aliphatic or alicyclic hydrocarbon that has less than the maximum number of hydrogen atoms for a given carbon structure.

hydrocele (hi'dro-sēl) a cystic accumulation of clear serous fluid in the tunica vaginalis testis. **h. mulie'bris,** watery dilatation of canal of Nuck.

hydrocelectomy (hi″dro-se-lek'to-me) excision of a lesion of the tunica vaginalis or of the canal of Nuck.

hydrocenosis (-se-no'sis) removal of dropsical fluid.

hydrocephalocele (-sef'ah lo-sēl″) hydroencephalocele.

hydrocephaloid (-sef'ah-loid) resembling hydrocephalus.

hydrocephalus (-sef'ah-lus) a condition characterized by abnormal accumulation of cerebrospinal fluid within the skull, with enlargement of the head, atrophy of the brain, mental weakness and convulsions. adj., **hydrocephal'ic. communicating h.,** that in which there is free access of fluid between the ventricles of the brain and the lumbar subarachnoid space. **h. ex vac'uo,** compensatory replacement by cerebrospinal fluid of volume of tissue lost in atrophy of the brain. **noncommunicating h.,** that in which cerebrospinal fluid enters neither cranial nor spinal subarachnoid space.

hydrocephaly (-sef'ah-le) hydrocephalus.

hydrochlorate (-klo'rāt) a salt of hydrochloric acid.

hydrochloretic (-klo-ret'ik) an agent which increases the volume of bile to a greater extent than the solids.

hydrochlorothiazide (-klo″ro-thi'ah-zīd) a

white, crystalline compound, $C_7H_8ClN_3O_4S_2$, used as a diuretic and antihypertensive agent.

hydrocholecystis (hi″dro-ko″le-sis′tis) distention of gallbladder with watery fluid.

hydrocholeretic (-ko″ler-et′ik) 1. pertaining to an increased output by the liver of bile of low specific gravity. 2. an agent that stimulates an increased output of bile of low specific gravity.

hydrocirsocele (-sir′so-sēl) hydrocele with varicocele.

hydrocodone (-ko′dōn) dihydrocodeinone.

hydrocolloid (-kol′loid) a colloid system in which water is the dispersion medium.

hydrocolpos (-kol′pos) collection of watery fluid in the vagina.

hydrocortamate (-kor′tah-māt) a compound used in treatment of dermatoses.

hydrocortisone (-kor′tī-sōn) an adrenocortical steroid used for its anti-inflammatory action.

Hydrocortone (-kor′tōn) trademark for preparations of hydrocortisone.

hydrocyst (hi′dro-sist) cyst with watery contents.

hydrocystoma (hi″dro-sis-to′mah) hidrocystoma.

hydrodipsia (-dip′se-ah) thirst for water.

Hydrodiuril (-di′u-ril) trademark for a preparation of hydrochlorothiazide.

hydroencephalocele (-en-sef′ah-lo-sēl) hernial protrusion of brain tissue containing a cavity communicating with the cerebral ventricles.

hydrogel (hi′dro-jel) a gel that contains water.

hydrogen (hi′dro-jen) chemical element (*see table*), at. no. 1, symbol H. **h. dioxide,** hydrogen peroxide. **h. disulfide,** ill-smelling gas, H_2S. **heavy h.,** hydrogen having double the mass of ordinary hydrogen. **h. monoxide,** water, H_2O. **h. peroxide,** H_2O_2, used in solution as an antibacterial agent. **h. sulfide,** ill-smelling, colorless, poisonous gas, H_2S.

hydrogenase (hi′dro-jen-ās″) an enzyme which reduces perhydrates.

hydrogenate (hi′dro-jen-āt″) to cause to combine with hydrogen.

hydrogenlyase (hi″dro-jen-li′ās) an adaptive enzyme formed by *Escherichia coli* which catalyzes the breakdown of formic acid to carbon dioxide and hydrogen.

Hydrogenomonas (hi-dro″jĕ-no-mo′nas) a genus of Schizomycetes (order Pseudomonadales, suborder Pseudomonadineae, family Methanomonadaceae).

hydrogymnastics (hi″dro-jim-nas′tiks) exercise performed under water.

hydrohymenitis (-hi″men-i′tis) inflammation of a serous membrane.

hydrokinesitherapy (-ki-ne″sī-ther′ah-pe) treatment by underwater exercise.

hydrokinetic (-ki-net′ik) relating to movement of water or other fluid, as in a whirlpool bath.

hydrokinetics (-ki-net′iks) the science treating of fluids in motion.

hydrolase (hi′dro-lās) an enzyme which catalyzes the hydrolysis of a compound.

hydrology (hi-drol′o-je) the study of water and its uses.

Hydrolose (hi′dro-lōs) trademark for a preparation of methylcellulose.

hydrolymph (hi′dro-limf) the thin blood of certain animals.

hydrolysis (hi-drol′ī-sis) the cleavage of a compound by the addition of water, the hydroxyl group being incorporated in one fragment and the hydrogen atom in the other. adj., **hydrolyt′ic.**

hydrolyst (hi′dro-list) an agent that promotes hydrolysis.

hydroma (hi-dro′mah) hygroma.

hydromeningitis (hi″dro-men″in-ji′tis) 1. meningitis with serous effusion. 2. descemetitis.

hydromeningocele (-mĕ-ning′go-sēl) protrusion of the meninges, containing fluid, through a defect in the skull or vertebral column.

hydrometer (hi-drom′ĕ-ter) an instrument for determining the specific gravity of a fluid.

hydrometra (hi″dro-me′trah) collection of watery fluid in the uterus.

hydrometrocolpos (-me″tro-kol′pos) collection of watery fluid in uterus and vagina.

hydrometry (hi-drom′ĕ-tre) measurement of specific gravity with a hydrometer.

hydromicrocephaly (hi″dro-mi″kro-sef′ah-le) smallness of the head with abnormal amount of cerebrospinal fluid.

hydromorphone (-mor′fon) a hydrogenated ketone of morphine; used as an analgesic. **h. hydrochloride,** a crystalline compound used as a narcotic analgesic.

hydromphalus (hi-drom′fah-lus) a cystic accumulation of watery fluid at the umbilicus.

hydromyelia (hi″dro-mi-e′le-ah) dilatation of the central canal of the spinal cord with an abnormal accumulation of fluid.

hydromyelomeningocele (-mi″ĕ-lo-mĕ-ning′-go-sēl) a defect of the spine marked by protrusion of the membranes and tissue of the spinal cord, forming a fluid-filled sac.

hydromyoma (-mi-o′mah) a cystic myoma containing fluid.

hydronephrosis (-ne-fro′sis) distention of the pelvis and calices of the kidney with urine, due to obstruction of the ureter, with atrophy of the kidney parenchyma.

hydropericarditis (-per″ī-kar-di′tis) pericarditis with watery effusion.

hydropericardium (-per″ī-kar′de-um) excessive amount of transudate in the pericardial cavity.

hydroperinephrosis (-per″ī-ne-fro′sis) collection of watery fluid around the kidney.

hydroperitoneum (-per″ī-to-ne′um) collection of watery fluid in the peritoneal cavity.

hydropexis (-pek′sis) the fixation or holding of water.

hydrophilia (-fil′e-ah) the property of absorbing water. adj., **hydrophil′ic, hydroph′ilous.**

hydrophobia (-fo′be-ah) rabies.

hydrophobophobia (-fo″bo-fo′be-ah) morbid dread of hydrophobia (rabies).

hydrophthalmia (hi″drof-thal′me-ah) distention of eyeball from watery effusion.

hydrophysometra (hi″dro-fi″so-me′trah) collection of fluid and gas in the uterus.

hydropic (hi-drop′ik) affected with dropsy.

hydroplasmia (hi″dro-plaz′me-ah) dilution of the blood plasma.

hydropneumatosis (-nu″mah-to′sis) collection of fluid and gas in the tissues.

hydropneumopericardium (-nu″mo-per″ĭ-kar′de-um) fluid and gas in the pericardium.

hydropneumoperitoneum (-per″ĭ-to-ne′um) fluid and gas in the peritoneal cavity.

hydropneumothorax (-tho′raks) the presence of both noninflammatory fluid and air or gas within the pleural cavity.

hydroponics (hi″dro-pon′iks) the soil-less cultivation of plants on liquid media containing the necessary nutrients.

hydroporphin (-por′fin) a partially or fully reduced porphyrin or porphin.

hydroposia (-po′ze-ah) the drinking of water.

hydropotherapy (-po-ther′ah-pe) therapeutic injection of ascitic fluid.

hydrops (hi′drops) [L.] abnormal accumulation of serous fluid in the tissues or in a body cavity; called also *dropsy*. **fetal h., h. feta′lis,** accumulation of fluid in the entire body of the newborn infant, in hemolytic disease due to antibodies present in the blood of the Rh-negative mother. **h. pericar′dii,** hydropericardium.

hydropyonephrosis (hi″dro-pi″o-ne-fro′sis) urine and pus in the kidney and its pelvis.

hydrorheostat (-re′o-stat) a rheostat in which water affords resistance.

hydrorrhea (-re′ah) a watery discharge. **h. gravida′rum,** watery discharge from the gravid uterus.

hydrosalpinx (-sal′pinks) accumulation of watery fluid in a uterine tube.

hydrosarcocele (-sar′ko-sēl) hydrocele and sarcocele together.

hydroscheocele (hi-dros′ke-o-sēl″) scrotal hernia containing fluid.

hydroscope (hi′dro-skōp) an instrument for detecting the presence of water.

hydrosis (hi-dro′sis) hidrosis.

hydrosol (hi′dro-sol) a colloid in which the dispersion medium is a liquid.

hydrosphere (hi′dro-sfēr) the aqueous phase of the earth's surface and atmosphere.

hydrostabile (hi″dro-sta′bil) tending to maintain constant weight under diet restrictions or in gastrointestinal disease.

hydrostat (hi′dro-stat) a device for regulating the height of a fluid in a column or reservoir.

hydrostatics (hi″dro-stat′iks) science of equilibrium of fluids.

hydrosudotherapy (-su″do-ther′ah-pe) hydrotherapy with induction of perspiration.

hydrosyringomyelia (-sī-ring″go-mi-e′le-ah) distention of central canal of spinal cord, with formation of cavities and degeneration.

hydrotaxis (-tak′sis) taxis in response to the influence of water or moisture.

hydrotherapy (-ther′ah-pe) use of water in any form, either externally or internally, in treatment of disease.

hydrothermic (hi″dro-ther′mik) relating to the temperature effects of water, as in hot baths.

hydrothionemia (-thi″o-ne′me-ah) hydrogen sulfide in the blood.

hydrothionuria (-thi″o-nu′re-ah) hydrogen sulfide in the urine.

hydrothorax (-tho′raks) the presence of noninflammatory serous fluid within the pleural cavity.

hydrotropism (hi-drot′ro-pizm) a growth response of a nonmotile organism to the presence of water or moisture.

hydrotympanum (hi″dro-tim′pah-num) watery fluid in the tympanic cavity.

hydroureter (-u-re′ter) distention of the ureter with fluid.

hydrovarium (-va′re-um) watery fluid in an ovary.

hydroxide (hi-drok′sīd) any compound of hydroxyl with another radical.

hydroxyacetanilide (hi-drok″se-as″ē-tan′ĭ-lid) acetaminophen.

hydroxyamphetamine (-am-fet′ah-min) a compound used as a sympathomimetic nasal decongestant, pressor and mydriatic.

hydroxyapatite (-ap′ah-tīt) a compound which is probably the main inorganic constituent of bone and teeth.

hydroxybenzene (hi-drok″sī-ben′zēn) phenol.

hydroxychloroquine (-klo′ro-kwin) a compound used as a suppressant for lupus erythematosus.

hydroxycorticosterone (-kor″tĭ-ko′stēr-ōn) cortisol.

hydroxydione (-di′ōn) a compound used as a basal anesthetic.

hydroxyl (hi-drok′sil) the univalent radical, HO.

hydroxylysine (hi-drok″sī-li′sēn) a naturally occurring amino acid.

hydroxyprogesterone (-pro-jes′ter-ōn) a long-acting progesterone used in treatment of corpus luteum deficiency.

hydroxyproline (-pro′lēn) a naturally occurring amino acid.

hydroxystilbamidine (-stil-bam′ĭ-dēn) a compound used in treatment of leishmaniasis and blastomycosis.

hydroxytetracycline (-tet″rah-si′klēn) oxytetracycline.

hydroxytryptamine (-trip′tah-mēn) serotonin.

hydroxyzine (hi-drok′sĭ-zēn) a compound used as a psychotherapeutic agent.

hydruria (hi-droo′re-ah) excretion of urine of low specific gravity.

hygeiophrontis (hi″je-o-fron′tis) anxious concern about one's own health; suggested to supplant hypochondriasis. adj., **hygeiophron′tis′tic.**

hygiene (hi′jēn) science of health and its preservation. adj., **hygien′ic. mental h.,** the science dealing with development of healthy mental and emotional reactions and habits. **oral h.,** the proper care of the mouth and teeth. **social h.,** the science dealing with prevention and cure of venereal disease.

hygienics (hi″je-en′iks) a system of principles for promoting health.

hygienist (hi'je-en"ist) a specialist in hygiene. **dental h.,** an auxiliary member of the dental profession, trained in the art of removing calcareous deposits and stains from surfaces of teeth and in providing additional services and information on prevention of oral disease.

hygienization (hi"je-en"i-za'shun) establishment of hygienic conditions.

hygro- (hi'gro) word element [Gr.], *moisture.*

hygroma (hi-gro'mah) an accumulation of fluid in a sac, cyst or bursa. adj., **hygrom'-atous. h. col'li,** a watery tumor of the neck. **cystic h., h. cys'ticum,** an endothelium-lined, fluid-containing lesion of lymphatic origin, encountered most often in infants and children and occurring in various regions of the body, most commonly in the posterior triangle of the neck, behind the sternocleidomastoid muscle *(hygroma colli cysticum).* **Fleischmann's h.,** enlargement of a bursa in the floor of the mouth, to the outer side of the genioglossus muscle.

hygrometer (hi-grom'ĕ-ter) instrument for measuring atmospheric moisture.

hygrometry (hi-grom'ĕ-tre) measurement of moisture in atmosphere.

hygroscope (hi'gro-skōp) instrument for showing variation in atmospheric moisture.

hygroscopic (hi"gro-skop'ik) readily absorbing moisture.

hygroscopy (hi-gros'ko-pe) hygrometry.

hygrostomia (hi"gro-sto'me-ah) excessive secretion of saliva.

Hygroton (hi'gro-ton) trademark for a preparation of chlorthalidone.

hyl(o)- (hi'lo) word element [Gr.], *matter (material; substance).*

hyle (hi'le) the primitive substance from which all matter is derived.

hylic (hi'lik) composed of embryonic pulp tissue.

hyloma (hi-lo'mah) a tumor of hylic tissues.

hylotropy (hi-lot'ro-pe) the ability of a substance to change from one physical form to another, e.g. solid to liquid, liquid to gas, without change in chemical composition.

hymen (hi'men) membranous fold partly closing the vaginal orifice. adj., **hy'menal.**

hymenectomy (hi"men-ek'to-me) excision of a membrane, especially of the hymen.

hymenitis (-i'tis) inflammation of the hymen.

hymenolepiasis (-o-lep-i'ah-sis) infection due to organisms of species of Hymenolepis.

Hymenolepis (hi"men-ol'ĕ-pis) a genus of tapeworms; three species, *H. diminuta, H. lanceolata* and *H. nana,* have been found in man.

hymenology (-ol'o-je) science of the membranes.

hymenotomy (-ot'o-me) incision of the hymen.

hyobasioglossus (hi"o-ba"se-o-glos'us) basal part of hyoglossus muscle.

hyoepiglottidean (-ep"ĭ-glo-tid'e-an) pertaining to hyoid bone and epiglottis.

hyoglossal (-glos'al) pertaining to hyoid bone and tongue.

hyoid (hi'oid) shaped like Greek letter *v.*

hyoscine (hi'o-sin) scopolamine. **h. hydrobromide,** scopolamine hydrobromide.

hyoscyamine (hi"o-si'ah-mēn) an alkaloid usually obtained from species of Hyoscyamus or other genera of the family Solanaceae. **h. sulfate,** a salt, $(C_{17}H_{23}NO_3)_2.H_2SO_4.2H_2O$; used as a parasympatholytic.

hyoscyamus (-si'ah-mus) the dried leaf of *Hyoscyamus niger;* used in tincture or extract to produce parasympathetic blockade.

hypacusia (hi"pah-ku'ze-ah) diminished acuteness of the sense of hearing.

hypalbuminosis (hi"pal-bu"mi-no'sis) deficiency of albumins in blood.

hypalgesia (-je'ze-ah) diminished sensibility to pain.

hypamnios (hi-pam'ne-os) deficiency of amniotic fluid.

hypanakinesis (hi"pan-ah-ki-ne'sis) defective motor (muscular) activity, as of the stomach.

hypaxial (hi-pak'se-al) beneath the axis of the vertebral column.

hyper- (hi'per) word element [Gr.], *abnormally increased; excessive.*

hyperacid (hi"per-as'id) abnormally or excessively acid.

hyperacidity (-ah-sid'ĭ-te) excessive acidity.

hyperactivity (-ak-tiv'ĭ-te) excessive activity.

hyperacusia (-ah-ku'ze-ah) abnormal acuteness of the sense of hearing.

hyperacute (-ah-kūt') extremely acute.

hyperadenosis (-ad"ĕ-no'sis) enlargement of glands.

hyperadiposis (-ad"ĭ-po'sis) extreme fatness.

hyperadrenalemia (ah-dre"nah-le'me-ah) increased amount of adrenal secretion in the blood.

hyperadrenalism (ah-dre'nal-izm) overactivity of the adrenal glands.

hyperadrenia (ah-dre'ne-ah) hyperadrenalism.

hyperadrenocorticalism (ah-dre"no-kor'tĭ-kal-izm") hyperadrenocorticism.

hyperadrenocorticism (-kor'tĭ-sizm) hypersecretion of the adrenal cortex.

hyperalbuminemia (hi"per-al-bu"mĭ-ne'me-ah) excessive albumin content of the blood.

hyperaldosteronemia (-al"do-stēr"on-e'me-ah) excess of aldosterone in the blood.

hyperaldosteronism (-al"do-stēr'ōn-izm) aldosteronism.

hyperaldosteronuria (-al"do-stēr"ōn-u're-ah) excess of aldosterone in urine.

hyperalgesia (-al-je'ze-ah) excessive sensitiveness to pain.

hyperalkalinity (-al"kah-lin'ĭ-te) excessive alkalinity.

hyperammoniemia (-ah-mo"ne-e'me-ah) excess of ammonia in the blood.

hyperammoniuria (-ah-mo"ne-u're-ah) excess of ammonia in the urine.

hyperanakinesia (-an"ah-ki-ne'ze-ah) excessive motor activity. **h. ventric'uli,** excessive motor activity of the stomach.

hyperandrogenism (-an'dro-jen-izm") excessive secretion of androgens.

hyperaphia (-a'fe-ah) abnormal acuteness of the sense of touch. adj., **hyperaph'ic.**

hyperazotemia (hi″per-az″o-te′me-ah) excess of nitrogenous matter in the blood.

hyperazoturia (-az″o-tu′re-ah) excess of nitrogenous matter in the urine.

hyperbaria (-bār′e-ah) disorder due to exposure to extremely high atmospheric pressure. adj., **hyperbar′ic.**

hyperbilirubinemia (-bil″i-roo″bī-ne′me-ah) excess of bilirubin in the blood.

hyperbrachycephalic (-brak″e-sĕ-fal′ik) having a cephalic index of 85.5 or more.

hyperbulia (-bu′le-ah) excessive wilfulness.

hypercalcemia (-kal-se′me-ah) excess of calcium in the blood. **idiopathic h.,** a condition of infants, associated with vitamin D intoxication, characterized by elevated serum calcium levels, increased density of the skeleton, mental deterioration and nephrocalcinosis.

hypercalciuria (-kal″se-u′re-ah) excess of calcium in the urine.

hypercapnia (-kap′ne-ah) excess of carbon dioxide in the blood. adj., **hypercap′nic.**

hypercarbia (-kar′be-ah) hypercapnia.

hypercatabolism (-kah-tab′o-lizm) abnormally increased catabolism. adj., **hypercatabol′ic.**

hypercatharsis (-kah-thar′sis) excessive purgation.

hypercellularity (-sel″u-lar′i-te) abnormal increase in the number of cells present, as in bone marrow. adj., **hypercell′ular.**

hypercementosis (-se″men-to′sis) excessive growth of tooth cement.

hypercenesthesia (-se″nes-the′ze-ah) an exaggerated feeling of well-being.

hyperchloremia (-klo-re′me-ah) excess of chlorides in the blood. adj., **hyperchlore′mic.**

hyperchlorhydria (-klōr-hi′dre-ah) excess of hydrochloric acid in the gastric juice.

hypercholesteremia (-ko-les″ter-e′me-ah) hypercholesterolemia.

hypercholesterolemia (-ko-les″ter-ol-e′me-ah) excess of cholesterol in the blood. adj., **hypercholesterole′mic.**

hypercholia (-ko′le-ah) excessive secretion of bile.

hyperchromasia (-kro-ma′ze-ah) hyperchromatism. adj., **hyperchromat′ic.**

hyperchromatism (-kro′mah-tizm) 1. excessive pigmentation. 2. increased staining capacity.

hyperchromatosis (-kro″mah-to′sis) excess of pigment in a part.

hyperchromemia (-kro me′me-ah) a high color index of the blood.

hyperchromia (-kro′me-ah) 1. hyperchromatism. 2. abnormal increase in the hemoglobin content of erythrocytes.

hyperchylia (-ki′le-ah) excessive secretion of gastric juice.

hyperchylomicronemia (-ki″lo-mi″kro-ne′me-ah) presence in the blood of an excessive number of particles of fat (chylomicrons).

hypercinesia (-si-ne′ze-ah) hyperkinesia.

hypercoagulability (-ko-ag″u-lah-bil′i-te) abnormally increased coagulability of the blood.

hypercorticism (-kor″tĭ-sizm) hyperadrenocorticism.

hypercrine (hi″per-krin′) due to endocrine hyperfunction.

hypercrinia (-krin′e-ah) hypercrinism.

hypercrinism (-kri′nizm) excessive secretion of an endocrine gland.

hypercryalgesia (-kri″al-je′ze-ah) excessive sensitiveness to cold.

hypercryesthesia (-kri″es-the′ze-ah) hypercryalgesia.

hypercupriuria (-ku″pre-u′re-ah) excess of copper in the blood.

hypercyanotic (-si″ah-not′ik) extremely cyanotic.

hypercyesis (-si-e′sis) superfetation.

hypererythemia (-si-the′me-ah) excess of red blood corpuscles.

hypercytosis (-si-to′sis) hyperleukocytosis.

hyperdactylia (-dak-til′e-ah) the presence of supernumerary digits on hand or foot.

hyperdiastole (-di-as′to-le) excessive cardiac diastole.

hyperdicrotic (-di-krot′ik) markedly dicrotic.

hyperdiploid (-dip′loid) 1. pertaining to or characterized by hyperdiploidy. 2. an individual or cell with more than the diploid number of chromosomes.

hyperdiploidy (-dip′loi-de) the state of having more than the diploid number of chromosomes ($>2n$).

hyperdipsia (-dip′se-ah) intense thirst of relatively brief duration.

hyperdistention (-dis-ten′shun) excessive distention.

hyperdiuresis (-di″u-re′sis) excessive secretion of urine.

hyperdontia (-don′she ah) a condition characterized by the presence of supernumerary teeth.

hyperdynamia (-di-na′me-ah) excessive power.

hypereccrisia (-e-kriz′e-ah) excessive excretion. adj., **hypereccrit′ic.**

hyperelectrolytemia (-e-lek″tro-li-te′me-ah) abnormally increased electrolyte content of the blood.

hyperemesis (-em′ĕ-sis) excessive vomiting. **h. gravida′rum,** the pernicious vomiting of pregnancy. **h. lacten′tium,** the vomiting of nursing babies.

hyperemia (-e′me-ah) excess of blood in a part. **active h.,** that due to local or general relaxation of arterioles. **arterial h.,** active hyperemia. **Bier′s passive h.,** induction of venous congestion by applying a thin rubber band. **constriction h.,** Bier′s passive hyperemia. **fluxionary h.,** active hyperemia. **leptomeningeal h.,** congestion of the pia-arachnoid. **passive h.,** that due to obstruction to flow of blood from the area. **reactive h.,** that due to increase in blood flow after its temporary interruption. **venous h.,** passive hyperemia.

hyperemotivity (-e″mo-tiv′ĭ-te) abnormally increased responsiveness to mild stimuli.

hyperencephalus (-en-sef′ah-lus) a monster fetus with the brain exposed.

hyperendocrinism (-en-dok′rĭ-nizm) excess of any internal secretion.

hypereosinophilia (hi″per-e″o-sin″o-fil′e-ah) excess of eosinophil leukocytes of the blood.

hyperephidrosis (-ef″ĭ-dro′sis) excessive sweating.

hyperepinephrinemia (-ep″ĭ-nef″rĭ-ne′me-ah) excessive adrenal secretion in the blood.

hypererethism (-er′ĕ-thizm) extreme irritability.

hyperergasia (-er-ga′ze-ah) excessive functional activity.

hyperergia (-er′je-ah) hyperergasia.

hyperergy (-er′je) increased capacity to react to a specific stimulus.

hypererythrocythemia (-ĕ-rith″ro-si-the′me-ah) excess of red corpuscles in the blood.

hyperesophoria (-es″o-fo′re-ah) deviation of visual axes upward and inward.

hyperesthesia (-es-the′ze-ah) a state of abnormally increased sensitivity to stimuli. adj., **hyperesthet′ic. acoustic h., auditory h.,** hyperacusia. **cerebral h.,** that which is due to a cerebral lesion. **gustatory h.,** hypergeusia. **muscular h.,** muscular oversensitiveness to pain or fatigue. **olfactory h.,** hyperosmia. **oneiric h.,** increase of sensitiveness or pain during sleep and dreams. **optic h.,** abnormal sensitiveness of the eye to light. **sexual h.,** abnormal increase of the sexual impulse. **tactile h.,** hyperaphia.

hyperestrinemia (-es″trĭ-ne′me-ah) excessive estrin in the blood.

hyperestrinism (-es′trin-izm) excessive secretion of estrin.

hyperestrogenemia (-es″tro-jĕ-ne′me-ah) excessive estrogen in the blood.

hyperestrogenism (-es′tro-jen-izm″) excessive secretion of estrogen.

hyperestrogenosis (-es″tro-jĕ-no′sis) an abnormally elevated level of estrogens in the body.

hyperexophoria (-ek″so-fo′re-ah) deviation of visual axes upward and outward.

hyperextension (-ek-sten′shun) excessive extension.

hyperferremia (-fĕ-re′me-ah) excess of iron in the blood. adj., **hyperferre′mic.**

hyperferricemia (-fer″ĭ-se′me-ah) hyperferremia.

hyperfunction (-funk′shun) excessive functioning of a part or organ.

hypergalactia (-gah-lak′she-ah) excessive secretion of milk. adj., **hypergalac′tous.**

hypergammaglobulinemia (-gam″ah-glob″u-lĭ-ne′me-ah) increased gamma globulins in the blood. adj., **hypergammaglobuline′mic.**

hypergenesis (-jen′ĕ-sis) excessive development.

hypergenitalism (-jen′ĭ-tal-izm) hypergonadism.

hypergeusia (-gu′ze-ah) abnormal acuteness of the sense of taste. adj., **hypergeu′sic.**

hypergia (hi-per′je-ah) hypersensitivity.

hypergigantosoma (hi″per-ji-gan″to-so′mah) excessive size of body.

hyperglandular (-glan′du-ler) marked by excessive glandular activity.

hyperglobulia (-glo-bu′le-ah) excess of red blood corpuscles.

hyperglobulinemia (hi″per-glob″u-lĭ-ne′me-ah) excess of globulin in the blood.

hyperglycemia (-gli-se′me-ah) excess of glucose in the blood. adj., **hyperglyce′mic.**

hyperglyceridemia (-glis″er-ĭ-de′me-ah) excess of glycerides in the blood.

hyperglycinemia (-gli″sĭ-ne′me-ah) excessive glycine in the blood.

hyperglycistia (-gli-sis′te-ah) excess of sugar in the tissues.

hyperglycogenolysis (-gli″ko-jĕ-nol′ĭ-sis) excessive splitting up of glycogen in the body.

hyperglycoplasmia (-plaz′me-ah) excessive sugar in the blood plasma.

hyperglycorrhachia (-ra′ke-ah) excessive sugar in the cerebrospinal fluid.

hyperglycosemia (-se′me-ah) hyperglycemia.

hyperglycosuria (-su′re-ah) excessive glycosuria.

hypergnosis (hi″per-no′sis) the projection of mental conflicts.

hypergonadism (-go′nad-izm) abnormally increased functional activity of the gonads, with excessive growth and precocious sexual development.

hyperhedonia (-he-do′ne-ah) morbid increase of enjoyment.

hyperhidrosis (-hĭ-dro′sis) abnormally increased secretion of sweat. adj., **hyperhidrot′-ic.**

hyperhormonism (-hŏr′mŏn-izm) excessive hormone secretion.

hyperhydration (-hi-dra′shun) abnormally increased water content of the body.

hyperidrosis (-ĭ-dro′sis) hyperhidrosis.

hyperinosemia (-in″o-se′me-ah) excess of fibrin in the blood.

hyperinsulinism (-in′su-lin-izm″) excessive secretion of insulin.

hyperinvolution (-in″vo-lu′shun) excessive involution.

hyperisotonia (-i″so-to′ne-ah) marked equality of tone.

hyperkalemia (-kah-le′me-ah) excess of potassium in the blood. adj., **hyperkale′mic.**

hyperkeratinization (-ker″ah-tin-i-za′shun) excessive development of keratin in the epidermis.

hyperkeratosis (-ker″ah-to′sis) 1. hypertrophy of cornea. 2. keratoglobus. 3. thickening of the horny layer of the skin.

hyperketonemia (-ke″to-ne′me-ah) increased concentration of ketone bodies in the blood.

hyperketonuria (-ke″to-nu′re-ah) excessive ketone in the urine.

hyperketosis (-ke-to′sis) excessive formation of ketone.

hyperkinemia (-ki-ne′me-ah) abnormally high cardiac output.

hyperkinesia (-ki-ne′ze-ah) abnormally increased motor function or activity. adj., **hyperkinet′ic.**

hyperlactation (-lak-ta′shun) lactation in greater than normal amount or for a longer than normal period.

hyperlecithinemia (-les″ĭ-thĭ-ne′me-ah) excessive lecithin in the blood.

hyperleukocytosis (hi″per-lu″ko-si-to′sis) excess of leukocytes in blood.

hyperlipemia (-li-pe′me-ah) excess of lipids in the blood.

hyperlipoproteinemia (-lip″o-pro″te-in-e′me-ah) excess of lipoproteins in the blood.

hyperliposis (-li-po′sis) excess of fat in the blood serum or tissues.

hyperlithuria (-li-thu′re-ah) excess of lithic (uric) acid in the urine.

hypermastia (-mas′te-ah) 1. excessive size of mammary gland. 2. polymastia.

hypermature (-mah-tūr′) past the stage of maturity.

hypermegasoma (-meg″ah-so′mah) excessive bodily development.

hypermelanotic (-mel″ah-not′ik) characterized by an excessive deposit of melanin.

hypermenorrhea (-men″ŏ-re′ah) excessive uterine bleeding occurring at regular intervals, the period of flow being of usual duration.

hypermetabolism (-mĕ-tab′o-lizm) increased metabolism. **extrathyroidal m.,** abnormally elevated basal metabolism unassociated with thyroid disease.

hypermetaplasia (-met″ah-pla′ze-ah) excessive metaplasia.

hypermetria (-me′tre-ah) excessive range of movement.

hypermetrope (-mĕ′trōp) hyperope.

hypermetropia (-me-tro′pe-ah) ametropia in which parallel rays come to a focus behind the retina, vision being better for distant objects.

hypermnesia (hi″perm-ne′ze-ah) extreme retentiveness of memory. adj., **hypermne′sic.**

hypermodal (hi″per-mo′dal) in statistics, relating to the values or items located to the right of the mode in a variations curve.

hypermorph (hi′per-morf) 1. a person who is tall, but of low sitting height. 2. in genetics, a hypermorphic mutant gene, i.e. one exaggerating or increasing normal activity. adj., **hypermor′phic.**

hypermyotonia (hi″per-mi″o-to′ne-ah) excessive muscular tonicity.

hypermyotrophy (-mi-ot′ro-fe) excessive development of muscular tissue.

hypernatremia (-na-tre′me-ah) excess of sodium in the blood. adj., **hypernatre′mic.**

hypernephroma (-ne-fro′mah) tumor derived from the adrenal cortex.

hypernitremia (-ni-tre′me-ah) excess of nitrogen in the blood.

hypernoia (-noi′ah) excessive mental activity.

hypernormal (-nor′mal) in excess of what is normal.

hypernormocytosis (-nor″mo-si-to′sis) excessive proportion of neutrophils in the blood.

hypernutrition (-nu-trish′un) overfeeding and its ill effects.

hyperonychia (-o-nik′e-ah) hypertrophy of the nails.

hyperope (hi′per-ōp) a person with hyperopia.

hyperopia (hi″per-o′pe-ah) a visual defect in which parallel light rays reaching the eye come to a focus behind the retina, vision being better for far objects than for near. **absolute h.,** that which can be partially corrected by accommodation. **axial h.,** that due to shortness of the anteroposterior diameter of the eye. **facultative h.,** that which can be entirely corrected by accommodation. **latent h.,** that part of the total hyperopia which is not corrected by accommodation. **manifest h.,** that which may be corrected by accommodation aided by convex lenses. **relative h.,** that in which vision is distinct only when excessive convergence is made. **total h.,** manifest and latent hyperopia combined.

hyperorchidism (hi″per-or′ki-dizm) excessive functional activity of the testes.

hyperorexia (-o-rek′se-ah) excessive appetite.

hyperosmia (-oz′me-ah) abnormal acuteness of the sense of smell. adj., **hyperos′mic.**

hyperosmolarity (-oz″mo-lar′ĭ-te) abnormally increased osmolar concentration.

hyperostosis (-os-to′sis) excessive growth of bony tissue. **h. cra′nii,** hyperostosis involving the cranial bones. **frontal internal h.,** thickening of the inner table of the frontal bone, with headache, fatigue and other symptoms. **infantile cortical h.,** hypertrophy of the cortex of bones, with swelling and tenderness of the overlying tissues. **Morgagni's h.,** frontal internal hyperostosis.

hyperovaria (-o-va′re-ah) excessive ovarian activity.

hyperoxaluria (-ok″sah-lu′re-ah) excess of oxalate in the urine. **primary h.,** a genetic disorder characterized by urinary excretion of oxalate, with nephrolithiasis, nephrocalcinosis and often a generalized deposit of calcium oxalate.

hyperoxemia (-ok-se′me-ah) excessive acidity of the blood.

hyperoxia (-ok′se-ah) an abnormally increased supply or concentration of oxygen. adj., **hyperox′ic.**

hyperpancreatism (-pan′kre-ah tizm″) excessive activity of the pancreas.

hyperpancreorrhea (pan″kre-o-re′ah) excessive secretion from the pancreas.

hyperparasite (-par′ah-sit) an individual or species parasitic on an organism that is itself parasitic upon a third species of organism. adj., **hyperparasit′ic.**

hyperparathyroidism (-par″ah-thi′roid-izm) excessive activity of the parathyroid glands.

hyperpepsinemia (-pep″si-ne′me-ah) abnormally high level of pepsin in the blood.

hyperpepsinia (-pep-sin′e-ah) excessive secretion of pepsin.

hyperpepsinuria (-pep″si-nu′re-ah) abnormally high level of pepsin in the urine.

hyperphalangism (-fal′an-jizm) presence of a supernumerary phalanx on a finger or toe.

hyperphasia (-fa′ze-ah) excessive talkativeness.

hyperphonesis (-fo-ne′sis) intensification of the sound in auscultation or percussion.

hyperphoria (-fo′re-ah) upward deviation of the visual axis of one eye when the other eye is covered and fusion is prevented.

hyperphosphatasia (hi″per-fos″fah-ta′ze-ah) excess of phosphatase in the body.

hyperphosphatemia (-te′me-ah) an excess of phosphates in the blood.

hyperphosphaturia (-tu′re-ah) an excess of phosphates in the urine.

hyperphrenia (hi″per-fre′ne-ah) 1. extreme mental excitement. 2. accelerated mental activity.

hyperpiesis (-pi-e′sis) abnormally high pressure, as blood pressure. adj., **hyperpiet′ic.**

hyperpituitarism (-pī-tu″ĭ-tar-izm″) excessive activity of the pituitary gland.

hyperplasia (-pla′ze-ah) increase in volume of a tissue or organ caused by the formation and growth of new cells. adj., **hyperplas′tic. chronic perforating h. of pulp,** internal resorption of a tooth. **lipoid h.,** increased formation of lipoid-containing cells.

hyperplasmia (-plaz′me-ah) 1. excess in the proportion of blood plasma to corpuscles. 2. increase in size of erythrocytes.

hyperplasminemia (-plaz″mĭ-ne′me-ah) excess of plasmin in the circulating blood.

hyperploid (hi′per-ploid) 1. characterized by hyperploidy. 2. an individual or cell characterized by hyperploidy.

hyperploidy (hi′per-ploi″de) the state of having more than the typical number of chromosomes in unbalanced sets.

hyperpnea (hi″perp-ne′ah) abnormal increase in depth and rate of respiration. adj., **hyperpne′ic.**

hyperponesis (hi″per-po-ne′sis) a feeling of being unduly weighed down by one's duties and responsibilities. adj., **hyperponet′ic.**

hyperporosis (-po-ro′sis) excessive callus formation.

hyperposia (-po′ze-ah) abnormally increased ingestion of fluids for relatively brief periods.

hyperpotassemia (-pot″ah-se′me-ah) hyperkalemia.

hyperpragic (-praj′ik) characterized by excessive activity.

hyperpraxia (-prak′se-ah) abnormal activity; restlessness.

hyperprochoresis (-pro″ko-re′sis) hyperperistalsis.

hyperprolinemia (-pro″lī-ne′me-ah) excessive proline in the blood.

hyperprosexia (-pro-sek′se-ah) occupation of the mind by one idea to the exclusion of all others.

hyperproteinemia (-pro″te-in-e′me-ah) excess of protein in the blood.

hyperproteinuria (-u′re-ah) excess of protein in the urine.

hyperproteosis (hi″per-pro″te-o′sis) excess of protein in the diet.

hyperpselaphesia (hi″perp-sel″ah-fe′ze-ah) increased tactile sensitiveness.

hyperpsychosis (hi″per-si-ko′sis) exaggeration of the function of thought.

hyperptyalism (-ti′al-izm) abnormally increased secretion of saliva.

hyperpyremia (-pi-re′me-ah) excess of carbonaceous matter in the blood.

hyperpyrexia (hi″per-pi-rek′se-ah) excessively high fever. adj., **hyperpyrex′ial, hyperpyret′ic.**

hyperreactor (-re-ak′tor) an individual showing greater than normal response to a stimulus. adj., **hyperreac′tive.**

hyperreflexia (-re-flek′se-ah) exaggeration of reflexes.

hyperresonance (-rez′o-nans) a sound elicited by percussion, of pitch lying between that of resonance and tympany.

hyperrhinolalia (-ri″no-la′le-ah) abnormal nasal quality of voice.

hypersalemia (-sah-le′me-ah) abnormally increased content of salt in the blood.

hypersalivation (-sal″ĭ-va′shun) ptyalism.

hypersecretion (-se-kre′shun) excessive secretion.

hypersegmentation (-seg″men-ta′shun) the appearance of being divided into multiple segments or lobes.

hypersegmented (-seg′ment-ed) divided into multiple segments or lobes.

hypersensibility (-sen″sĭ-bil′ĭ-te) exaggerated sensibility.

hypersensitivity (-sen″sĭ-tiv′ĭ-te) exaggerated susceptibility to a substance or stimulus.

hypersensitization (-sen″sĭ-ti-za′shun) creation of an abnormally sensitive condition.

hypersialosis (-si″ah-lo′sis) excessive secretion of the salivary glands.

hypersomnia (-som′ne-ah) pathologically excessive sleep.

hypersphyxia (-sfik′se-ah) increased activity of the circulation.

hypersplenism (-splen′izm) a morbid state resulting from hyperfunctioning of the spleen.

hypersthenia (-sthe′ne-ah) increased strength or tonicity. adj., **hypersthen′ic.**

hypersthenuria (-sthĕ-nu′re-ah) excretion of urine of abnormally high molecular concentration.

hypersystole (-sis′to-le) abnormal exaggeration of the systole. adj., **hypersystol′ic.**

hypertelorism (-te′lo-rizm) abnormally increased distance between two organs or parts. **ocular h., orbital h.,** increase in the interorbital distance, often associated with cleidocranial or craniofacial dysostosis and sometimes with mental deficiency.

hypertensin (-ten′sin) angiotensin.

hypertensinase (-ten′sĭ-nās) an enzyme which destroys hypertensin.

hypertensinogen (-ten-sin′o-jen) a globulin in the blood that is acted on by rennin to produce hypertensin.

hypertension (-ten′shun) abnormally high tension, especially a state of abnormally increased blood pressure with electrocardiographic evidence of cardioarterial derangement (left ventricular preponderance). **benign h.,** essential hypertension which exists for years without producing symptoms. **essential h.,** high blood pressure without known cause. **Goldblatt h.,** hypertension due to occlusion of the renal arteries. **malignant h.,** essential hypertension with acute stormy onset, neuroretinopathy, progressive course and poor prognosis. **pale h.,** malignant hypertension. **portal h.,** abnormally increased pressure in the portal circulation. **pulmonary h.,** abnormally increased pressure in the pulmonary circulation. **red h.,** benign hypertension. **vascular h.,** high blood pressure caused by an abnormal state of the blood vessels.

hypertensive (hi″per-ten′siv) 1. marked by increased blood pressure. 2. an individual with abnormally increased blood pressure.

hypertensor (-ten′sor) a substance that raises the blood pressure.

hypertetraploid (-tet′rah-ploid) having more than the tetraploid number of chromosomes in unbalanced sets (4n + x).

hyperthecosis (-the-ko′sis) hyperplasia and excessive luteinization of the cells of the inner stromal layer of the ovary.

hyperthelia (-the′le-ah) the presence of supernumerary nipples.

hyperthermalgesia (-ther″mal-je′ze-ah) abnormal sensitiveness to heat.

hyperthermia (-ther′me-ah) greatly increased temperature. adj., **hyperther′mal, hyperther′mic.**

hyperthermo-esthesia (-ther″mo-es-the′ze-ah) hyperthermalgesia.

hyperthermy (-ther′me) hyperthermia.

hyperthrombinemia (-throm″bi-ne′me-ah) excess of thrombin in the blood.

hyperthrombocytemia (-throm″bo-si-te′me-ah) excess of platelets in the blood.

hyperthymia (-thi′me-ah) excessive emotionalism.

hyperthymism (-thi′mizm) excessive thymus activity.

hyperthyroidism (-thi′roid-izm) morbid state produced by excessive secretion of the thyroid gland. adj., **hyperthy′roid.**

hypertonia (-to′ne-ah) abnormally increased tonicity or strength. adj., **hyperton′ic. h. oc′uli,** high intraocular pressure.

hypertonicity (-to-nis′ĭ-te) hypertonia.

hypertoxicity (-tok-sis′ĭ-te) an exaggerated or increased toxic quality.

hypertrichiasis (trĭ-ki′ah-sis) hypertrichosis.

hypertrichosis (-trĭ-ko′sis) excessive hairiness, which may be generalized or local, as on the pinna of the ear in males, a trait thought to be transmitted on the Y chromosome.

hypertriploid (-trip′loid) having more than the triploid number of chromosomes in unbalanced sets (3n + x).

hypertrophic (-trof′ik) characterized by hypertrophy.

hypertrophy (hi-per′tro-fe) increase in volume of a tissue or organ produced entirely by enlargement of existing cells. **ventricular h.,** hypertrophy of the myocardium of a ventricle, causing undue deviation of the axis of the electrocardiogram.

hypertropia (hi″per-tro′pe-ah) upward deviation of the visual axis of one eye when the other eye is fixing.

hyperuresis (-u-re′sis) polyuria.

hyperuricemia (-u″rĭ-se′me-ah) an excess of uric acid in the blood. adj., **hyperurice′mic.**

hypervascular (hi″per-vas′ku-ler) extremely vascular.

hypervegetative (-vej″ĕ-ta′tiv) denoting a constitutional body type in which the visceral, nutritional functions predominate.

hypervenosity (-ve-nos′ĭ-te) excessive development of veins.

hyperventilation (-ven″tĭ-la′shun) abnormally prolonged and deep breathing.

hyperviscosity (-vis-kos′ĭ-te) excessive viscosity.

hypervitaminosis (-vi″tah-mĭ-no′sis) a condition produced by ingestion of excessive amount of vitamin. adj., **hypervitaminot′ic.**

hypervolemia (-vo-le′me-ah) abnormally increased volume, as of the blood.

hypesthesia (hi″pes-the′ze-ah) abnormally diminished sensitiveness.

hypha (hi′fah), pl. *hy′phae* [L.] a filament composing the mycelium of a fungus.

hyphedonia (hĭp″he-do′ne-ah) diminution of power of enjoyment.

hyphema (hi-fe′mah) hemorrhage into the anterior chamber of the eye.

hyphemia (hi-fe′me-ah) 1. oligemia, or deficiency of blood. 2. hyphema.

hyphidrosis (hip″hĭ-dro′sis) too scanty perspiration.

Hyphomicrobiaceae (hi″fo-mi-kro″be-a′se-e) a family of Schizomycetes (order Hyphomicrobiales), including the genera Hyphomicrobium and Rhodomicrobium.

Hyphomicrobiales (-mi-kro″be-a′lēz) an order of Schizomycetes, including the families Hyphomicrobiaceae and Pasteuriaceae.

Hyphomicrobium (-mi-kro′be-um) a genus of Schizomycetes (order Hyphomicrobiales, family Hyphomicrobiaceae).

Hyphomycetes (-mi-se′tēz) a genus of fungi including the molds, etc.

hypinosis (hip″ĭ-no′sis) diminished fibrin in the blood.

hypn(o)- (hip′no) word element [Gr.], *sleep; hypnosis.*

hypnagogic (hip″nah-goj′ik) 1. producing sleep. 2. occurring during sleep.

hypnagogue (hip′nah-gog) 1. producing sleep. 2. an agent which produces sleep.

hypnalgia (hip-nal′je-ah) pain during sleep.

hypnoanalysis (hip″no-ah-nal′ĭ-sis) psychoanalysis with use of hypnosis to help uncover unconscious material.

hypnoanesthesia (-an″es-the′ze-ah) reduction of sensitivity to pain by hypnosis.

hypnodontics (-don′tiks) the application of hypnosis and controlled suggestion in the practice of dentistry.

hypnogenetic (-jĕ-net′ik) causing or producing sleep.

hypnoid (hip′noid) resembling hypnosis.

hypnoidization (hip″noi-di-za′shun) the production of light hypnosis.

hypnolepsy (hip′no-lep″se) abnormal sleepiness.

hypnology (hip-nol′o-je) scientific study of sleep or of hypnotism.

hypnonarcosis (hip″no-nar-ko′sis) light hypnosis combined with narcosis.

hypnosis (hip-no′sis) an artificially induced passive state in which there is increased amenability and responsiveness to suggestions and commands. adj., **hypnot′ic.**

hypnotherapy (hip″no-ther′ah-pe) treatment by hypnotism or by inducing sleep.

hypnotic (hip-not′ik) 1. pertaining to hypnosis or sleep. 2. an agent that induces sleep.

hypnotism (hip′no-tizm) the induction of hypnosis.

hypnotize (hip′no-tīz) to put into a condition of hypnosis.

hypnotoxin (hip″no-tok′sin) 1. a toxin which is supposed to accumulate during the waking hours until it is sufficient to inhibit the activity of the cortical cells and induce sleep. 2. a toxic substance derived from the tentacles of the hydrozoan Physalia, causing central nervous system depression, affecting both motor and sensory elements.

hypo (hi′po) 1. hypodermically. 2. sodium hyposulfite.

hypo- (hi′po) word element [Gr.], *abnormally decreased; deficient.*

hypoacidity (hi″po-ah-sid′ĭ-te) decreased acidity.

hypoadenia (-ah-de′ne-ah) diminished glandular activity.

hypoadrenalism (-ah-dre′nal-izm) deficiency of adrenal activity.

hypoadrenocorticism (-ah-dre″no-kor′tĭ-sizm) diminished activity of the adrenal cortex.

hypoaffectivity (-af″fek-tiv′ĭ-te) abnormally diminished sensitivity to superficial stimuli; abnormally decreased emotional reactivity.

hypoalbuminemia (-al-bu″mĭ-ne′me-ah) diminished albumin in the blood.

hypoaldosteronemia (-al″do-ster″o-ne′me-ah) abnormally low level of aldosterone in the blood.

hypoaldosteronism (-al″do-stēr′ōn-izm) aldosteronopenia.

hypoaldosteronuria (-al″do-stēr″o-nu′re-ah) abnormally low level of aldosterone in the urine.

hypoalimentation (-al″ĭ-men-ta′shun) insufficient nourishment.

hypoalkaline (-al′kah-līn) less alkaline than normal.

hypoalkalinity (-al″kah-lin′ĭ-te) decreased alkalinity.

hypoazoturia (-az″o-tu′re-ah) diminished nitrogenous material in the urine.

hypobaric (-bār′ik) characterized by less than normal pressure or weight; applied to gases under less than atmospheric pressure, or to solutions of lower specific gravity than another taken as a standard of reference.

hypobaropathy (-bār-op′ah-the) decompression sickness.

hypoblast (hi′po-blast) the entoderm. adj., **hypoblas′tic.**

hypobulia (hi″po-bu′le̱-ah) abnormal feebleness of will.

hypocalcemia (-kal-se′me-ah) diminished calcium in the blood.

hypocalcia (-kal′se-ah) deficiency of calcium.

hypocalciuria (hi″po-kal″se-u′re-ah) an abnormally diminished amount of calcium in the urine.

hypocapnia (-kap′ne-ah) diminished carbon dioxide in the blood. adj., **hypocap′nic.**

hypocarbia (-kar″be-ah) hypocapnia.

hypocatalasemia (-kat″ah-la-se′me-ah) diminished content of catalase in the blood.

hypocatalasia (-kat″ah-la′ze-ah) reduced level of catalase in all or most of the body tissues.

hypocellularity (-sel″u-lar′ĭ-te) abnormal decrease in the number of cells present, as in bone marrow. adj., **hypocell′ular.**

hypocenter (-sen′ter) the spot immediately beneath the exact site of explosion of an atomic bomb.

hypochloremia (-klo-re′me-ah) diminished chlorides in the blood.

hypochlorhydria (-klōr-hi′dre-ah) lack of hydrochloric acid in the gastric juice.

hypochlorization (-klōr″ĭ-za′shun) diminution of sodium chloride in the diet.

hypochloruria (-klōr-u′re-ah) diminished chloride content in the urine.

hypocholesteremia (-ko-les″ter-e′me-ah) diminished cholesterol in the blood.

hypocholesterolemia (-ko-les″ter-ol-e′me-ah) low level of cholesterol in the blood. adj., **hypocholesterole′mic.**

hypochondria (-kon′dre-ah) morbid anxiety about one's own health, with complaint of imaginary disorders.

hypochondriac (-kon′dre-ak) 1. situated under the lowest ribs. 2. a person affected with hypochondria.

hypochondriasis (-kon-dri′ah-sis) hypochondria.

hypochondrium (-kon′dre-um) the abdominal region on either side, just below the thorax.

hypochromasia (-kro-ma′ze-ah) hypochromatism. adj., **hypochromat′ic.**

hypochromatism (-kro′mah-tizm) 1. abnormally deficient pigmentation. 2. diminished staining capacity.

hypochromatosis (-kro″mah-to′sis) deficiency of pigmentation in a part.

hypochromemia (-kro-me′me-ah) abnormally low color index of the blood.

hypochromia (-kro′me-ah) 1. hypochromatism. 2. decrease of hemoglobin in the erythrocytes so that they are abnormally pale.

hypochromotrichia (-kro″mo-trik′e-ah) abnormally reduced pigmentation of the hair.

hypochromy (-kro′me) increase in the intensity of absorption of light.

hypochylia (-ki′le-ah) deficient secretion of gastric juice.

hypocitremia (-sit-re′me-ah) abnormally low content of citric acid in the blood.

hypocitruria (-sit-rú′re-ah) excretion of urine containing an abnormally small amount of citric acid.

hypocoagulability (-ko-ag″u-lah-bil′ĭ-te) abnormally decreased coagulability of the blood.

hypocondylar (-kon′dĭ-lar) below a condyle.

hypocorticism (-kor′tĭ-sizm) hypoadrenocorticism.

hypocrinism (hi″po-kri′nizm) deficient secretion of an endocrine gland.

hypocupremia (-ku-pre′me-ah) abnormally diminished concentration of copper in the blood.

hypocyclosis (-si-klo′sis) insufficient accommodation in the eye.

hypocythemia (-si-the′me-ah) deficiency in the number of erythrocytes in the blood.

hypocytosis (-si-to′sis) hypoleukocytosis.

hypodactylia (-dak-til′e-ah) less than the usual number of digits on hand or foot.

hypodermatic (-der-mat′ik) hypodermic.

hypodermic (-der′mik) beneath the skin; injected into subcutaneous tissues.

hypodermoclysis (-der-mok′li-sis) injection of fluids into subcutaneous tissues.

hypodiaphragmatic (-di″ah-frag-mat′ik) below the diaphragm.

hypodiploid (-dip′loid) 1. pertaining to or characterized by hypodiploidy. 2. an individual or cell with less than the diploid number of chromosomes.

hypodiploidy (-dip′loi-de) the state of having less than the diploid number of chromosomes ($<2n$).

hypodipsia (-dip′se-ah) abnormally diminished thirst.

hypodontia (-don′she-ah) partial anodontia.

hypodynamia (-di-na′me-ah) abnormally diminished power.

hypoeccrisia (-e-kriz′e-ah) diminished excretion. adj., **hypoeccrit′ic.**

hypoelectrolytemia (-e-lek″tro-li-te′me-ah) abnormally decreased electrolyte content of the blood.

hypoemotivity (-e″mo-tiv′ĭ-te) hypoaffectivity.

hypoendocrinism (-en-dok′ri-nizm) insufficiency of any internal secretion.

hypoeosinophilia (-e″o-sin″o-fil′e-ah) decrease of the eosinophil leukocytes of the blood.

hypoergasia (-er-ga′ze-ah) abnormally decreased functional activity.

hypoergia (-er′je-ah) 1. hypoergasia. 2. hyposensitivity to allergens.

hypoergic (-er′jik) 1. less energetic than normal. 2. pertaining to or characterized by hypoergy.

hypoergy (-er′je) abnormally diminished reactivity.

hypoesophoria (-es″o-fo′re-ah) deviation of visual axes downward and inward.

hypoesthesia (-es-the′ze-ah) a state of abnormally decreased sensitivity to stimuli. adj., **hypoesthet′ic. acoustic h., auditory h.,** hypacusis. **gustatory h.,** hypogeusesthesia. **olfactory h.,** hyposmia. **tactile h.,** hypopselaphesia.

hypoevolutism (-e-vol′u-tizm) abnormally retarded development.

hypoexophoria (-ek″so-fo′re-ah) deviation of visual axes downward and laterally when fusion is prevented.

hypoferremia (-fě-re′me-ah) deficiency of iron in the blood.

hypofibrinogenemia (-fi-brin″o-jě-ne′me-ah) deficiency of fibrinogen in the blood.

hypogammaglobulinemia (-gam″ah-glob″-u-lin-e′me-ah) deficiency of gamma globulins in the blood. adj., **hypogammaglobuline′mic.**

hypogastric (hi″po-gas′trik) pertaining to the hypogastrium.

hypogastrium (-gas′tre-um) the lowest middle abdominal region.

hypogenesis (-jen′ĕ-sis) defective development.

hypogenitalism (-jen′ĭ-tal-izm″) lack of sexual development because of deficient activity of the gonads.

hypogeusesthesia (-gūs″es-the′ze-ah) abnormally diminished acuteness of the sense of taste.

hypogeusia (-gu′ze-ah) hypogeuesthesia.

hypoglandular (-glan′du-ler) marked by decreased glandular (hormonal) activity.

hypoglobulia (-glo-bu′le-ah) decrease of red blood corpuscles.

hypoglossal (-glos′al) beneath the tongue.

hypoglottis (-glot′is) ranula.

hypoglycemia (-gli-se′me-ah) deficiency of sugar in the blood. adj., **hypoglyce′mic.**

hypoglycogenolysis (-gli″ko-gě-nol′ĭ-sis) defective glycogenolysis.

hypoglycorrhachia (-ra′ke-ah) abnormally low sugar content in the cerebrospinal fluid.

hypogonadism (hi″po-go′nad-izm) decreased functional activity of the gonads, with retardation of growth and sexual development.

hypogonadotropic (-gon″ah-do-trōp′ik) relating to or caused by deficiency of gonadotropin.

hypohidrosis (-hī-dro′sis) abnormally diminished secretion of sweat. adj., **hypohidrot′ic.**

hypohypnotic (-hip-not′ik) marked by light sleep or hypnosis.

hypoimmunity (-ĭ-mu′nĭ-te) lowered or diminished immunity.

hypoinosemia (-in″o-se′me-ah) diminished fibrin in the blood.

hypoinsulinism (-in′su-lin-izm″) deficient secretion of insulin.

hypoisotonic (-i″so-ton′ik) less than isotonic; said of a solution having a lesser osmotic power than another.

hypokalemia (-kah le′me-ah) deficiency of potassium in the blood. adj., **hypokale′mic.**

hypokinemia (-ki-ne′me-ah) abnormally low cardiac output.

hypokinesia (-ki-ne′ze-ah) abnormally diminished motor function or activity. adj., **hypokinet′ic.**

hypolarynx (-lar′inks) the part of the larynx below the glottis.

hypolemmal (-lem′al) located beneath a sheath, as the end-plates of motor nerves under the sarcolemma of muscle.

hypoleukocytosis (-lu″ko-si-to′sis) deficiency of leukocytes in blood.

hypoleydigism (-li′dig-izm) decreased secretion of the cells of Leydig.

hypomania (-ma′ne-ah) mania of a mild type. adj., **hypoman′ic.**

hypomastia (-mas′te-ah) abnormal smallness of mammary gland.

hypomelancholia (-mel″an-ko′le-ah) melancholia with slight mental disorder.

hypomenorrhea (hi″po-men″ŏ-re′ah) uterine bleeding of less than the normal amount occurring at regular intervals, the period of flow being of the same or less than usual duration.

hypomere (hi′po-mēr) 1. one of the ventrolateral portions of the fusing myotomes in embryonic development, forming muscles innervated by the ventral rami of the spinal nerves. 2. the part of the mesoderm which develops into the walls of the pleuroperitoneal cavity.

hypometabolism (hi″po-mē-tab′o-lizm) decreased metabolism.

hypometria (-me′tre-ah) diminished range of movement.

hypomineralization (-min″er-al-i-za′shun) abnormal decrease in mineral elements in the blood.

hypomnesia (hi″pom-ne′ze-ah) defective memory.

hypomorph (hi′po-morf) 1. a person short in standing height. 2. in genetics, a hypomorphic mutant gene, i.e. showing only a slight reduction of its effectiveness. adj., **hypomor′phic.**

hypomotility (hi″po-mo-til′ĭ-te) decreased motility.

hypomyotonia (-mi″o-to′ne-ah) deficient muscular tonicity.

hypomyxia (-mik′se-ah) decreased secretion of mucus.

hyponatremia (-na-tre′me-ah) deficiency of sodium in the blood.

hyponoia (-noi′ah) sluggish mental activity.

hyponychium (-nik′e-um) the thickened epidermis beneath the free distal end of the nail of a digit.

hypo-orchidism (-or′kĭ-dizm) defective activity of the testes.

hypo-ovaria (-o-va′re-ah) deficient ovarian activity.

hypopancreatism (-pan′kre-ah-tizm″) diminished activity of the pancreas.

hypoparathyroidism (-par″ah-thi′roid-izm) diminished activity of parathyroid glands, with hypocalcemia, hyperphosphatemia and tetany.

hypopepsinia (-pep-sin′e-ah) deficient pepsin secretion.

hypophalangism (-fah-lan′jizm) absence of a phalanx on a finger or toe.

hypophamine (hi-pof′ah-min) the active principle of the posterior lobe of the hypophysis. **alpha h.,** oxytocin. **beta h.,** vasopressin.

hypopharynx (hi″po-far′inks) the lower part of the pharynx.

hypophonesis (-fo-ne′sis) diminution of the sound in auscultation or percussion.

hypophoria (-fo′re-ah) downward deviation of the visual axis of one eye when the other eye is covered and fusion is prevented.

hypophosphatasia (-fos″fah-ta′ze-ah) deficiency of alkaline phosphatase in the body.

hypophosphate (-fos′fāt) a salt of hypophosphoric acid.

hypophosphatemia (-fos″fah-te′me-ah) deficiency of phosphates in the blood.

hypophosphite (-fos′fīt) any salt of hypophosphorous acid.

hypophrenia (hi″po-fre′ne-ah) feeblemindedness.

hypophrenic (-fren′ik) 1. below the diaphragm. 2. feebleminded.

hypophrenium (-fre′ne-um) the peritoneal space between the diaphragm and the transverse colon.

hypophrenosis (-fre-no′sis) feeblemindedness.

hypophysectomy (hi-pof″ĭ-sek′to-me) excision of the hypophysis cerebri.

hypophysin (hi-pof′ĭ-sin) a secretion from the hypophysis cerebri.

hypophysioprivic (hi″po-fiz″e-o-priv′ik) due to deficiency of the internal secretion of the hypophysis; dyspituitarism.

hypophysis (hi-pof′ĭ-sis), pl. *hypoph′yses* [Gr.] an important organ resting on the sphenoid bone and connected to the brain by a stalk. adj., **hypophys′eal. h. cer′ebri,** an epithelial body of dual origin at the base of the brain, attached by a stalk to the hypothalamus and composed of two main lobes, the *anterior lobe* (anterior pituitary), secreting several important hormones which regulate the proper functioning of the outer endocrine glands, and the *posterior lobe* (posterior pituitary), which is the source of a pressor and an oxytocic principle. **pharyngeal h.,** a mass in the pharyngeal wall with structure similar to that of the hypophysis. **h. sic′ca,** posterior pituitary.

hypophysitis (hi-pof″ĭ-si′tis) inflammation of the hypophysis cerebri.

hypophysoma (-so′mah) a tumor of the hypophysis cerebri.

hypopiesis (hi″po-pi-e′sis) abnormally low pressure, as low blood pressure. adj., **hypopiet′ic.**

hypopinealism (-pi′ne-al-izm″) diminished activity of the pineal gland.

hypopituitarism (-pĭ-tu′ĭ-tar-izm″) diminished activity of the pituitary gland. **fractional h.,** deficiency of only certain of the hormones secreted by the pituitary gland.

hypoplasia (-pla′ze-ah) incomplete development of an organ or tissue. adj., **hypoplas′tic. enamel h.,** incomplete or defective development of the enamel of the teeth. **enamel h., hereditary,** amelogenesis imperfecta. **h. of mesenchyme,** osteogenesis imperfecta.

hypoplasty (-po-plas″te) hypoplasia.

hypopnea (hi-pop′-ne-ah) abnormal decrease in depth and rate of respiration. adj., **hypopne′ic.**

hypoporosis (hi″po-po-ro′sis) deficient callus formation.

hypoposia (-po′ze-ah) abnormally diminished ingestion of fluids.

hypopotassemia (-pot″ah-se′me-ah) hypokalemia.

hypopraxia (-prak′se-ah) deficient activity.

hypoprosody (-pros′o-de) diminution of the normal variation of stress, pitch and rhythm of speech.

hypoproteinemia (-pro″te-ĕ-ne′me-ah) deficiency of protein in the blood.

hypoproteinia (-pro″te-in′e-ah) a subnormal protein status of the body.

hypoprothrombinemia (-pro-throm″bĭ-ne′me-ah) deficiency of prothrombin in the blood.

hypopselaphesia (hi″pop-sel″ah-fe′ze-ah) dulness of tactile sensitiveness.

hypopsychosis (hi″po-si-ko′sis) diminution of the function of thought.

hypoptyalism (-ti′ah-lizm) xerostomia.

hypopyon (hi-po′pe-on) pus in anterior chamber of the eye.

hyporeactor (hi″po-re-ak′tor) an individual showing less than normal response to a stimulus.

hyporeflexia (-re-flek′se-ah) diminution or weakening of reflexes.

hyposalemia (sah-le′me-ah) diminution of salts in the blood.

hyposalivation (-sal″ĭ-va′shun) xerostomia.

hyposarca (-sar′kah) anasarca.

hyposecretion (-se-kre′shun) diminished secretion.

hyposensitive (-sen′sĭ-tiv) less sensitive than normal.

hyposensitization (-sen″sĭ-ti-za′shun) reduction of sensitivity to a particular antigen, by appropriate treatment.

hyposmia (hi-poz′me-ah) diminished acuteness of the sense of smell.

hyposmolarity (hi-poz″mo-lar′ĭ-te) abnormally decreased osmolar concentration.

hyposomnia (hi″po-som′ne-ah) pathologically diminished sleep.

hypospadias (-spa′de-as) congenital defect of the anterior urethra, which opens ventrally and posteriorly to its normal site of opening. **female h.**, a developmental anomaly in the female in which the urethra opens into the vagina.

hyposphyxia (-sfik′se-ah) abnormally depressed circulation.

hypostasis (hi-pos′tah-sis) 1. deposit or sediment. 2. formation of a deposit. adj., **hypostat′ic.**

hyposteatolysis (hi″po-ste″ah-tol′ĭ-sis) inadequate hydrolysis of fats during digestion.

hyposthenia (hi″pos-the′ne-ah) diminished strength or tonicity. adj., **hyposthen′ic.**

hyposthenuria (-thě-nu′re-ah) decreased osmolality of the urine.

hypostomia (hi″po-sto′me-ah) a developmental anomaly characterized by abnormal smallness of the mouth, the slit being vertical instead of horizontal.

hypostypsis (-stip′sis) moderate astringency. adj., **hypostyp′tic.**

hyposulfite (-sul′fīt) any salt of hyposulfurous acid.

hyposynergia (-sĭ-ner′je-ah) defective coordination.

hyposystole (-sis′to-le) abnormal diminution of the systole.

hypotelorism (-te′lo-rizm) abnormally decreased distance between two organs or points. **ocular h., orbital h.,** abnormal decrease in the intraorbital distance.

hypotension (-ten′shun) diminished tension, especially low blood pressure.

hypotensive (-ten′siv) 1. marked by low blood pressure. 2. an individual with an abnormally low blood pressure.

hypotensor (hi″po-ten′sor) a substance that lowers blood pressure.

hypotetraploid (-tet′rah-ploid) having fewer than the tetraploid number of chromosomes in unbalanced sets (4n − x).

hypothalamotomy (-thal″ah-mot′o-me) production of lesions in the posterolateral part of the hypothalamus, in treatment of psychotic disorders.

hypothalamus (-thal′ah-mus) that part of the forebrain in the anterior part of the floor and adjacent lateral walls of the third ventricle; may be extended to include the optic chiasm, tuber cinereum, hypophysis and mamillary bodies.

hypothenar (hi-poth′ě-nar) the ridge on the palm along the bases of the fingers and the ulnar margin.

hypothermia (hi″po-ther′me-ah) greatly decreased temperature. adj., **hypother′mal, hypother′mic.**

hypothermy (-ther′me) hypothermia.

hypothesis (hi-poth′ě-sis) a supposition assumed as a basis of reasoning. **cardionector h.,** there are two pacemakers or cardionectors in the heart: one, the atrionector, controls the atria, and the other, the ventriculonector, the ventricles. **insular h.,** diabetes is due to disordered function of the islands of Langerhans in the pancreas. **lattice h.,** a theory of the nature of the antigen-antibody reaction which postulates reaction between multivalent antigen and divalent antibody to give an antigen-antibody complex of a lattice-like structure. **Makeham's h.,** death results from two coexisting factors: (1) chance, which is constant; (2) inability to withstand destruction, which progresses geometrically. **Planck's quantum h.,** energy is radiated or absorbed only in integral units equal to hn, in which h is Planck's constant and n is the frequency of vibration. **unitarian h.,** the theory that antibody is a single species of modified serum globulin regardless of the overt consequences of its reaction with homologous antigen, e.g. agglutination, precipitation, complement fixation.

hypothrombinemia (hi″po-throm″bĭ-ne′me-ah) diminution of thrombin in the blood.

hypothymia (-thi′me-ah) abnormally diminished emotionalism.

hypothymism (-thi′mizm) diminished thymus activity.

hypothyroidism (-thi′roi-dizm) morbid state produced by deficient secretion of the thyroid gland. adj., **hypothy′roid.**

hypotonia (-to′ne-ah) abnormally decreased tonicity or strength. adj., **hypoton′ic.**

hypotonic (-ton′ik) 1. marked by abnormally low tension. 2. less than isotonic. 3. a person affected with hypotonia.

hypotonicity (-to-nis′ĭ-te) the state or quality of being hypotonic.

hypotoxicity (-tok-sis′ĭ-te) abnormally reduced toxic quality.

hypotransferrinemia (-trans-fer″ĭ-ne′me-ah) deficiency of transferrin in the blood.

hypotrichosis (-trĭ-ko′sis) congenital absence

of body hair, which may be partial or complete.

hypotriploid (hi″po-trip′loid) having fewer than the triploid number of chromosomes in unbalanced sets (3n − x).

hypotrophy (hi-pot′ro-fe) 1. bacterial nutrition in which the organism is nourished by its host's nutrition. 2. abiotrophy.

hypotropia (hi″po-tro′pe-ah) downward deviation of the visual axis of one eye while the other is fixing.

hypotympanotomy (-tim″pah-not′o-me) surgical opening of the hypotympanum.

hypotympanum (-tim′pah-num) the lower part of the cavity of the middle ear, in the temporal bone.

hypouremia (-u-re′me-ah) an abnormally low level of urea in the blood.

hypouresis (-u-re′sis) oliguria.

hypovaria (-va′re-ah) hypo-ovaria.

hypovegetative (-vej′e-ta″tiv) denoting a constitutional body type in which somatic systems predominate in contrast to visceral organs.

hypovenosity (-ve-nos′ĭ-te) incomplete development of veins.

hypoventilation (-ven″tĭ-la′shun) decrease of air in lungs below the normal amount.

hypovitaminosis (-vi″tah-mĭ-no′sis) a condition produced by lack of an essential vitamin.

hypovolemia (-vo-le′me-ah) abnormally decreased volume of circulating fluid (plasma) in the body.

hypoxemia (hi″pok-se′me-ah) deficient oxygenation of the blood.

hypoxia (hi-pok′se-ah) an abnormally decreased supply or concentration of oxygen. adj., **hypox′ic. ambient h.,** deficiency of oxygen in the surrounding (environmental) atmosphere.

hyps(o)- (hip′so) word element [Gr.], *height.*

hypsarhythmia (hip″sah-rith′me-ah) random high-voltage slow waves and spikes arising from multiple foci and spreading to all cortical area, sometimes observed in electroencephalograms of infants.

hypsicephalic (hip″sī-sē-fal′ik) having a vertical index of 75.1 or more.

hypsiconchous (-kong′kus) having an orbital index over 85.

hypsochromy (hip″so-kro′me) a shift of the absorption band toward higher frequencies (shorter wavelengths) with lightening of color.

hypsokinesis (-ki-ne′sis) a backward swaying or falling in erect posture, seen in paralysis agitans and other forms of the amyostatic syndrome.

hypsonosus (hip-so′nŏ-sus) mountain sickness.

hypsophobia (hip″so-fo′be-ah) fear of great heights.

hypsotherapy (-ther′ah-pe) therapeutic use of high altitudes.

hysteralgia (his″tĕ-ral′je-ah) pain in the uterus.

hysterectomy (his″tĕ-rek′to-me) excision of the uterus. **abdominal h.,** excision of the uterus through an incision in the abdominal wall. **cesarean h.,** cesarean section followed by removal of the uterus, oviducts and ovaries. **complete h.,** panhysterectomy. **partial h.,** supracervical hysterectomy. **subtotal h.,** supracervical h.,** excision of the corpus of the uterus above the cervix. **total h.,** panhysterectomy. **vaginal h.,** excision of the uterus through the vagina.

hysteresis (his″tĕ-re′sis) the failure of coincidence of two associated phenomena, such as that exhibited in the differing temperatures of gelation and of liquefaction of a reversible colloid.

hystereurynter (his″ter-u-rin′ter) an instrument for dilating the os uteri.

hystereurysis (u″rĭ-sis) dilation of the os uteri.

hysteria (his-te′re-ah) a psychoneurosis with symptoms based on conversion and characterized by lack of control over acts and emotions, by morbid self-consciousness, by anxiety, by exaggeration of the effect of sensory impressions and by simulation of various disorders. adj., **hyster′ical. anxiety h.,** hysteria with recurring attacks of anxiety. **conversion h.,** hysteria in which psychic energy is converted into nervous stimuli, which give rise to physical symptoms. **fixation h.,** hysteria with symptoms based on those of an organic disease. **h. libidino′sa,** nymphomania. **h. ma′jor,** hysteria with sudden onset of dream states, stupors and paralyses. **h. mi′nor,** hysteria with mild convulsions in which consciousness is not lost. **monosymptomatic h.,** hysteria which manifests itself by one symptom only.

hysteriac (his-te′re-ak) a person affected with hysteria.

hysteritis (his″tĕ-ri′tis) inflammation of the uterus.

hysterocatalepsy (his″ter-o-kat′ah-lep″se) hysteria with cataleptic symptoms.

hysterocele (his′ter-o-sēl″) hernia of the gravid uterus.

hysterocleisis (his″ter-o-kli′sis) surgical closure of os uteri.

hysterocolpectomy (-kol-pek′to-me) vaginal hysterectomy with total colpectomy.

hysterodynia (-din′e-ah) pain in the uterus.

hysteroepilepsy (-ep″ĭ-lep′se) severe hysteria with epileptiform convulsions.

hysterogenic (-jen′ik) causing hysterical phenomena or symptoms.

hysterography (his″tĕ-rog′rah-fe) radiography of the uterus.

hysteroid (his′ter-oid) resembling hysteria.

hysterolith (his′ter-o-lith″) a uterine calculus.

hysterology (his″tĕ-rol′o-je) study of the uterus.

hysterolysis (-rol′ĭ-sis) freeing of the uterus from adhesions.

hysteromalacia (his″ter-o-mah-la′she-ah) softening of the uterus.

hysteromania (-ma′ne-ah) 1. hysterical mania. 2. nymphomania.

hysterometer (his″tĕ-rom′ē-ter) instrument for measuring the uterus.

hysterometry (-rom′ē-tre) measurement of the uterus.

hysteromyoma (his″ter-o-mi-o′mah) myoma of the uterus.

hysteromyomectomy (-mi″o-mek′to-me) local excision of fibroid tumor of the uterus.

hysteromyotomy (-mi-ot′o-me) incision of uterus for removal of a solid tumor.

hysteroneurosis (-nu-ro′sis) nervous disease due to uterine lesion.

hystero-oophorectomy (-o″of-o-rek′to-me) excision of uterus and ovaries.

hysteropathy (his″tĕ-rop′ah-the) any uterine disease.

hysteropexy (his′ter-o-pek″se) fixation of the uterus.

hysteropia (his″tĕ-ro′pe-ah) a hysterical disorder of vision.

hysteroptosis (his″ter-op-to′sis) prolapse of the uterus.

hysterorrhaphy (his″te-ror′ah-fe) 1. suture of the uterus. 2. hysteropexy.

hysterorrhexis (his″ter-o-rek′sis) rupture of the uterus.

hysterosalpingectomy (-sal″pin-jek′to-me) excision of the uterus and uterine tubes.

hysterosalpingography (-sal″ping-gog′rah-fe) radiography of uterus and uterine tubes.

hysterosalpingo-oophorectomy (-sal″ping-go-o″of-o-rek′to-me) excision of uterus, uterine tubes and ovaries.

hysterosalpingostomy (his″tĕ-ro-sal″ping-gos′to-me) anastomosis of a uterine tube to the uterus.

hysteroscope (his′ter-o-skōp″) endoscope used in direct visual examination of the canal of the uterine cervix and the cavity of the uterus.

hysterospasm (his′ter-o-spazm″) spasm of the uterus.

hysterotomy (his″tĕ-rot′o-me) incision of the uterus. **abdominal h.**, incision of the uterus through the wall of the abdomen. **vaginal h.**, incision of the uterus through the wall of the vagina.

hysterotrachelorrhaphy (his″ter-o-tra″kel-or′-rah-fe) suture of the uterus and uterine cervix.

hysterotrachelotomy (-tra″kel-ot′o-me) incision of the uterus and uterine cervix.

hysterotraumatism (-traw′mah-tizm) hysteric symptoms following injury.

hysterotubography (-tu-bog′rah-fe) hysterosalpingography.

hystriciasis (his″trĭ-si′ah-sis) 1. morbid erection of the hairs. 2. ichthyosis hystrix.

Hytakerol (hi-tak′er-ol) trademark for preparations of dihydrotachysterol.

hyzone (hi′zōn) triatomic form of hydrogen, H_3.

I

I chemical symbol, *iodine.*

I. intensity (of magnetism).

-ia (e′ah) word element, *state; condition; disease.*

IAEA International Atomic Energy Agency.

I.A.G.P. International Association of Geographic Pathology.

I.A.G.U.S. International Association of Genito-Urinary Surgeons.

I A M M International Association of Medical Museums.

ianthinopsia (i-an″thĭ-nop′se-ah) perversion of color vision in which objects are seen as violet.

I.A.P.B. International Association for Prevention of Blindness.

I.A.P.P. International Association for Preventive Pediatrics.

-iasis (i′ah-sis) word element [Gr.], *condition of.*

iateria (i″ah-te′re-ah) therapeutics.

iatr(o)- (i-at′ro) word element [Gr.], *medicine; physician.*

iatric (i-at′rik) pertaining to medicine or to a physician.

iatrochemistry (i-at″ro-kem′is-tre) 1. treatment of disease by chemical agents. 2. the early theory that all vital phenomena were chemical in essence.

iatrogenic (-jen′ik) resulting from an attitude or action of a physician.

iatrology (i″ah-trol′o-je) science of medicine.

iatrophysics (i-at″ro-fiz′iks) 1. treatment of disease by physical or mechanical means. 2. the early theory that all vital phenomena were controlled by laws of physics.

iatrotechnics (-tek′niks) practical application of therapeutic principles.

I.C.D. intrauterine contraceptive device.

ichor (i′kor) watery discharge from wounds or sores. adj., **i′chorous.**

ichorrhea (i″ko-re′ah) copious discharge of ichor.

ichthammol (ik-tham′ol) product of destructive distillation of certain bituminous schists, sulfonated and neutralized with ammonia, used in skin diseases.

ichthyismus (ik″the-iz′mus) disease caused by eating rancid or poisonous fish.

ichthyoacanthotoxin (ik″the-o-ah-kan″tho-tok′sin) the toxin secreted by venomous fishes.

ichthyohemotoxin (-he″mo-tok′sin) a toxic substance found in the blood of certain fishes.

ichthyoid (ik′the-oid) fishlike.

ichthyootoxin (ik″the-o″o-tok′sin) a toxic substance derived from the roe of certain fishes.

ichthyosarcotoxin (ik″the-o-sar″ko-tok′sin) a toxin found in the flesh of poisonous fishes.

ichthyosis (ik″the-o′sis) dryness, roughness and scaliness of the skin, resulting from failure of shedding of the keratin produced by the skin cells. adj., **ichthyot′ic. i. follicula′ris,** keratosis follicularis. **i. hys′trix,** a variety with dry, warty knobs. **i. seba′cea,** seborrhea. **i. sim′plex,** xeroderma.

ichthyotoxicology (ik″the-o-tok″sĭ-kol′o-je) the science of poisons derived from certain fish, their cause, detection and effects, and treatment of conditions produced by them.

ichthyotoxin (-tok′sin) a toxin derived from fish, including both ichthyoacanthotoxin and ichthyosarcotoxin.

I.C.N. International Council of Nurses.

ICRP International Commission on Radiological Protection.

ICRU International Commission on Radiological Units and Measurements.

I.C.S. International College of Surgeons.

ICSH interstitial cell-stimulating hormone.

icterogenic (ik″ter-o-jen′ik) causing jaundice.

icterohepatitis (-hep″ah-ti′tis) inflammation of the liver with marked jaundice.

icteroid (ik′ter-oid) resembling jaundice.

icterus (ik′ter-us) [L.] jaundice. adj., **icter′ic. cythemolytic i.,** icterus due to excessive formation of bile from destruction of red blood corpuscles. **febrile i., i. febri′lis,** an acute infectious jaundice. **i. gra′vis,** acute yellow atrophy of the liver. **i. me′las,** black jaundice. **i. neonato′rum,** jaundice in newborn children.

ictus (ik′tus) a stroke, blow or sudden attack. adj., **ic′tal.**

I.D. infective dose.

I.D.₅₀ median infective dose: that amount of pathogenic microorganisms which will produce infection in 50 per cent of the test subjects.

id (id) 1. the self-preservative tendencies and instincts of an individual as a totality; the true unconscious. 2. a skin eruption occurring as an allergic reaction to an agent causing primary lesions elsewhere.

-id (id) word element [Gr.], indicating a skin condition occurring secondarily to a primary infection.

idant (i′dant) a chromosome regarded as a factor in heredity.

-ide (īd) suffix indicating a binary compound.

idea (i-de′ah) a mental impression or conception. **autochthonous i.,** a strange idea which comes into the mind in some unaccountable way, but is not a hallucination. **compulsive i.,** an idea which persists despite reason and will. **dominant i.,** an impression that controls or colors every action and thought. **fixed i.,** an impression which stays in the mind and cannot be changed by reason. **i. of reference,** an idea that the words and actions of others refer to one's self.

ideal (i-de′al) a pattern or concept of perfection. **ego i.,** an ideal of perfection developed in childhood through identification with a loved person.

idealization (i-de″ah-li-za′shun) 1. a mental mechanism by which an object or person is unconsciously overvalued and emotionally aggrandized. 2. concentration upon and exaggeration of the liked attributes of a person. 3. the conscious or partly conscious process of building a person, principle or system into a standard of excellence.

ideation (i″de-a′shun) clear mental presentation of an object.

idée fixe (e-da′ fēks′) a psychopathologically fixed idea or belief of a delusional nature.

identification (i-den″tĭ-fĭ-ka′shun) the unconscious emulation and adoption of personality characteristics and values of another individual.

ideogenetic (i″de-o-jĕ-net′ik) induced by or related to vague sense impressions rather than organized images.

ideogenous (i″de-oj′ĕ-nus) aroused by an idea or thought.

ideology (i″de-ol′o-je, id″e-ol′o-je) 1. the science of the development of ideas. 2. the body of ideas characteristic of an individual or of a social unit.

ideomotion (i″de-o-mo′shun) muscular action induced by mental energy.

ideomotor (-mo′tor) transforming mental energy into motion.

ideophrenia (-fre′ne-ah) a morbid mental state characterized by perversion of ideas. adj., **ideophren′ic.**

idio- (id′e-o) word element [Gr.], *self; peculiar to substance or organism itself.*

idioblast (id′e-o-blast) early name for one of the submicroscopic particles in a cell which manifest specific functions.

idiocy (id′e-o-se) mental deficiency so severe as to render the patient incapable of guarding against common physical dangers, the intelligence quotient being less than 21. **amaurotic familial i.,** a familial condition characterized by subnormal mentality and blindness occurring without apparent lesion of the eye and due to a defect of lipid metabolism. **Aztec i.,** microcephalic idiocy. **cretinoid i.,** cretinism. **epileptic i.,** idiocy combined with epilepsy. **genetous i.,** idiocy dating from fetal life. **hydrocephalic i.,** idiocy combined with hydrocephalus. **microcephalic i.,** idiocy associated with microcephalia. **mongolian i.,** mongolism. **sensorial i.,** intellectual deficiency due to defect in a sense organ. **traumatic i.,** mental deficiency resulting from injury received at birth.

idioglossia (id″e-o-glos′e-ah) speech characterized by imprecise pronunciation of letters, creating virtually a new language peculiar to the individual.

idiogram (id′e-o-gram) a drawing or photograph of the chromosomes of a particular cell.

idiometritis (-me-tri′tis) inflammation of the uterine muscle.

idioneurosis (-nu-ro′sis) a neurosis arising from the nerves themselves.

idiopathic (-path′ik) self-originated; occurring without known cause.

idiopathy (id″e-op′ah-the) a morbid state arising without known cause.

idioplasm (id″e-o-plazm″) the self-reproducing portion of a cell; germ plasm.

idiosome (id′e-o-sōm″) 1. an ultimate element of living matter. 2. the centrosome of a spermatocyte, together with the surrounding Golgi apparatus and mitochondria.

idiosyncrasy (id″e-o-sin′krah-se) a qualitatively altered response to a stimulus occurring without obvious reason.

idiot (id'e-ot) a mentally defective person of the lowest order of intellectual potential (I.Q. less than 21). **i.-savant,** a person of subnormal intelligence who has a particular mental faculty developed to a high degree, e.g. mathematic ability, memory. **mongolian i.,** a term formerly applied to a patient with Down's syndrome and severe mental retardation.

idiotrophic (id"e-o-trof'ik) capable of selecting its own nourishment.

idioventricular (-ven-trik'u-ler) pertaining to cardiac ventricle alone.

I.D.S. Investigative Dermatological Society.

ignipuncture (ig"ni-pungk'tūr) therapeutic puncture with hot needles.

ignis (ig'nis) [L.] fire. **i. sa'cer,** 1. ergotism. 2. herpes zoster.

I.L.A. International Leprosy Association.

ile(o)- (il'e-o) word element [L.], *ileum.*

ileac (il'e-ak) pertaining to the ileum.

ileal (il'e-al) pertaining to the ileum.

ileectomy (il"e-ek'to-me) excision of the ileum.

ileitis (-i'tis) inflammation of the ileum. **regional i.,** inflammatory involvement of a portion of the ileum, the affected segment becoming inflexible and the lumen narrowed.

ileocecal (il"e-o-se'kal) pertaining to ileum and cecum.

ileocecostomy (-se-kos'to-me) anastomosis of the ileum to the cecum.

ileocolic (-kol'ik) pertaining to ileum and colon.

ileocolitis (-ko-li'tis) inflammation of ileum and colon. **i. ulcero'sa chron'ica,** chronic ileocolitis with fever, rapid pulse, anemia, diarrhea and right iliac pain.

ileocolostomy (-ko-los'to-me) anastomosis of the ileum to the colon.

ileocolotomy (-ko-lot'o-me) incision of ileum and colon.

ileocystoplasty (-sis'to-plas"te) repair of the wall of the urinary bladder with an isolated segment of the wall of the ileum.

ileocystostomy (-sis-tos'to-me) use of an isolated segment of ileum to create a passage from the urinary bladder to an opening in the abdominal wall.

ileoileostomy (-il"e-os'to-me) anastomosis between two parts of the ileum.

ileorectal (-rek'tal) pertaining to or communicating with the ileum and rectum.

ileorrhaphy (il"e-or'ah-fe) suture of the ileum.

ileosigmoidostomy (il"e-o-sig"moi-dos'to-me) anastomosis of ileum to sigmoid colon.

ileostomy (il"e-os'to-me) fistulization of the ileum.

ileotomy (-ot'o-me) incision of the ileum.

Iletin (il'ĕ-tin) trademark for preparations of insulin.

ileum (il'e-um) the distal portion of the small intestine, ending at the cecum. **duplex i.,** congenital duplication of the ileum.

ileus (il'e-us) intestinal obstruction. **adynamic i.,** that due to inhibition of bowel motility. **dynamic i., hyperdynamic i.,** spastic ileus. **mechanical i.,** intestinal obstruction due to mechanical causes. **meconium i.,** ileus in the newborn due to blocking of the bowel with thick meconium. **occlusive i.,** mechanical ileus. **paralytic i., i. paralyt'icus,** adynamic ileus. **spastic i.,** obstruction of the bowel due to contraction of the intestinal musculature.

ili(o)- (il'e-o) word element [L.], *ilium.*

iliac (il'e-ak) pertaining to the ilium.

iliadelphus (il"e-ah-del'fus) a twin monster joined at the pelvis.

Ilidar (il'ĭ-dar) trademark for a preparation of azapetine.

iliofemoral (il"e-o-fem'o-ral) pertaining to ilium and femur.

ilio-inguinal (-ing"gwĭ-nal) pertaining to iliac and inguinal regions.

iliolumbar (-lum'bar) pertaining to iliac and lumbar regions.

iliopectineal (-pek-tin'e-al) pertaining to ilium and pubes.

ilium (il'e-um) the lateral, flaring portion of the pelvic bone.

ill (il) 1. affected by disease. 2. disease. **quarter i.,** blackleg.

illness (il'nes) a condition marked by pronounced deviation from the normal healthy state; sickness. **compressed air i.,** decompression sickness. **radiation i.,** radiation sickness.

illumination (ĭ-lu"mĭ-na'shun) the lighting up of a part, organ or object for inspection. **axial i.,** light transmitted or reflected along the axis of a microscope. **direct i.,** light from a source in front of the object. **focal i.,** light thrown upon the focus of a lens or mirror. **oblique i.,** light from a source at one side of the object. **through i.,** light from a source behind and shining through the object.

illuminator (-na'tor) the source of light for viewing an object. **Abbe's i.,** Abbe's condenser.

illusion (ĭ-lu'zhun) a mental impression derived from misinterpretation of an actual sensory stimulus. adj., **illu'sional.**

Ilotycin (i"lo-ti'sin) trademark for preparations of erythromycin.

I.M. intramuscularly.

I.M.A. Industrial Medical Association.

image (im'ij) a picture or concept with more or less likeness to an objective reality. **aerial i.,** image in space seen with the ophthalmoscope. **body i.,** the organized cerebral model of all sensations originating within the body. **direct i., erect i.,** that from rays not yet focused. **false i.,** that formed by the deviating eye in strabismus. **inverted i.,** real image. **mirror i.,** 1. the image of light made visible by the reflecting surface of the cornea and lens when illuminated through the slit lamp. 2. an image with right and left relations reversed, as in the reflection of an object in a mirror. **motor i.,** the organized cerebral model of the possible movements of the body. **Purkinje's i's, Purkinje-Sanson i's,** three images of an object seen in observing the pupil of the eye: from the posterior and anterior surfaces of the lens, and the anterior surface of the cornea. **real i.,** one formed where the emanating rays are collected, in which the object is pictured as being inverted. **virtual i.,** direct image.

imago (ĭ-ma′go) 1. the adult or definitive form of an insect. 2. a childhood memory or fantasy of a loved person which persists in adult life.

imbalance (im-bal′ans) lack of balance; especially lack of balance between muscles, as in insufficiency of ocular muscles. **autonomic i.,** disturbance of the involuntary nervous system. **sympathetic i.,** vagotonia. **vasomotor i.,** autonomic imbalance.

imbecile (im′bē-sil) a mentally defective person of the second lowest order of intellectual potential (I.Q. 21–50), usually requiring custodial and complete protective care.

imbecility (im″bē-sil′ĭ-te) mental deficiency sufficient to render the patient incapable of managing himself or his own affairs, the intelligence quotient being between 21 and 50.

imbibition (im″bĭ-bish′un) absorption of a liquid.

imbricated (im′brĭ-kāt″ed) overlapping like shingles.

imidamine (im″id-am′in) antazoline.

imidazole (im″id-az′ōl) iminazole.

imide (im′īd) a monobasic acid ammonia in which two hydrogen atoms are replaced by an acid radical.

iminazole (im″in-az′ōl) a radical occurring in histidine.

imipramine (ĭ-mip′rah-mēn) a compound used as a psychic energizer.

immersion (ĭ-mer′shun) 1. the plunging of a body into a liquid. 2. the use of the microscope with the object and object glass both covered with a liquid.

immiscible (ĭ-mis′ĭ-bl) incapable of being mixed.

immobilization (ĭ-mo″bĭ-li-za′shun) the rendering of a part incapable of being moved.

immune (ĭ-mūn′) not susceptible to a particular disease.

immunifacient (ĭ-mu″nĭ-fa′shent) producing immunity.

immunity (ĭ-mu′nĭ-te) resistance of a body to the effects of a deleterious agent, such as a pathogenic microorganism. **acquired i.,** that which results from antibodies not normally present in the blood. **active i.,** immunity produced by natural or artificial stimulation of the antibody-producing mechanism. **cellular i.,** acquired immunity in which phagocytic cells have a predominant role. **herd i.,** the resistance of a group to attack by a disease to which a large proportion of the members are immune. **natural i.,** the resistance of the normal animal to infection. **passive i.,** acquired immunity produced by administration of preformed antibody.

immunization (im″u-ni-za′shun) the production of immunity.

immunochemistry (im″u-no-kem′is-tre) study of the chemistry of immunity.

immunoelectrophoresis (-e-lek″tro-fo-re′sis) a method of distinguishing proteins and other materials on the basis of their electrophoretic mobility and antigenic specificities.

immunogenetics (im″u-no-jĕ-net′iks) the scientific study of the interrelations of immune reactions and genetic constitution.

immunogenic (-jen′ik) producing immunity.

immunogenicity (-jĕ-nis′ĭ-te) the ability of a substance to induce specific resistance.

immunoglobulin (-glob′u-lin) a protein of animal origin having antibody activity and related proteins with similar antigenic specificity.

immunologist (im″u-nol′o-jist) a specialist in immunology.

immunology (-nol′o-je) the scientific study of immunity.

immunopolysaccharide (im″u-no-pol″e-sak′-ah-rīd) a polysaccharide which is responsible for the immunologic specificity of a microorganism.

immunosuppression (-su-presh′un) inhibition of the formation of antibodies to antigens that may be present. adj., **immunosuppres′-sive.**

immunotherapy (-ther′ah-pe) treatment by production of immunity.

immunotoxin (-tok′sin) an antitoxin.

immunotransfusion (-trans-fu′zhun) transfusion of blood from a donor previously immunized by vaccine prepared from the patient's serum or recently recovered from the same disease.

impaction (im-pak′shun) the condition of being wedged in firmly. **dental i.,** prevention of eruption, normal occlusion or routine removal of a tooth because of its being locked in position by bone, dental restoration or surfaces of adjacent teeth. **fecal i.,** a collection of hardened feces in the rectum or sigmoid.

impar (im′par) not even; unequal; unpaired.

impedance (im-pe′dans) obstruction or opposition to passage or flow, as of an electric current or other form of energy. **acoustic i.,** an expression of the opposition to passage of sound waves, being the product of the density of a substance and the velocity of sound in it.

impetigo (im″pē-ti′go) a bacterial, inflammatory skin disease with isolated pustules. adj., **impetig′inous. i. bullo′sa, bullous i.,** impetigo in which the developing vesicles do not rupture, but progress to form bullae, which collapse and become covered with crusts. **i. contagio′sa,** an exudative form with lesions principally on the head and extremities, caused by streptococci or staphylococci. **i. herpetifor′mis,** impetigo with symmetrically ringed, pustular lesions, occurring chiefly in pregnant women. **neonatal i., i neonato′-rum,** impetigo of newborn infants, caused by staphylococci or streptococci. **i. syphilit′ica,** a pustular eruption in syphilis. **i. vulga′ris,** impetigo contagiosa.

implant, 1. (im-plant′) to insert or graft. 2. (im′plant) material inserted or grafted into the body, or a small container holding radon or radium, for internal application of its radiation.

implantation (im″plan-ta′shun) imbedding of a material within the tissues, as of medication or of a device such as an artificial pacemaker, or of the fertilized ovum in the uterine lining.

impotence (im'po-tens) partial or complete inability of the male to perform the sexual act or to achieve orgasm.

impregnation (im″preg-na'shun) 1. fertilization of the ovum. 2. saturation.

impressio (im-pres'e-o), pl. *impressio′nes* [L.] impression.

impression (im-presh'un) 1. an indentation or dent. 2. an effect on the mind or senses produced by external objects. **basilar i.**, platybasia. **cardiac i.**, an impression made by the heart on another organ. **complete denture i.**, one made of the entire maxilla or mandible for the purpose of construction of a complete denture. **dental i.**, an impression of the jaw or teeth which is later filled in with plaster of Paris to produce a facsimile of the oral structures present. **mental i.**, an effect produced on the mind by stimuli from outside the body. **sensory i.**, an effect produced upon the mind as a result of stimuli from outside the body and received by a special sense organ.

impulse (im'puls) an instinctual urge.

impulsion (im-pul'shun) a state characterized by an instinctual urge to commit an unlawful or socially unacceptable act.

I.M.S. India Medical Service.

In chemical symbol, *indium*.

in- (in) word element [L.], *in; within; into*.

-in (in) [L.] suffix indicating a neutral carbohydrate, glucoside, protein or glyceride.

I.N.A. International Neurological Association.

inalimental (in″al-ĭ-men'tal) not nutritious.

inanition (in″ah-nish'un) lack of food; starvation.

inappetence (in-ap'ĕ-tens) lack of appetite or desire.

inarticulate (in″ar-tik'u-lāt) 1. without definite articulations. 2. incapable of articulate speech.

inassimilable (in″ah-sim'ĭ-lah-bl) not susceptible of being utilized as nutriment.

inbreeding (in'brēd-ing) the mating of closely related individuals or of individuals having closely similar genetic constitutions.

incarceration (in-kar″sĕ-ra'shun) abnormal confinement or constriction.

incest (in'sest) culturally prohibited sexual activity between persons of close blood relationship.

incidence (in'si-dens) the rate at which a certain event occurs, as the number of new cases of a specific disease occurring during a certain period.

incineration (in-sin″ĕ-ra'shun) the act of burning to ashes.

incision (-sizh'un) 1. a cut or wound. 2. the act of cutting. **relief i.**, one made to relieve tension or congestion.

incisive (-si'siv) 1. having the power or quality of cutting; sharp. 2. pertaining to the incisor teeth.

incisor (-si'zor) any one of the four front teeth of either jaw.

incisura (in″si-su'rah), pl. *incisu′rae* [L.] incisure.

incisure (in-si'zher) a cut, incision or notch.

i's of Schmidt and Lanterman, oblique slashes or lines on the sheath of the medullated nerve fibers.

inclination (in″kli-na'shun) a sloping or leaning; the angle of deviation from a particular line or plane of reference; in dentistry, the deviation of a tooth from the vertical. **i. of the pelvis,** the angle between the axis of the body and that of the pelvis.

inclusion (in-kloo'zhun) enclosure within something else. **cell i.,** a usually lifeless, often temporary, constituent in the cytoplasm of a cell. **dental i.,** a tooth which is so surrounded with bony material that it is unable to erupt. **intranuclear i's,** inclusion bodies.

incoagulability (in″ko-ag″u-lah-bil'ĭ-te) the state of being incapable of coagulation. adj., **incoag′ulable.**

incompatible (in″kom-pat'ĭ-bl) not suited for harmonious coexistence or simultaneous administration; not to be combined in the same preparation or taken concomitantly.

incompetent (in-kom'pĕ-tent) 1. not able to function properly. 2. not responsible for actions, usually because of severe emotional disorder.

incontinence (-kon'tĭ-nens) inability to refrain from yielding to normal impulses, as sexual desire or the urge to defecate or urinate. adj.; **incon′tinent. fecal i.,** inability to control the evacuation of feces. **stress i.,** involuntary escape of urine due to strain on the orifice of the bladder, as in coughing or sneezing. **urinary i.,** inability to control the voiding of urine.

incontinentia (-kon″tĭ-nen'she-ah) [L.] incontinence. **i. al'vi,** fecal incontinence. **i. pigmen'ti,** a pigmentary disorder marked by patches on the skin due to excessive deposit of melanin. **i. uri'nae,** urinary incontinence.

incoordination (in″ko-or″dĭ-na'shun) lack of normal adjustment of muscular motions; failure to work harmoniously.

incorporation (in-kor″po-ra'shun) 1. thorough mixing of a substance with another. 2. in psychiatry, a primitive mental mechanism whereby a person unconsciously and symbolically takes within himself another person, parts of another person, or other significant nonmaterial elements.

increment (in'kre-ment) increase or augmentative growth; the amount by which a value or quantity is increased.

incretion (in-kre'shun) an internal secretion. adj., **in′cretory.**

incrustation (in″krus-ta'shun) 1. the formation of a crust. 2. a crust or scab.

incubate (in'ku-bāt) 1. to provide proper conditions for growth and development, as to maintain optimum temperature for the growth of bacteria. 2. material that has been incubated.

incubation (in″ku-ba'shun) development, especially of pathogenic organisms within the body.

incubator (-ba'ter) an apparatus for maintaining optimal conditions (temperature, humidity, etc.) for growth and development, especially one used in the early care of premature infants.

incubus (in″ku-bus) 1. nightmare. 2. a heavy mental burden.

incudal (in″ku-dal) pertaining to the incus.

incudectomy (in″ku-dek′to-me) excision of the incus.

incudiform (in-ku′dĭ-form) anvil-shaped.

incudomalleal (in″ku-do-mal′e-al) pertaining to incus and malleus.

incudostapedial (-stah-pe′de-al) pertaining to incus and stapes.

incurable (in-kūr′ah-bl) 1. not susceptible of being cured. 2. a person with a disease which cannot be cured.

incyclophoria (in″si-klo-fo′re-ah) tendency of the upper segment of the eye to rotate toward the nasal side.

incyclotropia (-tro′pe-ah) rotation of the upper segment of the eye toward the nasal side.

Indecidua (in″de-sid′u-ah) a division of the class Mammalia, including the mammals without a decidua.

index (in′deks) 1. the second digit of the hand, or the forefinger. 2. the numerical ratio of measurement of any part in comparison with a fixed standard. **alveolar i.,** degree of prominence of jaws. **centromeric i.,** the ratio of the length of the shorter arm of a mitotic chromosome to the total length of the chromosome. **cephalic i.,** 100 times the maximum breadth of the skull divided by its maximum length. **cerebral i.,** ratio of greatest transverse to greatest anteroposterior diameter of the cranial cavity. **color i.,** the relative amount of hemoglobulin in a red blood corpuscle compared with that of a normal individual of the same age and sex. **dental i.,** 100 times the dental length, divided by the length of the basinasal line. **gnathic i.,** 100 times the basialveolar length divided by the basinasal length. **hand i.,** 100 times the breadth of the hand divided by the length of the hand. **hemolytic i.,** a formula for calculating increased erythrocyte destruction. **icteric i.,** the ratio of bilirubin in the blood. **length-breadth i.,** cephalic index. **length-height i.,** vertical index. **leukopenic i.,** any variation from the normal leukocyte count after ingestion of food to which a patient is allergic. **metacarpal i.,** the average of the figures obtained by dividing the lengths of the right second, third, fourth and fifth metacarpal bones by their respective breadths at the exact midpoint. **mitotic i.,** an expression of the number of mitoses found in a stated number of cells. **nasal i.,** 100 times the width of the nose, divided by its length. **opsonic i.,** the resisting power of the blood against bacilli, as compared with the normal. **orbital i.** (of Broca), 100 times the height of the opening of the orbit divided by its width. **pelvic i.,** 100 times the anteroposterior diameter of the pelvis divided by the maximum width across the inlet. **phagocytic i.,** the average number of bacteria ingested per leukocyte of the patient's blood. **refraction i., refractive i.,** the refracting power of any substance compared with air. **refractive i., absolute,** an expression of the ratio of the velocity of light in air to its velocity in a specific substance. **refractive i., relative,** an expression of the ratio of the absolute refractive indexes of two different optically dense substances. **sacral i.,** 100 times the breadth of the sacrum divided by the length. **thoracic i.,** the ratio of the anteroposterior diameter of the thorax to the transverse diameter. **uricolytic i.,** the percentage of uric acid oxidized to allantoin before being secreted. **ventilation i.,** the ratio of the residual volume of the lung to total lung capacity. **vertical i.,** 100 times the height of the skull divided by its length. **vital i.,** the ratio of births to deaths within a given time in a population. **volume i.,** the index indicating the size of the erythrocytes as compared to the normal.

indican (in′dĭ-kan) 1. yellow glycoside, $C_{26}H_3$, from indigo plants. 2. principle, $C_8H_7NSO_4$, from sweat and urine.

indicator (in″dĭ-ka′ter) a substance which makes manifest a condition of a solution (acid: alkaline), or the end-point of a reaction.

indigestible (in″dĭ-jes′tĭ-bl) not susceptible of digestion.

indigestion (-jes′chun) failure of digestive function. **acid i.,** hyperchlorhydria. **fat i.,** steatorrhea. **gastric i.,** indigestion from disorder of the stomach. **intestinal i.,** disorder of the digestive function of the intestine. **sugar i.,** fermentative diarrhea.

indigitation (in-dij″ĭ-ta′shun) intussusception.

indigotin (in″dĭ-go′tin) indigo blue.

indigotindisulfonate (in″dĭ-go″tin-di-sul′fo-nāt) a dye used in tests for measurement of kidney function.

indium (in′de-um) chemical element (see table), at. no. 49, symbol In.

individuation (in″dĭ-vid″u-a′shun) 1. the process of developing individual characteristics. 2. differential regional activity in the embryo occurring in response to organizer influence.

indole (in′dōl) a compound formed during the putrefaction of proteins, which contributes to the characteristic odor of feces.

indoxyl (in-dok′sil) an oily substance, C_8H_7NO, found in urine.

induction (-duk′shun) the process or act of inducing, or causing to occur, especially (1) the specific morphogenetic effect of a chemical stimulus transmitted from one part of the embryo to another, bringing about the orderly development of the various organs and body structures, or (2) the generation of electric phenomena in a body by influence of an electrified body near it.

inductor (-duk′tor) organizer.

inductotherm (-duk′to-therm) an apparatus for producing high body temperature by electric induction.

inductothermy (-duk′to-ther″me) production of artificial fever by the inductotherm.

indulin (in′du-lin) a coal tar dye used as a histologic stain.

indurated (in′du-rāt″ed) hardened; abnormally hard.

induration (in″du-ra′shun) quality of being hard; process of hardening; an abnormally hard spot. adj., **indura'tive. black i.**, hardening and pigmentation of lung, as in anthracosis. **brawny i.**, inflammatory hardening and thickening of tissues. **brown i.**, deposit of altered blood pigment in pneumonia. **cyanotic i.**, hardening of an organ from chronic venous congestion. **granular i.**, cirrhosis. **gray i.**, induration of lung tissue in or after pneumonia, without pigmentation. **red i.**, interstitial pneumonia in which the lung is red and congested.

inebriant (ĭ-ne'bre-ant) an intoxicating agent.

inelastic (in″e-las'tik) lacking elasticity.

inemia (in-e'me-ah) fibrin in the blood.

inert (in-ert') inactive.

inertia (-er'she-ah) [L.] inactivity. **colonic i.**, absence of efficient contraction of the muscular coat of the colon, leading to distention of the organ and constipation. **i. u'teri, uterine i.**, absence of effectual contraction of the muscular wall of the uterus, leading to prolonged labor.

in extremis (in ek-stre'mis) [L.] at the point of death.

infancy (in'fan-se) the first two years of life.

infant (in'fant) the human young from the time of birth to two years of age. **floppy i.**, one exhibiting severe generalized hypotonia. **immature i.**, one weighing between 17 ounces and 2⅕ pounds (500–999 gm.) at birth, with little chance of survival. **mature i.**, one weighing 5½ pounds (2500 gm.) or more at birth, with optimal chance of survival. **newborn i.**, the human young during the first two to four weeks after birth. **postmature i.**, one having an accurate history of a prolonged gestation period and weighing more than 9 pounds (4082 gm.) at birth. **premature i.**, one weighing between 2⅕ and 5½ pounds (1000–2499 gm.) at birth, with poor to good chance of survival.

infantile (in'fan-tīl) relating to the stage of infancy; having features or traits characteristic of early childhood.

infantilism (in-fan'tĭ-lizm) persistence of the characters of childhood in adult life, marked by mental retardation, underdevelopment of the sexual organs and often, but not always, by smallness of stature. **angioplastic i.**, that attributed to defective development of the vascular system. **cachectic i.**, that due to chronic infection or poisoning. **celiac i.**, that resulting from celiac disease. **dysthyroidal i.**, that due to defective thyroid activity. **hepatic i.**, that associated with hepatic cirrhosis. **hypophyseal i.**, a type of dwarfism, with retention of infantile characteristics, due to deficiency of hormones of the pituitary gland. **idiopathic i.**, infantilism of unknown causation. **lymphatic i.**, that associated with lymphatism. **myxedematous i.**, cretinism. **pancreatic i.**, delayed growth and development associated with atrophy of the pancreas and hepatomegaly. **partial i.**, arrested development of a single part or tissue. **renal i.**, renal osteodystrophy. **reversive i.**, infantilism beginning after bodily growth has been completed. **sexual i.**, retardation of sexual development, as in adiposogenital dystrophy. **symptomatic i.**, that due to general defective development of tissues. **tardy i.**, reversive infantilism. **universal i.**, general dwarfishness in stature, with absence of secondary sex characters.

infarct (in'farkt) a localized area of ischemic necrosis produced by occlusion of the arterial supply or the venous drainage of the part. **anemic i.**, one due to interruption of flow of arterial blood to the area. **bone i.**, an area of necrotic bone tissue due to loss of its arterial blood supply. **hemorrhagic i.**, that due to interruption of drainage of venous blood from the area. **pale i.**, anemic infarct. **red i.**, hemorrhagic infarct. **septic i.**, one in which the tissues have been invaded by pathogenic organisms. **white i.**, anemic infarct.

infarction (in-fark'shun) 1. engorgement or stoppage of a vessel. 2. development or presence of an infarct. **cardiac i.**, myocardial infarction. **cerebral i.**, an ischemic condition of the brain, causing a persistent focal neurologic deficit in the area affected. **intestinal i.**, occlusion of an artery or arteriole in the wall of the intestine, resulting in the formation of an area of coagulation necrosis. **myocardial i.**, formation of an infarct in the heart muscle, due to interruption of the blood supply to the area. **pulmonary i.**, infiltration of an airless area of lung with blood cells, due to obstruction of the pulmonary artery by an embolus or thrombus.

infection (-fek'shun) 1. a morbid state caused by multiplication of pathogenic microorganisms within the body. 2. the invasion of an organism (host) by any pathogenic (or nonpathogenic) organism, exclusive of the Arthropoda. **airborne i.**, infection by agents transmitted through the air. **consecutive i.**, secondary infection. **cross i.**, infection transmitted between patients infected with different pathogenic microorganisms. **cryptogenic i.**, infection without discoverable site of entrance or location of the infective agent. **droplet i.**, infection by microorganisms present in droplets of sputum expelled into the air during talking or by coughing or sneezing. **dust-borne i.**, infection by agents that have become affixed to particles of dust and are transmitted by that means. **ectogenous i.**, infection due to organisms that have gained entrance to the body from outside, as through surgical or accidental wounds, or a natural orifice. **endogenous i.**, a morbid state produced by organisms normally present in the body. **focal i.**, presence of microorganisms in circumscribed colonies, but causing general symptoms. **germinal i.**, transmission of infection to the child by means of the ovum or sperm of the parent. **latent i.**, persistence in the body of microorganisms which have ceased to multiply. **mixed i.**, infection with more than one kind of organism at the same time. **secondary i.**, infection by a bacterium following an infection by a bacterium of another kind. **septic i.**, true septicemia. **terminal i.**, an acute infection occurring near the end of a disease and causing death. **water-**

borne i., infection by microorganisms transmitted in water.

infectious (in-fek'shus) liable to be communicated by infection.

infertility (in″fer-til'ĭ-te) absence of ability to produce offspring. adj., **infer′tile.**

infestation (in″fes-ta'shun) invasion of the body by arthropods, including insects, mites and ticks.

infiltrate (in-fil'trāt) material deposited by infiltration.

infiltration (in″fil-tra'shun) the deposit or diffusion of a morbid solid or fluid in any tissue. **adipose i.**, fatty infiltration. **calcareous i.**, deposit of lime and earthy salts in the tissues. **cellular i.**, infiltration of tissues with round cells. **fatty i.**, the abnormal accumulation of fat within healthy cells as the result of a systemic metabolic derangement. **glycogenic i.**, deposit of glycogen in cells. **pigmentary i.**, deposits of pigment in tissues. **purulent i.**, presence of dispersed pus cells in a tissue. **serous i.**, abnormal presence of serum in a tissue. **urinous i.**, the extravasation of urine into a tissue. **waxy i.**, deposition of amyloid substance.

infirmary (in-fer'mah-re) a place for care of ill patients.

inflammation (in″flah-ma'shun) a protective tissue response to injury or destruction of the cells. adj., **inflam′matory. acute i.**, a tissue response usually of sudden onset and accompanied by the cardinal signs of heat, redness, swelling, pain and loss of function (calor, rubor, tumor, dolor and functio laesa). **catarrhal i.**, a condition characterized by out-pouring of large amounts of mucinous secretion, occurring only in tissues capable of secreting mucus. **chronic i.**, prolonged and persistent inflammation. **exudative i.**, a tissue response ordinarily of short duration, characterized by vascular congestion and exudation of fluids and white cells. **fibrinous i.**, a tissue response characterized by outpouring of large amounts of fibrinogen and precipitation of masses of fibrin. **granulomatous i.**, a tissue response, usually chronic, attended by formation of granulomas. **interstitial i.**, inflammation affecting primarily the materials between the essential structural elements. **parenchymatous i.**, inflammation affecting chiefly the essential structural elements. **productive i.**, one attended by a new growth of connective tissue. **pseudomembranous i.**, response characterized by formation on a mucosal surface of a false membrane composed of precipitated fibrin, necrotic epithelium and inflammatory white cells. **purulent i.**, suppurative inflammation. **reactive i.**, one occurring around a foreign body or a focus of degeneration. **serous i.**, inflammation marked by outpouring of watery, low-protein fluid derived from blood serum or secretions of serosal mesothelial cells. **simple i.**, one without pus or other specific inflammatory product. **specific i.**, one due to a particular microorganism. **subacute i.**, a condition intermediate between chronic and acute inflammation, exhibiting some of the characteristics of each. **suppurative i.**, that characterized by production of large amounts of pus or purulent exudate. **toxic i.**, one due to a poison. **traumatic i.**, one which follows a wound or injury. **ulcerative i.**, that in which necrosis on or near the surface leads to loss of tissue and creation of a local defect (ulcer).

inflation (in-fla'shun) distention with air, gas or fluid.

inflection (-flek'shun) the act of bending inward, or state of being bent inward.

influenza (in″floo-en'zah) an acute infectious, epidemic disease, marked by depression, distressing fever, acute catarrhal inflammation of the nose, larynx and bronchi, neuralgic and muscular pains, gastrointestinal disorder and nervous disturbances, and caused by a filterable virus. adj., **influen′zal. summer i. of Italy,** phlebotomus fever.

infra-axillary (in″frah-ak'si-ler″e) below the axilla.

infrabulge (in′frah-bulj) the surfaces of a tooth gingival to the height of contour, or sloping cervically.

infraclavicular (in″frah-klah-vik'u-lar) below the clavicle.

infracostal (-kos′tal) below a rib.

infradentale (-den-ta′le) a cephalometric landmark, being the highest anterior point on the gingiva between the mandibular medial incisors.

infrahyoid (-hi'oid) below the hyoid bone.

inframaxillary (-mak'si-ler″e) below the jaw.

infranuclear (-nu′kle-ar) below the nucleus.

infraocclusion (-ō-kloo'zhun) depression of a tooth below the line of occlusion.

infraorbital (-or′bĭ-tal) beneath the orbit.

infrapatellar (-pah-tel′ar) beneath the patella.

infraplacement (-plās′ment) downward displacement of a tooth.

infrapsychic (-si'kik) below the psychic level; automatic.

infrared (in″frah-red′) red end of the visible spectrum; noting rays with wavelengths between 7700 and 120,000 angstroms. **long-wave i.**, infra-red radiation furthest from the visible spectrum, with wavelengths between 15,000 and 120,000 angstroms. **short-wave i.**, infra-red radiation closest to the red end of the visible spectrum, with wavelengths between 7700 and 15,000 angstroms.

infrascapular (-skap'u-lar) beneath the scapula.

infrasonic (-son′ik) below the frequency range of the waves normally perceived as sound by the human ear.

infraspinous (-spi′nus) beneath the spine of the scapula.

infrasternal (-ster′nal) beneath the sternum.

infratrochlear (-trok′le-ar) beneath the trochlea.

infraversion (-ver′zhun) 1. downward deviation of the eye. 2. shortness of a tooth in relation to the plane of occlusion.

infundibuliform (in″fun-dib'u-lĭ-form″) shaped like a funnel.

infundibuloma (in″fun-dib″u-lo′mah) a tumor

of the stalk (infundibulum) of the hypophysis cerebri.

infundibulum (in″fun-dib′u-lum), pl. *infundib′ula* [L.] 1. any funnel-shaped passage. 2. conus arteriosus. adj., **infundib′ular. ethmoidal i.,** 1. a passage connecting the nasal cavity with anterior ethmoidal cells and frontal sinus. 2. a sinuous passage connecting the middle meatus of the nose with anterior ethmoidal cells and often with the frontal sinus. **i. of hypothalamus,** a hollow, funnel-shaped mass. **i. of uterine tube,** the distal, funnel-shaped portion of the uterine tube.

infusion (in-fu′zhun) 1. steeping of a substance in water to obtain its soluble principles. 2. a solution obtained by steeping a substance in water.

ingesta (-jes′tah) material taken into the body by mouth.

ingestant (-jes′tant) a substance that is or may be taken into the body by mouth or through the digestive system.

ingestion (jes′chun) the taking of nutrient material into the alimentary tract of the body.

ingravescent (in″grah-ves′ent) gradually becoming more severe.

inguen (in′gwen), pl. *in′guina* [L.] the groin.

inguinal (in′gwĭ-nal) pertaining to the groin.

INH trademark for preparations of isoniazid.

inhalant (in-ha′lant) a gaseous substance that is or may be taken into the body by way of the nose and trachea (through the respiratory system). **antifoaming i.,** an agent that is inhaled as a vapor to prevent the formation of foam in the respiratory passages of a patient with pulmonary edema.

inhalation (in″hah-la′shun) the drawing of air or other vapor into the lungs.

inhaler (in-ha′ler) instrument for administering a medicated vapor.

inheritance (-her′ĭ-tans) 1. the acquisition of characters or qualities by transmission from parent to offspring. 2. that which is transmitted from parent to offspring. **criss-cross i.,** inheritance by offspring of characters from the parent of the opposite sex. **cytoplasmic i.,** transmission of characters dependent on self perpetuating elements not nuclear in origin. **holandric i.,** inheritance by all the males, but not by the females. **maternal i.,** the transmission of characters that are dependent on peculiarities of the egg cytoplasm produced, in turn, by nuclear genes. **monofactorial i.,** the acquisition of a characteristic or quality whose transmission depends on a single gene. **multifactorial i.,** the acquisition of a characteristic or quality whose manifestation is subject to modification by a number of genes.

inhibition (in″ĭ-bish′un, in″hĭ-bish′un) the imposition of restraint, or arrest of a process. **competitive i.,** prevention of the action of an effector substance or agent by another substance or agent that enters into combination with the element on which the effector substance acts or which is essential to its action. **end-product i.,** inhibition by the ultimate product of a specific process, of the initial steps leading originally to its production. **false feed-back i.,** inhibition of the initial steps of a process by an analogue of the end-product of the specific process. **feed-back i.,** end-product inhibition. **serum i.,** antiplasmin.

inhibitor (in-hib′ĭ-tor) a substance or agent that depresses the activity of another substance or agent, particularly a substance which checks the action of an enzyme or a tissue organizer, or the growth of microorganisms. **competitive i.,** one which inhibits an action by combining with another substance necessary to the accomplishment of the action.

iniencephalus (in″e-en-sef′ah-lus) a fetus with a fissured occiput.

inion (in′e-on) the external occipital protuberance. adj., **in′ial.**

iniopagus (in″e-op′ah-gus) a twin monster joined at the occiput.

iniops (in′e-ops) a double-faced monster with the posterior face incomplete.

initis (i-ni′tis) inflammation of muscular substance.

injected (in-jek′ted) filled by injection; congested.

injection (-jek′shun) 1. introduction of a liquid directly into a body tissue, body cavity or tubular organ. 2. a solution intended for introduction directly into a body tissue or tubular organ, as intramuscularly or intravascularly. **adrenal cortex i.,** a preparation containing a mixture of the endocrine principles derived from the cortex of adrenal glands; used in treatment of adrenal insufficiency. **Brown-Séquard i.,** injection of testicular extract. **capillary i.,** a hyperemia which makes the small blood vessels visible. **circumcorneal i.,** dilatation of the conjunctival blood vessels close to the limbus, and diminishing toward the periphery. **dextrose i.,** a sterile solution of dextrose in water for injection; used as a fluid and nutrient replenisher. **fructose i.,** a sterile solution of fructose in water; used as a fluid and nutrient replenisher. **insulin i.,** a sterile solution of the active principle of the pancreas which affects the metabolism of glucose; a prompt-acting preparation used in treatment of diabetes mellitus. **liver i.,** a sterile preparation of the soluble thermostable fraction of mammalian livers that stimulates hematopoiesis in patients with pernicious anemia. **opacifying i.,** injection of a radiopaque substance into the vessels or into some body cavity for diagnostic radiologic study. **oxytocin i.,** a sterile solution of an oxytocic principle prepared by synthesis or obtained from the posterior lobe of the pituitary gland of domestic animals; used to stimulate contraction of smooth muscle, particularly the pregnant uterus. **parathyroid i.,** a sterile solution of water-soluble principles of parathyroid glands, administered intramuscularly to maintain blood calcium levels. **potassic saline i., lactated,** a sterile solution of potassium chloride, sodium chloride and sodium lactate in water for injection; used as a fluid and electrolyte replenisher. **protamine sulfate i.**, a sterile isotonic solution from sperm or mature testes of certain fish; used to counteract the action of heparin. **protein hydrolystate i.**, a sterile solution of amino acids and short-chain peptides; used as a parenteral nutrient. **radiochromate sodium i.**, a sterile solution of radioactive chromium; used in estimation of blood volume. **Ringer's i.**, a sterile solution of sodium chloride, potassium choride and calcium chloride in water for injection; used as a fluid and electrolyte replenisher. **sodium chloride i.**, a sterile isotonic solution of sodium chloride in water for injection; used as a fluid and electrolyte replenisher. **sodium chromate Cr.-51 i.**, a sterile solution containing radioactive chromium as sodium chromate; used in determination of blood volume. **sodium dehydrocholate i.**, a sterile solution of sodium dehydrocholate; used as a choleretic and in determination of circulation time. **sodium diatrizoate i.**, a sterile iodine-containing solution prepared with sodium hydroxide; used as a contrast medium in arteriography and urography. **sodium iodipamide i.**, a sterile solution of sodium iodipamide; used as a contrast medium in radiography of the biliary tract. **sodium iodohippurate I-131 i.**, a sterile solution of sodium iodohippurate in which some of the molecules contain radioactive iodine; used in tests of renal function. **sodium morrhuate i.**, a sterile solution of sodium salts of fatty acids of codliver oil; a sclerosing agent for venous varicosities. **vasopressin i.**, a sterile solution of the water-soluble, pressor principle of the posterior lobe of the pituitary gland of healthy domestic animals.

injury (in'ju-re) a specific impairment of body structure or function caused by an outside agent or force, which may be physical, chemical or psychic. **birth i.**, impairment of body function or structure due to adverse influences to which the infant has been subjected at birth. **Goyrand's i.**, pulled elbow. **whiplash i.**, injury to the spinal cord and spine due to rapid acceleration or deceleration of the body, as in sudden stopping or propulsion of a vehicle.

inlay (in'la) 1. a graft which is inserted into the substance of an organ or other body structure. 2. in dentistry, a filling first made to correspond with the form of a dental cavity and then cemented into the cavity.

inlet (in'let) a means or route of entrance. **pelvic i.**, the upper limit of the pelvic cavity.

innate (in'āt) inborn; hereditary; congenital.

innervation (in″er-va'shun) distribution of the nerves.

innidiation (ĭ-nid″e-a'shun) development of cells in a part to which they have been carried.

innocent (in'o-sent) not harmful or malignant.

innocuous (ĭ-nok'u-us) not hurtful.

innominate (-nom'ĭ-nāt) nameless or unnamed.

inoblast (in'o-blast) connective tissue cell in the formative stage.

inochondritis (in″o-kon-dri'tis) inflammation of a fibrocartilage.

inochondroma (-kon-dro'mah) fibrochondroma.

inoculability (ĭ-nok″u-lah-bil'ĭ-te) the state of being inoculable.

inoculable (ĭ-nok'u-lah-bl) 1. transmissible by inoculation. 2. not immune against a transmissible disease.

inoculation (ĭ-nok″u-la'shun) 1. introduction of pathogenic microorganisms into the body to stimulate the production of antibodies and immunity. 2. introduction of infectious material into culture medium in an effort to produce growth of the causative organism.

inoculum (ĭ-nok'u-lum) material used in inoculation.

inocystoma (in″o-sis-to'mah) fibrous tumor with cystic degeneration.

inocyte (in'o-sīt) a cell of fibrous tissue.

inogenesis (in″o-jen'ē-sis) the formation of fibrous tissue.

inogenous (in-oj'ē-nus) produced from or forming tissue.

inoperable (-op'er-ah-bl) not susceptible of being cured by surgery.

inorganic (in″or-gan'ik) 1. having no organs. 2. not of organic origin.

inosclerosis (in″o-skle-ro'sis) fibrous induration.

inose (in'ōs) inositol.

inosemia (in″o-se'me-ah) excess of fibrin in the blood.

inosite (in'o-sīt) inositol.

inositol (in-o'sī-tol) a compound found in many plants, microorganisms and animal tissues, capable of facilitating removal of fats from the liver.

inosituria (in″o-si-tu're-ah) inositol in the urine.

inotropic (in'o-trop″ik) affecting the force of cardiac contractions.

in ovo (in o'vo) [L.] in the egg, especially in a chick embryo.

insalubrious (in″sah-lu'bre-us) injurious to health.

insane (in-sān') mentally deranged.

insanity (-san'ĭ-te) legal term for disorder of the mental faculties. **circular i., cyclic i.**, manic-depressive psychosis. **doubting i.**, mental disorder characterized by morbid doubt, suspicion and indecision. **impulsive i.**, insane tendency to perform inappropriate acts. **moral i.**, a form marked by impairment of the moral sense. **perceptional i.**, a form marked by hallucination and illusions. **periodic i.**, a form recurring at regular intervals.

inscriptio (-skrip'she-o), pl. *incriptio'nes* [L.] inscription. **i. tendin'ea**, a fibrous band traversing the belly of a muscle and dividing it into two parts.

inscription (-skrip'shun) a writing, mark or line; that part of a prescription giving the name, size or strength, and quantity of the agent, or the name and amount of each of the ingredients to be combined.

Insecta (-sek'tah) a class of animals (phylum Arthropoda) characterized by division of the body into three distinct regions—head, thorax and abdomen.

insecticide (in-sek″tĭ-sīd) an agent which kills insects. adj., **insec′ticidal.**

Insectivora (in″sek-tiv′o-rah) an order of small, terrestrial and nocturnal mammals which feed on insects.

insectivore (in-sek′tĭ-vōr) an individual of the order Insectivora.

insemination (-sem″ĭ-na′shun) introduction of sperm into the female reproductive tract for the purpose of fertilization. **artificial i.,** instrumental introduction of semen into the female genital tract.

insensible (-sen′sĭ-bl) 1. devoid of sensibility or consciousness. 2. not perceptible to the senses.

insertion (-ser′shun) attachment, as the site of attachment of a skeletal muscle on the bone that is moved when the muscle contracts. **velamentous i.,** attachment of the umbilical cord to the membranes.

insight (in′sīt) recognition of the abnormality of one's own emotional reactions or motives.

in situ (in si′tu) [L.] in its normal place; confined to the site of origin.

insoluble (in-sol′u-bl) not susceptible of being dissolved.

insomnia (-som′ne-ah) inability to sleep; abnormal wakefulness.

insorption (-sorp′shun) movement of a substance into the blood, especially from the gastrointestinal tract into the circulating blood.

inspection (-spek′shun) visual examination for detection of features or qualities perceptible to the eye.

inspersion (-sper′shun) a sprinkling with powder.

inspiration (in″spĭ-ra′shun) the drawing of air into the lungs. adj., **inspi′ratory.**

inspissated (in-spis′āt-ed) thickened; made less fluid.

instability (in″stah-bil′ĭ-te) the quality of being unsteady or changeable. **emotional i.,** the quality of being too changeable in feeling tone.

instillation (in″stĭ-la′shun) the dropping of liquid into a cavity, as into the eye.

instinct (in′stinkt) an innate tendency to a certain action or mode of behavior. **death i.,** an unconscious drive toward dissolution and death. **herd i.,** the tendency to adopt the standards of thought and action of a group.

instrumentation (in″stroo-men-ta′shun) the use and care of instruments.

insufficiency (in″sŭ-fish′en-se) inability to perform properly an allotted function. **aortic i.,** inadequacy of the aortic valve, permitting blood to flow back into the left ventricle of the heart. **cardiac i.,** inability of the heart to perform its function properly. **coronary i.,** decrease in flow of blood through the coronary blood vessels. **i. of the externi,** deficient power in the externi muscles of the eye, resulting in esophoria. **ileocecal i.,** inability of the ileocecal valve to prevent backflow of

contents from the cecum into the ileum. **i. of the interni,** deficient power in the interni muscles of the eye, resulting in exophoria. **valvular i.,** failure of a cardiac valve to close perfectly, so that blood passes back through the orifice; named, according to the valve affected, *aortic, mitral, pulmonary* or *tricuspid.*

insufflation (in″su-fla′shun) the blowing of a powder, vapor or gas into a cavity. **perirenal i.,** injection of air around the kidney for roentgen examination of the adrenal glands. **tubal i.,** insufflation of air or gas through the uterus into the uterine tubes as a test of their patency.

insufflator (in″sŭ-fla′tor) an instrument for blowing gas or powder into a cavity.

insula (in′su-lah), pl. *in′sulae* [L.] a conical mass of cortical tissue lying at the bottom of the lateral fissure of the cerebral hemisphere. adj., **in′sular.**

insulation (in″sŭ-la′shun) the surrounding of a space or body with material designed to prevent the entrance or escape of radiant energy.

insulin (in′su-lin) a protein hormone secreted by cells of the islands of Langerhans of the pancreas into the blood, and concerned with carbohydrate metabolism; a sterile preparation of the active principle is used in treatment of hyperglycemia (diabetes). **globin zinc i.,** insulin modified by addition of zinc chloride and globin from beef blood. **i. lente,** a sterile suspension of insulin modified by the addition of zinc chloride. **NPH i.,** a neutral, crystalline protamine zinc insulin with a speedy and long-lasting action. **protamine zinc i.,** insulin modified by addition of zinc chloride and protamine from the sperm or mature testes of various genera of fish. **regular i.,** the active principle of the pancreas of slaughter-house animals (cattle or swine), used in sterile acidified solution.

insulinemia (in″su-lin c′me-ah) insulin in the blood.

insulinogenic (in″su lin″o-jen′ik) caused by insulin.

insulinoid (in′su-lin-oid″) resembling insulin.

insulitis (in″su-li′tis) cellular infiltration of the island of Langerhans, possibly in response to invasion by an infectious agent.

insuloma (in″su-lo′mah) adenoma of the islands of Langerhans of the pancreas.

insulopathic (in″su-lo-path′ik) pertaining to abnormal insulin secretion.

insusceptibility (in″sŭ-sep″tĭ-bil′ĭ-te) the state of being unaffected or uninfluenced.

intake (in′tāk) substance taken into the body by ingestion or parenterally, usually expressed quantitatively, as the amount of fluid or caloric intake.

integration (in″tĕ-gra′shun) assimilation into a common body or activity to achieve a common purpose. **biological i.,** the acquisition of functional coordination during embryonic development through humoral and nervous influences. **primary i.,** recognition by a child that his body is a unit apart from the environment. **secondary i.**, sublimation of the separate elements of the early sexual instinct into the mature psychosexual personality.

integument (in-teg'u-ment) the natural covering of the body; the skin. adj., **integumen'-tary.**

integumentum (in-teg″u-men'tum) [L.] integument.

in tela (in te'lah) [L.] in tissue; relating especially to stained histologic preparations.

intellect (in'tĕ-lekt) the mind, thinking faculty, or understanding.

intelligence (in-tel'ĭ-jens) the ability to comprehend or understand. **i. quotient,** a numerical expression of intellectual capacity obtained by multiplying the mental age of the subject by 100 and dividing by his chronologic age.

intensimeter (in″ten-sim'ĕ-ter) a device for measuring intensity of roentgen rays.

intention (in-ten'shun) the agglutination of the edges of a wound in healing.

inter- (in'ter) word element [L.], *between.*

interarticular (in″ter-ar-tik'u-ler) between articulating surfaces.

interatrial (-a'tre-al) between the atria of the heart.

interauricular (-aw-rik'u-ler) interatrial.

interbrain (in'ter-brān) diencephalon.

intercadence (in″ter-ka'dens) occurrence of an occasional extra beat between two pulse beats.

intercalary (in-ter'kah-ler″e) inserted between; interposed.

intercellular (in″ter-sel'u-lar) between the cells.

intercentral (-sen'tral) between, or connecting, nerve centers.

interchondral (-kon'dral) between cartilages.

intercilium (-sil'e-um) the space between the eyebrows.

interclavicular (-klah-vik'u-ler) between the clavicles.

intercondylar (-kon'dĭ-lar) between two condyles.

intercostal (-kos'tal) between two ribs.

intercostalis (-kos-ta'lis), pl. *intercosta'les* [L.] intercostal.

intercourse (in'ter-kōrs) interchange or communication between individuals. **sexual i.,** coitus.

intercricothyrotomy (in″ter-kri″ko-thi-rot'o-me) incision of the larynx through the cricothyroid membrane; inferior laryngotomy.

intercurrent (-kur'ent) occurring during the course of.

intercusping (-kusp'ing) the occlusion of the cusps of the teeth of one jaw with the depressions in the teeth of the other jaw.

interdental (-den'tal) between the proximal surfaces of adjacent teeth in the same dental arch.

interdentium (-den'she-um) the space between two contiguous teeth.

interdigital (-dij'ĭ-tal) between two digits (fingers or toes).

interdigitation (-dij″ĭ-ta'shun) 1. an interlocking of parts by finger-like processes. 2. one of a set of finger-like processes.

interfascicular (in″ter-fah-sik'u-lar) between adjacent fascicles.

interfemoral (-fem'o-ral) between the thighs.

interferon (-fēr'on) a protein produced by interaction of animal cells and viruses that is capable of inhibiting virus multiplication.

interfibrillary (-fib'rĭ-lār″e) between fibrils.

interfilar (-fi'lar) between the fibrils of a reticulum.

interganglionic (-gang″gle-on'ik) between ganglions.

intergenic (-jen'ik) occurring between two genes.

interictal (-ik'tal) occurring between attacks or paroxysms.

interlobar (-lo'bar) between lobes.

interlobitis (-lo-bi'tis) inflammation of pleura between lobes of the lung.

interlobular (-lob'u-lar) between lobules.

intermaxillary (-mak'sĭ-ler″e) between the maxillae.

intermedius (-me'de-us) [L.] intermediate.

intermeningeal (-mĕ-nin'je-al) between the meninges.

intermitotic (-mi-tot'ik) between successive mitoses.

intermural (-mu'ral) between the walls of an organ or organs.

intermuscular (-mus'ku-lar) between muscles.

intern (in'tern) a medical graduate serving and residing in a hospital preparatory to being licensed to practice medicine.

internalization (in-ter″nal-i-za'shun) a mental mechanism whereby certain external attributes, attitudes or standards are unconsciously taken within oneself.

internatal (in″ter-na'tal) between the nates, or buttocks.

interneuron (-nu'ron) a neuron between the primary afferent neuron and the final motor neuron.

internist (in-ter'nist) a specialist in diseases of the internal organs.

internode (in'ter-nōd) an interannular segment of a nerve fiber.

internship (in'tern-ship) the position of an intern in a hospital, or the term of service.

internuclear (in″ter-nu'kle-ar) between nuclei, or between nuclear layers of the retina.

internuncial (-nun'shal) transmitting impulses between two different parts.

internus (in-ter'nus) [L.] internal.

interocclusal (in″ter-ŏ-kloo'zal) situated between the occlusal surfaces of opposing teeth in the two dental arches.

interoceptive (-o-sep'tiv) receiving impulses from the viscera, or from the interior of the body.

interoceptor (-sep'tor) a sensory nerve terminal located in and transmitting impulses from the viscera.

interofective (-fek'tiv) affecting the interior of the organism — a term applied to the autonomic nervous system.

interogestate (-jes'tāt) 1. developing within

the uterus. 2. an infant developing within the uterus or during the period of interior gestation.

interoinferiorly (in″ter-o-in-fēr′e-or-le)   inwardly and downwardly.

interolivary (in″ter-ol′ĭ-var″e)   between the olivary bodies.

interorbital (-or′bĭ-tal) between the orbits.

interosseous (-os′e-us) between two bones.

interosseus (-os′e-us) pl. *interos'sei* [L.] interosseous.

interpalpebral (-pal′pĕ-bral) between the eyelids.

interparietal (-pah-ri′ē-tal) between the parietal bones.

interparoxysmal (-par″ok-siz′mal) between paroxysms.

interphase (in′ter-fāz) the stage in the life of a cell before it begins to divide mitotically, or between the first and second divisions in meiosis.

interplant (in′ter-plant) an embryonic part isolated by transference to an indifferent environment provided by another embryo.

interpolation (in-ter″po-la′shun) 1. surgical transplantation of tissue. 2. the determination of intermediate values in a series on the basis of observed values.

interproximal (in″ter-prok′sĭ-mal) between two adjoining surfaces.

interpubic (-pu′bik) between the pubic bones.

interpupillary (-pu′pĭ-ler″e) between the pupils.

interscapular (-skap′u-lar) between the scapulae.

intersectio (-sek′she-o), pl. *intersectio'nes* [L.] intersection.

intersection (-sek′shun) a site at which one structure cuts across another.

intersex (in′ter-seks) 1. intersexuality. 2. an individual showing one or more contradictions of the morphologic criteria of sex. **female i.**, one who has only female gonadal tissue and shows sex chromatin in the somatic cells. **male i.**, one who has only male gonadal tissue and shows no sex chromatin in the somatic cells. **true i.**, one who has both male and female gonadal tissue; the chromatin test may be either positive or negative in result.

intersexuality (in″ter-seks″u-al′ĭ-te) a blending of the characters of both sexes.

interspinalis (-spi-na′lis), pl. *interspina'les* [L.] between spines of the vertebrae.

interstice (in-ter′stis) an interval, space or gap in a tissue or structure. adj., **intersti'tial.**

intersystole (in″ter-sis′to-le) atriocarotid interval.

intertransversarius (-trans″ver-sa′re-us), pl. *intertransversa'rii* [L.] between transverse processes of the vertebrae.

intertrigo (-tri′go) erythema due to chafing of the skin.

intertubular (-tu′bu-lar) between tubules.

interureteral (-u-re′ter-al) interureteric.

interureteric (-u-re-ter′ik) between ureters.

intervaginal (-vaj′ĭ-nal) between sheaths.

interval (in′ter-val) the space between two objects or parts; the lapse of time between two

events. **a.-c. i.**, **atriocarotid i.**, **auriculocarotid i.**, the time between the beginning of the atrial and the beginning of the carotid waves in a jugular pulse tracing. **c.-a. i.**, **cardioarterial i.**, the time between the apex beat and arterial pulsation. **lucid i.**, a period of full possession of the faculties between periods of mental disturbance. **postsphygmic i.**, the time between beginning of dilation of the ventricles of the heart and opening of the atrioventricular valves. **presphygmic i.**, the time between the beginning of contraction of the ventricles of the heart and the opening of the arterial valves. **QRST i.**, the ventricular complex of the electrocardiogram.

intervalvular (in″ter-val′vu-lar) between valves.

intervascular (-vas′ku-lar) between blood vessels.

interventricular (-ven-trik′u-lar) between the ventricles of the heart.

intervertebral (-ver′tĕ-bral) between two vertebrae.

intestine (in-tes′tin) membranous tube extending from the pyloric opening of the stomach to the anus. adj., **intes'tinal. blind i.**, cecum. **empty i.**, jejunum. **large i.**, the distal portion of the intestine, from ileocecal valve to anus, about 5½ feet long and 2½ inches in diameter. **pancreatic i.**, duodenum. **segmented i.**, colon. **small i.**, the proximal portion of the intestine, from pyloric opening of the stomach to the cecum, about 20–22 feet long and 1½ inches in diameter. **straight i.**, rectum. **twisted i.**, ileum.

intestinum (in″tes-ti′num), pl. *intestin'na* [L.] intestine.

intima (in′tĭ-mah) the innermost coat of a blood vessel. adj., **in'timal.**

intima-pia (in″tĭ-mah-pi′ah) the combined intima of blood vessels and pia mater surrounding the arteries of the brain.

intimectomy (in″tĭ-mek′to-me) endarterectomy.

intimitis (-mi′tis) endarteritis.

Intocostrin (in″to-kos′trin) trademark for a preparation of *Chondodendron tomentosum* extract.

intorsion (in-tor′shun) tilting of the upper part of the vertical meridian of the eye toward the midline of the face.

intoxication (in-tok″sĭ-ka′shun) a morbid state resulting from the presence of toxins, especially that resulting from ingestion of alcohol. **acid i.**, a severe form of acidosis.

intra- (in′trah) word element [L.], *inside of; within.*

intra-abdominal (in″trah-ab-dom′ĭ-nal) within the abdomen.

intra-arterial (-ar-te′re-al) within an artery.

intra-articular (-ar-tik′u-lar) within a joint.

intracapsular (-kap′su-lar) within a capsule.

intracartilaginous (-kar″tĭ-laj′ĭ-nus) within a cartilage.

intracellular (-sel′u-lar) within a cell or cells.

intracervical (-ser′vĭ-kal) within the canal of the cervix uteri.

intracranial (-kra′ne-al) within the cranium.

intracutaneous (in″trah-ku-ta′ne-us) within the substance of the skin.

intracystic (-sis′tik) within the bladder or a cyst.

intrad (in′trad) inwardly.

intradermal (in″trah-der′mal) within the substance of the skin.

intraduodenal (-du″o-de′nal) within the duodenum.

intradural (-du′ral) within the dura mater.

intraerythrocytic (-ĕ-rith″ro-sit′ik) occurring or situated inside red blood cells (erythrocytes).

intrafebrile (-feb′ril) occurring in the febrile stage.

intragastric (-gas′trik) within the stomach.

intragenic (-jen′ik) within a gene.

intraictal (-ik′tal) occurring during an attack or seizure.

intralesional (-le′zhun-al) within a localized lesion.

intralocular (-lok′u-lar) within the loculi of a structure.

intralumbar (-lum′bar) within the lumbar portion of the spinal cord.

intraluminal (-lu″mĭ-nal) within the lumen of a tubular structure.

intramastoiditis (-mas″toi-di′tis) inflammation of the antrum and cells of the mastoid process.

intramural (-mu′ral) within the walls of an organ.

intramuscular (-mus′ku-lar) within the muscular substance.

intraocular (-ok′u-lar) within the eye.

intraoperative (-op′er-a″tiv) performed or occurring during a surgical operation.

intraparietal (-pah-ri′ĕ-tal) in the substance of a wall.

intrapartum (-par′tum) occurring during childbirth or during delivery.

intraperitoneal (-per″ĭ-to-ne′al) within the peritoneal sac.

intrapleural (-ploo′ral) within the pleura.

intrapolar (-po′lar) within the space between two poles.

intrapsychic (-si′kik) taking place within the mind.

intrapulmonary (-pul′mo-ner″e) within the substance of the lung.

intraspinal (-spi′nal) within the substance of the spinal cord.

intrathoracic (-tho-ras′ik) within the thorax.

intratracheal (-tra′ke-al) endotracheal.

intratympanic (-tim-pan′ik) within the tympanic cavity.

intrauterine (-u′ter-in) within the uterus.

intravasation (in-trav″ah-sa′shun) entrance of abnormal material into vessels.

intravenous (in″trah-ve′nus) within a vein.

intraventricular (-ven-trik′u-lar) within a ventricle.

intravital (-vi′tal) occurring during life.

intra vitam (in′trah vi′tam) [L.] during life.

intrinsic (in-trin′sik) of internal origin; innate.

introitus (in-tro′ĭ-tus), pl. *intro′itus* [L.] the entrance to a cavity or space.

introjection (in″tro-jek′shun) mental identification with another person or object.

intromission (in″tro-mish′un) the entrance of one part or object into another.

introspection (-spek′shun) contemplation or observation of one's own thoughts and feelings; self-analysis.

introsusception (-sŭ-sep′shun) intussusception.

introversion (-ver′zhun) 1. a turning inside out. 2. direction of one's energy and interests toward one's self and the inner world of experience.

introvert (in′tro-vert) a person whose interests are turned inward upon himself.

intubation (in″tu-ba′shun) the insertion of a tube, as into the larynx. **endotracheal i.,** insertion of a tube through the trachea to assure a clear airway and prevent entrance of foreign material into the tracheobronchial tree. **nasal i.,** insertion of a tube into the respiratory or gastrointestinal tract through the nose. **oral i.,** insertion of a tube into the respiratory or gastrointestinal tract through the mouth.

intuition (in″tu-ish′un) instinctual knowledge; awareness not gained through the use of conscious reasoning.

intumescence (in″tu-mes′ens) a normal or abnormal enlargement or swelling, such as the enlargement of the spinal cord in the cervical or lumbar region. adj., **intumes′cent.**

intumescentia (in-tu″mĕ-sen′she-ah) intumescence.

intussusception (in″tŭ-sŭ-sep′shun) the invagination of a portion of intestine into an adjacent portion.

intussusceptum (-sep′tum) a portion of intestine which has telescoped into another part.

intussuscipiens (-sip′e-ens) the portion of the intestine containing the intussusceptum.

inulin (in′u-lin) a starchlike substance found in many plants, which on hydrolysis yields fructose and a small amount of glucose.

inunction (in-unk′shun) 1. the rubbing of the skin with an ointment. 2. an ointment to be applied to the skin.

in utero (in u′ter-o) [L.] in the uterus; before delivery or birth.

invagination (in-vaj″ĭ-na′shun) the telescoping of an organ in the manner of a pouch.

Inversine (-ver′sēn) trademark for a preparation of mecamylamine.

inversion (-ver′zhun) 1. a turning inward, or other reversal of normal relationship of a part. 2. in genetics, the reunion of the middle segment in reverse position after breakage of a chromosome at two points. **carbohydrate i.,** hydrolysis of the complex carbohydrates to simple sugars. **sexual i.,** homosexuality. **i. of uterus,** a turning of the uterus inside out or upside down. **visceral i.,** the more or less complete right and left transposition of the viscera.

invert (in′vert) an individual who has adopted the attitudes and behavior of the opposite sex, manifested by overt homosexuality, transsexualism or transvestism.

invertase (in-ver′tās) an enzyme which converts cane sugar into invert sugar.

invertebrate (-ver′tĕ-brāt) 1. having no spinal

column. 2. an animal organism which has no spinal column.

invertin (in-ver'tin) invertase.

investment (-vest'ment) material in which a denture, tooth, crown or model for a dental restoration is enclosed for curing, soldering or casting, or the process of such enclosure.

inveterate (-vet'er-āt) confirmed and chronic; difficult to cure.

in vitro (in vit'ro) [L.] in glass; referring to studies performed on tissues removed from the living organism under artificial conditions in the laboratory.

in vivo (in vi'vo) [L.] in life; referring to studies performed on tissues not removed from the living organism.

involucrum (in"vo-lu'krum), pl. *involu'cra* [L.] a covering or sheath, as of a sequestrum.

involution (-lu'shun) 1. a rolling or turning inward. 2. retrograde change of the entire body or in a particular organ, as the retrogression of the uterus after expulsion of the fetus.

Io chemical symbol, *ionium.*

Iodamoeba (i-o"dah-me'bah) a genus of amebas, including *I. buetschlii*, parasitic in man, and *I. suis*, found in pigs.

iodate (i'o-dāt) a salt of iodic acid.

iodide (i'o-dīd) a binary compound of iodine.

iodination (i"o-din-a'shun) the incorporation or addition of iodine in a compound.

iodine (i'o-dīn) chemical elements *(see table)*, at. no. 53, symbol I. **protein-bound i.**, iodine firmly bound to protein in the body serum, determination of which constitutes one test of thyroid function.

iodinophilous (i"o-din-of'i-lus) easily stainable with iodine.

iodipamide (i"o-dip'ah-mīd) a compound used as a radiopaque medium in cholecystography.

iodism (i'o-dizm) ill health due to injudicious use of the iodides.

iodobrassid (i-o"do-bras'sid) a compound used in iodide therapy and as a radiopaque medium.

iodochlorhydroxyquin (i"o-do-klōr"hi-drok'se-kwin) a spongy, brownish yellow powder, containing 40–41.5 per cent of iodine and 11.9–12.2 per cent of chlorine; antiprotozoan and local anti-infective.

iododerma (-der'mah) skin eruption from use of iodides.

iodoform (i-o'do-form) a greenish yellow powder or lustrous crystals, CHI₃, local antibacterial.

iodoglobulin (i"o-do-glob'u-lin) a principle derived from the thyroid gland.

iodomethamate (i-o"do-meth'ah-māt) an acid compound used as a radiopaque medium for urography.

iodophilia (i"o-do-fil'e-ah) a condition in which potassium iodide staining produces brown discoloration of particles in the leukocytes.

iodophthalein (-thal'e-in) an iodine-containing compound. **i. sodium**, an odorless, blue-violet, crystalline powder with an astringent, saline taste; used as a radiopaque medium in cholecystography. **soluble i.**, iodophthalein sodium.

iodopyracet (i-o"do-pi'rah-set) a compound

used as a radiopaque medium for urography.

iodotherapy (i"o-do-ther'ah-pe) use of iodine and iodides as remedies.

iodoxyl (i"o-dok'sil) sodium iodomethamate.

iodum (i-o'dum) [L.] iodine.

ion (i'on) an atom or group of atoms carrying an electric charge and forming one of the elements of an electrolyte. **hydrogen i.**, the positively charged hydrogen atom (H⁺), which is the positive ion of all acids. **hydroxyl i.**, the negatively charged group, OH⁻, present to excess in alkaline solutions.

ionium (i-o'ne-um) a radioactive isotope of thorium, which is transformed into radium; symbol, Io.

ionization (i"on-i-za'shun) the breaking up of molecules into their component ions.

ionogen (i-on'o-jen) a substance which may be ionized. adj., **ionogen'ic.**

ionometer (i"o-nom'ē-ter) an instrument for measuring the intensity or quantity of roentgen rays.

ionotherapy (i"o-no-ther'ah-pe) iontophoresis.

iontophoresis (i-on"to-fo-re'sis) the introduction of ions into the body for therapeutic purposes.

iontotherapy (-ther'ah-pe) 1. iontophoresis. 2. treatment with violet rays.

iophendylate (i"o-fen'dī-lāt) a compound used as a radiopaque medium for roentgenography of the spine and of the biliary tract.

iophobia (-fo'be-ah) morbid fear of poisons.

iothiouracil (-thi"o-u'rah-sil) a compound used in preparation for thyroidectomy and in treatment of hyperthyroidism.

I.P. International Pharmacopoeia, a publication of the World Health Organization, presenting a uniform terminology and establishing uniform standards of strength and composition of drugs.

I.P.A.A. International Psychoanalytical Association.

ipecac (ip'ē-kak) the dried rhizome and roots of *Cephaelis ipecacuanha* or *Cephaelis acuminata*; used as an emetic or expectorant.

ipomea (i"po me'ah) the dried root of *Ipomaea orizabensis*; used as a cathartic.

IPPB intermittent positive-pressure breathing.

Ipral (ip'ral) trademark for preparations of probarbital.

iproniazid (i"pro-ni'ah-zid) a compound used as a psychic energizer, antituberculotic and antihypertensive.

ipsi- (ip'se) word element [L.], *same; self.*

ipsilateral (ip"sī-lat'er-al) pertaining to or situated on the same side.

I.Q. intelligence quotient.

Ir chemical symbol, *iridium.*

Ircon (ir'kon) trademark for a preparation of ferrous fumarate.

iridal (i'rĭ-dal) pertaining to the iris.

iridalgia (i"rī-dal'je-ah) pain in the iris.

iridauxesis (ir"id-awk-se'sis) thickening of the iris.

iridectasis (ir"ī-dek'tah-sis) dilatation of the iris, or pupil of the eye.

iridectomesodialysis (ir"ī-dek"to-me"so-di-al'-ī-sis) excision and separation of adhesions around the inner edge of the iris to form an artificial pupil.

iridectomize (ir″ĭ-dek′to-mīz) to subject to iridectomy.

iridectomy (-dek′to-me) excision of part of the iris.

iridectopia (ir″id-ek-to′pe-ah) displacement of the iris of the eye.

iridemia (ir″ĭ-de′me-ah) hemorrhage from the iris.

iridencleisis (ir″ĭ-den-kli′sis) strangulation of a slip of the iris in a corneal incision.

irideremia (ir″ĭ-der-e′me-ah) absence of the iris.

iridesis (i-rĭd′ĕ-sis) formation of artificial iris.

iridic (i-rid′ik) pertaining to the iris.

iridium (ĭ-rid′e-um, i-rid′e-um) chemical element (*see table*), at. no. 77, symbol Ir.

irido-avulsion (ir″ĭ-do-ah-vul′shun) tearing away of the iris.

iridocapsulitis (-kap″su-li′tis) inflammation of iris and lens capsule.

iridocele (i-rid′o-sēl) hernial protrusion of a slip of the iris.

iridochoroiditis (ir″ĭ-do-ko″roi-di′tis) inflammation of iris and choroid.

iridocoloboma (-kol″o-bo′mah) fissure of the iris.

iridoconstrictor (-kon-strik′tor) a muscle element or an agent which acts to constrict the pupil of the eye.

iridocyclectomy (-si-klek′to-me) excision of iris and ciliary body.

iridocyclitis (-si-kli′tis) inflammation of the iris and ciliary body. **recurrent i.,** periodic ophthalmia.

iridocyclochoroiditis (-si″klo-ko″roi-di′tis) inflammation of the iris, ciliary body and choroid.

iridocystectomy (-sis-tek′to-me) a plastic operation on the iris.

iridodesis (ir″ĭ-dod′ĕ-sis) formation of artificial pupil by ligating the iris.

iridodialysis (ir″ĭ-do-di-al′ĭ-sis) separation or loosening of the iris from its attachments, as in the surgical creation of a new pupil (coredialysis).

iridodilator (-di-la′tor) a muscle element or an agent which acts to dilate the pupil of the eye.

iridodonesis (-do-ne′sis) hippus.

iridokeratitis (-ker″ah-ti′tis) inflammation of iris and cornea.

iridokinesis (-ki-ne′sis) contraction and expansion of the iris.

iridoleptynsis (-lep-tin′sis) thinning of the iris.

iridology (ir″ĭ-dol′o-je) the study of the iris as associated with disease.

iridolysis (-dol′ĭ-sis) surgical release of adhesions from the iris.

iridomalacia (-mah-la′she-ah) softening of the iris.

iridomesodialysis (-me″so-di-al′ĭ-sis) loosening of adhesions around the inner edge of the iris.

iridomotor (-mo′tor) pertaining to movements of the iris.

iridoncus (ir″ĭ-dong′kus) tumor of the iris.

iridoparalysis (ir″ĭ-do-pah-ral′ĭ-sis) paralysis of the pupil.

iridoperiphakitis (-per″ĭ-fah-ki′tis) inflammation of the lens capsule.

iridoplegia (-ple′je-ah) paralysis of the pupil.

iridoptosis (ir″ĭ-dop-to′sis) prolapse of the iris.

iridorhexis (ir″ĭ-do-rek′sis) 1. rupture of iris. 2. tearing away of iris.

iridosclerotomy (-skle-rot′o-me) puncture of the sclera and of the edge of the iris.

iridosteresis (-stē-re′sis) removal of all or part of the iris.

iridotasis (ir″ĭ-dot′ah-sis) stretching of the iris for glaucoma.

iridotomy (-dot′o-me) incision of the iris.

I.R.I.S. International Research Information Service.

iris (i′ris) the circular pigmented membrane behind the cornea, perforated by the pupil.

iritis (i-ri′tis) inflammation of the iris. adj., **irit′ic.**

iritoectomy (ir″ĭ-to-ek′to-me) excision of part of the iris.

iritomy (i-rit′o-me) iridotomy.

irium (ir′e-um) sodium lauryl sulfate.

iron (i′ern) chemical element (*see table*), at. no. 26, symbol Fe. **i. choline citrate,** ferrocholinate. **i. gluconate,** ferrous gluconate. **i. protosulfate,** ferrous sulfate. **reduced i.,** grayish black powder produced by action of hydrogen upon ferric oxide.

Ironate (i′ron-āt) trademark for a preparation of ferrous sulfate.

Irosul (i′ro-sul) trademark for preparations of ferrous sulfate.

irotomy (i-rot′o-me) iridotomy.

irradiate (ĭ-ra′de-āt) to treat with radiant energy.

irradiation (ĭ-ra″de-a′shun) application of radiant energy (heat, light, roentgen ray, radium) for therapeutic or diagnostic purposes.

irrespirable (ir″e-spīr′ah-bl) not to be breathed with safety.

irrigation (ir″ĭ-ga′shun) washing of a body cavity or wound by a stream of water or other solution.

irritability (ir″ĭ-tah-bil′ĭ-te) 1. ability of an organism or a specific tissue to react to the environment. 2. the state of being overexcitable or unduly sensitive. **faradic i.,** condition in which a faradic current will produce a muscular response. **galvanic i.,** condition in which a galvanic current will cause a muscular response. **muscular i.,** the normal contractile quality of muscle. **nervous i.,** the ability of a nerve to transmit impulses. **tactile i.,** responsiveness to stimulation arising from touching an object.

irritable (ir′ĭ-tah-bl) 1. capable of reacting to a stimulus. 2. abnormally sensitive to stimuli.

irritant (ir′ĭ-tant) 1. causing irritation. 2. an agent causing irritation.

irritation (ir″ĭ-ta′shun) 1. the act of stimulating. 2. a state of overexcitation and undue sensitiveness. adj., **ir′ritative.**

I.S.A. Instrument Society of America.

ischemia (is-ke′me-ah) deficiency of blood in a part, due to functional constriction or actual obstruction of a blood vessel. adj., **ische′mic**.
myocardial i., deficiency of blood supply to the heart muscle, due to obstruction or constriction of the coronary arteries.

ischi(o)- (is′ke-o) word element [Gr.], *ischium*.

ischiadic (is″ke-ad′ik) ischiatic.

ischial (is′ke-al) ischiatic.

ischiatic (is″ke-at′ik) pertaining to the ischium.

ischidrosis (is″ki-dro′sis) suppression of secretion of sweat.

ischiobulbar (is″ke-o-bul′bar) pertaining to ischium and bulb of urethra.

ischiocele (is′ke-o-sēl″) hernia at the sacrosciatic notch.

ischiodidymus (is″ke-o-did′ĭ-mus) conjoined twins united at the pelvis.

ischiodymia (-dim′e-ah) the condition seen in an ischiodidymus.

ischiodynia (-din′e-ah) pain in the ischium.

ischiofemoral (-fem′o-ral) pertaining to the ischium and femur.

ischiofibular (-fib′u-lar) pertaining to ischium and fibula.

ischiohebotomy (-he-bot′o-me) ischiopubiotomy.

ischioneuralgia (-nu-ral′je-ah) sciatica.

ischiopagus (is″ke-op′ah-gus) a twin fetal monster united at the pelvis, the axes of the bodies forming a straight line.

ischiopubic (is″ke-o-pu′bik) pertaining to ischium and pubes.

ischiopubiotomy (-pu″be-ot′o-me) transection of the bar of bone constituting the lower margin of the obturator foramen and formed by the conjoined rami of the ischium and pubis.

ischiorectal (-rek′tal) pertaining to ischium and rectum.

ischium (is′ke-um) the posterior, heavy portion of the pelvic bone.

ischo- (is′ko) word element [Gr.], *suppression; deficiency.*

ischochymia (is″ko-ki′me-ah) suppression of gastric digestion.

ischomenia (-me′ne-ah) suppression of the menstrual flow.

ischuria (is-ku′re-ah) retention or suppression of the urine. adj., **ischuret′ic**.

I.S.C.P. International Society of Comparative Pathology.

iseikonia (is″i-ko′ne-ah) equality in size of the two retinal images. adj., **iseikon′ic**.

I.S.G.E. International Society of Gastro-Enterology.

I.S.H. International Society for Hematology.

island (i′land) an isolated mass of tissue.
blood i., a group of cells in the mesoderm of the early embryo, from which the blood vessels and blood corpuscles are later derived.
i's of Langerhans, masses in the pancreas composed of cells smaller than the ordinary cells, concerned in carbohydrate metabolism.
i. of Reil, isolated part of the cerebral cortex in the fissure of Sylvius.

islet (i′let) an island. **i's of Langerhans,** islands of Langerhans.

I.S.M. International Society of Microbiologists.

Ismelin (is′me-lin) trademark for a preparation of guanethidine.

I.S.O. International Standards Organization.

iso- (i′so) word element [Gr.], *equal.*

isoagglutinin (i″so-ah-gloo′tĭ-nin) an agglutinin acting on cells of animals of the same species as that from which it is derived.

isoamyl nitrite (-am′il ni-trīt) amyl nitrite.

isoanaphylaxis (-an″ah-fi-lak′sis) anaphylaxis produced by serum from an individual of the same species.

isoantibody (-an″tĭ-bod′e) an antibody combining with an antigen present in tissues of some, but not all, individuals of the same species as the antibody producer.

isoantigen (-an″tĭ-jen) an antigen present in tissues of some, but not all, individuals of the same species as the antibody producer; best known are the blood group antigens of man and animals.

isobar (i′so-bahr) one of several nuclides having the same number of nucleons, but different combinations of protons and neutrons, i.e. the same mass number, but different atomic numbers.

isobornyl thiocyanoacetate (i″so-bor′nil thi″o-si″ah-no-as′ĕ-tāt) a compound used as a pediculicide.

isobutanol (-bu″tah-nol″) isobutyl alcohol.

isocaloric (-kah-lo′rik) providing the same number of calories.

isocarboxazid (-kar-bok′sah-zid) a compound used as a psychic energizer and to reduce pain of angina pectoris.

isocellular (-sel′u-lar) made up of identical cells.

isochromatic (-kro-mat′ik) of the same color throughout.

isochromatophil (-kro-mat′o-fil) staining alike with the same stain.

isochromosome (-kro′mo-sōm) one whose two arms are exact duplicates, formed by division of a chromosome on a plane perpendicular to rather than parallel with its long axis, so that each resulting chromosome contains a duplication of material on one arm, but no material of the other arm of the original chromosome.

isochronic (-kron′ik) 1. passing through the same phases at the same time. 2. performed in the same period of time.

isochronous (i-sok′ro-nus) isochronic.

isocoria (i″so-ko′re-ah) equality of size of the pupils of the two eyes.

isocortex (-kor′teks) that portion of the cerebral cortex made up of layers developing between the sixth and eighth fetal months.

isocytolysin (-si-tol′ĭ-sin) a cytolysin acting on cells of animals of the same species as that from which it is derived.

isocytosis (-si-to′sis) equality in size of red blood corpuscles.

isodactylism (-dak′tĭ-lizm) relatively even length of the fingers.

isodiametric (-di″ah-met′rik) measuring the same in all diameters.

isodontic (-don′tik) having all the teeth alike.

isodose (i′so-dōs) a radiation dose of the same number of roentgens.

isoelectric (i″so-e-lek′trik) showing no variation of electric potential.

isoenergetic (-en″er-jet′ik) exhibiting equal energy.

isoenzyme (-en′zīm) one of the many forms of a protein catalyst, differing chemically, physically and/or immunologically.

isoflurophate (-floo′ro-fāt) a compound used as an anticholinesterase inhibitor and as a miotic in glaucoma.

isogamety (-gam′ē-te) production by an individual of one sex of gametes identical with respect to the sex chromosome. adj., **isogamet′ic.**

isogamy (i-sog′ah-me) the conjugation of gametes identical in size and structure to form the zygote from which the new organism develops. adj., **isog′amous.**

isogeneic (i″so-jĕ-ne′ik) having the same genetic constitution.

isogeneric (-jĕ-ner′ik) of the same kind; belonging to the same species.

isogenesis (-jen′ē-sis) identity in development.

isograft (i′so-graft) a graft of tissue from a donor of the same genotype as the recipient.

isohemagglutination (i″so-hem″ah-gloo″tī-na′shun) agglutination of erythrocytes of one individual when mixed with normal serum of another individual of the same species and incubated at body temperature.

isohemagglutinin (-hem″ah-gloo′tĭ-nin) an agglutinin capable of agglutinating the erythrocytes of other individuals of the same species as that in which it is found.

isohemolysin (-he-mol′ĭ-sin) a hemolysin acting on the blood of animals of the same species as that from which it is derived.

isohemolysis (-he-mol′ĭ-sis) hemolysis produced by serum from an animal of the same species.

isohypercytosis (-hi″per-si-to′sis) increase of leukocytes with normal proportions of neutrophil cells.

isohypocytosis (-hi″po-si-to′sis) decrease of leukocytes with normal proportion of neutrophil cells.

isoimmunization (-im″u-ni-za′shun) development of antibodies in response to antigens from individuals of the same species.

isolate (i′so-lāt) 1. to separate from others, or set apart. 2. a group of individuals prevented by geographic, genetic, ecologic or social barriers from interbreeding with others of their kind.

isolateral (i″so-lat′er-al) 1. equilateral. 2. ipsilateral.

isolation (-la′shun) the act of separating or setting apart, or state of being set apart, e.g. the segregation of patients with a communicable disease or, in psychology, failure to connect behavior with its motives, or contradictory attitudes and behavior with each other.

isoleucine (-lu′sēn) a naturally occurring amino acid, one of those essential for human metabolism.

isologous (i-sol′o-gus) characterized by an identical genotype.

isolysis (i-sol′ĭ-sis) isohemolysis. adj., **isolyt′-ic.**

isomer (i′so-mer) one of two or more nuclides having the same mass number and atomic number, but existing in the excited state with a higher energy and other properties differing from those of the ground state nuclide.

isomerase (i-som′er-ās) an enzyme that catalyzes the process of isomerization, such as the interconversion of aldoses and ketoses.

isomerism (i-som′ē-rizm) the existence of two or more compounds (isomers) having the same number and kinds of atoms in the molecule, and the same molecular weight, but differing in other characteristics. **geometric i.,** a type of stereoisomerism in which no compound is optically active. **optical i.,** a type of stereoisomerism determined by the effect on polarized light. **structural i.,** isomerism in which the difference results from the different order in which the atoms are attached to each other, such as different skeletal linkages (skeletal isomers), a different position of another element or group (position isomers) or even greater differences, giving rise to different functional groups (functional isomers).

isometheptene (i″so-meth′ep-tēn) a compound used as a sympathomimetic and antispasmodic.

isometric (-met′rik) maintaining, or pertaining to, the same measure or length.

isometropia (-mĕ-tro′pe-ah) equality in refraction of the two eyes.

isomorphism (-mor′fizm) identity in form; in genetics, referring to genotypes of polyploid organisms which produce similar gametes even though containing genes in different combinations on homologous chromosomes. adj., **isomor′phous.**

isoniazid (-ni′ah-zid) an antibacterial compound used in treatment of tuberculosis.

isonicotinoylhydrazine (-nik″o-tin″o-il-hi′-drah-zēn) isoniazid.

isopathy (i-sop′ah-the) treatment by administering the agent producing the disease.

isopepsin (i″so-pep′sin) pepsin changed by heat.

isophoria (-fo′re-ah) correspondence of the visual axes of the two eyes.

Isophrine (i′so-frin) trademark for a preparation of phenylephrine.

isoplastic (i′so-plas″tik) taken from an animal of the same species.

isoprecipitin (i″so-pre-sip′ĭ-tin) a precipitin acting on serum of animals of the same species as that from which it is derived.

isopregnenone (-preg′ne-nōn) a compound used as a progestational agent and as a test of pregnancy.

isoprenaline (-pren′ah-lēn) isoproterenol.

isopropamide (-pro′pah-mīd) a compound used in parasympathetic blockade and as an antispasmodic.

isopropanol (-pro′pah-nol) isopropyl alcohol.

isopropyl meprobamate (-pro′pil mep″ro-bam′āt) carisoprodol.

isoproterenol (-pro″tĕ-re′nol) an odorless,

white, crystalline powder used as a sympathomimetic, cardiac stimulant and antispasmodic, and in relief of bronchospasm.

isopter (i-sop'ter) a curve representing areas of equal visual acuity in the field of vision.

isopyknosis (i"so-pik-no'sis) 1. the quality of showing uniform density throughout. 2. uniformity of condensation observed in comparison of different chromosomes or in different areas of the same chromosome. adj., **isopyknot'ic.**

Isordil (i'sor-dil) trademark for preparations of isosorbide dinitrate.

isorrhea (i"so-re'ah) a steady equilibrium between the intake and output, by the body, of water and/or solutes. adj , **isorrhe'ic.**

isosexual (-sek'su-al) pertaining to or characteristic of the same sex.

isosmotic (i"sos-mot'ik) having the same osmotic pressure.

isosorbide dinitrate (i"so-sor'bīd di-ni'trāt) a compound used in treatment of coronary insufficiency.

Isospora (i-sos'po-rah) a genus of sporozoan parasites found in birds, amphibians, reptiles and various mammals, including man.

isospore (i'so-spōr) a spore that develops directly into an adult.

isosthenuria (i"sos-thē-nu're-ah) maintenance of a constant osmolality of the urine, regardless of changes in osmotic pressure of the blood.

isostimulation (i"so-stim"u-la'shun) stimulation of an animal with antigenic material from other animals of the same species.

isotherapy (-ther'ah-pe) isopathy

isotherm (i'so-therm) a line on a map or chart depicting the boundaries of an area in which the temperature is the same.

isothermal (i"so-ther'mal) having the same temperature.

isothiazine (-thi'ah-zēn) ethopropazine.

isothipendyl (-thi'pen-dil) a compound used as an antihistaminic.

isotone (i'so-tōn) one of several nuclides having the same number of neutrons, but differing in number of protons in their nuclei.

isotonic (i"so-ton'ik) of the same tonicity or strength; of a solution, having the same concentration as the solution of reference.

isotope (i'so-tōp) a chemical element having the same atomic number as another (i.e. the same number of nuclear protons), but having a different atomic mass (i.e. a different number of nuclear neutrons); now usually indicated by the conventional chemical symbol with the atomic mass number in the left superscript position. **radioactive i.,** one transmuted into another element with emission of corpuscular or radiomagnetic radiations. **stable i.,** one that does not transmute into another element with emission of corpuscular or electromagnetic radiations.

isotopology (i"so-to-pol'o-je) the scientific study of isotopes and of their uses and applications.

isotropic (-trop'ik) transmitting light equally in all directions.

isotropy (i-sot'ro-pe) the quality or condition of being isotropic. ˚

isotypical (i"so-tip'e-kal) belonging to the same type.

isoxsuprine (i-sok'su-prēn) a compound proposed as a vasodilator and uterine relaxant.

isozyme (i'so-zīm) isoenzyme.

issue (ish'ū) a suppurating sore, made and kept open by inserting an irritant substance.

isthmectomy (is-mek'to-me) excision of an isthmus, especially of the isthmus of the thyroid.

isthmitis (is-mi'tis) inflammation of isthmus faucium.

isthmoparalysis (is"mo-pah-ral'ĭ-sis) isthmoplegia.

isthmoplegia (-ple'je-ah) paralysis of the isthmus faucium.

isthmospasm (is'mo-spazm) spasm of an isthmus.

isthmus (is'mus) a narrow strip of tissue or narrow passage connecting two larger parts. adj., **isth'mian. i. of eustachian tube,** the narrowest part of the eustachian tube. **i. fau'cium,** the passage between the mouth and fauces. **i. rhombenceph'ali,** that part of the embryonic hindbrain comprising the anterior medullary velum, the superior cerebellar peduncles and uppermost part of the fourth ventricle. **i. of thyroid,** the band of tissue joining the lobes of the thyroid. **i. of uterine tube,** the narrower, thicker-walled portion of the uterine tube closest to the uterus.

I.S.U. International Society of Urology.

Isuprel (i'su-prel) trademark for a preparation of isoproterenol.

isuria (i-su're-ah) excretion of urine at a uniform rate.

I.T.A. International Tuberculosis Association.

itch (ich) 1. a skin disease attended with itching. 2. scabies. **Aujesky's i.,** mad itch. **bakers' i.,** eczema of the hands from irritation by yeast. **barbers' i.,** tinea barbae. **barley i.,** grain itch. **cow-lot i., dew i.,** ground itch. **dhobie i.,** a contact dermatitis in India, caused by marking fluid used by native washermen (dhobie). **foot i.,** ground itch. **grain i.,** itching dermatitis due to a mite parasitic on various plants, which bites human beings who come in close contact with the host plants. **grocers' i.,** an eczema of the hands said to be sometimes due to a sugar mite. **ground i.,** an itching eruption caused by the presence of larval forms of Uncinaria. **mad i.,** a disease of cattle due to a filterable virus, and marked by severe pruritus, convulsions and coma; called also *bovine pseudorabies*. **mattress i., millers' i.,** grain itch. **miners' i.,** ground itch. **Moeller's i., Norway i.,** an itch caused by a species of Sarcoptes parasitic on wolves. **seven-year i.,** scabies. **straw i.,** grain itch. **swamp i.,** ground itch. **swimmers' i., water i.,** schistosome dermatitis. **washerman's i.,** dhobie itch. **winter i.,** pruritus hiemalis.

itching (ich'ing) a teasing irritation of the skin, arousing the desire to scratch.

iter (i'ter) a tubular passage. adj., **i'teral. i. ad infundib'ulum,** the passage from the third ventricle to the infundibulum (1). **i. a ter'tio ad quar'tum ventric'ulum,** aqueduct of Sylvius. **i. den'tium,** the passage through which a permanent tooth erupts through the gums.

iteroparity (it″er-o-par'ĭ-te) the state, in an individual organism, of reproducing repeatedly, or more than once in a lifetime. adj., **iterop'arous.**

-itides (it'ĭ-dēz) plural of *-itis.*

-itis (i'tis) word element, *inflammation.*

ITP idiopathic thrombocytopenic purpura.

Itrumil (it'roo-mil) trademark for a preparation of iothiouracil.

I.U. immunizing unit; International unit.

IUCD intrauterine contraceptive device.

IUD intrauterine contraceptive device.

I.V. intravenously.

I.V.T. intravenous transfusion.

Ixodes (ik-so'dēz) a genus of arthropods (family Ixodidae).

ixodiasis (ik″so-di'ah-sis) fever caused by bites of ticks of the genus Ixodes.

ixodic (ik-sod'ik) pertaining to, or caused by, ticks.

Ixodidae (ik-sod'ĭ-de) a family of arthropods (class Arachnoidea, order Acarina, suborder Ixodides), including the hard-bodied ticks.

Ixodides (ik-sod'i-dēz) a suborder of arthropods (class Arachnoidea, order Acarina), including the ticks.

J

J symbol, *Joule's equivalent.*

jacket (jak'et) an encasement or covering for the thorax. **plaster-of-Paris j.,** a casing of plaster of Paris enveloping the body, for the purpose of giving support or correcting deformities. **Sayre's j.,** a plaster-of-Paris jacket used as a support for the vertebral column. **strait j.,** a contrivance for restraining the arms of a violently disturbed person.

jackscrew (jak'skroo) a device for expanding the arch in regulating teeth.

jactitation (jak″tĭ-ta'shun) restless tossing to and fro in acute illness.

janiceps (jan'ĭ-seps) a fetal monster with one head and two opposite faces.

jaundice (jawn'dis) yellowness of skin and eyes from bile pigments. **acathectic j.,** jaundice from pathologic changes in the liver cells, which become unable to retain their secretion. **acholuric familial j.,** hemolytic jaundice. **acute febrile j., acute infectious j., catarrhal j.,** infectious hepatitis. **hematogenous j., hemolytic j.,** a rare, chronic and generally hereditary disease with periods of excessive hemolysis, splenic enlargement and jaundice. **hemorrhagic j.,** leptospiral jaundice. **hepatogenous j.,** a form caused by obstruction of the bile ducts. **homologous serum j.,** jaundice resulting from injection of human serum. **infective j.,** infectious hepatitis; leptospiral jaundice. **leptospiral j.,** an acute infectious disease with nephritis, jaundice, fever, muscular pain and enlargement of liver and spleen. **malignant j.,** acute yellow atrophy of the liver. **mechanical j.,** obstructive jaundice. **j. of the newborn,** icterus neonatorum. **obstructive j.,** jaundice due to blocking of the bile flow. **retention j.,** obstructive jaundice. **spirochetal j.,** leptospiral jaundice.

jaw (jaw) one of the two opposing rigid structures of the mouth of animals, for seizing prey, for biting or for masticating food. **lumpy j.,** actinomycosis. **rubber j.,** a softened condition of the jaw in animals, due to resorption and replacement of the bone by fibrous tissue, occurring in association with renal osteodystrophy.

jaw-winking (jaw-wingk'ing) elevation of a congenitally ptotic eyelid when the mouth is opened, giving the appearance of constant winking.

jejunectomy (je″joo-nek'to-me) excision of the jejunum.

jejunitis (-ni'tis) inflammation of the jejunum.

jejunocecostomy (je-joo″no-se-kos'to-me) anastomosis of the jejunum to the cecum.

jejunocolostomy (-ko-los'to-me) anastomosis of the jejunum to the colon.

jejunoileitis (-il″e-i'tis) inflammation of jejunum and ileum.

jejunoileostomy (-il'e-os'to-me) anastomosis of the jejunum to the ileum.

jejunojejunostomy (-je″joo-nos'to-me) surgical creation of an anastomosis between two portions of the jejunum.

jejunorrhaphy (je″joo-nor'ah-fe) suture of the jejunum.

jejunostomy (-nos'to-me) fistulization of the jejunum.

jejunotomy (-not'o-me) incision of the jejunum.

jejunum (je-joo'num) second portion of small intestine, between the duodenum and the ileum. adj., **jeju'nal.**

jelly (jel'e) an elastic, homogeneous mass. **cardiac j.,** a jelly present between the endothelium and myocardium of the embryonic heart that transforms into the connective tissue of the endocardium. **contraceptive j.,** a nongreasy jelly used in the vagina for prevention of conception. **enamel j.,** the soft material from which dental enamel is developed. **Wharton's j.,** the substance of the umbilical cord.

jennerian (jĕ-ne're-an) relating to Edward Jenner, who developed vaccination.

jerk (jerk) a spasmodic muscular movement. **ankle j.,** ankle clonus. **biceps j.,** biceps reflex.

elbow j., involuntary flexion of the elbow on striking the tendon of the biceps or triceps muscle. **jaw j.,** jaw reflex. **knee j.,** quadriceps reflex. **tendon j.,** tendon reaction. **triceps surae j.,** a twitchlike contraction of the triceps surae muscle elicited by sharply tapping the muscle or the Achilles tendon.

joint (joint) the site of junction or union between two or more bones, especially one that admits of motion of one or more of the components. **amphidiarthrodial j.,** anphidiarthrosis. **arthrodial j.,** plane joint. **ball-and-socket j.,** one in which the rounded head of one bone fits in a cup-shaped depression in another. **biaxial j.,** one with two chief axes of movement, at right angles to each other. **bilocular j.,** one which has two cavities. **Brodie's j.,** hysteric joint. **cartilaginous j.,** one in which the bones are united by cartilage. **Charcot's j.,** neurogenic arthropathy. **Chopart's j.,** the union of the os calcis and astragalus with the remaining bones of the tarsus. **cochlear j.,** a form of hinge joint which permits of some lateral motion. **composite j., compound j.,** one in which several bones articulate. **condyloid j.,** a ball-and-socket joint in which rotation around a vertical axis is prevented. **diarthrodial j.,** a special form of articulation permitting more or less free movement. **ellipsoid j.,** one of the ball-and-socket type, the articular surfaces being ellipsoidal instead of spheroidal. **enarthrodial j.,** spheroidal joint. **false j.,** a site of abnormal mobility between segments of bone that should be in rigid continuity. **fibrocartilaginous j.,** one in which the participating elements are united by fibrocartilage, usually separated from the bones by thin plates of hyaline cartilage; called also *symphysis* and *secondary cartilaginous joint.* **fibrous j.,** one between bones which have arisen in membrane or have been preceded by cartilaginous models, and in which the primitive membranous connection has persisted. **flail j.,** an unusually mobile joint. **ginglymoid j.,** ginglymus. **gliding j.,** plane joint. **hinge j.,** ginglymus. **hip j.,** the articulation of the femur and pelvis. **hysteric j.,** a condition that resembles arthritis, but is of psychic origin. **immovable j.,** synarthrosis. **intercarpal j's,** articulations between the carpal bones in relation to each other. **irritable j.,** one which is subject to attacks of inflammation without known cause. **knee j.,** the compound joint between the femur, patella and tibia. **Lisfranc's j.,** the articulation between the tarsal and metatarsal bones. **mixed j.,** one combining features of different types of joints. **multiaxial j.,** one permitting movement in each of the assumed three mutually perpendicular axes, or having three degrees of freedom. **pivot j.,** one allowing motion around a vertical axis, a cylindrical surface articulating with a ring of bone and tendon. **plane j.,** a type of synovial joint in which the opposed surfaces are flat or only slightly curved. **polyaxial j.,** multiaxial joint. **rotary j.,** pivot joint. **saddle j.,** one having two saddle-shaped surfaces at right angles to each other. **simple j.,** the articulation between two bones. **spheroidal j.,** a type of synovial joint in which a spheroidal surface on one bone ("ball") moves within a concavity ("socket") on the other bone. **spiral j.,** cochlear joint. **stifle j.,** the articulation in quadrupeds corresponding with the knee joint of man, consisting of two joints, that between the femur and tibia and that between the femur and patella. **synarthrodial j.,** synarthrosis. **synovial j.,** a special form of articulation permitting more or less free movement. **trochoid j.,** pivot joint. **uniaxial j.,** one which moves on one axis only. **unilocular j.,** one having only one cavity.

joule (jōol) the M.K.S. unit of work energy, i.e. the work done in moving a body a distance of 1 meter against a force of 1 newton, or the energy expended by a current of 1 ampere flowing for 1 second through a resistance of 1 ohm.

jugal (joo′gal) pertaining to the cheek or cheek bone.

jugale (joo-ga′le) the point at the angle of the zygomatic bone.

jugged (jugd) having glanderous swellings; said of a horse.

jugular (jug′u-lar) pertaining to the neck.

jugum (joo′gum), pl. *ju′ga* [L.] a depression or ridge connecting two structures. **j. pe′nis,** a forceps for compressing the penis.

juice (joos) any fluid from animal or plant tissue. **cherry j.,** fluid expressed from fresh ripe fruit of *Prunus cerasus,* used in preparing flavored vehicles for medicinal agents. **gastric j.,** the secretion of glands in the wall of the stomach. **intestinal j.,** the liquid secretion of glands in the intestinal lining. **pancreatic j.,** enzyme-containing fluid secreted by the pancreas and conducted through its ducts to the duodenum. **raspberry j.,** fluid expressed from fresh ripe fruit of *Rubus idaeus* or *R. strigosus,* used as a flavoring agent.

jumping (jump′ing) Gilles de la Tourette's disease.

junction (junk′shun) the place of meeting or coming together. adj., **junc′tional. amelodentinal j.,** dentinoenamel junction **dentinocemental j.,** the line of meeting of the dentin and cementum. **dentinoenamel j.,** the plane of meeting between dentin and enamel on the crown of a tooth. **mucogingival j.,** the scalloped line marking the separation of the gingiva from the oral mucosa overlying the dental alveoli. **myoneural j.,** the site of termination of an efferent neuron on a muscle fiber. **sclerocorneal j.,** the line of union of sclera and cornea.

junctura (junk-tu′rah), pl. *junctu′rae* [L.] a junction or joint.

jurisprudence (joor″is-proo′dens) the science of the law. **medical j.,** the science of the law as applied to the practice of medicine.

jury-mast (joor′e mast) upright bar used in supporting the head in cases of Pott's disease.

juvantia (joo-van'she-ah) adjuvant and palliative medicines.

juvenile (ju'vĕ-nīl) a young organism or individual of adult form, having passed through the various developmental (larval) stages.

juxta-articular (juks"tah-ar-tik'u-lar) in the region of a joint.

juxtapyloric (-pi-lor'ik) near the pylorus.

juxtaspinal (-spi'nal) near the spinal column.

K

K chemical symbol, *potassium* (L. *kalium*).

K. cathode; electrostatic capacity.

Ka *(Kathode)* cathode.

kainophobia (ki"no-fo'be-ah) morbid fear of new things.

kak- for words beginning thus, see also those beginning *cac-*.

kakidrosis (kak"ī-dro'sis) excretion of foul-smelling perspiration.

kakosmia (kak-oz'me-ah) an offensive odor.

kala-azar (kah"lah-ah-zar') a fatal epidemic fever of tropical Asia, resembling malarial fever, caused by *Leishmania donovani*.

kalemia (kah-le'me-ah) the presence of potassium in the blood.

kaliemia (ka"le-e'me-ah) kalemia.

kaligenous (kah-lij'ĕ-nus) producing potash.

kalimeter (kah-lim'ē-ter) alkalimeter.

kaliopenia (ka"le-o-pe'ne-ah) deficiency of potassium in the body. adj., **kaliope'nic.**

kalium (ka'le-um) [L.] potassium (symbol K).

kaliuresis (ka"le-u-re'sis) excretion of potassium in the urine.

kaliuretic (-ret'ik) 1. pertaining to or promoting kaliuresis. 2. an agent that promotes kaliuresis.

kallak (kal'ak) a pustular dermatitis occurring among Eskimos.

kallidin (kal'li-din) a type of kinin liberated by the action of kallikrein on a globulin of blood plasma.

kallikrein (kal"li-kre'in) a type of enzyme present in pancreas, saliva, urine, blood plasma, etc., which liberates kallidin from a globulin of blood plasma and hence has vasodilator and whealing actions.

kallikreinogen (-kri'no-jen) the inactive precursor of kallikrein which is normally present in blood.

kanamycin (kan"ah-mi'sin) a broad-spectrum antibiotic derived from *Streptomyces kanamyceticus.*

kansasiin (kan-sas'e-in) a product prepared from *Mycobacterium kansasii,* comparable to tuberculin, used in a cutaneous test of hypersensitivity.

Kantrex (kan'treks) trademark for preparations of kanamycin.

kaolin (ka'o-lin) native hydrated aluminum silicate, powdered and freed from gritty particles by elutriation; adsorbent.

kaolinosis (ka"o-lin-o'sis) pneumonoconiosis from inhaling particles of kaolin.

Kappadione (kap"pah-di'ōn) trademark for preparation of menadiol sodium diphosphate.

karyo- (kar'e-o) word element [Gr.], *nucleus.*

karyoblast (kar'e-o-blast") a cell at the beginning of the erythrocyte series.

karyochromatophil (kar"e-o-kro-mat'o-fil) 1. having a stainable nucleus. 2. a cell with an easily staining nucleus.

karyochrome (kar'e-o-krōm") nerve cell with an easily staining nucleus.

karyoclasis (kar"e-ok'lah-sis) the breaking down of a cell nucleus. adj., **karyoclas'tic.**

karyocyte (kar'e-o-sīt") 1. a nucleated cell. 2. an early normoblast.

karyogamy (kar"e-og'ah-me) cell conjugation with union of nuclei.

karyogenesis (kar"e-o-jen'ĕ-sis) the formation of a cell nucleus. adj., **karyogen'ic.**

karyokinesis (-ki-ne'sis) division of the nucleus of a cell in the formation of daughter cells.

karyolymph (kar'e-o-limf") the fluid portion of the nucleus of a cell, in which the other elements are dispersed.

karyolysis (kar"e-ol'ĭ-sis) the dissolution of the nucleus of a cell. adj., **karyolyt'ic.**

karyomegaly (kar"e-o-meg'ah-le) abnormal enlargement of the nucleus of a cell, not caused by polyploidy.

karyomere (kar'e-o-mēr") 1. chromomere (1). 2. a vesicle containing only a small portion of the typical nucleus, usually after abnormal mitosis.

karyomit (kar'e-o-mit) chromosome.

karyomitome (kar"e-om'ī-tōm) nuclear chromatin network.

karyomitosis (kar"e-o-mi-to'sis) mitosis.

karyomorphism (-mor'fizm) the shape of a cell nucleus.

karyon (kar'e-on) the nucleus of a cell.

karyonide (kar'e-o-nīd") a clone all of whose nuclei are derived from a single nucleus by vegetative reproduction.

karyophage (kar'e-o-fāj") an intracellular sporozoon.

karyoplasm (kar'e-o-plazm") the protoplasm of a cell contained within the nuclear membrane.

karyoplastin (kar"e-o-plas'tin) the substance of a mitotic spindle; the parachromatin.

karyopyknosis (-pik-no'sis) shrinkage of a cell nucleus, with condensation of the chromatin. adj., **karyopyknot'ic.**

karyorrhexis (-rek'sis) fragmentation of the nucleus of a cell. adj., **karyorrhec'tic.**

karyosome (kar′e-o-sōm″) a spherical mass of chromatin in the cell nucleus.

karyostasis (kar″e-os′tah-sis) the so-called resting stage of the nucleus between mitotic divisions.

karyotheca (kar″e-o-the′kah) nuclear membrane.

karyotype (kar′e-o-tīp″) the chromosomal element typical of a cell, arranged according to the Denver classification and drawn in their true proportions, based on the average of measurements determined in a number of cells.

kat(a)- (kat′ah) word element [Gr.], *down; against.* See also words beginning *cat(a)-*.

katathermometer (kat″ah-ther-mom′ĕ-ter) a thermometer for showing decrease in temperature.

kc. kilocycle.

kc.p.s. kilocycles per second.

kelis (ke′lis) 1. keloid. 2. morphea.

keloid (ke′loid) a new growth of the skin consisting of whitish ridges, nodules, and plaques of dense tissue. **Addison′s k.**, morphea.

keloidosis (ke″loi-do′sis) a condition marked by the formation of keloids.

keloma (ke-lo′ma) a keloid.

keloplasty (ke′lo-plas″te) any plastic operation on a scar.

kelosomus (ke″lo-so′mus) a fetal monster with eventration or fissure or absence of the sternum.

kelotomy (ke-lot′o-me) relief of hernial strangulation by cutting.

Kemadrin (kem′ah-drin) trademark for a preparation of tricyclamol.

Kenacort (ken′ah-kort) trademark for preparations of triamcinolone.

Kenalog (ken′ah-log) trademark for preparations of triamcinolone acetonide.

keno- (ken′o) word element [Gr.], *empty.*

kenophobia (ke″no-fo′be-ah) morbid dread of large open spaces.

kenotoxin (-tok′sin) a toxin produced by muscular contraction.

kerasin (ker′ah-sin) a cerebroside containing lignoceric acid.

kerat(o)- (ker′ah-to) word element [Gr.], *horny tissue; cornea.*

keratalgia (ker″ah-tal′je-ah) pain in the cornea.

keratectasia (-tek-ta′ze-ah) protrusion of the cornea.

keratectomy (-tek′to-me) excision of a portion of the cornea.

keratiasis (-ti′ah-sis) presence of horny warts on the skin.

keratic (kĕ-rat′ik) pertaining to horn; horny.

keratin (ker′ah-tin) a scleroprotein in various animal tissues, e.g. horn, nails, hoofs and feathers.

keratinization (ker″ah-tin″i-za′shun) formation of microscopic fibrils of keratin in the keratinocytes.

keratinocyte (kĕ-rat′ĭ-no-sīt) the cell of the epidermis that synthesizes keratin, known in its successive stages in the various layers of the skin as basal cell, prickle cell and granular cell.

keratinous (kĕ-rat′ĭ-nus) composed of keratin.

keratitis (ker″ah-ti′tis) inflammation of the cornea. **k. bullo′sa**, presence of large or small blebs upon the cornea. **interstitial k.**, chronic keratitis with deposits in the cornea, which becomes hazy. **lattice k.**, familial degeneration of the cornea with lattice-like areas. **neuroparalytic k.**, that which follows disease of the trifacial nerve. **phlyctenular k.**, a variety marked by formation of pustules or papules on the cornea. **punctate k.**, descemetitis. **purulent k.**, that in which pus is formed. **sclerosing k.**, keratitis with scleritis. **trachomatous k.**, pannus. **traumatic k.**, that which results from a wound of the cornea.

keratoacanthoma (ker″ah-to-ak″an-tho′mah) a rapidly growing papular lesion with a superficial crater filled with a keratin plug, usually on the face.

keratocele (ker′ah-to-sēl″) corneal protrusion of Descemet′s membrane.

keratocentesis (ker″ah-to-sen-te′sis) puncture of the cornea.

keratoconjunctivitis (-kon-junk″ti-vi′tis) inflammation of the cornea and conjunctiva. **epidemic k.**, an acute viral infection of the eye, with systemic symptoms and occurring in epidemics. **k. sic′ca**, a condition marked by hyperemia of the conjunctiva, thickening and drying of the corneal epithelium, itching and burning of the eye. **virus k.**, epidemic keratoconjunctivitis.

keratoconus (-ko′nus) conical protrusion of the central part of the cornea.

keratocyte (ker′ah-to-sīt″) one of the flattened connective tissue cells between the lamellae of fibrous tissue composing the cornea, with branching processes that intercommunicate with those of other cells.

keratoderma (ker″ah-to-der′mah) hypertrophy of the horny layer of the skin. **k. blennorrha′gica**, a symptom complex characterized by peculiar crusted, hornlike lesions on hands and feet and sometimes elsewhere. **k. climacter′icum, endocrine k.**, circumscribed hyperkeratosis of palms and soles, occurring in menopausal women.

keratodermatitis (-der″mah-ti′tis) inflammation of stratum corneum of the skin.

keratodermia (-der′me-ah) keratoderma.

keratogenous (ker″ah-toj′ĕ-nus) producing horny tissue, or keratin.

keratoglobus (ker″ah-to-glo′bus) prominent globular protrusion of the cornea.

keratohelcosis (-hel-ko′sis) ulceration of the cornea.

keratoid (ker′ah-toid) resembling horn; hornlike.

keratoiditis (ker″ah-toi-di′tis) keratitis.

kerato-iridoscope (ker″ah-to-i-rid′o-skōp) a compound microscope used for examining the eye.

kerato-iritis (-i-ri′tis) inflammation of the cornea and iris.

keratoleptynsis (-lep-tin′sis) removal of the anterior thickness of the cornea and covering the denuded area with bulbar conjunctiva.

keratoleukoma (ker″ah-to-lu-ko′mah) white opacity of the cornea.

keratolysis (ker″ah-tol′ĭ-sis) separation of the horny layer of the epidermis.

keratolytic (ker″ah-to-lit′ik) 1. pertaining to or promoting keratolysis. 2. an agent that promotes keratolysis.

keratoma (ker″ah-to′mah) any growth of horny tissue.

keratomalacia (ker″ah-to-mah-la′she-ah) softening of cornea.

keratome (ker′ah-tōm) a knife for incising the cornea.

keratometer (ker″ah-tom′ĕ-ter) an instrument for measuring the curves of the cornea.

keratometry (-tom′ĕ-tre) measurement of corneal curves. adj., **keratomet′ric.**

keratomycosis (ker″ah-to-mi-ko′sis) fungus disease of the cornea. **k. lin′guae,** black tongue.

keratonosis (-no′sis) any disease of the horny structure of the epidermis.

keratonyxis (-nik″sis) puncture of the cornea.

keratopathy (ker″ah-top′ah-the) noninflammatory disease of the cornea. **band k.,** a condition characterized by an abnormal circumcorneal band.

keratoplasty (ker′ah-to-plas″te) plastic surgery of the cornea. **optic k.,** transplantation of corneal material to replace scar tissue which interferes with vision. **tectonic k.,** transplantation of corneal material to replace tissue which has been lost.

keratoprotein (ker″ah-to-pro′te-in) the protein of the horny tissues of the body, such as the hair, nails and epidermis.

keratorhexis (-rek′sis) rupture of the cornea.

keratoscleritis (-skle-ri′tis) inflammation of cornea and sclera.

keratoscope (ker′ah-to-skōp″) instrument for examining the cornea.

keratoscopy (ker″ah-tos′ko-pe) 1. inspection of the cornea. 2. skiascopy.

keratosis (ker″ah-to′sis) formation of horny growth or tissue. **k. blennorrha′gica,** keratoderma blennorrhagica. **k. follicula′ris,** a rare hereditary condition manifested by areas of crusting, verrucous papular growths, usually occurring symmetrically on the trunk, axillae, neck, face, scalp and retroauricular areas. **gonorrheal k.,** keratoderma blennorrhagica. **k. lin′guae,** leukoplakia linguae. **k. ni′gricans,** acanthosis nigricans. **k. palma′ris et planta′ris,** a disease marked by thickening of the skin of the palms and soles. **k. pharynge′us,** horny projections from the tonsils and pharyngeal walls. **k. pila′ris,** formation of a hard elevation around each hair follicle. **k. puncta′ta,** keratosis occurring as small spots or points. **seborrheic k., k. seborrhe′-ica,** formation of a small, sharply marginated, yellowish or brownish lesion, covered by a thin, greasy scale. **k. seni′lis,** a harsh, dry state of skin in old age.

keratotomy (ker″ah-tot′o-me) incision of the cornea.

keratotorus (ker″ah-to-to′rus) a toric or vaultlike protrusion of the cornea.

keraunophobia (kĕ-raw″no-fo′be-ah) morbid dread of lightning.

kerectomy (kĕ-rek′to-me) removal of a part of the cornea.

kerion (ke′re-on) a pustular disease of the scalp.

kerma (ker′mah) the energy initially imparted to secondary electrons per unit mass of absorbing material through photon interaction.

kernicterus (ker-nik′ter-us) a condition with severe neural symptoms, associated with high levels of bilirubin in the blood.

keto- (ke′to) word element, *ketone group.*

ketogenesis (ke″to-jen′ĕ-sis) the production of ketones (ketone bodies). adj., **ketogenet′ic.**

ketogenic (-jen′ik) conducive to the production of ketones (ketone bodies).

ketolysis (ke-tol′ĭ-sis) the splitting up of ketone (acetone) bodies. adj., **ketolyt′ic.**

ketone (ke′tōn) a chemical compound characterized by the presence of the bivalent carbonyl group ($>C:O$).

ketonemia (ke″to-ne′me-ăh) presence of ketone bodies in the blood.

ketonuria (-nu′re-ah) presence of excessive amounts of ketone bodies in the urine.

ketose (ke′tōs) a sugar that contains the ketone radical ($>C:O$).

ketosis (ke-to′sis) accumulation of excessive amounts of ketone bodies in body tissues and fluids. adj., **ketot′ic.**

ketosteroid (ke″to-stēr′oid) a steroid that contains the ketone radical ($>C:O$). **17-k.,** a steroid with a ketone radical on the seventeenth carbon atom; normally found in human urine and occurring in excessive amounts in certain pathologic conditions.

ketosuria (-su′re-ah) ketose in the urine.

kev kilo (1000) electron volts (3.82×10^{-17} gramcalories, or 1.6×10^{-9} ergs).

kg. kilogram.

kg.-m. kilogram-meter.

kidney (kid′ne) one of two glandular bodies in the lumbar region that secrete urine. **amyloid k.,** one affected with amyloid degeneration. **artificial k.,** an extracorporeal device through which blood may be circulated for removal of elements that normally are excreted in the urine. **cicatricial k.,** a shriveled, irregular and scarred kidney due to suppurative pyelonephritis. **cirrhotic k., contracted k.,** granular kidney. **definite k.,** metanephros. **doughnut k.,** one formed by polar or mesial fusion of the renal anlagen in the embryo, before rotation begins. **fatty k.,** one affected with fatty degeneration. **floating k.,** one which is loosened and displaced. **fused k.,** a single anomalous organ developed as a result of fusion of the renal anlagen. **granular k.,** one affected with chronic interstitial inflammation. **head k.,** pronephros. **horseshoe k.,** an anomalous organ resulting from fusion of the corresponding poles of the renal anlagen. **lump k.,** a solid, irregularly lobed organ of bizarre shape resulting from fusion of the kidney anlagen in the embryo. **medullary sponge k.,** a large, smooth kidney with dilated collecting tubules. **middle k.,** mesonephros. **polycystic k.,** a congenital condition of nodular (cystic) enlargement, usually involving both kidneys. **primordial k.,** pronephros. **red contracted k.,** granular kidney. **sigmoid k.,** an organ produced by fusion of the lower poles of one renal anlage with the upper pole of the other. **small white k.,** atrophied and degenerated state following chronic interstitial nephritis. **sponge k.,** medullary sponge kidney. **wandering k.,** floating kidney. **waxy k.,** amyloid kidney.

killeen (kil'lēn) chondrus.

kilo- (kil'o) word element [Gr.], *one thousand* (10³), used in naming units of measurement.

kilogram (kil'o-gram) a unit of mass (weight) of the metric system, 1000 grams; equivalent to 15,432 grains, or 2.205 pounds (avoirdupois) or 2.679 pounds (apothecaries' weight).

kilogram-meter (kil'o-gram-me'ter) a unit of work, representing the energy required to raise 1 kg. of weight 1 meter vertically against gravitational force, equivalent to about 7.2 foot pounds and to 1000 gram-meters.

kiloliter (kil'o-le'ter) one thousand liters; 264 gallons.

kilomegacycle (kil'o-meg''ah-si'kl) a unit of 1000 megacycles; applied to the frequency of electromagnetic waves.

kilometer (kil'o-me'ter) one thousand meters; five-eighths of a mile.

kilounit (kil''o-u'nit) a quantity equivalent to one thousand (10³) units.

kilovolt (kil'o-volt) one thousand volts.

kinanesthesia (kin''an-es-the'ze-ah) loss of power of perceiving sensations of movement.

kinase (ki'nās) 1. an enzyme that catalyzes the transfer of a high-energy group of a donor to an acceptor. 2. an enzyme that activates a zymogen. **bacterial k.,** an enzyme of bacterial origin that activates a precursor (plasminogen) of a plasma protease (plasmin). **creatine k.,** an enzyme that catalyzes the transfer of a high-energy phosphate group from a donor to creatine, producing phosphocreatine. **insulin k.,** an enzyme assumed to exist in the liver which activates insulin. **phosphoglycerate k.,** an enzyme that catalyzes the transfer of a high-energy phosphate group from a donor to D-3-phosphoglycerate, producing D-1,3-diphosphoglycerate. **tissue k.,** fibrinokinase.

kine- (kine') word element [Gr.], *movement.* See also words beginning *cine-.*

kinematics (kin''e-mat'iks) that phase of mechanics which deals with the possible motions of a material body.

kinematograph (-mat'o-graf) an instrument for showing pictures of objects in motion.

kinemia (ki-ne'me-ah) the blood output of the heart. adj., **kine'mic.**

kineplasty (kin'e-plas''te) utilization of the stump of an amputated extremity for producing motion of the prosthesis.

kinergety (kin-er'jĕ-te) the capacity for kinetic energy.

kinesalgia (kin''ĕ-sal'je-ah) pain on muscular exertion.

kinescope (kin'ĕ-skōp) an instrument for ascertaining ocular refraction.

kinesi(o)- (ki-ne'se-o) word element [Gr.], *movement.*

kinesia (ki-ne'se-ah) motion sickness.

kinesialgia (ki-ne''se-al'je-ah) kinesalgia.

kinesiatrics (-at'riks) kinesitherapy.

kinesimeter (kin''e-sim'ĕ-ter) instrument for quantitative measurement of motions.

kinesiology (ki-ne''se-ol'o-je) scientific study of movement of body parts.

kinesioneurosis (ki-ne''se-o-nu-ro'sis) disordered movements from nervous disease.

-kinesis (ki-ne'sis) word element, *movement.*

kinesitherapy (ki-ne''si-ther'ah-pe) treatment of disease by movements.

kinesthesia (kin''es-the'ze-ah) the sense by which one is aware of position and movement of various body parts. adj., **kinesthet'ic.**

kinesthesiometer (-the''ze-om'ĕ-ter) an apparatus for testing kinesthesia.

kinesthesis (-the'sis) kinesthesia.

kinetia (ki-ne'te-ah) kinetosis.

kineticist (ki-net'ĭ-sist) a specialist in kinetics.

kinetics (ki-net'iks) the scientific study of the turnover, or rate of change, of a specific factor in the body, commonly expressed as units of amount per unit time. **chemical k.,** scientific study of the rates at which chemical reactions occur.

kinetocardiogram (ki-ne''to-kar'de-o-gram) the record produced by kinetocardiography.

kinetocardiography (-kar''de-og'rah-fe) the graphic recording of slow vibrations of the chest wall in the region of the heart, representing the absolute motion at a given point on the chest.

kinetochore (ki-ne'to-kōr) centromere.

kinetogenic (ki-ne''to-jen'ik) causing or producing movement.

kinetoplasm (ki-ne'to-plazm) the chromophilic matter of the nervous system.

kinetoplast (ki-ne'to-plast) an accessory body, often called the micronucleus, found in many protozoa, and consisting of two parts, the blepharoplast and parabasal body, united by a delicate fibril.

kinetosis (ki''ne-to'sis) any disorder due to unaccustomed motions.

kinetosome (ki-ne'to-sōm) basal body.

kinetotherapy (ki-ne''to-ther'ah-pe) kinesitherapy.

kingdom (king'dum) one of the three major categories into which natural objects are usually classified: the animal (including all animals), plant (including all plants) and mineral (including all substance and objects without life).

kinin (ki'nin) an endogenous peptide that acts on blood vessels, smooth muscles and nociceptive nerve endings. **venom k.,** a peptide found in the venom of insects.

kink (kingk) a bend or twist. **ileal k., Lane's k.,** obstruction of the small intestine due to kinking of Lane's band.

kinocilium (ki''no-sil'e-um), pl. *kinocil'ia,* a motile, protoplasmic filament on the free surface of a cell.

kinoplasm (ki'no-plazm) the substance giving

origin to the spindle fiber of cytoplasm. adj., **kinoplas'tic.**

kinosphere (kin'o-sfēr) aster.

kinotoxin (ki"no-tok'sin) a toxin produced as a result of fatigue.

kinship (kin'ship) a group of individuals of varying degrees of descent from a common ancestor.

kiotomy (ki-ot'o-me) excision of the vulva.

kl. kiloliter.

Klebsiella (kleb"se-el'ah) a genus of Schizomycetes (order Eubacteriales, family Enterobacteriaceae, tribe Escherichieae) frequently found in the respiratory or intestinal tract in man. **K. friedlän'deri, K. pneumo'niae,** an organism occurring in patients with lobar pneumonia and other infections of the respiratory tract.

kleptomania (klep"to-ma'ne-ah) compulsive stealing, the objects taken usually having a symbolic value of which the subject is unconscious, rather than an intrinsic value.

km. kilometer.

kMc. kilomegacycle.

kMc.p.s. kilomegacycles per second.

knee (ne) the point of articulation of the femur with the tibia. **housemaid's k.,** inflammation of the bursa of the patella.

knife (nīf) a sharp instrument for cutting. **Beer's k.,** one with a triangular blade, for incising the cornea.

knock-knee (nok'ne) a deformity in which the space between the knees is abnormally reduced and that between the ankles is increased.

knot (not) a knoblike structure or an entanglement, as of two ends of a thread or suture. **net k.,** karyosome. **primitive k.,** a mass of cells at the forward end of the primitive streak in the early embryo.

knuckle (nuk'l) the dorsal aspect of any phalangeal joint, or any similarly bent structure.

knuckling (nuk'ling) upward and forward displacement of the fetlock joint of a horse.

koilo- (koi'lo) word element [Gr.], *hollowed; depressed.*

koilonychia (koi"lo-nik'e-ah) a disorder of the nails, which are abnormally thin and concave from side to side, with the edges turned up.

koilorrhachic (-rak'ik) having a vertebral column in which the lumbar curvature is anteriorly concave.

koilosternia (-ster'ne-ah) congenital chondrosternal depression.

koinotropic (koi"no-trop'ik) having a well balanced personality with normal social outlook.

kolp- for words beginning thus, see those beginning *colp-.*

Konakion (kon"ah-ki'on) trademark for a preparation of vitamin K.

konometer (ko-nom'ĕ-ter) an apparatus for counting the dust particles in the air.

Konsyl (kon'sil) trademark for a preparation of plantago ovata coating.

kopiopia (ko"pe-o'pe-ah) copiopia.

koumiss (koo'mis) fermented drink prepared from milk.

Kr chemical symbol, *krypton.*

kraurosis (kraw-ro'sis) a dried, shriveled condition. **k. vul'vae,** shrivelling and dryness of the vulva.

Krebs cycle (krebz si'kl) tricarboxylic acid cycle.

kreo- for words beginning thus, see also those beginning *creo-.*

kreotoxism (kre"o-tok'sizm) poisoning by meat.

krypton (krip'ton) chemical element *(see table),* at. no. 36, symbol Kr.

Kurthia (kur'the-ah) a genus of Schizomycetes (order Eubacteriales, family Brevibacteriaceae) found in decomposing material.

kuru (koo'roo) a chronic, progressive disorder involving the central nervous system, observed in Melanesian natives of one region of the Australian Trust Territory of New Guinea.

kv. kilovolt.

kvp. kilovolt peak.

kw. kilowatt.

kwashiorkor (kwash"e-or'kor) a syndrome due to severe protein deficiency, with characteristic changes in pigmentation of the skin and hair. **marasmic k.,** a condition in which there is deficiency of both calories and protein, with severe tissue wasting, loss of subcutaneous fat and usually dehydration.

Kwell (kwel) trademark for preparations of lindane.

kyestein (ki-es'te-in) an albuminoid which floats on decomposing urine.

kymatism (ki'mah-tizm) myokymia.

kymogram (ki'mo-gram) the graphic record (tracing or film) produced by kymography.

kymograph (ki'mo-graf) instrument for recording motion or changes in density.

kymography (ki-mog'rah-fe) the recording of the movement of the silhouette of an organ.

kymoscope (ki'mo-skōp) device used in observing the blood current.

Kynex (ki'neks) trademark for preparations of sulfamethoxypyridazine.

kynocephalus (ki"no-sef'ah-lus) a monster with a head like that of a dog.

kynurenine (kin"u-re'nin) a metabolite of tryptophan found in the urine of normal mammals; a precursor of kynurenic acid.

kyogenic (ki-o-jen'ik) producing pregnancy.

kyphos (ki'fos) the hump in the spine in kyphosis.

kyphoscoliosis (ki"fo-sko"le-o'sis) kyphosis blended with scoliosis.

kyphosis (ki-fo'sis) abnormally increased convexity in the curvature of the thoracic spine as viewed from the side. adj., **kyphot'-ic. k. dorsa'lis juvenil'lis, juvenile k., Scheuermann's k.,** osteochondritis of the vertebrae.

kyrtorrhachic (kir"to-rak'ik) having a vertebral column in which the lumbar curvature is anteriorly convex.

kyto- (ki'to) for words beginning thus, see those beginning *cyto-.*

L

L. Latin; left; length; libra *(pound, balance),* licentiate; light sense; limes *(boundary),* liter; lumbar; coefficient of induction.

L₀ Ehrlich's symbol for a toxin-antitoxin mixture which is completely neutralized and will not kill an animal.

L+ Ehrlich's symbol for a toxin-antitoxin mixture which contains one fatal dose in excess and which will kill the experimental animal.

l- prefix, *levo-.*

La chemical symbol, *lanthanum.*

labialism (la′be-ah-lizm″) defective speech with use of labial sounds.

labile (la′bil) subject to free and rapid change.

lability (la-bil′ĭ-te) a state of being extremely susceptible to change.

labio-alveolar (la″be-o-al-ve′o-lar) pertaining to the labial side of a dental alveolus.

labiocervical (-ser′vĭ-kal) pertaining to the labial surface of the neck of a tooth.

labiochorea (-ko-re′ah) a choreic affection of the lips, with stammering.

labioclination (-kli-na′shun) deviation of an anterior tooth from the vertical, in the direction of the lips.

labiogingival (-jin-ji′val) pertaining to or formed by the labial and gingival walls of a tooth cavity.

labioglossolaryngeal (-glos″o-lah-rin′je-al) pertaining to lips, tongue and larynx.

labioglossopharyngeal (-fah-rin′je-al) pertaining to lips, tongue and pharynx.

labiograph (la′be-o-graf″) an instrument for registering movements of the lips.

labioincisal (la″be-o-in-si′sal) pertaining to or formed by the labial and incisal surfaces of a tooth.

labiology (la″be-ol′o-je) the study of the movements of the lips. adj., **labiolog′ic.**

labiomancy (la′be-o-man″se) lip-reading.

labiomental (la″be-o-men′tal) pertaining to lips and chin.

labiopalatine (-pal′ah-tīn) pertaining to lips and palate.

labioplacement (-plās′ment) displacement of a tooth toward the lip.

labioplasty (la′be-o-plas″te) cheiloplasty.

labioversion (la″be-o-ver′zhun) labial displacement of a tooth from the line of occlusion.

labium (la′be-um), pl. *la′bia* [L.] a border or edge; a lip. adj., **la′bial. l. ma′jus** (pl. *la′bia majo′ra),* hairy fold of skin on either side of the vulva. **l. mi′nus** (pl. *la′bia mino′ra),* fold of mucous membrane within the labia majora.

labor (la′bor) the function of the female organism by which the product of conception is expelled through the vagina to the outside world. **artificial l.,** induced labor. **dry l.,** that in which the bag of waters ruptures before contraction of the uterus begins. **false l.,** false pains. **induced l.,** that which is brought on by extraneous means. **instrumental l.,** delivery facilitated by use of instruments. **missed l.,** retention of the dead fetus in utero after normal time of delivery. **postponed l.,** that occurring later than the expected date. **precipitate l.,** delivery accomplished with undue celerity. **premature l.,** expulsion of a viable infant before the normal end of gestation; usually applied to interruption of pregnancy between the twenty-eighth and thirty-seventh weeks. **spontaneous l.,** delivery occurring without artificial aid.

laboratory (lab′o-rah-tor″e) a place for making tests or doing experimental work.

labrale (lah-bra′le) an anthropometric land mark on the border of the lip.

labrum (la′brum), pl. *la′bra* [L.] an edge, rim or lip.

labyrinth (lab′ĭ-rinth) the internal ear, made up of the vestibule, cochlea and canals. adj., **labyrin′thine. bony l.,** the bony part of the internal ear. **membranous l.,** a system of communicating epithelial sacs and ducts within the bony labyrinth, containing the endolymph. **osseous l.,** bony labyrinth.

labyrinthectomy (lab″ĭ-rin-thek′to-me) excision of the labyrinth.

labyrinthitis (-thi′tis) inflammation of the labyrinth.

labyrinthotomy (-thot′o-me) incision of the labyrinth.

labyrinthus (lab″ĭ-rin′thus), pl. *labyrin′thi* [L.] labyrinth.

lac (lak), pl. *lac′ta* [L.] milk.

laceration (las″ĕ-ra′shun) a wound produced by tearing.

lacertus (lah-ser′tus), pl. *lacer′ti* [L.] a name given certain fibrous attachments of muscles because of a fancied resemblance to a lizard.

lachry- (lak′re) for words beginning thus, see those beginning *lacri-.*

lacrimal (lak′rĭ-mal) pertaining to tears.

lacrimase (lak′rĭ-mās) an enzyme from the lacrimal secretion.

lacrimation (lak″rĭ-ma′shun) secretion and discharge of tears.

lacrimonasal (lak″rĭ-mo-na′zal) pertaining to the lacrimal sac and nose.

lacrimotomy (lak″rĭ-mot′o-me) incision of lacrimal gland, duct or sac.

lactacidase (lak-tas′ĭ-dās) the enzyme of lactic acid bacteria.

lactacidemia (lak-tas″ĭ-de′me-ah) lactic acid in the blood.

lactaciduria (-du′re-ah) lactic acid in the urine.

lactagogue (lak′tah-gog) galactagogue.

lactalase (lak′tah-lās) an enzyme which changes dextrose into lactic acid.

lactalbumin (lak″tal-bu′min) the albumin from milk.

lactase (lak′tās) an enzyme that catalyzes the conversion of lactose into glucose and galactose.

lactate (lak'tāt) a salt of lactic acid.

lactation (lak-ta'shun) secretion of milk.

lacteal (lak'te-al) pertaining to milk.

lactescence (lak-tes'ens) resemblance to milk.

lacticemia (lak″tĭ-se'me-ah) lactic acid in the blood.

lactiferous (lak-tif'er-us) conveying milk.

lactifuge (lak'tĭ-fūj) an agent which lessens the secretion of milk.

lactigenous (lak-tij'ĕ-nus) producing milk.

lactigerous (lak-tij'er-us) lactiferous.

lactin (lak'tin) lactose.

lactivorous (lak-tiv'o-rus) subsisting upon milk.

Lactobacillaceae (lak″to-bas″il-la'se-e) a family of Schizomycetes (order Eubacteriales).

Lactobacilleae (-bah-sil'le-e) a tribe of Schizomycetes (order Eubacteriales, family Lactobacillaceae).

Lactobacillus (-bah-sil'lus) a genus of Schizomycetes (order Eubacteriales, family Lactobacillaceae, tribe Lactobacilleae), some of which are considered to be etiologically related to dental caries, but are otherwise nonpathogenic.

lactobacillus (-bah-sil'us), pl. *lactobacil'li* [L.] an organism of the genus Lactobacillus.

lactocele (lak'to-sēl) galactocele.

lactoflavin (lak″to-fla'vin) riboflavin.

lactoglobulin (-glob'u-lin) a globulin occurring in milk. **immune l's,** antibodies occurring in the colostrum of animals.

lactolase (lak'to-lās) an enzyme which produces lactic acid.

lactometer (lak-tom'ĕ-ter) instrument for measuring specific gravity of milk.

lactone (lak'tōn) an aromatic liquid from lactic acid.

lactophosphate (lak″to-fos'fāt) a salt of lactic and phosphoric acids.

lactoprecipitin (-pre-sip'ĭ-tin) a precipitin which precipitates the casein of milk.

lactoprotein (-pro'te-in) a protein derived from milk.

lactorrhea (-re'ah) galactorrhea.

lactose (lak'tōs) a sugar derived from milk, $C_{12}H_{22}O_{11}$.

lactoserum (lak″to-se'rum) the serum of an animal into which milk has been injected.

lactosum (lak-to'sum) [L.] lactose.

lactosuria (lak″to-su're-ah) lactose in urine.

lactotherapy (-ther'ah-pe) treatment by milk diet.

lactotoxin (-tok'sin) a toxin found in milk.

lactovegetarian (-vej″ĕ-ta're-an) a person who subsists on a diet of milk or milk products and vegetables.

lacuna (lah-ku'nah), pl. *lacu'nae* [L.] a small pit or hollow cavity; an area where substance is lacking. adj. **lacu'nar. absorption l.,** a pit or groove in developing bone that is undergoing resorption; frequently found to contain osteoclasts. **Howship's l.,** absorption lacuna. **intervillous l.,** a blood space of the placenta in which the fetal villi are found. **l. mag'na,** largest of the orifices of the glands of Littre. **l. pharyn'gis,** depression at the pharyngeal

end of the eustachian tube. **trophoblastic l.,** intervillous lacuna.

lacunule (lah-ku'nūl) a minute lacuna.

lacus (la'kus), pl. *la'cus* [L.] lake. **l. lacrima'lis,** the triangular space at the inner canthus between the two eyelids.

lae- for words beginning thus, see also those beginning *le-*.

laeve (le've) [L.] nonvillous.

lag (lag) 1. the time elapsing between application of a stimulus and the resulting reaction. 2. the early period after inoculation of bacteria into a culture medium, in which the growth is slow.

lagena (lah-je'nah) a part of the upper extremity of the scala media.

lageniform (lah-jen'ĭ-form) flask shaped.

lagnosis (lag-no'sis) excessive sexual desire, especially in the male; satyriasis.

lagophthalmos (lag″of-thal'mos) inability to shut the eyes completely.

laiose (li'ōs) a syrupy compound, $C_6H_{12}O_6$, found in urine in diabetes.

lake (lāk) 1. a lacuna. 2. to undergo separation of hemoglobin from the erythrocytes. **lacrimal l.,** the space deep to the margin of the eyelids which contains the fluid secreted by the lacrimal glands.

lal(o)- (lal'o) word element [Gr.], *speech; babbling.*

laliatry (lal-i'ah-tre) the study and treatment of disorders of speech.

lallation (lah-la'shun) babbling, semi-infantile speech.

lalognosis (lal″og-no'sis) the understanding of speech.

laloneurosis (lal″o-nu-ro'sis) speech disorder of nervous or central origin.

lalopathology (-pah-thol'o-je) the branch of medicine dealing with disorders of speech.

lalopathy (lah-lop'ah-the) any speech disorder.

lalophobia (lal″o-fo'be-ah) dislike of speaking, often with extreme stuttering.

laloplegia (-ple'je-ah) paralysis of the organs of speech.

lalorrhea (-re'ah) an abnormal flow of words.

lambda (lam'dah) point of union of lambdoid and sagittal sutures.

lambdacism (lam'dah-sizm) inability to utter the *l* sound.

lambdoid (lam'doid) shaped like the Greek letter lambda, Λ.

Lamblia (lam'ble-ah) a former name of the genus Giardia.

lambliasis (lam-bli'ah-sis) giardiasis.

lame (lām) incapable of normal locomotion.

lamella (lah-mel'ah), pl. *lamel'lae* [L.] 1. a thin scale or plate. 2. a thin gelatin disk to be placed under the eyelid, containing medication acting on the eye. adj. **lamel'lar. circumferential l.,** one of the bony plates that underlie the periosteum and endosteum. **concentric l.,** haversian lamella. **endosteal l.,** one of the bony plates lying beneath the endosteum. **ground l.,** interstitial lamella. **haversian l.,** one of the concentric bony plates surrounding a haversian canal. **intermediate l.,** inter-

stitial l., one of the bony plates that fill in between the haversian systems. **triangular l.,** a layer joining the choroid plexuses of the third ventricle. **vitreous l.,** lamina basalis.

lamina (lam'ĭ-nah), pl. *lam'inae* [L.] a thin, flat plate or layer; used in anatomic nomenclature to designate such a structure, or a specific portion of a composite structure. **l. basa'lis,** one of the pair of longitudinal zones of the embryonic neural tube, from which develop the ventral gray columns of the spinal cord and the motor centers of the brain. **l. basila'ris,** a membrane which with the lamina spiralis forms the partition between the scala tympani and scala vestibuli. **Bowman's l.,** Bowman's membrane. **l. cine'rea,** layer of gray matter between the callosum and optic chiasm. **l. cribro'sa.** 1. the fascia covering the saphenous opening. 2. either of the perforated spaces in the brain. 3. part of sclera perforated for passage of optic nerve. **dental l.,** a thickened epithelial band along the margin of the gum in the embryo, from which the enamel organs are developed. **elastic l.,** Descemet's membrane. **epithelial l.,** the layer of ependymal cells covering the choroid plexus. **l. fus'ca,** the pigmentary layer of the sclera. **l. pro'pria.** 1. the connective tissue layer of mucous membrane. 2. the middle or fibrous layer of the tympanic membrane. **l. reticula'ris,** the perforated hyaline membrane which covers the organ of Corti. **l. spira'lis,** a small bony plate projecting from the wall of the cochlea. **vitreous l., vitreal l.,** Bruch's membrane.

laminagraphy (lam''ĭ-nag'rah-fe) laminography.

laminar (lam'ĭ-nar) made up of laminae or layers; pertaining to a lamina.

Laminaria (lam''i-na're-ah) a genus of seaweeds, various species of which are used as sources of alginates.

laminated (lam'ĭ-nāt''ed) made up of laminae or layers.

lamination (lam''i-na'shun) 1. laminar structure or arrangement. 2. the slicing of the fetal head in embryotomy.

laminectomy (-nek'to-me) excision of a lamina of a vertebra.

laminography (-nog'rah-fe) a special technique of body section roentgenography.

laminotomy (-not'o-me) transection of a lamina of a vertebra.

lamp (lamp) an apparatus for furnishing artificial light. **annealing l.,** an alcohol lamp for heating gold leaf for tooth fillings. **carbon arc l.,** an open flame lamp with carbon arcs; used in artificial light therapy. **Gullstrand's slit l.,** an apparatus for projecting a narrow, flat beam of intense light into the eye. **Kromayer's l.,** a quartz or mercury vapor lamp used in treating skin diseases with actinic rays. **mercury vapor l.,** a lamp in which the arc is in mercury vapor, enclosed in a quartz burner; used in light therapy; it may be air-cooled or water-cooled. **quartz l.,** a mercury vacuum lamp made of melted quartz glass embedded in a running water bath; used for applying light treatment. **slit l.,** Gullstrand's slit lamp. **tungsten arc l.,** a lamp having highly compressed tungsten electrodes. **zoalite l.,** a device for producing radiant heat for therapeutic purposes.

lampas (lam'pas) swelling of the mucous membrane over the hard palate, projecting in a ridge behind the upper incisors of horses.

lampblack (lamp'blak) powdered carbon from combustion of oil or tar.

Lamprocystis (lam''pro-sis'tis) a genus of Schizomycetes (order Pseudomonadales, suborder Rhodobacteriineae, family Thiorhodaceae).

lamprophonia (-fo'ne-ah) clearness of voice. adj., **lamprophon'ic.**

lamziekte (lam'zēk-te) a disease of cattle in South Africa, characterized by motor paralysis and due to ingestion by phosphorus-deficient animals of bones contaminated by toxin produced by *Clostridium botulinum.*

lanatoside (lah-nat'o-sīd) a precursor of a cardiac glycoside obtained from the leaf of *Digitalis lanata.* **l. C,** a poisonous crystalline compound used as a heart stimulant.

lancet (lan'set) a small, pointed, two-edged surgical knife.

lancinating (lan'sĭ-nāt''ing) tearing, darting or sharply cutting.

lanolin (lan'o-lin) purified, fatlike substance from the wool of sheep, *Ovis aries,* used as a water-absorbable ointment base. **anhydrous l.,** lanolin that contains not more than 0.25 per cent of water.

Lanoxin (lah-nok'sin) trademark for preparations of digoxin.

lanthanin (lan'thah-nin) oxychromatin.

lanthanum (lan'thah-num) chemical element (*see table*), at. no. 57, symbol La.

lanugo (lah-nu'go) fine hair, such as that covering the body of the fetus.

laparo- (lap'ah-ro) word element [Gr.], *loin or flank; abdomen.*

laparorrhaphy (lap''ah ror'ah fe) suture of the abdominal wall.

laparotomaphilia (lap''ah-rot''o-mah-fil'e-ah) a morbid desire to undergo abdominal surgery for simulated symptoms.

laparotomy (lap''ah-rot'o-me) incision of the abdominal wall.

laparotrachelotomy (lap''ah ro tra''kĕ lot'o me) low cervical cesarean section.

lapis (la'pis, lap'is) [L.] stone.

laqueus (lak'we-us) lemniscus.

lard (lard) purified internal fat of the abdomen of the hog; emollient, used in ointments and cerates. **benzoinated l.,** a mixture of benzoin and lard.

lardacein (lar-da'se-in) a protein found in amyloid degeneration.

lardaceous (lar-da'shus) 1. resembling lard. 2. containing lardacein.

Largon (lar'gon) trademark for a preparation of propiomazine hydrochloride.

larithmics (lah-rith'miks) the study dealing with population in its quantitative aspects.

larixin (la-rik'sin) laricic acid.

larva (lar'vah), pl. *lar'vae* [L.] the first or worm-

like stage of an insect on issuing from the egg.
l. mi′grans, a peculiar eruption occurring in a changing pattern on the skin, due to migration beneath its surface of a fly larva or helminth.
l. mi′grans, visceral, a condition due to prolonged migration of larvae of animal nematodes in human tissue other than skin.

larval (lar′val) 1. pertaining to larvae. 2. larvate.

larvate (lar′vāt) masked; concealed.

larvicide (lar′vī-sīd) 1. destructive to larvae. 2. an agent destructive to larvae.

larvivorous (lar-viv′o-rus) feeding on or consuming larvae, especially larvae of mosquitoes.

laryng(o)- (lah-ring′go) word element [Gr.], *larynx.*

laryngalgia (lar″in-gal′je-ah) pain in the larynx.

laryngeal (lah-rin′je-al) pertaining to the larynx.

laryngectomee (lar″in-jek′to-me) a person whose larynx has been removed.

laryngectomy (-jek′to-me) excision of the larynx.

laryngismus (-jiz′mus) spasm of the larynx. **l. paralyt′icus,** roaring. **l. strid′ulus,** sudden laryngeal spasm with crowing inspiration.

laryngitis (-ji′tis) inflammation of the larynx. **atrophic l.,** inflammation of the larynx leading to atrophic changes in the mucosa. **subglottic l.,** inflammation of the under surface of the vocal cords.

laryngocele (lah-ring′go-sēl) protrusion of mucous membrane across the cricothyroid space.

laryngocentesis (lah-ring″go-sen-te′sis) puncture of the larynx, with aspiration.

laryngofissure (-fish′er) median laryngotomy.

laryngogram (lah-ring′go-gram) a roentgenogram of the larynx.

laryngography (lar″ing-gog′rah-fe) radiography of the larynx.

laryngology (-gol′o-je) sum of what is known about the larynx.

laryngopathy (-gop′ah-the) any disorder of the larynx.

laryngophantom (lah-ring″go-fan′tom) an artificial model of the larynx.

laryngopharyngeal (-fah-rin′je-al) pertaining to larynx and pharynx.

laryngopharyngectomy (-far″in-jek′to-me) excision of larynx and pharynx.

laryngopharyngitis (-far″in-ji′tis) inflammation of larynx and pharynx.

laryngopharynx (-far′inks) the lower portion of the pharynx.

laryngophony (lar″ing-gof′o-ne) sound heard in auscultating the larynx.

laryngoplasty (lah-ring′go-plas″te) plastic repair of the larynx.

laryngoplegia (lah-ring″go-ple′je-ah) paralysis of the larynx.

laryngoptosis (-to′sis) lowering and mobilization of the larynx.

laryngorhinology (-ri-nol′o-je) the science of the larynx and nose and their diseases.

laryngorrhagia (lah-ring″go-ra′je-ah) hemorrhage from the larynx.

laryngorrhaphy (lar″ing-gor′ah-fe) suture of the larynx.

laryngorrhea (lah-ring″go-re′ah) excessive secretion of mucus from the larynx.

laryngoscleroma (-skle-ro′mah) scleroma of the larynx.

laryngoscope (lah-ring′go-skōp) an endoscope for examining the larynx.

laryngoscopy (lar″in-gos′ko-pe) visual examination of the larynx. **direct l.,** examination of the larynx with use of a speculum or laryngoscope. **indirect l., mirror l.,** examination of the larynx by observing its reflection in a mirror.

laryngospasm (lah-ring′go-spazm) laryngismus stridulus.

laryngostenosis (lah-ring″go-ste-no′sis) narrowing of the larynx.

laryngostomy (lar″ing-gos′to-me) fistulization of the larynx.

laryngotomy (-got′o-me) incision of the larynx. **inferior l.,** incision of the larynx between the thyroid and cricoid cartilages. **median l.,** incision of the larynx through the thyroid cartilage.

laryngotracheitis (lah-ring″go-tra″ke-i′tis) inflammation of the larynx and trachea.

laryngotracheotomy (-tra″ke-ot′o-me) incision of the larynx and trachea.

laryngoxerosis (-ze-ro′sis) dryness of the throat.

larynx (lar′inks) air passage between the pharynx and trachea, containing the vocal cords.

laser (la′zer) a device which produces an extremely intense, small and nearly nondivergent beam of monochromatic radiation in the visible region, with all the waves in phase.

latency (la′ten-se) the state of being latent.

latent (la′tent) dormant or concealed; not manifest.

laterad (lat′er-ad) toward the lateral aspect.

lateral (lat′er-al) pertaining to or situated at the side.

lateralis (lat″er-a′lis) [L.] lateral.

laterality (-al′ĭ-te) a tendency to use preferentially the organs (hand, foot, ear, eye) of the same side in voluntary motor acts. **crossed l.,** the preferential use of heterolateral members of the different pairs of organs in voluntary motor acts, e.g. right eye and left hand. **dominant l.,** the preferential use of ipsilateral members of the different pairs of organs in voluntary motor acts, e.g. right (dextrality) or left (sinistrality) ear, eye, hand and leg.

lateroflexion (lat″er-o-flek′shun) flexion to one side.

lateroversion (-ver′zhun) abnormal turning to one side.

latex (la′teks) a viscid, milky juice secreted by some seed plants.

lathyrism (lath′ĭ-rizm) a morbid condition following ingestion of seeds of plants of the genus Lathyrus. adj., **lathyrit′ic.**

lathyrogenic (lath″ĭ-ro-jen′ik) causing symptoms similar to those of lathyrism.

latissimus (lah-tis''ĭ-mus) [L.] widest.

latrodectism (lat''ro-dek'tizm) intoxication due to venom of spiders of the genus Latrodectus.

latus (la'tus) [L.] 1. broad, wide. 2. the side or flank.

laugh (laf) the movement of facial muscles and utterance of vocal sounds, usually expressive of amusement. **sardonic l.**, risus sardonicus.

Lauron (law'ron) trademark for a preparation of aurothioglycanide.

lavage (lah-vahzh') a washing out or irrigation. **intestinal l.**, vividialysis by instillation and withdrawal of a rinsing fluid in the intestine for the removal, through the intestinal mucosa, of elements not being excreted by the kidneys. **peritoneal l.**, vividialysis by instillation and withdrawal of a rinsing fluid in the peritoneal cavity.

Lavema (lah-ve'mah) trademark for preparations of oxyphenisatin.

law (law) a uniform or constant fact or principle. **all-or-none l.**, the heart muscle, under whatever stimulus, will contract to the fullest extent or not at all. **Allen's l.**, the more carbohydrate a diabetic takes, the less he utilizes. **l's of articulation**, a set of rules formulated by R. L. Hanau, to be followed in arranging teeth to produce a balanced articulation. **Avogadro's l.**, equal volumes of perfect gases at the same temperature and pressure contain the same number of molecules. **Behring's l.**, blood and serum of an immunized person when transferred to another subject will render the latter immune. **Bell's l.**, anterior roots of spinal nerves are motor, posterior roots sensory. **Berthollet's l.**, if two salts in solution by double decomposition can produce a salt less soluble than either, such a salt will be produced. **biogenetic l.**, ontogeny is a recapitulation of phylogeny. **Boyle's l.**, at a constant temperature the volume of a perfect gas varies inversely as the pressure, and the pressure varies inversely as the volume. **Charles's l.**, at a constant pressure the volume of a given mass of a perfect gas varies directly with the absolute temperature. **Colles's l.**, a child affected with congenital syphilis, the mother showing no signs of the disease, will not infect the mother. **Dalton's l.**, the pressure exerted by a mixture of nonreacting gases is equal to the sum of the partial pressures of the separate components. **Donders's l.**, the rotation of the eye around the line of sight is not voluntary. **Fechner's l.**, the sensation produced by a stimulus varies as the logarithm of the stimulus. **Galton's l.**, each parent contributes, on an average, one fourth, or $(0.5)^2$, of an individual's heritage, each grandparent one sixteenth, or $(0.5)^4$, and so on, the occupier of each ancestral place in the nth degree contributing $(0.5)^{2n}$ of the heritage. **Gay-Lussac's l.**, Charles's law. **Graham's l.**, the rate of diffusion of a gas through porous membranes varies inversely with the square root of its density. **Henry's l.**, the solubility of a gas in a liquid solution is proportionate to the partial pressure of the gas. **Hellin's l.**, one in about 80 pregnancies ends in the birth of twins; one in about 6400, of triplets; one in about 512,000, of quadruplets. **Hilton's l.**, a nerve trunk which supplies any given joint also supplies the muscles which move the joint and the skin over the insertion of such muscles. **l. of independent assortment**, the members of gene pairs segregate independently during miosis. **Koch's l.**, the specificity of a given organism requires the fulfilment of the following conditions: 1, the microorganism is present in every case of the disease; 2, it is to be cultivated in pure culture; 3, inoculation of such culture must produce the disease in susceptible animals; 4, it must be obtained from such animals, and again grown in a pure culture. **Listing's l.**, when the eyeball is moved from a resting position, the rotational angle in the second position is the same as if the eye were turned about a fixed axis perpendicular to the first and second positions of the visual line. **Malthusian l.**, the hypothesis that the human population tends to outrun the means available to sustain it. **Mariotte's l.**, Boyle's law. **Mendel's l.**, **mendelian l.**, offspring are not intermediate in type between the two parents, but the type of one or the other is predominant according to a fixed ratio. **Minot's l.**, organisms age fastest when young. **Müller-Haeckel l.**, biogenetic law. **Nernst's l.**, the current required to stimulate a muscle varies as the square root of its frequency. **Nysten's l.**, rigor mortis affects first the muscles of mastication, next those of the face and neck, then those of the trunk and arms, and last those of the legs and feet. **Ohm's l.**, strength of an electric current varies directly as the electromotive force and inversely as the resistance. **Profeta's l.**, a nonsyphilitic child born of syphilitic parents is immune. **psychophysical l.**, Weber-Fechner law. **Rault's l.**, 1. (for freezing points) the depression of the freezing point for the same type of electrolyte dissolved in a given solvent is proportional to the molecular concentration of the solute. 2. (for vapor pressures) a, the vapor pressure of a volatile substance from a liquid solution is equal to the mole fraction of that substance times its vapor pressure in the pure state. b, when a nonvolatile nonelectrolyte is dissolved in a solvent, the decrease in vapor pressure of that solvent is equal to the mole fraction of the solute times the vapor pressure of the pure solvent. **l. of retaliation**, the principle of retribution in kind, i.e. an "eye for an eye and a tooth for a tooth." **Ritter-Valli l.**, the primary increase and secondary loss of irritability in a nerve produced by a section which separates it from the nerve center, travel in a peripheral direction. **l. of sines**, the sine of the angle of incidence is equal to the sine of the angle of reflection multiplied by a constant quantity. **Tait's l.**, exploratory laparotomy should be performed in every case of abdominal or pelvic disease ruining health or endangering life, except when it is known to be malignant. **Talbot's l.**, when complete fusion occurs and the sensation is uniform, the intensity is the same as it would be were the same amount of light spread uniformly over the disk. **van't Hoff's l.**, the velocity of chemical reactions is increased twofold or more for each rise of 10 degrees in temperature. **Weber's l.**, the variation of stimulus which causes the smallest appreciable change in sensation maintains an approximately fixed ratio to the whole stimulus. **Weber-Fechner l.**, for a sensation to increase by arithmetical progression, the stimulus must increase by geometrical progression. **Wolff's l.**, all changes in the form and function of bones are attended by definite changes in their internal structure.

lawrencium (law-ren'se-um) chemical element (*see table*), at. no. 103, symbol Lw.

laxative (lak'sah-tiv) 1. mildly cathartic. 2. an agent that acts mildly to promote defecation. **bulk l.**, an agent that increases evacuation of the bowel by increasing the volume of the intestinal contents.

laxator (lak-sa'tor) that which slackens or relaxes.

laxoin (lak'so-in) phenolphthalein.

layer (la'er) a stratum of nearly uniform thickness. **ameloblastic l.**, the inner layer of cells of the enamel organ, which forms the enamel prisms. **bacillary l.**, the rod and cone layer of the retina. **Bernard's glandular l.**, the stratum of cells lining the acini of the pancreas. **blastodermic l.**, germ layer. **columnar l.**, 1. layer of rods and cones. 2. mantle layer. **compact l.**, stratum compactum. **cortical l.**, the cortex of an organ, as of the brain or ovary. **cuticular l.**, a striate border of modified cytoplasm at the free end of some columnar cells. **enamel l.**, the outermost layer of cells of the enamel organ. **ganglionic l.**, a stratum of angular cells in the cerebral cortex. **germ l.**, one of the three primary layers of cells formed in the early development of the embryo: ectoderm, entoderm and mesoderm. **half-value l.**, that thickness of a filter (copper or aluminum) which will reduce the original intensity of a roentgen-ray beam by half. **Haller's l.**, the portion of the vascular layer of the choroid made up of large vessels. **Henle's l.**, the outermost layer of the inner root sheath of the hair follicle. **horny l.**, stratum corneum. **Langhans' l.**, cytotrophoblast. **malpighian l.**, the deep part of the epidermis. **mantle l.**, the middle layer of the wall of the primitive neural tube, containing primitive nerve cells and later forming the gray substance of the central nervous system. **nerve fiber l.**, a layer of the retina between the ganglion cell layer and the internal limiting membrane. **nervous l.**, all of the retina except the pigment layer; the inner layer of the optic cup. **neuroepidermal l.**, ectoblast. **odontoblastic l.**, the epithelioid layer of odontoblasts in contact with the dentin of teeth. **Oehl's l.**, stratum corneum. **osteogenetic l.**, the innermost layer of the periosteum. **palisade l.**, the basal layer of the stratum mucosum. **prickle cell l.**, stratum spinosum. **Rauber's l.**, the external layer of flat cells covering the ectoderm of the blastodermic vesicle at an early stage. **l. of rods and cones**, a layer of the retina immediately beneath the pigment epithelium, between it and external limiting membrane, containing the rods and cones. **subendocardial l.**, the layer

of loose fibrous tissue uniting the endocardium and myocardium. **trophic l., vegetative l.**, entoderm.

lb. [L.] *li'bra* (pound).

L.D. lethal dose; light difference (difference in light perception between the two eyes).

L.D.$_{50}$ median lethal dose.

LDH lactic dehydrogenase.

L.E. left eye; lupus erythematosus.

lead[1] (led) chemical element (*see table*), at. no. 82, symbol Pb. **l. acetate**, $C_4H_6O_4Pb.3H_2O$; irritant and astringent. **black l.**, graphite. **l. monoxide**, PbO; used in preparations for local application. **sugar of l.**, lead acetate.

lead[2] (lēd) a specific array (pair) of electrodes used in recording changes in electric potential, created by activity of an organ, such as the heart (electrocardiography) or brain (electroencephalography); applied also to the particular segment of the tracing produced by the potential registered through the specific electrodes; in electrocardiography lead I records the potential differences between the two arms, lead II between the right arm and left leg, lead III between the left arm and left leg, and lead V from various sites of the precordium. **bipolar l.**, an array involving two electrodes which experience significant variations in potential. **esophageal l.**, difference in potential recorded with one electrode inserted in the esophagus. **limb l's**, differences in potential recorded with electrodes placed on the arms and left leg. **precordial l's**, leads recording electric potential from various sites of the precordium, designated V with subscript numeral indicating exact site: V_1, fourth intercostal space immediately to right of sternum; V_2, fourth intercostal space immediately to left of sternum; V_3, midway between V_2 and V_4; V_4, fifth intercostal space in midclavicular line; V_5, left anterior axillary line at same horizontal level as V_4; V_6, left midaxillary line at same horizontal level as V_4 and V_5. **unipolar l.**, an array of two electrodes, only one of which experiences considerable potential variation.

lechopyra (lek"o-pi'rah) puerperal fever.

lecithin (les'i-thin) a phospholipid consisting of glycerophosphoric acid esters of oleic, stearic or other fatty acid combined with choline, found in many animal tissues and plants.

lecithinase (les'ī-thin-ās) an enzyme which splits up lecithin.

lecitho- (les'ī-tho) word element [Gr.] denoting relationship to the yolk of an egg or ovum.

lecithoblast (les'ī-tho-blast") the primitive entoderm of a two-layered blastodisk.

lectin (lek'tin) a term applied to hemagglutinating substances extracted from certain plant seeds.

L.E.D. lupus erythematosus disseminatus.

Ledercillin (led"er-sil'lin) trademark for preparations of penicillin G procaine.

leech (lēch) an aquatic annelid, *Hirudo medicinalis*, formerly used for drawing blood. **artificial l., Heurteloup's l.**, a cupping glass or other apparatus for drawing blood by suction.

leeching (lēch'ing) 1. the application of a leech for the withdrawal of blood. 2. leeches.

left-handedness (left-hand'ed-nes) preferential or more skillful use of the left hand than the right hand in voluntary motor acts.

leg (leg) the lower extremity, especially the part between knee and ankle. **Anglesey l.,** a jointed artificial leg. **baker's l.,** knock-knee, or genu valgum. **bandy l.,** genu varum. **Barbados l.,** elephantiasis. **bayonet l.,** ankylosis of the knee after backward displacement of the tibia and fibula. **black l.,** symptomatic anthrax. **bow l.,** genu varum. **deck l's,** edema of lower legs occurring in passengers aboard ship in the tropics. **elephant l.,** elephantiasis. **milk l.,** phlegmasia alba dolens. **scissor l.,** deformity with crossing of the legs. **tropical l's,** deck legs.

Legio (le'je-o) a genus of viruses (order Virales, suborder Zoophagineae, family Erronaceae) proposed to include the viruses of the poliomyelitis group.

legumin (lē-gu'min) a globulin characteristically found in the seeds of leguminous plants.

leiodermia (li″o-der'me-ah) abnormal smoothness and glossiness of the skin.

leiomyoma (-mi-o'mah) myoma of the nonstriated muscle fibers.

leiomyosarcoma (-mi″o-sar-ko'mah) a sarcoma containing cells of unstriped muscle.

leiphemia (li-fe'me-ah) thinness of the blood.

Leishmania (lēsh-ma'ne-ah) a genus of protozoan organisms, including L. brasiliensis, the cause of American leishmaniasis, L. donovani, the cause of kala-azar, and L. tropica, the cause of cutaneous leishmaniasis. **L. cani'num,** a species infecting dogs and children in the Mediterranean basin. **L. infan'tum,** a species found in children in China.

leishmaniasis (lēsh″mah-ni'ah-sis) any disease due to infection with Leishmania. **American l.,** infection of the mucous membranes of the nose and throat by L. brasiliensis. **cutaneous l.,** chronic ulcerative granuloma caused by L. tropica. **visceral l.,** kala-azar.

lemic (le'mik) pertaining to an epidemic disease, as the plague.

lemmoblastic (lem″o-blas'tik) developing into neurilemma tissue.

lemmoblastoma (-blas-to'mah) spongioblastoma.

lemmocyte (lem'o-sit) a cell which develops into a neurilemma cell.

lemniscus (lem-nis'kus), pl. lemnis'ci [L.] a band or ribbon-like structure, applied especially to collections of nerve fibers in the central nervous system.

lemography (le-mog'rah-fe) a treatise on the plague or on epidemic diseases.

lemology (le-mol'o-je) the study of epidemic disease, especially the plague.

length (length) the distance between two extremities or poles. **basialveolar l.,** the distance from the basion to the lower end of the intermaxillary suture. **basinasal l.,** the distance from the basion to the center of the suture between the frontal and nasal bones. **crown-heel l.,** the distance from the crown of the head to the heel in embryos, fetuses and infants; the equivalent of standing height in older subjects. **crown-rump l.,** the distance from the crown of the head to the breech in embryos, fetuses and infants; the equivalent of sitting height in older subjects. **dental l.,** the distance between the mesial surface of the first premolar and the distal surface of the third molar of the upper jaw. **focal l.,** the distance between a lens and an object from which all rays of light are brought to a focus.

lens (lenz) 1. a glass for refracting light. 2. the transparent, biconvex body separating the posterior chamber and vitreous body, and constituting part of the refracting mechanism of the eye. **achromatic l.,** a lens corrected for chromatic aberration. **acrylic l.,** an artificial lens of methacrylate, sometimes used as a prosthesis after removal of the crystalline lens of the eye. **apochromatic l.,** one corrected for chromatic and spheric aberration. **artificial l.,** one made of appropriate material, to be inserted in the eyeball after removal of the natural lens. **biconcave l.,** one concave on both faces. **biconvex l.,** one convex on both faces. **bifocal l.,** one made up of two segments, the upper for far vision and the lower for near vision. **concave l.,** dispersing lens. **concavoconcave l.,** biconcave lens. **contact l.,** a thin, curved shell of glass or plastic that is applied directly to the cornea to correct refractive errors. **converging l.,** **convex l.,** one which focuses light. **convexoconcave l.,** one which has one convex and one concave face. **crystalline l.,** the transparent lenticular organ behind the pupil of the eye. **cylindrical l.,** one which has one surface plane and another concave or convex. **decentered l.,** one in which the visual line does not pass through the center. **dispersing l.,** one which disperses light. **omnifocal l.,** a spectacle lens whose power increases regularly in a downward direction, avoiding the discontinuity in field and power inherent in bifocal and trifocal lenses. **orthoscopic l.,** one which gives a flat and undistorted field of vision. **periscopic l.,** a concavoconvex or concavoconcave lens. **prosthetic l.,** artificial lens. **spectacle l.,** one that is held in an appropriate frame before the eyes to correct refractive errors and improve vision. **spherical l.,** one which has a surface which is the segment of a sphere. **Stokes's l's,** apparatus used in diagnosis of astigmatism. **trial l's,** lenses used in determining visual acuity. **trifocal l.,** one made up of three segments, the upper for distant, the middle for intermediate, and the lower for near vision.

lentectomize (len-tek'to-mīz) to deprive of the crystalline lens by surgical excision.

lentectomy (-tek'to-me) excision of the lens of the eye.

lenticonus (len″ti-ko'nus) a conical protrusion of the substance of the lens of the eye.

lenticular (len-tik'u-ler) having the form of a lens.

lenticulostriate (len-tik″u-lo-stri'āt) pertaining to lenticular nucleus and corpus striatum.

lentiform (len'tĭ-fôrm) lens-shaped.

lentigines (len-tij'ĭ-nēz) plural of *lentigo*.

lentiginosis (len-tij"ĭ-no'sis) a condition marked by multiple lentigines.

lentiglobus (len"tĭ-glo'bus) exaggerated curvature of the lens of the eye, producing a spherical bulging.

lentigo (len-ti'go), pl. *lentig'ines* [L.] a brownish pigmented spot on the skin due to increased deposition of melanin and an increased number of melanocytes. **l. malig'na,** a specialized type that tends to become malignant.

lentitis (len-ti'tis) inflammation of the eye lens.

lentoptosis (len"to-to'sis) hernia of the lens of the eye.

leontiasis (le"on-ti'ah-sis) form of leprosy with lion-like expression about the face.

leotropic (le"o-trop'ik) running spirally from right to left.

leper (lep'er) a patient with leprosy; the term is officially disapproved of.

lepidic (lĕ-pid'ik) pertaining to, or made up of, scales.

lepidosis (lep"ĭ-do'sis) a scaly eruption.

lepocyte (lep'o-sīt) a nucleated cell having a cell wall.

lepothrix (lep'o-thriks) a condition in which the hairs become covered with scales.

lepra (lep'rah) leprosy; prior to about 1850, psoriasis.

leprid (lep'rid) cutaneous lesion or lesions of tuberculoid leprosy: hypopigmented or erythematous macules or plaques, lacking bacilli.

leprology (lep-rol'o-je) the study of leprosy.

leproma (lep-ro'mah) a superficial granulomatous nodule, rich in bacilli, the characteristic lesion of lepromatous leprosy.

lepromin (lep'ro-min) a repeatedly boiled, autoclaved, gauze-filtered suspension of finely ground lepromatous tissue devised for performing the skin test for tissue resistance to leprosy.

leprosarium (lep"ro-sa're-um) a hospital or colony for treatment and isolation of patients with leprosy.

leprosy (lep'ro-se) a chronic communicable disease due to an acid-fast bacillus, *Mycobacterium leprae*, and characterized by the production of granulomatous lesions of the skin, upper respiratory and ocular mucous membranes, peripheral nerves and the testes, and small, subclinical granulomas throughout the reticuloendothelial system. adj., **lep'rous. Asturian l.,** pellagra. **borderline l.,** an unstable form in which the lesions are inflammatory and granulomatous and often present concentric annular formations or mimic lepromas, with many bacilli. **cutaneous l.,** lepromatous leprosy. **dimorphous l.,** indeterminate or borderline leprosy. **indeterminate l.,** an unstable form with hypopigmented or erythematous macules, often with a few bacilli in the tissue. **Italian l.,** pellagra. **lazarine l.,** properly, the pure, diffuse, leproma-less variant of lepromatous leprosy; loosely, any bullous and ulcerating lesion of leprosy. **lepromatous l.,** that form in which bacilli are abundant from the beginning, nerve damage occurs only slowly, and the skin

reaction to lepromin is negative; the only form which may regularly serve as a source of infection. **Lombardy l.,** pellagra. **macular l., maculoanesthetic l.,** tuberculoid leprosy with hypopigmented macular skin lesions. **neural l.,** tuberculoid leprosy. **nodular l.,** lepromatous leprosy. **reactional l.,** leprosy during one of the recurring phases of acute exacerbation of lesions, accompanied in the lepromatous form by fever and often erythema multiforme. **trophoneurotic l.,** leprosy lesions due to the effects of denervation of tissues by leprous neuritis. **tuberculoid l.,** the "polar" type of leprosy in which bacilli are few or lacking by ordinary methods of examination and nerve damage occurs early; the patient is only rarely a source of infection to others.

leptazol (lep'tah-zol) pentylenetetrazol.

lepto- (lep'to) word element [Gr.], *slender; thin*.

leptocephalus (lep"to-sef'ah-lus) fetus with a very small head.

leptochromatic (-kro-mat'ik) having a fine chromatin network.

leptocyte (lep'to-sīt) an erythrocyte characterized by a hemoglobinated border surrounding a clear area containing a center of pigment.

leptocytosis (lep"to-si-to'sis) leptocytes in the blood.

leptodactyly (-dak'tĭ-le) abnormal slenderness of the digits. adj., **leptodac'tylous.**

leptodermic (-der'mik) having a thin skin.

leptomeninges (-mē-nin'jēz) the two more delicate components of the meninges: the pia mater and arachnoid.

leptomeningitis (-men"in-ji'tis) inflammation of the leptomeninges.

leptomeningopathy (-men"ing-gop'ah-the) any disease of the leptomeninges.

leptopellic (-pel'ik) having a narrow pelvis.

leptophonia (-fo'ne-ah) weakness or feebleness of the voice. adj., **leptophon'ic.**

leptorrhine (lep'to-rīn) having a nasal index below 48.

leptoscope (lep'to-skōp) an apparatus by which the thickness and composition of an extremely thin layer or membrane can be determined.

Leptospira (lep"to-spi'rah) a genus of Schizomycetes (order Spriochaetales, family Treponemataceae) pathogenic for man and other mammals.

leptospire (lep'to-spīr) an individual organism of the genus Leptospira.

leptospirosis (lep"to-spi-ro'sis) infection with Leptospira.

leptostaphyline (-staf'ĭ-līn) having a high, narrow palate.

leptothricosis (-thrĭ-ko'sis) leptotrichosis.

Leptothrix (lep'to-thriks) a genus of Schizomycetes (order Chlamydobacteriales, family Chlamydobacteriaceae) usually found in fresh water.

leptotrichosis (lep"to-trĭ-ko'sis) infection with Leptothrix.

Leritine (ler'ĭ-tēn) trademark for preparations of anileridine.

lesbianism (lez'be-ah-nizm") homosexual behavior in the female.

lesion (le'zhun) a site of structural or functional change in body tissues produced by disease or injury. **central l.**, a lesion present in the central nervous system. **discharging l.**, a brain lesion attended with sudden liberation of energy. **focal l.**, a lesion of small area and definite limits. **Ghon's l.**, a bean-shaped shadow in the roentgenogram of the lung of children with pulmonary tuberculosis. **primary l's**, the original lesions manifesting a disease.

lethal (le'thal) deadly; fatal.

lethargy (leth'ar-je) stupor, or coma, resulting from disease or hypnosis. **African l.**, African trypanosomiasis.

leucine (lu'sēn) a naturally occurring amino acid, one of those essential for human metabolism.

leucinuria (lu″sin-u're-ah) leucine in the urine.

leucismus (lu-siz'mus) whiteness. **l. pilo'rum**, an abnormal streak or spot of white hairs among the hair of the scalp.

leucitis (lu-si'tis) scleritis.

leuco- (lu'ko) for words beginning thus, see also those beginning *leuko-*.

Leuconostoc (lu″ko-nos'tok) a genus of Schizomycetes (order Eubacteriales, family Lactobacillaceae, tribe Streptococceae) found in milk and fruit juices. **L. citrovo'rum**, an organism found in milk and milk products, frequently used in the study of nutritional requirements in bacteria.

leucovorin (-vo'rin) a derivative of folic acid; used in megaloblastic anemia.

leuko(o)- (lu'ko) word element [Gr.], *white.*

leukapheresis (lu″kah-fē-re'sis) the selective removal of leukocytes from withdrawn blood, which is then retransfused into the patient.

leukasmus (lu-kaz'mus) leukoderma.

leukemia (lu-ke'me-ah) fatal disease, with marked increase in number of leukocytes. adj , **leuke'mic. aleukemic l.**, leukemia in which the leukocyte count is normal or below normal. **aplastic l.**, leukemia with diminution of red and white cells and an increase of the proportion of large, atypical leukocytes. **basophilic l., basophilocytic l.**, leukemia in which many basophilic granulocytes (mast cells) are present in the blood. **embryonal l.**, stem cell leukemia. **eosinophilic l.**, leukemia in which eosinophils are the predominating cells. **granulocytic l.**, myelocytic leukemia. **histiocytic l.**, monocytic leukemia. **leukopenic l.**, aleukemic leukemia. **lymphatic l., lymphoblastic l., lymphocytic l., lymphogenous l., lymphoid l.**, leukemia associated with hyperplasia and overactivity of the lymphoid tissue, in which the leukocytes are lymphocytes or lymphoblasts. **lymphosarcoma cell l.**, a form of lymphocytic or lymphoblastic lymphoma characterized by the presence of neoplastic lymphocytes in the peripheral blood. **megakaryocytic l.**, hemorrhagic thrombocythemia. **monocytic l.**, leukemia in which the predominating leukocytes are monocytes. **myeloblastic l.**, leukemia in which myeloblasts predominate. **myelocytic l., myelogenous l., myeloid granulocytic l.**, leukemia arising from myeloid tissue in which the granular polymorphonuclear leukocytes predominate. **stem cell l.**, leukemia in which the predominating cell is so immature and primitive that its classification is difficult. **subleukemic l.**, aleukemic leukemia.

leukemid (lu-ke'mid) a nonspecific skin lesion of leukemia which does not represent cutaneous infiltrations with leukemic cells.

leukemogen (lu-ke'mo-jen) any substance which produces leukemia. adj., **leukemogen'ic.**

leukemoid (lu-ke'moid) exhibiting blood and sometimes clinical findings resembling those of true leukemia.

leukencephalitis (lūk″en-sef″ah-li'tis) inflammation of the white matter of the brain.

leukergy (lu'ker-je) appearance in blood of peculiar leukocytes characterized by adhesiveness and tendency to agglomerate; a defense mechanism in infections and other forms of stress. adj., **leuker'gic.**

leuko-agglutinin (lu″ko-ah-gloo'ti-nin) an agglutinin which acts upon leukocytes.

leukoblast (lu'ko-blast) an immature leukocyte. **granular l.**, premyelocyte.

leukoblastosis (lu″ko-blas-to'sis) proliferation of immature leukocytes.

leukocidin (-si'din) a substance destructive to leukocytes.

leukocyte (lu'ko-sīt) a colorless blood corpuscle capable of ameboid movement, whose chief function is to protect the body against microorganisms causing disease and which may be one of five types: lymphocytes, monocytes, neutrophils, eosinophils and basophils. adj., **leukocyt'ic. agranular l's, nongranular l's, lymphoid l's** (agranulocytes or lymphocytes), 1. lymphocytes with a round, chromatic nucleus. 2. monocytes with a nucleus indented at the poles. **granular l's** (granulocytes), 3. polymorphonuclear or polynuclear neutrophil leukocytes (heterophil leukocytes) with an irregularly lobed nucleus. 4. eosinophil leukocytes with a bilobed nucleus. 5. basophil leukocytes with a bent lobed nucleus. **hyaline l.**, monocyte. **leukergic l's**, leukocytes that appear in the blood in leukergy. **mast l.**, the basophil of the circulating blood. **transitional l.**, monocyte.

leukocythemia (lu″ko-si-the'me ah) leukemia.

leukocytoblast (-si'to-blast) a cell which develops into a leukocyte.

leukocytogenesis (si″to-jen'ē-sis) the formation of leukocytes.

leukocytology (-si tol'o-je) the study of leukocytes.

leukocytolysin (-si-tol'ĭ-sin) a lysin which destroys leukocytes.

leukocytolysis (-si-tol'ĭ-sis) disintegration of leukocytes. adj., **leukocytolyt'ic.**

leukocytoma (-si-to'mah) tumor-like mass of leukocytes.

leukocytopenia (-si″to-pe'ne-ah) leukopenia.

leukocytophagy (-si-tof'ah-je) ingestion and destruction of leukocytes by cells of the reticuloendothelial system.

leukocytoplania (-si″to-pla'ne-ah) wandering of leukocytes; passage of leukocytes through a membrane.

leukocytopoiesis (-poi-e'sis) the formation of leukocytes.

leukocytosis (lu″ko-si-to′sis) increase in number of leukocytes in the blood. **mononuclear l.,** mononucleosis. **pathologic l.,** that due to some morbid reaction, e.g. infection or trauma.

leukocytotaxis (-si″to-tak′sis) leukotaxis.

leukocytotoxin (-tok′sin) a toxin which destroys leukocytes.

leukocytotropic (-trop′ik) having a selective affinity for leukocytes.

leukocyturia (lu″ko-si-tu′re-ah) leukocytes in the urine.

leukoderma (-der′mah) an acquired condition with localized loss of pigmentation of the skin. **l. acquisi′tum centrif′ugum,** depigmentation of the skin around a pigmented nevus.

leukoedema (-ĕ-de′mah) an abnormality of buccal mucosa, consisting of an increase in thickness of the epithelium, with intracellular edema of the spinous or malpighian layer.

leukoencephalopathy (-en-sef″ah-lop′ah-the) disease of the white substance of the brain.

leukogram (lu′ko-gram) tabulation of different types of leukocytes in a blood specimen.

leukokeratosis (lu″ko-ker″ah-to′sis) leukoplakia.

leukokinesis (-ki-ne′sis) the movement of the leukocytes within the circulatory system. adj., **leukokinet′ic.**

leukokinetics (-ki-net′iks) study of the production, circulation and destruction of leukocytes in the body.

leukokoria (-ko′re-ah) appearance of a whitish reflex or mass in the pupillary area behind the lens.

leukokraurosis (-kraw-ro′sis) kraurosis vulvae.

leukolymphosarcoma (-lim″fo-sar-ko′mah) lymphosarcoma cell leukemia.

leukolysin (lu-kol′ĭ-sin) leukocytolysin.

leukolysis (lu-kol′ĭ-sis) leukocytolysis.

leukoma (lu-ko′mah) 1. white corneal opacity. 2. leukosarcoma. adj., **leukom′atous. l. adhae′rens,** a white tumor of the cornea enclosing a prolapsed adherent iris.

leukomaine (lu′ko-mān) an alkaloid derived from living animal tissue.

leukomyelitis (lu″ko-mi″ĕ-li′tis) inflammation of white substance of the brain or spinal cord.

leukomyelopathy (-mi″ĕ-lop′ah-the) disease of the white matter of the spinal cord.

leukomyoma (-mi-o′mah) lipomyoma.

leukon (lu′kon) the leukocytes and leukocyte-forming tissues of the body.

leukonuclein (lu″ko-nu′kle-in) nuclein from digested leukocytes.

leukonychia (-nik′e-ah) abnormal whiteness of the nails, either total or in spots or streaks.

leukopathia (-path′e-ah) leukoderma. **l. un′-guium,** leukonychia.

leukopedesis (-pĕ-de′sis) diapedesis of leukocytes.

leukopenia (-pe′ne-ah) deficiency in number of leukocytes in the blood. adj., **leukope′nic. malignant l., pernicious l.,** agranulocytosis.

leukophagocytosis (-fag″o-si-to′sis) leukocytophagy.

leukophlegmasia (-fleg-ma′ze-ah) phlegmasia alba dolens.

leukoplakia (lu″ko-pla′ke-ah) white patches on mucous membrane, a precancerous condition.

leukoplasia (-pla′ze-ah) leukoplakia.

leukoplastid (-plas′tid) any one of the white granules of plant cells whence the starch-forming elements are formed.

leukopoiesis (-poi-e′sis) the production of leukocytes. adj., **leukopoiet′ic.**

leukoprecipitin (-pre-sip′ĭ-tin) a precipitin specific for leukocytes.

leukoprotease (-pro′te-ās) an enzyme in the leukocytes which splits up protein.

leukopsin (lu-kop′sin) a visual white derived from rhodopsin by bleaching on exposure to light.

leukorrhagia (lu″ko-ra′je-ah) profuse leukorrhea.

leukorrhea (-re′ah) a whitish discharge from the vagina.

leukosarcoma (-sar-ko′mah) an uncolored or colorless sarcoma.

leukosis (lu-ko′sis) proliferation of leukocyte-forming tissue. **avian l., fowl l.,** a neoplastic disease chiefly affecting chickens, but found occasionally in other birds and thought to be of viral origin.

leukotaxis (lu″ko-tak′sis) cytotaxis of leukocytes; the tendency of leukocytes to collect in regions of injury and inflammation.

Leukothrix (lu′ko-thriks) a genus of Schizomycetes (order Beggiatoales, family Leukotrichaceae).

leukothrombin (lu″ko-throm′bin) a fibrin factor formed by leukocytes in the blood.

leukotomy (lu-kot′o-me) incision of the white matter of the frontal lobe of the brain.

leukotoxic (lu″ko-tok′sik) destructive to leukocytes.

leukotoxicity (-tok-sis′ĭ-te) toxicity for leukocytes.

leukotoxin (-tok′sin) a toxin which destroys leukocytes.

Leukotrichaceae (-tri-ka′se-e) a family of Schizomycetes (order Beggiatoales).

leukotrichia (-trik′e-ah) whiteness of the hair.

leuko-urobilin (-u″ro-bi′lin) a transformation product of urobilin found in colorless stools.

levallorphan (lev″al-lor′fan) a compound used as an antagonist to narcotics.

levarterenol (lev″ar-tĕ-re′nol) norepinephrine. **l. bitartrate,** a compound used as a sympathomimetic and as a pressor agent.

levator (lĕ-va′tor), pl. *levato′res* [L.] that which lifts or elevates.

levigation (lev″ĭ-ga′shun) the grinding of moist substances.

levo- (le′vo) word element [L.], *left.*

levocardia (le″vo-kar′de-ah) location of the heart in the left hemithorax, with the apex pointing to the left, associated with transposition of the abdominal viscera, congenital structural anomaly of the heart and usually with absence of the spleen.

Levo-dromoran (dro′mo-ran) trademark for preparations of levorphanol tartrate.

levoduction (-duk′shun) movement of an eye to the left.

levogram (le′vo-gram) an electrocardiographic tracing showing left axis deviation, indicative of left ventricular hypertrophy.

levogyration (le″vo-ji-ra′shun) rotation to the left.

levogyrous (-ji′rus) levorotatory.

levonordefrin (-nor′dĕ-frin) a compound used as a vasoconstrictor.

Levophed (lev′o-fed) trademark for a preparation of levarterenol.

levophobia (le″vo-fo′be-ah) fear of objects on the left side of the body.

levopropoxyphene (-pro-pok′sĭ-fēn) a compound used as an antitussive.

levorotation (-ro-ta′shun) a turning to the left.

levorotatory (-ro′tah-to″re) turning the plane of polarization to the left.

levorphanol (lēv-or′fah-nol) a compound used as a narcotic analgesic.

levothyroxine (le″vo-thi-rok′sin) the levorotatory isomer of thyroxine. **sodium l.,** the sodium salt of levothyroxine.

levotorsion (-tor′shun) a twisting toward the left.

levoversion (-ver′zhun) a turning toward the left.

levulose (lev′u-lōs) a sugar, $C_6H_{12}O_6$, from fruits, honey and the intestines.

leydigarche (li″dig-ar′ke) establishment or beginning of gonadal function in the male.

L.F.A. left frontoanterior (position of the fetus).

L.F.P. left frontoposterior (position of the fetus).

L.H. luteinizing hormone.

Li chemical symbol, *lithium.*

libido (lĭ-bi′do) instinctual energy or drive, often used with special reference to the motive power of the sex life.

libra (li′brah) [L.] 1. pound. 2. balance.

Librium (lib′re-um) trademark for preparations of chlordiazepoxide.

licentiate (li-sen′she-āt) one holding a license entitling him to practice a particular profession.

lichen (li′ken) 1. an individual organism formed by the intimate combination of an alga and a fungus; usually placed in a separate taxonomic category, a separate class of the phylum Eumycophyta. 2. papular skin disease of many kinds. **l. al′bus,** lichen sclerosus et atrophicus. **l. amyloido′sus,** a condition characterized by localized cutaneous amyloidosis. **l. annula′ris,** granuloma annulare. **l. chron′icus sim′plex,** localized neurodermatitis. **l. fibromucinoido′sus,** lichen myxedematosus. **l. lepro′sus,** a manifestation of lepromatous leprosy, with lichenoid papules appearing in groups. **l. myxedemato′sus,** a skin condition characterized by abnormal deposits of mucin and widespread eruption of soft, pale red or yellowish papules. **l. nit′idus,** a rare skin disease with small, usually flat, sharply margined papules scarcely raised above the level of the skin, pale red or yellowish brown. **l. pila′ris,** lichen spinulosus. **l. planopila′ris,** a variant of lichen planus characterized by formation of acuminate horny papules around the hair follicles, in addition to the typical lesions of ordinary lichen planus. **l. pla′nus,** an inflammatory skin disease with wide flat papules, often in circumscribed patches. **l. pla′nus et acu-**

mina′tus atroph′icans, cicatricial alopecia with an eruption of follicular spinous papules. **l. ru′ber monilifor′mis,** a variant of lichen simplex chronicus. **l. ru′ber pla′nus,** lichen planus. **l. sclero′sus et atroph′icus,** a skin disorder characterized by cicatricial alopecia and papules. **l. scrofulo′sus,** a form consisting of reddish papules, peculiar to persons of a tuberculous diathesis. **l. sim′plex chron′icus,** localized neurodermatitis. **l. spinulo′sus,** a condition in which there is a horn or spine in the center of each hair follicle. **l. stria′tus,** a condition characterized by a linear lichenoid eruption, usually in children. **l. trop′icus,** miliaria. **l. urtica′tus,** papular urticaria.

lichenification (li-ken″ĭ-fi-ka′shun) thickening and hardening of the skin.

lichenoid (li′kĕ-noid) resembling lichen.

licorice (lik′or-is) glycyrrhiza.

lidocaine (li′do-kān) a compound used as a local anesthetic.

lien (li′en) [L.] spleen. adj., **lie′nal. l. accesso′rius,** an accessory spleen. **l. mo′bilis,** an abnormally movable spleen.

lien(o)- (li-e′no) word element [L.], *spleen.*

lienectomy (li″en-ek′to-me) excision of the spleen.

lienitis (li″en-i′tis) splenitis.

lienocele (li-e′no-sēl) hernia of the spleen.

lienography (li″ĕ-nog′rah-fe) roentgen examination of the spleen.

lienomalacia (li-e″no-mah-la′she-ah) softening of the spleen.

lienomedullary (-med′u-ler″e) pertaining to spleen and bone marrow.

lienomyelogenous (-mi″e-loj′ĕ-nus) originating in spleen and bone marrow.

lienomyelomalacia (-mi″ĕ-lo-mah-la′she-ah) softening of spleen and bone marrow.

lienopancreatic (-pan″kre-at′ik) pertaining to spleen and pancreas.

lienopathy (li″ĕ-nop′ah-the) any disease of the spleen.

lienorenal (li″ĕ-no-re′nal) pertaining to spleen and kidney.

lienotoxin (-tok′sin) splenotoxin.

lientery (li′en-ter″e) diarrhea with passage of undigested food. adj., **lienter′ic.**

lienunculus (li″en ung′ku-lus) a detached mass of splenic tissue; an accessory spleen.

L.I.F. left iliac fossa.

ligament (lig′ah-ment) a tough band connecting bones or supporting viscera. adj., **ligamen′tous. accessory l.,** one which strengthens or supplements another. **adipose l.,** the mucous ligament of the knee. **alar l's,** the two folds of synovial membrane on either side of the adipose ligament. **alveolodental l.,** periodontium. **appendiculo-ovarian l.,** a fold of mesentery extending between the appendix and the broad ligament. **arcuate l's,** the arched ligaments which connect the diaphragm with the lowest ribs and the first lumbar vertebra. **Bardinet's l.,** the posterior portion of the annular ligament of the elbow. **Barkow's l.,** anterior and posterior ligaments of elbow joint. **Bérard's l.,** suspensory ligament of pericardium. **Bertin's l., Bigelow's**

l., the iliofemoral ligament. **broad l.**, a broad fold of peritoneum extending from the side of the uterus to the wall of the pelvis; it consists of three parts: supporting the uterus (mesometrium), uterine tube (mesosalpinx) and ovary (mesovarium). **Brodie's l.**, the transverse humeral ligament. **Burns's l.**, the falciform process of the fascia lata. **Campbell's l.**, suspensory ligament of axilla. **Camper's l.**, the deep perineal fascia. **capsular l.**, the tough fibrous framework surrounding every joint. **Carcassonne's l.**, triangular ligament of urethra. **cardinal l.**, part of a thickening of the visceral pelvic fascia beside the cervix and vagina, passing laterally to merge with the upper fascia of the pelvic diaphragm. **central l.**, filum terminale. **costopericardiac l.**, a ligament joining the upper costosternal articulation with the pericardium. **cotyloid l.**, a ring of fibrocartilage connected with the rim of the acetabulum. **cruciform l.**, the transverse ligament of the atlantoaxoid joint. **crural l.**, Poupart's ligament. **cutaneophalangeal l's**, ligamentous fibers from the sides of the phalanges near the joints to the skin. **cysticoduodenal l.**, an anomalous fold of peritoneum extending between the gallbladder and the duodenum. **deltoid l.**, the internal lateral ligament of the ankle joint. **diaphragmatic l.**, the involuting urogenital ridge that becomes the suspensory ligament of the ovary. **falciform l.**, the broad ligament of the liver. **false l.**, any suspensory ligament that is a peritoneal fold and not of true ligamentous structure. **Flood's l.**, the superior glenohumeral ligament. **Gimbernat's l.**, triangular expanse of the aponeurosis of the external oblique muscle, anteriorly joined to Poupart's ligament, and going to the iliopectineal line. **glenoid l.**, 1. a ring of fibrocartilage connected with the rim of the glenoid fossa. 2. the anterior ligaments of the metacarpophalangeal joints. **Helmholtz's l.**, part of the anterior ligament of the malleus. **hepatic l's**, folds of peritoneum extending from the liver to adjacent structures. **Hey's l's**, a falciform expansion of the fascia lata. **iliotrochanteric l.**, a portion of the articular capsule of the hip joint. **interarticular l.**, any ligament situated within the capsule of a joint. **interprocess l.**, a ligament that connects two processes on the same bone. **lienorenal l.**, a fold of peritoneum connecting the spleen and the left kidney. **mesenteriomesocolic l.**, mesenteriomesocolic fold. **nephrocolic l.**, fasciculi from the fatty capsule of the kidney passing down on the right side to the posterior wall of the ascending colon and on the left side to the posterior wall of the descending colon. **pancreaticosplenic l.**, a fold of peritoneum extending from the pancreas to the spleen. **Petit's l.**, uterosacral ligament. **Poupart's l.**, lower border of aponeurosis of external oblique muscle between anterior spine of ilium and the spine of the pubis. **reinforcing l's**, ligaments that serve to reinforce joint capsules. **rhomboid l.**, ligament connecting cartilage of the first rib to under surface of clavicle. **round l.**, 1. a broad

ligament arising from the fatty cushion of the acetabulum and inserted on the head of the femur. 2. a fibrous cord from the navel to anterior border of liver. 3. either of two cords from cornua of uterus to the mons veneris. **Schlemm's l's**, two ligamentous bands of the capsule of the shoulder joint. **spring l.**, the ligament joining the calcaneus and navicular bone. **subflavous l.**, a yellowish ligament between the laminae of a vertebra. **suspensory l.**, Zinn's zonule. **suspensory l. of axilla**, a layer ascending from the axillary fascia and ensheathing the pectoralis minor muscle. **sutural l.**, a band of fibrous tissue between the opposed bones of a suture or immovable joint. **synovial l.**, a large synovial fold. **tendinotrochanteric l.**, a portion of the capsule of the hip joint. **uteropelvic l's**, expansions of muscular tissue in the broad ligament of the uterus, radiating from the fascia over the obturator internus to the side of the uterus and the vagina. **uterosacral l.**, a part of the thickening of the visceral pelvic fascia beside the cervix and vagina. **ventricular l.**, a false vocal cord. **vesicoumbilical l.**, urachus. **vesicouterine l.**, a ligament that extends from the anterior aspect of the uterus to the bladder. **vocal l's**, the true vocal cords. **Y l.**, 1. part of the capsular ligament of the hip joint. 2. a ligament of the ankle connecting the calcaneus, and cuboid and navicular bones. **Zinn's l.**, Zinn's zonule.

ligamentopexy (lig″ah-men′to-pek″se) fixation of the uterus by shortening the ligaments supporting it.

ligamentum (lig″ah-men′tum), pl. *ligamen'ta* [L.] ligament.

ligase (li′gās) an enzyme that catalyzes the joining together of two molecules.

ligation (li-ga′shun) application of a ligature.

ligature (lig′ah-tūr) 1. material such as thread or wire, used for tying a part. 2. a constricting band or knot. **provisional l.**, a constricting band applied at the beginning of an operation, but removed before its close.

light (līt) a form of radiant energy capable of stimulating the special sense organ and giving rise to the sensation of sight. **axial l., central l.**, light whose rays are parallel to each other and to optic axis. **diffused l.**, light whose rays have been scattered by reflection and refraction. **Finsen l.**, sunlight passed through a lens containing a solution of copper sulfate in ammonia, which absorbs the yellow, red and infra-red rays, leaving the violet; used in treatment of lupus. **Minin l.**, a lamp for therapeutic administration of ultraviolet light. **oblique l.**, light falling obliquely on a surface. **polarized l.**, light of which the vibrations are made over one plane or in circles or ellipses. **reflected l.**, light whose rays have bent out of their original course by passing through a transparent medium. **transmitted l.**, light which passes or has passed through an object. **white l.**, that produced by a mixture of all wavelengths of electromagnetic energy perceptible as light. **Wood l.**, see under *filter*.

lightening (līt′en-ing) descent of the uterus into the pelvic cavity, two or three weeks before labor begins.

lignocaine (lig'no-kān) lidocaine.

ligula (lig'u-lah) a strip of white substance near the lateral border of the fourth ventricle.

limb (lim) 1. an arm or leg, including all its component parts. 2. a structure or part resembling an arm or leg. **anacrotic l.**, the ascending portion of a tracing of the pulse wave obtained by sphygmography. **catacrotic l.**, the descending portion of a tracing of the pulse wave obtained by sphygmography. **pectoral l.**, the arm, or a homologous part. **pelvic l.**, the leg, or a homologous part. **phantom l.**, a model of an absent part of an arm or leg, subjectively perceived as real and active. **thoracic l.**, pectoral limb.

limberneck (lim'ber-nek) a disease of fowl due to ingestion of food contaminated with *Clostridium botulinum*, and characterized by a flaccid paralysis.

limbic (lim'bik) pertaining to a limbus, or margin.

limbus (lim'bus), pl. *lim'bi* [L.] an edge or border; used in anatomic nomenclature to designate the edge of the cornea, where it joins the sclera (*lim'bus cor'neae*), and other margins in the body. **1. conjuncti'vae**, the edge of conjunctiva overlapping the margin of the cornea. **l. cor'neae**, the edge of the cornea where it joins the sclera. **l. lam'inae spira'-lis**, crista spiralis. **l. lu'teus**, macula lutea.

lime (līm) 1. calcium oxide, a compound occurring in hard white or grayish white masses or granules, or as a white or grayish white powder. 2. the acid fruit of *Citrus aurantifolia*. **l. arsenate**, a solution of white arsenic and soda in water, used as an insecticide. **chlorinated l.**, white or grayish granular powder with odor of chlorine; used as a decontaminant. **slaked l.**, calcium hydroxide. **soda l.**, a mixture of calcium hydroxide with sodium or potassium hydroxide; used to absorb exhaled carbon dioxide. **sulfurated l.**, a preparation of lime and sublimed sulfur, used in solution in acute acne vulgaris.

limen (li'men), pl. *lim'ina* [L.] a threshold or boundary. **l. na'si**, the upper limit of the vestibule of the nose. **l. of two-ness**, the distance between two points of contact on the skin necessary for their recognition as giving rise to separate stimuli.

liminal (lim'ĭ-nal) barely perceptible; pertaining to a threshold.

limitans (lim'ĭ-tanz) [L.] limiting.

limitation (lim"ĭ-ta'shun) the act of limiting or the quality of being limited. **eccentric l.**, a circumscribed condition of the visual field, greater at some parts of the periphery than at others. **genetic l.**, the necessity that all cells react in accordance with the standards of the particular species to which they belong.

limosis (li-mo'sis) extreme or abnormal hunger.

limp (limp) 1. without normal tonus or turgor. 2. a defect of walking characterized by uneven distribution of weight on or unequal length of the two extremities. **protective l.**, one adopted as a means of avoiding pain due to walking in the normal way.

lincomycin (lin'ko-mi''sin) an antibiotic with a narrow antimicrobial spectrum, useful in certain staphylococcal infections in patients sensitive to penicillin.

lindane (lin'dān) a compound used in treatment of scabies and pediculosis, and to rid animals of ectoparasites.

line (līn) a stripe, streak, mark or narrow ridge; often an imaginary line connecting different anatomic landmarks (linea). adj., **lin'ear**. **abdominal l's**, lines on abdomen, indicating the boundaries of muscles. **absorption l's**, dark lines in the spectrum due to absorption of light by the substance through which the light has passed. **alveobasilar l.**, from nasion to alveolar point. **alveolonasal l.**, from alveolar to nasal point. **angular l.**, an irregular, jagged line dividing the anterior surface of the iris into two regions. **anocutaneous l.**, pectinate line. **auriculobregmatic l.**, from auricular point to bregma. **base l.**, from infraorbital ridge to external auditory meatus and to middle line of occiput. **basinasal l.**, from the basion to the nasion. **basiobregmatic l.**, from basion to bregma. **Beau's l's**, transverse lines on the fingernails, seen after wasting disease. **biauricular l.**, from one auditory meatus over the vertex to the other. **bi-iliac l.**, one joining the most prominent points of the iliac crests. **blood l.**, a line of direct descent through several generations. **blue l.**, characteristic line on gums showing chronic lead poisoning. **cement l.**, a line visible in microscopic examination of bone in cross section, marking the boundary of an osteon (haversian system). **cervical l.**, an anatomic landmark determined by the junction of the enamel- and cementum-covered portions of a tooth (cementoenamel junction). **cleavage l's**, linear clefts in the skin indicative of direction of the fibers. **costoarticular l.**, from sternoclavicular joint to point of eleventh rib. **costoclavicular l.**, line midway from nipple line and border of sternum. **dentate l.**, pectinate line. **facial l.**, a straight line connecting the nasion and pogonion. **Fraunhofer's l's**, dark lines on the solar spectrum. **Frommann's l's**, black lines produced on axons by silver nitrate. **genal l.**, one of Jadelot's lines, from malar surface to nasal line. **gingival l.**, 1. a line determined by the level to which the gingiva extends on a tooth. 2. any linear mark visible on the surface of the gingiva. **gum l.**, gingival line (1). **heave l.**, a groove along the costal arch coincidental with forced contraction of the abdominal muscles after the normal passive expiratory movement in an animal with heaves. **Hensen's l.**, a light line in the middle of the dark band of a sarcomere. **Hilton's white l.**, pectinate line. **iliopectineal l.**, ridge on ilium and pubes showing the brim of the true pelvis. **incremental l's**, lines supposedly showing the successive layers deposited in a tissue. **intertrochanteric l's** (anterior and posterior), traces on anterior and posterior surfaces of femur between the trochanters. **isothermal l's,** lines on a map or chart indicating areas of uniform temperature. **Jadelot's l's,** lines of the face in young children, considered indicative of disease. **Krause's l.,** a line passing through white bands of a muscle fibril. **Langer's l's,** cleavage lines. **lead l.,** a bluish line at the edge of the gums in lead poisoning. **lip l.,** a line at the level to which the margin of either lip extends on the teeth. **magnetic l's of force,** lines indicating the direction of magnetic force in a magnetic field. **mammary l.,** 1. a line from one nipple to the other. 2. milk line. **median l.,** a vertical line dividing the body equally into right and left parts. **milk l.,** the line of thickened epithelium in the embryo along which the mammary glands are developed. **mylohyoid l.,** a ridge on inner surface of lower jaw. **nasobasilar l.,** line through basion and nasal point. **Nélaton's l.,** from anterior superior process of ilium to most prominent part of tuberosity of ischium. **nipple l.,** mammary line. **parasternal l.,** costoclavicular line. **pectinate l.,** one marking the junction of the rectal mucosa and the skin lining the anus. **Poupart's l.,** an imaginary line on the surface of the abdomen, passing perpendicularly through the midpoint on Poupart's ligament. **primitive l.,** primitive streak. **quadrate l.,** line on posterior surface of femur. **respiratory l.,** line which connects bases of upstrokes in a sphygmogram. **Retzius' l's,** brownish lines in the enamel of a tooth. **scapular l.,** vertical downward line from lower angle of scapula. **sternal l.,** midline of sternum. **sternomastoid l.,** a line from the heads of the sternomastoid to the mastoid process. **subcostal l.,** a transverse line on the surface of the abdomen at the level of the lower edge of the tenth costal cartilage. **supraorbital l.,** line across forehead above root of external angular process of frontal bone. **trapezoid l.,** mark of attachment of trapezoid ligament to the clavicle. **triradiate l's,** the stars of the embryonic lens. **visual l.,** line from object seen through nodal point of eye to macula lutea. **white l.,** linea alba. **l's of Zahn,** laminations visible in antemortem blood clots, due to alternating layers of gray-white fibrin interspersed with narrow zones of apparent red-blue clot.

linea (lin'e-ah), pl. *lin'eae* [L.] a narrow ridge or streak on a surface, as of the body or a bone or other organ. **l. al'ba,** tendinous mesial line down the front of the belly. **lin'eae albican'-tes,** white abdominal lines seen after pregnancy. **l. as'pera,** a rough longitudinal line on the back of the femur. **lin'eae atroph'icae,** fine reddish lines on the abdomen in Cushing's syndrome. **l. cor'neae seni'lis,** a horizontal brown line on the lower part of the cornea in senile degeneration. **l. epiphysia'lis,** a line on the surface of an adult bone marking the site of junction of the epiphysis and diaphysis. **l. ni'gra,** a band of pigmentation seen on the median line of the abdomen during pregnancy. **l. splen'dens,** fibrous band down the anterior surface of the pia mater of the spinal cord.

liner (līn'er) material applied to the inside of the walls of a cavity or container for protection or insulation of the surface. **cavity l.,** a substance applied to the tooth surface exposed by caries, to protect the dentin and insulate the pulp.

lingua (ling'gwah), pl. *lin'guae* [L.] tongue. adj., **lin'gual. l. geograph'ica,** geographic tongue. **l. ni'gra,** black tongue.

linguale (ling-gwa'le) the upper end of the lingual surface of the symphysis of the lower jaw.

Linguatula (lin-gwat'u-lah) a genus of arthropods frequently parasitic in the respiratory tract and lungs of vertebrates. **L. rhina'ria,** a common parasite of livestock, sometimes parasitic in man. **L. serra'ta,** the most common species, found in cats and dogs.

lingula (ling'gu-lah), pl. *lin'gulae* [L.] a small, tonguelike structure, such as the projection from the lower portion of the upper lobe of the left lung *(lin'gula pulmo'nis sin'istra)*. **l. of sphenoid,** ridge between the body and greater wing of the sphenoid.

linguo- (ling'gwo) word element [L.], *tongue.*

linguoaxial (ling"gwo-ak'se-al) pertaining to or formed by the lingual and axial walls of a tooth cavity.

linguocervical (-ser'vĭ-kal) 1. pertaining to the lingual surface of the neck of a tooth. 2. linguogingival.

linguoclusion (-kloo'zhun) malocclusion in which the tooth is lingual to the line of the normal dental arch.

linguodistal (-dis'tal) pertaining to or formed by the lingual and distal surfaces of a tooth, or the lingual and distal walls of a tooth cavity.

linguogingival (-jin'jĭ-val) pertaining to the tongue and gingiva; pertaining to or formed by the lingual and gingival walls of a tooth cavity.

linguopapillitis (-pap"ĭ-li'tis) small painful ulcers around the papillae of the tongue.

linguoversion (-ver'zhun) displacement of a tooth lingually to the line of occlusion.

liniment (lin'ĭ-ment) a solution of an irritant drug in an oily, soapy or alcoholic vehicle, intended to be rubbed on the skin as a counter-irritant. **camphor l.,** a preparation of camphor and cottonseed oil used as a local irritant. **camphor and soap l.,** a mixture of green soap, camphor, rosemary oil, alcohol and purified water, used as a local irritant. **chloroform l.,** a mixture of chloroform with camphor and soap liniment, used as a local irritant. **medicinal soft soap l.,** a preparation of medicinal soft soap, lavender oil and alcohol; used as a detergent.

linin (li'nin) substance of the achromatic nuclear reticulum of the cell.

Liniola (li-ne'o-lah) a genus of Schizomycetes (order Caryophanales, family Caryophanaceae).

linitis (lī-ni'tis) inflammation of gastric cellular tissue. **plastic l.,** linitis resulting in hypertrophy of the connective tissue around the stomach.

linkage (lingk'ij) an existing connection; in genetics, the relation between genes located on a single chromosome, which are ordinarily transmitted as a group.

linked (linkt) united; in genetics, referring to characters which are united so as invariably to be inherited together.

linseed (lin'sēd) dried ripe seed of *Linum usitatissimum;* used as a protective.

liothyronine (li″o-thī'ro-nēn) levorotatory isomer of triiodothyronine; used in treatment of hypothyroidism. **sodium l.,** sodium salt of triiodothyronine, used in thyroid replacement therapy.

lip (lip) 1. the upper or lower fleshy margin of the mouth. 2. a marginal part. **cleft l.,** harelip. **double l.,** redundancy on the submucous tissue and mucous membrane of the lip on either side of the median line. **Hapsburg l.,** a thick, overdeveloped lower lip that often accompanies a Hapsburg jaw.

lip(o)- (lip'o) word element [Gr.], *fat; lipid.*

lipacidemia (lip″as-ĭ-de'me-ah) fatty acid in the blood.

lipaciduria (-du're-ah) fatty acid in the urine.

liparomphalus (lip″ah-rom'fah-lus) fatty tumor of the navel.

liparthritis (li″par-thri'tis) arthritis caused by cessation of ovarian function.

lipase (li'pās, lip'ās) an enzyme which catalyzes the decomposition of fats into glycerol and fatty acids.

lipectomy (li-pek'to-me) excision of fatty tissue or of a lipoma.

lipedema (lip″ē-de'mah) an accumulation of excess fat and fluid in subcutaneous tissues.

lipemia (li-pe'me-ah) fat or oil in the blood. **alimentary l.,** that occurring after ingestion of food. **l. retina'lis,** a high level of lipids in the blood, manifested by a milky appearance of the veins and arteries of the retina.

lipfanogen (lip-fan'o-jen) a substance that produces visible fat.

lipid (lip'id) one of a group of naturally occurring substances consisting of the higher fatty acids, their naturally occurring compounds, and substances found naturally in chemical association with them.

lipiduria (lip″i-du're-ah) the presence of lipids in the urine.

lipo-arthritis (lip″o-ar thri'tis) inflammation of fatty tissue of the joints.

lipo-atrophia (-ah-tro'fe-ah) atrophy of fatty tissues of the body.

lipoblast (lip'o-blast) a connective tissue cell which develops into a fat cell.

lipoblastoma (lip″o-blas-to'mah) lipoma.

lipocaic (-ka'ik) a substance extracted from pancreas which prevents deposit of fat in the liver after pancreatectomy.

lipocardiac (-kar'de-ak) pertaining to fatty degeneration of the heart.

lipocatabolic (-kat″ah-bol'ik) pertaining to the catabolism of fat.

lipochondrodystrophy (-kon″dro-dis'tro-fe) abnormal endochondral ossification due to defective metabolism of polysaccharides, as observed in Hurler's syndrome.

lipochondroma (-kon-dro'mah) a chondroma containing fatty elements.

lipochrome (lip'o-krōm) a yellow-brown, granu-

lar pigment containing small amounts of lipid, thought to be a metabolic waste product.

lipoclasis (li-pok'lah-sis) lipolysis. adj., **lipoclas'tic.**

lipocorticoid (lip″o-kor'tĭ-koid) a corticoid effective in causing deposition of fat, especially in the liver.

lipocyte (lip'o-sīt) a fat cell.

lipodieresis (lip″o-di-er'ĕ-sis) the splitting or destruction of fat. adj., **lipodieret'ic.**

lipodystrophy (-dis'tro-fe) disturbance of fat metabolism. **intestinal l.,** a condition marked by deposits of fats in the intestinal lymphatic tissue, with fatty diarrhea, arthritis and loss of weight.

lipofibroma (-fi-bro'mah) lipoma with fibrous elements.

lipofuscin (-fus'in) a brown pigment similar to melanin, found in various organs in brown atrophy and in nerve cells of senile persons.

lipogenesis (-jen'ĕ-sis) the formation of fat. adj., **lipogenet'ic.**

lipogenic (-jen'ik) producing fat or fatness.

lipoid (lip'oid) 1. fatlike. 2. lipid.

lipoidemia (lip″oi-de'me-ah) lipids in the blood.

lipoidosis (-do'sis) lipids in a tissue.

lipoiduria (-du're-ah) lipids in the urine.

lipolipoidosis (lip″o-lip″oi-do'sis) both fats and lipids in a tissue.

Lipo-lutin (li″po-lu'tin) trademark for preparations of progesterone.

lipolysis (li-pol'ĭ-sis) the splitting up of fat. adj., **lipolyt'ic.**

lipoma (li-po'mah) a fatty tumor.

lipomatosis (lip″o-mah-to'sis) 1. excessive fat in the tissues. 2. the presence of lipomas. adj., **lipomatous.**

lipomatous (li-po'mah-tus) affected with lipoma.

lipomeria (li″po-me're-ah) congenital absence of a limb.

lipometabolism (lip″o-mĕ-tab'o-lizm) metabolism of fat. adj., **lipometabol'ic.**

lipomicron (-mi'kron) a microscopic fat particle in the blood.

lipomyxoma (-mik-so'mah) lipoma with myxomatous elements.

liponephrosis (-ne-fro'sis) lipoid nephrosis.

lipopenia (-pe'ne-ah) diminution of the fats in the blood.

lipopeptid (-pep'tid) a compound of an amino acid and a fatty acid.

lipopexia (-pek'se-ah) accumulation of fat in the tissues. adj., **lipopec'tic.**

lipophage (lip'o-fāj) a cell which absorbs or ingests fat.

lipophagia (lip″o-fa'je-ah) 1. destruction of fat. 2. eating of fat. adj., **lipopha'gic. l. granulomato'sis,** intestinal lipodystrophy.

lipophagy (li-pof'ah-je) lipophagia.

lipophil (lip'o-fil) an element which has an affinity for fat.

lipophilia (lip″o-fil'e-ah) affinity for fat. adj., **lipophil'ic.**

lipophore (lip'o-for) xanthophore.

lipophrenia (li″po-fre'ne-ah) failure of mental powers.

lipoprotein (-pro'te-in) a combination of a

lipid and a protein, having the general properties (e.g. solubility) of proteins.

liposarcoma (lip″o-sar-ko′mah) sarcoma containing fatty elements.

liposin (li-po′sin) a fat-splitting enzyme in the blood.

liposis (li-po′sis) lipomatosis.

liposoluble (lip″o-sol′u-bl) soluble in fats.

liposome (lip′o-sōm) one of the particles of lipoid matter held emulsified in the tissues in the form of invisible foci.

lipothymia (li″po-thi′me-ah) syncope.

lipotrophy (li-pot′ro-fe) increase of bodily fat. adj., **lipotroph′ic.**

lipotropism (li-pot′ro-pizm) affinity for fat or fatty tissue, especially that of certain agents that are capable of decreasing the deposits of fat in the liver. adj., **lipotrop′ic.**

lipotrophy (li-pot′ro-pe) lipotropism. adj., **lipotrop′ic.**

lipovaccine (lip″o-vak′sēn) a vaccine in a vegetable oil vehicle.

lipoxeny (li-pok′sē-ne) desertion of the host by a parasite.

lipoxidemia (lip″ok-sī-de′me-ah) lipacidemia.

lipping (lip′ing) development of a bony lip in osteoarthritis.

lip reading (lip′rēd-ing) perception of speech through the sense of sight, by recognition of the words formed from movement of the lips.

lipsotrichia (lip″so-trik′e-ah) falling of the hair.

lipuria (li-pu′re-ah) fat or oil in the urine.

Liquaemin (lik′wah-min) trademark for preparations of heparin.

Liquamar (lik′wah-mar) trademark for a preparation of phenprocoumon.

liquefacient (lik″wĕ-fa′shent) 1. producing or pertaining to liquefaction. 2. an agent that produces liquefaction.

liquefaction (-fak′shun) conversion into a liquid form.

liquescent (li-kwes′ent) tending to become liquid or fluid.

liquor (lik′er, li′kwor) 1. a liquid. 2. a solution of nonvolatile substance in water. **l. am′nii,** amniotic fluid. **l. cotun′nii,** perilymph. **l. follic′uli,** the fluid in the cavity of a developing graafian follicle. **Morgagni's l.,** fluid between the eye lens and its capsule. **mother l.,** the liquid remaining after removal of crystals from a solution. **l. pu′ris,** the more liquid or sanious portion of pus. **l. san′guinis,** the fluid portion of the blood. **l. scar′pae,** endolymph.

Lissencephala (lis″en-sef′ah-lah) a group of placental mammals characterized by having a brain that is smooth or marked by only a few shallow gyri.

lissencephalia (-sē-fa′le-ah) absence of gyri on the surface of the brain. adj., **lissencephal′ic.**

lissive (lis′iv) relieving muscle spasm without interfering with function.

Listerella (lis-ter-el′ah) Listeria.

Listeria (lis-te′re-ah) a genus of Schizomycetes (order Eubacteriales, family Corynebacteriaceae).

listeriosis (lis-tēr″e-o′sis) infection due to organisms of the genus Listeria.

listerism (lis′ter-izm) the principles and practice of antiseptic and aseptic surgery.

liter (le′ter) the basic unit of capacity of the metric system, the equivalent of 1.0567 quarts liquid measure.

lith(o)- (lith′o) word element [Gr.], *stone; calculus.*

lithagogue (lith′ah-gog) 1. expelling calculi. 2. an agent which expels calculi.

lithectasy (li-thek′tah-se) removal of calculi by perineal incision.

lithectomy (li-thek′to-me) lithotomy.

lithemia (li-the′me-ah) excess of uric acid in the blood.

lithiasis (li-thi′ah-sis) the formation of concretions in any hollow structure of the body.

lithium (lith′e-um) chemical element (*see table*), at. no. 3, symbol Li. **l. bromide,** pinkish white granular powder; sedative hypnotic.

lithocenosis (lith″o-se-no′sis) litholapaxy.

lithoclast (lith′o-klast) an instrument for crushing calculi.

lithocystotomy (lith″o-sis-tot′o-me) incision of the bladder for removal of stone.

lithodialysis (-di-al′i-sis) the dissolution or crushing of a calculus.

lithogenesis (-jen′ē-sis) formation of calculi.

litholapaxy (li-thol′ah-pak′se) the crushing of a stone in the bladder and washing out of the fragments.

lithology (li-thol′o-je) the scientific study of calculi.

litholysis (li-thol′i-sis) dissolution of calculi.

lithometra (lith″o-me′trah) ossification of the uterus.

lithonephrotomy (-ne-frot′o-me) excision of a renal calculus.

lithopedion (-pe′de-on) a stony or petrified fetus.

lithophone (lith′o-fōn) device for detecting calculi in the bladder.

lithoscope (lith′o-skōp) instrument for detecting calculi in the bladder.

lithosis (li-tho′sis) disease of lungs from inhaling fine particles of stone.

lithosphere (lith′o-sfēr) the solid portion of the earth.

lithotomy (li-thot′o-me) incision of an organ for removal of calculi.

lithotresis (lith″o-tre′sis) the drilling or boring of holes in a calculus.

lithotripsy (lith′o-trip″se) the crushing of calculi in the body.

lithotriptic (lith′o-trip″tik) 1. dissolving vesical calculi. 2. an agent which dissolves vesical calculi.

lithotrite (lith′o-trīt) instrument for crushing calculi.

lithotrity (li-thot′ri-te) lithotripsy.

lithous (lith′us) pertaining to a calculus.

lithoxiduria (lith″ok-sī-du′re-ah) xanthic oxide in the urine.

lithuresis (lith″u-re′sis) passage of gravel in the urine.

lithuria (li-thu′re-ah) excess of uric acid or urates in the urine.

litmus (lit′mus) a stain prepared by enzymatic fermentation of coarsely powdered lichens; used as a pH indicator.

Litomosoides (lit″o-mo-soi′dēz) a genus of nematode parasites of the superfamily Filarioidea. **L. cari′nii,** a species parasitic in the pleural cavity of the cotton rat, and a worm commonly used in research laboratories as an experimental animal.

litter (lit′er) 1. a stretcher for carrying sick or wounded. 2. the offspring produced at one birth by a multiparous animal.

livedo (li-ve′do) a discolored patch on the skin. **l. annula′ris, l. racemo′sa, l. reticula′ris,** permanent mottling of the skin.

liver (liv′er) a large red gland situated in the upper part of the abdomen on the right side. **albuminoid l., amyloid l.,** one with albuminoid or amyloid degeneration. **fatty l.,** one affected with fatty degeneration and infiltration. **feuerstein l.,** a smooth cirrhotic liver seen chiefly in children with congenital syphilis. **floating l.,** wandering liver. **hobnail l.,** liver whose surface is marked with nail-like points from atrophic cirrhosis. **iron l.,** the condition of the liver in hepatic siderosis. **lardaceous l.,** amyloid liver. **wandering l.,** a displaced and movable liver. **waxy l.,** albuminoid liver.

livid (liv′id) discolored, as from a contusion or bruise.

lividity (li-vid′i-te) discoloration, as from a bruise or congestion. **postmortem l.,** livor mortis.

livor (li′vor) discoloration. **l. mor′tis,** discoloration on dependent parts of the body after death.

lixiviation (liks″iv-e-a′shun) separation of soluble from insoluble material by use of an appropriate solvent, and drawing off the solution.

L.L.L. left lower lobe.

L.M. Licentiate in Midwifery.

L.M.A. left mentoanterior (position of the fetus).

L.M.P left mentoposterior (position of the fetus).

L.O.A. left occipitoanterior (position of the fetus).

Loa (lo′ah) a genus of nematode parasites of the superfamily Filarioidea. **L. lo′a,** a species commonly found in subcutaneous tissues of man and baboons in Central and South Africa; frequently seen in the eyeball in its migration about the body.

loaiasis (lo″ah-i′ah-sis) infestation with Loa loa.

lobate (lo′bāt) divided into lobes.

lobe (lōb) a more or less well defined portion of an organ or gland. adj., **lo′bar. azygos l.,** a small accessory or anomalous lobe at the apex of the right lung. **caudate l.,** a small lobe of the liver between the inferior vena cava on the right and the left lobe. **cuneate l.,** cuneus. **frontal l.,** the rostral (anterior) portion of the cerebral hemisphere. **hepatic l.,** one of the lobes of the liver, designated the right and left and the caudate and quadrate.

linguiform l., Riedel′s lobe. **occipital l.,** the most posterior portion of the cerebral hemisphere, forming a small part of its dorsolateral surface. **parietal l.,** the upper central portion of the cerebral hemisphere, between the frontal and occipital lobes, and above the temporal lobe. **quadrate l.,** a small lobe of the liver, between the gallbladder on the right and the left lobe. **Riedel′s l.,** an anomalous tongue-shaped mass of tissue projecting from the right lobe of the liver. **spigelian l.,** caudate lobe. **temporal l.,** a long, tongue-shaped process constituting the lower lateral portion of the cerebral hemisphere.

lobectomy (lo-bek′to-me) excision of a lobe, as of the lung, brain or liver.

lobelia (lo-be′le-ah) the dried leaves and tops of Lobelia inflata, a herb with properties resembling those of nicotine.

lobitis (lo-bi′tis) inflammation of a lobe, as of the lung.

lobocyte (lo′bo-sīt) a granulocyte with a segmented nucleus.

lobopodium (lo″bo-po′de-um), pl. lobopo′dia [Gr.] a blunt pseudopodium composed of both ectoplasm and endoplasm, or of ectoplasm alone.

lobostomy (lo-bos′to-me) incision of a lobe of the lung with drainage.

lobotomy (lo-bot′o-me) cutting of nerve fibers connecting the frontal lobes of the brain with the thalamus.

lobulated (lob′u-lāt″ed) made up of lobules.

lobule (lob′ūl) a small segment or lobe, especially one of the smaller divisions making up a lobe. adj., **lob′ular. falciform l.,** cuneus.

lobulus (lob′u-lus), pl. lob′uli [L.] a lobule.

lobus (lo′bus), pl. lo′bi [L.] lobe.

localization (lo″kah-li-za′shun) limitation to a particular area. **cerebral l.,** determination of areas of the cortex involved in performance of certain functions. **germinal l.,** the location on a blastoderm of prospective organs. **selective l.,** the tendency of a microorganism to infect a specific variety of tissue.

locator (lo-ka′tor) a device for determining the site of foreign objects within the body. **electroacoustic l.,** a device which amplifies into an audible click the contact of the probe with a solid object.

lochia (lo′ke-ah) discharge from the reproductive tract occurring after childbirth. adj., **lo′chial. l. al′ba,** that of the final phase after childbirth, containing little blood, but many microorganisms and degenerating cells. **l. cruen′ta,** lochia rubra. **l. purulen′ta,** lochia alba. **l. ru′bra,** that occurring immediately after childbirth, consisting almost entirely of blood. **l. sero′sa,** that of the second phase after childbirth, containing blood and mucus and wound exudation.

lochiocolpos (lo″ke-o-kol′pos) distention of the vagina by retained lochia.

lochiometra (-me′trah) distention of the uterus by retained lochia.

lochiometritis (-me-tri′tis) puerperal metritis.

lochiopyra (-pi′rah) puerperal fever.

lochiorrhagia (-ra′je-ah) lochiorrhea.

lochiorrhea (lo″ke-o-re′ah) abnormally free lochial discharge.

lochioschesis (lo″ke-os′kĕ-sis) retention of the lochia.

lockjaw (lok′jaw) inability to open the jaws, as seen in trismus or tetanus.

locomotion (lo″ko-mo′shun) movement from one place to another. adj., **locomo′tor. brachial l.,** brachiation.

locular (lok′u-lar) containing loculi.

loculus (lok′u-lus), pl. *loc′uli* [L.] 1. a small space or cavity. 2. a local enlargement of the uterus in some mammals, containing an embryo.

locum (lo′kum) [L.] place. **l. ten′ens, l. ten′ent,** a practitioner who temporarily takes the place of another.

locus (lo′kus), pl. *lo′ci* [L.] place; in genetics, the specific site of a gene on a chromosome.

löffleria (lef-le′re-ah) presence of the diphtheria bacillus without the ordinary symptoms of diphtheria.

logadectomy (log″ah-dek′to-me) excision of a portion of the conjunctiva.

logaditis (-di′tis) inflammation of the sclera.

logagnosia (log″ag-no′ze-ah) central word defect, as aphasia.

logagraphia (log″ah-graf′e-ah) inability to express ideas in writing.

logamnesia (log″am-ne′ze-ah) sensory aphasia.

logaphasia (log″ah-fa′ze-ah) motor aphasia.

logasthenia (log″as-the′ne-ah) disturbance of the mental processes necessary to speech.

logogram (log′o-gram) the graphic record of the symptoms and signs exhibited by a patient, charted by means of the logoscope.

logoklony (log′o-klon″e) spasmodic repetition of the end-syllables of words.

logokophosis (log″o-ko-fo′sis) word deafness.

logomania (-ma′ne-ah) talkative manic-depressive psychosis.

logoneurosis (-nu-ro′sis) any neurosis with speech disorder.

logopathy (log-op′ah-the) any disorder of speech due to derangement of the central nervous system.

logopedia (log″o-pe′de-ah) logopedics.

logopedics (-pe′diks) the study and treatment of speech defects.

logoplegia (-ple′je-ah) 1. any paralysis of speech organs. 2. inability to speak, while words are remembered.

logorrhea (-re′ah) excessive or abnormal volubility.

logoscope (log′o-skōp) a device in slide-rule form designed to facilitate identification of the diseases in which certain signs and symptoms occur.

logoscopy (lo-gos′ko-pe) the use of a logoscope for determining the differential diagnostic possibilities in a case exhibiting certain signs and symptoms.

logospasm (log′o-spazm) the spasmodic utterance of words.

-logy word element [Gr.], *science; treatise; sum of knowledge in a particular subject.*

loin (loin) part of back between thorax and pelvis.

Lomotil (lo′mo-til) trademark for preparations of diphenoxylate hydrochloride.

longiradiate (lon″jī-ra′de-āt) having long radiations.

longissimus (lon-jis′ī-mus) [L.] longest.

longitudinalis (lon″jī-tu″dī-na′lis) [L.] lengthwise.

longus (long′gus) [L.] long.

loop (lōōp) a turn or sharp curve in a cordlike structure. **capillary l′s,** minute endothelial tubes that carry blood in the papillae of the skin. **Henle's l.,** the U-shaped loop of the uriniferous tubule of the kidney.

L.O.P. left occipitoposterior (position of the fetus).

lophotrichous (lo-fot′rī-kus) having a tuft of flagella at one end; said of microorganisms.

lordoma (lor-do′mah) lordosis.

lordoscoliosis (lor″do-sko″le-o′sis) lordosis complicated with scoliosis.

lordosis (lor-do′sis) abnormally increased concavity in the curvature of the lumbar spine.

Lorfan (lor′fan) trademark for preparations of levallorphan.

lotio (lo′she-o) [L.] lotion. **l. al′ba, l. sulfura′ta,** white lotion.

lotion (lo′shun) a liquid suspension or dispersion for external application to the body. **benzyl benzoate l.,** a preparation of benzyl benzoate, triethanolamine, oleic acid and water. **calamine l.,** a mixture of calamine, zinc oxide, glycerin, bentonite magma and calcium hydroxide solution. **calamine l., phenolated,** calamine lotion with liquefied phenol added. **hydrocortisone l.,** hydrocortisone in an aqueous vehicle for topical application. **white l.,** a preparation of zinc sulfate and sulfurated potash in purified water; astringent and protectant.

Lotusate (lo′tu-sāt) trademark for a preparation of talbutal.

louse (lows), pl. *lice* [L.] a small wingless insect. **body l.,** *Pediculus humanus* var. *corporis.* **chicken l.,** *Dermanyssus.* **clothes l.,** *Pediculus humanus* var. *corporis.* **crab l.,** *Phthirus pubis.* **head l.,** *Pediculus humanus* var. *capitis.* **horse l.,** *Trichodectes pilosus.*

loxoscelism (lok-sos′sĕ-lizm) poisoning due to the bite of a spider of the genus Loxosceles.

loxotic (lok-sot′ik) slanting.

loxotomy (lok-sot′o-me) oblique amputation.

lozenge (loz′enj) a medicated troche.

L.P.N. Licensed Practical Nurse.

L.R.C.P. Licentiate of Royal College of Physicians.

L.R.C.S. Licentiate of Royal College of Surgeons.

L.S.A. left sacroanterior (position of the fetus).

L.Sc.A. left scapuloanterior (position of the fetus).

L.Sc.P. left scapuloposterior (position of the fetus).

LSD a compound (lysergic acid diethylamide) derived from ergot and having consciousness-expanding (hallucinogenic or psychotomimetic) effects.

L.S.P. left sacroposterior (position of the fetus).

L.S.T. left sacrotransverse (position of the fetus).

LTH luteotropic hormone.

Lu chemical symbol, *lutetium.*

lubb (lub) a syllable used to express the first sound of the heart in auscultation, a dull, prolonged, low sound.

lubb-dupp (lub'dup) syllables used to express the two sounds which mark a complete heart cycle in auscultation.

luciferase (lu-sif'er-ās) an enzyme that catalyzes the bioluminescent reaction in certain animals capable of luminescence.

luciferin (lu-sif'er-in) a heat-stable compound which, when acted on by an enzyme (luciferase), produces bioluminescence.

lucifugal (lu-sif'u-gal) repelled by bright light.

lucipetal (lu-sip'ĕ-tal) attracted by bright light.

lues (lu'ēz) syphilis. adj., **luet'ic.**

L.U.L. left upper lobe.

Lullamin (lul'ah-min) trademark for a preparation of methapyrilene.

lumbo(o)- (lum'bo) word element [L.], *loin.*

lumbago (lum-ba'go) rheumatic pain in the lumbar region.

lumbar (lum'bar) pertaining to the loins.

lumbarization (lum"bar-i za'shun) coalescence of the first sacral vertebra with the transverse processes of the fifth lumbar vertebra.

lumbocostal (lum"bo-kos'tal) pertaining to loin and ribs.

lumbodynia (-din'e-ah) lumbago.

lumboinguinal (-ing'gwi-nal) pertaining to loin and groin.

lumbosacral (-sa'kral) pertaining to the lumbar and sacral region, or to the lumbar vertebrae and sacrum.

lumbricide (lum'bri-sīd) an agent which destroys lumbrici.

lumbricosis (lum"bri-ko'sis) infection with worms.

Lumbricus (lum-bri'kus), pl. *lumbri'ci* [L.] 1. the earthworm. 2. ascaris. adj., **lum'bricoid.**

lumbus (lum'bus) [L.] loin.

lumen (lu'men), pl. *lu'mina* [L.] 1. the cavity or channel within a tube or tubular organ. 2. the unit of light flux, also known as *meter candle.* **residual l.,** the remains of Rathke's pouch, between the pars distalis and pars intermedia of the hypophysis.

luminal (lu'mi-nal) pertaining to a lumen.

luminescence (lu"mi-nes'ens) the property of giving off light.

luminophore (lu"mi-no-fōr") a chemical group which gives the property of luminescence to organic compounds.

lunate (lu'nāt) 1. moon-shaped or crescentic. 2. the lunate (semilunar) bone.

lung (lung) either of the pair of thoracic organs which serve for the aeration of the blood. **coalminer's l.,** anthracosis. **farmer's l.,** a morbid condition due to inhalation of moldy hay dust. **iron l.,** a mechanical device for maintaining artificial respiration for long periods of time. **white l.,** white pneumonia.

lungworm (lung'werm) a worm parasitic in the air passages of animals, including various species of roundworms and one of flatworms.

lunula (lu'nu-lah), pl. *lu'nulae* [L.] a small, crescentic or moon-shaped area or structure, e.g. the white area at the base of the nail of a finger or toe, or one of the segments of the valve guarding the opening of the heart into the aorta or the pulmonary trunk.

lupiform (lu'pĭ-form) 1. resembling lupus. 2. resembling a wen.

lupus (lu'pus) tuberculosis of the skin marked by the formation of brownish nodules on the corium; called also *lupus vulgaris.* adj., **lu'pous. l. erythemato'sus,** inflammation of the skin with disklike patches having raised reddish edges and depressed centers and covered with scales or crusts which exfoliate, leaving dull white cicatrices. **l. erythemato'-sus dissemina'tus, disseminated l. erythemato'sus,** an acute or subacute, remitting, febrile disease principally of young women, with widespread collagen damage in many organs and systems. **l. vulga'ris,** lupus.

lusus (lu'sus) [L.] a game, sport. **l. natu'rae,** a sport or freak of nature; a minor congenital anomaly.

luteal (lu'te-al) pertaining to corpus luteum.

luteectomy (lu"te-ek'to-me) excision of the corpus luteum.

lutein (lu'te-in) a pigment found in nature. **serum l.,** a yellow coloring matter from serum.

luteinic (lu"te-in'ik) pertaining to the corpus luteum or to lutein.

luteohormone (lu"te-o-hor'mōn) progesterone.

luteoma (lu"te-o'mah) thecoma.

luteotrophic (lu"te-o-trof'ik) luteotropic.

luteotropic (-trop'ik) stimulating formation of the corpus luteum.

luteotropin (-trop'in) a hormone of the anterior pituitary gland which stimulates formation of the corpus luteum

lutetium (lu-te'she-um) chemical element (*see table*), at. no. 71, symbol Lu.

Lutocylol (lu"to-si'lol) trademark for preparations of ethisterone.

Lutrexin (lu-trek'sin) trademark for a preparation of lututrin.

Lutromone (lu'tro-mōn) trademark for a preparation of progesterone.

lututrin (loo'tu-trin) a protein or polypeptide substance from the corpus luteum of sow ovaries; used as a uterine relaxant in treatment of functional dysmenorrhea.

lux (luks) the unit of illumination, being one lumen per square meter.

luxation (luk-sa'shun) dislocation. **Malgaigne's l.,** pulled elbow.

luxus (luk'sus) [L.] excess.

Lw chemical symbol, *lawrencium.*

lyase (li'ās) an enzyme that catalyzes the removal of a group of atoms from the substrate.

lycanthropy (li-kan'thro-pe) delusion in which patient believes himself a wolf.

lycomania (li"ko-ma'ne-ah) lycanthropy.

lycopodium (-po'de-um) spores of *Lycopodium*

clavatum; used chiefly in pharmaceutical manipulations.

lying-in (li′ing-in) the puerperal state; childbed.

lymph (limf) 1. a clear, colorless fluid, derived from and closely resembling the blood, carried by an independent system of vessels, constituting the lymph system, which serves to return fluid from the tissues to the heart. 2. any clear watery liquid resembling typical lymph. **humanized l.,** vaccine virus from the human subject. **inflammatory l.,** lymph produced by inflammation, as in wounds. **Koch's l.,** tuberculin. **plastic l.,** that from which embryonic tissue is formed. **tissue l.,** lymph derived from body tissues.

lympha (lim′fah) [L.] lymph.

lymphadenectasis (lim-fad″ĕ-nek′tah-sis) dilatation of a lymph node.

lymphadenectomy (-nek′to-me) excision of a lymph node.

lymphadenia (lim″fah-de′ne-ah) overgrowth of lymphatic tissue. **l. os′sea,** multiple myeloma.

lymphadenitis (lim-fad″ĕ-ni′tis) inflammation of lymph nodes.

lymphadenocyst (lim-fad′ĕ-no-sist″) a degenerated lymph node.

lymphadenogram (lim-fad′ĕ-no-gram″) the film produced by lymphadenography.

lymphadenography (lim″fad-ĕ-nog′rah-fe) radiography of lymph nodes after injection of a contrast medium in a lymph vessel.

lymphadenoleukopoiesis (lim-fad″ĕ-no-lu″-ko-poi-e′sis) production of leukocytes by lymphatic tissues.

lymphadenoma (-no′mah) lymphoma.

lymphadenomatosis (-no-mah-to′sis) lymphomatosis.

lymphadenopathy (lim-fad″ĕ-nop′ah-the) disease of the lymph nodes. **giant follicular l.,** a disorder of the lymphatic system, with multiple proliferative follicle-like nodules occurring in the lymph nodes.

lymphadenosis (lim-fad″ĕ-no′sis) proliferation of lymphatic tissue, producing lymphatic anemia.

lymphadenotomy (lim-fad″ĕ-not′o-me) incision of a lymph node.

lymphagogue (lim′fah-gog) an agent promoting production of lymph.

lymphangiectasis (lim-fan″je-ek′tah-sis) dilatation of a lymphatic vessel.

lymphangiectomy (-ek′to-me) excision of a lesion of a lymphatic vessel.

lymphangiitis (-i′tis) lymphangitis.

lymphangioadenography (lim-fan″je-o-ad″ĕ-nog′rah-fe) lymphography.

lymphangioendothelioma (-en″do-the″le-o′-mah) endothelioma arising from lymph channels.

lymphangiofibroma (-fi-bro′mah) fibroma containing lymphangiomatous tissue.

lymphangiogram (lim-fan″je-o-gram″) the film produced by lymphangiography.

lymphangiography (lim-fan″je-og′rah-fe) radiography of lymphatic channels after introduction of a contrast medium. **pedal l.,** radiography of the lymphatic channels of the lower extremity after injection of contrast medium into the first and second interdigital spaces of the foot.

lymphangiology (lim-fan″je-ol′o-je) the scientific study of the lymphatic system.

lymphangioma (lim-fan″je-o′mah) a benign lesion of a lymphatic channel, creating well formed channels. **cavernous l.,** one in which the lymph spaces are large and cavernous.

lymphangiophlebitis (lim-fan″je-o-fle-bi′tis) inflammation of lymphatic channels and veins.

lymphangioplasty (lim-fan′je-o-plas″te) surgical restoration of lymphatic channels.

lymphangiosarcoma (lim-fan″je-o-sar-ko′-mah) lymphangioma combined with sarcoma.

lymphangiotomy (lim-fan″je-ot′o-me) incision of a lymphatic vessel.

lymphangitis (lim″fan-ji′tis) inflammation of a lymphatic vessel.

lymphatic (lim-fat′ik) 1. pertaining to lymph. 2. a lymphatic vessel.

lymphaticostomy (lim-fat″ĭ-kos′to-me) fistulization of the thoracic duct.

lymphatism (lim′fah-tizm) hyperplasia of the lymphatic organs.

lymphatitis (lim″fah-ti′tis) lymphangitis.

lymphatogenous (-toj′ĕ-nus) transmitted through lymph channels or by means of lymph.

lymphatolysin (-tol′ĭ-sin) a toxin which acts on lymphatic tissue.

lymphatolysis (-tol′ĭ-sis) destruction of lymphatic tissue. adj., **lymphatolyt′ic.**

lymphectasia (lim″fek-ta′ze-ah) distention with lymph.

lymphedema (lim″fĕ-de′mah) swelling of subcutaneous tissues due to the presence of excessive lymph fluid. **congenital l.,** Milroy's disease.

lymphemia (lim-fe′me-ah) presence of lymphocytes in blood.

lymphendothelioma (lim″fen-do-the″le-o′mah) overgrowth of the endothelium of lymphatics.

lymphenteritis (lim″fen-ter-i′tis) enteritis with serous infiltration.

lympho-adenoma (lim″fo-ad″ĕ-no′mah) a form of tumor of the uterus.

lymphoblast (lim′fo-blast) a cell of the lymphocytic series having a fine chromatin structure in the nucleus.

lymphoblastoma (lim″fo-blas-to′mah) malignant lymphoma in which the predominant cell resembles the lymphoblast.

lymphoblastomatosis (-blas″to-mah-to′sis) the condition produced by the presence of lymphoblastomas.

lymphoblastosis (-blas-to′sis) excess of lymphoblasts in the blood.

lymphocele (lim′fo-sēl) a tumor containing lymph.

lymphocyst (lim′fo-sist) lymphocele.

lymphocystosis (lim″fo-sis-to′sis) formation of cysts containing lymph.

lymphocyte (lim′fo-sīt) a variety of leukocyte that arises in reticular tissue of lymph nodes, generally described as nongranular and including small and large varieties. adj., **lymphocyt′ic.**

lymphocytoblast (lim″fo-si′to-blast) a lymphoblast.

lymphocytoma (-si-to′mah) malignant lymphoma in which the predominant cell is the mature type of lymphocyte. adj., **lymphocyto′matous.**

lymphocytopenia (-si″to-pe′ne-ah) reduction of the number of lymphocytes in the blood.

lymphocytopoiesis (-poi-e′sis) the formation of lymphocytes. adj., **lymphocytopoiet′ic.**

lymphocytorrhexis (lim″fo-si″to-rek′sis) the rupture or bursting of lymphocytes.

lymphocytosis (-si-to′sis) increase in lymphocytes in the blood.

lymphocytotoxin (-si″to-tok′sin) a toxin which destroys lymphocytes.

lymphodermia (-der′me-ah) any disease of the skin lymphatics.

lymphoduct (lim′fo-dukt) a lymphatic vessel.

lymphogenous (lim-foj′ĕ-nus) producing lymph.

lymphoglandula (lim″fo-glan′du lah) pl. *lymphoglan′dulae* [L.] a lymph node.

lymphogonia (-go′ne-ah) large lymphocytes with a large nucleus, seen in lymphatic leukemia.

lymphogram (lim′fo-gram) a roentgenogram of the lymphatic channels and lymph nodes.

lymphogranuloma (-gran″u-lo′mah) Hodgkin's disease. **l. inguina′le, venereal l., l. vene′reum,** a venereal infection due to a virus, and characterized by headache, fever and joint pains, swelling of regional lymph nodes, rectal stricture and elephantiasis of external genitalia.

lymphogranulomatosis (-gran″u-lo″mah-to′sis) 1. infectious granuloma of the lymphatic system. 2. Hodgkin's disease.

lymphography (lim-fog′rah-fe) roentgenography of the lymphatic channels and lymph nodes, after injection of radiopaque material in a lymphatic vessel.

lymphoid (lim′foid) 1. resembling lymph. 2. adenoid.

lymphoidectomy (lim″foi-dek′to-me) excision of lymphoid tissue.

lymphoidocyte (lim-foi′do-sīt) a term applied to the early form of various blood cells.

lymphokinesis (lim″fo-ki-ne′sis) movement of endolymph in the semicircular canals.

lympholeukocyte (-lu′ko-sīt) a large mononuclear leukocyte.

lymphology (lim-fol′o-je) the study of the lymphatics.

lymphoma (lim-fo′mah) 1. a primary tumor of lymphoid tissue. 2. a collection of lymph in the body, producing a tumor-like swelling or mass. **clasmocytic l.,** reticulum cell sarcoma. **giant follicular l.,** giant follicular lymphadenopathy. **granulomatous l.,** Hodgkin's disease. **lymphoblastic l.,** lymphoblastoma. **lymphocytic l.,** lymphocytoma.

lymphomatosis (lim″fo-mah-to′sis) the formation of multiple lymphomas in the body. **avian l., l. of fowl,** a group of diseases of chickens characterized by lymphomatous tumors or infiltration of various organs by lymphoid cells; it may affect the nerves, bones, viscera, or iris of the eye.

lymphomatous (lim-fo′mah-tus) pertaining to, or of the nature of, lymphoma.

lymphopathia (lim″fo-path′e-ah) lymphopathy. **l. vene′reum,** lymphogranuloma venereum.

lymphopathy (lim-fop′ah-the) any disease of the lymphatic system.

lymphopenia (lim″fo-pe′ne-ah) decrease in the lymphocytes of the blood.

lymphoplasm (lim′fo-plazm) spongioplasm.

lymphoplasmia (lim″fo-plaz′me-ah) absence of hemoglobin from red blood corpuscles.

lymphopoiesis (-poi-e′sis) the development of lymphocytes or of lymphatic tissue. adj., **lymphopoiet′ic.**

lymphoproliferative (-pro-lif′er-ah″tiv) pertaining to or characterized by proliferation of lymphoid tissue.

lymphoreticulosis (-re-tik″u-lo′sis) proliferation of the reticuloendothelial cells of the lymph nodes. **benign l.,** cat-scratch disease.

lymphorrhagia (-ra′je-ah) lymphorrhea.

lymphorrhea (-re′ah) flow of lymph from cut or ruptured lymph vessels.

lymphorrhoid (lim′fo-roid) a localized dilatation of a perianal lymph channel, resembling a hemorrhoid.

lymphosarcoma (lim″fo-sar-ko′mah) a general term applied to malignant neoplastic disorders of lymphoid tissue, but not including Hodgkin's disease.

lymphosarcomatosis (-sar″ko-mah-to′sis) a condition characterized by the presence of multiple lesions of lymphosarcoma.

lymphostasis (lim-fos′tah-sis) stoppage of lymph flow.

lymphotomy (lim-fot′o-me) the anatomy of lymphatics.

lymph-vascular (limf-vas′ku-ler) pertaining to lymphatic vessels.

Lynoral (lin′or-al) trademark for a preparation of ethinyl estradiol.

lyochrome (li′o-krōm) a cell pigment soluble in water and sensitive to light.

lyoenzyme (li′o-en′zim) an enzyme dissolved directly in the protoplasm, the extraction of which is relatively easy.

lyophil (li′o-fil) a lyophilic substance.

lyophile (li′o-fil) 1. lyophil. 2. lyophilic.

lyophilic (li″o-fil′ik) having an affinity for or stable in solution.

lyophilization (li-of″ĭ-li-za′shun) the creation of a stable preparation of a biological substance by rapid freezing and dehydration of the frozen product under high vacuum.

lyophobe (li′o-fōb) repelling liquids.

lyophobic (li″o-fo′bik) not having an affinity for or unstable in solution.

lyotropic (-trop′ik) readily soluble.

lypothymia (li″po-thi′me-ah) melancholia.

lyra (li′rah) a name applied to certain anatomic structures because of their fancied resemblance to a lute.

lysemia (li-se′me-ah) disintegration of the blood.

lysin (li′sin) a substance that causes lysis; an antibody that causes dissolution of cells or other material.

lysine (li'sēn) a naturally occurring amino acid, one of those essential for human metabolism.

lysinogen (li-sin'o-jen) a substance which produces lysins.

lysis (li'sis) 1. destruction or decomposition, as of a cell or other substance, under influence of a specific agent. 2. solution or separation, as of adhesions binding different anatomic structures. 3. gradual abatement of the symptoms of a disease. adj., **lyt'ic.**

-lysis (li'sis) word element [Gr.], *dissolution.* adj., **-lyt'ic.**

lysogen (li'so-jen) an antigen causing the formation of lysin.

lysogenesis (li″so-jen'ĕ-sis) 1. the production of lysis or lysins. 2. lysogenicity.

lysogenicity (-jĕ-nis'i-te) 1. the ability to produce lysins or cause lysis. 2. the potentiality of a bacterium to produce phage. 3. symbiosis of a bacterium with a phage.

lysogeny (li-soj'ĭ-ne) lysogenicity.

Lysol (li'sol) a proprietary solution containing phenol derivatives; used as a disinfectant and antiseptic.

lysokinase (li″so-ki'nās) a substance of the fibrinolytic system that activates plasma proactivators.

lysosome (li'so-sōm) a minute body occurring in a cell and containing various enzymes, mainly hydrolytic.

lysotype (li'so-tīp) 1. he type of a microorganism as determined by its reactions to specific phages. 2. a taxonomic subdivision of bacteria based on their reactions to specific phages, or a formula expressing the reactions on which such a subdivision is based.

lysozyme (li'so-zīm) a bacteriolytic substance present in animal and vegetable tissues.

lyssa (lis'ah) rabies. adj., **lys'sic.**

lyssoid (lis'oid) resembling rabies.

lyssophobia (lis″o-fo'be-ah) morbid fear of rabies.

lytic (lit'ik) pertaining to lysis or a lysin.

lyze (līz) to cause or produce lysis.

M

M a symbol used in general chemical formulas to represent a metal.

M. macerate; member; L. meri'dies *(noon);* meter; L. mil'le *(thousand);* minim; L. mis'ce *(mix);* L. mistu'ra *(mixture);* molar; L. mus'culus *(muscle);* myopia.

m- meta-.

μ symbol, *micron.*

M.A. Master of Arts; meter angle.

ma. milliampere.

maceration (mas″ĕ-ra'shun) the softening of a solid by soaking; in obstetrics, the degenerative changes and eventual disintegration of a fetus retained in the uterus after its death.

machine (mah-shēn') a mechanical contrivance for doing work or generating energy.

macies (ma'she-ēz) [L.] wasting.

Macracanthorhynchus (mak″rah-kan″tho-ring'kus) a genus of parasites of the class Acanthocephala. **M. hirudina'ceus,** a species parasitic in swine in the United States.

macr(o)- (mak'ro) word element [Gr.], *large size of.*

macrencephalia (mak″ren-sĕ-fa'le-ah) hypertrophy of the brain.

macroanalysis (mak″ro-ah-nal'ĭ-sis) chemical analysis using 0.1 to 0.2 gm. of the substance under study.

macrobiota (-bi-o'tah) the macroscopic living organisms of a region. adj., **macrobiot'ic.**

macroblast (mak'ro-blast) an abnormally large, nucleated red blood cell; a large young normoblast; a megaloblast.

macrocardius (mak″ro-kar'de-us) a fetus with an extremely large heart.

macrocephalous (-sef'ah-lus) having an abnormally large head.

macrocephalus (-sef'ah-lus) megalocephaly.

macrocephaly (-sef'ah-le) abnormal enlargement of the cranium.

macrocheilia (-ki'le-ah) excessive size of lip.

macrocheiria (-ki're-ah) excessive size of the hands.

macrocolon (-ko'lon) excessive size of the colon.

macrocoly (-ko'le) macrocolon.

macrocrania (-kra'ne-ah) abnormal increase in size of the skull in relation to the face.

macrocyte (mak'ro-sīt) a red blood corpuscle of largest type.

macrocythemia (mak″ro-si-the'me-ah) macrocytosis.

macrocytosis (-si-to'sis) presence of abnormally large erythrocytes in the blood.

macrodactylia (-dak-til'e-ah) abnormal largeness of fingers or toes.

macrodont (mak'ro-dont) macrodontic.

macrodontia (mak″ro-don'she-ah) abnormal increase in size of the teeth. adj., **macrodon'tic.**

macrodystrophia (-dis-tro'fe-ah) overgrowth of a part. **m. lipomato'sa progres'siva,** partial gigantism with tumor-like overgrowth of adipose tissue.

macroecology (-e-kol'o-je) study of the relations between parasites and the external environment, either directly or indirectly.

macrofauna (-faw'nah) the macroscopic animal organisms of a region.

macroflora (-flo'rah) the macroscopic vegetable organisms of a region.

macrogamete (-gam'ēt) the larger, female gamete.

macrogametocyte (-gah-me'to-sīt) the cell producing macrogametes.

macrogammaglobulin (mak″ro-gam″mah-glob′u-lin) a gamma globulin of extremely high molecular weight.

macrogammaglobulinemia (-glob″u-lī-ne′me-ah) presence in the blood of gamma globulins of extremely high molecular weight.

macrogenitosomia (mak″ro-jen″ĭ-to-so′me-ah) excessive bodily development, with unusual enlargement of the genital organs. **m. pre′cox,** macrogenitosomia occurring at an early age.

macroglia (mak-rog′le-ah) astroglia.

macroglobulin (mak″ro-glob′u-lin) a protein (globulin) of unusually high molecular weight, in the range of 1,000,000.

macroglobulinemia (-glob″u-lī-ne′me-ah) presence in the blood serum of macroglobulins. **Waldenström's m.,** a form of macroglobulinemia observed chiefly in males past age 50.

macroglossia (-glos′e-ah) hypertrophy of the tongue.

macrognathia (-nath′e-ah) abnormal overgrowth of the mandible. adj., **macrognath′ic.**

macrogyria (-ji′re-ah) moderate reduction in the number of sulci of the cerebrum, sometimes with increase in the brain substance, resulting in excessive size of the gyri.

macrolabia (-la′be-ah) macrocheilia.

macrolecithal (-les′ĭ-thal) having a large amount of yolk.

macromastia (-mas′te-ah) excessive size of the breasts.

macromelia (-me′le-ah) enlargement of one or more extremities.

macromelus (mak-rom′ĕ-lus) fetus with abnormally large limbs.

macromere (mak′ro-mēr) one of the larger cells formed in unequal cleavage of the fertilized ovum (at the vegetal pole).

macromethod (mak′ro-meth″od) a chemical test in which normal quantities are used.

macromolecular (mak″ro-mo-lek′u-lar) composed of large molecules.

Macromonas (-mo′nas) a genus of Schizomycetes (order Pseudomonadales, suborder Pseudomonadineae, family Thiobacteriaceae).

macromonocyte (-mon′o-sīt) a giant monocyte.

macronormoblast (-nor′mo-blast) an early form of the erythrocytic series.

macronormocyte (-nor′mo-sīt) a giant red blood corpuscle.

macronucleus (-nu′kle-us) the larger of two nuclei of a unicellular organism, associated with nutrition of the cell.

macronychia (-nik′e-ah) abnormally enlarged nails.

macrophage (mak′ro-fāj) a large phagocytic cell. **fixed m.,** a quiescent phagocyte. **free m.,** an ameboid phagocyte at the site of inflammation. **inflammatory m.,** free macrophage.

macrophthalmia (mak″rof-thal′me-ah) abnormal enlargement of the eyeball.

macropodia (mak″ro-po′de-ah) excessive size of the feet.

macropolycyte (-pol′ĭ-sīt) a hypersegmented polymorphonuclear leukocyte of greater than normal size.

macroprosopia (mak″ro-pro-so′pe-ah) excessive size of the face.

macropsia (mah-krop′se-ah) a disorder of visual perception in which objects appear larger than their actual size.

macrorrhinia (mak″ro-rin′e-ah) excessive size of the nose.

macroscelia (-se′le-ah) excessive size of the legs.

macroscopic (-skop′ik) of large size; visible to the unaided eye.

macroscopy (mah-kros′ko-pe) examination with the unaided eye.

macrosigma (mak″ro-sig′mah) macrosigmoid.

macrosigmoid (-sig′moid) excessive size of the sigmoid.

macrosomatia (-so-ma′she-ah) great bodily size.

macrosomia (-so′me-ah) macrosomatia.

macrostomia (-sto′me-ah) excessive size of the mouth.

macrotia (mak-ro′she-ah) abnormal enlargement of the pinna of the ear.

macula (mak′u-lah), pl. *mac′ulae* [L.] a stain or spot. adj., **mac′ular. mac′ulae acus′ticae,** terminations of acoustic nerve in utricle and saccule. **m. atroph′ica,** a white atrophic patch on the skin. **cerebral m.,** tache cérébrale. **m. ceru′lea,** a blue patch on the skin seen in pediculosis. **m. cor′neae,** a circumscribed opacity of the cornea. **m. cribro′sa,** a perforated spot or area; an area in the wall of the vestibule of the ear through which branches of the vestibulocochlear nerve pass to the saccule, utricle and semicircular canals. **m. den′sa,** a zone of heavily nucleated cells in the distal renal tubule. **m. fla′va,** a yellow nodule at one end of a vocal cord. **m. follic′-uli,** the point on the surface of a vesicular ovarian follicle where rupture occurs. **m. germinati′va,** germinal area. **m. lu′tea,** a pigment area of the retina on the temporal side of the optic disk. **m. ret′inae,** an irregular yellowish depression on the retina, lateral to and slightly below the optic disk. **m. sola′ris,** a freckle.

maculate (mak′u-lāt) spotted or blotched.

macule (mak′ūl) a macula.

maculocerebral (mak″u-lo-ser′ĕ-bral) pertaining to macula lutea and cerebrum.

maculopapule (-pap′ūl) a papule developed on a macule.

madarosis (mad″ah-ro′sis) loss of eyelashes or eyebrows.

maduromycosis (mah-du″ro-mi-ko′sis) a chronic fungus disease affecting various body tissues, including the hands, legs and feet.

mafenide (maf′en-īd) compound used in the topical treatment of superficial infections.

magenta (mah-jen′tah) fuchsin or other salt of rosaniline.

maggot (mag′ot) the soft-bodied larva of an insect.

magma (mag′mah) 1. a suspension of finely divided material in a small amount of water. 2. a thin, pastelike substance composed of organic material. **bentonite m.,** a preparation of bentonite and purified water, used as a suspending agent. **bismuth m.**, a water suspension of bismuth hydroxide and bismuth subcarbonate, used as an astringent and antacid. **magnesia m.**, magnesium hydroxide; used as a laxative and antacid.

Magnacort (mag'nah-kort) trademark for a preparation of hydrocortamate.

magnesia (mag-ne'zhe-ah) magnesium oxide, MgO; aperient and antacid.

magnesium (mag-ne'ze-um) chemical element (*see table*), at. no. 12, symbol Mg. **m. carbonate**, an odorless, stable compound used as an antacid. **m. citrate**, a mild cathartic. **m. hydroxide**, a bulky white powder used as an antacid and cathartic. **m. oxide**, a white powder used as an antacid and cathartic. **m. phosphate, dibasic**, a salt used as a mild saline laxative. **m. phosphate, tribasic**, a white, odorless, tasteless powder used as an antacid. **m. salicylate**, a colorless or slightly reddish crystalline powder used as an intestinal antiseptic. **m. stearate**, a combination of magnesium with stearic and palmitic acids. **m. sulfate**, a crystalline compound used as a cathartic and anticonvulsant. **m. trisilicate**, a combination of magnesium oxide and silicon dioxide with varying proportions of water; used as a gastric antacid.

magnet (mag'net) an object having polarity and capable of attracting iron.

magneto-electricity (mag-ne"to-e"lek-tris'ĭ-te) electric current induced by a magnet.

magnetotherapy (-ther'ah-pe) treatment of disease by magnetic currents.

magnetropism (mag-net'ro-pizm) a growth response in a nonmotile organism under the influence of a magnet.

magnification (mag"nĭ-fĭ-ka'shun) apparent increase of the size of an object by means of a lens or a system of lenses.

main (mān) [Fr.], hand. **m. en griffe** (ma-nongrif') clawhand.

make (māk) closure and completion of an electric circuit.

makro- (mak'ro) for words beginning thus, see those beginning *macro-*.

mal (mal) [Fr.] illness; disease. **m. de caderas,** a disease of horses, mules and dogs in South America due to *Trypanosoma equinum.* **grand m.**, a generalized convulsive seizure attended by loss of consciousness. **m. de mer,** seasickness. **petit m.**, momentary loss of consciousness without convulsive movements. **m. de los pintos,** pinta.

mala (ma'lah) 1. the cheek. 2. the zygomatic bone. adj., **ma'lar.**

malacia (mah-la'she-ah) 1. morbid softening of a part. 2. morbid craving for highly spiced foods.

malacoma (mal"ah-ko'mah) malacia.

malacoplakia (mal"ah-ko-pla'ke-ah) a circumscribed area of softening on the membrane lining a hollow organ, as the ureter, urethra or kidney pelvis. **m. vesi'cae,** a flat yellow growth on the bladder mucosa.

malacosarcosis (-sar-ko'sis) softness of muscular tissue.

malacosis (mal"ah-ko'sis) malacia.

malacosteon (mal"ah-kos'te-on) softening of the bones; osteomalacia.

malacotic (mal"ah-kot'ik) soft.

malacotomy (mal"ah-kot'o-me) incision of the abdominal wall.

malady (mal'ah-de) a disease or illness.

malaise (mal-āz') [Fr.] a feeling of uneasiness or indisposition.

malalignment (mal"ah-līn'ment) displacement of the teeth from their normal relation to the line of the dental arch.

malanders (mal'an-derz) psoriasis at the bend of the knee of the foreleg in the horse.

malaria (mah-lār'e-ah) a febrile disease caused by a parasite (Plasmodium), transmitted by mosquitoes of the genus Anopheles, marked by a chill followed by fever, and attended with general symptoms, terminating in a sweating phase. adj., **malar'ial. cerebral m.**, a falciparum malaria with delirium or coma. **estivoautumnal m., falciparum m.**, the most serious form of malaria, due to *Plasmodium falciparum,* with severe constitutional symptoms and sometimes causing death. **hemolytic m.**, blackwater fever. **hemorrhagic m.**, falciparum malaria with hemorrhages. **ovale m.**, a mild form due to *Plasmodium ovale,* with recurring tertian febrile paroxysms and a tendency to end in spontaneous recovery. **pernicious m.**, falciparum malaria. **quartan m.**, malaria in which the febrile paroxysms occur every fourth day (every three days); due to *Plasmodium malariae.* **quotidian m.**, that in which the febrile paroxysms occur daily. **tertian m.**, that in which the febrile paroxysms occur every third day (every other day). **vivax m.**, that due to *Plasmodium vivax,* in which the febrile paroxysms commonly occur every other day (tertian malaria), but may occur daily (quotidian malaria).

malariacidal (mah-lār"e-ah-si'dal) destructive to malarial plasmodia.

malariologist (-ol'o-jist) a specialist in malariology.

malariology (-ol'o-je) the study of malaria.

malariotherapy (mah-lār"e-o-ther'ah-pe) treatment of paresis by infecting the patient with the parasite of tertian malaria.

Malassezia (mal"ah-se'ze-ah) a genus of pathogenic fungi. **M. fur'fur,** the causative agent of tinea versicolor. **M. trop'ica,** the causative agent of tinea flava.

malassimilation (mal"ah-sim"ĭ-la'shun) defective or faulty assimilation.

malate (ma'lāt) a salt of malic acid.

malaxate (mal'ak-sāt) to knead, as in making pills.

malaxation (mal"ak-sa'shun) an act of kneading.

male (māl) an individual of the sex that produces spermatozoa or begets young.

maleruption (mal"e-rup'shun) eruption of a tooth out of its normal position.

malformation (mal"for-ma'shun) defective formation.

malignancy (mah-lig'nan-se) tendency to progress in virulence.

malignant (mah-lig′nant) progressing in virulence.

malingerer (mah-ling′ger-er) one who is guilty of malingering.

malingering (mah-ling′ger-ing) willful, deliberate and fraudulent feigning or exaggeration of the symptoms of illness or injury to attain a consciously desired end.

malleoincudal (mal″e-o-ing′ku-dal) pertaining to malleus and incus.

malleolus (mah-le′o-lus), pl. *malle′oli* [L.] either of the two rounded prominences on either side of the ankle joint, at the lower end of the fibula *(external, lateral* or *outer malleolus)* or of the tibia *(inner, internal* or *medial malleolus),* adj., **malle′olar.**

malleotomy (mal″e-ot′o-me) 1. division of the malleus. 2. operative separation of the malleoli.

malleus (mal′e-us) 1. the largest of the auditory ossicles. 2. glanders.

malnutrition (mal″nu-trish′un) any disorder of nutrition.

malocclusion (mal″o-kloo′zhun) absence of proper relations of apposing teeth when the jaws are in contact.

malonal (mal′o-nal) barbital.

malposition (mal″po-zish′un) abnormal placement.

malpractice (mal-prak′tis) wrong or injurious treatment.

malpresentation (mal″prez-en-ta′shun) faulty fetal presentation.

malrotation (mal″ro-ta′shun) abnormal or pathologic rotation.

maltase (mawl′tās) an enzyme which catalyzes the decomposition of maltose to glucose.

maltodextrin (mawl″to-dek′strin) a dextrin convertible into maltose.

maltose (mawl′tōs) a glucose from malt or digested starch.

malum (ma′lum) [L.] disease. **m. articulo′rum seni′lis,** a painful degenerative state of a joint as a result of aging. **m. cox′ae seni′lis,** osteoarthritis of the hip joint. **m. per′forans pe′dis,** perforating ulcer of the foot.

malunion (mal-ūn′yon) faulty union of the fragments of a fractured bone.

mamila (mah-mil′ah), pl. *mamil′lae* [L.] 1. the nipple of the breast. 2. a nipple-like prominence. adj., **mam′illary.**

mamillated (mam″ĭ-lāt′ed) having nipple-like projections or prominences.

mamillation (-la′shun) 1. the condition of being mamillated. 2. a nipple-like elevation or projection.

mamilliform (mah-mil′ĭ-form) shaped like a nipple.

mamilliplasty (mah-mil′ĭ-plas″te) theleplasty.

mamillitis (mam″ĭ-li′tis) inflammation of the nipple.

mamm(o)- (mam′o) word element [L.], *breast, mammary gland.*

mamma (mam′ah), pl. *mam′mae* [L.] the milk-secreting gland of the female; mammary gland.

mammalgia (mah-mal′je-ah) pain in the mammary gland.

mammaplasty (mam′ah-plas″te) mammoplasty.

mammary (mam′ar-e) pertaining to the mammary gland.

mammectomy (mah-mek′to-me) mastectomy.

mammilla (mah-mil′ah) mamilla.

mammillated (mam″ĭ-lāt′ed) mamillated.

mammilliplasty (mah-mil′ĭ-plas″te) theleplasty.

mammillitis (mam″ĭ-li′tis) thelitis.

mammiplasia (mam″ĭ-pla′ze-ah) mammoplasia.

mammiplasty (mam′ĭ-plas″te) mammoplasty.

mammitis (mah-mi′tis) mastitis.

mammography (mah-mog′rah-fe) radiography of the mammary gland.

mammoplasia (mam″-o-pla′ze-ah) development of breast tissue.

mammoplasty (mam′o-plas″te) plastic surgery of the breast. **augmentation m.,** plastic surgery to increase the size of the female breast. **reduction m.,** plastic surgery to decrease the size of the female breast.

mammose (mam′ōs) having unusually large mammary glands.

mammotomy (mah-mot′o-me) mastotomy.

mammotrophic (mam″o-trof′ik) mammotropic.

mammotropic (-trop′ik) having a stimulating effect on the mammary gland.

mammotropin (-trōp′in) a hormone of the anterior pituitary which stimulates the mammary gland.

M and B 693 sulfapyridine.

mandible (man′dĭ-bl) the lower jaw. adj., **mandib′ular.**

mandibula (man-dib′u-lah), pl. *mandib′ulae* [L.] mandible.

mandrel (man′drel) the shaft on which a dental tool is held in the dental handpiece, for rotation by the dental engine.

mandrin (man′drin) a metal guide for a flexible catheter.

maneuver (mah-noo′ver) a skillful or dextrous procedure. **Müller's m.,** an inspiratory effort with a closed glottis after expiration, used during fluoroscopic examination to cause a negative intrathoracic pressure with engorgement of intrathoracic vascular structures. **Scanzoni's m.,** double application of forceps blades for delivery of a fetus in the occiput posterior position. **Valsalva's m.,** increase of intrapulmonic pressure by forcible exhalation against the closed glottis.

manganese (man′gah-nēs) chemical element *(see table),* at. no. 25, symbol Mn. **m. butyrate,** a red powder, used in treatment of some skin diseases. **m. citrate,** soluble, pale orange powder. **m. dioxide,** black oxide of manganese. **m. glycerophosphate,** odorless white powder; hematinic and nerve tonic. **m. sulfate,** a purgative and cholagogue.

mange (mānj) skin disease of domestic animals, due to mites.

mania (ma′ne-ah) disordered mental state of extreme excitement. adj., **mani′acal. acute hallucinatory m.,** Ganser's syndrome.

maniac (ma'ne-ak) one affected with mania.

manic-depressive (man″ik-de-pres'iv) marked by alternating periods of elation and depression.

manikin (man'ĭ-kin) a model to illustrate anatomy or on which to practice surgical or other manipulations.

manipulation (mah-nip″u-la-shun) skilful or dextrous treatment by the hands.

mannitol (man'ĭ-tol) a sugar occurring widely in nature, especially in fungi; used originally in diagnostic tests of kidney function and now therapeutically. **m. hexanitrate,** a crystalline compound; vasodilator.

manometer (mah-nom'ĕ-ter) instrument for ascertaining the pressure of liquids.

Mansonella (man″so-nel'ah) a genus of nematode parasites of the superfamily Filarioidea. **M. ozzar'di,** a species found in man, usually in adipose tissues surrounding organs in the body cavities.

Mansonia (man-so'ne-ah) a genus of mosquitoes comprising some 55 species, distributed primarily in tropical regions; important as vectors of microfilariae and viruses.

mantle (man'tl) the cortex of the brain.

manubrium (mah-nu'bre-um), pl. *manu'bria* [L.] 1. the uppermost portion of the sternum *(manu'brium ster'ni).* 2. the largest process of the malleus, giving attachment to the tendon of the tensor tympanic muscle *(manu'-brium mal'lei).*

manudynamometer (man″u-di″nah-mom'ĕ-ter) an apparatus for measuring the force of the thrust of an instrument.

manus (ma'nus), pl. *ma'nus* [L.] hand.

map (map) a two-dimensional graphic representation of arrangement in space. **chromosome m.,** a diagram showing the location of particular genes on a chromosome. **fate m.,** a graphic representation of a blastula or other early stage of an embryo, showing prospective significance of certain areas in normal development. **genetic m.,** a graphic representation of the chromosomes constituting a karyotype and the genes located thereon.

Mapharsen (mah-far'sen) trademark for a preparation of oxophenarsine hydrochloride.

marasmus (mah-raz'mus) progressive wasting, especially in young infants. adj., **maran'tic, maras'mic.**

Marezine (mar'e-zēn) trademark for a preparation of cyclizine hydrochloride.

marfanil (mar'fah-nil) a white crystalline compound, for topical application.

margarine (mar'jah-rin) a food product containing 80 per cent of fat, primarily refined cottonseed and soybean oils, and fortified with vitamin A.

margin (mar'jin) an edge or border. adj., **mar'ginal. dentate m.,** pectinate line. **gingival m., gum m.,** the border of the gingiva surrounding, but unattached to, the substance of the teeth.

margo (mar'go), pl. *mar'gines* [L.] border; margin.

marihuana (mar″ĭ-wahn'ah) the leaves and tops of *Cannabis sativa,* a habit-forming intoxicating agent, usually used in cigarettes by addicts.

maritonucleus (mar″ĭ-to-nu'kle-us) nucleus of the ovum after the sperm cell has entered it.

mark (mark) a spot or blemish. **mother's m.,** mulberry m., nevus. **strawberry m.,** hemangioma congenitale.

Marplan (mar'plan) trademark for a preparation of isocarboxazid.

marrow (mar'o) soft organic material, especially that filling the cavities of the bones. **spinal m.,** the spinal cord.

marsupialization (mar-su″pe-ah-li-za'shun) conversion of a closed cavity into an open pouch, by incising it and suturing the edges of its wall to the edges of the wound.

marsupium (mar-su'pe-um), pl. *marsu'pia* [L.] pouch; the scrotum.

masculation (mas″ku-la'shun) the development of male characteristics.

masculine (mas'ku-lin) pertaining to the male sex.

masculinity (mas″ku-lin'ĭ-te) the possession of masculine qualities.

masculinization (-lin-ĭ-za'shun) the induction or development of male secondary sex characters in the female.

masculinize (mas'ku-lĭ-nīz″) to produce masculine qualities in women.

masculinovoblastoma (mas″ku-lin-o″vo-blas-to'mah) an ovarian tumor which causes masculinization.

masculonucleus (mas″ku-lo-nu'kle-us) arsenoblast.

maser (ma'zer) a device which produces an extremely intense, small and nearly nondivergent beam of monochromatic radiation in the microwave region, with all the waves in phase.

mask (mask) 1. to cover or conceal; in audiometry, to obscure or diminish a sound by the presence of another sound of different frequency. 2. an appliance for shading, protecting or medicating the face. **ecchymotic m.,** traumatic asphyxia. **Esmarch's m.,** a frame of metal over which strips of gauze are stretched; used for administering ether or chloroform by inhalation. **Hutchinson's m.,** a sensation as if the skin of the face were compressed by a mask, often a symptom of tabes dorsalis. **luetic m.,** a brownish, blotchy pigmentation over the forehead, temples and cheeks, sometimes occurring in tertiary syphilis. **Mikulicz's m.,** a wire frame covered with gauze for covering the surgeon's nose and mouth while operating. **Ombrédanne m.,** a mask for administering ether in exact dosage. **m. of pregnancy,** brown pigmentation of the forehead, cheeks and nose, occurring in pregnancy.

masochism (mas'o-kizm) 1. the derivation of sexual gratification through the suffering of pain. 2. the passive acceptance of pain. adj., **masochis'tic.**

masochist (mas'o-kist) a person exhibiting or characterized by masochism.

mass (mas) 1. a lump or collection of cohering particles. 2. that characteristic of matter which gives it inertia. **atomic m.,** the mass of a neutral atom of a nuclide, usually expressed as atomic mass units (amu). **body cell m.,** the total weight of the cells of the body, constituting the total mass of oxygen-utilizing, carbohydrate-burning and energy-exchanging cells of the body; regarded as proportional to total exchangeable potassium in the body. **ferrous carbonate m.,** a soft, greenish-gray mass, containing 36–41 per cent ferrous carbonate, formerly used in chlorosis and simple anemia. **inner cell m.,** an internal cluster of cells at one pole of the distended blastocyst which develops into the body of the embryo. **intermediate cell m.,** nephrotome. **lean body m.,** that part of the body including all its components except neutral storage lipid; in essence, the fat-free mass of the body. **tigroid m's,** Nissl bodies. **Vallet's m.,** ferrous carbonate mass. **rest m.,** the mass of a particle at rest, such as that of a nuclear particle when the atom is neither emitting nor absorbing energy. **Stent's m.,** a plastic resinous material which sets into a very hard substance; used in dentistry for making impressions of oral structures and in surgery for molds to hold grafts in place.

massa (mas'ah), pl. *mas'sae* [L.] mass (1).

massage (mah-sahzh') systematic stroking or kneading. **auditory m.,** massage of the tympanic membrane. **cardiac m.,** intermittent compression of the heart by pressure applied over the sternum (*closed cardiac massage*) or directly to the heart through an opening in the chest wall (*open cardiac massage*). **electrovibratory m.,** massage by means of an electric vibrator. **vibratory m.,** massage by rapidly repeated light percussion with a vibrating hammer or sound.

masseur (mah-ser') [Fr.] a man who performs massage.

masseuse (mah-suhz') [Fr.] a woman who performs massage.

massotherapy (mas″o-ther′ah-pe) treatment of disease by massage.

mastadenitis (mas″tad-e-ni′tis) inflammation of a mammary gland.

mastalgia (mas-tal′je-ah) pain in the breast.

mastatrophy (mas-tat′ro-fe) atrophy of the breast.

mastectomy (mas-tek′to-me) excision of the breast. **radical m.,** amputation of the breast with wide excision of the pectoral muscles and axillary lymph nodes.

mastication (mas″ti-ka′shun) the act of chewing.

masticatory (mas″ti-kah-tor″e) 1. pertaining to mastication. 2. a substance to be chewed, but not swallowed.

Mastigophora (mas″ti-gof′o-rah) a subphylum of protozoa, including all those that have one or more flagella in their trophozoite form; many are parasitic in both invertebrates and vertebrates, including man.

mastigote (mas′ti-gōt) a flagellate animal microorganism.

mastitis (mas-ti′tis) inflammation of the breast. **m. neonato′rum,** an abnormal condition of the breast in the newborn. **periductal m.,** inflammation of tissues about the ducts of the mammary gland. **plasma cell m.,** mastitis with infiltration of the breast stroma with plasma cells.

masto- (mas′to) word element [Gr.], *mammary gland; breast.*

mastocyte (mas′to-sīt) a mast cell.

mastocytoma (mas″to-si-to′mah) a tumor containing mast cells.

mastocytosis (-si-to′sis) urticaria pigmentosa.

mastodynia (-din′e-ah) mastalgia.

mastography (mas-tog″rah-fe) radiography of the breast.

mastoid (mas′toid) 1. nipple-shaped. 2. the portion of the temporal bone lying behind the meatus of the ear (*pars mastoidea*), or more specifically the conical projection from it (*mastoid process*).

mastoidale (mas″toi-da′le) the lowest point of the mastoid process.

mastoidalgia (mas″toi-dal′je-ah) pain in the mastoid region.

mastoidea (mas-toi′de-ah) the mastoid process of the temporal bone.

mastoidectomy (mas″toi-dek′to-me) excision of the mastoid cells.

mastoideocentesis (mas-toi″de-o-sen-te′sis) paracentesis of the mastoid cells.

mastoiditis (mas″toi-di′tis) inflammation of the mastoid antrum and cells.

mastoidotomy (-dot′o-me) incision of the mastoid antrum.

mastology (mas-tol′o-je) study of the mammary gland.

mastoncus (mas-tong′kus) a tumor or swelling of the breast.

masto-occipital (mas″to-ok-sip′ĭ-tal) pertaining to mastoid process and occipital bone.

mastopathy (mas-top′ah-the) disease of the mammary gland.

mastopexy (mas′to-pek″se) surgical fixation of a pendulous breast.

mastoplasia (mas″to-pla′ze-ah) hyperplasia of breast tissue.

mastoplasty (mas′to-plas″te) mammoplasty.

mastoptosis (mas″to-to′sis) a pendulous condition of the breast.

mastorrhagia (-ra′je-ah) hemorrhage from the mammary gland.

mastoscirrhus (-skir′us) hardening of the mammary gland.

mastosis (mas-to′sis) degeneration of breast tissue, with painful nodular swellings. adj., **mastot′ic.**

mastotomy (mas-tot′o-me) incision of a mammary gland.

masturbation (mas″ter-ba′shun) induction of orgasm by self-stimulation of the genital organs.

matching (mach′ing) comparison for the purpose of selecting objects having similar or identical characteristics. **m. of blood,** comparing the blood of a contemplated donor with that of the recipient to ascertain whether their bloods belong to the same group. **cross m.,** determination of the compatibility of the blood of a donor and that of a recipient before transfusion.

materia (mah-tēr'e-ah) [L.] material; substance. **m. med'ica,** pharmacology.

material (mah-te're-al) substance or elements from which a concept may be formulated, or an object constructed. **genetic m.,** that transmitted from an organism to those of succeeding generations and responsible for the features characteristic of the species, as well as for the heritable difference between individuals.

maternal (mah-ter'nal) pertaining to the female parent.

mating (māt'ing) pairing of individuals of opposite sexes, especially for reproduction. **assortative m., assorted m., assortive m.,** the mating of individuals having similar qualities or constitutions. **random m.,** the mating of individuals without regard to any similarity between them.

matrix (ma'triks), pl. *mat'rices* [L.] 1. uterus. 2. a generative structure, such as the organs from which grow the hair and nail. **interterritorial m.,** a paler staining region among the darker territoral matrices. **nail m.,** matrix unguis. **territorial m.,** basophilic matrix about groups of cartilage cells. **m. un'guis,** the end of the nail bed.

matroclinous (mat″ro-kli'nus) resembling the maternal species rather than the paternal; said of a hybrid.

matter (mat'er) physical material having form and weight under ordinary conditions of gravity.

maxilla (mak-sil'ah), pl. *maxil'lae* [L.] the bone of the upper jaw. adj., **max'illary. inferior m.,** the mandible.

maxillectomy (mak″sĭ-lek'to-me) removal of the maxilla.

maxillitis (mak″sĭ-li'tis) inflammation of the maxillary gland.

maximum (mak'sĭ-mum) 1. the greatest quantity or value possible or achieved under given circumstances. 2. the acme of a disease or process. adj., **max'imal.**

Maxitate (mak'sĭ-tāt) trademark for preparations of mannitol hexanitrate.

maze (māz) a complicated system of intersecting paths used in intelligence tests and in demonstrating learning in experimental animals.

mazopexy (ma'zo-pek″se) mastopexy.

mazoplasia (ma″zo-pla'ze-ah) mastoplasia.

M.B. Bachelor of Medicine.

M.C. [L.] Ma'gister Chirur'giae (*Master of Surgery*); Medical Corps.

Mc megacurie; megacycle.

mc. millicurie.

μc. microcurie.

mcg. microgram.

MCH mean corpuscular hemoglobin (hemoglobin × 10 ÷ number of red cells).

μc.h. microcurie hour.

MCHC mean corpuscular hemoglobin concentration (hemoglobin × 100 ÷ hematocrit determination).

Mc.p.s. megacycles per second.

M.C.S.P. Member of the Chartered Society of Physiotherapists (Brit.).

MCV. mean corpuscular volume (hematocrit determination × 10 ÷ number of red cells). 2. mean clinical value (obtained by assigning a numerical value to the response noted in a number of patients receiving a specific treatment, adding these numbers and dividing by the number of patients treated).

M.D. Doctor of Medicine.

Md chemical symbol, *mendelevium.*

M.D.S. Master of Dental Surgery.

meal (mēl) a portion of food or foods taken at some particular and usually stated or fixed time. **bismuth m.,** a meal containing some preparation of bismuth as the opaque constituent. **opaque m.,** a meal containing some substance opaque to roentgen rays, permitting visualization of the gastrointestinal tract. **Oslo m.,** a meal for school children consisting of a third of a liter of unskimmed milk, wholemeal bread with margarine and goat's-milk cheese, half an orange, half an apple, and a raw carrot.

mean (mēn) an average; a numerical value intermediate between two extremes. **arithmetical m.,** the arithmetical average. **geometrical m.,** the antilogarithm of the arithmetical mean of the logarithm of a series of values.

measles (me'zelz) an acute infectious, highly communicable childhood disease, characterized by a generalized exanthem. **black m.,** a severe form in which the eruption is very dark and petechial. **German m.,** rubella. **hemorrhagic m.,** black measles.

meatorrhaphy (me″ah-tor'ah-fe) suture of a meatus.

meatoscopy (-tos'ko-pe) examination of the ureteral orifices by cystoscopy.

meatotomy (-tot'o-me) incision of a meatus.

meatus (me-a'tus), pl. *mea'tus* [L.] an opening or passage. adj., **mea'tal. acoustic m., m. acus'ticus,** a passage in the ear, one leading to the ear drum (*mea'tus acus'ticus exter'nus*) and one for passage of nerves and blood vessels (*mea'tus acus'ticus inter'nus*). **m. audito'rius, auditory m.,** acoustic meatus. **m. of nose,** one of the three portions of the nasal cavity on either side of the septum, inferior, middle or superior (*mea'tus na'si infe'rior, me'dius, supe'rior*). **m. urina'rius, urinary m.,** the opening of the urethra on the body surface through which urine is discharged.

Mebaral (meb'ah-ral) trademark for a preparation of mephobarbital.

mebutamate (meb'u-tam″āt) a compound used to reduce blood pressure and as a mild tranquilizer.

mecamine (mek'ah-min) mecamylamine.

mecamylamine (mek″ah-mil'ah-min) a compound used in blockade of autonomic ganglia and as an antihypertensive.

mechanicoreceptor (mē-kan″ĭ-ko-re-sep'tor) a receptor for mechanical stimuli.

mechanics (mē-kan'iks) the science dealing with the motions of material bodies. **animal m.,** biomechanics. **body m.,** the application of kinesiology to use of the body in daily life activities and to the prevention and correction of problems related to posture. **development m.**, experimental embryology.

mechanocyte (mek′ah-no-sīt″) fibroblast.

mechanology (mek″ah-nol′o-je) the science of mechanics or of machines.

mechanoreceptor (mek″ah-no-re-sep′tor) a nerve ending sensitive to mechanical stimuli, e.g. changes in tension or pressure.

mechanotherapy (-ther′ah-pe) use of mechanical apparatus in treatment of disease or its results, especially in therapeutic exercises.

mechanothermy (-ther′me) therapeutic heat produced by massage, exercise, etc.

mechlorethamine (mē″klōr-eth′ah-mēn) a compound used as a neoplastic suppressant.

Mecholyl (me′ko-lil) trademark for preparations of methacholine.

meclizine (mek′lī-zēn) a compound used as an antinauseant.

meconate (mek′o-nāt) a salt of meconic acid.

meconism (mek′o-nizm) opium poisoning.

meconium (mē-ko′ne-um) dark green mucilaginous material in the intestine of the full-term fetus.

media (me′de-ah) middle.

medial (me′de-al) pertaining to or situated toward the midline.

medialecithal (me″de-ah-les′ī-thal) having a moderate amount of yolk.

medialis (me″de-a′lis) [L.] medial.

median (me′de-an) pertaining to or situated in the midline.

medianus (me″de-a′nus) [L.] median.

mediastinitis (me″de-as″ti-ni′tis) inflammation of mediastinum.

mediastinogram (me″de-as-ti′no-gram) a roentgenogram of the mediastinum.

mediastinography (me″de-as″tī-nog′rah-fe) radiography of the structures of the mediastinum.

mediastinopericarditis (me″de-as″tī-no-per″-ī-kar-di′tis) inflammation of mediastinum and pericardium.

mediastinoscopy (-nos′ko-pe) endoscopic examination of the mediastinum.

mediastinotomy (-not′o-me) incision of the mediastinum.

mediastinum (me″de-ah-sti′num), pl. *mediasti′na* [L.] 1. a median septum or partition 2. the mass of tissues and organs separating the sternum in front and the vertebral column behind, commonly considered to have three divisions: anterior, middle and superior. adj., **mediasti′nal. m. tes′tis**, a partial septum of the testis formed near its posterior border by a continuation of the tunica albuginea.

mediate (me′de-āt) indirect; accomplished by means of a medium.

medical (med′ī-kal) pertaining to medicine.

medicament (mē-dik′ah-ment, med′ī-kah-ment) a medicinal agent.

medicated (med′ī-kāt″ed) imbued with a medicinal substance.

medication (med″ī-ka′shun) 1. administration of remedies. 2. a medicinal agent. **dialytic m.**, treatment by internal use of artificial

mineral waters, as dilute aqueous solutions of salt. **ionic m.**, the application of medicines by cataphoresis, the ions of the drugs passing from one pole of the battery to the other through the body.

medicinal (mē-dis′ī-nal) having healing qualities.

medicine (med′ī-sin) 1. a drug or remedy. 2. the art of healing disease. **aviation m.**, that branch of medicine which deals with the physiologic, medical, psychologic and epidemiologic problems involved in flying. **clinical m.**, study of medicine at the bedside. **experimental m.**, study of the science of healing diseases based on experimentation in animals. **forensic m.**, medical jurisprudence. **internal m.**, that dealing especially with diagnosis and medical treatment of diseases and disorders of internal structures of the body. **ionic m.**, treatment by electrochemical means, such as cataphoresis, iontophoresis. **legal m.**, medical jurisprudence. **oral m.**, that dealing especially with diseases of the mouth. **patent m.**, a remedy whose manufacture is protected by letters patent. **physical m.**, physiatrics. **preclinical m.**, the subjects studied in medicine before the student observes actual diseases in patients. **preventive m.**, science aimed at preventing disease. **proprietary m.**, a remedy whose formula is owned exclusively by the manufacturer and which is marketed usually under a name registered as a trademark. **psychosomatic m.**, the study of the interrelations between bodily processes and emotional life. **socialized m.**, the control and direction of the practice of medicine by the government. **space m.**, that branch of aviation medicine concerned with conditions to be encountered in space. **state m.**, 1. that which deals with the public health, sanitation, etc. 2. socialized medicine. **tropical m.**, medical science as applied to diseases ordinarily occurring only in hot or tropical countries. **veterinary m.**, the diagnosis and treatment of the diseases of animals.

medicolegal (med″ī-ko-le′gal) pertaining to medical jurisprudence.

medicus (med′ī-kus) [L.] physician.

medionecrosis (me″de-o-ne-kro′sis) focal areas of destruction of the elastic tissue and smooth muscle of the middle coat of the aorta or of its major branches.

mediopontine (-pon′tin) pertaining to the center of the pons.

mediotarsal (-tar′sal) pertaining to the center of the tarsus.

medium (me′de-um), pl. *mediums, me′dia* [L.] 1. conditions and environment of the body. 2. an agent by which something is accomplished. 3. a substance providing the proper nutritional environment for the growth of microorganisms. **clearing m.**, a substance for rendering histologic specimens transparent. **contrast m.**, radiopaque substance used in roentgenography to permit visualization of body structures. **culture m.**, a substance used to support the growth of microorganisms or other

cells. **dioptric media,** refracting media.
disperse m., dispersion m., the continuous
phase of a colloid system; the medium in
which a colloid is dispersed, corresponding to
the solvent in a true solution. **nutrient m.,**
a culture medium to which nutrient materials
have been added. **refracting media,** the
transparent tissues and fluid in the eye
through which light rays pass and by which
they are refracted and brought to a focus on
the retina.

medius (me′de-us) [L.] situated in the middle.

Medomin (med′o-min) trademark for a preparation of heptabarbital.

Medrol (med′rol) trademark for a preparation
of methylprednisolone.

medroxyprogesterone (med-rok″sĭ-pro-jes′-
ter-ōn) a compound used as a progestational
agent.

medulla (mĕ-dul′ah), pl. *medul′lae* [L.] the
middle; marrow; applied to the marrow of
bones *(medul′la os′sium),* the spinal cord
(medul′la spinalis) and the central portion
of such organs as the adrenal gland and the
kidney *(medul′la re′nis).* adj., **med′ullary.**
adrenal m., the highly vascular mass of
chromaffin tissue forming the center of an
adrenal gland. **m. neph′rica,** the pyramids of
the kidneys collectively. **m. oblonga′ta,** that
part of the hindbrain lying between the pons
above and the spinal cord below. **m. os′sium,**
bone marrow. **m. spina′lis,** spinal cord.

medullispinal (mĕ-dul″ĭ-spi′nal) pertaining
to the spinal cord.

medullitis (med″u-li′tis) 1. myelitis. 2. osteomyelitis.

medullization (-li-za′shun) abnormal enlargement of marrow spaces in cancellous bone.

medulloadrenal (mĕ-dul″o-ah-dre′nal) pertaining to the adrenal medulla.

medulloblast (mĕ-dul′o-blast) an undifferentiated cell of the neural tube which may develop into either a neuroblast or spongioblast.

medulloblastoma (mĕ-dul″o-blas-to′mah) a
cerebral tumor composed of medulloblasts.

medulloepithelioma (-ep″ĭ-the″le-o′-mah) a
tumor of primitive retinal epithelium and
neuroepithelium.

mega- (meg′ah) word element [Gr.], *large;*
used in naming units of measurement to designate an amount 10^6 (one million) times
the size of the unit to which it is joined, as
megacuries (10^6 curies); symbol M.

megabacterium (meg″ah-bak-te′re-um) a
large bacterium.

megabladder (-blad′er) permanent overdis-
tention of the bladder.

megacaryocyte (-kar′e-o-sīt) megakaryocyte.

megacecum (-se′kum) enlargement of the
cecum.

megacephaly (-sef′ah-le) megalocephaly.

megacoccus (-kok′us) a coccus of large size.

megacolon (-ko′lon) excessive dilatation of the
colon. **acquired m.,** dilatation of the colon,
of unknown etiology, occurring in an adult.
aganglionic m., a congenital condition characterized by great dilatation of the colon
proximal to a narrowed segment in which

myenteric plexus ganglion cells are absent.
congenital m., massive dilatation of the colon
proximal to an area which lacks autonomic
ganglia.

megacoly (meg′ah-ko″le) megacolon.

megacurie (meg″ah-ku′re) a unit of radioactivity, being one million (10^6) curies; abbreviated Mc.

megadont (meg′ah-dont) having very large
teeth.

megadyne (meg′ah-dīn) one million dynes.

megaesophagus (meg″ah-e-sof′ah-gus) dilatation and muscular hypertrophy of most of
the esophagus, above a constricted, often
atrophied, distal segment.

megakaryoblast (-kar′e-o-blast″) any cell of
the thrombocytic series with fine chromatin
structure in the nucleus.

megakaryocyte (-kar′e-o-sīt″) any nucleated
cell of the thrombocytic series in which nucleoli are not discernible.

megakaryocytosis (-kar″e-o-si-to′sis) megakaryocytes in the blood.

megakaryophthisis (-thi′sis) deficiency of
megakaryocytes in bone marrow or blood.

megal(o)- (meg′ah-lo) word element [Gr.]
large; abnormal enlargement.

megalencephaly (meg″ah-len-sef′ah-le) mac-
rencephaly.

megalecithal (meg″ah-les′ĭ-thal) containing
a large amount of yolk.

megalgia (meg-al′je-ah) a severe pain.

megaloblast (meg′ah-lo-blast″) a name given
early forms of the erythrocytic series.

megalocardia (meg″ah-lo-kar′de-ah) cardiomegaly.

megalocephaly (-sef′ah-le) abnormally increased size of the head. adj., **megalocephal′-
ic.**

megalocheiria (-ki′re-ah) abnormal largeness of the hands.

megalocornea (-kor′ne-ah) abnormal enlargement of the cornea.

megalocyte (meg′ah-lo-sīt″) an extremely large
erythrocyte.

megalodactyly (meg″ah-lo-dak′tĭ-le) excessive
size of fingers or toes. adj., **megalodac′tyl-
ous.**

megalodontia (-don′she-ah) abnormal largeness of the teeth.

megaloenteron (-en′ter-on) enlargement of
the intestine.

megaloesophagus (-e-sof′ah-gus) megaesophagus.

megalogastria (-gas′tre-ah) enlargement of
the stomach.

megaloglossia (-glos′e-ah) macroglossia.

megalohepatia (-he-pat′e-ah) enlargement of
the liver.

megalokaryoblast (-kar′e-o-blast″) megakaryoblast.

megalokaryocyte (-kar′e-o-sīt″) megakaryocyte.

megalomania (-ma′ne-ah) a mental state
characterized by delusions of exaggerated
personal importance, wealth or power.

megalomelia (-me′le-ah) abnormal largeness
of the limbs.

megalonychosis (meg"ah-lo-nī-ko'sis) hypertrophy of the nails and their matrices.

megalopenis (-pe'nis) abnormal largeness of the penis.

megalophthalmos (meg"ah-lof-thal'mos) buphthalmos.

megalopodia (meg"ah-lo-po'de-ah) abnormal largeness of the feet.

megalopsia (meg"ah-lop'se-ah) macropsia.

megaloscope (meg'ah-lo-skōp") a magnifying speculum.

megalosplenia (meg"ah-lo-sple'ne-ah) enlargement of the spleen.

megalosyndactyly (-sin-dak'tĭ-le) a condition in which the digits are large and webbed together.

megaloureter (-u-re'ter) enlargement of the ureter.

-megaly (meg'ah-le) word element [Gr.], *enlargement.*

megarectum (meg"ah-rek'tum) enlargement of the rectum.

megaseme (meg'ah-sēm) having an orbital index of more than 89.

megavolt (meg'ah-volt) one million volts.

Megimide (meg'ĭ-mīd) trademark for a preparation of bemegride.

megohm (meg'ōm) one million ohms.

megophthalmos (meg"of-thal'mos) buphthalmos.

megrim (me'grim) migraine.

meibomianitis (mi-bo"me-ah-ni'tis) inflammation of the meibomian glands.

meiogenic (mi"o-jen'ik) promoting meiosis.

meiosis (mi-o'sis) a special method of cell division occurring in maturation of sex cells, each daughter nucleus receiving half the number of chromosomes typical of the somatic cells of the species. adj., **meiot'ic.**

mel (mel) [L.] honey.

melalgia (mel-al'je-ah) neuralgic pain in the limbs.

melan(o)- (mel'ah-no) word element [Gr.], *black.*

melancholia (mel"an-ko'le-ah) a mental state characterized by extreme sadness. **acute m.,** severe melancholia marked by loss of appetite, emaciation, insomnia and subnormal temperature. **affective m.,** melancholia corresponding to the depressive phase of manic-depressive psychosis. **agitated m., m. agita'ta,** melancholia with constant motion and signs of great emotional excitement. **m. atton'ita,** stuporous melancholia. **m. with delirium,** a form with distressing delusions and hallucinations. **m. hypochon-dri'aca,** extreme hypochondria. **involution m.,** melancholia developing in advanced life during senile involution. **recurrent m.,** melancholia occurring at more or less regular intervals. **m. sim'plex,** a mild form without delusions or great excitement. **stuporous m.,** a form in which the patient lies motionless and silent, with fixed eyes and indifference to surroundings, sometimes with hallucinations.

melanedema (-ĕ-de'mah) anthracosis.

melanephidrosis (mel"an-ef"ĭ-dro'sis) discharge of black sweat.

mélangeur (ma-lan-zher') [Fr.] an instrument for drawing and diluting specimens of blood for examination.

melaniferous (mel"ah-nif'er-us) containing melanin.

melanin (mel'ah-nin) the pigment normally found in the skin, adrenal glands, pia, and choroid of the eye, which contributes to the color of those structures.

melanism (mel'ah-nizm) excessive deposit of melanin in the skin.

melanoameloblastoma (mel"ah-no-ah-mel"o-blas-to'mah) ameloblastoma with bluish-black discoloration due to melanin granules.

melanoblast (mel'ah-no-blast") a cell originating from the neural crest, which develops into a melanophore.

melanoblastoma (mel"ah-no-blas-to'mah) a tumor composed of melanoblasts.

melanocarcinoma (-kar"sĭ-no'mah) melanoma.

melanocyte (mel'ah-no-sit", mē-lan'o-sīt) a cell of the epidermis that synthesizes melanin.

melanoderma (-der'mah) an increased amount of melanin in the skin.

melanodermatitis (-der"mah-ti'tis) dermatitis with a deposit of melanin in the skin.

melanogen (mē-lan'o-jen) a colorless chromogen, convertible into melanin, which may occur in the urine in certain diseases.

melanogenesis (mel"ah-no-jen'ē-sis) the production of melanin.

melanoglossia (-glos'e-ah) black tongue.

melanoid (mel'ah-noid) resembling melanosis, or melanin.

melanoidin (mel"ah-noi'din) a melanin obtained from the albumins.

melanoleukoderma (mel"ah-no-lu"ko-der'-mah) a mottled appearance of the skin. **m. col'li,** a mottled appearance of the skin of the neck and adjacent regions, a rare manifestation of syphilis.

melanoma (mel"ah-no'mah) a tumor or malignant growth characterized by dark pigmentation.

melanomatosis (mel"ah-no-mah-to'sis) the formation of melanomas throughout the body.

melanonychia (-nik'e-ah) blackness of the nails.

melanopathy (mel"ah-nop'ah-the) excess of skin pigmentation.

melanophore (mel'ah-no-fōr") a pigment cell containing melanin.

melanoplakia (mel"ah-no-pla'ke-ah) pigmented patches on the mucous membrane of the mouth.

melanosarcoma (-sar-ko'mah) melanoma.

melanosis (mel"ah-no'sis) condition characterized by dark pigmentary deposits. **m. co'li,** brown-black discoloration of the mucosa of the colon, due to accumulation of a melanin-like pigment in the phagocytic mononuclear cells. adj., **melanot'ic.**

melanotrichia (mel"ah-no-trik'e-ah) abnormal hyperpigmentation of hair.

melanuria (mel″ah-nu′re-ah) the discharge of darkly stained urine.

melasma (mĕ-laz′mah) dark pigmentation of the skin. **m. addiso′nii,** Addison's disease. **m. gravida′rum,** discoloration of the skin in pregnancy.

melatonin (mel″ah-to′nin) a compound found in the pineal body which has a molecular structure similar to that of serotonin.

Meleda disease (mĕ′la-dah) familial hyperkeratosis palmaris et plantaris.

melena (mĕ-le′nah) darkening of feces by blood pigments.

melenemesis (mel″ĕ-nem′e-sis) vomiting of black matter.

meletin (mel′ĕ-tin) quercetin.

melioidosis (mel″e-oi-do′sis) a glanders-like disease of rodents, transmissible to man, and caused by *Malleomyces pseudomallei.*

melitagra (mel″ĭ-tag′rah) eczema with honeycomb crusts.

melitemia (-te′me-ah) excessive sugar in the blood.

melitococcosis (mel″ĭ-to-kŏ-ko′sis) brucellosis.

melitoptyalism (-ti′al-izm) secretion of saliva containing glucose.

melituria (mel″ĭ-tu′re-ah) diabetes mellitus.

Mellaril (mel′ah-ril) trademark for preparations of thioridazine hydrochloride.

melodidymus (mel″o-did′ĭ-mus) a person with a supernumerary limb.

melomelus (mĕ-lom′ĕ-lus) a fetal monster with supernumerary limbs.

meloplasty (mel′o-plas″te) 1. plastic surgery of a cheek. 2. plastic surgery of the extremities.

melorheostosis (mel″o-re″os-to′sis) a form of osteosclerosis, with linear tracks extending through the long bones.

melotia (mĕ-lo′she-ah) congenital displacement of the auricle of the ear.

membrana (mem-bra′nah), pl. *membra′nae* [L.] membrane.

membrane (mem′brān) a thin layer of tissue which covers a surface or divides an organ. adj., **mem′branous. abdominal m.,** peritoneum. **accidental m.,** false membrane. **alveolodental m.,** periodontium. **animal m.,** a thin diaphragm of membrane, as of bladder, used as a dialyzer. **aponeurotic m.,** aponeurosis. **arachnoid m.,** arachnoid. **Ascherson's m.,** the covering of casein enclosing the milk globules. **asphyxial m.,** hyaline membrane (3). **Baer's m.,** chromicized pig's bladder. **basement m.,** delicate layer underlying epithelium. **basilar m.,** the lower boundary of the scala media of the ear. **birth m's,** the amnion and placenta. **Bowman's m.,** the basement membrane that underlies the epithelium of the cornea. **Bruch's m.,** inner layer of choroid coat. **cell m.,** the condensed protoplasm which forms the enveloping capsule of a cell. **chromatic m.,** a continuous layer of chromatin substance situated on the internal surface of a nuclear membrane. **Corti's m.,** membrane over Corti's organ. **croupous m.,** false membrane of true croup. **Débove's m.,** delicate layer between the epithelium and tunica propria of bronchial, vesicular and intestinal mucous membrane. **dentinoenamel m.,** a continuous, thin membrane laid down by ameloblasts adjoining the basement membrane separating them from the dentin in an early developing tooth. **Descemet's m.,** posterior lining membrane of the cornea. **diphtheritic m.,** the peculiar false membrane characteristic of diphtheria. **drum m.,** tympanic membrane. **elastic m.,** a membrane made up largely of elastic fibers. **endoneural m.,** neurilemma. **false m.,** membranous exudate, like that of diphtheria. **fenestrated m.,** one of the perforated elastic plates of the tunica intima and tunica media of arteries. **fetal m's,** the membranes that protect the embryo and provide for its nutrition, respiration and excretion: the yolk sac (umbilical vesicle), allantois, amnion, chorion, decidua and placenta. **germinal m.,** the blastoderm. **homogeneous m.,** one covering the placental villi. **Huxley's m.,** cellular membrane of root sheath and proximal end of a hair. **hyaline m.,** 1. a membrane between outer root sheath and inner fibrous layer of hair follicle. 2. basement membrane. 3. a homogeneous eosinophilic membrane lining alveolar ducts and alveoli, frequently found at necropsy in premature infants. **hymenal m.,** hymen. **hyoglossal m.,** a fibrous lamina connecting the under surface of the tongue with the hyoid bone. **impermeable m.,** one which does not permit passage through it of any substance. **Jackson's m.,** a web of adhesions sometimes covering the cecum and causing obstruction of the bowel. **Jacob's m.,** bacillary layer. **keratogenous m.,** matrix unguis. **Krause's m.,** membrane supposed to separate disks of sarcous matter in muscle. **limiting m.,** one which constitutes the border of some tissue or structure. **medullary m.,** endosteum. **mucous m.,** membrane covered with epithelium lining canals and cavities which communicate with exterior of the body. **Nasmyth's m.,** membrane covering enamel of an unworn tooth. **nictitating m.,** a transparent fold of skin, the so-called third eyelid of various animals. **nuclear m.,** the outer layer of the nucleoplasm. **olfactory m.,** the olfactory portion of the mucous membrane lining the nasal fossa. **oronasal m.,** a thin epithelial plate separating the nasal pits from the oral cavity of the embryo. **ovular m.,** vitelline membrane. **peridental m., periodontal m.,** periodontium. **permeable m.,** one permitting free passage of substances through it. **placental m.,** the semipermeable membrane which separates the fetal from the maternal blood in the placenta. **plasma m.,** the surrounding membrane of a cell. **pulmonary hyaline m.,** hyaline membrane (3). **Reissner's m.,** a thin membrane between the cochlear canal and the scala vestibuli. **Ruysch's m., ruyschian m.,** lamina choriocapillaris. **Scarpa's m.,** the membrane closing the fenestra rotunda. **schneiderian m.,** mucous membrane lining the nose. **semipermeable m.,** one permitting passage through it of some but not all substances. **serous m.,** the lining membrane of the cavities which have no communication with the exterior of the body. **Shrapnell's m.**, the thin upper part of the tympanic membrane. **striated m.**, zona pellucida. **subepithelial m.**, basement membrane. **synaptic m.**, the layer separating the neuroplasm of an axon from that of the body of the nerve cell with which it makes synapsis. **synovial m.**, vascular connective tissue lining the articular capsule of diarthrodial joints, bursae and tendon sheaths. **tectorial m.**, Corti's membrane. **tendinous m.**, aponeurosis. **Tenon's m.**, vaginae bulbi. **tympanic m.**, the membrane marking the inner termination of the external ear canal, separating it from the middle ear. **undulating m.**, a protoplasmic membrane running like a fin along the bodies of certain protozoa. **vernix m.**, hyaline membrane (3). **virginal m.**, hymen. **vitelline m.**, the external envelope of the ovum. **vitreous m.**, Descemet's membrane; hyaline membrane (1). **yolk m.**, vitelline membrane.

membraniform (mem-bran'i-form) resembling a membrane.

membranocartilaginous (mem″brah-no-kar″-tĭ-laj'ĭ-nus) pertaining to membrane and cartilage.

membranoid (mem′brah-noid) resembling a membrane.

membrum (mem′brum), pl. *mem'bra* [L.] a limb or member of the body; an entire arm or leg. **m. mulie'bre**, clitoris. **m. viri'le**, penis.

menacme (mĕ-nak′me) the period of a woman's life which is marked by menstrual activity.

menadiol (men″ah-di′ol) a vitamin K analogue. **m. sodium diphosphate**, a compound used to promote the formation of prothrombin.

menadione (-di′ōn) a compound used as a prothrombinogenic vitamin.

menaphthene (men-af′thēn) menadione.

menaphthone (men-af′thōn) menadione.

menarche (mĕ-nar′ke) establishment or beginning of the menstrual function. adj., **menar'-chial**.

mendelevium (men″dĕ-le′ve-um) chemical element (*see table*), at. no. 101, symbol Md.

Menformon (men′for-mon) trademark for a preparation of estrone.

mening(o)- (mĕ-ning′go) word element [Gr.], *meninges*.

meningeal (mĕ-nin′je-al) pertaining to the meninges.

meningeorrhaphy (mĕ-nin″je-or′ah-fe) suture of membranes.

meninges (mĕ-nin′jēz) (plural of *meninx*) the three membranes covering the brain and spinal cord: dura mater, arachnoid and pia mater. adj., **menin'geal**.

meningioma (mĕ-nin″je-o′mah) a tumor of the meninges. **angioblastic m.**, angioblastoma.

meningism (men′in-jizm) meningismus.

meningismus (men″in-jiz′mus) a noninfective state resembling meningitis.

meningitis (-ji′tis), pl. *meningit'ides* [Gr.] inflammation of the meninges, with both mental and motor symptoms. adj., **meningit'ic**. **basal m.**, inflammation of the meninges at the base of the brain. **cerebral m.**, inflamma-tion of the membranes of the brain. **cerebrospinal m.**, inflammation of meninges of brain and spinal cord. **epidemic cerebrospinal m.**, an acute infectious disease attacking children especially, and caused by the meningococcus. **m. ossif'icans**, ossification of the meninges. **septicemic m.**, that due to septic blood poisoning. **serous m.**, meningitis marked by serous exudation into the cerebral ventricles. **spinal m.**, inflammation of the membranes of spinal cord. **tubercular m.**, acute hydrocephalus.

meningocele (mĕ-ning′go-sēl) hernial protrusion of meninges through a defect in the cranium or vertebral column.

meningocerebritis (mĕ-ning″go-ser″e-bri′tis) inflammation of brain and meninges.

meningococcemia (-kok-se′me-ah) presence of meningococci in the blood, producing an acute fulminating disease or an insidious disorder persisting for months or years. **acute fulminating m.**, Waterhouse-Friderichsen syndrome.

meningococcidal (-kok-si′dal) destroying meningococci.

meningococcus (-kok′us), pl. *meningococ'ci* [Gr.] *Neisseria meningitidis*.

meningocortical (-kor′tĭ-kal) pertaining to meninges and cortex.

meningocyte (mĕ-ning′go-sīt) a histiocyte of the meninges.

meningoencephalitis (mĕ-ning″go-en-sef″ah-li′tis) inflammation of brain and meninges.

meningoencephalocele (-en-sef′ah-lo-sēl″) hernial tissue through a defect in the cranium.

meningoencephalomyelitis (-en-sef″ah-lo-mi″ĕ-li′tis) inflammation of meninges, brain and spinal cord.

meningoencephalomyelopathy (-mi″ĕ-lop′ah-the) disease involving meninges, brain and spinal cord.

meningoencephalopathy (mĕ-ning″go-en-sef″ah-lop′ah-the) noninflammatory disease of the cerebral meninges and brain.

meningomalacia (-mah-la′she-ah) softening of a membrane.

meningomyelitis (-mi″ĕ-li′tis) inflammation of spinal cord and membranes.

meningomyelocele (-mi′ĕ-lo-sēl″) hernial protrusion of the meninges and spinal cord through a defect in the vertebral column.

meningomyeloradiculitis (-mi″ĕ-lo-rah-dĭk″u-li′tis) inflammation of meninges, spinal cord and spinal nerve roots.

meningopathy (men″in-gop′ah-the) any disease of the meninges.

meningorhachidian (mĕ-ning″go-rah-kid′e-an) pertaining to spinal cord and meninges.

meningorrhagia (-ra′je-ah) hemorrhage from cerebral or spinal membranes.

meningorrhea (-re′ah) effusion of blood on the meninges.

meningosis (men″in-go′sis) attachment of bones by membrane.

meningothelioma (mĕ-ning″go-the″le-o′mah) meningioma.

meninx (me′ninks), pl. *menin'ges* [Gr.] a membrane, especially one of the membranes of the brain or spinal cord—the dura mater, arachnoid and pia mater.

meniscectomy (men″ĭ-sek′to-me) excision of a meniscus, as of the knee joint.

meniscitis (-si′tis) inflammation of a semilunar cartilage of the knee joint.

meniscocyte (mĕ-nis′ko-sīt) a crescent- or sickle-shaped red blood corpuscle.

meniscocytosis (mĕ-nis″ko-si-to′sis) sickle cell anemia.

meniscus (mĕ-nis′kus), pl. *menis′ci* [L.] something of crescent shape, as the concave or convex surface of a column of liquid in a pipet or buret, or a crescent-shaped fibrocartilage in the knee joint.

meno- (men′o) word element [Gr.], *menstruation.*

menolipsis (men″o-lip′sis) temporary cessation of menstruation.

menometastasis (-mĕ-tas′tah-sis) vicarious menstruation.

menometrorrhagia (-met″ro-ra′je-ah) excessive uterine bleeding at and between menstrual periods.

menopause (men′o-pawz) cessation of menstruation. adj., **men′opausal.**

menorrhagia (men″o-ra′je-ah) excessive menstruation.

menorrhalgia (-ral′je-ah) pain during menstruation.

menoschesis (mĕ-nos′kĕ-sis, men″o-ske′sis) suppression of menstruation.

menostasis (mĕ-nos′tah-sis) menoschesis.

menostaxis (men″o-stak′sis) a prolonged menstrual period.

menotoxin (-tok′sin) a toxic substance in the body fluid during menstruation. adj., **menotox′ic.**

menses (men′sēz) menstruation. adj., **men′strual.**

menstruation (men″stroo-a′shun) the cyclic, physiologic discharge of blood from the nonpregnant uterus, occurring usually at approximately four-week intervals in the human and a few other primates. **anovular m., anovulatory m.,** periodic uterine bleeding without preceding ovulation. **vicarious m.,** bleeding from extragenital mucous membrane at the time one would normally expect the menstrual period.

menstruum (men′stroo-um) a solvent medium.

mensuration (men″su-ra′shun) the process of measuring.

mentagra (men-tag′rah) sycosis.

mental (men′tal) 1. pertaining to the mind. 2. pertaining to the chin.

menthol (men′thol) an alcohol from various mint oils or produced synthetically, used locally to relieve itching.

menticide (men′tĭ-sīd) destruction of the mind of an individual.

mentum (men′tum) [L.] chin.

mepacrine (mep′ah-krin) quinacrine hydrochloride.

mepazine (mep′ah-zēn) a phenothiazine derivative used as a sedative in psychoses and severe neuroses.

mepenzolate (me-pen′zo-lāt) a compound used in parasympathetic blockade and as an antispasmodic.

meperidine (mĕ-per′ĭ-dēn) a fine, white crystalline powder used as a narcotic analgesic.

mephenamine (mĕ-fen′ah-mēn) orphenadrine.

mephenesin (mĕ-fen′ĕ-sin) a white crystalline powder used as a skeletal muscle relaxant.

mephenoxalone (mef″en-ok′sah-lōn) a compound used as an antianxiety and calming agent.

mephentermine (mĕ-fen′ter-mēn) a compound used as a sympathomimetic and as a pressor substance.

mephitibiosis (mĕ-fit″ĭ-bi-o′sis) the capacity of certain bacteria to grow better under increased carbon dioxide tension. adj., **mephitibiot′ic.**

mephitic (mĕ-fit′ik) noxious; foul.

mephobarbital (mef″o-bar′bĭ-tal) a white crystalline powder used as an anticonvulsant with a slight hypnotic action.

Mephyton (mef′ĭ-ton) trademark for preparations of vitamin K₁.

Meprane (me′prān) trademark for preparations of promethestrol.

meprobamate (mĕ-pro′bah-māt, mep″ro-bam′āt) a bitter white powder used as a tranquilizer.

meprylcaine (mep′ril-kān) a compound used as a local anesthetic.

mepyramine (me-pir′ah-mēn) pyrilamine.

mEq. milliequivalent.

meralluride (mer-al′lu-rīd) a white or slightly yellow powder used as a diuretic.

meralgia (mĕ-ral′je-ah) pain in the thigh. **m. paresthet′ica,** a disease marked by disturbance of sensation in the outer surface of the thigh.

Meratran (mer′ah-tran) trademark for a preparation of pipradrol hydrochloride.

merbromin (mer-bro′min) an antibacterial compound occurring as iridescent green scales or granules.

mercaptan (mer-kap′tan) an alcohol in which oxygen is replaced by sulfur.

mercaptomerin (mer-kap″to-mer′in) an organic mercurial diuretic. **sodium m.,** a compound used parenterally as a diuretic.

mercaptopurine (-pu′rēn) a yellow crystalline compound used as a neoplastic suppressant.

Mercodinone (mer″ko-di′nōn) trademark for a preparation of dihydroxodeinone.

Mercuhydrin (mer″ku-hi′drin) trademark for preparations of meralluride.

mercuramide (mer-kūr′ah-mīd) mersalyl.

mercurial (mer-ku′re-al) 1. pertaining to mercury. 2. a preparation containing mercury.

mercurialism (mer-ku′re-al-izm″) chronic poisoning from mercury.

mercuric (mer-ku′rik) pertaining to mercury in its higher valency; containing divalent mercury. **m. chloride,** mercury bichloride. **m. iodide, red,** mercury biniodide, used as an antibacterial agent. **m. oxide, red,** orange-red crystalline powder; antiseptic. **m. oxide, yellow,** a yellow to orange-yellow, heavy, impalpable powder used as a local antibacterial agent. **m. salicylate,** slightly yellow or pink odorless powder; used in treatment of syphilis.

Mercurochrome (mer-ku′ro-krōm) trademark for preparations of merbromin.

mercurophylline (mer″ku-ro-fil′lin) a white

to slightly yellow, odorless powder used as a diuretic.

mercurous (mer'ku-rus) pertaining to mercury in its lower valency; containing monovalent mercury. **m. chloride,** a white, odorless, tasteless powder used in pills or tablets as a cathartic or, in an ointment, as a local antibacterial agent. **m. iodide, yellow,** strong, yellowish-orange amorphous powder; antisyphilitic.

mercury (mer'ku-re) chemical element (*see table*), at. no. 80, symbol Hg. **ammoniated m.,** a compound occurring in white, pulverulent pieces or amorphous powder, used as a local anti-infective. **m. bichloride,** a poisonous compound occurring as heavy, odorless crystals, crystalline masses or white powder; used as a disinfectant. **m. chloride, mild,** mercurous chloride. **m. oleate,** yellowish-brown, ointment-like substance, yellow mercuric oxide in oleic acid; used locally in various skin diseases. **m. perchloride,** mercury bichloride.

mere (mēr) one of the parts into which a zygote divides.

merergastic (mer"er-gas'tik) pertaining to the simplest type of disorder of psychic function, marked by emotional instability and anxiety.

merethoxylline (mer"ĕ-thok'sĭ-lēn) a compound used as a diuretic.

meridian (mĕ-rid'e-an) an imaginary line on the surface of a globe or sphere, connecting the opposite ends of its axis.

meridianus (mĕ-rid"e-a'nus), pl. *meridia'ni* [L.] meridian. adj., **morid'ional.**

meroblastic (mer-o-blas'tik) partially dividing; undergoing cleavage in which only part of the egg participates.

merocele (mer'o-sēl) femoral hernia.

merocoxalgia (mer"o-kok-sal'je-ah) pain in the thigh and hip.

merocrine (mer'o-krin) discharging only the secretory product and maintaining the secretory cell intact (e.g. salivary glands, pancreas).

merogenesis (mer"o-jen'ĕ-sis) cleavage of an ovum. adj., **merogenet'ic.**

merogony (mĕ-rog'o-ne) the development of a portion only of an ovum. adj., **merogon'ic. diploid m.,** development of a fragment of an ovum containing the fused male and female pronuclei. **parthenogenetic m.,** development of an enucleated portion of an ovum under the influence of an artificial stimulus.

meromicrosomia (mer"o-mi"kro-so'me-ah) unusual smallness of some part of the body.

meronecrosis (-ne-kro'sis) necrosis affecting only limited areas of cells.

meroparesthesia (-par"es-the'ze-ah) alteration of the tactile sense in the extremities.

meropia (mĕ-ro'pe-ah) partial blindness.

merorhachischisis (me"ro-rah-kis'kĭ-sis) fissure of part of the spinal cord.

merosmia (mĕ-roz'me-ah) inability to perceive certain odors.

merostotic (mer"os-tot'ik) affecting only part of a bone.

merosystolic (me"ro-sis-tol'ik) pertaining to part of the systole.

merotomy (mĕ-rot'o-me) a cutting into segments.

merozoite (mer"o-zo'ĭt) one of the organisms formed by multiple fission (schizogony) of a sporozoite within the body of the host.

Merphene (mer'fēn) trademark for preparations of phenylmercuric nitrate.

Merphenyl (mer'fen-il) trademark for preparations of phenylmercuric compounds.

mersalyl (mer'sah-lil) white crystalline powder; mercurial diuretic.

Merthiolate mer-thi'o-lāt trademark for preparations of thimerosal.

merycism (mer'ĭ-sizm) the regurgitation of food from the stomach and chewing it again.

mes(o)- (mes'o) word element [Gr.], *middle.*

mesad (me'sad) mesiad.

mesal (me'sal) mesial.

Mesantoin (mē-san'to-in) trademark for methylphenylethyl hydantoin.

mesaortitis (mes"a-or-ti'tis) inflammation of the middle (muscular) coat of the aorta.

mesaraic (mes"ah-ra'ik) mesenteric.

mesarteritis (mes"ar-ter-i'tis) inflammation of the middle coat of an artery.

mesati- word element, *midmost.*

mesaticephalic (mes-at"ĭ-se-fal'ik) having a cephalic index of 75–80.

mesatipellic (-pel'ik) having a pelvic index between 90 and 95.

mescaline (mes'kah-lēn) a poisonous alkaloid derived from a Mexican cactus, which produces hallucinations of sound and color.

mescalism (mes'kah-lizm) intoxication due to mescal buttons or mescaline.

mesectoderm (mĕ-sek'to-derm) migratory cells derived from the neural crest of the head that contribute to the formation of the meninges and become pigment cells.

mesencephalitis (mes"en-sef"ah-li'tis) inflammation of the mesencephalon.

mesencephalon (-sef'ah-lon) the midbrain.

mesencephalotomy (-sef"ah-lot'o-me) surgical production of lesions in the midbrain for the relief of intractable pain.

mesenchyma (mē-seng'kĭ-mah) the meshwork of embryonic connective tissue in the mesoderm from which are formed the connective tissues of the body and also the blood vessels and lymphatic vessels. adj., **mesen'chymal.**

mesenchyme (mes'eng-kīm) mesenchyma.

mesenchymoma (mes"en-ki-mo'mah) a mixed mesenchymal tumor composed of two or more cellular elements.

mesenterectomy (mes"en-tĕ-rek'to-me) excision of the mesentery.

mesenteriopexy (-ter'e-o-pek"se) fixation of a torn mesentery.

mesenteriorrhaphy (-ter"e-or'ah-fe) suture of the mesentery.

mesenteriplication (mes"en-ter"ĭ-pli-ka'shun) the operation of taking a tuck in the mesentery to shorten it.

mesenteritis (mes"en-te-ri'tis) inflammation of the midgut.

mesenterium (-te're-um) mesentery.

mesenteron (mes-en'ter-on) the part of the primitive body cavity from which the alimentary canal, lungs, liver and pancreas are derived.

mesentery (mes'en-ter"e) fold of peritoneum

attaching the intestine to the posterior abdominal wall. adj., **mesenter'ic.**

mesiad (me'ze-ad) toward the middle or center.

mesial (me'ze-al) situated in the middle.

mesially (me'ze-al″e) toward the median line.

mesiobuccal (me″ze-o-buk'kal) pertaining to or formed by the mesial and buccal surfaces of a tooth, or the mesial and buccal walls of a tooth cavity.

mesioclination (-kli-na'shun) deviation of a tooth from the vertical, toward the tooth next mesial to it in the dental arch.

mesioclusion (-kloo'zhun) malocclusion in which the teeth of the mandible are mesial to their opposite numbers in the maxilla.

mesiodens (me'ze-o-dens) a small, supernumerary tooth between the maxillary central incisors.

mesion (me'ze-on) the plane dividing the body into right and left symmetrical halves.

mesioversion (me″ze-o-ver'zhun) displacement of a tooth along the dental arch toward the midline of the face.

mesmerism (mes'mer-izm) hypnotism.

mesoappendix (mes″o-ah-pen'diks) peritoneal fold connecting the appendix to the ileum.

mesoarium (mes″o-a're-um) mesovarium.

mesobacterium (-bak-te're-um), pl. *mesobacte'ria* [L.] a rod-shaped microorganism of medium size.

mesoblast (mes'o-blast) mesoderm.

mesobronchitis (mes″o-brong-ki'tis) inflammation of middle coat of bronchi.

mesocardia (-kar'de-ah) location of the heart in the middle line of the thorax.

mesocardium (-kar'de-um) a membrane connecting the embryonic heart with the body wall.

mesocecum (-se'kum) the mesentery of the cecum.

mesocephalic (-sĕ-fal'ik) 1. pertaining to the mesencephalon. 2. mesaticephalic.

mesocephalon (-sef'ah-lon) mesencephalon.

mesococcus (-kok'us), pl. *mesococ'ci* [L.] a spherical microorganism of medium size.

mesocoelia (-se'le-ah) the aqueduct of Sylvius.

mesocolon (-ko'lon) the peritoneal process attaching the colon to the posterior abdominal wall. **pelvic m., sigmoid m.,** the peritoneum attaching the sigmoid colon to the posterior abdominal wall. **transverse m.,** peritoneum attaching the transverse colon to the posterior abdominal wall.

mesocolopexy (-ko'lo-pek″se) mesocoloplication.

mesocoloplication (-ko″lo-pli-ka'shun) the taking of a tuck in the mesocolon to shorten it.

mesoconchous (-kong'kus) having an orbital index of 76–84.9.

mesocord (mes'o-kord) an umbilical cord adherent to the placenta.

mesocyst (mes'o-sist) peritoneal fold attaching the gallbladder to the liver.

mesocytoma (mes″o-si-to'mah) a connective tissue tumor.

mesodens (mes'o-dens) mesiodens.

mesoderm (mes'o-derm) an intermediate layer of cells developing between the ecto-

derm and entoderm; from it are formed all types of muscle, connective tissue, bone marrow, blood, lymphoid tissue, and the epithelium of body and joint cavities, blood vessels, etc. adj., **mesoder'mal, mesoder'-mic. somatic m.,** the outer layer of the developing mesoderm. **splanchnic m.,** the inner layer of the developing mesoderm.

mesodmitis (mes″od-mi'tis) inflammation of the mediastinum.

mesoduodenum (mes″o-du″o-de'num) the mesentery of the duodenum.

meso-epididymis (-ep″ĭ-did'ĭ-mis) a fold of tunica vaginalis connecting the epididymis and testis.

mesogaster (-gas'ter) mesogastrium.

mesogastric (-gas'trik) 1. pertaining to mesogastrium. 2. pertaining to the umbilical region.

mesogastrium (-gas'tre-um) the portion of the primitive mesentery which encloses the stomach and from which the greater omentum develops.

mesoglia (me-sog'le-ah) oligodendroglia.

mesoglioma (mes″o-gli-o'mah) a tumor of the oligodendroglia.

mesognathion (mes″og-na'the-on) the lateral center of ossification in the incisive bone for the lateral incisor tooth.

mesognathous (mĕ-sog'nah-thus) having a gnathic index of 98–103.

mesohyloma (mes″o-hi-lo'mah) a tumor developed from the mesothelium.

meso-ileum (-il'e-um) the mesentery of the ileum.

mesojejunum (-je-ju'num) the mesentery of the jejunum.

mesolecithal (-les'ĭ-thal) having a moderate amount of yolk.

mesolymphocyte (-lim'fo-sīt) a medium-sized lymphocyte.

mesomere (mes'o-mēr) 1. a blastomere of size intermediate between a macromere and a micromere. 2. a midzone of the mesoderm between the epimere and hypomere.

mesomerism (mĕ-som'er-izm) the existence of organic chemical structures differing only in the position of electrons rather than atoms. adj., **mesomer'ic.**

mesometritis (mes″o-me-tri'tis) inflammation of the broad ligament.

mesometrium (-me'tre-um) the broad ligament.

mesomorph (mez'o-morf, mes'o-morf) a person exhibiting mesomorphy.

mesomorphy (mes″o-mor'fe) a type of body build in which tissues derived from the mesoderm predominate; a somatotype in which the bone, muscle and connective tissue are highly developed. adj., **mesomor'phic.**

meson (me'zon, mes'on) 1. mesion. 2. any elementary particle having a rest mass intermediate between the mass of the electron and that of the proton.

mesonephroma (mez″o-ne-fro'mah) a tumor arising from the mesonephron.

mesonephron (-nef'ron) mesonephros. adj., **mesoneph'ric.**

mesonephros (-nef'ros), pl. *mesoneph'roi* [Gr.] the excretory organ of the embryo, arising

THE HUMAN BODY

SKELETAL MUSCLES

Frontalis

Temporalis

Orbicularis oculi

Masseter

Sternocleido-mastoid

Trapezius

Deltoid

Pectoralis major

Biceps brachii

Latissimus dorsi

Pronator teres

Flexor carpi radialis

Palmaris longus

Tensor fascia lata

Rectus abdominis (beneath rectus sheath)

Iliotibial band

Vastus lateralis

Patella

Peroneus longus

Tibialis anterior

Soleus

Tibia

Medial malleolus (tibia)

Orbicularis oris

Clavicle

Sternum

Triceps brachii

Brachialis

Brachioradialis

Extensor carpi radialis longus

Serratus anterior

Ext. oblique

Crest of iliac bone

Inguinal ligament

Iliopsoas

Pectineus

Adductor longus

Gracilis

Rectus femoris

Sartorius

Vastus lateralis

Vastus medialis

Tendon of quadriceps femoris muscle group

Patella

Patellar ligament

Gastrocnemius

Soleus

BONES

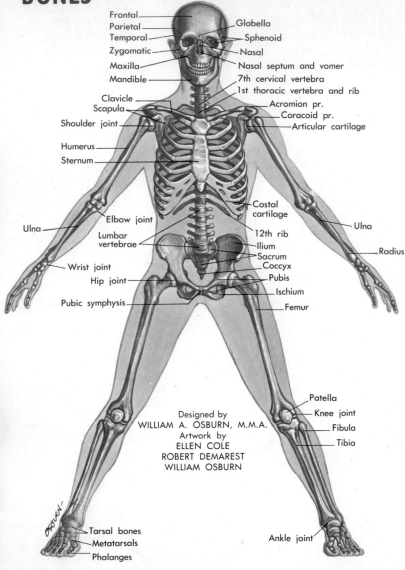

Frontal
Parietal
Temporal
Zygomatic
Maxilla
Mandible
Glabella
Sphenoid
Nasal
Nasal septum and vomer
7th cervical vertebra
1st thoracic vertebra and rib
Clavicle
Scapula
Shoulder joint
Acromion pr.
Coracoid pr.
Articular cartilage
Humerus
Sternum
Costal cartilage
Ulna
Elbow joint
Lumbar vertebrae
12th rib
Ilium
Sacrum
Coccyx
Ulna
Radius
Wrist joint
Hip joint
Pubic symphysis
Pubis
Ischium
Femur
Patella
Knee joint
Fibula
Tibia

Designed by
WILLIAM A. OSBURN, M.M.A.
Artwork by
ELLEN COLE
ROBERT DEMAREST
WILLIAM OSBURN

Tarsal bones
Metatarsals
Phalanges
Ankle joint

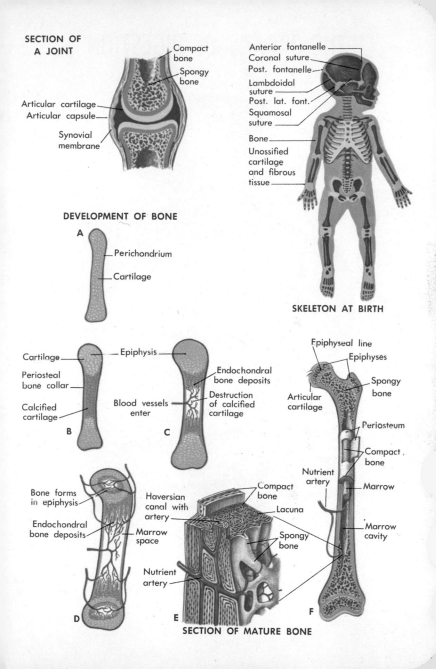

SECTION OF A JOINT

Compact bone
Spongy bone
Articular cartilage
Articular capsule
Synovial membrane

Anterior fontanelle
Coronal suture
Post. fontanelle
Lambdoidal suture
Post. lat. font.
Squamosal suture
Bone
Unossified cartilage and fibrous tissue

SKELETON AT BIRTH

DEVELOPMENT OF BONE

A
Perichondrium
Cartilage

B
Cartilage
Periosteal bone collar
Calcified cartilage
Epiphysis

C
Endochondral bone deposits
Blood vessels enter
Destruction of calcified cartilage

D
Bone forms in epiphysis
Endochondral bone deposits
Marrow space

E
Haversian canal with artery
Compact bone
Lacuna
Spongy bone
Nutrient artery

SECTION OF MATURE BONE

F
Epiphyseal line
Epiphyses
Spongy bone
Articular cartilage
Periosteum
Compact bone
Nutrient artery
Marrow
Marrow cavity

THE ORGANS OF DIGESTION

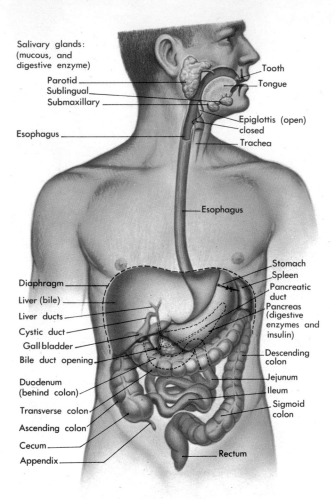

Salivary glands:
(mucous, and
digestive enzyme)

Parotid
Sublingual
Submaxillary

Tooth
Tongue

Esophagus

Epiglottis (open)
closed
Trachea

Esophagus

Diaphragm
Liver (bile)
Liver ducts
Cystic duct
Gall bladder
Bile duct opening

Duodenum
(behind colon)

Transverse colon
Ascending colon
Cecum
Appendix

Stomach
Spleen
Pancreatic
duct
Pancreas
(digestive
enzymes and
insulin)

Descending
colon

Jejunum
Ileum
Sigmoid
colon

Rectum

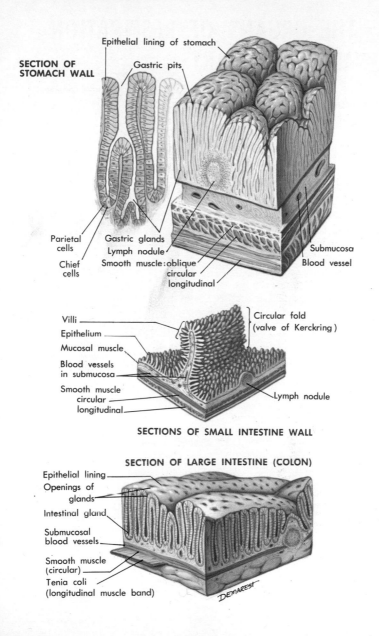

SECTION OF STOMACH WALL

Epithelial lining of stomach

Gastric pits

Parietal cells

Chief cells

Gastric glands

Lymph nodule

Smooth muscle: oblique
circular
longitudinal

Submucosa

Blood vessel

Villi

Epithelium

Mucosal muscle

Blood vessels in submucosa

Smooth muscle
circular
longitudinal

Circular fold
(valve of Kerckring)

Lymph nodule

SECTIONS OF SMALL INTESTINE WALL

SECTION OF LARGE INTESTINE (COLON)

Epithelial lining

Openings of glands

Intestinal gland

Submucosal blood vessels

Smooth muscle (circular)

Tenia coli
(longitudinal muscle band)

DEMAREST

THE ORGANS OF RESPIRATION AND THE HEART

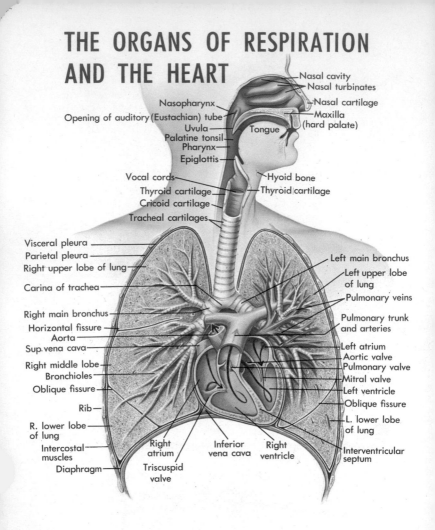

Nasal cavity
Nasal turbinates
Nasal cartilage
Maxilla (hard palate)
Nasopharynx
Opening of auditory (Eustachian) tube
Uvula
Tongue
Palatine tonsil
Pharynx
Epiglottis
Vocal cords
Hyoid bone
Thyroid cartilage
Thyroid cartilage
Cricoid cartilage
Tracheal cartilages
Visceral pleura
Parietal pleura
Right upper lobe of lung
Left main bronchus
Left upper lobe of lung
Carina of trachea
Pulmonary veins
Right main bronchus
Pulmonary trunk and arteries
Horizontal fissure
Aorta
Sup. vena cava
Left atrium
Aortic valve
Pulmonary valve
Right middle lobe
Mitral valve
Bronchioles
Left ventricle
Oblique fissure
Oblique fissure
Rib
L. lower lobe of lung
R. lower lobe of lung
Intercostal muscles
Interventricular septum
Diaphragm
Right atrium
Inferior vena cava
Right ventricle
Triscuspid valve

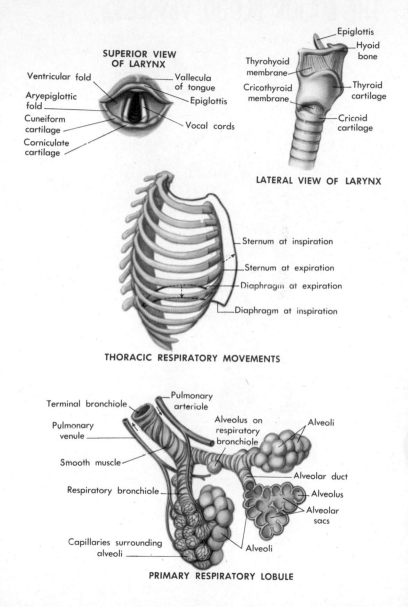

SUPERIOR VIEW OF LARYNX

Ventricular fold
Aryepiglottic fold
Cuneiform cartilage
Corniculate cartilage
Vallecula of tongue
Epiglottis
Vocal cords

Epiglottis
Hyoid bone
Thyrohyoid membrane
Cricothyroid membrane
Thyroid cartilage
Cricoid cartilage

LATERAL VIEW OF LARYNX

Sternum at inspiration
Sternum at expiration
Diaphragm at expiration
Diaphragm at inspiration

THORACIC RESPIRATORY MOVEMENTS

Terminal bronchiole
Pulmonary arteriole
Pulmonary venule
Alveolus on respiratory bronchiole
Alveoli
Smooth muscle
Respiratory bronchiole
Alveolar duct
Alveolus
Alveolar sacs
Capillaries surrounding alveoli
Alveoli

PRIMARY RESPIRATORY LOBULE

THE MAJOR BLOOD VESSELS

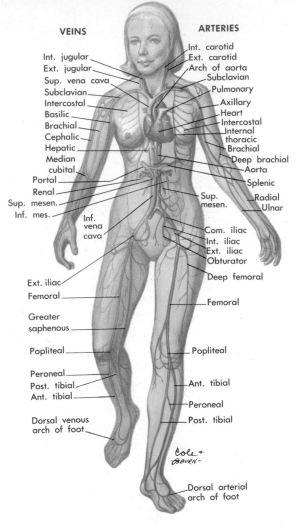

VEINS

- Int. jugular
- Ext. jugular
- Sup. vena cava
- Subclavian
- Intercostal
- Basilic
- Brachial
- Cephalic
- Hepatic
- Median cubital
- Portal
- Renal
- Sup. mesen.
- Inf. mes.
- Inf. vena cava
- Ext. iliac
- Femoral
- Greater saphenous
- Popliteal
- Peroneal
- Post. tibial
- Ant. tibial
- Dorsal venous arch of foot

ARTERIES

- Int. carotid
- Ext. carotid
- Arch of aorta
- Subclavian
- Pulmonary
- Axillary
- Heart
- Intercostal
- Internal thoracic
- Brachial
- Deep brachial
- Aorta
- Splenic
- Sup. mesen.
- Radial
- Ulnar
- Com. iliac
- Int. iliac
- Ext. iliac
- Obturator
- Deep femoral
- Femoral
- Popliteal
- Ant. tibial
- Peroneal
- Post. tibial
- Dorsal arterial arch of foot

Cole & OSBURN

DETAILS OF CIRCULATORY STRUCTURES

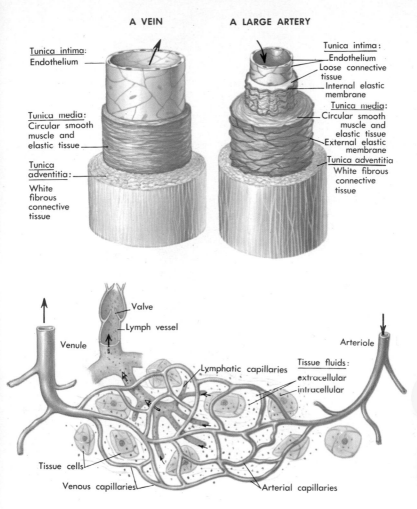

A CAPILLARY BED

THE BRAIN AND SPINAL NERVES

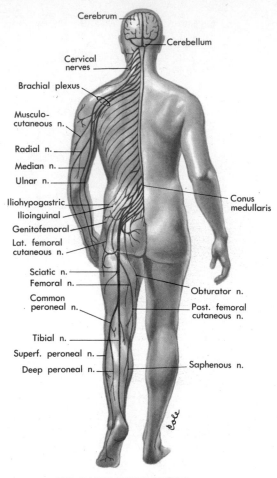

Cerebrum

Cerebellum

Cervical nerves

Brachial plexus

Musculo-cutaneous n.

Radial n.

Median n.

Ulnar n.

Iliohypogastric

Ilioinguinal

Genitofemoral

Lat. femoral cutaneous n.

Sciatic n.

Femoral n.

Common peroneal n.

Tibial n.

Superf. peroneal n.

Deep peroneal n.

Conus medullaris

Obturator n.

Post. femoral cutaneous n.

Saphenous n.

THE MAJOR SPINAL NERVES

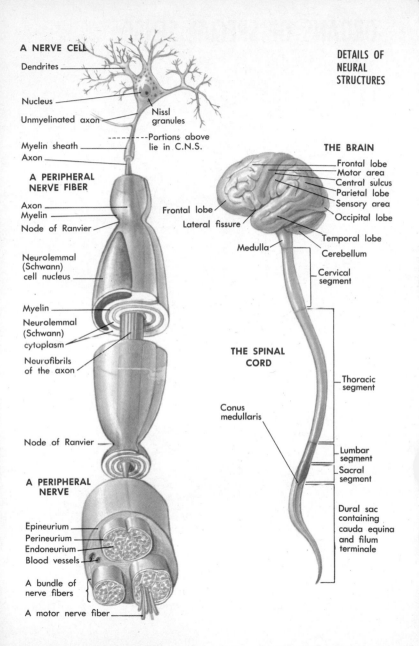

A NERVE CELL

Dendrites

Nucleus

Unmyelinated axon

Nissl granules

Myelin sheath

Portions above lie in C.N.S.

Axon

A PERIPHERAL NERVE FIBER

Axon

Myelin

Node of Ranvier

Neurolemmal (Schwann) cell nucleus

Myelin

Neurolemmal (Schwann) cytoplasm

Neurofibrils of the axon

Node of Ranvier

A PERIPHERAL NERVE

Epineurium

Perineurium

Endoneurium

Blood vessels

A bundle of nerve fibers

A motor nerve fiber

DETAILS OF NEURAL STRUCTURES

THE BRAIN

Frontal lobe

Motor area

Central sulcus

Parietal lobe

Sensory area

Occipital lobe

Frontal lobe

Lateral fissure

Temporal lobe

Medulla

Cerebellum

Cervical segment

THE SPINAL CORD

Thoracic segment

Conus medullaris

Lumbar segment

Sacral segment

Dural sac containing cauda equina and filum terminale

ORGANS OF SPECIAL SENSE THE EAR

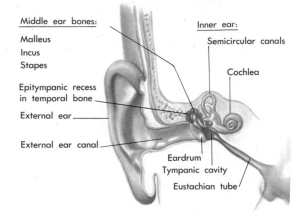

Middle ear bones:

Malleus
Incus
Stapes

Epitympanic recess
in temporal bone

External ear

External ear canal

Inner ear:

Semicircular canals

Cochlea

Eardrum
Tympanic cavity
Eustachian tube

THE ORGAN OF HEARING

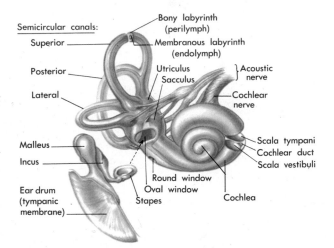

Semicircular canals:

Superior

Posterior

Lateral

Malleus

Incus

Ear drum
(tympanic
membrane)

Bony labyrinth
(perilymph)

Membranous labyrinth
(endolymph)

Utriculus
Sacculus

Acoustic
nerve

Cochlear
nerve

Scala tympani
Cochlear duct
Scala vestibuli

Round window
Oval window
Stapes

Cochlea

THE MIDDLE EAR AND INNER EAR

THE LACRIMAL APPARATUS AND THE EYE

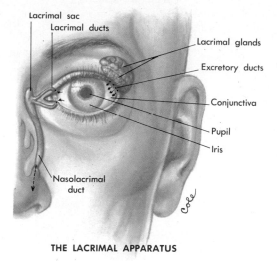

Lacrimal sac
Lacrimal ducts
Lacrimal glands
Excretory ducts
Conjunctiva
Pupil
Iris
Nasolacrimal duct

THE LACRIMAL APPARATUS

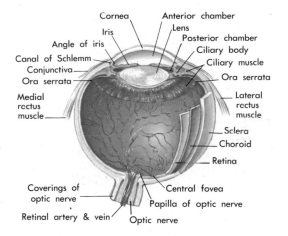

Cornea
Iris
Angle of iris
Canal of Schlemm
Conjunctiva
Ora serrata
Medial rectus muscle
Anterior chamber
Lens
Posterior chamber
Ciliary body
Ciliary muscle
Ora serrata
Lateral rectus muscle
Sclera
Choroid
Retina
Coverings of optic nerve
Retinal artery & vein
Optic nerve
Central fovea
Papilla of optic nerve

HORIZONTAL SECTION OF THE EYE

STRUCTURAL DETAILS

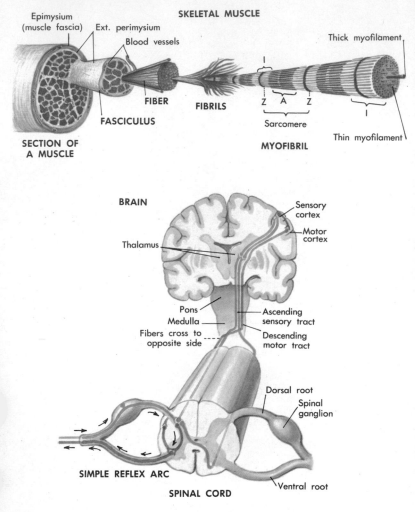

SKELETAL MUSCLE

Epimysium (muscle fascia)
Ext. perimysium
Blood vessels
Thick myofilament
FIBER
FIBRILS
FASCICULUS
Thin myofilament
SECTION OF A MUSCLE
MYOFIBRIL
Z A Z
Sarcomere

BRAIN

Sensory cortex
Motor cortex
Thalamus
Pons
Medulla
Fibers cross to opposite side
Ascending sensory tract
Descending motor tract
Dorsal root
Spinal ganglion
SIMPLE REFLEX ARC
Ventral root
SPINAL CORD

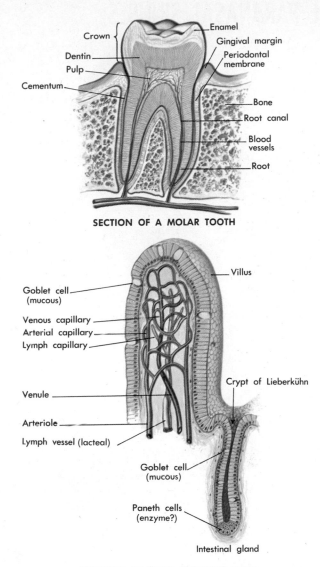

SECTION OF A MOLAR TOOTH

Crown
Dentin
Pulp
Cementum
Enamel
Gingival margin
Periodontal membrane
Bone
Root canal
Blood vessels
Root

Villus
Goblet cell (mucous)
Venous capillary
Arterial capillary
Lymph capillary
Venule
Arteriole
Lymph vessel (lacteal)
Crypt of Lieberkühn
Goblet cell (mucous)
Paneth cells (enzyme?)
Intestinal gland

SECTIONS OF SMALL INTESTINE WALL

THE PARANASAL SINUSES

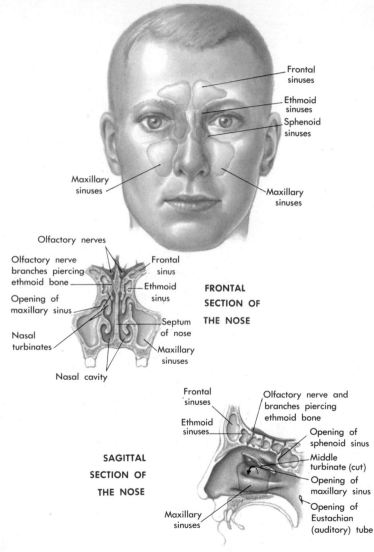

Frontal sinuses

Ethmoid sinuses

Sphenoid sinuses

Maxillary sinuses

Maxillary sinuses

Olfactory nerves

Olfactory nerve branches piercing ethmoid bone

Frontal sinus

Ethmoid sinus

Opening of maxillary sinus

Nasal turbinates

Septum of nose

Maxillary sinuses

Nasal cavity

FRONTAL SECTION OF THE NOSE

SAGITTAL SECTION OF THE NOSE

Frontal sinuses

Ethmoid sinuses

Olfactory nerve and branches piercing ethmoid bone

Opening of sphenoid sinus

Middle turbinate (cut)

Opening of maxillary sinus

Opening of Eustachian (auditory) tube

Maxillary sinuses

caudad to the pronephros and using its duct.

mesoneuritis (mez"o-nu-ri'tis) 1. inflammation of the substance of a nerve. 2. inflammation of the lymphatics of a nerve.

mesopallium (mes"o-pal'e-um) the portion of the pallium with stratification and organization that is transitional between archipallium and neopallium.

mesopexy (mes'o-pek"se) repair of the mesentery.

mesopharynx (mes"o-făr'inks) the oral portion of the pharynx.

mesophil (mes'o-fil) an organism which grows best at 20–55° C. adj., **mesophil'ic**.

mesophlebitis (mes"o-fle-bi'tis) inflammation of the middle coat of a vein.

mesophryon (mes-of're-on) central point of the glabellum

Mesopin (mes'o-pin) trademark for a preparation of homatropine methylbromide.

mesopneumon (mes"o-nu'mon) fold of pleura which attaches the lung.

mesoporphyrin (-por'fi-rin) a crystalline iron-free porphyrin from hematin obtained by a process of reduction.

mesorchium (mes-or'ke-um) peritoneal fold holding the fetal testis in place.

mesorectum (mes"o-rek'tum) the fold of peritoneum connecting the upper portion of the rectum with the sacrum.

mesoretina (-ret'i-nah) the middle layer of the retina.

mesoropter (-rop'ter) the normal position of the eyes with their muscles at rest.

mesorrhaphy (mes-or'ah-fe) suture of the mesentery.

mesorrhine (mes'o-rin) having a nasal index of 48–53.

mesosalpinx (mes"o-sal'pinks) the peritoneal fold investing the uterine tube.

mesoseme (mes'o-sēm) having an orbital index of 84–89.

mesosigmoid (mes"o-sig'moid) the mesentery of the sigmoid flexure.

mesosigmoidopexy (-sig-moi'do-pek"se) fixation of the mesosigmoid for prolapse of the rectum.

mesosternum (-ster'num) the middle piece or body of the sternum.

mesotendineum (-ten-din'e-um) the connective tissue sheath attaching a tendon to its fibrous sheath.

mesotendon (-ten'don) mesotendineum.

mesothelial (-the"le-al) pertaining to the mesothelium.

mesothelioma (-the"le-o'mah) a tumor made up of cells derived from the mesothelium.

mesothelium (-the'le-um) part of mesoderm from which the serous cavities and muscles are developed.

mesothenar (mes-oth'e-nar) the adductor pollicis muscle.

mesotron (mes'o-tron) meson (2).

mesoturbinate (mes"o-ter'bi-nāt) the middle turbinate body.

mesovarium (-va're-um) portion of the broad ligament enclosing and holding the ovary in place.

met (met) a unit of measure of metabolic heat, the quantity produced by a resting-sitting subject, or 50 kilogram-calories per square meter per hour.

meta- (met'ah) word element [Gr.], (1) *change; transformation; exchange;* (2) *after; next;* (3) the 1,3-position in derivatives of benzene.

metabasis (mě-tab'ah-sis) change of disease or place.

metabiosis (met"ah-bi-o'sis) dependence of one organism upon a preceding organism, influencing the environment.

metabolism (mě-tab'o-lizm) the sum total of the physical and chemical processes by which an organism converts simpler compounds into living, organized substance (constructive metabolism, substance metabolism, anabolism) and then reconverts such material into simpler compounds with release of energy for its use (destructive metabolism, energy metabolism, retrograde metabolism, catabolism). adj., **metabol'ic. basal m.** the measure of metabolism of the body in the resting state, determined by the amount of oxygen utilized or of heat produced. **constructive m.,** the processes by which simpler compounds are converted into complex, living, organized substances in the body. **destructive m.,** the conversion of complex material into simpler compounds for release of energy or to facilitate its elimination from the body. **energy m.,** the vital processes by which energy is derived from substances taken into the body. **retrograde m.,** the reconversion of complex material into simpler compounds. **substance m.,** constructive metabolism.

metabolite (mě-tab'o-līt) any compound produced during metabolism.

metabolodispersion (mě-tab"o-lo-dis-per'zhun) the dispersion of colloids of the body.

metabutethamine (met"ah-bu-teth'ah-min) a compound used as a local anesthetic.

metabutoxycaine (-bu-tok'si-kān) a compound used as a local anesthetic.

metacarpal (-kar'pal) pertaining to the metacarpus.

metacarpectomy (-kar-pek'to-me) excision of a metacarpal bone.

metacarpus (-kar'pus) the proximal part of the hand, or the five (metacarpal) bones composing it.

metacentric (-sen'trik) having the centromere almost at the middle of the replicating chromosome.

metacercaria (-ser ka're-ah), pl. *metacerca'riae,* the encysted resting or maturing stage of a trematode parasite in the tissues of an intermediate host.

metachromasia (-kro-ma'ze-ah) 1. failure to stain true with a given stain. 2. the different coloration of different tissues produced by the same stain. 3. change of color produced by staining. adj., **metachromat'ic**.

metachromatin (-kro'mah-tin) the basophil part of the chromatin.

metachromatism (-kro'mah-tizm) metachromasia.

metachromophil (-kro'mo-fil) not staining normally.

metachromosome (-kro'mo-sōm) one of two small chromosomes which conjugate only in the last phase of the spermatocyte division.

metachronous (mĕ-tak′ro-nus) occurring at different times.

metachrosis (met″ah-kro′sis) change of color in animals.

metacinesis (-si-ne′sis) separation of daughter stars from each other.

metacoele (met′ah-sēl) 1. the fourth ventricle. 2. metacoeloma.

metacoeloma (met″ah-se-lo′mah) that part of the embryonic coelom which develops into the pleuroperitoneal cavity.

metacone (met′ah-kōn) the distobuccal cusp of an upper molar tooth.

metaconid (met″ah-ko′nid) the mesiolingual cusp of a lower molar tooth.

metaconule (-ko′nūl) the distal intermediate cusp of an upper molar tooth.

metacortandracin (-kor-tan′drah-sin) prednisone.

metacortandralone (-kor-tan′drah-lōn) prednisolone.

metacyesis (-si-e′sis) extrauterine pregnancy.

metagaster (-gas′ter) the permanent intestinal canal of the embryo.

metagenesis (-jen′ĕ-sis) alternation of generation.

metagglutinin (-gloo′tĭ-nin) an agglutinin which acts on closely related organisms.

metagranulocyte (-gran′u-lo-sīt″) metamyelocyte.

metakaryocyte (-kar′e-o-sīt″) metarubricyte.

metal (met′al) a chemical element or substance marked by luster, malleability, ductility, and conductivity of electricity and heat. adj., **metal′lic. alkali m′s,** the monovalent elements of the first group of the periodic system: lithium, potassium, sodium, rubidium, cesium. **Babbitt m.,** an alloy used in dentistry.

metalbumin (met″al-bu′min) a proteid found in ovarian cysts.

metalloid (met′ah-loid) 1. a nonmetallic element. 2. having some properties resembling those of a typical metal.

metallophobia (met″al-o-fo′be-ah) morbid fear of metallic objects.

metallurgy (-er′je) the science and art of using metals.

metamer (met′ah-mer) a compound exhibiting, or capable of exhibiting, metamerism.

metamere (met′ah-mēr) one of a series of homologous segments of the body of an animal.

metamerism (mĕ-tam′er-izm) 1. a type of structural isomerism in which different radicals of the same chemical type are attached to the same polyvalent element and yet give rise to compounds having identical molecular formulas. 2. arrangement into metameres by the serial repetition of a structural pattern. adj., **metamer′ic.**

Metamine (met′ah-mēn) trademark for preparations of trolnitrate.

metamorphopsia (met″ah-mor-fop′se-ah) defective vision, with distortion of the shape of objects looked at.

metamorphosis (-mor′fo′-sis) change of structure or shape. **fatty m.,** fatty degeneration. **platelet m., structural m., viscous m.,** a series of progressive, irreversible structural alterations that platelets undergo during coagulation, dependent on the presence of divalent metallic ions. **retrograde m.,** conversion into a simpler or more primitive form.

Metamucil (met″ah-mu′sil) trademark for a preparation of psyllium hydrophilic mucilloid.

metamyelocyte (-mi′e-lo-sīt) a polymorphonuclear leukocyte in which the nuclear element is a single fragment no longer containing a definite nucleolus.

Metandren (mĕ-tan′dren) trademark for preparations of methyltestosterone.

metanephron (met″ah-nef′ron) metanephros.

metanephros (-nef′ros), pl. *metaneph′roi* [Gr.] the permanent embryonic kidney, developing later than and caudad to the mesonephros.

metaneutrophil (-nu′tro-fil) a cell not staining normally with neutral stains. adj., **metaneutrophil′ic.**

metaphase (met′ah-fāz) the second stage of division of the nucleus of a cell in either meiosis or mitosis.

Metaphedrin (met″ah-fed′rin) trademark for a preparation of nitromersol and ephedrine.

Metaphen (met′ah-fen) trademark for preparations of nitromersol.

metaphrenia (met″ah-fre′ne-ah) a switching of the libido toward the practical interests of life.

metaphysis (mĕ-taf′ĭ-sis), pl. *metaph′yses* [Gr.] the wider part at the end of the shaft of a long bone, adjacent to the epiphyseal disk. adj., **metaphys′eal.**

metaplasia (met″ah-pla′ze-ah) a reversible change in which one adult cell type is replaced by another adult cell type. adj., **metaplas′tic. myeloid m., agnogenic,** a condition characterized by foci of extramedullary hematopoiesis and by immature red and white cells in the peripheral blood and mild to moderate anemia.

metaplasm (met′ah-plazm) the inanimate particles of protoplasm.

metaplexus (met″ah-plek′sus) the choroid plexus of the fourth ventricle.

metapneumonic (-nu-mon′ik) following pneumonia.

metapodialia (-po″de-a′le-ah) the bones of the metacarpus and metatarsus.

metapophysis (-pof′ĭ-sis) any tubercle on the superior articular processes of a vertebra.

metapore (met′ah-pōr) the foramen of Magendie.

metaprotein (met″ah-pro′te-in) a product of the action of an acid or an alkali on a protein.

metaraminol (-ram′ĭ-nol) an ephedrine compound used as a sympathomimetic and pressor agent.

metargon (met-ar′gon) a name given an isotope of argon, atomic weight 38.

metarubricyte (met″ah-roo′brĭ-sīt) a red cell containing a pyknotic, contracted nucleus, the last stage in erythrocyte development.

metastable (-sta′bl) capable of undergoing change.

metastasis (mĕ-tas′tah-sis) 1. transfer of disease from one organ or part of the body to another. 2. (pl. *metas′tases*) a secondary lesion developing at some distance from the site of a primary lesion, the causative agent having been conveyed by the blood or lymph. adj., **metastat'ic.**

metastasize (mĕ-tas'tah-sīz) to move from one organ or part of the body to another.

metasternum (met"ah-ster'num) the xiphoid process.

metatarsal (-tar'sal) pertaining to the metatarsus.

metatarsalgia (-tar-sal'je-ah) pain in the metatarsus.

metatarsectomy (-tar-sek'to-me) excision of a metatarsal bone.

metatarsophalangeal (-tar"so-fah-lan'je-al) pertaining to a metatarsal bone and a phalanx.

metatarsus (-tar'sus) the anterior segment of the foot or, collectively, the five (metatarsal) bones composing it. **m. pri'mus va'rus,** angulation of the first metatarsal bone toward the midline of the body, producing an angle sometimes of 20 degrees or more between its base and that of the second metatarsal bone.

metathalamus (-thal'ah-mus) the part of the thalamencephalon composed of the medial and lateral geniculate bodies.

metathesis (mĕ-tath'ĕ-sis) 1. artificial transfer of a morbid process. 2. replacement of molecular atoms by other atoms.

metatrophic (met"ah-trof'ik) utilizing organic matter for food.

Metazoa (-zo'ah) a phylum of the animal kingdom which includes the multicellular animals, i.e. all animals except the Protozoa. adj., **metazo'al, metazo'an.**

metazoon (met"ah-zo'on), pl. *metazo'a* [Gr.] an individual organism of the phylum Metazoa.

metencephalon (met"en-sef'ah-lon), pl. *metenceph'ala* [Gr.] 1. part of the central nervous system comprising the pons and cerebellum. 2. the anterior of two vesicles formed by specialization of the rhombencephalon in the developing embryo.

meteorism (me'te-o-rizm") tympanites.

meteorology (me"te-o-rol'o-je) the science of the atmosphere and its phenomena.

meteorophobia (me"te-o-ro-fo'be-ah) morbid fear of meteors.

meteorotropic (-o-trop'ik) influenced by the weather.

meteorotropism (me"te-o-rot'ro-pizm) response to influence by meteorologic factors noted in certain biological events. adj., **meteorotrop'ic.**

meter (me'ter) the basic unit of linear measure of the metric system, being the equivalent of 39.371 inches.

-meter (me'ter) word element [Gr.], *instrument for measuring.*

metestrus (met-es'trus) the period of subsiding follicular function following estrus in female mammals.

methacholine chloride (meth"ah-ko'lēn klo'-rīd) colorless or white crystals; a parasympathomimetic used in cardiovascular disease.

methacrylate (meth-ak'rĭ-lāt") an acrylic resin widely used in denture bases.

methadone (meth'ah-dōn) a synthetic compound with pharmacologic properties qualitatively similar to those of morphine.

methallenestril (meth"al-lĕ-nes'tril) a nonsteroid estrogenic compound.

methamphetamine hydrochloride (meth"am-fet'ah-mēn hi"dro-klo'rīd) white crystalline powder; vasoconstrictor, used for raising blood pressure and stimulating cerebral activity.

methandriol (meth-an'dre-ol) a compound used as an anabolic stimulant.

methandrostenolone (-an"dro-sten'o-lōn) a compound used as an anabolic hormone.

methane (meth'ān) a gas from decayed organic matter.

Methanobacterium (meth"ah-no-bak-te're um) a genus of Schizomycetes (order Pseudomonadales, suborder Pseudomonadineae, family Spirillaceae).

Methanococcus (-kok'us) a genus of Schizomycetes (order Eubacteriales, family Micrococcaceae).

methanol (meth'ah-nol) a mobile, colorless liquid widely used as a solvent.

Methanomonadaceae (meth"ah-no-mo"nah-da'se-e) a family of Schizomycetes (order Pseudomonadales, suborder Rhodobacteriineae) found in soil and water.

Methanomonas (-mo'nas) a genus of Schizomycetes (order Pseudomonadales, suborder Pseudomonadineae, family Methanomonadaceae) found in soil.

methantheline (mĕ-than'thĕ-lin) an odorless, bitter, white or nearly white powder used in parasympathetic blockade and to depress gastric activity.

methapyrilene (meth"ah-pir'ĭ-lēn) an antihistaminic substance for treatment of allergic symptoms attributed to histamine.

metharbital (meth-ar'bĭ-tal) a long-acting barbiturate used as a central nervous system depressant with anticonvulsant action.

methdilazine (-di'lah-zēn) a phenothiazine compound used as an antihistaminic.

Methedrine (meth'ĕ-drin) trademark for preparations of methamphetamine.

methemoglobin (met-he"mo-glo'bin) a compound formed from hemoglobin by oxidation of the ferrous to the ferric state with essential ly ionic bonds.

methemoglobinemia (-glo"bī-ne'me-ah) methemoglobin in the blood.

methemoglobinuria (-nu're-ah) methemoglobin in the urine.

methenamine (meth"en-am'in) white crystalline powder; urinary antiseptic. **m. mandelate,** a salt of methenamine and mandelic acid, used in infections of the urinary tract.

Methergine (meth'er-jin) trademark for preparations of methylergonovine.

methexenyl (meth-ek'sĕ-nil) hexobarbital.

methicillin (meth"ĭ-sil'in) dimethoxyphenyl penicillin, a semisynthetic penicillin which is highly resistant to inactivation by penicillinase. **sodium m.,** an antibacterial compound for parenteral administration.

methimazole (meth-im'ah-zōl) a white to pale buff, crystalline powder, used as a thyroid inhibitor.

methiodal (meth-i'o-dal) an iodine-containing compound. **sodium m.,** an odorless, white, crystalline powder with a slightly saline taste, used as a radiopaque medium in excretory urography.

methionine (mě-thi'o-nin) a sulfur-bearing amino acid essential for optimal growth in infants and for nitrogen equilibrium in adults; used therapeutically as a dietary supplement with lipotropic action.

Methium (meth'e-um) trademark for preparations of hexamethonium.

methocarbamol (meth"o-kar'bah-mol) a compound used as a skeletal muscle relaxant.

method (meth'od) a manner of procedure, or course of action. **Abbott's m.,** correction of lateral spinal curvature with a series of plaster casts. **Altmann-Gersch m.,** a method of preparing tissue for histologic study by freeze drying. **closed-plaster m.,** treatment of wounds, fractures or osteomyelitis by enclosing the limb in an immobilizing plaster cast. **Credé's m.,** 1. instillation of two drops of 1 per cent silver nitrate solution in each eye to prevent ophthalmia neonatorum. 2. expulsion of the placenta by kneading and pressing the uterus. **Fahraeus m.,** one for determination of the rate of sedimentation of erythrocytes. **Orr m.,** treatment of compound fractures and osteomyelitis by drainage with petrolatum gauze and immobilization in a plaster cast until the discharge has softened the plaster. **Whipple's m.,** use of liver in pernicious anemia.

methodology (meth"o-dol'o-je) the science dealing with principles of procedure in research and study.

methohexital (-hek'si-tal) an ultrashort-acting barbiturate. **sodium m.,** a compound used intravenously to produce general anesthesia.

methopromazine (-pro'mah-zēn) methoxypromazine.

methotrexate (-trek'sāt) a poisonous, orange-brown crystalline compound used as an antineoplastic agent.

methoxamine (mě-thok'sah-mēn) a compound used as a sympathomimetic and pressor agent.

methoxsalen (mě-thok'sah-len) an acrylic acid compound used with ultraviolet light in treatment of idiopathic vitiligo.

methoxyflurane (mě-thok"se-floo'rān) a compound used as a general anesthetic administered by inhalation.

methoxyphenamine (-fen'ah-mēn) a compound used as a sympathomimetic drug with predominant bronchodilator action.

methoxypromazine (-pro'mah-zēn) a phenothiazine derivative used as a tranquilizer.

methscopolamine (meth"sko-pol'ah-min) a compound used in parasympathetic blockade.

methsuximide (meth-suk'si-mīd) a white to grayish-white crystalline powder used as an anticonvulsant to treat petit mal and psychomotor epilepsy.

methyl (meth'il) the monovalent radical, —CH₃. **m. salicylate,** a colorless, yellowish or reddish liquid obtained from leaves of *Gualtheria procumbens* or bark of *Betula lenta,* or produced synthetically; flavoring agent.

methylamine (meth"il-am'in) gaseous ptomaine from decaying fish and from cultures of *Vibrio comma.*

methylate (meth'i-lāt) a compound of methyl alcohol and a base.

methylbenzethonium (meth"il-ben"zě-tho'ne-um) an ammonium compound used as a local anti-infective.

methylcellulose (-sel'u-lōs) a methyl ester of cellulose; used as a bulk laxative and a suspending agent for drugs.

methylcytosine (-si'to-sin) a pyrimidine occurring in deoxyribonucleic acid.

methylene blue (meth'i-lēn blu) a synthetic dyestuff used as a stain in pathology and bacteriology, and as an antiseptic.

methylergonovine (meth"il-er"go-no'vin) a compound used as an oxytocic.

methylglucamine (-gloo'kah-min) a compound prepared from D-glucose and methylamine, used in the synthesis of pharmaceuticals. **m. diatrizoate,** a compound used as a contrast medium for roentgenography.

methylhexaneamine (-hek-sān'ah-min) a compound used as an inhalant to relieve nasal congestion.

methylmelubrin (-mel'u-brin) dipyrone.

methylparaben (-par'ah-ben) a compound used as a preservative for drug solutions.

methylparafynol (-par"ah-fi'nol) a compound used as a hypnotic and sedative.

methylphenidate (-fen'i-dāt) a compound used as a mild psychomotor stimulant.

methylprednisolone (-pred-nis'o-lōn) a white, odorless, crystalline powder, an adrenocortical steroid of the glucogenic type, having an anti-inflammatory action similar to that of prednisolone.

methylrosaniline chloride (-ro-zan'i-lēn klo'rīd) gentian violet.

methyltestosterone (-tes-tos'ter-ōn) an orally effective form of testosterone.

methylthionine chloride (-thi'o-nin klo'rīd) methylene blue.

methylthiouracil (-thi"o-u'rah-sil) a white, odorless, crystalline powder, used as a thyroid inhibitor.

methyprylon (meth"i-pri'lon) a white, crystalline powder used as a sedative and hypnotic.

Meticortelone (met"i-kor'tě-lōn) trademark for preparations of prednisolone.

Meticorten (-kor'ten) trademark for a preparation of prednisone.

metmyoglobin (met-mi"o-glo'bin) a compound formed from myoglobin by oxidation of the ferrous to the ferric state with essentially ionic bonds.

metopagus (mě-top'ah-gus) conjoined twins united at the forehead.

metopic (mě-top'ik) pertaining to the forehead.

metopion (mě-to'pe-on) point in midline of the forehead, between the frontal eminences.

Metopon (met-o'pon) trademark for a preparation of methyldihydromorphinone hydrochloride.

metopon (met-o'pon) the anterior metopic lobule of the brain.

metoxenous (mě-tok'sě-nus) requiring two hosts for the entire life cycle.

metoxeny (mě-tok'sě-ne) the condition of being metoxenous.

metra (me'trah) the uterus.

metralgia (me-tral'je-ah) pain in the uterus.

metrapectic (me"trah-pek'tik) transmitted by the mother, who remains unaffected.

metratonia (-to'ne-ah) uterine atony.

metratrophia (-tro'fe-ah) atrophy of the uterus.

Metrazol (met'rah-zol) trademark for preparations of pentylenetetrazol.

metrectasia (me"trek-ta'ze-ah) dilatation of the uterus.

metreurynter (me"troo-rin'ter) an inflatable bag for dilating the cervical canal of the uterus.

metreurysis (me-troo'rĭ-sis) dilation of the cervix uteri by means of the metreurynter.

metric (met'rik) 1. pertaining to measures or measurement. 2. having the meter as a basis.

metriocephalic (me"tre-o-sĕ-fal'ik) having a vertical index of 72–77.

metritis (me-tri'tis) inflammation of the uterus. **m. dis'secans,** metritis with necrosis of portions of the uterine wall.

metrocarcinoma (me"tro-kar"sĭ-no'mah) carcinoma of the uterus.

metrocele (me'tro-sēl) hernia of the uterus.

metrocolpocele (me"tro-kol'po-sēl) hernia of uterus with vaginal prolapse.

metrocystosis (-sis-to'sis) formation of cysts in the uterus.

metrocyte (me'tro-sīt) a mother cell.

metrodynia (me"tro-din'e-ah) pain in the uterus.

metrofibroma (-fi-bro'mah) fibroma of uterus.

metroleukorrhea (-lu"ko-re'ah) leukorrhea of uterine origin.

metrology (me-trol'o-je) the science dealing with measurements.

metromalacoma (me"tro-mal"ah-ko'mah) morbid softening of the uterus.

metroparalysis (-pah-ral'ĭ-sis) paralysis of the uterus.

metropathia (-path'e-ah) disorder of the uterus. **m. haemorrha'gica,** essential uterine hemorrhage.

metropathy (me-trop'ah-the) any uterine disorder. adj., **metropath'ic.**

metroperitoneal (me"tro-per"ĭ-to-ne'al) pertaining to uterus and peritoneum.

metroperitonitis (-per"ĭ-to-ni'tis) inflammation of uterus and peritoneum.

metrophlebitis (-fle-bi'tis) inflammation of uterine veins.

Metropine (met'ro-pin) trademark for preparations of methyl atropine nitrate.

metroptosis (me"tro-to'sis) prolapse of the uterus.

metrorrhagia (-ra'je-ah) uterine hemorrhage.

metrorrhea (-re'ah) abnormal uterine discharge.

metrorrhexis (-rek'sis) rupture of the uterus.

metrorthosis (me"tror-tho'sis) correction of uterine displacement.

metrosalpingitis (me"tro-sal"pin-ji'tis) inflammation of uterus and oviducts.

metrosalpingography (-sal"ping-gog'rah-fe) hysterosalpingography.

metroscope (me'tro-skōp) instrument for examining the uterus.

metrostaxis (me"tro-stak'sis) slow loss of blood from the uterus.

metrostenosis (-ste-no'sis) stenosis of the uterus.

metrotomy (me-trot'o-me) hysterotomy.

-metry, word element [Gr.], *measurement.*

Metubine (mĕ-tu'bin) trademark for a preparation of dimethyl tubocurarine.

Metycaine (met'ĭ-kān) trademark for preparations of piperocaine.

mev million electron volts.

M.F.D. minimum fatal dose.

Mg chemical symbol, *magnesium.*

mg. milligram.

micaceous (mi-ka'shus) pertaining to or resembling mica; occurring in silvery gray flakes.

mication (mi-ka'shun) a quick motion, such as winking.

micr(o)- (mi'kro) word element [Gr.], *small;* used in naming units of measurement to designate an amount 10^{-6} (one millionth) the size of the unit to which it is joined, e.g. microcuries.

micrangiopathy (mi-kran"je-op'ah-the) disease of the capillaries.

micrencephaly (mi"kren-sef'ah-le) abnormal smallness and underdevelopment of the brain.

microabscess (mi"kro-ab'ses) an abscess visible only under a microscope.

microaerobic (-a"er-o'bik) thriving best or surviving only in the presence of a limited amount of molecular oxygen.

microaerophilic (-a"er-o-fil'ik) growing best in the presence of very little free oxygen.

microanalysis (-ah-nal'ĭ-sis) the chemical analysis of minute quantities of material.

microanatomy (-ah-nat'o-me) histology.

microaneurysm (-an'u-rizm) a minute aneurysm occurring on a vessel of small size, as one in the retina of the eye.

microangiopathy (-an"je-op'ah-the) a disorder involving the small blood vessels. adj., **microangiopath'ic. thrombotic m.,** a condition characterized by fever, hemolytic anemia, thrombocytopenic purpura and neurologic disturbances.

Microbacterium (-bak-te're-um) a genus of Schizomycetes (order Eubacteriales, family Corynebacteriaceae) found in dairy products.

microbar (mi'kro-bahr) a unit of pressure, being one millionth (10^{-6}) bar.

microbe (mi'krōb) a vegetable microorganism. adj., **micro'bial, micro'bic.**

microbicidal (mi-kro"bī-si'dal) destroying microbes.

microbicide (mi-kro'bī-sīd) an agent that destroys microbes.

microbioassay (mi"kro-bi"o-as'a) determination of the active power of a nutrient or other factor by noting its effect on the growth of a microorganism, as compared with the effect of a standard preparation.

microbiologist (-bi-ol'o-jist) a specialist in microbiology.

microbiology (-bi-ol'o-je) study of minute living organisms, including bacteria, molds and pathogenic protozoa.

microbiota (mi″kro-bi-o′tah) the microscopic living organisms of a region.

microblast (mi′kro-blast) an erythroblast of 5 microns or less in diameter.

microblepharism (mi″kro-blef′ah-rizm) abnormal smallness of eyelids.

microbody (mi′kro-bod″e) a spherical or ovoid organelle surrounded by a single membrane, found in the cytoplasm of certain cells.

microbrachius (mi″kro-bra′ke-us) fetus with abnormally small arms.

microburet (-bu-ret′) a buret with a capacity of the order of 0.1 to 10 ml., with graduated intervals of 0.001 to 0.02 ml.

microcalorie (-kal′o-re) small calorie; the heat required to raise 1 cc. of distilled water from 0 to 1°C.

microcardia (-kar′de-ah) abnormal smallness of the heart.

microcentrum (-sen′trum) centrosome.

microcephalus (-sef′ah-lus) an idiot or fetus with a very small head.

microcephaly (-sef′ah-le) small size of head in relation to the rest of the body. adj., **microcephal′ic.**

microcheilia (-ki′le-ah) abnormal smallness of lip.

microcheiria (-ki′re-ah) abnormal smallness of the hands.

microchemistry (-kem′is-tre) chemistry concerned with exceedingly small quantities of chemical substances.

microcinematography (-sin″e-mah-tog′rah-fe) moving picture photography of microscopic objects.

Micrococcaceae (-kok-a′se-e) a family of Schizomycetes (order Eubacteriales).

Micrococcus (-kok′us) a genus of Schizomycetes (order Eubacteriales, family Micrococcaceae) found in soil, water, etc.

micrococcus (-kok′us), pl. *micrococ′ci*, a small bacterium occurring predominantly as a single cell rather than in groups or aggregates.

microcolon (-ko′lon) abnormal smallness of the colon.

microcoria (-ko′re-ah) smallness of the pupil.

microcornea (-kor′ne-ah) unusual smallness of the cornea.

microcoulomb (-koo′lomb) one millionth of a coulomb.

microcrania (-kra′ne-ah) abnormal smallness of the skull in relation to the face.

microcrith (mi′kro-krith) the weight of one atom of hydrogen.

microcrystalline (mi″kro-kris′tah-lin) made up of minute crystals.

microcurie (-ku′re) one millionth (10^{-6}) curie; abbreviated μc.

microcurie-hour (mi′kro-ku″re-owr″) a unit of dose equivalent to that obtained by exposure for one hour to radioactive material disintegrating at the rate of 3.7×10^4 atoms per second; abbreviated μc-hr.

Microcyclus (mi″kro-si′klus) a genus of Schizomycetes (order Pseudomonadales, suborder Pseudomonadineae, family Spirillaceae).

microcyst (mi′kro-sist) a cyst visible only under a microscope.

microcyte (mi′kro-sīt) an erythrocyte 5 microns or less in diameter.

microcythemia (mi″kro-si-the′me-ah) microcytosis.

microcytosis (-si-to′sis) presence of abnormally small erythrocytes in the blood.

microdactylia (-dak-til′e-ah) abnormal smallness of fingers or toes.

microdetermination (-de-ter″mī-na′shun) chemical examination of minute quantities of substance.

microdissection (-dī-sek′shun) dissection of tissue or cells under the microscope.

microdont (mi′kro-dont) having a dental index below 42.

microdontia (mi″kro-don′she-ah) abnormal smallness of the teeth.

microecology (-e-kol′o-je) the branch of the ecology of parasites concerned with the relations of the organisms and the environment provided by the hosts.

microecosystem (-e″ko-sis′tem) a miniature ecologic system, occurring naturally or produced in the laboratory for experimental purposes.

microembolus (-em′bo-lus), pl. *microem′boli* [L.] an embolus of microscopic size.

micro-erythrocyte (-ĕ-rith′ro-sīt) microcyte.

microfarad (-far′ad) one millionth (10^{-6}) farad; abbreviated μf.

microfauna (-faw′nah) the microscopic animal organisms of a special region.

microfibril (-fi′bril) an extremely small fibril.

microfilaremia (-fil″ah-re′me-ah) presence of microfilariae in the circulating blood.

Microfilaria (-fi-la′re-ah) a genus name formerly given larval forms of nematode parasites of the superfamily Filarioidea.

microfilaria (-fi-la′re-ah), pl. *microfila′riae* [L.] a larva of an organism of the superfamily Filarioidea, present in the blood of the infected host.

microfilm (mi′kro-film) 16- or 35-mm. film used in high-speed automatic machines to photograph books, documents, forms or other material for preservation in small space.

microflora (mi″kro-flo′rah) the microscopic vegetable organisms of a special region.

microgamete (-gam′ēt) the smaller, male gamete.

microgametocyte (-gah-me′to-sīt) the cell producing microgametes.

microgastria (-gas′tre-ah) congenital smallness of the stomach.

microgenia (-je′ne-ah) abnormal smallness of the chin.

microgenitalism (-jen′ī-tal-izm) smallness of the external genitals.

microglia (mi-krog′le-ah) non-neural cells forming part of the adventitial structure of the central nervous system.

microglossia (mi″kro-glos′e-ah) abnormal smallness of the tongue.

micrognathia (-nath′e-ah) abnormal smallness of the lower jaw. adj., **micrognath′ic.**

microgram (mi′kro-gram) one millionth (10^{-6}) gram, or one thousandth (10^{-3}) milligram; abbreviated μg. or mcg.

micrograph (mi′kro-graf) a permanent reproduction of the appearance of an object as observed through a microscope. **electron m.,**

a graphic reproduction of an object as viewed with an electron microscope.

micrography (mi-krog'rah-fe) 1. account of microscopic objects. 2. use of the micrograph.

microgyria (mi"kro-ji're-ah) abnormal smallness of the cerebral convolutions.

microhematocrit (-he-mat'o-krit) rapid determination of packed red cell volume in whole blood, by high-speed centrifugation of a small quantity of blood in a capillary tube.

microhepatia (-he-pat'e-ah) smallness of the liver.

microhm (mi'krōm) one millionth (10^{-6}) ohm.

microincineration (mi"kro-in-sin"er-a'shun) the oxidation of a small quantity of material, to eliminate organic matter and leave only the ash.

microlecithal (mi"kro-les'ĭ-thal) having a small amount of yolk.

microlesion (mi'kro-le"zhun) a minute lesion.

microliter (mi'kro-le"ter) one millionth part of a liter, or one thousandth of a milliliter; abbreviated μl.

microlith (mi'kro-lith) a minute concretion or calculus.

microlithiasis (mi"kro-lĭ-thi'ah-sis) the formation of minute concretions in an organ. **m. alveola'ris pulmo'num, pulmonary alveolar m.,** a condition simulating pulmonary tuberculosis, with deposition of minute calculi in the alveoli of the lungs.

micrology (mi-krol'o-je) the science of microscopy.

micromandible (mi"kro-man'dĭ-bl) extreme smallness of the mandible.

micromastia (-mas'te-ah) abnormal smallness of the mammary gland.

micromelia (-me'le-ah) abnormal smallness of one or more extremities.

micromelus (mi-krom'ē-lus) fetus with abnormally small limbs.

micromere (mi'kro-mēr) one of the small blastomeres formed by unequal cleavage of a fertilized ovum.

micrometeorology (mi"kro-me"te-or-ol'o-je) that branch of meteorology dealing with the effects on living organisms of the extraorganic aspects of the physical environment within a few inches of the surface of the earth.

micrometer (mi-krom'ē-ter) instrument for making minute measurements.

micromethod (mi'kro-meth"od) a technique dealing with exceedingly small quantities of material.

micrometry (mi-krom'ē-tre) measurement of microscopic objects.

micromicro- (mi"kro-mi'kro) word element designating 10^{-6} (one millionth) of 10^{-6} (one millionth), or 10^{-12} (one trillionth), part of the unit to which it is joined.

micromicrocurie (-mi"kro-ku're) one millionth (10^{-6}) microcurie, or 10^{-12} curie; abbreviated $\mu\mu c$.

micromicrogram (-mi"kro-gram) one millionth (10^{-6}) microgram, or 10^{-12} gram; abbreviated $\mu\mu g$. or $\mu\gamma$.

micromicron (-mi'kron) one millionth micron

(10^{-9} mm., or 10^{-2} angstroms); abbreviated $\mu\mu$.

micromillimeter (mi"kro-mil'ĭ-me"ter) 1. micron. 2. one millionth of a millimeter; abbreviated μmm.

micromolecular (-mo-lek'u-lar) composed of small molecules.

Micromonospora (-mo-nos'po-rah) a genus of Schizomycetes (order Actinomycetales, family Streptomycetaceae) found in soil and water.

micromyelia (-mi-e'le-ah) abnormal smallness of the spinal cord.

micron (mi'kron) a unit of linear measurement of the metric system, equivalent to 10^{-3} mm., or 10^4 angstroms; abbreviated μ.

micronucleus (mi"kro-nu'kle-us) the smaller of two nuclei of a unicellular organism, associated with reproduction of the cell.

micronutrient (-nu'tre-ent) a dietary element essential only in small quantities.

microorganism (-or'gah-nizm) a microscopic animal or plant.

micropathology (-pah-thol'o-je) 1. the sum of what is known about minute pathologic change. 2. pathology of diseases caused by microorganisms.

microphage (mi'kro-fāj) a neutrophilic granulocyte.

microphakia (mi"kro-fa'ke-ah) abnormal smallness of the crystalline lens.

microphallus (-fal'us) abnormal smallness of the penis.

microphobia (-fo'be-ah) morbid dread of microbes.

microphone (mi'kro-fōn) a device to pick up sound for purposes of amplification or transmission.

microphonia (mi"kro-fo'ne-ah) marked weakness of voice.

microphotograph (-fo'to-graf) a photograph of small size.

microphthalmos (mi"krof-thal'mos) abnormal smallness of the eyeball.

microphysics (mi"kro-fiz'iks) the science of the ultimate structure of matter.

microphyte (mi'kro-fīt) a microscopic plant.

micropipet (mi"kro-pi-pet') a pipet for handling small quantities of liquids (0.1 to 1 ml.).

micropodia (-po'de-ah) abnormal smallness of the feet.

micropredator (-pred'ah-tor) an organism that derives elements essential for its existence from other species of organisms, larger than itself, without destroying them.

micropsia (mi-krop'se-ah) a disorder of visual perception in which objects appear smaller than their actual size.

micropyle (mi'kro-pīl) an opening through which a spermatozoon enters the ovum.

microradiography (mi"kro-ra"de-og'rah-fe) radiography under conditions which permit subsequent microscopic examination or enlargement of the radiograph up to several hundred linear magnifications.

microrhinia (-rin'e-ah) abnormal smallness of the nose.

Microscilla (-sil'ah) a genus of Schizomycetes

(order Beggiatoales, family Vitreoscillaceae).

microscope (mi′kro-skōp) an instrument used to obtain an enlarged image of small objects and reveal details of structure not otherwise distinguishable. **binocular m.**, one with two eyepieces, permitting use of both eyes simultaneously. **compound m.**, one consisting of two lens systems. **electron m.**, one in which electrons, instead of light rays, are used to produce an image which may be viewed on a fluorescent screen or photographed. **light m.**, one in which the specimen is viewed under ordinary illumination. **operating m.**, one designed for use in performance of delicate surgical procedures, e.g. on the middle ear or small vessels of the heart. **simple m.**, one that consists of a single lens. **stereoscopic m.**, a binocular microscope modified to give a three-dimensional view of the specimen. **x-ray m.**, one in which x-rays are used instead of light, the image usually being reproduced on film.

microscopic (mi″kro-skop′ik) of extremely small size; visible only by aid of a microscope.

microscopical (-skop′ĭ-kal) pertaining to a microscope or to microscopy.

microscopy (mi-kros′ko-pe) examination with a microscope. **television m.**, a special technique in which a magnified image produced by a microscope is projected on a television screen.

microseme (mi′kro-sēm) having an orbital index of less than 83.

microsome (mi′kro-sōm) one of the microscopic particles in the cytoplasm of a cell.

microsomia (mi″kro-so′me-ah) abnormally small size of the body.

microspectroscope (-spek′tro-skōp) spectroscope and microscope combined.

microsphere (mi′kro-sfēr) a rounded mass of microscopic size.

microspherocyte (mi″kro-sfe′ro-sīt) an erythrocyte whose diameter is less than normal, but whose thickness is increased.

microspherocytosis (-sfe′ro-si-to′sis) the presence in the blood of an excessive number of microspherocytes.

microsphygmia (-sfig′me-ah) that condition of the pulse in which it is perceived with difficulty by the finger.

microsphyxia (-sfik′se-ah) microsphygmia.

microsplenia (-sple′ne-ah) smallness of the spleen.

Microsporon (-spo′ron) Microsporum.

Microsporum (-spo′rum) a genus of fungi which cause various diseases of skin and hair, including the species *M. audouini, M. canis (lanosum)* and *M. fulvum (gypseum).*

microstat (mi′kro-stat) the stage and finder of a microscope.

microstomia (mi″kro-sto′me-ah) abnormally decreased size of the mouth.

microsurgery (-ser′jer-e) dissection of minute structures under the microscope, with the use of extremely small instruments.

Microtatobiotes (-ta″to-bi-o′tēz) a class of vegetable organisms (division Protophyta), including the orders Rickettsiales and Virales, dependent on other living organisms for growth and multiplication.

microthrombosis (mi″kro-throm-bo′sis) presence of many small thrombi in capillaries and other small blood vessels.

microthrombus (-throm′bus) a small thrombus in a capillary or other small blood vessel.

microtia (mi-kro′she-ah) abnormal smallness of the pinna of the ear.

microtome (mi′kro-tōm) instrument for making thin sections for microscopic study. **freezing m.**, one for cutting frozen tissues. **rotary m.**, one in which wheel action is translated into a back and forth movement of the specimen being sectioned. **sliding m.**, one in which the specimen being sectioned is made to slide on a track.

microtomy (mi-krot′o-me) the cutting of thin sections.

microtransfusion (mi″kro-trans-fu′zhun) introduction into the circulation of a small quantity of blood of another individual.

microtrauma (-traw′mah) a microscopic lesion or injury.

microtubule (-tu′bul) a straight, hollow-appearing structure in the cytoplasm of a cell.

microvillus (-vil′us) a minute process or protrusion from the free surface of a cell.

microvolt (mi′kro-volt) one millionth of a volt; symbol μv.

microwave (mi′kro-wāv) a wave typical of electromagnetic radiation between far infrared and radio waves, generally regarded as extending from 300,000 to 100 megacycles (wavelength of 1 mm. to 30 cm.).

micturate (mik′tu-rāt) urinate.

micturition (mik″tu-rish′un) urination.

midbrain (mid′brān) the portion of the brain developed from the middle of the three primary brain vesicles of the early embryo, situated between the forebrain and hindbrain.

midfoot (mid′foot) the middle portion of the foot, comprising the region of the navicular, cuboid and cuneiform bones.

midgut (mid′gut) an intermediate region in the embryo between the foregut and hindgut, which is of only brief duration in man.

Midicel (mid′ĭ-sel) trademark for preparations of sulfamethoxypyridazine.

midwife (mid′wīf) a woman who assists at childbirth.

migraine (mi′grān) a form of headache usually occurring episodically and commonly involving only one side of the head.

Mikedimide (mi-ked′ĭ-mīd) trademark for a preparation of bemegride.

mikro- for words beginning thus, see those beginning *micro-.*

mil (mil) milliliter.

miliaria (mil″e-a′re-ah) a cutaneous condition with retention of sweat, which is extravasated at different levels in the skin. **m. ru′bra**, a condition due to obstruction of the sweat glands.

miliary (mil′e-er″e) 1. like millet seeds. 2. characterized by lesions resembling millet seeds.

Milibis (mil′ĭ-bis) trademark for preparations of glycobiarsol.

milieu (me-lyuh′) [Fr.], surroundings; environment. **m. exté′rieur,** external environment.

m. inté′rieur, internal environment; the blood and lymph in which the cells are bathed.

milium (mil′e-um), pl. *mil′ia* [L.] a small, whitish or yellowish nodule in the skin.

milk (milk) 1. a nutrient fluid produced by many animals for nourishment of the young. 2. a liquid (emulsion or suspension) resembling the secretion of the mammary gland. **acidophilus m.,** milk fermented with cultures of *Lactobacillus acidophilus;* used in gastrointestinal disorders to modify the bacterial flora of the intestinal tract. **m. of bismuth,** bismuth magma. **Budd m., buddeized m.,** milk sterilized by adding hydrogen dioxide and heating, so as to decompose the dioxide and liberate the oxygen. **casein m.,** a prepared milk containing very little salts and sugars and a large amount of fat and casein. **certified m.,** milk whose purity is certified by a committee of physicians or a medical milk commission. **condensed m.,** milk which has been partly evaporated and sweetened with sugar. **diabetic m.,** milk containing a small percentage of lactose. **dialyzed m.,** milk with sugar removed by dialysis through a parchment membrane. **evaporated m.,** milk prepared by evaporation of half of its water content. **fortified m.,** milk made more nutritious by addition of cream or vitamins. **homogenized m.,** milk treated so that the fats form a permanent emulsion. **m. of magnesia,** a suspension containing 7–8.5 per cent of magnesium hydroxide, used as an antacid. **modified m.,** cow's milk made to correspond to composition of human milk. **protein m.,** milk modified to have a relatively low content of carbohydrate and fat and a relatively high protein content. **m. of sulfur,** precipitated sulfur. **vitamin A m.,** cow's milk fortified by addition of vitamin A. **vitamin D m.,** cow's milk fortified by addition of vitamin D. **witch's m.,** milk secreted in the breast of the newborn infant.

milli- (mil′e) word element [Fr.], *one thousandth;* used in naming units of measurement to designate an amount 10^{-3} the size of the unit to which it is joined, e.g. milligram (0.001 gm.).

milliampere (mil″e-am′per) one thousandth of an ampere.

milliampere-minute (-min′ut) a unit of electricity equivalent to that delivered by a current of 1 milliampere strength acting for one minute.

millicoulomb (mil″i koo′lom) one thousandth (10^{-3}) coulomb; abbreviated mcoul.

millicurie (-ku′re) one thousandth (10^{-3}) curie; abbreviated mc.

millicurie-hour (-owr) a unit of dose equivalent to that obtained by exposure for one hour to radioactive material disintegrating at the rate of 3.7×10^7 atoms per second; abbreviated mc.-hr.

milliequivalent (mil″e-e-kwiv′ah-lent) one thousandth of the equivalent weight of a substance; symbol, mEq.

milligram (mil′i-gram) one thousandth of a gram; equivalent of 0.015432 grain avoirdupois or apothecaries' weight; abbreviated mg.

milliliter (mil′i-le″ter) one thousandth of a liter; equivalent of 16.23 minims; abbreviated ml.

millimeter (mil′i-me″ter) one thousandth of a meter; equivalent of 0.039 inch; abbreviated mm.

millimicro- (mil″li-mi′kro) word element designating 10^{-3} (one thousandth) of 10^{-6} (one millionth), or 10^{-9} (one billionth), part of the unit to which it is joined.

millimicrocurie (-mi″kro-ku′re) one thousandth (10^{-3}) microcurie, or 10^{-9} curie; abbreviated mμc.

millimicrogram (-mi′kro-gram) one thousandth (10^{-3}) microgram, or 10^{-9} gram; abbreviated mμg.

millimicron (-mi′kron) one thousandth of a micron (10^{-6} mm., or 10 angstroms); abbreviated mμ.

milliosmole (-os′mol) one thousandth of an osmole.

millirad (mil′i-rad) a unit of absorbed radiation dose, 10^{-3} rad; abbreviated mrad.

milliroentgen (mil″i-rent′gen) a unit of dose equal to one thousandth (10^{-3}) roentgen; abbreviated mr.

milliunit (-u′nit) one thousandth part of a unit (10^{-3}).

millivolt (mil′i-volt) one thousandth of a volt; abbreviated mv.

Milontin (mi-lon′tin) trademark for preparations of phensuximide.

Milpath (mil′path) trademark for a preparation of meprobamate and tridihexethyl chloride.

Miltown (mil′town) trademark for a preparation of meprobamate.

milt (milt) the male reproductive glands of fish or the fluid filling them at breeding season.

milt-sickness (milt′sik-nes) disease of the spleen in cattle.

min. minim; minimum; minute.

Mincard (min′kard) trademark for a preparation of aminometradine.

mind (mind) the faculty by which one is aware of surroundings and by which he is able to remember, reason and make decisions.

mineral (min′er-al) a nonorganic homogeneous substance.

mineralocorticoid (min″er-al-o-kor′ti koid) a corticoid effective in causing the retention of sodium and loss of potassium.

minim (min′im) a unit of volume in the English system, equivalent to 0.0616 cc.

miocardia (mi″o-kar′de-ah) the contraction of the heart; systole.

miopus (mi′o-pus) fetal monster with two fused heads, one face being rudimentary.

miosis (mi-o′sis) excessive contraction of pupil.

miotic (mi-ot′ik) 1. causing the pupil to contract. 2. an agent that causes contraction of the pupil.

miracidium (mi″rah-sid′e-um), pl. *miracid′ia* [Gr.] the free-swimming larva of a trematode parasite which emerges from an egg and penetrates the body of a snail host.

mire (mer) [Fr.] a figure on the arm of an ophthalmometer the image of which is reflected on the cornea.

mirror (mir'or) a polished surface that reflects light or creates visible images of objects in front of it. **concave m.**, one with a concave reflecting suface. **convex m.**, one with a convex reflecting surface. **dental m.**, mouth mirror. **frontal m., head m.**, a circular mirror strapped to the head; used especially for laryngoscopy or rhinoscopy. **Glatzel m.**, a plate of cold metal held below the nostrils; the patch of moisture deposited by breathing on its surface indicates the patency or nonpatency of the nasal passages. **mouth m.**, a small mirror used by dentists. **nasographic m.**, Glatzel mirror. **plane m.**, one with a flat reflecting surface.

miscarriage (mis-kar'ij) loss of the products of conception from the uterus before the fetus is viable; abortion.

miscible (mis'i-bl) susceptible of being mixed.

misocainia (mis"o-ki'ne-ah) aversion to new ideas.

misogamy (mĭ-sog'ah-me) morbid aversion to marriage.

misogyny (mĭ-soj'ĭ-ne) aversion to women.

misologia (mis"o-lo'je-ah) morbid dread of mental application.

misopedia (-pe'de-ah) morbid dislike of children.

mite (mīt) an arthropod of the order Acarina, characterized by minute size, usually transparent or semitransparent body, and other features distinguishing them from organisms of the suborder Ixodides; they may be free-living or parasitic on animals or plants. **harvest m.**, chigger. **itch m., mange m.**, *Sarcoptes scabiei.*

mithridatism (mith'rĭ-da"tizm) acquisition of immunity to a poison by ingestion of gradually increasing amounts of it.

miticide (mi'tĭ-sid) an agent destructive to mites.

mitochondrion (mi"to-kon'dre-on), pl. *mitochon'dria* [Gr.] a filamentous or granular component (organelle) of cytoplasm, the principal site of oxidative reactions by which the energy in foodstuff is made available for endergonic processes in the cell.

mitogen (mi'to-jen) an agent that induces mitosis. adj., **mitogen'ic.**

mitogenesis (mi"to-jen'ĕ-sis) the induction of mitosis in a cell. adj., **mitogenet'ic.**

mitome (mi'tōm) thready network of protoplasm.

mitosis (mi-to'sis) a method of indirect cell division in which the two daughter nuclei normally receive identical complements of the number of chromosomes characteristic of the somatic cells of the species. adj., **mitot'ic.**

mitosome (mi'to-sōm) a body formed from the spindle fibers of the preceding mitosis; a spindle remnant.

mitral (mi'tral) shaped like a miter; pertaining to the valve between the left atrium and ventricle.

mittelschmerz (mit'el-shmerts) pain midway between the menstrual periods.

mixotrophic (mik"so-trof'ik) having nutritional characters of both animals and plants.

mixture (miks'tūr) a combination of different drugs or ingredients, as a fluid with other fluids or solids, or of a solid with a liquid. **brown m.**, a preparation of glycyrrhiza fluidextract, antimony potassium tartrate, paregoric, alcohol, glycerin and purified water; used as an expectorant. **chalk m.**, prepared chalk, with bentonite magma, cinnamon water and saccharin sodium; used as an antacid. **kaolin m. with pectin**, a preparation containing kaolin, pectin, powdered tragacanth, benzoic acid, saccharin sodium, glycerin and peppermint oil in purified water; used as an antacid and demulcent.

Miyagawanella (mi"yah-gah"wah-nel'ah) a genus of Microtatobiotes (order Rickettsiales, family Chlamydiaceae).

M.K.S. meter-kilogram-second, indicating a system of measurements based on these units as standards of length, mass and time.

M.L. Licentiate in Medicine.

M.L.A. Medical Library Association.

ml. milliliter.

M.L.D. minimum lethal dose.

mm. millimeter; muscles.

mμ millimicron.

Mn chemical symbol, *manganese.*

mnemonics (ne-mon'iks) cultivation of the memory.

M.O. Medical Officer.

Mo chemical symbol, *molybdenum.*

mobilization (mo"bĭ-li-za'shun) the rendering of a fixed part movable. **stapes m.**, surgical correction of immobility of the stapes in treatment of deafness.

mock-knee (mok'ne) a large swelling on the knees of horses and cattle, caused by injury.

modality (mo-dal'ĭ-te) 1. a physical agent used therapeutically. 2. a condition which modifies a drug action (homeopathy).

Moderil (mod'er-il) trademark for a preparation of rescinnamine.

modiolus (mo-di'o-lus) central pillar or columella of the cochlea.

Modumate (mod'u-māt) trademark for a preparation of arginine and glutamic acid.

M.O.H. Medical Officer of Health.

mol (mol) mole (3).

molality (mo-lal'ĭ-te) the number of moles of a solute per kilogram of pure solvent.

molar (mo'lar) 1. pertaining to a mass. 2. pertaining to a mole. 3. a tooth adapted for grinding.

molarity (mo-lar'ĭ-te) the number of moles of a solute per liter of solution.

mold (mōld) 1. a true fungus or Eumycetes. 2. a matrix or cavity in which something is shaped. 3. to shape, or give form to.

mole (mōl) 1. a fleshy mass formed in the uterus by abortive development of an ovum. 2. a pigmented fleshy growth or blemish on the skin. 3. that amount of a chemical compound whose mass in grams is equivalent to its formula mass. **hairy m.**, hairy nevus. **hydatid m., hydatidiform m., hydatiform m.**, myxoma formed by cystic degeneration of villi of the chorion. **pigmented m.**, nevus pigmentosus.

molecule (mol'ē-kūl) a very small mass of matter; an aggregation of atoms composing the smallest unit of a compound possessing its characteristic properties.

molimen (mo-li′men) the monthly effort of the menstrual flow.

mollities (mo-lish′e-ēz) abnormal softening. **m. os′sium,** osteomalacia.

molluscacide (mŏ-lusk′ah-sīd) an agent that destroys snails and other molluscs.

molluscum (mŏ-lus′kum) a soft growth. adj., **mollus′cous. m. contagio′sum,** disease with rounded skin tubercles containing a semifluid. **m. fibro′sum, m. sim′plex,** multiple fibroma of the skin.

mol. wt. molecular weight.

molybdenum (mo-lib′dĕ-num) chemical element (*see table*), at. no. 42, symbol Mo.

momentum (mo-men′tum) quantity of motion; product of mass by velocity.

monad (mo′nad) 1. a single-celled protozoon. 2. a univalent radical or element.

monarthritis (mon″ar-thri′tis) inflammation of a single joint.

monarticular (-tik′u-ler) pertaining to one joint.

monaster (mon-as′ter) the single star-shaped figure in mitosis.

monathetosis (-ath″ĕ-to′sis) athetosis of one part of the body.

monatomic (mon″ah-tom′ik) 1. containing one atom. 2. univalent.

monecious (mon-e′shus) requiring only one host for completion of the entire life cycle.

monesthetic (mon″es-thet′ik) affecting a single sense of sensation.

mongolism (mon′go-lizm) Down's syndrome; a congenital condition associated with a chromosomal defect and characterized by small, flattened skull, short, flat-bridged nose and mental retardation.

monilethrix (mo-nil′ĕ-thriks) disease in which the hair becomes brittle and beaded.

Monilia (mo-nil′e-ah) former name of a genus of parasitic fungi, now called Candida.

moniliasis (mo″nĭ-li′ah-sis) candidiasis.

moniliform (mo-nil′ĭ-form) beaded.

monitor (mon′ĭ-tor) 1. to check constantly on a given condition or phenomenon, e.g. blood pressure or heart or respiratory rate. 2. an apparatus by which certain conditions or phenomena can be constantly observed.

mono- (mon′o) word element [Gr.], *one.*

monobasic (mon″o-ba′sik) having but one atom of replaceable hydrogen.

monobenzone (bĕn′zōn) a white, crystalline powder used as a hypopigmenting agent.

monoblast (mon′o-blast) the cell which is the precursor of the mature monocyte.

monoblastoma (mon″o-blas-to′mah) a tumor containing monoblasts and monocytes.

monoblepsia (-blep′se-ah) blindness to all colors but one.

monobrachius (-bra′ke-us) fetus with but one arm.

monobulia (-bu′le-ah) concentrated wishing on one thing only.

monocellular (-sel′u-lar) unicellular.

monocephalus (-sef′ah-lus) fetal monster with two bodies and one head.

monochlorothymol (mon″o-klo″ro-thi′mol) chlorothymol.

monochorea (-ko-re′ah) chorea affecting but one part.

monochorial (-ko′re-al) pertaining to or characterized by the presence of a single chorion.

monochorionic (-ko″re-on′ik) monochorial.

monochromatic (-kro-mat′ik) pertaining to a single color.

monococcus (-kok′us) a form of coccus consisting of single cells.

monocontaminated (-kon-tam′ĭ-nāt″ed) infected by only one species of microorganisms or a single contaminating agent.

monocular (mon-ok′u-lar) pertaining to one eye.

monoculus (-ok′u-lus) 1. a bandage for one eye. 2. a cyclops.

monocyclic (mon″o-si′klik) in chemistry, having an atomic structure containing only one ring.

monocyesis (-si-e′sis) pregnancy with a single fetus.

monocyte (mon′o-sīt) the largest of the leukocytes, 9–12 microns in diameter, with a considerably dented nucleus normally constituting 5–10 per cent of the leukocytes of the blood. adj., **monocyt′ic.**

monocytopenia (mon″o-si″to-pe′ne-ah) deficiency of monocytes in the blood.

monocytosis (-si-to′sis) excess of monocytes in the blood.

monodactylism (-dak′tĭ-lizm) only one finger or toe on a hand or foot.

monodal (mon-o′dal) having connection with one terminal of a resonator or a grounded solenoid.

monodiplopia (mon″o-dĭ-plo′pe-ah) double vision in one eye.

Monodral (mon′o-dral) trademark for preparations of penthienate.

monoecious (mon-e′shus) 1. having reproductive organs typical of both sexes in a single individual. 2. requiring only one host for completion of the entire life cycle.

monogenesis (mon″o-jen′ĕ-sis) nonsexual reproduction.

monogenic (-jen′ik) pertaining to or influenced by a single gene.

monogenous (mon-oj′ĕ-nus) produced asexually.

monogerminal (mon″o-jer′mĭ-nal) developed from one ovum.

monoglyceride (-glis′er-īd) a compound consisting of one molecule of fatty acid esterified to glycerol.

monoiodotyrosine (-i-o″do-ti′ro-sēn) a derivative of tyrosine containing one atom of iodine, found in the thyroid gland.

monolayer (-la′er) pertaining to or consisting of a single layer.

monolocular (-lok′u-lar) having but one cavity.

monomania (-ma′ne-ah) a logical system of delusions based on a single false premise.

monomastigote (-mas′tĭ-gōt) having a single flagellum.

monomelic (-mel′ik) affecting one limb.

monomer (mon'o-mer) a simple molecule of relatively low molecular weight. **fibrin m.,** the material resulting from the action of thrombin on fibrinogen, which then polymerizes to form fibrin.

monomeric (mon″o-mer′ik) pertaining to a single segment.

monometallic (-mĕ-tal′ik) having one atom of a metal in a molecule.

monomicrobic (-mi-kro′bik) pertaining to or caused by a single variety of pathogenic microorganisms.

monomorphic (-mor′fik) existing in only one form.

monomphalus (mon-om′fah-lus) a double fetal monster joined at the navel.

monomyoplegia (mon″o-mi″o-ple′je-ah) paralysis of a single muscle.

monomyositis (-mi″o-si′tis) inflammation of a single muscle.

mononeural (-nu′ral) supplied by a single nerve.

mononeuritis (-nu-ri′tis) inflammation of a single nerve.

monont (mon′ont) schizont.

mononuclear (mon″o-nu′kle-ar) having only one nucleus.

mononucleosis (-nu″kle-o′sis) excess of mononuclear leukocytes in the blood. **infectious m.,** a disease characterized by lymphadenopathy and lymphocytosis, and elevated titer of sheep cell agglutinins in the serum.

mononucleotide (-nu′kle-o-tīd″) a compound of phosphoric acid and a glucoside or pentoside, obtained by the digestion or hydrolytic decomposition of nucleic acid.

monoparesis (-par′ĕ-sis) paresis of a single part.

monoparesthesia (-par″es-the′ze-ah) paresthesia of a single part.

monopathy (mo-nop′ah-the) a disease affecting a single part.

monophthalmus (mon″of-thal′mus) a fetus with one eye.

monophyletic (mon″o-fi-let′ik) descended from a single source.

monoplegia (-ple′je-ah) paralysis of a single part.

monopolar (mon′o-po″lar) having a single pole.

monops (mon′ops) a fetus with a single eye.

monopus (mon′o-pus) a fetus with only one foot.

monorchis (mon-or′kis) a person having only one testis in the scrotum.

monorchism (mon′or-kizm) the condition of having only one descended testis.

monosaccharide (mon″o-sak′ah-rīd) a carbohydrate that cannot be broken down to simpler substances by acid hydrolysis.

monosexual (-sek′su-al) showing characteristics or traits of one sex only.

monosomy (-so′me) existence in a cell of only one instead of the normal diploid pair of a particular chromosome. adj., **monoso′mic.**

monostotic (mon″os-tot′ik) affecting a single bone.

monostratal (mon″o-stra′tal) pertaining to a single layer or stratum.

monosubstituted (mon″o-sub′stī-tūt″ed) having only one atom in the molecule replaced.

monosymptomatic (-simp″to-mat′ik) having only one symptom.

monosynaptic (-sĭ-nap′tik) pertaining to or passing through a single synapse.

monoterminal (-ter′mĭ-nal) using one terminal only in giving electric treatment.

Monotheamin (-the′ah-min) trademark for preparations of theophylline monoethanolamine.

monothermia (-ther′me-ah) identity of body temperature morning and evening.

monotrichous (mon-ot′rĭ-kus) having a single flagellum.

monotropic (mon″o-trop′ik) affecting only one kind of bacteria or one variety of tissue.

monovalent (-va′lent) 1. having a valency of one. 2. capable of binding one complement only.

monoxenic (-zen′ik) associated with a known single species of microorganisms.

monoxenous (mo-nok′sĕ-nus) requiring only one host to complete the life cycle.

monoxide (mon-ok′sīd) an oxide with one oxygen atom in the molecule.

monozygotic (mon″o-zi-got′ik) pertaining to or derived from a single zygote (fertilized ovum).

mons (mons), pl. *mon′tes* [L.] a prominence. **m. pu′bis,** the rounded fleshy prominence over the symphysis pubis. **m. ven′eris,** a name given the mons pubis in the female.

monster (mon′ster) a fetus which shows such developmental anomalies as to be grotesque and nonviable. **autositic m.,** one capable of independent life. **compound m.,** a monster made up of parts of more than one individual. **double m.,** twin monster. **emmenic m.,** an infant that menstruates. **endocymic m.,** a monster which never comes to birth, but is retained and forms the basis of a dermoid tumor. **parasitic m.,** an imperfect fetus attached to another and unable to exist alone. **triplet m.,** a monster containing parts of three individuals. **twin m.,** a monster consisting of two individuals joined at some point.

monstriparity (mon″strĭ-par′ĭ-te) the act of giving birth to a monster.

monstrosity (mon-stros′ĭ-te) 1. great congenital deformity. 2. a monster or teratism.

monticulus (mon-tik′u-lus), pl. *montic′uli* [L.] a small eminence. **m. cerebel′li,** projecting part of superior vermiform process of cerebellum.

mood (mōod) a prevailing emotional tone or feeling.

Moraxella (mo-rak-sel′ah) a genus of Schizomycetes (order Eubacteriales, family Brucellaceae) found as parasites and pathogens in warm-blooded animals.

morbid (mor′bid) 1. pertaining to, characteristic of or characterized by disease or abnormality. 2. pathologic or abnormal.

morbidity (mor-bid′ĭ-te) 1. condition of being diseased. 2. proportion of disease to health in a community.

morbific (mor-bif′ik) causing or inducing disease.

morbilli (mor-bil′i) [L.] measles.

morbilliform (mor-bil′ĭ-form) resembling measles.

morbus (mor′bus) [L.] disease. **m. cadu′cus,** epilepsy. **m. caeru′leus,** severe cyanosis, resulting from congenital malformation of the heart. **m. coxa′rius,** hip joint disease. **m. hemorrhag′icus neonato′rum,** hemorrhagic disease of the newborn. **m. maculo′- sus werlhof′ii, m. werlhof′ii,** idiopathic thrombocytopenic purpura.

morcellation (mor″se-la′shun) division of a tumor or organ, with removal by piecemeal.

mordant (mor′dant) 1. a substance used to fix a stain or dye. 2. to treat with a substance which can be fixed to a fiber or other structure and later can be dyed.

moria (mo′re-ah) a morbid tendency to joke.

moribund (mor′ĭ-bund) in a dying state.

Mornidine (mor′nĭ-dēn) trademark for preparations of pipamazine.

moron (mo′ron) a mentally defective person with an I.Q. between 50 and 69, usually requiring special training and supervision.

moronity (mo-ron′ĭ-te) the condition of being a moron.

morphallaxis (mor″fah-lak′sis) renewal of a lost tissue or part by reorganization of the remaining part of the body of an animal. adj., **morphallac′tic.**

morphea (mor-fe′ah) disease marked by pinkish patches bordered by a purplish areola.

morpheme (mor′fēm) a meaningful unit of sound.

morphine (mor′fēn) an opium alkaloid, a narcotic analgesic usually used as *morphine sulfate*. **m. hydrochloride,** white, silky, glistening substance; analgesic, respiratory sedative.

morphinism (mor′fĭ niẑm) morbid state due to morphine.

morphinomania (mor″fĭ-no-ma′ne-ah) morbid and habitual craving for morphine.

morphium (mor′fe-um) morphine.

morphodifferentiation (mor″fo-dif″er-en″she-a′shun) arrangement of formative cells so as to establish the future shape and size of an organ.

morphogenesis (-jen′ĕ-sis) the developmental change occurring in the shape and organization of the body and its parts. adj., **morphogenet′ic.**

morphology (mor-fol′o-jc) science of organic forms and structure.

morphometry (mor-fom′ĕ-tre) the measurement of forms.

mors (mōrs) [L.] death.

morsus (mor′sus) [L.] bite. **m. diab′oli,** the fimbriated end of an oviduct.

mortal (mor′tal) 1. destined to die. 2. causing or terminating in death.

mortality (mor-tal′ĭ-te) 1. the quality of being mortal. 2. the frequency of death in a certain population or caused by a particular disease. **perinatal m.,** the mortality of infants between the end of the twenty-eighth week of gestation and the end of the first week after birth.

mortalogram (mor-tal′o-gram) a graphic presentation in grid form of crude and age-standardized mortality rates and the numerical distribution of deaths for a given cause according to the time period, age and sex, and the median age at death.

mortar (mor′tar) a vessel with rounded internal surface, used with a pestle, for reducing a solid to a powder or producing a homogeneous mixture of solids.

morula (mor′u-lah) a solid mass of cells resembling a mulberry, formed by cleavage of a fertilized ovum.

mosaic (mo-za′ik) a pattern made of numerous small pieces fitted together; in genetics, occurrence in an individual of two or more cell populations each having a different chromosome complement.

mosaicism (mo-za′i-sizm) presence in an individual of cells derived from the same zygote, but differing in chromosomal constitution.

mosquito (mos-ke′to) a blood-sucking dipterous insect, chiefly of the genus Aedes, Anopheles, Culex or Stegomyia.

mosquitocide (mos-ke′to-sid) 1. destructive to mosquitoes. 2. an agent that kills mosquitoes. adj., **mosquitoci′dal.**

motor (mo′tor) 1. pertaining to motion. 2. a muscle, nerve or center that affects movements.

mottling (mot′ling) discoloration in irregular areas.

moulage (moo-lahzh′) [Fr.] a wax model of a structure or lesion.

moulding (mōld′ing) the shaping of a child's head to the size and shape of the birth canal.

mounding (mownd′ing) the rising in a lump of a wasting muscle when struck.

mount (mownt) to prepare specimens and slides for study.

mouse (mows) a small rodent, various species of which are used in laboratory experiments. **joint m.,** a movable fragment of cartilage or other body within a joint. **peritoneal m.,** a free body in the peritoneal cavity, probably a small detached mass of omentum, sometimes visible radiographically.

mouth (mowth) an opening, especially the anterior opening of the alimentary canal, the cavity containing the tongue and teeth. **trench m.,** necrotizing ulcerative gingivitis.

mouthwash (mowth′wawsh) a solution for rinsing the mouth, as the official N.F. preparation of potassium bicarbonate, sodium borate, thymol, eucalyptol, methyl salicylate, amaranth solution, alcohol, glycerin and purified water.

movement (mōōv′ment) an act of moving; motion. **ameboid m.,** movement like that of an ameba, accomplished by protrusion of cytoplasm of the cell. **angular m.,** movement which changes the angle between two bones. **associated m.,** movement of parts which act together, as the eyes. **brownian m.,** the peculiar, rapid, oscillatory movement of fine particles suspended in a fluid medium. **communicated m.,** that produced by a force acting from without. **compulsory m's, forced m's,** involuntary coordinated movements due to injury of a nerve center. **index m.,** a movement of the cephalic part of the body about the fixed caudal part. **molecular m.**, brownian movement. **passive m.**, a movement of the body or of the extremities of a patient performed by another person without voluntary motion on the part of the patient. **vermicular m's**, the wormlike movements of the intestines in peristalsis.

M.P.D. maximum permissible dose: that amount of ionizing radiation that is not expected to lead to bodily injury.

M.P.H. Master of Public Health.

M.Phys.A. Member of the Physiotherapists' Association (Brit.)

mr. milliroentgen.

M.R.C. Medical Reserve Corps.

M.R.C.P. Member of Royal College of Physicians.

M.R.C.S. Member of Royal College of Surgeons.

M.R.D. minimum reacting dose.

M.R.L. Medical Record Librarian.

mRNA messenger RNA.

M.S. Master of Science; Master of Surgery.

MSH melanocyte-stimulating hormone.

M.T. Medical Technologist.

M.U. Maché unit; mouse unit.

μ micron.

μc. microcurie.

muciferous (mu-sif'er-us) secreting mucus.

muciform (mu'sĭ-form) resembling mucus.

mucigen (mu'sĭ-jen) substance convertible into mucin and mucus.

mucilage (mu'sĭ-lij) an aqueous solution of a gummy substance, used as a vehicle or demulcent. **acacia m.**, a preparation of acacia and benzoic acid in purified water. **tragacanth m.**, a preparation of tragacanth, benzoic acid, glycerin and purified water.

mucilloid (mu'sil-loid) a preparation of a mucilaginous substance. **psyllium hydrophilic m.**, a powdered preparation of the mucilaginous portion of blond psyllium seeds, used in treatment of constipation.

mucin (mu'sin) a mixture of proteins which is the chief constituent of mucus. **gastric m.**, a preparation from the linings of hog's stomach; used in treating peptic ulcer.

mucinase (mu'sĭ-nās) an enzyme which acts upon mucin.

mucinogen (mu-sin'o-jen) a precursor of mucin.

mucinoid (mu'sĭ-noid) resembling mucin.

mucinosis (mu"si-no'sis) a state with abnormal deposits of mucin in the skin, often associated with hypothyroidism (myxedema). **follicular m.**, a disease of unknown cause, characterized by plaques of folliculopapules and usually alopecia.

muciparous (mu-sip'ah-rus) producing mucin.

mucocele (mu'ko-sēl) 1. dilatation of a cavity with mucous secretion. 2. a mucous polyp.

mucocutaneous (mu"ko-ku-ta'ne-us) pertaining to mucous membrane and skin.

muco-enteritis (-en"tĕ-ri'tis) acute catarrhal enteritis.

mucofibrous (-fi'brus) composed of mucous and fibrous tissues.

mucoglobulin (-glob'u-lin) any one of the class of proteids to which plastin belongs.

mucoid (mu'koid) 1. resembling mucus. 2. a conjugated protein of animal origin, differing from mucin in solubility.

mucomembranous (mu"ko-mem'brah-nus) composed of mucous membrane.

mucopolysaccharide (-pol"ĭ-sak'ah-rīd) a group of polysaccharides which contains hexosamine, which may or may not be combined with protein and which, dispersed in water, form many of the mucins.

mucoprotein (-pro'te-in) a compound present in all connective and supporting tissues, containing, as prosthetic groups, mucopolysaccharides; soluble in water and relatively resistant to denaturation.

mucopurulent (-pu'roo-lent) marked by an exudate containing both mucus and pus.

mucopus (mu'ko-pus) mucus blended with pus.

Mucor (mu'kor) a genus of saprophytic mold fungi.

mucormycosis (mu"kor-mi-ko'sis). a mycosis due to fungus of the genus Mucor; it is usually a pulmonary infection, but metastatic abscesses may form in various organs.

mucosa (mu-ko'sah), pl. *muco'sae* [L.] mucous membrane. adj., **muco'sal.**

mucosanguineous (mu"ko-sang-gwin'e-us) composed of mucus and blood.

mucoserous (-se'rus) composed of mucus and serum.

mucosin (mu-ko'sin) a form of mucin found in tenacious mucus.

mucosocutaneous (mu-ko"so-ku-ta'ne-us) pertaining to a mucous membrane and the skin.

mucoviscidosis (mu"ko-vis"ĭ-do'sis) cystic fibrosis; so called because of the abnormal viscosity of the secretions of certain exocrine glands.

mucus (mu'kus) the free slime of the mucous membrane, composed of its secretion, mucin, and various salts and body cells. adj., **mu'-cous.**

μg. microgram.

μl. microliter.

multangular (mul-tang'gu-lar) having many angles or corners.

multi- (mul'tĭ) word element [L.], *many.*

multiallelic (mul"te-ah-lel'ik) pertaining to or made up of a number of alleles.

multi-articular (-ar-tik'u-lar) pertaining to many joints.

multibacillary (-bas'ĭ-la"re) pertaining to or made up of a number of bacilli.

multicellular (-sel'u-lar) composed of many cells.

multicontaminated (-kon-tam'ĭ-nāt"ed) infected by many species of microorganisms or known contaminating agents.

multicuspidate (-kus"pĭ-dāt) having numerous cusps.

multifactorial (-fak-to're-al) 1. of or pertaining to, or arising through the action of, many factors. 2. in genetics, arising as the result of the interaction of several genes.

multifid (mul'tĭ-fid) cleft into many parts.

multifocal (mul"tĭ-fo'kal) arising from or pertaining to many foci.

multiform (mul'tĭ-form) occurring in many forms.

multiglandular (mul"tĭ-glan'du-lar) affecting several glands.

multigravida (-grav'ĭ-dah) a woman who has had three or more previous pregnancies. **grand m.**, a woman who has had six or more previous pregnancies.

multilobular (-lob'u-lar) having many lobules.

multilocular (-lok'u-lar) having many loculi.

multinodular (-nod'u-lar) having many nodules.

multinuclear (-nu'kle-ar) having many nuclei.

multipara (mul-tip'ah-rah) a woman who has had more than two pregnancies which resulted in viable offspring. adj., **multip'arous. grand m.**, a woman who has had seven or more pregnancies that resulted in viable offspring.

multiparity (mul"tĭ-par'ĭ-te) the condition of being a multipara.

multipolar (-po'lar) having more than two poles or processes.

multisynaptic (-sĭ-nap'tik) pertaining to or relayed through two or more synapses.

multiterminal (-ter'mĭ-nal) having several sets of terminals so that several electrodes may be used.

multivalent (-va'lent) combining with several univalent atoms.

μmm. micromillimeter.

mummying (mum'e-ing) a form of physical restraint in which the entire body is enclosed in a sheet or blanket, leaving only the head exposed.

mumps (mumps) epidemic parotitis.

μμg. micromicrogram.

mural (mu'ral) pertaining to a wall.

Murel (mu'rel) trademark for preparations of valethamate bromide.

murine (mu'rēn) pertaining to mice or rats.

murmur (mer'mer) a gentle, blowing auscultatory sound. **accidental m.**, one due to some temporary and insignificant circumstance. **anemic m.**, one due to anemia. **aneurysmal m.**, one due to an aneurysm. **aortic m.**, a sound indicative of disease of the aortic valve. **apex m.**, one heard over the apex of the heart. **arterial m.**, one in an artery, sometimes aneurysmal and sometimes hemic. **blood m.**, one due to an abnormal, commonly anemic, condition of the blood. **cardiac m.**, any adventitious sound heard over the region of the heart. **cardiopulmonary m.**, one produced by the impact of the heart against the lung. **crescendo m.**, a heart murmur increasing in pitch and force. **diastolic m.**, one at diastole, due to mitral obstruction or to aortic or pulmonary regurgitation. **direct m.**, one due to a roughened endocardium and contracted valvular orifice. **Duroziez m.**, double murmur heard on compression of the femoral artery with the stethoscope, in aortic regurgitation and other conditions. **dynamic m.**, one caused by irregular pulsation of the heart. **endocardial m.**, one produced within the heart cavities. **exocardial m.**, a heart murmur produced outside the heart's cavities. **Flint's m.**, a peculiar murmur at the apex in aortic regurgitation. **friction m.**, one due to the rubbing together of two serous surfaces. **functional m.**, cardiac murmur from excited action of heart or from anemia. **Gibson m.**, a long, rumbling sound occupying most of systole and diastole, usually localized in the second left interspace near the sternum, and pathognomonic of patent ductus arteriosus. **Graham Steell m.**, one due to relative pulmonary insufficiency. **heart m.**, cardiac murmur. **hemic m.**, blood murmur. **indirect m.**, one caused by reversal of the direction of blood current. **innocent m.**, functional murmur. **inorganic m.**, one not due to valvular lesions. **machinery m.**, a continuous, loud, rough murmur heard in the second left space in patent ductus arteriosus. **mitral m.**, one due to diseased mitral valve. **musical m.**, one with a musical quality. **organic m.**, one due to structural change in the heart. **pericardial m.**, one produced in the pericardium. **prediastolic m.**, one occurring just before diastole. **presystolic m.**, one before systole, from mitral or tricuspid obstruction. **pulmonic m.**, one due to disease of the valves of the pulmonary artery. **regurgitant m.**, one due to a dilated valvular orifice. **seagull m.**, a musical murmur resembling the call of a seagull, frequently heard in aortic insufficiency. **systolic m.**, one at systole, from mitral, aortic, tricuspid or pulmonary obstruction. **tricuspid m.**, one caused by disease of the tricuspid valve. **vesicular m.**, the murmur of normal breathing.

murrain (mur'in) any destructive cattle plague.

murrina (moo-re'nah) a form of trypanosomiasis among mules and horses in the Canal Zone.

Musca (mus'kah) a genus of flies, including the common housefly, M. domes'tica.

musca (mus'kah), plural mus'cae [L.] a fly. **mus'cae volitan'tes**, specks seen as floating before the eyes.

muscarine (mus'kah-rin) a deadly alkaloid first obtained from the mushroom, Amanita muscaria.

muscle (mus'l) an organ which by contraction produces movement of an animal organism (see table of muscles). adj., **mus'cular. agonistic m.**, one opposed in action by another muscle, called the antagonist. **antagonistic m.**, one that counteracts the action of another muscle. **antigravity m's**, those that by their tone resist the constant pull of gravity in the maintenance of normal posture. **appendicular m.**, one of the muscles of a limb. **articular m.**, one that has one end attached to the synovial capsule of a joint. **Bell's m.**, the muscular strands between the ureteric orifices and the uvula vesicae, bounding the trigone of the urinary bladder. **Brücke's m.**, the longitudinal fibers of the ciliary muscle. **cardiac m.**, the muscle of the heart, composed of striated muscle fibers. **cutaneous m.**, striated muscle that inserts into the skin. **epimeric m.**, one derived from an epimere and innervated by a posterior ramus of a spinal nerve. **extraocular m's**, the extrinsic muscles of the eye. **extrinsic m.**, one which originates in

TABLE OF MUSCLES

NA TERM	ORIGIN	INSERTION	INNERVATION	ACTION
m. abductor digiti minimi manus	pisiform bone, flexor carpi ulnaris tendon	medial side of base of proximal phalanx of little finger	ulnar	abducts little finger
m. abductor digiti minimi pedis	lateral tubercle of calcaneus	lateral side of base of proximal phalanx of little toe	lateral plantar	abducts little toe
m. abductor hallucis	medial tubercle of calcaneus, plantar aponeurosis	medial side of base of proximal phalanx of great toe	medial plantar	abducts, flexes great toe
m. abductor pollicis brevis	tubercles of scaphoid and trapezium flexor retinaculum	lateral side of base of proximal phalanx of thumb	median	abducts thumb
m. abductor pollicis longus	posterior surfaces of radius and ulna	lateral side of base of first metacarpal bone and trapezium	posterior interosseous	abducts thumb
m. adductor brevis	body and inferior ramus of pubis	upper part of linea aspera of femur	obturator	adducts, flexes thigh
m. adductor hallucis	oblique head from long plantar ligament; transverse head from plantar ligaments	lateral side of base of proximal phalanx of great toe; sheath of flexor hallucis longus	lateral plantar	flexes and adducts great toe
m. adductor longus	body of pubis	linea aspera of femur	obturator	adducts, flexes thigh
m. adductor magnus	*adductor part* – inferior ramus of pubis, ramus of ischium; *extensor part* – ischial tuberosity	*adductor part* – linea aspera of femur; *extensor part* – adductor tubercle of femur	*adductor part* – obturator; *extensor part* – sciatic	*adductor part* – adducts thigh; *extensor part* – extends thigh
m. adductor pollicis	*oblique head* from second metacarpal, capitate and trapezoid; *transverse head* from front of third metacarpal	medial side of base of proximal phalanx of thumb	ulnar	adducts thumb
m. anconeus	back of lateral epicondyle of humerus	olecranon and posterior surface of ulna	radial	extends forearm
m. antitragicus	antitragus	caudate process of helix	temporal, posterior auricular branches of facial	
m. arrectores pilorum	dermis	hair follicles	sympathetic	elevate hairs
m. articularis cubiti	a name applied to a few fibers of the deep surface of the triceps brachii that insert into the posterior ligament and synovial membrane of the elbow joint			
m. articularis genus	lower part of anterior surface of shaft of femur	suprapatellar bursa	femoral	raises capsule of knee joint

Muscle	Description	Nerve	Action
m. aryepiglotticus	a name applied to inconstant fibers of oblique arytenoid muscle, from apex of arytenoid cartilage to lateral margin of epiglottis	recurrent laryngeal	closes inlet of larynx
m. arytenoideus obliquus	muscular process of arytenoid cartilage to apex of opposite arytenoid cartilage	recurrent laryngeal	approximates arytenoid cartilages
m. arytenoideus transversus	medial surface of arytenoid cartilage to medial surface of opposite arytenoid cartilage	recurrent laryngeal	approximates arytenoid cartilages
m. auricularis anterior	galea aponeurotica to cartilage of ear	facial	may draw auricle forward
m. auricularis posterior	mastoid process to cartilage of ear	facial	may draw auricle backward
m. auricularis superior	galea aponeurotica to cartilage of ear	facial	may raise auricle
m. biceps brachii	*long head* – supraglenoid tubercle of scapula; *short head* – apex of coracoid process to tuberosity of radius and antebrachial fascia	musculocutaneous	flexes and supinates forearm
m. biceps femoris	*long head* – ischial tuberosity; *short head* – linea aspera of femur to head of fibula, lateral condyle of tibia	sciatic	flexes and rotates leg laterally, extends thigh
m. brachialis	anterior aspect of humerus to coronoid process of ulna	musculocutaneous, radial	flexes forearm
m. brachioradialis	lateral supracondylar ridge of humerus to lateral surface of lower end of radius	radial	flexes forearm
m. bronchoesophageus	A name applied to muscle fibers arising from wall of left bronchus, reinforcing musculature of esophagus		
m. buccinator	alveolar processes of maxilla and mandible, pterygomandibular raphe to orbicularis oris and lips	buccal branch of facial	compresses cheek
m. bulbocavernosus. *See* m. bulbospongiosus			
m. bulbospongiosus	tendinous center of perineum, median raphe of bulb to fascia of penis or of clitoris	pudendal	constricts urethra in male, vagina in female
m. caninus. *See* m. levator anguli oris			
m. ceratocricoideus	a name applied to muscle fibers from cricoid cartilage to inferior horn of thyroid cartilage		
m. chondroglossus	lesser horn and body of hyoid bone to substance of tongue	hypoglossal	depresses, retracts tongue
m. ciliaris	*longitudinal division* (Brücke's muscles) – junction of cornea and sclera; *circular division* (Müller's muscle) – sphincter of ciliary body to outer layers of choroid and ciliary processes	short ciliary	makes lens more convex in visual accommodation

TABLE OF MUSCLES (Continued)

NA TERM	ORIGIN	INSERTION	INNERVATION	ACTION
m. coccygeus	ischial spine	lower part of lateral border of sacrum, coccyx	third and fourth sacral	supports and raises coccyx
m. constrictor pharyngis inferior	arch of cricoid, oblique line of thyroid cartilages	median raphe of posterior wall of pharynx	pharyngeal plexus, and external and recurrent laryngeal	constricts pharynx
m. constrictor pharyngis medius	horns of hyoid bone, stylo-hyoid ligament	median raphe of posterior wall of pharynx	pharyngeal plexus of vagus, glossopharyngeal	constricts pharynx
m. constrictor pharyngis superior	pterygoid hamulus, pterygo-mandibular raphe, mylo-hyoid line of mandible, mucous membrane of mouth	median raphe of posterior wall of pharynx	pharyngeal plexus of vagus	constricts pharynx
m. coracobrachialis	coracoid process of scapula	medial border of humerus	musculocutaneous	flexes arm
m. corrugator supercilii	medial end of superciliary arch	skin of eyebrow	facial	draws eyebrow downward and medially
m. cremaster	inferior margin of internal oblique muscle of abdomen	pubic tubercle	genital branch of genito-femoral	elevates testis
m. cricoarytenoideus lateralis	arch of cricoid cartilage	muscular process of arytenoid cartilage	recurrent laryngeal	approximates vocal folds
m. cricoarytenoideus posterior	back of lamina of cricoid cartilage	muscular process of arytenoid cartilage	recurrent laryngeal	separates vocal folds
m. cricothyroideus	arch of cricoid cartilage	lamina and inferior horn of thyroid cartilage	external laryngeal	tenses vocal folds
m. deltoideus	clavicle, acromion, spine of scapula	deltoid tuberosity of humerus	axillary	abducts and flexes or extends arm
m. depressor anguli oris	external surface of mandible	angle of mouth	facial	pulls down angle of mouth
m. depressor labii inferioris	external surface of mandible	orbicularis oris and skin of lower lip	facial	depresses lower lip
m. depressor septi nasi	incisive fossa of maxilla	ala and septum of nose	facial	constricts nostril and depresses ala
m. depressor supercilii	a name applied to a few fibers of orbital part of orbicularis oculi that are inserted into the eyebrow		facial	lowers eyebrow
detrusor urinae	a collective name applied to muscular coat of urinary bladder			
diaphragma	back of xiphoid process, inner surfaces of lower 6 costal cartilages and lower 4 ribs, medial and lateral arcuate ligaments, bodies of upper lumbar vertebrae	central tendon of diaphragm	phrenic	increases volume of thorax in inspiration

396

Muscle	Origin	Insertion	Nerve	Action
m. digastricus	*anterior belly*—digastric fossa or lower border of mandible near symphysis; *posterior belly*—mastoid notch of temporal bone	by middle tendon to hyoid bone	*anterior belly*—mylohyoid branch of inferior alveolar; *posterior belly*—facial	lowers jaw
m. dilator pupillae	a name applied to fibers extending radially from free to attached margin of iris		sympathetic through ciliary	enlarges pupil of eye
m. epicranius	a name applied to muscular covering of scalp, including occipitofrontalis and temporoparietalis muscles, and galea aponeurotica			
m. erector spinae	a name applied to fibers of more superficial of deep muscles of back, originating from sacrum, spines of lumbar and eleventh and twelfth thoracic vertebrae, and iliac crest; it splits into iliocostalis longissimus and spinalis muscles			
m. extensor carpi radialis brevis	lateral epicondyle of humerus, radial collateral ligament	backs of base of second and third metacarpal bones	radial or its deep branch	extends, abducts hand
m. extensor carpi radialis longus	lateral supracondylar ridge of humerus	base of second metacarpal bone	radial	extends, abducts hand
m. extensor carpi ulnaris	*humeral head*—lateral epicondyle of humerus; *ulnar head*—posterior border of ulna	base of fifth metacarpal bone	deep branch of radial	extends, adducts hand
m. extensor digiti minimi manus	lateral epicondyle of humerus	extensor aponeurosis of little finger	deep branch of radial	extends little finger
m. extensor digitorum manus	lateral epicondyle of humerus	extensor expansion of 4 medial fingers	deep branch of radial	extends distal phalanges
m. extensor digitorum brevis pedis	upper surface of calcaneus	extensor tendons of first, second, third, fourth toes	deep peroneal	extends toes
m. extensor digitorum longus pedis	anterior surface of fibula, lateral condyle of tibia, interosseous membrane	extensor expansions of 4 lateral toes	deep peroneal	extends toes
m. extensor hallucis brevis	a name applied to portion of short extensor muscle of toes that goes to great toe	base of distal phalanx of great toe	deep peroneal	extends great toe, dorsiflexes foot
m. extensor hallucis longus	front of fibula, interosseous membrane	extensor expansion of index finger	posterior interosseous	extends index finger
m. extensor indicis	posterior surface of ulna, interosseous membrane	back of proximal phalanx of thumb	posterior interosseous	extends thumb
m. extensor pollicis brevis	posterior surface of radius	back of distal phalanx of thumb	posterior interosseous	extends, adducts thumb
m. extensor pollicis longus	posterior surface of ulna and interosseous membrane			
m. fibularis. *Official alternative for* m. peroneus				

NA TERM	ORIGIN	INSERTION	INNERVATION	ACTION
m. flexor carpi radialis	medial epicondyle of humerus	bases of second and third metacarpal bones	median	flexes, abducts hand
m. flexor carpi ulnaris	*humeral head*—medial epicondyle of humerus; *ulnar head*—olecranon and posterior border of ulna	pisiform bone, hook of hamate bone, base of fifth metacarpal bone	ulnar	flexes, adducts hand
m. flexor digiti minimi brevis manus	hook of hamate bone	medial side of proximal phalanx of little finger	ulnar	flexes little finger
m. flexor digiti minimi brevis pedis	sheath of peroneus longus	lateral surface of base of proximal phalanx of little toe	lateral plantar	flexes little toe
m. flexor digitorum brevis pedis	medial tuberosity of calcaneus	middle phalanges of 4 lateral toes	medial plantar	flexes toes
m. flexor digitorum longus pedis	posterior surface of shaft of tibia	distal phalanges of 4 lateral toes	tibial	flexes toes
m. flexor digitorum profundus manus	shaft of ulna, coronoid process, interosseous membrane	bases of distal phalanges of 4 medial fingers	anterior interosseous, ulnar	flexes distal phalanges
m. flexor digitorum sublimis. *See* m. flexor digitorum superficialis.				
m. flexor digitorum superficialis manus	*humeroulnar head*—medial epicondyle of humerus, coronoid process of ulna; *radial head*—anterior border of radius	sides of middle phalanges of 4 medial fingers	median	flexes middle phalanges
m. flexor hallucis brevis	ligaments of sole	both sides of base of proximal phalanx of great toe	medial plantar	flexes great toe
m. flexor hallucis longus	posterior surface of fibula	base of distal phalanx of great toe	tibial	flexes great toe
m. flexor pollicis brevis	tubercle of trapezium, flexor retinaculum	lateral side of base of proximal phalanx of thumb	median	flexes thumb
m. flexor pollicis longus	anterior surface of radius, medial epicondyle of humerus, coronoid process of ulna	base of distal phalanx of thumb	anterior interosseous	flexes thumb
m. gastrocnemius	*medial head*—popliteal surface of femur, upper part of medial condyle; *lateral head*, lateral condyle	aponeurosis unites with tendon of soleus to form tendo calcaneus	tibial	plantar flexes foot, flexes knee joint

398

m. gemellus inferior	tuberosity of ischium	obturator internus tendon	nerve to quadratus femoris	rotates thigh laterally
m. gemellus superior	spine of ischium	obturator internus tendon	nerve to obturator internus	rotates thigh laterally
m. genioglossus	superior genial tubercle	hyoid bone, under surface of tongue	hypoglossal	protrudes and depresses tongue
m. geniohyoideus	inferior genial tubercle	body of hyoid bone	a branch of first cervical nerve through hypoglossal	draws hyoid bone forward
m. glossopalatinus. *See* m. palatoglossus.				
m. gluteus maximus	dorsal aspect of ilium, dorsal surface of sacrum and coccyx, sacrotuberous ligament	iliotibial tract band of fascia lata, gluteal tuberosity of femur	inferior gluteal	extends thigh or trunk
m. gluteus medius	dorsal aspect of ilium between anterior and posterior gluteal lines	greater trochanter of femur	superior gluteal	abducts, rotates thigh medially
m. gluteus minimus	dorsal aspect of ilium between anterior and inferior gluteal lines	greater trochanter of femur	superior gluteal	abducts, rotates thigh medially
m. gracilis	body and inferior ramus of pubis	medial surface of shaft of tibia	obturator	adducts thigh
m. helicis major	spine of helix	anterior border of helix	temporal, posterior auricular branches of facial	tenses skin of acoustic meatus
m. helicis minor	anterior rim of helix	concha	temporal, posterior auricular branches of facial	
m. hyoglossus	body and greater horn of hyoid bone	side of tongue	hypoglossal	depresses, retracts tongue
m. iliacus	iliac fossa, ala of sacrum	psoas major tendon, lesser trochanter of femur	femoral	flexes thigh or trunk
m. iliococcygeus	a name applied to posterior portion of levator ani muscle, including fibers originating as far forward as obturator canal, and inserting on side of coccyx and in anococcygeal ligaments		third and fourth sacral	*see* m. levator ani
m. iliocostalis	a name applied to lateral division of erector spinae muscle			
m. iliocostalis cervicis	angles of third, fourth, fifth and sixth ribs	transverse processes of lower cervical vertebrae	cervical	extends cervical spine
m. iliocostalis lumborum	iliac crest	angles of lower ribs	thoracic and lumbar	extends lumbar spine
m. iliocostalis thoracis	upper borders of angles of 6 lower ribs	angles of upper ribs and transverse process of seventh cervical vertebra	thoracic	keeps thoracic spine erect
m. iliopsoas	a name applied collectively to iliacus and psoas major muscles			
incisive mm., superior and inferior	incisive fossae of maxilla and mandible	angle of mouth	facial	make vestibule of mouth shallow

TABLE OF MUSCLES (Continued)

NA TERM	ORIGIN	INSERTION	INNERVATION	ACTION
m. incisurae helicis	a name applied to inconstant slips of fibers continuing forward from muscle of tragus to bridge notch of cartilaginous part of meatus			
m. infraspinatus	infraspinous fossa of scapula	greater tubercle of humerus	suprascapular	rotates arm laterally
mm. intercostales externi	inferior border of rib	superior border of rib below	intercostal	elevate ribs in inspiration
mm. intercostales interni	inferior border of rib and costal cartilage	superior border of rib and costal cartilage below	intercostal	act on ribs in expiration
mm. intercostales	a name applied to the layer of muscle fibers separated from the internal intercostal muscles by the intercostal nerves and vessels			
mm. interossei dorsales manus	each by two heads from adjacent sides of metacarpal bones	extensor tendons of second, third and fourth fingers	ulnar	abduct, flex proximal, extend middle and distal phalanges
mm. interossei dorsales pedis	sides of adjacent metatarsal bones	base of proximal phalanges of second, third and fourth toes	lateral plantar	flex toes
mm. interossei palmares	sides of first, second, fourth and fifth metacarpal bones	extensor tendons of first, second, fourth and fifth fingers	ulnar	adduct, flex proximal, extend middle and distal phalanges
mm. interossei plantares	medial side of third, fourth and fifth metatarsal bones	medial side of base of proximal phalanges of third, fourth and fifth toes	lateral plantar	flex toes
mm. interspinales	a name applied to muscular bands extending on each side between spinous processes of contiguous vertebrae		spinal	extend vertebral column
mm. intertransversarii	a name applied to small muscles passing between transverse processes of adjacent vertebrae		spinal	bend vertebral column laterally
m. ischiocavernosus	ramus of ischium	crus penis or crus clitoridis	perineal branches of pudendal	maintains erection of penis or clitoris
m. latissimus dorsi	spines of lower thoracic vertebrae, thoracolumbar fascia, iliac crest, lower ribs, inferior angle of scapula	floor of intertubercular groove of humerus	thoracodorsal	adducts, extends and rotates humerus medially
m. levator anguli oris	canine fossa of maxilla	orbicularis oris, skin at angle of mouth	facial	raises angle of mouth
m. levator ani	a name applied collectively to important muscular components of pelvic diaphragm, arising mainly from back of body of pubis and running backward toward coccyx; includes pubococcygeal (levator prostatae in the male and pubovaginalis in the female), puborectalis and iliococcygeus muscles		third and fourth sacral	helps to support pelvic viscera and resist increases in intra-abdominal pressure

400

mm. levatores costarum	transverse processes of seventh cervical and first 11 thoracic vertebrae	medial to the angle of the rib below	intercostal	aid elevation of ribs in respiration
m. levator glandulae thyroideae	isthmus or pyramical lobule of thyroid gland	body of hyoid bone	external laryngeal	
m. levator labii superioris	lower margin or orbit	musculature of upper lip	facial	raises upper lip
m. levator labii superioris alaeque nasi	frontal process of maxilla	skin and cartilage of ala of nose, upper lip	infraorbital branch of facial	raises upper lip, dilates nostril
m. levator palpebrae superioris	sphenoid bone above optic canal	skin and tarsal plate of upper eyelid	oculomotor	raises upper eyelid
m. levator prostatae	a name applied to part of anterior portion of pubococcygeus muscle, which in male is inserted into prostate and tendinous center of perineum		sacral, pudendal	supports and compresses prostate, helps control micturition
m. levator scapulae	transverse processes of 4 upper cervical vertebrae	vertebral border of scapula	third and fourth cervical	raises scapula
m. levator veli palatini	apex of petrous portion of temporal bone and cartilage of auditory tube	aponeurosis of soft palate	pharyngeal plexus	raises and draws back soft palate
m. longissimus capitis	transverse processes of 4 or 5 upper thoracic vertebrae, articular processes of 3 or 4 lower cervical vertebrae	mastoid process of temporal bone	cervical	draws head backward, rotates head
m. longissimus cervicis	transverse processes of 4 or 5 upper thoracic vertebrae	transverse processes of second or third to sixth cervical vertebrae	lower cervical and upper thoracic	extends cervical vertebrae
m. longissimus thoracis	transverse and articular processes of lumbar vertebrae and thoracolumbar fascia	transverse processes of all thoracic vertebrae, 9 or 10 lower ribs	lumbar and thoracic	extends thoracic vertebrae
m. longitudinalis inferior linguae	under surface of tongue at base	tip of tongue	hypoglossal	changes shape of tongue in mastication and deglutition
m. longitudinalis superior linguae	submucosa and septum of tongue	margins of tongue	hypoglossal	changes shape of tongue in mastication and deglutition
m. longus capitis	transverse processes of third to sixth cervical vertebrae	basilar portion of occipital bone	cervical	flexes head
m. longus colli	superior oblique portion—transverse processes of third to fifth cervical vertebrae; inferior oblique portion—bodies of first to third thoracic vertebrae; vertical portion—bodies of 3 upper thoracic and 3 lower cervical vertebrae	superior oblique portion—tubercle of anterior arch of atlas; inferior oblique portion—transverse processes of fifth and sixth cervical vertebrae; vertical portion—bodies of second to fourth cervical vertebrae	cervical	flexes and supports cervical vertebrae

TABLE OF MUSCLES (*Continued*)

NA TERM	ORIGIN	INSERTION	INNERVATION	ACTION
mm. lumbricales manus	tendons of flexor digitorum profundus	extensor tendons of 4 lateral fingers	median, ulnar	flex proximal, extend middle and distal phalanges
mm. lumbricales pedis	tendons of flexor digitorum longus	medial side of base of proximal phalanges of 4 lateral toes	medial and lateral plantar	aid in flexing proximal phalanges
m. masseter	*superficial part* – zygomatic process of maxilla, lower border of zygomatic arch; *deep part* – lower border and medial surface of zygomatic arch	*superficial part* – angle and ramus of mandible; *deep part* – upper half of ramus and lateral surface of coronoid process of mandible	masseteric, from mandibular	raises mandible, closes jaws
m. mentalis	incisive fossa of mandible	skin of chin	facial	wrinkles skin of chin
m. multifidus	sacrum, sacroiliac ligament, mamillary processes of lumbar, transverse processes of thoracic and articular processes of cervical vertebrae	spines of contiguous vertebrae above	spinal	extends, rotates vertebral column
m. mylohyoideus	mylohyoid line of mandible	body of hyoid bone, median raphe	mylohyoid branch of inferior alveolar	elevates hyoid bone, supports floor of mouth
m. nasalis	maxilla	*alar part* – ala of nose; *transverse part* – by aponeurotic expansion with fellow of opposite side	facial	*alar part* – aids in widening nostril; *transverse part* – depresses cartilage of nose
m. obliquus auriculae	cranial surface of concha	cranial surface of auricle above concha	posterior auricular, temporal branches of facial	rotates atlas and head
m. obliquus capitis inferior	spinous process of axis	transverse process of atlas	spinal	extends and moves head laterally
m. obliquus capitis superior	transverse process of atlas	occipital bone	spinal	
m. obliquus externus abdominis	lower 8 ribs at costal cartilages	crest of ilium, linea alba through rectus sheath	lower thoracic	flexes, rotates vertebral column, compresses abdominal viscera
m. obliquus inferior bulbi	orbital surface of maxilla	sclera	oculomotor	abducts, elevates and rotates eyeball laterally
m. obliquus internus abdominis	thoracolumbar fascia, iliac crest, fascia iliaca	lower 3 or 4 costal cartilages, linea alba, conjoined tendon to pubis	lower thoracic	flexes, rotates vertebral column, compresses abdominal viscera

402

m. obliquus superior bulbi	lesser wing of sphenoid above optic canal	sclera	trochlear	abducts, depresses and rotates eyeball
m. obturatorius externus	pubis, ischium, external surface of obturator membrane	trochanteric fossa of femur	obturator	rotates thigh laterally
m. obturatorius internus	pelvic surface of hip bone and obturator membrane, margin of obturator foramen	greater trochanter of femur	fifth lumbar, first and second sacral	rotates thigh laterally
m. occipitofrontalis	*frontal belly*–galea aponeurotica; *occipital belly*–highest nuchal line of occipital bone	*frontal belly*–skin of eyebrow, root of nose; *occipital belly*–galea aponeurotica	*frontal belly* – temporal branch of facial; *occipital belly* – posterior auricular branch of facial	*frontal belly*–raises eyebrow; *occipital belly*–draws scalp backward
m. omohyoideus	superior border of scapula	body of hyoid bone	ansa cervicalis	depresses hyoid bone
m. opponens digiti minimi manus	hook of hamate bone	front of fifth metacarpal	ulnar	draws fifth metacarpal forward
m. opponens pollicis	tubercle of trapezium, flexor retinaculum	lateral side of first metacarpal bone	median	opposes thumb
m. orbicularis oculi	*orbital part*–medial margin of orbit, including frontal process of maxilla; *palpebral part*–medial palpebral ligament; *lacrimal part*–posterior lacrimal crest	*orbital part*–near origin after encircling orbit; *palpebral part*–orbital tubercle of zygomatic bone; *lacrimal part* – lateral palpebral raphe	facial	closes eyelids, wrinkles forehead, compresses (or dilates?) lacrimal sac
m. orbicularis oris	a name applied to complicated sphincter muscle of mouth, comprising 2 parts: *labial part*–consisting of fibers restricted to lips; *marginal part*–consisting of fibers blending with those of adjacent muscles		facial	closes lips
m. orbitalis	bridges inferior orbital fissure		sympathetic fibers	possibly protrudes eye
m. palatoglossus	under surface of soft palate	side of tongue	pharyngeal plexus	elevates tongue, constricts fauces
m. palatopharyngeus	soft palate, bony palate	aponeurosis of pharynx, posterior border of thyroid cartilage	pharyngeal plexus	constricts pharynx
m. palmaris brevis	palmar aponeurosis	skin of medial border of hand	ulnar	assists in deepening hollow of palm
m. palmaris longus	medial epicondyle of humerus	flexor retinaculum, palmar aponeurosis	median	tenses palmar aponeurosis
mm. papillares	a name applied to conical muscular projections from walls of cardiac ventricles, attached to cusps of atrioventricular valves by chordae tendineae			steady and strengthen atrioventricular valves and prevent eversion of their cusps
mm. pectinati	a name applied to small muscular ridges projecting from inner walls of auricles of heart, and extending in right atrium from auricle to crista terminalis			

TABLE OF MUSCLES (Continued)

NA TERM	ORIGIN	INSERTION	INNERVATION	ACTION
m. pectineus	pectineal line of pubis	pectineal line of femur	femoral, obturator	flexes, adducts thigh
m. pectoralis major	clavicle, sternum, 6 upper costal cartilages, aponeurosis of external oblique m. of abdomen	greater tubercle of humerus	lateral and medial pectoral	adducts, rotates arm medially
m. pectoralis minor	second, third, fourth and fifth ribs	coracoid process of scapula	medial pectoral	draws shoulder downward
m. peroneus brevis	lateral surface of fibula	tuberosity of fifth metatarsal bone	superficial peroneal	everts foot
m. peroneus longus	lateral condyle of tibia, lateral surface of fibula	medial cuneiform bone, first metatarsal bone	superficial peroneal	plantar flexes and everts foot
m. peroneus tertius	anterior surface of fibula	fascia or base of fifth metatarsal bone	deep peroneal	aids extensor digitorum longus
m. piriformis	ilium, second to fourth sacral vertebrae	greater trochanter of femur	first and second sacral	rotates thigh laterally
m. plantaris	popliteal surface of femur	tendo calcaneus or back of calcaneus	tibial	aids triceps surae
platysma	a name applied to a platelike muscle originating from the fascia of cervical region and inserting on mandible, and skin around mouth		cervical branch of facial	wrinkles skin of neck, depresses jaw
m. pleuroesophageus	a name applied to a bundle of smooth muscle fibers, usually connecting esophagus with left mediastinal pleura			
m. popliteus	lateral condyle of femur, lateral meniscus	posterior surface of tibia	tibial	rotates leg medially
m. procerus	fascia over nasal bones	skin of forehead	facial	draws eyebrows down
m. pronator quadratus	anterior surface and border of distal third or fourth of shaft of ulna	anterior surface and border of distal fourth of shaft of radius	anterior interosseous	pronates forearm
m. pronator teres	*humeral head*—medial epicondyle of humerus; *ulnar head*—coronoid process of ulna	lateral surface of radius	median	pronates and flexes forearm
m. psoas major	lumbar vertebrae	lesser trochanter of femur	second and third lumbar	flexes thigh or trunk
m. psoas minor	last thoracic and first lumbar vertebrae	arcuate line of hip bone	first lumbar	assists psoas major
m. pterygoideus lateralis	*upper head*—infratemporal surface of greater wing of	neck of mandible, capsule of temporomandibular joint	mandibular	protrudes mandible, opens jaws, moves mandible from

			side to side
	sphenoid, infratemporal crest; *lower head*–lateral surface of lateral pterygoid plate	mandibular	closes jaws
m. pterygoideus medialis	medial surface of lateral pterygoid plate, tuber of maxilla	medial surface of ramus and angle of mandible	
m. pubococcygeus	a name applied to anterior portion of levator ani muscle, originating in front of obturator canal and inserting in anococcygeal ligament and side of coccyx	third and fourth sacral	
m. puboprostaticus	a name applied to smooth muscle fibers contained within medial puboprostatic ligament, which pass from prostate anteriorly to pubis		
m. puborectalis	a name applied to portion of levator ani muscle, with a more lateral origin from pubic bone, and continuous posteriorly with corresponding muscle of opposite side	third and fourth sacral	
m. pubovaginalis	a name applied to part of anterior portion of pubococcygeal muscle which in female is inserted in walls of urethra and vagina	sacral and pudendal	helps control micturition
m. pubovesicalis	a name applied to smooth muscle fibers extending from neck of urinary bladder to pubis		
m. pyramidalis	linea alba		
m. pyramidalis auriculae	a name applied to inconstant prolongation of fibers of tragicus to spina helicis	last thoracic	tenses abdominal wall
m. quadratus femoris	tuberosity of ischium	intertrochanteric crest and quadrate tubercle of femur	fourth and fifth lumbar, first sacral	rotates thigh laterally
m. quadratus labii inferioris. *See* m. depressor labii inferioris.			
m. quadratus labii superioris. *See* m. levator labii superioris			
m. quadratus lumborum	twelfth rib, transverse processes of lumbar vertebrae	iliac crest, thoracolumbar fascia	first and second lumbar, twelfth thoracic	flexes trunk laterally
m. quadratus plantae	tendons of flexor digitorum longus	calcaneus, plantar fascia	lateral plantar	aids in flexing toes
m. quadriceps femoris	a name applied collectively to rectus femoris, and vasti intermedius, lateralis and medialis, inserting by a common tendon that surrounds patella and ends on tuberosity of tibia		femoral	extends leg
m. rectococcygeus	a name applied to smooth muscle fibers originating from anterior surface of second and third coccygeal vertebrae and inserting on posterior surface of rectum		autonomic	retracts, elevates rectum

405

TABLE OF MUSCLES (*Continued*)

NA TERM	ORIGIN	INSERTION	INNERVATION	ACTION
m. rectourethralis	a name applied to band of smooth muscle fibers in male, extending from perineal flexure of rectum to membranous part of urethra			
m. rectouterinus	a name applied to band of fibers in female, running between cervix uteri and rectum, in rectouterine fold			
m. rectovesicalis	a name applied to band of fibers in male, connecting longitudinal musculature of rectum with external muscular coat of bladder			
m. rectus abdominis	pubic crest and symphysis	xiphoid process, fifth, sixth and seventh costal cartilages	lower thoracic	flexes lumbar vertebrae, supports abdomen
m. rectus capitis anterior	lateral mass of atlas	basilar part of occipital bone	first and second cervical	flexes, supports head
m. rectus capitis lateralis	transverse process of atlas	jugular process of occipital bone	first and second cervical	flexes, supports head
m. rectus capitis posterior major	spinous process of axis	occipital bone	suboccipital, greater occipital	extends head
m. rectus capitis posterior minor	posterior tubercle of atlas	occipital bone	suboccipital, greater occipital	extends head
m. rectus femoris	anterior inferior iliac spine, rim of acetabulum	base of patella, tuberosity of tibia	femoral	extends leg, flexes thigh
m. rectus inferior bulbi	common tendinous ring	sclera	oculomotor	adducts, depresses and rotates eyeball laterally
m. rectus lateralis bulbi	common tendinous ring	sclera	abducens	abducts eyeball
m. rectus medialis bulbi	common tendinous ring	sclera	oculomotor	adducts eyeball
m. rectus superior bulbi	common tendinous ring	sclera	oculomotor	adducts, elevates and rotates eyeball medially
m. rhomboideus major	spinous processes of second, third, fourth and fifth thoracic vertebrae	vertebral margin of scapula	dorsal scapular	retracts and fixes scapula
m. rhomboideus minor	spinous processes of seventh cervical and first thoracic vertebrae, lower part of ligamentum nuchae	vertebral margin of scapula at root of spine	dorsal scapular	retracts and fixes scapula
m. risorius	fascia over masseter	skin at angle of mouth	buccal branch of facial	draws angle of mouth laterally
mm. rotatores	a name applied to a series of small muscles deep in groove between spinous and transverse processes of vertebrae		spinal	extend and rotate vertebral column toward opposite side
m. sacrococcygeus dorsalis	a name applied to muscular slip passing from dorsal surface of sacrum to coccyx			

m. sacrococcygeus ventralis	a name applied to musculotendinous slip passing from lower sacral vertebrae to coccyx			
m. sacrospinalis. See m. erector spinae				
m. salpingopharyngeus	cartilage of auditory tube	posterior part of palatopharyngeus	pharyngeal plexus	raises pharynx
m. sartorius	anterior superior iliac spine	upper part of medial surface of tibia	femoral	flexes thigh and leg
m. scalenus anterior	transverse processes of third to sixth cervical vertebrae	scalene tubercle of first rib	second to seventh cervical	raises first rib, flexes cervical vertebrae laterally
m. scalenus medius	transverse processes of first to seventh cervical vertebrae	upper surface of first rib	second to seventh cervical	raises first rib, flexes cervical vertebrae laterally
m. scalenus minimus	a name applied to muscular band occasionally found between anterior and middle scalene muscles			
m. scalenus posterior	transverse processes of fourth to sixth cervical vertebrae	second rib	second to seventh cervical	raises first and second ribs, flexes cervical vertebrae laterally
m. scalenus pleuralis. See m. scalenus minimus				
m. semimembranosus	tuberosity of ischium	lateral condyle of femur, medial condyle and border of tibia	sciatic	flexes leg, extends thigh
m. semispinalis capitis	transverse processes of upper thoracic and lower cervical vertebrae	occipital bone	suboccipital, greater occipital, branches of cervical	extends head
m. semispinalis cervicis	transverse processes of upper thoracic vertebrae	spinous processes of second to fifth (or fourth) cervical vertebrae	branches of cervical	extends, rotates vertebral column
m. semispinalis thoracis	transverse processes of lower thoracic vertebrae	spinous processes of lower cervical and upper thoracic vertebrae	spinal	extends, rotates vertebral column
m. semitendinosus	tuberosity of ischium	upper part of medial surface of tibia	sciatic	flexes and rotates leg medially, extends thigh
m. serratus anterior	8 upper ribs	vertebral border of scapula	long thoracic	draws scapula forward, rotates scapula to raise shoulder in abduction of arm
m. serratus posterior inferior	spines of lower thoracic and upper lumbar vertebrae	4 lower ribs	ninth to twelfth (or eleventh) thoracic	perhaps lowers ribs in expiration
m. serratus posterior superior	ligamentum nuchae, spinous processes of upper thoracic vertebrae	second, third, fourth and fifth ribs	upper 4 thoracic	perhaps raises ribs in inspiration

407

TABLE OF MUSCLES (Continued)

NA TERM	ORIGIN	INSERTION	INNERVATION	ACTION
m. soleus	fibula, tendinous arch, tibia	calcaneus by tendo calcaneus	tibial	plantar flexes foot
m. sphincter ampullae hepatopancreaticae	a name applied to annular band of muscle fibers investing hepatopancreatic ampulla			
m. sphincter ani externus	tip of coccyx, anococcygeal ligament	tendinous center of perineum	inferior rectal, perineal branch of fourth sacral	closes anus
m. sphincter ani internus	a name applied to a thickening of circular layer of muscular tunic at caudal end of rectum			
m. sphincter ductus choledochi	a name applied to annular sheath of muscle fibers investing bile duct within wall of duodenum			
m. sphincter pupillae	a name applied to circular fibers of iris		parasympathetic through ciliary	constricts pupil
m. sphincter pylori	a name applied to a thickening of middle layer of stomach musculature around pylorus			
m. sphincter urethrae	inferior ramus of pubis	median raphe behind and in front of urethra	perineal	compresses urethra, at least in male
m. sphincter vesicae urinariae	a name applied to circular layer of fibers surrounding internal urethral orifice		vesical	closes internal orifice of urethra
m. spinalis capitis	spinous processes of upper thoracic and lower cervical vertebrae	occipital bone	spinal	extends head
m. spinalis cervicis	spinous process of seventh cervical vertebra, ligamentum nuchae	spinous processes of axis	branches of cervical	extends vertebral column
m. spinalis thoracis	spinous processes of upper lumbar and lower thoracic vertebrae	spinous processes of upper thoracic vertebrae	branches of spinal	extends vertebral column
m. splenius capitis	lower half of ligamentum nuchae, spinous processes of seventh cervical and upper thoracic vertebrae	mastoid part of temporal bone, occipital bone	cervical	extends, rotates head
m. splenius cervicis	spinous process of upper thoracic vertebrae	transverse processes of upper cervical vertebrae	cervical	extends, rotates head and neck
m. stapedius	interior of pyramidal eminence of tympanic cavity	neck of stapes	facial	dampens movement of stapes
m. sternalis	a name applied to muscular band occasionally found parallel to sternum on sternocostal head of pectoralis major			
m. sternocleidomastoideus	sternal head – manubrium;	mastoid process, superior	accessory and cervical	flexes vertebral column, ro-

408

muscle	origin	insertion	plexus	action
	clavicular head – medial third of clavicle	nuchal line of occipital bone		tates head to opposite side
m. sternocostalis. See m. transversus thoracis				
m. sternohyoideus	manubrium sterni and/or clavicle	body of hyoid bone	ansa cervicalis	depresses hyoid bone and larynx
m. sternothyroideus	manubrium sterni	lamina of thyroid cartilage	ansa cervicalis	depresses thyroid cartilage
m. styloglossus	styloid process	margin of tongue	hypoglossal	raises and retracts tongue
m. stylohyoideus	styloid process	body of hyoid bone	facial	draws hyoid bone and tongue upward and backward
m. stylopharyngeus	styloid process	thyroid cartilage, side of pharynx	glossopharyngeal	raises, dilates pharynx
m. subclavius	first rib and its cartilage	lower surface of clavicle	nerve to subclavius	depresses lateral end of clavicle
mm. subcostales	lower border of ribs	upper border of second or third rib below	intercostal	raise ribs in inspiration
m. subscapularis	subscapular fossa of scapula	lesser tubercle of humerus	subscapular	rotates arm medially
m. supinator	lateral epicondyle of humerus, ligaments of elbow	radius	deep branch of radial	supinates forearm
m. supraspinatus	supraspinous fossa of scapula	greater tubercle of humerus	suprascapular	abducts arm
m. suspensorius	a name applied to flat band of smooth muscle fibers originating from left crus of diaphragm and inserting continuous with muscular coat of duodenum at its junction with jejunum			
m. tarsalis inferior	inferior rectus muscle	tarsal plate of lower eyelid	sympathetic	widens palpebral fissure
m. tarsalis superior	levator palpebrae superioris	tarsal plate of upper eyelid	sympathetic	widens palpebral fissure
m. temporalis	temporal fossa and fascia	coronoid process of mandible	mandibular	closes jaws
m. temporoparietalis	temporal fascia above ear	galea aponeurotica	temporal branches of facial	tightens scalp
m. tensor fasciae latae	iliac crest	iliotibial tract of fascia lata	superior gluteal	flexes, rotates thigh medially
m. tensor tympani	cartilaginous portion of auditory tube	handle of malleus	mandibular	tenses tympanic membrane
m. tensor veli palatini	scaphoid fossa and spine of sphenoid	aponeurosis of soft palate, wall of auditory tube	mandibular	tenses soft palate, opens auditory tube
m. teres major	inferior angle of scapula	crest of lesser tubercle of humerus	lower subscapular	adducts arm
m. teres minor	lateral margin of scapula	greater tubercle of humerus	axillary	rotates arm laterally
m. thyroarytenoideus	medial surface of lamina of thyroid cartilage	muscular process of arytenoid cartilage	recurrent laryngeal	shortens vocal folds
m. thyroepiglotticus	lamina of thyroid cartilage	epiglottis	recurrent laryngeal	closes inlet to larynx
m. thyrohyoideus	lamina of thyroid cartilage	greater horn of hyoid bone	ansa cervicalis	raises larynx
m. tibialis anterior	lateral condyle and surface of tibia, interosseous membrane	medial cuneiform, base of first metatarsal	deep peroneal	dorsiflexes and inverts foot

NA TERM	ORIGIN	INSERTION	INNERVATION	ACTION
m. tibialis posterior	tibia, fibula, interosseous membrane	bases of second to fourth metatarsal bones and tarsal bones, except talus	tibial	inverts foot
m. trachealis	a name applied to transverse smooth muscle fibers filling gap at back of each cartilage of trachea		autonomic	lessens caliber of trachea
m. tragicus	a name applied to short, flattened, vertical band on lateral surface of tragus		temporal, posterior auricular branches of facial	
m. transversospinalis	a name applied collectively to semispinalis, multifidus and rotatores muscles			
m. transversus abdominis	lower 6 costal cartilages, thoracolumbar fascia, iliac crest	linea alba through rectus sheath, conjoined tendon to pubis	lower thoracic	compresses abdominal viscera
m. transversus auriculae	cranial surface of auricle	circumference of auricle	posterior auricular branch of facial	retracts helix
m. transversus linguae	median septum of tongue	dorsum and margins of tongue	hypoglossal	changes shape of tongue in mastication
m. transversus menti	a name applied to superficial fibers of depressor anguli oris which turn medially and cross to opposite side			
m. transversus nuchae	a name applied to small muscle often present, passing from occipital protuberance to posterior auricular muscle; it may be either superficial or deep to trapezius			
m. transversus perinei profundus	ramus of ischium	tendinous center of perineum	perineal	fixes tendinous center of perineum
m. transversus perinei superficialis	ramus of ischium	tendinous center of perineum	perineal	fixes tendinous center of perineum
m. transversus thoracis	posterior surface of body of sternum and of xiphoid process	second to sixth costal cartilages	intercostal	perhaps narrows chest
m. trapezius	occipital bone, ligamentum nuchae, spinous processes of seventh cervical and all thoracic vertebrae	clavicle, acromion, spine of scapula	accessory, cervical plexus	elevates shoulder, rotates scapula to raise shoulder in abduction of arm, draws scapula backward
m. triangularis. See m. depressor anguli oris				
m. triceps brachii	long head—infraglenoid tubercle of scapula; lateral head—posterior surface of	olecranon of ulna	radial	extends forearm

Name	Origin	Insertion	Nerve	Action
m. triceps surae	humerus; *medial head*—posterior surface of humerus below groove for radial nerve; a name applied collectively muscles	to gastrocnemius and soleus		
m. uvulae	posterior nasal spine of palatine bone and aponeurosis of soft palate	uvula	pharyngeal plexus	raises uvula
m. vastus intermedius	anterior and lateral surfaces of femur	patella, common tendon of quadriceps femoris	femoral	extends leg
m. vestus lateralis	lateral aspect of femur	patella, common tendon of quadriceps femoris	femoral	extends leg
m. vastus medialis	medial aspect of femur	patella, common tendon of quadriceps femoris	femoral	extends leg
m. verticalis linguae	dorsal fascia of tongue	sides and base of tongue	hypoglossus	changes shape of tongue in mastication and deglutination
m. vocalis	angle between laminae of thyroid cartilage	vocal process of arytenoid cartilage	recurrent laryngeal	causes local variations in tension of vocal fold
m. zygomaticus major	zygomatic bone	angle of mouth	facial	draws angle of mouth upward and laterally
m. zygomaticus minor	zygomatic bone	orbicularis oris, levator labii superioris	facial	draws upper lip upward and laterally

411

another part than that of its insertion, as those originating outside the eye, which move the eyeball. **fixation m's, fixator m's,** accessory muscles that serve to steady a part. **fusiform m.,** a spindle-shaped muscle. **Gavard's m.,** the oblique muscular elements of the stomach wall. **hamstring m's,** the muscles of the back of the thigh. **Houston's m.,** fibers of the bulbocavernosus muscle compressing the dorsal vein of the penis. **hypomeric m.,** one derived from a hypomere and innervated by an anterior ramus of a spinal nerve. **inspiratory m's,** muscles that act in inspiration. **intraocular m's,** the intrinsic muscles of the eyeball. **intrinsic m.,** one whose origin and insertion are both in the same part or organ, as those entirely within the eye. **involuntary m.,** one that is not under the control of the will. **iridic m's,** those controlling the iris. **Landström's m.,** minute muscle fibers in the fascia around and behind the eyeball, attached in front to the anterior orbital fascia and eyelids. **Langer's m.,** muscular fibers from the insertion of the pectoralis major muscle over the bicipital groove to the insertion of the latissimus dorsi. **Lushka's m's,** the uterosacral ligaments which contain muscular tissue. **Müller's m.,** the circular fibers of the ciliary muscle. **nonstriated m.,** a type of muscle without transverse striations on its constituent fibers; such muscles are almost always involuntary. **Ochsner's m.,** Ochsner's ring. **orbicular m.,** one that encircles a body opening, e.g. the eye or mouth. **organic m.,** visceral muscle. **Phillips's m.,** a muscular slip from the radial collateral ligament of the wrist and the styloid process of the radius to the phalanges. **postaxial m.,** one on the dorsal side of an extremity. **preaxial m.,** one on the ventral side of an extremity. **red m.,** the darker-colored muscle tissue of some mammals, composed of fibers rich in sarcoplasm, but with only faint cross-striping. **Reisseisen's m.,** the smooth muscle fibers of the smallest bronchi. **rider's m's,** the adductor muscles of the thigh. **Rouget's m.,** the circular portion of the ciliary muscle. **Ruysch's m.,** the muscular tissue of the fundus uteri. **skeletal m's,** striated muscles attached to bones, which cross at least one joint. **smooth m.,** nonstriated, involuntary muscle. **striated m., striped m.,** any muscle whose fibers are divided by transverse bands into striations; such muscles are voluntary. **synergic m's, synergistic m's,** those that assist one another in action. **thenar m's,** the abductor and flexor muscles of the thumb. **unstriated m.,** nonstriated muscle. **vestigial m.,** one that is rudimentary in man, but well developed in some other mammals. **visceral m.,** muscle fibers associated chiefly with the hollow viscera. **voluntary m.,** any muscle that is normally under the control of the will. **white m.,** the paler muscle tissue of some mammals, composed of fibers with little sarcoplasm and prominent cross-striping. **yoked m's,** those that normally act simultaneously and equally, as in moving the eyes.

muscularis (mus″ku-la′ris) [L.] relating to

muscle, specifically a muscular layer (lamina muscularis) or coat (tunica muscularis).

musculature (mus′ku-lah-tūr) the muscular system of the body, or the muscles of a particular region.

musculocutaneous (mus″ku-lo-ku-ta′ne-us) pertaining to muscle and skin.

musculomembranous (-mem′brah-nus) pertaining to muscle and membrane.

musculophrenic (-fren′ik) pertaining to (chest) muscles and diaphragm.

musculoskeletal (-skel′ē-tal) pertaining to muscle and skeleton.

musculotendinous (-ten′dĭ-nus) pertaining to muscle and tendon.

musculotropic (-trop′ik) exerting its principal effect upon muscle.

musculus (mus′ku-lus), pl. *mus′culi* [L.] muscle.

musicotherapy (mu″ze-ko-ther′ah-pe) treatment of disease by music.

musophobia (mu″so-fo′be-ah) morbid fear of mice.

mustard (mus′tard) an irritant compound derived from dried ripe seed of *Brassica nigra* or *B. juncea*. **nitrogen m's,** highly toxic compounds used in treatment of neoplastic disease. **sulfur m.,** a synthetic compound with vesicant and other toxic properties.

Mustargen (mus′tar-jen) trademark for a preparation of mechlorethamine.

mutacism (mu′tah-sizm) improper pronunciation of sounds of mute letters.

mutagen (mu′tah-jen) an agent which induces genetic mutation.

mutagenesis (mu″tah-jen′ē-sis) the induction of genetic mutation.

mutagenic (-jen′ik) pertaining to a mutagen; capable of inducing genetic mutation.

mutagenicity (-jĕ-nis′ĭ-te) the property of being able to induce genetic mutation.

mutant (mu′tant) a sport or variation which breeds true.

mutarotation (mu″tah-ro-ta′shun) the change with time of the rotation of an optically active compound in solution.

mutase (mu′tās) 1. an enzyme which produces rearrangement of molecules. 2. a vegetable food preparation rich in proteins.

mutation (mu-ta′shun) change; especially an alteration in a gene which produces a change in later generations of the organism. **chromosomal m.,** one accompanied by a visible change in the structure of the chromosome. **induced m.,** a genetic mutation caused by external factors experimentally or accidentally produced. **point m.,** one not accompanied by a visible change in the structure of the chromosome and presumably occurring at the molecular level. **somatic m.,** a genetic mutation occurring in a somatic cell, providing the basis for a mosaic condition.

mute (mūt) 1. unable or unwilling to speak. 2. a person who is unable to speak.

mutism (mu′tizm) inability or refusal to speak. **akinetic m.,** a state in which the person makes no spontaneous movement or vocal sound. **deaf m.,** inability to speak due to deafness. **hysterical m.**, hysterical inability to utter words.

muton (mu'ton) a gene when specified as the smallest hereditary element that can be altered by mutation.

mutualism (mu'tu-al-izm") the biologic association of two individuals or populations of different species, both of which are benefited by the relationship and sometimes unable to exist without it.

mutualist (mu'tu-al-ist) one of the organisms or species living with another in a mutually beneficial relationship.

M.V. [L.] *Medicus Veterinarius* (veterinary physician).

Mv chemical symbol, *mendelevium.*

mv. millivolt.

M.W.I.A. Medical Women's International Association.

my(o)- (mi'o) word element [Gr.], *muscle.*

myalgia (mi-al'je-ah) muscular pain.

Myanesin (mi-an'ĕ-sin) trademark for mephenesin.

myasthenia (mi"as-the'ne-ah) muscular debility or weakness. adj., **myasthen'ic. angiosclerotic m.**, excessive muscular fatigue due to vascular changes. **m. gas'trica,** weakness and loss of tone in the muscular coats of the stomach; atony of the stomach. **m. gra'vis, m. gra'vis pseudoparalyt'ica,** a chronic progressive muscular paralysis without atrophy.

myatonia (mi"ah-to'ne-ah) defective muscular tone. **m. congen'ita,** amyotonia congenita.

myatrophy (mi-at'ro-fe) atrophy of a muscle.

myc(o) (mi'ko) word element [Gr.], *fungus.*

mycelium (mi-se'le-um) the filamentary part of a fungus.

mycetismus (mi"sĕ-tiz'mus) mushroom poisoning.

mycetogenic (mi-se"to-jen'ik) caused by fungi.

mycetoma (mi"sĕ-to'mah) a chronic disease caused by a variety of fungi, affecting the feet, hands, legs and other parts; the most common form is that of the foot *(Madura foot* or *fungus foot),* characterized by sinus formation, necrosis and swelling.

Mycobacteriaceae (mi"ko-bak-te"re-a'se-e) a family of Schizomycetes (order Actinomycetales) found in soil and dairy products.

Mycobacterium (-bak-te're-um) a genus of Schizomycetes (order Actinomycetales, family Mycobacteriaceae). **M. kansas'ii,** the etiologic agent of a tuberculosis-like disease in man. **M. lep'rae,** a species considered to be the etiologic agent of leprosy. **M. tuberculo'-sis,** the causative agent of tuberculosis in man.

mycobacterium (-bak-te're-um), pl. *mycobacte'ria* [L.] 1. an individual organism of the genus Mycobacterium. 2. a slender, acid-fast microorganism resembling the bacillus that causes tuberculosis.

Mycococcus (-kok'us) a genus of Schizomycetes (order Actinomycetales, family Mycobacteriaceae) found in soil and water.

mycodermatitis (-der"mah-ti'tis) inflammation of a mucous membrane.

mycogastritis (mi"ko-gas-tri'tis) inflammation of mucous membrane of stomach.

mycologist (mi-kol'o-jist) a specialist in mycology.

mycology (mi-kol'o-je) the study of fungi and fungus diseases.

mycomyringitis (mi"ko-mir"in-ji'tis) fungus inflammation of drum membrane.

Myconostoc (mi"ko-nos'tok) a genus of Schizomycetes (order Pseudomonadales, suborder Pseudomonadineae, family Spirillaceae).

mycopathology (-pah-thol'o-je) scientific study of morbid changes caused by fungi.

mycophylaxin (-fi-lak'sin) any phylaxin that destroys microbes.

Mycoplana (-pla'nah) a genus of Schizomycetes (order Pseudomonadales, suborder Pseudomonadineae, family Pseudomonadaceae) found in the soil.

Mycoplasma (-plaz'mah) a genus of Schizomycetes (order Mycoplasmatales, family Mycoplasmataceae). **M. mycoi'des,** a microorganism causing pleuropneumonia in cattle.

mycoplasma (-plaz'mah), pl. *mycoplas'mas, mycoplas'mata* [Gr.] a microorganism of the genus Mycoplasma.

Mycoplasmataceae (-plaz"mah-ta'se-e) a family of Schizomycetes (order Mycoplasmatales).

Mycoplasmatales (-plaz"mah-ta'lēz) an order of Schizomycetes.

mycosis (mi-ko'sis) any disease caused by fungi. **m. favo'sa,** favus. **m. fungoi'des,** a fatal skin disease, with fungous tumors, cachexia and much pain. **m. interdigita'lis,** dermatophytosis.

mycosozin (mi"ko-so'zin) any sozin that destroys fungi.

mycostasis (mi-kos'tah-sis) prevention of growth and multiplication of fungi. adj., **mycostat'ic.**

mycostat (mi'ko-stat) an agent which inhibits the growth of fungi.

mycotoxicosis (mi"ko-tok-si-ko'sis) poisoning due to a fungus.

mydriasis (mī-dri'ah-sis) great dilatation of the pupil.

mydriatic (mid"re-at'ik) 1. dilating the pupil. 2. a drug that dilates the pupil.

myectomy (mi-ek'to-me) excision of a muscle

myectopia (mi"ek-to'pe-ah) displacement of a muscle.

myel(o) (mi'el-o) word element [Gr.], *spinal cord; bone marrow.*

myelalgia (mi"ĕ-lal'je-ah) pain in the spinal cord.

myelapoplexy (mi"el-ap'o-plek"se) hemorrhage in the spinal cord.

myelatelia (-ah-te'le-ah) imperfect development of spinal cord.

myelatrophy (-at'ro-fe) atrophy of the spinal cord.

myelemia (-e'me-ah) presence of myelocytes or neutrophil leukocytes in the blood.

myelencephalon (-en-sef'ah-lon) 1. the part of the central nervous system comprising the medulla oblongata and lower part of the fourth ventricle. 2. the posterior of the two brain vesicles formed by specialization of the rhombencephalon in the developing embryo.

myelin (mi'ĕ-lin) 1. the soft material surrounding the axon of a medullated nerve fiber. 2. a lipoid substance found in the body, especially in certain degenerations. adj., **myelin'ic.**

myelination (mi"ĕ-lĭ-na'shun) myelinization.

myelinization (mi"ĕ-lin"ĭ-za'shun) production of myelin around an axon.

myelinoma (mi"ĕ-lĭ-no'mah) a tumor of the myelin.

myelinopathy (-nop'ah-the) degeneration of white matter of brain or spinal cord.

myelinosis (-no'sis) fatty degeneration, with formation of myelin.

myelitis (mi"ĕ-li'tis) inflammation of spinal cord or bone marrow (osteomyelitis). adj., **myelit'ic. ascending m.,** that moving cephalad along the cord. **bulbar m.,** that involving the oblongata. **cavitary m.,** a type accompanied by formation of cavities. **central m.,** affecting chiefly the gray substance of the cord. **disseminated m.,** that which has several distinct foci. **focal m.,** myelitis affecting a small area. **transverse m.,** inflammation affecting the entire cross section of the cord.

myeloarchitecture (mi"ĕ-lo-ar"kĭ-tek"tūr) the organization of the nerve tracts in the spinal cord.

myeloblast (mi'ĕ-lo-blast") one of the large mononuclear, nongranular cells of bone marrow which develop into myelocytes and also into erythroblasts, according to some hematologists.

myeloblastemia (mi"ĕ-lo-blas-te'me-ah) myeloblasts in the blood.

myeloblastoma (-blas-to'mah) a focal malignant tumor observed in chronic or acute myelocytic leukemia.

myeloblastomatosis (-blas"to-mah-to'sis) the presence of many myeloblastomas.

myeloblastosis (-blas-to'sis) excess of myeloblasts in the blood.

myelocele (mi'ĕ-lo-sel") 1. hernial protrusion of the spinal cord through a defect in the vertebral column. 2. the central canal of the spinal cord.

myelocyst (mi'ĕ-lo-sist") cyst developed from rudimentary medullary canals.

myelocystocele (mi"ĕ-lo-sis'to-sēl) hernial protrusion of cystic spinal cord through a defect in the vertebral column.

myelocystomeningocele (-sis"to-mĕ-ning'go-sēl) protrusion of cystic spinal cord and covering membranes through a defect in the vertebral column.

myelocyte (mi'ĕ-lo-sīt") one of the typical cells of red bone marrow, giving rise to the granular leukocytes of the blood. adj., **myelocyt'ic.**

myelocytoma (mi"ĕ-lo-si-to'mah) plasma cell myeloma.

myelocytosis (-si-to'sis) increase of myelocytes in the blood.

myelodiastasis (-di-as'tah-sis) disintegration of spinal marrow.

myelodysplasia (-dis-pla'ze-ah) defective development of the spinal cord.

myelo-encephalic (-en"sĕ-fal'ik) pertaining to spinal cord and brain.

myelo-encephalitis (mi"ĕ-lo-en-sef"ah-li'tis) inflammation of spinal cord and brain.

myelofibrosis (-fi-bro'sis) replacement of bone marrow by fibrous tissue.

myelogenesis (-jen'ĕ-sis) development of the central nervous system.

myelogenic (-jen'ik) myelogenous.

myelogenous (mi"ĕ-loj'ĕ-nus) produced in bone marrow.

myelogeny (-loj'ĕ-ne) development of myelin sheaths of nerve fibers.

myelogone (mi'ĕ-lo-gōn") a primitive cell of the myeloid series. adj., **myelogon'ic.**

myelography (mi"ĕ-log'rah-fe) radiography of the spinal cord.

myeloid (mi'ĕ-loid) 1. pertaining to, derived from or resembling bone marrow. 2. pertaining to the spinal cord. 3. having the appearance of myelocytes, but not derived from bone marrow.

myeloidosis (mi"ĕ-loi-do'sis) formation of myeloid tissue.

myelolymphocyte (mi"ĕ-lo-lim'fo-sīt) a small abnormal lymphocyte.

myeloma (mi"ĕ-lo'mah) a tumor composed of cells of the type normally found in the bone marrow. **multiple m., plasma cell m.,** a malignant neoplasm containing plasma cells, arising in bone marrow, and characterized by destructive lesions in the bones of the trunk and Bence Jones protein in the urine.

myelomalacia (mi"ĕ-lo-mah-la'she-ah) morbid softening of spinal cord.

myelomatosis (-mah-to'sis) 1. simultaneous presence of many myelomas. 2. any leukemic disease in which myeloblasts are abundant in the blood.

myelomeningitis (-men"in-ji'tis) inflammation of spinal cord and meninges.

myelomeningocele (-mĕ-ning'go-sēl) meningomyelocele

myelon (mi'ĕ-lon) the spinal cord. adj., **myelon'ic.**

myeloneuritis (mi"ĕ-lo-nu-ri'tis) inflammation of spinal cord and peripheral nerves.

myeloparalysis (-pah-ral'ĭ-sis) spinal paralysis.

myelopathy (mi"ĕ-lop'ah-the) any disease of the spinal cord.

myelopetal (mi"ĕ-lop'ĕ-tal) moving toward the spinal cord.

myelophage (mi'ĕ-lo-fāj") a macrophage which digests myelin.

myelophthisis (mi"ĕ-lo-thi'sis) wasting of the spinal cord.

myeloplast (mi"ĕ-lo-plast") any leukocyte of the bone marrow

myeloplax (mi'ĕ-lo-plaks) a multinuclear giant cell of bone marrow.

myeloplegia (mi"ĕ-lo-ple'je-ah) spinal paralysis.

myelopoiesis (-poi-e'sis) the formation of marrow or myelocytes.

myeloproliferative (-pro-lif"er-ah"tiv) pertaining to or characterized by proliferation of myeloid tissue.

myeloradiculitis (-rah-dik"u-li'tis) inflammation of spinal cord and spinal nerve roots.

myeloradiculodysplasia (-rah-dik"u-lo-dis-pla'ze-ah) abnormal development of spinal cord and spinal nerve roots.

myeloradiculopathy (mi″ĕ-lo-rah-dik″u-lop'ah-the) disease of spinal cord and spinal nerve roots.

myelorrhagia (-ra'je-ah) spinal hemorrhage.

myelorrhaphy (mi″ĕ-lor'ah-fe) suture of the spinal cord.

myelosarcoma (mi″ĕ-lo-sar-ko'mah) a sarcomatous growth made up of myeloid tissue or bone marrow cells.

myeloscintogram (-sin'to-gram) the graphic record of particles counted by a scintillation counter after injection into the subarachnoid space of a solution containing a radioactive isotope.

myelosclerosis (-skle-ro'sis) 1. sclerosis of the spinal cord. 2. obliteration of the marrow cavity by small spicules of bone.

myelosis (mi″ĕ-lo'sis) 1. proliferation of myelocytes. 2. formation of a tumor of the spinal cord. **erythremic m.,** a condition characterized by overgrowth of erythroid and reticuloendothelial cells in bone marrow.

myelospongium (mi″ĕ-lo-spun'je-um) a network developing into the neuroglia.

myelotomy (mi″ĕ-lot'o-me) severance of nerve fibers in the spinal cord.

myelotoxin (mi″ĕ-lo-tok'sin) a toxin which destroys marrow cells. adj., **myelotox'ic.**

myenteron (mi-en'ter-on) the muscular coat of the intestine. adj., **myenter'ic.**

myesthesia (mi″es-the'ze-ah) muscle sensibility.

myiasis (mi-i'ah-sis) invasion of the body by the larvae of flies, characterized as cutaneous (subdermal tissue), gastrointestinal, nasopharyngeal, ocular or urinary, depending on the region invaded.

myitis (mi-i'tis) inflammation of muscle.

myko- (mi'ko) for words beginning thus, see those beginning myco-.

Myleran (mil'er-an) trademark for a preparation of busulfan.

mylohyoid (mi″lo-hi'oid) pertaining to hyoid bone and molar teeth.

myoalbumin (mi″o-al-bu'min) an albumin in muscle tissue.

myoalbumose (-al'bu-mōs) a protein from muscle juice.

myoarchitectonic (-ar″ki-tek-ton'ik) pertaining to structural arrangement of muscle fibers.

myoatrophy (-at'ro-fe) muscular atrophy.

myoblast (mi'o-blast) an embryonic cell which becomes a cell of muscle fiber.

myoblastoma (mi″o-blas-to'mah) a tumor of muscle made up of cells resembling myoblasts. **granular cell m.,** a benign, circumscribed tumor of the mucosa of the lips or other oral structures, made up of large granular cells with small, round nuclei.

myobradia (-bra'de-ah) slow reaction of muscle to stimulation.

myocardiograph (-kar'de-o-graf″) instrument for making tracings of heart movements.

myocardiopathy (-kar″de-op'ah-the) nonspecific disease of the myocardium.

myocarditis (mi″o-kar-di'tis) inflammation of the myocardium. **Fiedler's m.,** acute myocarditis due to unknown cause.

myocardium (-kar'de-um) the muscular substance of the heart. adj., **myocar'dial.**

myocardosis (-kar-do'sis) any myocardial disorder which is not due to an inflammatory condition, but is the result of hypertension, coronary sclerosis and hyperthyroidism.

myocele (mi'o-sēl) hernia of muscle through its sheath.

myocellulitis (mi″o-sel″u-li'tis) myositis with cellulitis.

myocerosis (-se-ro'sis) waxy degeneration of muscle.

myochrome (mi'o-krōm) any member of a group of muscle pigments.

Myochrysine (mi″o-kri'sin) trademark for a preparation of gold sodium thiomalate.

myoclonus (mi″o-klo'nus) shocklike contractions of part of a muscle, an entire muscle or a group of muscles. adj., **myoclon'ic. palatal m.,** a condition characterized by a rapid rhythmic movement of one side of the palate.

myocyte (mi'o-sīt) a cell of muscular tissue.

myocytolysis (mi″o-si-tol'ĭ-sis) disintegration of muscle fibers. **focal m. of the heart,** a miliary lesion characterized by loss of muscular syncytium, preservation of stroma, absence of inflammatory reaction, and eventual necrosis.

myocytoma (-si-to'mah) a tumor composed of myocytes.

myodemia (-de'me-ah) fatty degeneration of muscle.

myodiastasis (-di-as'tah-sis) separation of muscle fibers.

myodynia (-din'e-ah) myalgia.

myodystrophy (-dis'tro-fe) muscular dystrophy; myotonia atrophica.

myo-edema (-ē-de'mah) 1. mounding. 2. edema of a muscle.

myo-electric (-e-lek'trik) pertaining to electric properties of muscle.

myo-endocarditis (-en″do-kar-di'tis) combined myocarditis and endocarditis.

myoepithelial (-ep″ĭ-the'le-al) pertaining to smooth muscle cells of epithelial origin, occurring in certain glands.

myofascitis (-fah-si'tis) inflammation of a muscle and its fascia.

myofibril (-fi'bril) one of the finer elements making up a muscle fiber.

myofibroma (-fi-bro'mah) myoma combined with fibroma.

myofibrosis (-fi-bro'sis) replacement of muscle tissue by fibrous tissue.

myofibrositis (-fi″bro-si'tis) inflammation of the sheath of muscle fiber.

myofilament (-fil'ah-ment) 1. a myofibril of a smooth muscle cell. 2. one of the ultramicroscopic threadlike structures occurring in bundles in the myofibrils of striated muscle fibers.

myogelosis (-je-lo'sis) hardening of muscle substance.

myogen (mi'o-jen) a protein occurring in muscle plasma.

myogenesis (mi″o-jen'ĕ-sis) the formation of

muscle fibers and muscles in embryonic development. adj., **myogenet′ic.**

myogenic (mi″o-jen′ik) producing muscle fibers and muscles.

myogenous (mi-oj′ĕ-nus) originating in muscular tissue.

myoglia (mi-og′le-ah) a fibrillar substance formed by muscle cells.

myoglobin (mi″o-glo′bin) a substance present in muscle which contributes to its color and acts as a storehouse of oxygen.

myoglobulin (-glob′u-lin) a globulin from muscle serum.

myogram (mi′o-gram) a record produced by myography.

myograph (mi′o-graf) apparatus for recording effects of muscular contraction.

myography (mi-og′rah-fe) 1. the use of a myograph. 2. description of muscles.

myohemoglobin (mi″o-he″mo-glo′bin) the hemoglobin of muscle tissue.

myoid (mi′oid) resembling muscle.

myoidema (mi″oi-de′mah) mounding.

myoischemia (mi″o-is-ke′me-ah) local deficiency of blood supply in muscle.

myokinesimeter (-kin″ĕ-sim′ĕ-ter) an apparatus for measuring muscular contraction from electrical stimulation.

myokinesis (-ki-ne′sis) 1. muscular movement. 2. operative displacement of muscle fibers. adj., **myokinet′ic.**

myokymia (-ki′me-ah) persistent quivering of the muscles.

myolemma (-lem′ah) the sarcolemma.

myolipoma (-li-po′mah) myoma with fatty elements.

myologia (-lo′je-ah) myology.

myology (mi-ol′o-je) scientific study or description of the muscles and accessory structures (bursae and synovial sheath).

myolysis (mi-ol′ĭ-sis) degeneration of muscular tissue.

myoma (mi-o′mah) a tumor formed of muscular tissue. adj., **myom′atous.**

myomagenesis (mi″o-mah-jen′ĕ-sis) the development of myomas.

myomalacia (-mah-la′she-ah) morbid softening of a muscle.

myomatosis (-mah-to′sis) the formation of myomas throughout the body.

myomectomy (-mek′to-me) excision of a myoma.

myomelanosis (-mel″ah-no′sis) melanosis of muscle.

myomere (mi′o-mēr) a protovertebra, or embryonic muscular segment.

myometer (mi-om′ĕ-ter) apparatus for measuring muscle contraction.

myometritis (mi″o-me-tri′tis) inflammation of the myometrium.

myometrium (-me′tre-um) the smooth muscle coat of the uterus. adj., **myome′trial.**

myoneme (mi′o-nēm) a fine contractile fiber found in the cytoplasm of certain protozoa.

myoneuralgia (mi″o-nu-ral′je-ah) neuralgic pain in a muscle.

myoneure (mi′o-nūr) a nerve cell supplying a muscle.

myoneuroma (mi″o-nu-ro′mah) a neuroma containing muscular tissue.

myoneurosis (-nu-ro′sis) any neurosis of muscle.

myopachynsis (-pah-kin′sis) hypertrophy of muscle.

myoparalysis (-pah-ral′ĭ-sis) paralysis of a muscle.

myopathy (mi-op′ah-the) any disease of a muscle. adj., **myopath′ic.**

myope (mi′ōp) a person affected with myopia.

myopericarditis (mi″o-per″ĭ-kar-di′tis) inflammation of both myocardium and pericardium.

myopia (mi-o′pe-ah) ametropia in which parallel rays come to a focus in front of the retina, vision being better for near objects than for far. adj., **miop′ic. curvature m.,** myopia due to changes in curvature of the refracting surfaces of the eye. **index m.,** myopia due to abnormal refractivity of the media of the eye. **malignant m., pernicious m.,** progressive myopia with disease of the choroid, leading to retinal detachment and blindness. **progressive m.,** myopia that continues to increase in adult life.

myoplasty (mi′o-plas″te) plastic surgery on muscle. adj., **myoplas′tic.**

myopsychosis (mi″o-si-ko′sis) any neuromuscular affection associated with mental disorder.

myoreceptor (-re-sep′tor) a receptor situated in skeletal muscle and stimulated by muscular contraction.

myorrhaphy (mi-or′ah-fe) suture of a muscle.

myorrhexis (mi″o-rek′sis) rupture of a muscle.

myosalpinx (-sal′pinks) the muscular tissue of the oviduct.

myosarcoma (-sar-ko′mah) myoma blended with sarcoma.

myoschwannoma (-shwan-no′mah) schwannoma.

myosclerosis (-skle-ro′sis) hardening of muscle.

myosin (mi′o-sin) one of the two proteins involved in contraction of muscle fibers.

myosinose (mi-os′ĭ-nōs) an albumose produced by digestion of myosin.

myositis (mi″o-si′tis) inflammatory disease of muscle tissue. **multiple m.,** dermatomyositis. **m. ossif′icans,** myositis marked by bony deposits.

myospasm (mi′o-spazm) spasm of a muscle.

myosteoma (mi-os″te-o′mah) a bony tumor in muscle.

myosynizesis (mi″o-sin″i-ze′sis) adhesion of muscles.

myotactic (-tak′tik) pertaining to the muscular sense of touch.

myotasis (mi-ot′ah-sis) stretching of muscle. adj., **myotat′ic.**

myotenositis (mi″o-te″no-si′tis) inflammation of a muscle and tendon.

myotenotomy (-te-not′o-me) surgical division of the tendon of a muscle.

myotome (mi′o-tōm) 1. instrument for dividing muscles. 2. the dorsomesial portion of a somite, from which the skeletal muscles are developed.

myotomy (mi-ot'o-me) cutting or dissection of muscular tissue or of a muscle.

myotonia (mi″o-to'ne-ah) increased tone or tension of muscle. adj., **myoton'ic. m. atroph'-ica,** dystrophia myotonica. **m. congen'ita,** a hereditary disease marked by tonic spasm and rigidity of certain muscles when attempts are made to move them. **m. dystroph'-ica,** dystrophia myotonica.

myotonometer (-to-nom'ĕ-tcr) instrument for measuring muscular tonus.

myotonus (mi-ot'o-nus) tonic spasm of a muscle or a group of muscles.

myotrophic (mi'o-tro″fik) 1. increasing weight of muscle. 2. pertaining to myotrophy.

myotrophy (mi-ot'ro-fe) nutrition of muscle.

myotropic (mi″o-trop'ik) having a special affinity for muscle.

myovascular (-vas'ku-ler) pertaining to muscle and blood vessels.

myria- (mir'e-ah) word element [Gr.] used in naming units of measurement to indicate a multiple (10^4) of the unit designated by the root with which it is connected.

Myriapoda (mir″e-ap'o-dah) a class of arthropods, including the millipedes and centipedes.

myriapodiasis (mir″e-ah-po-di'ah-sis) infestation with organisms of the class Myriapoda.

myringa (mĭ-ring'gah) the tympanic membrane.

myringectomy (mir″in-jek'to-me) excision of the tympanic membrane.

myringitis (-ji'tis) inflammation of tympanic membrane. **bullous m., m. bullo'sa,** a form of viral otitis media in which serous or hemorrhagic blebs appear on the tympanic membrane and adjacent wall of the auditory meatus.

myringomycosis (mĭ-ring″go-mi-ko'sis) fungus disease of the tympanic membrane.

myringoplasty (mĭ-ring'go-plas″te) surgical reconstruction of the tympanic membrane.

myringorupture (mĭ-ring″go-rup'chŭr) rupture of the tympanic membrane.

myringoscope (mĭ-ring'go-skōp) an instrument for inspecting the tympanic membrane.

myringostapediopexy (mi-ring″go-stah-pe'de-o-pek″se) fixation of the pars tensa of the tympanic membrane to the head of the stapes.

myringotomy (mir″ing-got'o-me) incision of the tympanic membrane.

myrrh (mer) the oleo-gum-resin from *Commiphora molmol* or other species, used as a protective agent.

Mysoline (mi'so-lēn) trademark for preparations of primidone.

mysophobia (mi″so-fo'be-ah) morbid dread of contamination and filth.

mytacism (mi'tah-sizm) too free use of *m* sound in speaking.

Mytelase (mi'tĕ-lās) trademark for a preparation of ambenonium.

mythomania (mith″o-ma'ne-ah) morbid tendency to lie or exaggerate.

mythophobia (mith″o-fo'be-ah) morbid fear of stating an untruth.

mytilotoxin (mit″ĭ-lo-tok'sin) a poisonous principle from mussels.

myx(o) (mik'so) word element [Gr.], *mucus; slime.*

myxadenitis (mik″sad-ĕ-ni'tis) inflammation of a mucous gland.

myxadenoma (-sad-ĕ-no'mah) an epithelial tumor with the structure of a mucous gland.

myxasthenia (-sas-the'ne-ah) deficient secretion of mucus.

myxedema (mik″sĕ de'mah) a dry, waxy type of swelling with abnormal deposits of mucin in the skin, often associated with hypothyroidism. adj., **myxedem'atous. congenital m.,** cretinism. **papular m.,** lichen myxedematosus.

Myxobacterales (mik″so-bak-tē-ra'lēz) an order of Schizomycetes.

myxoblastoma (-blas-to'mah) a tumor of mucous connective tissue cells.

myxochondroma (-kon-dro'mah) myxoma blended with chondroma.

Myxococcaceae (-kok-ka'se-e) a family of Schizomycetes (order Myxobacterales) found in soil and decaying organic matter.

Myxococcus (-kok'us) a genus of Schizomycetes (order Myxobacterales, family Myxococcaceae) found in decaying organic matter.

myxocystoma (-sis-to'mah) a cystic tumor with mucoid contents.

myxocyte (mik'so-sīt) one of the cells of mucous tissue.

myxofibroma (mik″so-fi-bro'mah) myxoma blended with fibroma.

myxoid (mik'soid) resembling mucus.

myxolipoma (mik″so-lĭ-po'mah) myxoma blended with lipoma.

myxoma (mik-so'mah) a tumor composed of mucous tissue. **odontogenic m.,** an uncommon tumor of the jaw, possibly produced by myxomatous degeneration of an odontogenic fibroma.

myxomatosis (mik″so-mah-to'sis) 1. the development of multiple myxomas. 2. myxomatous degeneration.

Myxomycetes (-mi-se'tēz) a group of fungoid organisms now classified as Myxobacterales.

myxomyoma (-mi-o'mah) myxoma that has undergone mucous degeneration.

myxoneuroma (-nu-ro'mah) myxoma blended with neuroma.

myxopapilloma (-pap″ĭ-lo'mah) myxoma combined with papilloma.

myxopoiesis (-poi-e'sis) the formation of mucus.

myxorrhea (-re'ah) a flow of mucus. **m. intestina'lis,** excessive secretion of intestinal mucus.

myxosarcoma (-sar-ko'mah) sarcoma that has partly undergone mucous degeneration.

myxospore (mik'so-spōr) a spore embedded in a jelly-like mass.

Myxosporidia (mik″so-spo-rid'e-ah) an order of parasitic sporozoans.

myxovirus (mik″so-vi′rus) a virus of the influenza, parainfluenza, mumps, Newcastle disease or a related group, characteristically causing agglutination of chicken erythrocytes.

Myzomyia (mi″zo-mi′yah) a genus of mosquitoes, several species of which act as carriers of malarial parasites.

Myzorhynchus (mi″zo-ring′kus) a genus of mosquitoes, several species of which act as carriers of malarial parasites.

N

N chemical symbol, *nitrogen*.

N. nasal; north.

n. 1. symbol: *index of refraction; normal* (of chemical compounds). 2. [L.] *nervus* (nerve).

NA Nomina Anatomica, official anatomic terminology approved by the International Congress of Anatomists.

Na chemical symbol, *sodium* (L. *natrium*).

nacreous (na′kre-us) having a pearl-like luster.

Nacton (nak′ton) trademark for a preparation of poldine methylsulfate.

nae- for words beginning thus, see also those beginning *ne-*.

naepaine (ne′pān) a compound used as a local anesthetic.

nagana (nah-gah′nah) a trypanosome disease of horses and cattle in Central Africa.

nail (nāl) horny dorsal plate on the distal phalanx of a finger or toe. **fracture n.,** a steel nail for fastening together the fragments of a broken bone. **hang n.,** a shred of epidermis at one side of a nail. **ingrowing n., ingrown n.,** overlapping of the anterior corners of a nail by the flesh of the digit. **Smith-Petersen n.,** a flanged nail for fixing the head of the femur in fracture of the femoral neck. **spoon n.,** a nail with a concave surface.

Nalline (nal′lēn) trademark for a preparation of nalorphine.

nalorphine (nal′or-fēn) a semisynthetic congener of morphine, used as a narcotic antagonist.

nandrolone (nan′dro-lōn) a compound used as an anabolic agent.

nanism (na′nizm) dwarfishness.

nano- (na′no) word element [Gr.], *dwarf; small size;* used in naming units of measurement to designate an amount 10^{-9} (one billionth) the size of the unit to which it is joined, e.g. nanocurie.

nanocephalous (na″no-sef′ah-lus) having a very small head.

nanocormia (-kor′me-ah) abnormal smallness of the body or trunk.

nanocurie (-ku′re) a unit of radioactivity, being 10^{-9} curie, or the quantity of radioactive material in which the number of nuclear disintegrations is 3.7×10, or 37, per second; abbreviated nc.

nanogram (na′no-gram) one billionth (10^{-9}) gram.

nanoid (na′noid) dwarfish.

nanomelus (na-nom′ĕ-lus) a fetus with stunted limbs.

nanoplankton (na″no-plank′ton) plankton of extremely minute size.

nanosomia (-so′me-ah) dwarfishness of body.

nanounit (-u′nit) one billionth (10^{-9}) part of a unit.

nanous (na′nus) dwarfed.

nanus (na′nus) 1. a dwarf. 2. stunted; dwarfish.

nape (nāp) the back of the neck.

naphazoline (naf-az′o-lēn) white crystalline powder; vasoconstrictor and nasal decongestant.

naphtha (naf′thah) benzine.

naphthalene (naf′thah-lēn) a hydrocarbon from coal tar oil; antiseptic.

naphthol (naf′thol) a crystalline antiseptic substance occurring in two forms, alphanaphthol and betanaphthol.

N.A.P.N.E. National Association for Practical Nurse Education.

Naqua (nak′wah) trademark for a preparation of trichlormethiazide.

narcissism (nar′si-sizm) dominant interest in one's self. adj., **narcissis′tic.**

narcoanalysis (nar″ko-ah-nal′ĭ-sis) psychoanalysis with use of sedative drugs to help uncover unconscious material.

narcoanesthesia (-an″es-the′ze-ah) anesthesia by injection of scopolamine and morphine.

narcohypnia (-hip′ne-ah) numbness felt on waking from sleep.

narcolepsy (nar′ko-lep″se) recurrent uncontrollable desire for sleep. adj., **narcolep′tic.**

narcomania (nar″ko-ma′ne-ah) a morbid craving for narcotics.

narcose (nar′kōs) 1. somewhat narcotic. 2. drowsy.

narcosine (nar′ko-sēn) noscapine.

narcosis (nar-ko′sis) a sleeplike, stuporous state induced by a sedative drug. **basal n., basis n.,** narcosis with complete unconsciousness and analgesia.

narcosynthesis (nar″ko-sin′thĕ-sis) treatment of neuroses by inducing a seminarcosis in which the patient recalls his suppressed memories and synthesizes his emotions.

narcotic (nar-kot′ic) 1. producing stupor or sleep. 2. a drug which produces sleep or stupor.

narcotine (nar′ko-tin) noscapine.

narcotism (nar′ko-tizm) addiction to a narcotic drug.

narcotize (nar'ko-tīz) to put under the influence of a narcotic.

Nardil (nar'dil) trademark for a preparation of phenelzine dihydrogen sulfate.

naris (na'ris), pl. *na'res* [L.] an opening into the nasal cavity on the exterior of the body (*anterior* or *external naris*) or into the nasopharynx (*posterior naris*).

Narone (nar'ōn) trademark for a preparation of dipyrone.

NASA National Aeronautics and Space Administration.

nasal (na'zal) pertaining to the nose.

nascent (nas'ent, na'sent) being born, or just coming into being; applied especially to a substance or element just escaping from a chemical combination.

N.A.S.E. National Association for the Study of Epilepsy.

nasion (na'ze-on) the middle point of the frontonasal suture.

nasitis (na-zi'tis) inflammation of the nose.

NAS-NRC National Academy of Sciences—National Research Council.

naso-antritis (na"zo-an-tri'tis) inflammation of the nose and antrum of Highmore.

nasofrontal (-frun'tal) pertaining to nasal and frontal bones.

nasolacrimal (-lak'rĭ-mal) pertaining to nose and lacrimal apparatus.

nasopalatine (-pal'ah-tīn) pertaining to nose and palate.

nasopharyngitis (-far"in-ji'tis) inflammation of the nasopharynx.

nasopharynx (-far'inks) part of pharynx above the soft palate. adj., **nasopharyn'geal.**

nasoseptitis (-sep-ti'tis) inflammation of the nasal septum.

nasosinusitis (-si"nŭ-si'tis) inflammation of the accessory sinuses of the nose.

nasospinale (-spi-na'le) the point at which the midsagittal plane intersects a line tangent to the lower margin of the nasal apertures.

nasus (na'sus) nose.

natal (na'tal) 1. pertaining to birth. 2. pertaining to the nates (buttocks).

natality (na-tal'ĭ-te) the birth rate.

nates (na'tēz) (pl.) 1. the buttocks. 2. the anterior pair of corpora quadrigemina.

natimortality (na"te-mor-tal'ĭ-te) the proportion of stillbirths to the general birth rate.

Natolone (nat'o-lōn) trademark for a preparation of pregnenolone.

natremia (na-tre'me-ah) the presence of sodium in the blood.

natrium (na'tre-um) [L.] sodium (symbol Na).

natriuresis (na"tre-u-re'sis) the excretion of sodium in the urine.

natriuretic (-u-ret'ik) 1. pertaining to or promoting natriuresis. 2. an agent that promotes natriuresis.

natron (na'tron) native sodium carbonate.

natruresis (nat"roo-re'sis) natriuresis.

natruretic (-ret'ik) natriuretic.

Naturetin (nat"u-re'tin) trademark for preparations of bendroflumethiazide.

naturopath (na'tūr-o-path") a practitioner of naturopathy.

naturopathy (na"tūr-op'ah-the) a drugless system of healing by the use of physical methods.

Naumanniella (naw-man"ne-el'lah) a genus of Schizomycetes (order Pseudomonadales, suborder Pseudomonadineae, family Siderocapsaceae) found in iron-containing water.

nausea (naw'ze-ah) tendency to vomit. **n. gravida'rum,** the morning sickness of pregnancy. **n. mari'na, n. nava'lis,** seasickness.

nauseant (naw'ze-ant) 1. inducing nausea. 2. an agent causing nausea.

nauseous (naw'shus, naw'ze-us) producing nausea or disgust.

navel (na'vel) the umbilicus.

navicular (nah-vik'u-ler) boat-shaped.

Nb chemical symbol, *niobium.*

N.B.S. National Bureau of Standards.

nc. nanocurie.

N.C.I. National Cancer Institute.

N.C.M.H. National Committee for Mental Hygiene.

N.C.N. National Council of Nurses.

NCRP National Committee on Radiation Protection and Measurements.

Nd chemical symbol, *neodymium.*

N.D.A. National Dental Association.

Ne chemical symbol, *neon.*

nearsightedness (nēr-sīt'ed-nes) myopia.

nearthrosis (ne"ar-thro'sis) a false or artificial joint.

nebula (neb'u-lah) 1. slight corneal opacity. 2. cloudiness in urine.

nebulization (neb"u-li-za'shun) dispersal of a bulk liquid in a fine mist, all large particles being removed.

nebulizer (neb'u-līz"er) an apparatus for dispersing bulk liquid in a fine mist.

Necator (ne-ka'tor) a genus of nematode parasites. **N. america'nus,** a species widely distributed in southern United States, Central and South America and the Caribbean area; the New World, or American, hookworm.

necatoriasis (ne-ka"to-ri'ah-sis) infestation with organisms of the genus Necator.

neck (nek) 1. part between head and thorax. 2. the narrow part near the extremity of an organ or bone. **anatomic n.,** constriction of the humerus just below its proximal articular surface. **big n.,** goiter. **Madelung's n.,** a neck affected with diffuse symmetrical lipoma. **surgical n. of humerus,** constricted part of humerus just below the tuberosities. **n. of a tooth,** the narrowed part of a tooth between the crown and the root. **uterine n., n. of uterus,** cervix uteri. **webbed n.,** obliteration of the usual angle between the neck and shoulders by an abnormal expanse of tissue. **wry n.,** torticollis.

necklace (nek'las) a structure encircling the neck. **Casal's n.,** an eruption in pellagra, encircling the lower part of the neck.

necrectomy (ne-krek'to-me) excision of necrosed tissue.

necro- (nek'ro) word element [Gr.], *death.*

necrobacillosis (nek"ro-bas"ĭ-lo'sis) a disease of animals caused by *Actinomyces necrophorus.*

necrobiosis (-bi-o'sis) the physiologic death of

cells; the modifications taking place in a living organism prior to death, when its occurrence is slow and gradual. adj., **necrobiot'ic. n. lipoi'dica diabetico'rum,** degeneration of the elastic and connective tissue of the skin occurring in diabetes.

necrocytosis (nek″ro-si-to'sis) death and decay of cells.

necrology (ně-krol'o-je, ne-krol'o-je) statistics or records of death.

necromania (nek″ro-ma'ne-ah) morbid interest in death or dead persons.

necroparasite (-par'ah-sīt) an organism which lives in dead tissue.

necrophagous (ne-krof'ah-gus) feeding upon carrion.

necrophilia (nek″ro-fil'e-ah) morbid attraction to death or to dead bodies; sexual intercourse with a dead body.

necrophobia (-fo'be-ah) morbid dread of death or of dead bodies.

necropneumonia (-nu-mo'ne-ah) gangrene of lung.

necropsy (nek'rop-se) examination of a body after death.

necrose (ne-krōs') to become affected with necrosis.

necrosin (ne-kro'sin) a toxic substance occurring in inflammatory exudates.

necrosis (ně-kro'sis, ne-kro'sis) death of a cell as the result of disease or injury. adj., **necrot'ic. aseptic n., avascular n.,** necrosis occurring as a result of isolation of a part from its blood supply. **Balser's fatty n.,** necrosis of pancreas, spleen and omentum. **caseous n.,** necrosis in which the tissue is soft, dry and cheesy. **central n.,** necrosis affecting the central portion of an affected bone, cell or lobule of the liver. **cheesy n.,** caseous necrosis. **coagulation n., coagulative n.,** death of cells, the protoplasm of the cells becoming fixed and opaque by coagulation of the protein elements, the cellular outline persisting for a long time. **colliquative n.,** liquefactive necrosis. **dry n.,** that in which the necrotic tissue becomes dry. **fat n.,** necrosis of fatty tissue in small white areas. **gangrenous n.,** cell death caused by a combination of ischemia and superimposed bacterial infection, combining the features of coagulative and liquefactive necrosis. **liquefactive n.,** necrosis in which the necrotic material becomes softened and liquefied. **mercurial n.,** necrosis due to mercurial poisoning. **moist n.,** necrosis in which the dead tissue is wet and soft. **phosphorus n.,** necrosis in the upper jaw, from exposure to fumes of phosphorus. **septic n.,** necrosis resulting from bacterial infection. **superficial n.,** necrosis affecting the surface of a bone. **n. ustilagin'ea,** dry gangrene from ergot poisoning.

necrospermia (nek″ro-sper'me-ah) a condition in which the spermatozoa are dead. adj., **necrosper'mic.**

necrotizing (nek'ro-tīz″ing) causing necrosis.

necrotomy (ne-krot'o-me) 1. dissection of a dead body. 2. excision of a sequestrum.

necrotoxin (nek″ro-tok'sin) a factor or substance produced by certain staphylococci which kills tissue cells.

needle (ne'dl). sharp instrument for sewing or puncturing. **aneurysm n.,** one used in ligating blood vessels. **artery n., aspirating n.,** a long, hollow needle for removing fluid from a cavity. **cataract n.,** one designed for operating upon the cataractous lens. **discission n.,** a special form of cataract needle. **exploring n.,** one used in exploratory puncture. **Hagedorn's n.,** a form of flat suture needle. **hypodermic n.,** a hollow, sharp-pointed needle to be attached to a hypodermic syringe for subcutaneous injection of solutions. **knife n.,** a cutting-edged needle used in operation. **Silverman n.,** one designed for removal of tissue from an internal organ for study under the microscope. **stop n.,** one with a disk which prevents too deep penetration.

Negatan (neg'ah-tan) trademark for a preparation of negatol.

negative (neg'ah-tiv) having a value of less than zero; indicating lack or absence, as chromatin-negative; characterized by denial or opposition.

negativism (neg'ah-tī-vizm″) opposition and resistance to suggestion or advice; behavior opposite to that appropriate to a specific situation.

negatol (neg'ah-tol) a colloidal product used as a parasiticide, germicide and bacteriostatic, for topical application to the cervix.

negatron (neg'ah-tron) a negatively charged electron.

neighborwise (na'bor-wīz) developing in accordance with the region to which it is transplanted, characteristic of tissue from a young amphibian gastrula.

Neisseria (ni-se're-ah) a genus of Schizomycetes (order Eubacteriales, family Neisseriaceae). **N. gonorrhoe'ae,** the etiologic agent of gonorrhea. **N. meningi'tidis,** a prominent cause of meningitis and the specific etiologic agent of meningococcal meningitis.

neisseriaceae (ni-se″re-a'se-e) a family of Schizomycetes (order Eubacteriales).

neisserian (ni-se're-an) pertaining to or caused by organisms of the genus *Neisseria,* usually *N. gonorrhoea.*

Nema (ne'mah) trademark for a preparation of tetrachloroethylene.

nematoblast (nem'ah-to-blast″) spermatid.

nematocide (nem'ah-to-sīd″) 1. destroying nematodes. 2. an agent which destroys nematodes.

Nematoda (nem″ah-to'dah) a class of roundworms, some of which are parasitic in man.

nematode (nem'ah-tōd) 1. like a thread. 2. an individual organism of the class Nematoda.

nematodiasis (nem″ah-to-di'ah-sis) infestation by a nematode.

Nembutal (nem'bu-tal) trademark for preparations of pentobarbital.

neo- (ne'o) word element [Gr.], *new.*

Neo-antergan (ne″o-an'ter-gan) trademark for a preparation of pyrilamine maleate.

neo-arthrosis (ne″o-ar-thro′sis) nearthrosis.

neoblastic (-blas′tik) originating in new tissue.

neocerebellum (-ser″ĕ-bel′um) the more newly developed part of the cerebellum, comprising the lateral lobes.

neocinchophen (-sin′ko-fen) white to yellow crystalline powder; analgesic and antipyretic.

neocinetic (-si-net′ik) neokinetic.

neocortex (-kor′teks) neopallium.

neocyte (ne′o-sīt) an immature form of leukocyte.

neocytosis (ne″o-si-to′sis) presence of neocytes in the blood.

neodiathermy (-di″ah-ther′me) short-wave diathermy.

Neo-diloderm (-di′lo-derm) trademark for a preparation of dichlorisone containing neomycin sulfate.

neodymium (-dim′e-um) chemical element (*see table*), at. no. 60, symbol Nd.

neogenesis (-jen′ĕ-sis) tissue regeneration. adj., **neogenet′ic.**

Neohetramine (-he′trah-min) trademark for a preparation of thonzylamine hydrochloride.

Neo-hombreol (-hom′bre-ol) trademark for preparations of testosterone propionate.

Neohydrin (-hi′drin) trademark for a preparation of chlormerodrin.

Neo-iopax (-i′o-paks) trademark for a preparation of sodium iodomethamate.

neokinetic (-ki-net′ik) pertaining to the nervous motor mechanism regulating voluntary muscular control.

neologism (ne-ol′o-jizm) a newly coined word; in psychiatry, a new word whose meaning may be known only to the patient using it.

neomembrane (ne″o-mem′brān) a false membrane.

neomycin (-mi′sin) an antibacterial substance produced by growth of *Streptomyces fradiae*; used as an intestinal antiseptic and in treatment of systemic infections due to gramnegative microorganisms.

neon (ne′on) chemical element (*see table*), at. no. 10, symbol Ne.

neonatal (ne″o-na′tal) pertaining to the newborn.

neonate (ne′o-nāt) a newborn infant, variously considered to be up to two to four weeks old.

neonatologist (ne″o na-tol′o-jist) a physician whose primary concern is in the specialty of neonatology.

neonatology (-na-tol′o-je) the art and science of diagnosis and treatment of disorders of the newborn infant.

neopallium (-pal′le-um) that part of the pallium showing stratification and organization of the most highly evolved type.

neopathy (ne-op′ah-the) a new disease or a new complication in a disease.

neophilism (ne-of′ĭ-lizm) abnormal love of new things.

neophobia (ne″o-fo′be-ah) morbid dread of new things.

neoplasia (-pla′ze-ah) a condition characterized by the presence of new growths (tumors).

neoplasm (ne′o-plazm) a mass of newly formed tissue; a new growth (tumor).

neoplastic (ne″o-plas′tik) 1. pertaining to neoplasia or neoplasm. 2. pertaining to neoplasty.

neoplasty (ne′o-plas″te) replacement of lost parts by plastic methods.

Neorickettsia (ne″o-ri-ket′sī-ah) a genus of Microtatobiotes (order Rickettsiales, family Rickettsiaceae, tribe Ehrlichieae).

neostigmine (-stig′min) a cholinergic drug used to improve muscle function in myasthenia gravis. **n. bromide,** white, crystalline powder; parasympathomimetic. **n. methylsulfate,** white crystalline powder; parasympathomimetic, used parenterally.

neostomy (ne-os′tu-me) creation of a new opening into an organ or between two organs.

neostriatum (ne″o-stri-a′tum) the more recently developed part of the corpus striatum.

Neo-synephrine (-sī-nef′rin) trademark for preparations of phenylephrine.

neothalamus (-thal′ah-mus) the more lateral, cortical part of the thalamus.

Neothylline (-thil′lin) trademark for preparations of dyphylline.

neoteny (ne-ot′ĕ-ne) the maintenance of larval form in a sexually mature organism. adj., **neoten′ic.**

nephelometer (nef″ĕ-lom′ĕ-ter) an apparatus for measuring minute degrees of turbidity of a solution.

nephelometry (-lom′ĕ-tre) measurement of the concentration of a suspension by means of a nephelometer.

nephralgia (ne-fral′je-ah) pain in a kidney.

nephrectasia (nef″rek-ta′ze-ah) dilatation of a renal pelvis.

nephrectomy (ne-frek′to-me) excision of a kidney.

nephrelcosis (nef″rel-ko′sis) ulceration of the kidney.

nephremphraxis (nef″rem-frak′sis) obstruction of the vessels of the kidney.

nephric (nef′rik) pertaining to the kidney.

nephridium (ne-frid′e-um), pl. *nephrid′ia* [L.] a rudimentary excretory organ, as found in lower animals, or the embryonic tube from which the kidney develops.

nephrism (nef′rizm) cachexia due to kidney disease.

nephritis (ne-fri′tis), pl. *nephrit′ides* [Gr.] inflammation of the kidney. adj., **nephrit′ic. diffuse n.,** nephritis affecting both parenchyma and stroma. **fibrous n.,** nephritis affecting the stroma. **glomerular n.,** nephritis affecting the glomeruli. **interstitial n.,** nephritis with increase of interstitial tissue and thickening of vessel walls and malpighian corpuscles. **parenchymatous n.,** nephritis affecting the parenchyma of kidney. **saturnine n.,** nephritis due to chronic lead poisoning. **scarlatinal n.,** an acute nephritis due to scarlet fever. **suppurative n.,** a form accompanied by abscess of kidney. **tubular n.,** nephritis especially affecting the tubules.

nephritogenic (ne-frit″o-jen′ik) causing nephritis.

nephroblastoma (nef″ro-blas-to′mah) a kidney neoplasm containing embryonic tissue.

nephrocalcinosis (-kal″sĭ-no′sis) deposition of calcium phosphate in the renal tubules.

nephrocardiac (-kar′de-ak) pertaining to kidney and heart.

nephrocele (nef′ro-sēl) hernia of a kidney.

nephrocolic (nef″ro-kol′ik) 1. pertaining to kidney and colon. 2. renal colic.

nephrocoloptosis (-ko″lop-to′sis) downward displacement of the kidney and colon.

nephrogenic (-jen′ik) producing kidney tissue.

nephrogenous (nĕ-froj′ĕ-nus) arising in a kidney.

nephrography (nĕ-frog′rah-fe) roentgenography of the kidney.

nephroid (nef′roid) resembling a kidney.

nephrolith (nef′ro-lith) a calculus in a kidney.

nephrolithiasis (nef″ro-lĭ-thi′ah-sis) presence of renal calculi.

nephrolithotomy (-lĭ-thot′o-me) incision of kidney for removal of calculi.

nephrology (nĕ-frol′o-je) scientific study of the kidney.

nephrolysine (nĕ-frol′ĭ-sin) nephrotoxin.

nephrolysis (nĕ-frol′ĭ-sis) 1. freeing of a kidney from adhesions. 2. destruction of kidney substance.

nephroma (nĕ-fro′mah) a tumor of kidney tissue.

nephromegaly (nef″ro-meg′ah-le) enlargement of kidney.

nephron (nef′ron) the structural and functional unit of the kidney, numbering a million or more in the parenchyma of the organ.

nephropathy (nĕ-frop′ah-the) disease of the kidneys.

nephropexy (nef′ro-pek″se) surgical fixation of a freely movable kidney.

nephroptosis (nef″rop-to′sis) downward displacement of a kidney.

nephropyelitis (nef″ro-pi″ĕ-li′tis) nephritis complicated with pyelitis.

nephropyelography (-pi″ĕ-log′rah-fe) radiography of the kidney.

nephropyosis (-pi-o′sis) suppuration of a kidney.

nephrorrhagia (-ra′je-ah) hemorrhage from the kidney.

nephrorrhaphy (nef-ror′ah-fe) suture of the kidney.

nephrosclerosis (nef″ro-skle-ro′sis) hardening of the kidney. **arteriolar n.,** nephritis characterized by thickening of arterioles, degeneration of renal tubules and thickening of glomeruli.

nephrosis (nĕ-fro′sis) pl. *nephro′ses* [Gr.] any disease of the kidney, especially disease characterized by degenerative lesions of the renal parenchyma. adj., **nephrot′ic. amyloid n.,** chronic nephrosis with amyloid degeneration of the renal epithelium. **lower nephron n.,** a condition of renal insufficiency leading to uremia, blocking the tubular lumens of this region.

nephrostoma (nĕ-fros′to-mah) the internal orifice of the nephridium.

nephrostomy (nĕ-fros′to-me) creation of a permanent fistula leading into the pelvis of the kidney.

nephrotome (nef′ro-tōm) a short plate of cells extending ventrolaterally from each somite, which in series will develop the urogenital glands and their ducts.

nephrotomography (nef″ro-to-mog′rah-fe) body-section roentgenography for visualization of the kidney. adj., **nephrotomograph′ic.**

nephrotomy (nĕ-frot′o-me) incision of a kidney.

nephrotoxicity (nef″ro-tok-sis′ĭ-te) the quality of being toxic or destructive to kidney cells.

nephrotoxin (-tok′sin) a toxin destructive to kidney tissue.

nephrotropic (-trop′ik) having a special affinity for kidney tissue.

neptunium (nep-tu′ne-um) chemical element (*see table*), at. no. 93, symbol Np.

nerve (nerv) a cordlike structure composed of highly specialized tissue by which impulses are conveyed between a part of the central nervous system and another part of the body. For names of specific nerves, see *table of nerves*. **accelerator n's,** the cardiac sympathetic nerves, which, when stimulated, accelerate action of the heart. **afferent n.,** a nerve which transmits impulses from the periphery toward the central nervous system. **anabolic n's,** nerves which control constructive metabolic processes. **association n.,** an occasional branch of the abducens nerve running to the nerve of the pterygoid canal. **calorific n.,** any nerve stimulation of which causes an increase in body temperature. **centrifugal n.,** efferent nerve. **centripetal n.,** afferent nerve. **cerebral n.,** **cranial n.,** one of the twelve pairs of nerves arising from the brain. **depressor n.,** 1. any afferent nerve whose stimulation depresses a motor center. 2. a nerve that lessens activity of an organ. **efferent n.,** a nerve which transmits impulses from the central nervous system toward the periphery. **exciter n.,** one that transmits impulses resulting in an increase in functional activity. **excitoreflex n.,** a visceral nerve that produces reflex action. **frigorific n.,** any nerve whose stimulation causes a decrease in body temperature. **furcal n.,** the fourth lumbar nerve. **gangliated n.,** any nerve of the sympathetic nervous system. **inhibitory n.,** one that transmits impulses resulting in a decrease in functional activity. **Jacobson's n.,** tympanic nerve. **Langley's n's,** pilomotor nerves. **mixed n.,** one composed of both sensory and motor fibers. **motor n.,** one that contains motor fibers. **pain n.,** a sensory nerve whose function is the conduction of stimuli which produce the sensation of pain. **pilomotor n's,** those that supply the arrectores pilorum muscles. **pressor n.,** an afferent nerve irritation of which stimulates a vasomotor center and increases intravascular tension. **secretory n.,** an efferent nerve whose stimulation increases vascular activity. **sensory n.,** a peripheral nerve that conducts impulses from a sense organ to the

COMMON NAME [MODALITY]	NA TERM	ORIGIN	BRANCHES	DISTRIBUTION
abducent n. (6th cranial) [motor]	n. abducens	lower border of pons		lateral rectus muscle of eye
accessory n. (11th cranial) [motor]	n. accessorius	medulla oblongata and cervical segments of spinal cord		sternocleidomastoid and trapezius muscles
acoustic n. *See* vestibulocochlear n.				
alveolar n., inferior [motor, general sensory]	n. alveolaris inferior	mandibular n.	inferior dental and inferior gingival branches; mylohyoid and mental n's	teeth and gums of lower jaw, skin of chin and lower lip, mylohyoid muscle and anterior belly of digastric muscle
alveolar nn., superior	nn. alveolares superiores	superior alveolar branches (anterior, middle and posterior) that arise from infraorbital and maxillary nerves, innervating teeth of upper jaw and maxillary sinus, and forming superior dental plexus		
ampullary n., anterior	n. ampullaris anterior	branch of vestibular part of eighth cranial (vestibulocochlear) nerve that innervates ampulla of anterior semicircular duct, ending around hair cells of ampullary crest		
ampullary n., inferior. *See* ampullary n., posterior				
ampullary n., lateral	n. ampullaris lateralis	branch of vestibular part of eighth cranial (vestibulocochlear) nerve that innervates ampulla of lateral semicircular duct, ending around hair cells of ampullary crest		
ampullary n., posterior	n. ampullaris posterior	branch of vestibular part of eighth cranial (vestibulocochlear) nerve that innervates ampulla of posterior semicircular duct, ending around hair cells of ampullary crest		
ampullary n., superior. *See* ampullary n., anterior				
anococcygeal nn. [general sensory]	nn. anococcygei	coccygeal plexus	/	skin region of coccyx
auditory n. *See* vestibulocochlear n.				
auricular nn., anterior [general sensory]	nn. auriculares anteriores	auriculotemporal n.		skin of anterosuperior part of external ear
auricular n., great [general sensory]	n. auricularis magnus	cervical plexus — C2-C3	anterior and posterior branches	skin of side of head

423

COMMON NAME [MODALITY]	NA TERM	ORIGIN	BRANCHES	DISTRIBUTION
auricular n., posterior [motor, general sensory]	n. auricularis posterior	facial n.	occipital branch	posterior auricular and occipito-frontal muscles, skin of external acoustic meatus
auriculotemporal n. [general sensory, para-sympathetic]	n. auriculotemporalis	mandibular n.	anterior auricular n., n. of external acoustic meatus, parotid and superficial temporal branches, branch to tympanic membrane, communicating branch with facial n.	parotid gland, scalp in temporal region, tympanic membrane. See also auricular n., anterior, and n. of external acoustic meatus
axillary n. [motor, general]	n. axillaris	brachial plexus—C5–C6 through posterior cord	lateral superior brachial cutaneous n., muscular branches	deltoid and teres minor muscles, skin over shoulder
brachial plexus	plexus brachialis	fibers from spinal nerves C5–C8, T1		
buccal n. [general sensory]	n. buccalis	mandibular n.		skin of cheek, mucosa of floor of mouth
cardiac n., cervical inferior [sympathetic (accelerator), visceral afferent]	n. cardiacus cervicalis inferior	cervicothoracic ganglion		heart via cardiac plexus
cardiac n., cervical, middle [sympathetic (accelerator), visceral afferent]	n. cardiacus cervicalis medius	middle cervical ganglion		heart
cardiac n., cervical, superior [sympathetic (accelerator)]	n. cardiacus cervicalis superior	superior cervical ganglion		heart
cardiac n., inferior. See cardiac n., cervical, inferior				
cardiac n., middle. See cardiac n., cervical, middle				
cardiac n., superior. See cardiac n., cervical, superior				
cardiac nn., thoracic [sympathetic (accelerator), visceral afferent]	nn. cardiaci thoracici	ganglia T2–T5 of sympathetic trunk		heart

English term	Latin term	Description	Supply/Distribution
caroticotympanic mm. [sympathetic]	mm. caroticotympanici	superior cervical sympathetic ganglion	tympanic region, parotid gland
carotid nn., external [sympathetic]	mm. carotici externi	superior cervical ganglion	cranial blood vessels and glands via external carotid plexus
carotid n., internal [sympathetic]	n. caroticus internus	superior cervical ganglion	cranial blood vessels and glands via internal carotid plexus
cavernous nn. of clitoris [parasympathetic, sympathetic, visceral afferent]	mm. cavernosi clitoridis	uterovaginal plexus	erectile tissue of clitoris
cavernous nn., of penis [sympathetic, parasympathetic, visceral afferent]	mm. cavernosi penis	prostatic plexus	erectile tissue of penis
cervical nn.	mm. cervicales	the 8 pairs of nerves that arise from cervical segments of spinal cord and, except last pair, leave vertebral column above correspondingly numbered vertebra; the ventral branches of upper four, on either side, unite to form cervical plexus; those of lower four contribute most of brachial plexus	
cervical n., transverse [general sensory]	n. transversus colli	cervical plexus – C2–C3	skin and subcutaneous tissue in anterior cervical region
cervical plexus	plexus cervicalis	fibers from spinal nerves C1–C4	superior and inferior branches
chorda tympani [parasympathetic, special sensory]	chorda tympani	facial n. (n. intermedius)	submandibular and sublingual glands, anterior two thirds of tongue
ciliary nn., long [general sensory]	nn. ciliares longi	nasociliary n., from ophthalmic n.	intraocular structures
ciliary nn., short [parasympathetic, and sympathetic and general sensory from communicating branches with trigeminal n.]	nn. ciliares breves	ciliary ganglion from oculomotor n.	smooth muscle of eye
clunial nn., inferior [general sensory]	nn. clunium inferiores	posterior femoral cutaneous n.	skin of inferior gluteal region
clunial nn., middle [general sensory]	nn. clunium medii	lateral branch of dorsal branch of sacral n.	skin of middle gluteal region
clunial nn., superior [general sensory]	nn. clunium superiores	lateral branch of dorsal branch of lumbar n.	skin of superior gluteal region
coccygeal n. [general sensory]	n. coccygeus	either of the thirty-first pair of spinal nerves, arising from coccygeal segment of spinal cord	
coccygeal plexus	plexus coccygeus	fibers from spinal nerves S4–S5, Co 1	

425

TABLE OF NERVES (Continued)

COMMON NAME [MODALITY]	NA TERM	ORIGIN	BRANCHES	DISTRIBUTION
cochlear n. *See* vestibular cochlear n.				
cranial nn.	nn. craniales	the 12 pairs of nerves connected with brain, including olfactory (I), optic (II), oculomotor (III), trochlear (IV), trigeminal (V), abducens (VI), facial (VII), vestibulocochlear (VIII), glossopharyngeal (IX), vagus (X), accessory (XI) and hypoglossal (XII) nerves		
cubital n. *See* ulnar n.				
cutaneous n. of arm, lateral, inferior [general sensory]	n. cutaneus brachii lateralis inferior	radial n.		skin of back of arm
cutaneous n. of arm, lateral, superior [general sensory]	n. cutaneus brachii lateralis superior	axillary n.		skin of back of arm
cutaneous n. of arm, medial [general sensory]	n. cutaneus brachii medialis	T1 through medial cord		skin on medial and posterior aspects of arm
cutaneous n. of arm, posterior [general sensory]	n. cutaneus brachii posterior	radial n.		skin on dorsal surface of arm
cutaneous n. of calf, lateral [general sensory]	n. cutaneus surae lateralis	common peroneal n.	sural n.	skin of lower dorsal aspect of leg and lateral aspect of foot
cutaneous n. of calf, medial [general sensory]	n. cutaneus surae medialis	tibial n.	sural n.	skin of lower dorsal aspect of leg and lateral aspect of foot
cutaneous n. of foot, dorsal, intermediate [general sensory]	n. cutaneus dorsalis intermedius pedis	superficial peroneal n.	dorsal digital nn. of foot	skin of lateral side of foot and ankle; adjacent sides of third and fourth and of fourth and fifth toes
cutaneous n. of foot, dorsal, lateral [general sensory]	n. cutaneus dorsalis lateralis pedis	sural n.		adjacent sides of fourth and fifth toes, lateral side of fifth toe
cutaneous n. of foot, dorsal, medial [general sensory]	n. cutaneus dorsalis medialis pedis	superficial peroneal n.		skin of medial side of foot and adjacent sides of second and third toes
cutaneous n. of forearm, lateral [general sensory]	n. cutaneus antebrachii lateralis	musculocutaneous n.		skin over radial part of forearm

426

Common name [modality]	Latin	Origin	Branches	Distribution
cutaneous n. of forearm, medial [general sensory]	n. cutaneus antebrachii medialis	brachial plexus—C8–T1 through medial cord	anterior and ulnar branches	skin of front, medial and posteromedial aspects of forearm
cutaneous n. of forearm, posterior [general sensory]	n. cutaneus antebrachii posterior	radial n.		skin of dorsal aspect of lower half of arm and of forearm
cutaneous n. of thigh, lateral [general sensory]	n. cutaneus femoris lateralis	lumbar plexus—L2–L3		skin of lateral aspect and front of thigh
cutaneous n. of thigh, posterior [general sensory]	n. cutaneus femoris posterior	sacral plexus—S1–S3	inferior clunial mm., perineal branches	skin of inferior gluteal region, back of thigh and leg, external genitalia
digital nn., dorsal, radial. See digital nn. of radial n., dorsal				
digital nn., dorsal, ulnar. See digital nn. of ulnar n., dorsal				
digital nn. of foot, dorsal [general sensory]	nn. digitales dorsales pedis	intermediate dorsal cutaneous n.		adjacent sides of third and fourth, and of fourth and fifth toes
digital nn. of lateral plantar n., plantar, common [general sensory]	nn. digitales plantares communes nervi plantaris lateralis	superficial branch of lateral plantar n.	proper plantar digital nn. of lateral plantar n.	(see distribution of nerves listed under branches)
digital nn. of lateral plantar n., plantar, proper [general sensory]	nn. digitales plantares proprii nervi plantaris lateralis	common plantar digital nn. of lateral plantar n.		lateral plantar surface of foot; plantar and adjacent surfaces of fourth and fifth toes
digital nn. of lateral surface of great toe and of medial surface of second toe, dorsal [general sensory, motor]	nn. digitales dorsales hallucis lateralis et digiti secundi medialis	deep peroneal n.		dorsal interosseous muscles, articulations of ankle and foot, skin of adjacent sides of great and second toes
digital nn. of medial plantar n., plantar, common [general sensory]	nn. digitales plantares communes nervi plantaris medialis	medial plantar n.	proper plantar digital nn. of medial plantar n.	(see distribution of nerves listed under branches)
digital nn. of medial plantar n., plantar, proper [general sensory]	nn. digitales plantares proprii nervi plantaris medialis	common planter digital nn. of medial plantar n.		medial plantar surface of foot; plantar and adjacent surfaces of great and second, and of second and third toes
digital nn. of median n., palmar, common [general sensory]	nn. digitales palmares communes nervi mediani	median n.	proper palmar digital nn. of median n.	(see distribution of nerves listed under branches)
digital nn. of median n., palmar, proper [general sensory]	nn. digitales palmares proprii nervi mediani	common palmar digital nn. of median n.		skin on palmar surface and sides of digits

COMMON NAME [MODALITY]	NA TERM	ORIGIN	BRANCHES	DISTRIBUTION
digital nn. of radial n., dorsal [general sensory]	nn. digitales dorsales nervi radialis	superficial branch of radial n.		ulnar side of thumb, radial side of second finger; adjacent sides of second and third, and of third and fourth fingers
digital nn. of ulnar n., dorsal [general sensory]	nn. digitales dorsales nervi ulnaris	dorsal branch of ulnar n.		skin of ulnar sides of third, fourth and fifth, and of radial sides of fourth and fifth fingers
digital nn. of ulnar n., palmar, common [general sensory]	nn. digitales palmares communes nervi ulnaris	superficial branch of palmar branch of ulnar n.	proper palmar digital nn. of ulnar n.	(see distribution of nerves listed under branches)
digital nn. of ulnar n., palmar, proper [general sensory]	nn. digitales palmares proprii nervi ulnaris	common palmar digital nn. and superficial branch of palmar branch of ulnar n.		skin of adjacent sides of fourth and fifth fingers
dorsal n. of clitoris [general sensory, motor]	n. dorsalis clitoridis	perineal nn.		deep transverse perineal muscle, sphincter muscle of urethra, clitoris
dorsal n. of penis [general sensory, motor]	n. dorsalis penis	perineal nn.		deep transverse perineal muscle, sphincter muscle of urethra, skin of penis
dorsal scapular n. [motor]	n. dorsalis scapulae	brachial plexus—ventral branch of C5		levator scapulae and rhomboid muscles
ethmoidal n., anterior [general sensory]	n. ethmoidalis anterior	nasociliary n., from ophthalmic n.	internal, external, lateral and medial nasal branches	mucosa of nasal septum, lateral wall of nasal cavity, skin of bridge and tip of nose
ethmoidal n., posterior [general sensory]	n. ethmoidalis posterior	nasociliary n., from ophthalmic n.		mucosa of posterior ethmoid cells and of sphenoidal sinus
n. of external acoustic meatus [general sensory]	n. meatus acustici	auriculotemporal n.	branch to tympanic membrane	skin of external acoustic meatus, tympanic membrane
facial n. (7th cranial) [motor, parasympathetic, general sensory, special sensory]	n. facialis	inferior border of pons, between olive and inferior cerebellar peduncle	n. to stapedius; greater petrosal and posterior auricular n.; parotid plexus; digastric, temporal, zygomatic, buccal, lingual, marginal, mandibular and cervical branches, and communicating branch with tympanic plexus	various structures of face, head and neck (see also distribution of individual nerves listed under branches)

English name [modality]	Latin equivalent	Origin	Branches	Distribution
...ossa n. [general sensory]		lumbar plexus—L2-L4	saphenous n., muscular and anterior cutaneous branches	anterior thigh muscles, skin on front and medial aspect of thigh and patella (see also distribution of saphenous n.)
fibular n. See entries under peroneal n.	n. fibularis (official alternative for n. peroneus)			
frontal n. [general sensory]	n. frontalis	ophthalmic n.	supraorbital and supratrochlear nn.	(see distribution of nerves listed under branches)
genitofemoral n. [general sensory, motor]	n. genitofemoralis	lumbar plexus—L1-L2	genital and femoral branches	cremaster muscle, skin of scrotum or labium majus and of adjacent area of thigh and femoral triangle
glossopalatine n. See intermediate n.				
glossopharyngeal n. (9th cranial) [parasympathetic, general sensory, special sensory, visceral sensory]	n. glossopharyngeus	medulla oblongata, lateral to olive	tympanic n., pharyngeal, stylopharyngeal, tonsillar and lingual branches, communicating branch with auricular branch of vagus n.	mucosa of oropharynx, stylopharyngeus muscle, mucosa of palatine tonsil and of adjacent part of soft palate, posterior third of tongue, carotid sinus, carotid body (see also distribution of tympanic n.)
gluteal n., inferior [motor]	n. gluteus inferior	sacral plexus—L5-S2		gluteus maximus muscle
gluteal n., superior [motor]	n. gluteus	sacral plexus—L4-S1		gluteal muscles
hemorrhoidal nn., inferior. See inferior rectal nn., inferior				
hypogastric n.	n. hypogastricus (dexter et sinister)	a nerve trunk situated on either side (right and left), interconnecting superior and inferior hypogastric plexuses		
hypoglossal n. (12th cranial) [motor]	n. hypoglossus	lingual branches between pyramid and olive		styloglossus, hyoglossus and genioglossus muscles, intrinsic muscles of tongue
hypoglossal n., lesser. See lingual n.				
iliohypogastric n. [general sensory]	n. iliohypogastricus	lumbar plexus—T12	lateral and anterior cutaneous branches	skin over side of buttock and over pubis
ilioinguinal n. [general sensory]	n. ilioinguinalis	lumbar plexus—T12-L1	anterior scrotal branches or anterior labial branches	anterior scrotal or anterior labial region
infraoccipital n. See suboccipital n.				

TABLE OF NERVES (Continued)

COMMON NAME [MODALITY]	NA TERM	ORIGIN	BRANCHES	DISTRIBUTION
infraorbital n. [general sensory]	n. infraorbitalis	maxillary n.	middle and anterior superior alveolar, inferior palpebral, internal and external nasal and superior labial branches	incisor, canine and premolar teeth of upper jaw, skin and conjunctiva of lower eyelid, mobile septum and skin of side of nose, mucous membrane of mouth, skin of upper lip
infratrochlear n. [general sensory]	n. infratrochlearis	nasociliary n., from ophthalmic n.	palpebral branches	root and bridge of nose, conjunctiva and skin of lower eyelid, lacrimal duct
intercostobrachial nn. [general sensory]	nn. intercostobrachiales	second and third intercostal nn.		skin on back and medial aspect of arm
intermediate n. [parasympathetic, special sensory]	n. intermedius	a name given to a small part of facial n., between remainder of facial n. and vestibulocochlear n.	greater petrosal n., chorda tympani	lacrimal, nasal, palatine, submandibular and sublingual glands, and anterior two thirds of tongue
interosseous n. of forearm, anterior [motor]	n. interosseous antebrachii anterior	median n.		deep muscles on anterior aspect of forearm
interosseous n. of forearm, posterior [motor]	n. interosseous antebrachii posterior	deep branch of radial n.		abductor pollicis longus, extensor muscles of thumb and second finger
interosseous n. of leg [general sensory]	interosseous cruris	tibial n.		inferior tibiofibular joint, interosseous membrane
ischiadic n. See sciatic n.				
jugular n.	n. jugularis	a name given to sympathetic fibers originating from the superior cervical ganglion and distributed to glossopharyngeal and vagus nn.		
labial nn., anterior [general sensory]	nn. labiales anteriores	ilioinguinal n.		skin of anterior labial region
labial nn., posterior [general sensory]	nn. labiales posteriores	perineal nn.		labium majus
lacrimal n. [general sensory]	n. lacrimalis	ophthalmic n.		lacrimal gland, conjunctiva, lateral commissure of eye, skin of upper eyelid
laryngeal n., inferior [motor]	n. laryngeus inferior	recurrent laryngeal n.		intrinsic muscles of larynx, except cricothyroid muscle

Name	Latin	Origin	Branches	Distribution
laryngeal n., recurrent [parasympathetic, visceral afferent, motor]	n. laryngeus recurrens	vagus n.	inferior laryngeal, tracheal, esophageal and inferior cardiac branches,	tracheal mucosa, esophagus, cardiac plexus (see also distribution of laryngeal n., inferior)
laryngeal n., superior [motor, general sensory; visceral afferent, parasympathetic]	n. laryngeus superior	vagus n.	external and internal branches, branch communicating with inferior laryngeal n.	cricothyroid muscle and inferior constrictor of pharynx, mucosa of epiglottis, base of tongue, larynx
lingual n. [general sensory]	n. lingualis	mandibular n.	sublingual n., lingual branches, branch to isthmus of fauces, branch communicating with hypoglossal n. and chorda tympani	anterior two thirds of tongue, adjacent areas of mouth, gums, isthmus of fauces
lumbar nn.	nn. lumbales	the 5 pairs of nerves that arise from lumbar segments of spinal cord, each pair leaving vertebral column below correspondingly numbered vertebrae; ventral branches of these nerves participate in formation of lumbosacral plexus		
lumbar plexus	plexus lumbalis	fibers from spinal nerves L1–L4		
mandibular n. (third division of trigeminal n.) [general sensory, motor]	n. mandibularis	trigeminal ganglion	meningeal branch, masseteric, deep temporal, lateral and medial pterygoid, buccal, auriculotemporal, lingual and inferior alveolar nn.	meningeal branch—accompanies middle meningeal artery to supply dura mater, helps innervate mucosa of mastoid air cells (see also distribution of other nerves listed under branches)
masseteric n. [motor, general sensory]	n. massetericus	mandibular n.		masseter muscle, temporomandibular joint
maxillary n. (second division of trigeminal n.) [general sensory]	n. maxillaris	trigeminal ganglion	middle meningeal branch, zygomatic n., posterior superior alveolar branches, infraorbital n., pterygopalatine n., nasopalatine n. and other branches of pterygopalatine nn. and ganglion	middle meningeal branch – accompanies middle meningeal artery to supply dura mater; posterior superior alveolar branches – maxillary sinus, molar teeth of upper jaw (see also distribution of other nerves listed under branches)
median n. [general sensory]	n. medianus	brachial plexus – C6–T1 through lateral and medial cords	anterior interosseous n. of forearm, common palmar digital nn., and muscular and palmar branches	muscular branches—most of flexor muscles on front of forearm, most of short muscles of thumb; palmar branch—skin of palm (see also distribution of other nerves listed under branches)

COMMON NAME [MODALITY]	NA TERM	ORIGIN	BRANCHES	DISTRIBUTION
mental n. [general sensory]	n. mentalis	inferior alveolar n.	mental and inferior labial branches	skin of chin, lower lip
musculocutaneous n. [general sensory, motor]	n. musculocutaneus	brachial plexus – C5–C7 through lateral cord	lateral cutaneous n. of forearm, muscular branches	biceps and brachialis muscles, skin of radial side of forearm
mylohyoid n. [motor]	n. mylohyoideus	inferior alveolar n.		mylohyoid muscle, anterior belly of digastric muscle
nasociliary n. [general sensory]	n. nasociliaris	ophthalmic n.	long ciliary, posterior ethmoidal, anterior ethmoidal and infratrochlear nn.	(see distribution of nerves listed under branches)
nasopalatine n. [general sensory]	n. nasopalatinus	pterygopalatine ganglion		mucosa of most of nasal septum and anterior part of hard palate
obturator n. [general sensory, motor]	n. obturatorius	lumbar plexus – L3–L4	anterior and posterior branches	gracilis, adductor brevis and longus muscles, sometimes pectineus; skin of medial side of thigh and leg; knee joint, obturator externus and adductor magnus muscles
occipital n., greater [general sensory, motor]	n. occipitalis major	medial branch of dorsal branch of C2		medial portion of scalp of back of head, semispinalis muscle of head
occipital n., lesser [general sensory]	n. occipitalis minor	cervical plexus – C2–C3		lateral portion of scalp of back of head
occipital n., third [general sensory]	n. occipitalis tertius	medial branch of dorsal branch of C3		skin of upper part of back of neck
oculomotor n. (3rd cranial) [motor, proprioceptive, parasympathetic]	n. oculomotorius	midbrain, at medial border of cerebral peduncle	superior and inferior branches	medial and inferior rectus and inferior oblique muscles of eyeball, ciliary muscles, sphincter of pupil; superior rectus muscle, levator muscle of upper eyelid
olfactory nn. (1st cranial) [special sensory]	nn. olfactorii	olfactory bulb		nasal mucosa
ophthalmic n. (first division of trigeminal n.) [general sensory]	n. ophthalmicus	trigeminal ganglion	tentorial branches, frontal, lacrimal, nasociliary nn.	tentorial branches – dura mater of tentorium cerebelli and falx cerebri (see also distribution of other nerves listed under branches)

Nerve [modality]	Latin term	Origin	Branches	Distribution
optic n. (2nd cranial) [special sensory]	n. opticus	optic chiasm		retina
palatine n., anterior. See palatine n., greater				
palatine n., greater [general sensory]	n. palatinus major	pterygopalatine ganglion	posterior inferior lateral nasal n.	gums, mucosa of soft and hard palates, and of inferior concha
palatine nn., lesser [general sensory]	nn. palatini minores	pterygopalatine ganglion		soft palate, uvula, tonsil
perineal nn. [general sensory, motor]	nn. perineales	pudendal n.	posterior scrotal nn., dorsal n. of penis; posterior labial nn., dorsal n. of clitoris	muscles of urogenital diaphragm, skin of external genitalia
peroneal n., common [general sensory, motor]	n. peroneus communis	sciatic n.	lateral cutaneous n. of calf, superficial and deep peroneal nn.	(see distribution of nerves listed under branches)
peroneal n., deep [general sensory, motor]	n. peroneus profundus	common peroneal n.	muscular branches, dorsal digital nn. of lateral surface of great toe and medial surface of second toe	muscular branches – tibialis anterior, extensor hallucis longus, extensor digitorum longus, peroneus tertius
peroneal n., superficial [general sensory, motor]	n. peroneus superficialis	common peroneal n.	muscular branches, medial and intermediate dorsal cutaneous nn. of foot	muscular branches – peroneus longus and brevis muscles (see also distribution of nerves listed under branches)
petrosal n., deep [sympathetic]	n. petrosus profundus	superior cervical sympathetic ganglion		lacrimal, nasal and palatine glands via internal carotid plexus, nerve of pterygoid canal, and branches of pterygopalatine ganglion
petrosal n., greater [parasympathetic, general sensory]	n. petrosus major	n. intermedius via geniculate ganglion		lacrimal, nasal and palatine glands and nasopharynx via pterygopalatine ganglion and its branches
petrosal n., lesser [parasympathetic]	n. petrosus minor	tympanic plexus of glossopharyngeal n.		otic ganglion and, through communicating branch with auriculotemporal n., parotid gland
phrenic n. [general sensory, motor]	n. phrenicus	cervical plexus – C3-C5	pericardial and phrenico-abdominal branches	diaphragm, pericardium
phrenic nn., accessory	nn. phrenici	contributions of fifth cervical n. to phrenic n. when fifth cervical n. runs separately from rest of phrenic n. throughout a large part of its course		
plantar n., lateral [general sensory]	n. plantaris lateralis	tibial n.	superficial and deep branches	various structures of foot
plantar n., medial [general sensory, motor]	n. plantaris medialis	tibial n.	common plantar digital nn. of medial plantar n.	(see distribution of nerves listed under branches)

COMMON NAME [MODALITY]	NA TERM	ORIGIN	BRANCHES	DISTRIBUTION
pneumogastric n. See vagus n.				
n. to lateral pterygoid [motor]	n. pterygoideus lateralis	mandibular n.		lateral pterygoid muscle
n. to medial pterygoid [motor]	n. pterygoideus	mandibular n.		medial pterygoid muscle
n. of pterygoid canal [parasympathetic, sympathetic, general sensory]	n. canalis pterygoidei	formed by union of deep and greater petrosal nn.		pterygopalatine ganglion and branches
pterygopalatine nn. [general sensory]	nn. pterygopalatini	maxillary n.	nasopalatine and greater and lesser palatine nn., n. of pterygoid canal, orbital, pharyngeal, posterior superior nasal and posterior inferior nasal branches	connect pterygopalatine ganglion with maxillary division of trigeminal n.; branches are usually called "branches of pterygo-palatine ganglion"
pudendal n. [general sensory, motor, parasympathetic]	n. pudendus	sacral plexus – S2–S4	inferior rectal and perineal nn., parasympathetic branches to pelvic viscera	organs of pelvis (see also distribution of nerves listed under branches)
radial n. [general sensory, motor]	n. radialis	brachial plexus – C6–C8, and sometimes C5 and T1, through posterior cord	posterior cutaneous and inferior lateral cutaneous nn. of arm, posterior cutaneous n. of forearm, muscular, deep and superficial branches	arm, forearm and hand (see also distribution of nerves listed under branches)
rectal nn., inferior [general sensory, motor]	nn. rectales inferiores	pudendal n.		sphincter ani externus muscle, skin around anus, lining of anal canal
recurrent n. See laryngeal n., recurrent				
saccular n.	n. saccularis	the branch of vestibular part of eighth cranial (vestibulo-cochlear) nerve that innervates macula of saccule		
sacral nn.	nn. sacrales	the 5 pairs of nerves that arise from sacral segments of spinal cord; the ventral branches of first 4 pairs participate in formation of sacral plexus		
sacral plexus	plexus sacralis	fibers from spinal nerves L4–L5, S1–S4		

Name	Latin	Origin	Branches	Distribution
saphenous n. [general sensory]	n. saphenus	femoral n.	infrapatellar and medial crural cutaneous branches	skin of medial aspect of leg and foot
sciatic n. [general sensory]	n. ischiadicus	sacral plexus – L4-S3	common peroneal and tibial nn.	(see distribution of nerves listed under branches)
scrotal nn., anterior [general sensory]	mn. scrotales anteriores	ilioinguinal r.		skin of anterior scrotal region
scrotal nn., posterior [general sensory]	mn. scrotales posteriores	perineal nn.		skin of scrotum
spinal nn. [general sensory]	mn. spinales	the 31 pairs of nerves that arise from spinal cord, including 8 cervical, 12 thoracic, 5 lumbar, 5 sacral and one coccygeal		
splanchnic n., greater [preganglionic sympathetic, visceral afferent]	n. splanchnicus major	thoracic ganglia T5-T10 of sympathetic trunk		celiac ganglion
splanchnic n., lesser [preganglionic sympathetic, visceral afferent]	n. splanchnicus minor	ganglia T9, T10 of sympathetic trunk	renal branch	aorticorenal ganglion
splanchnic n., lowest [sympathetic, visceral afferent]	n. splarchnicus imus	last ganglion of sympathetic trunk, or lesser splanchnic n.		renal plexus
splanchnic nn., lumbar [preganglionic sympathetic, visceral afferent]	mn. splanchnici lumbales	lumbar ganglia of sympathetic trunk		celiac, mesenteric and hypogastric plexuses
splanchnic nn., pelvic [preganglionic, parasympathetic, visceral afferent]	nn. splanchnici pelvini	S2-S4		terminal ganglia in pelvic viscera
splanchnic nn., sacral [preganglionic sympathetic, visceral afferent]	nn. splarchnici sacrales	sacral part of sympathetic trunk		inferior hypogastric plexus
n. to stapedius [motor]	n. to stapedius	facial n.		stapedius muscle
subclavian n. [motor, general sensory]	n. subclavius	brachial plexus – C5-C6 through superior trunk		subclavius muscle, sternoclavicular joint
subcostal n. [generally sensory, motor]	n. subcostalis	twelfth thoracic n.		abdominal muscles, skin of lower part of abdomen and gluteal region
sublingual n. [general sensory]	n. sublingualis	lingual n.		region of sublingual gland
suboccipital n. [motor]	n. suboccipitalis	C1		straight and oblique muscles of neck

TABLE OF NERVES (*Continued*)

COMMON NAME [MODALITY]	NA TERM	ORIGIN	BRANCHES	DISTRIBUTION
subscapular n. [motor]	n. subscapularis	brachial plexus–C5 through posterior cord		subscapularis and teres major muscles
supraclavicular nn., anterior. *See* supraclavicular nn., medial				
supracavicular nn., intermediate [general sensory]	mn. supraclaviculares intermedii	cervical plexus–C3–C4		skin over pectoral and deltoid regions
supraclavicular nn., lateral [general sensory]	mn. supraclaviculares laterales	cervical plexus–C3–C4		skin of superior and posterior aspects of shoulder
supraclavicular nn., medial [general sensory]	mn. supraclaviculares mediales	cervical plexus–C3–C4		skin of medial infraclavicular region
supraclavicular nn., middle. *See* supraclavicular nn., intermediate				
supraclavicular nn., posterior. *See* supraclavicular nn., lateral				
supraorbital n. [general sensory]	n. supraorbitalis	frontal n., from ophthalmic n.	lateral and medial branches	skin of upper eyelid, forehead, anterior part of scalp (to vertex), mucosa of frontal sinus
suprascapular n. [motor, general sensory]	n. suprascapularis	brachial plexus–C5–C6 through superior trunk		supraspinatus and infraspinatus muscles, shoulder joint
supratrochlear n. [general sensory]	n. supratrochlearis	frontal n., from ophthalmic n.		medial part of forehead, root of nose, medial commissure of eye, conjunctiva, upper eyelid
sural n. [general sensory]	n. suralis	medial and lateral cutaneous nn.	lateral dorsal cutaneous n. of foot, lateral calcanean branches	skin on back of leg and lateral side of foot and heel
temporal nn., deep [motor]	mn. temporales profundi	mandibular n.		temporal muscles
n. to tensor tympani [motor]	n. tensoris tympani	mandibular n. via otic ganglion		tensor tympani muscle
n. to tensor veli palatini [motor]	n. tensoris veli palatini	mandibular n. via otic ganglion		tensor veli palatini muscle
thoracic nn.	mn. thoracici	the 12 pairs of spinal nerves that arise from thoracic segments of spinal cord, each pair leaving vertebral column below corresponding vertebra		body wall of thorax and upper part of abdomen

thoracic n., long [motor]	n. thoracicus longus	brachial plexus – ventral branches of C5–C7	serratus anterior muscle
thoracodorsal n. [motor]	n. thoracodorsalis	brachial plexus – C7–C8 through posterior cord	latissimus dorsi muscle
tibial n. [general sensory, motor]	n. tibialis	sciatic n.	interosseous n. of leg, medial cutaneous n. of calf, sural and medial and lateral plantar nn., and muscular and medial calcanean branches — leg and foot
trigeminal n. (5th cranial)	n. trigeminus	emerges from lateral surface of pons as a motor and a sensory root, the latter expanding into trigeminal ganglion, from which the 3 divisions of nerve arise (see mandibular n., maxillary n. and ophthalmic n.)	
trochlear n. (4th cranial) [motor, proprioceptive]	n. trochlearis	midbrain, below colliculus	superior oblique muscle of eyeball
tympanic n. [general sensory, parasympathetic]	n. tympanicus	glossopharyngeal n	helps form tympanic plexus — tympanic cavity, tympanic membrane, mastoid air cells, auditory tube
ulnar n. [general sensory, motor]	n. ulnaris	brachial plexus – C7–T1 through medial and lateral cords	muscular, palmar cutaneous, dorsal, palmar, superficial and deep branches — arm and hand
utricular n.	n. utricularis	the branch of vestibular part of eighth cranial (vestibulocochlear) nerve that innervates macula of utricle	
utriculoampullary n.	n. utriculoampullaris	a nerve that arises by peripheral division of vestibular part of eighth cranial (vestibulocochlear) nerve, and supplies utricle and ampullae of semicircular ducts	
vaginal nn. [sympathetic, parasympathetic]	nn. vaginales	uterovaginal plexus from sacral part of sympathetic trunk and parasympathetic branches from pudendal n.	vagina
vagus n. (10th cranial) [parasympathetic, visceral afferent, motor, general sensory]	n. vagus (L. "wandering")	medulla oblongata, lateral to olive	superior and recurrent laryngeal nn., meningeal, auricular, pharyngeal, inferior and superior cardiac, bronchial, anterior and posterior gastric, hepatic, celiac and renal branches — various organs (see also distribution of nerves listed under branches)
vertebral n. [sympathetic]	n. vertebralis	cervicothoracic ganglion	posterior cranial fossa via vertebral plexus

437

TABLE OF NERVES (Concluded)

COMMON NAME [MODALITY]	NA TERM	ORIGIN	BRANCHES	DISTRIBUTION
vestibular n. See vestibulo- cochlear n. vestibulocochlear n. (8th cranial)	n. vestibulocochlearis	emerges from brain between pons and medulla oblongata, be- hind facial nerve; it consists of 2 sets of fibers, the vestib- ular part and the cochlear part, and is connected with the brain by corresponding superior and inferior roots		
vidian n. See n. of pterygoid canal vidian n., deep. See petrosal n., deep zygomatic n. [general sensory]	n. zygomaticus	maxillary n.	zygomaticofacial and zygo- maticotemporal branches	skin over zygomatic bone and in anterior temporal region

spinal cord or brain. **somatic n's,** the sensory and motor nerves. **spinal n.,** one of the 31 pairs of nerves arising from the spinal cord and passing out between the vertebrae, including eight cervical, twelve thoracic, five lumbar, five sacral and one coccygeal. **splanchnic n's,** those of the blood vessels and viscera. **sudomotor n's,** those that control sweating. **sympathetic n.,** any nerve of the sympathetic system. **thermic n., thermogenic n.,** calorific nerve. **trisplanchnic n.,** a general name for the system of sympathetic nerves. **trophic n.,** one concerned with regulation of nutrition. **vasoconstrictor n.,** one whose stimulation contracts blood vessels. **vasodilator n.,** one whose stimulation dilates blood vessels. **vasomotor n.,** one concerned in controlling the caliber of vessels. **vasosensory n.,** any nerve supplying sensory fibers to the vessels.

nervimotor (ner″vĭ-mo′tor) pertaining to a motor nerve.

nervone (ner′vōn) a cerebroside containing nervonic acid.

nervous (ner′vus) 1. pertaining to a nerve or nerves. 2. unduly excitable.

nervousness (ner′vus-nes) morbid or undue excitability.

nervus (ner′vus), pl. *ner′vi* [L.] nerve.

Nesacaine (nes′ah-kān) trademark for preparations of chloroprocaine.

network (net′werk) a structure formed by interlacing fibers. **Gerlach's n.,** a fibrous structure in the gray substance of the cord.

neur(o)- (nu′ro) word element [Gr.], *nerve.*

neurad (nu′rad) toward the neural axis or aspect.

neural (nu′ral) pertaining to nerves.

neuralgia (nu-ral′je-ah) pain in a nerve. adj., **neural′gic. alveolar n.,** pain in an alveolus from which the tooth has been extracted. **degenerative n.,** neuralgia occurring in advanced age, and marked by signs of degeneration in the central nervous system. **epileptiform n.,** trifacial neuralgia. **n. facia′lis ve′ra,** geniculate neuralgia. **Fothergill's n.,** neuralgia of the trigeminal nerve. **geniculate n.,** neuralgia involving the geniculate ganglion. **Hunt's n.,** geniculate neuralgia. **idiopathic n.,** neuralgia not accompanied by any structural change. **intercostal n.,** neuralgia of the intercostal nerves, causing pain in the side. **mammary n.,** neuralgic pain in the breast. **Morton's n.,** metatarsalgia. **nasociliary n.,** pain in the eyes, brow, and root of the nose. **otic n.,** geniculate neuralgia. **red n.,** erythromelalgia. **trifacial n., trigeminal n.,** neuralgia due to involvement of the trigeminal nerve, and marked by pain along the course of the nerve. **vidian n.,** neuralgia affecting the vidian nerve.

neuranagenesis (nu″ran-ah-jen′e-sis) regeneration of nerve tissue.

neurapophysis (nu″rah-pof′ĭ-sis) structure forming either side of the neural arch.

neurapraxia (-prak′se-ah) a nerve lesion producing paralysis in the absence of peripheral degeneration.

neurarthropathy (nūr″ar-throp′ah-the) combined disease of joints and nerves.

neurasthenia (nu″ras-the′ne-ah) excessive fatigue of neurotic origin. **cerebral n.,** a form characterized by mental and visual disturbances and other head symptoms. **gastric n.,** a form marked by functional stomach complications. **sexual n.,** a form associated with disorders of sexual function. **traumatic n.,** neurasthenia following shock or injury.

neurataxia (nu″rah-tak′se-ah) neurasthenia.

neuratrophia (-tro′fe-ah) impaired nutrition of nervous system.

neuraxis (nu-rak′sis) 1. the cerebrospinal axis. 2. axon.

neuraxitis (nu-rak-si′tis) encephalitis. **epidemic n.,** epidemic encephalitis.

neuraxon (nu-rak′son) axon.

neure (nūr) a neuron.

neurectasia (nu″rek-ta′ze-ah) stretching of a nerve, to relieve pain.

neurectasis (nu-rek′tah-sis) neurectasia.

neurectomy (nu-rek′to-me) excision of a nerve.

neurectopia (nu″rek-to′pe-ah) displacement of a nerve.

neurergic (nu-rer′jik) pertaining to nerve action.

neurexeresis (nūr″ek-ser-e′sis) the tearing out of a nerve.

neurilemma (nu″rĭ-lem′ah) the sheath of a nerve fiber.

neurilemmitis (-le-mi′tis) inflammation of neurilemma.

neurilemoma (-le-mo′mah) a tumor of a peripheral nerve sheath.

neurinoma (-no′mah) a nodular enlargement or tumor on a peripheral nerve.

neurinomatosis (-no″mah-to′sis) the presence of multiple neurinomas.

neurite (nu′rīt) axon.

neuritis (nu-ri′tis) pl. *neurit′ides,* inflammation of a nerve. adj., **neurit′ic. ascending n.,** that which progresses toward the central nervous system. **axial n.,** inflammation of central part of a nerve. **degenerative n.,** neuritis marked by degeneration of the parenchyma. **descending n.,** that which progresses toward the periphery. **endemic n.,** beriberi. **facial n.,** Bell's palsy. **interstitial n.,** inflammation of the connective tissue of a nerve trunk. **multiple n.,** neuritis affecting several nerves at once. **optic n.,** inflammation of the optic nerve. **parenchymatous n.,** neuritis affecting primarily the medullary substance and axons. **peripheral n.,** neuritis of the terminal nerves. **postocular n., retrobulbar n.,** inflammation of that part of the optic nerve posterior to the eyeball. **toxic n.,** neuritis due to some poison. **traumatic n.,** neuritis due to injury.

neuroanastomosis (nu″ro-ah-nas″to-mo′sis) surgical anastomosis of one nerve to another.

neuroanatomy (-ah-nat′o-me) anatomy of the nervous system.

neuroarthropathy (-ar-throp′ah-the) joint disease associated with disease of the central nervous system.

neurobiology (nu″ro-bi-ol′o-je) biology of the nervous system.

neurobiotaxis (-bi″o-tak′sis) the alleged tendency of bodies and dendrites of nerve cells to grow toward the source of their stimulation. adj., **neurobiotac′tic.**

neuroblast (nu′ro-blast) an embryonic cell from which nervous tissue is formed.

neuroblastoma (nu″ro-blas-to′mah) a tumor made up of neuroblasts. **n. sympath′icum,** a tumor of sympathetic nerve cell origin.

neurobrucellosis (-broo″sĕ-lo′sis) brucellosis with severe neurologic complications.

neurocanal (-kah-nal′) the central canal of the spinal cord.

neurocardiac (-kar′de-ak) pertaining to the nerves of the heart.

neurocele (nu′ro-sēl) the neural canal.

neurocentrum (nu″ro-sen′trum) one of the embryonic vertebral elements from which the spinous processes of the vertebrae develop. adj., **neurocen′tral.**

neuroceptor (nu′ro-sep″tor) one of the terminal elements of a dendrite which receives the stimulus from the neuromittor of the adjoining neuron.

neurochemistry (nu″ro-kem′is-tre) scientific study of chemical processes taking place in the nervous system.

neurochondrite (-kon′drīt) an embryonic cartilaginous element which develops into the neural arch of the vertebra.

neurochorioretinitis (-ko″re-o-ret″ĭ-ni′tis) inflammation of optic nerve, choroid and retina.

neurochoroiditis (-ko″roi-di′tis) inflammation of the optic nerve and choroid.

neurocirculatory (-cer′ku-lah-to″re) pertaining to the nervous and circulatory systems.

neurocladism (nu-rok′lah-dizm) the formation of new branches by the process of a neuron.

neuroclonic (nu″ro-klon′ik) marked by nervous spasm.

neurocranium (-kra′ne-um) the part of the cranium enclosing the brain. adj., **neurocra′nial.**

neurocutaneous (-ku-ta′ne-us) pertaining to nerves and skin.

neurocyte (nu′ro-sīt) a nerve cell of any kind.

neurocytology (nu″ro-si-tol′o-je) scientific study of cellular components of the nervous system.

neurocytoma (-si-to′mah) a brain tumor consisting of undifferentiated nerve cells of nervous origin (neural epithelium).

neurodendrite (-den′drīt) dendrite.

neurodendron (-den′dron) dendrite.

neurodermatitis (-der″mah-ti′tis), pl. *neurodermatit′ides* [Gr.] a chronic, itching, lichenoid eruption of the skin due to emotional disorder. **n. dissemina′ta,** atopic eczema.

neurodermatosis (-der″mah-to′sis) a skin disease of nervous origin.

neurodiagnosis (-di″ag-no′sis) diagnosis of neurologic diseases.

neurodynamic (-di-nam′ik) pertaining to nervous energy.

neurodynia (nu″ro-din′e-ah) pain in a nerve.

neuroelectricity (-e″lek-tris′ĭ-te) electric current generated in the nervous system.

neuroencephalomyelopathy (-en-sef″ah-lo-mi″ĕ-lop′ah-the) disease involving nerves, brain and spinal cord.

neuroepithelioma (-ep″ĭ-the″le-o′mah) neurocytoma.

neuroepithelium (-ep″ĭ-the′le-um) epithelium containing cells that receive and transmit nerve impulses.

neurofibril (-fi′bril) one of the delicate threads traversing the cytoplasm of nervous cells in every direction.

neurofibrilla (-fi-bril′ah) neurofibril.

neurofibroma (-fi-bro′mah) a connective tissue tumor of the nerve fiber fasciculus.

neurofibromatosis (-fi″bro-mah-to′sis) a familial condition characterized by developmental changes in the nervous system, muscles, bones and skin, and marked by the formation of neurofibromas over the entire body associated with areas of pigmentation.

neurofibrositis (-fi″bro-si′tis) inflammation of muscle fibers involving sensory nerve filaments.

neurogenesis (-jen′ĕ-sis) formation of the nervous system in embryonic development.

neurogenic (-jen′ik) forming nervous tissue, or generating nervous energy.

neurogenous (nu-roj′ĕ-nus) arising from the nervous system.

neuroglia (nu-rog′le-ah) the supporting structure of the brain and spinal cord.

neurogliocyte (nu-rog′le-o-sīt″) one of the cells composing the neuroglia.

neuroglioma (nu″ro-gli-o′mah) glioma in which there are nerve cells. **n. gangliona′re,** glioma in which ganglion cells are embedded.

neurogliosis (nu-rog″le-o′sis) a condition marked by numerous neurogliomas.

neurogram (nu′ro-gram) the imprint left on the brain by past mental experiences.

neurohistology (nu″ro-his-tol′o-je) histology of the nervous system.

neurohormone (nu′ro-hor″mōn) a hormone stimulating the neural mechanism.

neurohumor (nu″ro-hu′mor) a chemical substance secreted by a neuron. adj., **neurohu′-moral.**

neurohypophysis (-hi-pof′ĭ-sis) the pars nervosa, or main part of the posterior lobe of the hypophysis cerebri. adj., **neurohypophys′eal.**

neuroid (nu′roid) resembling a nerve.

neuro-induction (nu″ro-in-duk′shun) mental suggestion.

neurokeratin (-ker′ah-tin) a scleroprotein present in neuroglia fibrils (supporting elements) of nervous tissue.

neurolemma (-lem′ah) a thin membrane spirally enwrapping myelin layers of myelinated nerves or axons of unmyelinated nerves.

neurolemmitis (-lĕ-mi′tis) inflammation of the neurolemma.

neurolemmoma (-lĕ-mo′mah) a tumor of a peripheral nerve sheath.

neuroleptic (nu″ro-lep′tik) 1. producing symptoms resembling those of disorders of the nervous system. 2. an agent that produces symptoms resembling those of nervous system disorders.

neurolipomatosis (-lĭ-po″mah-to′sis) a condition characterized by the formation of multiple fat deposits, with involvement of the nervous system because of pressure on the nerves. **n. doloro′sa,** adiposis dolorosa.

neurologist (nu-rol′o-jist) a specialist in neurology.

neurology (nu-rol′o-je) scientific study of the nervous system, its functions and its disorders. adj., **neurolog′ic. clinical n.,** that especially concerned with the diagnosis and treatment of disorders of the nervous system.

neurolysis (nu-rol′i-sis) 1. liberation of a nerve from adhesions. 2. relief of tension upon a nerve obtained by stretching. 3. exhaustion of nervous energy. adj., **neurolyt′ic.**

neuroma (nu-ro′mah) a bulbous enlargement on a nerve made up of a tangled skein of interlacing fibers. adj., **neurom′atous. amputation n.,** one formed at the end of a nerve severed in amputation of a limb. **amyelinic n.,** one containing only nonmedullated nerve fibers. **n. cu′tis,** neuroma in the skin. **cystic n.,** a false neuroma, or a neuroma which has become cystic. **false n.,** one which does not contain genuine nerve fibers. **ganglionated n., ganglionic n.,** one composed of true nerve cells. **myelinic n.,** one containing medullated nerve fibers. **plexiform n.,** one marked by multiple nodular enlargements along the course of the cutaneous nerves. **n. telangiecto′des,** one containing an excess of blood vessels.

neuromalacia (nu″ro-mah-la′she-ah) softening of the nerves.

neuromechanism (-mek′ah-nizm) the nervous regulation of the function of an organ.

neuromere (nu′ro-mēr) one of the segments of the cerebrospinal axis in the developing embryo.

neuromittor (nu″ro-mit′or) one of the terminal ends of a neuron which transfers a stimulus to the neuroceptor of the adjoining neuron.

neuromuscular (-mus′ku-ler) pertaining to the nerves and muscles.

neuromyal (-mi′al) neuromuscular.

neuromyelitis (-mi″ĕ-li′tis) inflammation of the nerves and spinal cord.

neuromyositis (-mi″o-si′tis) neuritis blended with myositis.

neuron (nu′ron) one of the units making up the nervous system, having a cell body, nucleus and cell membrane. adj., **neuro′nal, neuron′ic. afferent n.,** one which conducts a nervous impulse from a receptor to a center. **connector n.,** one whose dendrites and axon both synapse with other neurons. **efferent n.,** one which conducts a nervous impulse from a center to an organ of response. **motor n.,** any neuron having a motor function; an efferent neuron conveying motor impulses. **sensory n.,** any neuron having a sensory function; an afferent neuron conveying sensory impulses.

neuronitis (nu″ro-ni′tis) inflammation of a neuron.

neuronophage (nu-ron′o-fāj) a phagocyte which destroys nerve cells.

neuronophagia (nu″ron-o-fa′je-ah) phagocytic destruction of nerve cells.

neuronyxis (nu″ro-nik′sis) surgical puncture of a nerve.

neuropapillitis (-pap″ĭ-li′tis) optic neuritis.

neuroparalysis (-pah-ral′ĭ-sis) paralysis due to disease of a nerve or nerves.

neuropathogenicity (-path″o-jĕ-nis′ĭ-te) the quality of producing or the ability to produce pathologic changes in nerve tissue.

neuropathology (pah-thol′o-je) pathology of diseases of the nervous system.

neuropathy (nu-rop′ah-the) any disease of the nervous system, especially a degenerative (noninflammatory) disease of a nerve or nerves. adj., **neuropath′ic. diabetic n.,** a disease of the posterior nerve roots and posterior columns of the spinal cord occurring in diabetes. **ischemic n.,** nerve degeneration due to circulatory obstruction. **progressive hypertrophic interstitial n.,** a familial disease characterized by chronic interstitial neuritis, hypertrophy of the peripheral nerves and posterior roots and sclerosis of the posterior columns.

neurophage (nu′ro-fāj) neuronophage.

neuropharmacology (nu″ro-far″mah-kol′o-je) scientific study of the effects of drugs on the nervous system.

neurophthisis (nu-rof′thĭ-sis) wasting of nerve tissue.

neurophysiology (nu″ro-fiz″e-ol′o-je) physiology of nervous system.

neuropil (nu′ro-pīl) a feltwork in nerve tissue formed by interlacing arborizations of dendrites and telodendria.

neuroplasm (nu′ro-plazm) the protoplasm of a nerve cell. adj., **neuroplas′mic.**

neuroplasty (nu′ro-plas″te) plastic repair of a nerve.

neuropodium (nu″ro-po′de-um) a bullous termination of an axon in a synapse.

neuropore (nu′ro-pōr) an opening in the neural tube of the developing embryo. **anterior n.,** the embryonic opening in the anterior portion of the forebrain, which closes at the 20-somite stage. **posterior n.,** the embryonic opening at the posterior end of the neural tube, which closes by about the 25-somite stage.

neuropotential (nu″ro-po-ten′shal) nerve energy; nerve potential.

neuropsychiatrist (-si-ki′ah-trist) a specialist in neuropsychiatry.

neuropsychiatry (-si-ki′ah-tre) a branch of medicine combining neurology and psychiatry.

neuropsychopathy (-si-kop′ah-the) a combined nervous and mental disease.

neuropsychosis (-si-ko′sis) nervous disease complicated with mental disorder; a psychosis.

neuroradiology (nu″ro-ra″de-ol′o-je) the branch of radiography concerned especially with visualization of the contents of the skull and vertebral column.

neurorecidive (-res″ĭ-dēv′) neurorelapse.

neurorecurrence (-re-ker′ens) neurorelapse.

neuroregulation (-reg″u-la′shun) regulation and control of nervous activity.

neurorelapse (nu″ro-re-laps″) acute nervous symptoms following treatment for syphilis.

neuroretinitis (nu″ro-ret″ĭ-ni′tis) inflammation of optic nerve and retina.

neuroretinopathy (-nop′ah-the) pathologic involvement of the optic disk and retina.

neurorrhaphy (nu-ror′ah-fe) suture of a divided nerve.

neuroroentgenography (nu″ro-rent″gen-og′rah-fe) neuroradiology.

neurosarcoma (-sar-ko′mah) a sarcoma with neuromatous elements.

neurosclerosis (-skle-ro′sis) hardening of nerve tissue.

neurosecretion (-se-kre′shun) secretory activities of nerve cells.

neurosensory (-sen′so-re) pertaining to a sensory nerve.

neurosis (nu-ro′sis) a mild emotional disturbance characterized by severe anxiety or exaggerated defenses, with personality and contact with reality relatively intact. adj., **neurot′ic. accident n.,** a neurosis with hysterical symptoms caused by accident or injury. **anxiety n.,** a chronic reaction pattern of emotional illness, characterized primarily by direct subjective experiencing of anxiety. **cardiac n.,** neurocirculatory asthenia. **character n.,** a neurosis in which certain personality traits have become exaggerated or overdeveloped. **combat n.,** a neurosis resulting from battle experiences and conditions of military life. **compensation n.,** a neurosis following injury and motivated in part by prospects of financial compensation. **compulsive n.,** an urge to perform unacceptable or senseless acts. **conversion n.,** a neurosis characterized by disorders of the motility, sensation or other organic systems of the body. **experimental n.,** a neurosis produced by deliberate exposure to biological or psychologic stress. **obsessional n.,** compulsive neurosis. **occupational n.,** a neurosis in which the symptoms are related to the patient's occupation and interfere with its pursuit. **traumatic n.,** a neurosis resulting from an injury. **vegetative n.,** erythredema polyneuropathy. **Westphal's n.,** hysteria with symptoms simulating multiple sclerosis.

neuroskeletal (nu″ro-skel′ĕ-tal) pertaining to nervous tissue and skeletal muscular tissue.

neuroskeleton (-skel′ĕ-ton) endoskeleton.

neurosome (nu′ro-sōm) 1. the body of a nerve cell. 2. a small particle in the ground substance of the protoplasm of neurons.

neurospasm (nu′ro-spazm) nervous twitching of a muscle.

neurospongioma (nu″ro-spun″je-o′mah) neuroglioma.

neurospongium (-spun′je-um) 1. the fibrillar component of neurons. 2. a meshwork of nerve fibrils.

Neurospora (nu-ros′po-rah) a genus of molds capable of converting tryptophan to nicotinic acid.

neurosurgery (nu″ro-ser′jer-e) surgery of the nervous system.

neurosuture (nu′ro-su″tūr) neurorrhaphy.

neurosyphilis (nu″ro-sif′ĭ-lus) syphilis of the nervous system. **paretic n.,** dementia paralytica.

neurotension (-ten′shun) neurectasia.

neurothecitis (-the-si′tis) inflammation of a nerve sheath.

neurotherapy (-ther′ah-pe) 1. the treatment of nervous disorders. 2. psychotherapy.

neurothlipsis (-thlip′sis) pressure on a nerve.

neuroticism (nu-rot′ĭ-sizm) perverted or excessive nervous action.

neurotization (nu-rot″ĭ-za′shun) regeneration of a nerve after its division.

neurotmesis (nu″rot-me′sis) damage to a nerve, producing complete division of all the essential structures.

neurotomy (nu-rot′o-me) dissection or cutting of nerves.

neurotony (nu-rot′o-ne) stretching of a nerve.

neurotoxicity (nu″ro-tok-sis′ĭ-te) the quality of exerting a destructive or poisonous effect upon nerve tissue. adj., **neurotox′ic.**

neurotoxin (-tok′sin) an exotoxin characterized by a marked affinity for nerve tissue.

neurotrauma (-traw′mah) wounding of a nerve.

neurotripsy (nu′ro-trip″se) crushing or bruising of a nerve.

neurotrophy (nu-rot′ro-fe) nutrition of nerve tissue. adj., **neurotroph′ic.**

neurotropism (nu-rot′ro-pizm) 1. the quality of having a special affinity for nervous tissue. 2. the alleged tendency of regenerating nerve fibers to grow toward specific portions of the periphery. adj., **neurotrop′ic.**

neurovascular (nu″ro-vas′ku-ler) both nervous and vascular.

neurovirulence (-vir′u-lens) the competence of an infectious agent to produce pathologic effects on the nervous system. adj., **neurovir′ulent.**

neurovisceral (-vis′er-al) pertaining to the cerebrospinal and the parasympathetic nervous system.

neurula (nu′roo-lah) the third stage of development in the embryo, marked by first appearance of elements of the nervous system.

neurulation (nu″roo-la′shun) formation in the early embryo of the neural plate, followed by its closure with development of the neural tube.

neutral (nu′tral) neither basic nor acid.

neutralism (nu′tral-izm) the absence of interaction between coexisting organisms of different species.

neutralize (nu′tral-īz) to counteract and thereby destroy acid or alkaline qualities.

Neutrapen (nu′trah-pen) trademark for a lyophilized preparation of penicillinase.

neutrino (nu-tre′no) a hypothetical elementary

particle with an extremely small mass and no electric charge.

neutrocyte (nu'tro-sīt) a neutrophil leukocyte.

neutrocytopenia (nu"tro-si"to-pe'ne-ah) neutropenia.

neutrocytophilia (-fil'e-ah) neutrophilia.

neutrocytosis (nu"tro-si-to'sis) neutrophilia.

neutroflavine (-fla'vin) acriflavine.

neutron (nu'tron) an elementary particle of neutral or zero electrical charge and of mass number 1; considered to be a constituent particle of all nuclei of mass number greater than 1.

neutropenia (nu"tro pe'ne-ah) diminished number of neutrophils in the blood. **chronic n. of childhood,** a condition in which granulocytopenia, recurrent infections, lymphadenopathy and hepatosplenomegaly may be present for a considerable time, with subsequent spontaneous remission. **chronic hypoplastic n.,** a syndrome resembling primary splenic neutropenia, but with hypocellular bone marrow. **cyclic n.,** diminution or disappearance of neutrophils of circulating blood occurring at regular intervals. **hypersplenic n.,** deficiency of neutrophils in the blood as the result of increased peripheral destruction. **periodic n.,** cyclic neutropenia. **idiopathic n., malignant n.,** agranulocytosis. **peripheral n.,** decrease of neutrophils in the circulating blood. **primary splenic n.,** a syndrome marked by splenomegaly, destruction of granular leukocytes of the blood, and overactive bone marrow.

neutrophil (nu'tro-fil) a medium-sized leukocyte, with a three- to five-lobed nucleus, and cytoplasm containing small granules which stain a pale lavender, normally constituting 60-70 per cent of the leukocytes of the blood. **filamented n.,** a neutrophilic leukocyte which has two or more lobes connected by a filament of chromatin. **nonfilamented n.,** a neutrophilic leukocyte whose lobes are connected by thick strands of chromatin. **rod n., stab n.,** a neutrophilic leukocyte whose nucleus is not divided into segments.

neutrophilia (nu"tro-fil'e-ah) 1. the quality of being neutrophilic. 2. increase in the neutrophilic leukocytes of the blood.

neutrophilic (-fil'ik) 1. stainable by neutral dyes. 2. neither anthropophilic nor zoophilic; said of certain mosquitoes.

nevoid (ne'void) resembling a nevus.

nevoxanthoendothelioma (ne"vo-zan"tho-en"do-the"le-o'mah) a condition in which groups of yellow-brown papules or nodules occur on the extensor surfaces of the extremities of infants.

Nevskia (nev'ske-ah) a genus of Schizomycetes (order Pseudomonadales, suborder Pseudomonadineae, family Caulobacteraceae).

nevus (ne'vus), pl. *ne'vi* [L.] a small, flat, elevated or pedunculated tumor of the skin, pigmented or nonpigmented, and with or without hair growth, characterized by a specific type of cell. **n. arachnoi'deus, n. araneo'sus, n. ara'neus,** one composed of dilated blood vessels radiating from a point in branches resembling the legs of a spider. **blue n.,** a papular to nodular solitary growth composed of masses of dermal melanoblasts in the cutis, developing in childhood, and occurring on the face, forearms or hands. **capillary n.,** one that involves the skin capillaries. **n. caverno'sus,** cavernous angioma, **n. flam'meus,** a single or multiple, localized or extensive, dull red, nonraised lesion, characterized by dilatation and increase in number of capillaries in the dermis. **hairy n.,** a more or less pigmented nevus with hairs growing from its surface. **n. lipomato'sus,** one which contains a mass of fat. **n. of Ota,** dermal melanocytic pigmentation of the side of the face, involving also the sclera, ocular muscles, retrobulbar fat and sometimes the periosteum of the orbit. **n. pigmento'sus,** a congenital dark-colored spot on the skin. **sebaceous n.,** a benign sebaceous tumor with highly differentiated cells, found after middle age and sometimes simulating early basal cell carcinoma. **sebaceous n. of Jadassohn,** a congenital tumor of sebaceous glands, present at birth and appearing as a single, slightly raised, firm, yellow plaque on the face or scalp. **spider n.,** nevus arachnoideus. **n. spi'lus,** a smooth, flat mole. **n. spongio'sus al'bus,** a white spongy nevus. **n. uni'us latera'lis,** an epithelial nevus occurring as a transverse band around one side of the trunk. **n. vasculo'sus,** an elevated nodule, usually soft, bright red, and from a few millimeters to several centimeters in diameter, apparent soon after birth. **venous n.,** one composed mainly of veins.

N.F. National Formulary, a publication of the American Pharmaceutical Association, revised at five-year intervals, establishing official standards for therapeutically useful drugs; National Foundation.

N.F.L.P.N. National Federation for Licensed Practical Nurses.

ng. nanogram.

N.H.I. National Heart Institute.

N.H.M.R.C. National Health and Medical Research Council.

Ni chemical symbol, *nickel.*

niacin (ni'ah-sin) nicotinic acid.

niacinamide (ni"ah-sin-am'mīd) a white, crystalline powder, the amide of nicotinic acid; used in prophylaxis and prevention of pellagra.

NIAID National Institute of Allergy and Infectious Diseases.

nialamide (ni-al'ah-mīd) a monoamine oxidase inhibitor with antidepressive action, used in psychoses.

NIAMD National Institute of Arthritis and Metabolic Diseases.

Niamid (ni'ah-mid) trademark for a preparation of nialamide.

niche (nich) a small recess, depression or indentation, especially a recess in the wall of a hollow organ which tends to retain contrast media, as revealed by roentgenography. **Barclay's n.,** a deformity of the cap in the roentgenogram in duodenal ulcer. **ecologic n.,** the place of an organism within its community or ecosystem. **enamel n.,** either of two depressions between the dental lamina and the developing tooth germ, one pointing distally (*distal enamel niche*) and the other mesially (*mesial enamel niche*). **Haudek's n.,** a budlike deformity of the stomach contour in the roentgenogram in perforating gastric ulcer.

NICHHD National Institute of Child Health and Human Development.

nickel (nik'el) chemical element (*see table*), at. no. 28, symbol Ni.

Niconyl (ni'ko-nil) trademark for a preparation of isoniazid.

nicotinamide (nik″o-tin'ah-mīd) niacinamide.

nicotine (nik'o-tēn, nik'o-tin) a poisonous alkaloid from tobacco, which may also be produced synthetically.

nicotinism (nik'o-tin-izm″) poisoning by tobacco or by nicotine.

nicoumalone (ni-koo'mah-lōn) acenocoumarol.

nictitation (nik″tī-ta'shun) the act of winking.

nidation (ni-da'shun) implantation of the fertilized ovum (zygote) in the endometrium of the uterus in pregnancy.

NIDR National Institute of Dental Research.

nidus (ni'dus), pl. *ni'di* [L.] a nest; point of origin or focus of a morbid process. **n. hirun'dinis** [L., swallow's nest], a depression in the cerebellum between the posterior velum and uvula.

nifuroxime (ni″fūr-ok'sim) a white to yellow crystalline powder used as local antibacterial and antiprotozoan agent.

nightshade (nīt'shād) a plant of the genus Solanum. **deadly n.,** belladonna leaf.

NIGMS National Institute of General Medical Sciences.

nigra (ni'grah) [L., black] substantia nigra. adj., **ni'gral.**

nigrities (ni-grish'e-ēz) blackness. **n. lin'guae,** black tongue.

N.I.H. National Institutes of Health.

nihilism (ni'ē-lizm) 1. a doctrine of meaninglessness or nothingness. 2. a delusion of nonexistence of the self or part of the self.

nikethamide (nī-keth'ah-mīd) clear colorless to yellowish crystals; analeptic and respiratory stimulant.

Nilevar (ni'le-var) trademark for preparations of norethandrolone.

NIMH National Institute of Mental Health.

nimiety (nī-mi'ē-te) repletion or excess; the state of having too much.

NINDB National Institute of Neurological Diseases and Blindness.

ninhydrin (nin-hi'drin) a chemical compound used as a test for amino acids.

niobium (ni-o'be-um) chemical element (*see table*), at. no. 41, symbol Nb.

Nionate (ni'o-nāt) trademark for a preparation of ferrous gluconate.

niperyt (ni'per-it) pentaerythritol tetranitrate.

niphablepsia (nif″ah-blep'se-ah) snow blindness.

nipple (nip'l) the conical organ of the mammary gland in the female which gives outlet to the milk, or the homologous structure in the male.

Nisentil (ni'sen-til) trademark for a preparation of alphaprodine.

Nisulfazole (ni-sul'fah-zōl) trademark for a preparation of para-nitrosulfathiazole.

nisus (ni'sus) [L.] an effort or striving, especially the annual procreative urge occurring in birds in the spring.

nit (nit) the egg of a louse.

nitavirus (ni″tah-vi'rus) a minute infectious agent, probably consisting of deoxyribonucleic acid and generally associated with an eosinophilic body occupying most of the central area of the affected cell.

niter (ni'ter) potassium nitrate.

niton (ni'ton) radon.

Nitranitol (ni'trah-ni″tol) trademark for preparations of mannitol hexanitrate.

nitrate (ni'trāt) a salt of nitric acid.

nitre (ni'ter) potassium nitrate.

nitremia (ni-tre'me-ah) excess of nitrogen in the blood.

Nitretamin (ni-tre'tah-min) trademark for preparations of trolnitrate.

nitric (ni'trik) pertaining to or containing nitrogen in one of its higher valences.

nitrification (ni″trī-fī-ka'shun) the oxidation of nitrites into nitrates.

nitrify (ni'trī-fi) to oxidize nitrites into nitrates.

nitrile (ni'trīl) a compound containing the monovalent −CN radical.

nitrite (ni'trīt) a salt of nitrous acid.

Nitrobacter (ni″tro-bak'ter) a genus of Schizomycetes (order Pseudomonadales, suborder Pseudomonadineae, family Nitrobacteraceae) which oxidize nitrites to nitrates.

Nitrobacteraceae (-bak″te-ra'se-e) a family of Schizomycetes (order Pseudomonadales, suborder Rhodobacteriineae), known informally as the nitrifying bacteria.

nitrobacteria (-bak-te're-ah) bacteria capable of oxidizing ammonia into nitrogen acids.

nitrobenzene (-ben'zēn) a poisonous benzol derivative.

nitrocellulose (-sel'u-lōs) pyroxylin.

Nitrocystis (-sis'tis) a genus of Schizomycetes (order Pseudomonadales, suborder Pseudomonadineae, family Nitrobacteraceae) which oxidize nitrites to nitrates.

nitrofurantoin (-fu-ran'to-in) an antibacterial agent used in treatment of urinary tract infections.

nitrofurazone (-fu'rah-zōn) an odorless, lemon-yellow, crystalline powder used as a local antibacterial.

nitrogen (ni'tro-jen) chemical element (*see table*), at. no. 7, symbol N. **alloxuric n.,** nitrogen in the form of alloxur bases. **amide n., amino n.,** that portion of the nitrogen in protein that exists in the form of acid amides. **authentic n.,** legitimate nitrogen. **filtrate n.,** nonprotein nitrogen. **illegitimate n.,** that part of administered nitrogen not found in the excreta and the retention of which in the organism is not justifiable. **justifiable n., legitimate n.,** that part of administered nitrogen used by the organism in building up its own tissues or excreted. **n. monoxide,** nitrous oxide. **n. mustards,** see under *mustard.* **nomadic n.,** free nitrogen from the air which enters into plant and animal growth. **nonprotein n.,** the nitrogenous constituents of the blood exclusive of the protein bodies, consisting of the nitrogen of urea, uric acid, creatinc, creatinine, amino acids, polypeptides and an undetermined part known as *rest nitrogen.* **n. pentoxide,** a crystalline compound, nitric anhydride, which combines with water to form nitric acid. **n. peroxide, n. tetroxide,** a poisonous volatile liquid, giving off brownish irritant fumes.

nitrogenous (ni-troj′ĕ-nus) containing nitrogen.

nitroglycerin (ni″tro-glis′er-in) glyceryl trinitrate.

Nitroglyn (ni′tro-glin) trademark for a preparation of glyceryl trinitrate.

Nitrol (ni′trol) trademark for preparations of glyceryl trinitrate.

nitromannite (ni″tro-man′īt) mannitol hexanitrate.

nitromersol (-mer′sol) brownish yellow to yellow granules or powder used as a local antibacterial.

nitrosification (ni-tro″sī-fī-ka′shun) the oxidation of ammonia into nitrites.

nitrosify (ni-tro′sī-fi) to oxidize ammonia into nitrites.

nitrosobacterium (ni-tro″so-bak-te′re-um), pl. *nitrosobacte′ria* [L.] a microorganism which oxidizes nitrites to nitrates.

Nitrosococcus (ni″tro-so-kok′us) a genus of Schizomycetes (order Pseudomonadales, suborder Pseudomonadineae, family Nitrobacteraceae) which oxidize ammonia to nitrite.

Nitrosocystis (-so-sis′tis) a genus of Schizomycetes (order Pseudomonadales, suborder Pseudomonadineae, family Nitrobacteraceae) which oxidize ammonia to nitrite.

Nitrosogloea (-so-gle′ah) a genus of Schizomycetes (order Pseudomonadales, suborder Pseudomonadineae, family Nitrobactcraceae) which oxidize ammonia to nitrite.

Nitrosomonas (-so-mo′nas) a genus of Schizomycetes (order Pseudomonadales, suborder Pseudomonadineae, family Nitrobacteraceae) which oxidize ammonia to nitrite.

Nitrosospira (-so-spi′rah) a genus of Schizomycetes (order Pseudomonadales, suborder Pseudomonadineae, family Nitrobacteraceae) which oxidize ammonia to nitrite.

nitrous (ni′trus) pertaining to or containing nitrogen in one of its lower valences. **n. oxide,** a colorless gas used by inhalation as a general anesthetic.

Nitrovas (ni′tro-vas) trademark for a preparation of glyceryl trinitrate.

N.L.N. National League for Nursing.

N.L.N.E. National League of Nursing Education.

N.M.A. National Malaria Association; National Medical Association.

N.M.R.I. Naval Medical Research Institute, part of the National Naval Medical Center.

N.M.S.S. National Multiple Sclerosis Society.

nn. nervi (L. pl.), *nerves.*

N.N.D. New and Nonofficial Drugs, an annual publication of the American Medical Association, describing and stating the actions, uses, dosage and trade names of drugs evaluated by the Council on Pharmacy and Chemistry.

No chemical symbol, *nobelium.*

nobelium (no-be′le-um) chemical element (*see table*), at. no. 102, symbol No.

Nocardia (no-kar′de-ah) a genus of Schizomycetes (order Actinomycetales, family Actinomycetaceae).

nocardiosis (no-kar″de-o′sis) infection with Nocardia.

noci- (no′se) word element [L.], *harm; injury.*

noci-association (no″se-ah-so″se-a′shun) unconscious discharge of nervous energy under the stimulus of injury.

nociceptor (-sep′tor) a receptor organ sensitive to stimuli capable of causing harm or injury, such stimuli giving rise to the sensation of pain. adj., **nocicep′tive.**

noci-influence (-in′floo-ens) injurious or traumatic influence.

nociperception (-per-sep′shun) the perception of traumatic stimuli.

noctalbuminuria (nok″tal-bu″mĭ-nu′re-ah) excess of albumin in urine secreted at night.

Noctec (nok′tek) trademark for preparations of chloral hydrate.

noctiphobia (nok″tĭ-fo′be-ah) morbid dread of night.

nocuity (nok-u′ĭ-te) injuriousness; harmfulness.

node (nōd) a swelling, knot or protuberance. adj., **no′dal. n. of Aschoff and Tawara,** atrioventricular node. **atrioventricular n., auriculoventricular n.,** fibers at the base of the interauricular septum, and forming the beginning of the atrioventricular bundle or bundle of His. **Bouchard's n's,** nodules on the second joints of the fingers, considered symptomatic of gastrectasis. **Delphian n.,** a lymph node encased in the fascia in the midline just above the thyroid isthmus, so called because it is exposed first at operation and, if diseased, is indicative of the condition to be found in the thyroid gland. **Dürck's n's,** granulomatous perivascular infiltrations in the cerebral cortex in trypanosomiasis. **Ewald n.,** sentinel node. **Fereol's n's,** subcutaneous nodes in acute rheumatism. **Flack's n.,** sinoatrial node. **gouty n.,** one due to gouty inflammation. **Haygarth's n's,** joint swellings in arthritis deformans. **Heberden's n's,** nodular protrusions on the phalanges at the distal interphalangeal joints of the fingers in osteoarthritis. **Hensen's n.,** primitive knot. **Keith's n., Keith-Flack n.,** sinoatrial node. **Legendre's n's,** Bouchard's nodes. **lymph n.,** one of the accumulations of lymphatic tissue organized as lymphatic organs along the course of lymphatic vessels, consisting of an outer cortical and an inner medullary part.

Meynet's n's, nodules in the capsules of joints and in tendons in rheumatic conditions, especially in children. **Osler's n's,** small, raised, swollen, tender areas, bluish or sometimes pink or red, occurring commonly in the pads of the fingers or toes, in the thenar or hypothenar eminences or the soles of the feet; they are practically pathognomonic of subacute bacterial endocarditis. **Parrot's n.,** a syphilitic node on the outer table of the skull. **piedric n's,** nodes seen on the hair in piedra. **n's of Ranvier,** the periodic interruptions in the myelin sheath of myelinated nerve fibers. **Rotter's n's,** lymph nodes occasionally found between the pectoralis major and minor muscles which often contain metastases from mammary cancer. **Schmidt's n.,** the medullated interannular segment of a nerve fiber. **Schmorl's n.,** an irregular or hemispherical bone defect in the upper or lower margin of the body of a vertebra. **sentinel n., signal n.,** a firm node just above the left clavicle, behind inserting fibers of the sternocleidomastoid muscles, evidencing metastases from a visceral carcinoma. **singer's n.,** a small, white nodule on the vocal cord in chorditis nodosa. **sinoatrial n., sinoauricular n.,** a collection of atypical muscle fibers in the wall of the right atrium by which the rhythm of cardiac contraction is usually established. **syphilitic n.,** a swelling upon a bone due to syphilitic periostitis. **n. of Tawara,** atrioventricular node. **teacher's n.,** singer's node. **Troisier's n., Virchow's n.,** sentinel node. **vital n.,** the respiratory center.

nodose (no'dōs) having nodes or projections.

nodosity (no-dos'i-te) 1. a node. 2. the quality of being nodose.

nodular (nod'u-ler) marked with, or resembling, nodules.

nodule (nod'ūl) 1. a small node or boss. 2. anterior segment of the inferior vermis of the cerebellum in the fourth ventricle. 3. a circumscribed, usually solid lesion, often deep in the skin or subcutaneous tissues, or in another organ of the body. **Albini's n's,** gray nodules of the size of sago grains, sometimes seen on the free edges of the atrioventricular valves of infants; they are remains of fetal structures. **apple jelly n's,** cutaneous nodules of apple-jelly color in lupus vulgaris. **Bianchi's n.,** Arantius' body. **epicardial n's,** nodules over the vessels of the epicardium, probably due to high pressure. **Gamna n's,** brown or yellow pigmented nodules seen in the spleen in Gamna disease. **Jeanselme's n's,** nodules on the limbs near the joints due to treponemal infection. **juxta-articular n's,** Jeanselme's nodes. **Kerckring's n., Köster's n.,** tubercle composed of one giant cell enclosed by a double layer of cells. **Leishman's n's,** the pinkish nodules seen in the nonulcerative keloid-like type of oriental sore. **lymphatic n's,** a term applied to lymph nodes, as well as to one of the small collections of lymphatic tissue situated deep to epithelial surfaces, and also to temporary small accumulations of lymphocytes in the cortex of a lymph node. **Morgagni's n.,** Arantius'

body. **pearly n.,** one of the nodules of bovine tuberculosis. **pulp n.,** a mass of dentin found in the pulp cavity of a tooth. **n. tabac,** Gamna nodes. **triticeous n.,** a nodule in the thyrohyoid ligament. **warm n.,** a nodule in the thyroid gland which shows the same I^{131} uptake as the rest of the gland; normally not carcinomatous.

nodulus (nod'u-lus), pl. *nod'uli* [L.] nodule.

nodus (no'dus), pl. *no'di* [L.] node.

Noguchia (no-goo'che-ah) a genus of Schizomycetes (order Eubacteriales, family Brucellaceae) found in the conjunctiva of man and animals having a follicular type of disease.

Noludar (nol'u-dar) trademark for preparations of methyprylon.

noma (no'mah) a condition characterized by destruction of tissue, such as gangrenous stomatitis or dermatitis. **n. puden'di, n. vul'vae,** destructive ulceration of the external genitalia in the female.

nomen (no'men), pl. *no'mina* [L.] name. **No'mina Anatom'ica,** the official body of anatomic nomenclature.

nomenclature (no'men-kla″chūr) system of technical terms; terminology. **anatomic n.,** a scheme presenting the names of all the structures of the body. **binomial n.,** a scheme of designating living organisms, based on use of both the genus and the species names. **taxonomic n.,** a scheme presenting the names of taxa into which living organisms are grouped in the different kingdoms.

nomogram (nom'o-gram) the graphic representation produced in nomography.

nomography (no-mog'rah-fe) a graphic method of representing the relation between any number of variables.

nonan (no'nan) recurring every ninth day.

nonapeptide (non″ah-pep'tīd) a peptide containing nine amino acids.

non compos mentis (non kom'pos men'tis) [L.] not of sound mind.

nonconductor (non″kon-duk'tor) a substance that does not readily transmit electricity, light or heat.

nondisjunction (non″dis-junk'shun) failure of a pair of chromosomes to separate during meiosis.

nonelectrolyte (non″e-lek'tro-līt) a compound which, dissolved in water, does not separate into charged particles and is incapable of conducting an electric current.

nonphotochromogen (non″fo-to-kro'mo-jen) a microorganism that is not conspicuously affected in color by exposure to light.

nonsecretor (non″se-kre'tor) a person with A or B type blood whose body secretions do not contain the particular (A or B) substance.

nontaster (non-tās'ter) a person unable to taste a particular substance, such as phenylthiocarbamide, which is used in certain genetic studies.

nonunion (-un'yun) failure of the ends of a fractured bone to unite.

nonviable (-vi'ah-bl) not capable of living.

noopsyche (no'o-si″ke) the intellectual processes of the mind.

noothymopsychic (no″o-thi″mo-si'kik) pertaining to intellectual and affective processes of the mind.

N.O.P.H.N. National Organization for Public Health Nursing.

noradrenalin (nor″ah-dren′ah-lin) levarterenol.

noramidopyrine (nor-am″i-do-pi′rēn) dipyrone.

norandrostenolone (nor-an″dro-sten′o-lōn) nandrolone.

nordefrin (nor′dĕ-frin) a compound used as a sympathomimetic agent.

norepinephrine (nor″ep-ĭ-nef′rin) a hormone secreted by the adrenal medulla in response to splanchnic stimulation; also prepared synthetically and used as a sympathomimetic and pressor agent.

norethandrolone (nor″eth-an′dro-lōn) a synthetic androgen equal to testosterone in anabolic activity, but having less androgenic activity.

norethindrone (nor-eth′in-drōn) a compound used as a progestational agent.

Norisodrine (-i′so-drin) trademark for preparations of isoproterenol.

Norlutin (-lu′tin) trademark for a preparation of norethindrone.

norm (norm) a fixed or ideal standard.

norm(o)- (nor′mo) word element [L.], *normal; usual; conforming to the rule.*

normoblast (nor′mo-blast) a late stage in the development of a red blood corpuscle characterized by a pyknotic nucleus and abundant hemoglobin in the cytoplasm. **intermediate n.,** polychromatophilic erythroblast.

normocalcemia (nor″mo-kal-se′me-ah) a normal level of calcium in the blood. adj., **normocalce′mic.**

normocapnia (-kap′ne-ah) a normal level of carbon dioxide in the blood. adj., **normocap′nic.**

normocholesterolemia (-ko-les″ter-ol-e′me-ah) a normal level of cholesterol in the blood. adj., **normocholesterole′mic.**

normochromasia (-kro-ma′ze-ah) normal staining reaction in a cell or tissue.

normochromia (-kro′me-ah) normal color of erythrocytes.

normochromocyte (-kro′mo-sīt) an erythrocyte having the normal amount of hemoglobin.

normocyte (nor′mo-sīt) erythrocyte.

Normocytin (nor″mo-si′tin) trademark for preparations of concentrated crystalline vitamin B_{12}.

normocytosis (-si-to′sis) a normal state of the blood corpuscles.

normoglycemia (-gli-se′me-ah) normal sugar content of the blood. adj., **normoglyce′mic.**

normokalemia (-kah-le′me-ah) a normal level of potassium in the blood. adj., **normokale′mic.**

normotension (-ten′shun) normal tone, tension or pressure.

normotensive (-ten′siv) 1. characterized by normal tension or blood pressure. 2. a person with normal blood pressure.

normothermia (-ther′me-ah) a normal state of temperature. adj., **normother′mic.**

normotonia (-to′ne-ah) normal tone or tension. adj., **normoton′ic.**

normotopic (nor″mo-top′ik) normally located.

normotrophic (-trof′ik) of normal development; not exhibiting either hypertrophy or hypotrophy.

normovolemia (-vo-le′me-ah) normal blood volume.

Norodin (nor′o-din) trademark for a preparation of methamphetamine hydrochloride.

norsulfazole (nor-sul′fah-zōl) sulfathiazole.

nos(o)- (nos′o) word element [Gr.], *disease.*

noscapine (nos′kah-pēn) an alkaloid present in opium; used as a nonaddictive antitussive.

nosebleed (nōz′blēd) bleeding from the nose; epistaxis.

Nosema (no-se′mah) a genus of sporozoan parasites. **N. bom′bycis,** a parasite of silkworms.

nose (nōz) the special organ of the sense of smell. **saddle n.,** a nose with a sunken bridge.

nosencephalus (no″sen-sef′ah-lus) a fetus with defective cranium and brain.

nosepiece (nōz′pēs) the portion of a microscope nearest to the stage, which bears the objective or objectives.

nosocomial (nos″o-ko′me-al) pertaining to a hospital or infirmary.

nosogeny (no-soj′ĕ-ne) pathogenesis.

nosography (no-sog′rah-fe) a description of diseases.

nosology (no-sol′o-je) the science of the classification of diseases. adj., **nosolog′ic.**

nosomania (nos″o-ma′ne-ah) insane belief that one is diseased.

nosomycosis (-mi-ko′sis) a disease caused by a parasitic fungus.

nosonomy (no-son′o-me) the classification of diseases.

nosoparasite (nos″o-par′ah-sīt) an organism found in a disease which it is able to modify, but not to produce.

nosophilia (-fil′e-ah) morbid desire to be sick.

nosophobia (-fo′be-ah) morbid dread of sickness.

nosopoietic (poi-et′ik) causing disease.

Nosopsyllus (-sīl′us) a genus of fleas. **N. fasciatus,** rat flea, a carrier of murine typhus and plague.

nosotaxy (nos′o-tak″se) the classification of disease.

nosotherapy (nos″o-ther′ah-pe) the treatment of one disease by means of another.

nostril (nos′tril) either aperture of the nose.

nostrum (nos′trum) a quack, patent or secret remedy.

Nostyn (nos′tin) trademark for a preparation of ectylurea.

notal (no′tal) dorsal.

notalgia (no-tal′je-ah) pain in the back.

notancephalia (no″tan-sĕ-fa′le-ah) absence of back of skull.

notch (noch) an indentation on the edge of a bone or other organ. **aortic n.,** dicrotic notch. **craniofacial n.,** an opening in the bony partition between the orbital and nasal cavities. **dicrotic n.,** the depression on the sphygmogram due to closure of the aortic valves. **parotid n.,** the notch between the ramus of the mandible and the mastoid process of the temporal bone. **preoccipital n.,** one on the lower edge of the external surface of a cerebral hemisphere, between the occipital and temporal lobes. **Sibson's n.**, an inward bend of the left upward limit of precordial dullness in acute pericardial effusion. **trigeminal n.**, one in the superior border of the petrosal portion of the temporal bone, near the apex, for transmission of the trigeminal nerve.

notencephalocele (no"ten-sef'ah-lo-sēl") hernial protrusion of brain at the back of the head.

notencephalus (no"ten-sef'ah-lus) fetus affected with notencephalocele.

notifiable (no"ti-fi'ah-bl) necessary to be reported to the board of health.

notochord (no'to-kord) a cylindrical cord of cells on the dorsal side of an embryo, marking its longitudinal axis.

notomelus (no-tom'ĕ-lus) a fetus with accessory limbs attached to the back.

not-self (not'self) a name given antigen constituents foreign to an organism, which is thereby stimulated to create antibodies against them to achieve their elimination.

noumenal (noo'mē-nal) pertaining to pure thought, independent of sensory perception.

Novaldin (no-val'din) trademark for preparations of dipyrone.

novobiocin (no"vo-bi'o-sin) an antibacterial substance produced by growth of species of Streptomyces.

Novocaine (no'vo-kān) trademark for preparations of procaine hydrochloride.

Novrad (nov'rad) trademark for preparations of levopropoxyphene.

noxa (nok'sah) an injurious agent, act or influence.

noxious (nok'shus) hurtful; injurious.

Np chemical symbol, *neptunium.*

N.P.N. nonprotein nitrogen.

N.S.A. Neurosurgical Society of America.

N.S.C.C. National Society for Crippled Children.

N.S.N.A. National Student Nurse Association.

N.S.P.B. National Society for the Prevention of Blindness.

N.T.A. National Tuberculosis Association.

nucha (nu'kah) the nape of the neck.

nuclease (nu'kle-ās) an enzyme which decomposes nucleic acids.

nucleated (nu'kle-āt"ed) having a nucleus or nuclei.

nuclein (nu'kle-in) a protein found in cell nuclei.

nucleofugal (nu"kle-of'u-gal) moving away from a nucleus.

nucleohistone (nu"kle-o-his'tōn) a complex nucleoprotein made up of deoxyribonucleic acid and a histone, found in the nucleus of various cells.

nucleolonema (nu"kle-o"lo-ne'mah) a threadlike element appearing as a tangled skein within the nucleolus of a cell.

nucleolus (nu-kle'o-lus), pl. *nucle'oli* [L.] a rounded, basophilic body, rich in RNA, within the nucleus of a cell.

nucleolymph (nu'kle-o-limf'") karyolymph.

nucleomitophobia (nu"kle-o-mi"to-fo'be-ah) morbid fear of an atomic explosion.

nucleon (nu'kle-on) a particle of an atomic nucleus; a proton or neutron, the total number of which constitutes the mass number of the isotope.

nucleopetal (nu"kle-op'ĕ-tal) moving toward a nucleus.

nucleophilic (nu"kle-o-fil'ik) having an affinity for nuclei.

nucleoplasm (nu'kle-o-plazm") karyoplasm.

nucleoprotamine (nu"kle-o-pro-tam'in) a combination of protamine and a nucleic acid of the deoxyribose type, found chiefly in fish sperm.

nucleoprotein (-pro'te-in) one of a class of conjugated proteins, the prosthetic groups of which are nucleic acids.

nucleosidase (-si'dās) an intracellular enzyme which is capable of causing the decomposition of nucleosides.

nucleoside (nu'kle-o-sīd") one of a class of compounds produced by hydrolysis of nucleotides, consisting of a sugar and a nitrogenous base.

nucleotide (nu'kle-o-tīd") one of a group of compounds obtained by hydrolysis of nucleic acids, consisting of purine or pyrimidine bases linked to sugars, which in turn are esterified with phosphoric acid. **diphosphopyridine n.**, one which on hydrolysis yields two molecules of phosphoric acid, a coenzyme widely distributed in nature and involved in many enzymatic reactions. **triphosphopyridine n.**, one which on hydrolysis yields three phosphate units instead of two, a coenzyme similar to diphosphopyridine nucleotide, but involved in a smaller number of reactions.

nucleotoxin (nu"kle-o-tok'sin) a toxin from cell nuclei, or one which affects cell nuclei.

nucleus (nu'kle-us), pl. *nu'clei* [L.] 1. a spheroid body within a cell; the core or center of a cell. 2. a mass of gray matter in the central nervous system, especially such a mass marking the central termination of a cerebral nerve. adj., **nu'clear. n. ambig'uus**, nucleus of glossopharyngeal nerve in medulla oblongata. **atomic n., n. of atom**, the central core of an atom, constituting most of its mass, but only a small part of its volume, and containing an excess of electricity. **caudate n., n. cauda'tus**, a long, horseshoe-shaped mass of gray substance which forms part of the corpus striatum and is closely related to the lateral ventricle. **central n. of thalamus, n. centra'lis thal'ami**, a collection of cells close to the wall of the third ventricle, between the medial and posterior ventral nuclei of the thalamus. **cervical n.**, one in the spinal cord opposite the origin of the third and fourth cervical nerves. **cleavage n.**, segmentation nucleus. **compact n.**, one with an inconspicuous nuclear membrane and minute chromatin granules throughout its substance. **conjugation n.**, fertilization nucleus. **cuneate n., n. cunea'tus**, a gray mass in the medulla oblongata within which the fibers of the fasciculus cuneatus of the spinal cord end. **daughter n.**, a new nucleus formed in mitosis by the diaster. **Deiters' n.**, lateral vestibular nucleus. **dentate n.**, **n. denta'tus**, a crumpled mass of gray matter in each cerebellar hemisphere. **diploid n.**, a cell nucleus containing the number of chromosomes typical of the somatic cells of the particular species. **end nuclei**, terminal nuclei. **n. fasti'gii**, flat mass of gray matter in cerebellum, over roof of fourth ventricle. **fertilization n.**, one produced by fusion of the male and female pronuclei in the fertilized ovum. **free n.**, a cell nucleus from which the other elements of the cell have disappeared. **germ n.**, **germinal n.**, pronucleus. **gonad n.**, the reproductive nucleus of a cell. **n. gra'cilis**, a gray mass in the medulla oblongata, within which the fibers of the fasciculus gracilis of the spinal cord end. **gray n.**, gray substance of spinal cord. **haploid n.**, a cell nucleus containing half of the number of chromosomes typical of the somatic cells of a particular species. **hypoglossal n.**, nucleus of hypoglossal nerve in the medulla oblongata. **intraventricular n.**, nucleus caudatus. **Kölliker's n.**, gray mass around canal of cord. **large cell n.**, nucleus ambiguus. **laryngeal n.**, nucleus of origin of nerve fibers to larynx. **lenticular n.**, **lentiform n.**, part of corpus striatum external to the third ventricle. **motion n.**, kinetoplast. **motor n.**, any collection of cells in the central nervous system giving origin to a motor nerve. **nerve n.**, a collection of cells in the nervous system directly related to a peripheral nerve. **nutrition n.**, macronucleus. **n. of origin**, any collection of nerve cells giving origin to the fibers, or a part of the fibers, of a peripheral nerve. **polymorphic n.**, a cell nucleus that assumes an irregular form or splits up into lobes. **n. pulpo'sus**, pulpy mass in center of an intervertebral disk. **pyramidal n.**, inner accessory olivary nucleus. **red n.**, nucleus ruber. **reproductive n.**, micronucleus. **ring nuclei**, **ringed nuclei**, ringlike nuclei in the polymorphonuclear leukocytes in the stools of patients with bacillary dysentery. **roof n.**, nucleus fastigii. **n. ruber**, an oval mass of gray matter in the anterior part of the tegumentum and extending into the posterior part of the subthalamic region. **sacral n.**, a mass of gray substance in the spinal cord opposite the site of origin of the second and third sacral nerves. **segmentation n.**, the fertilization nucleus after cleavage has begun. **sensory n.**, the nucleus of termination of the afferent (sensory) fibers of a peripheral nerve. **somatic n.**, macronucleus. **sperm n.**, the male pronucleus. **striate n.**, corpus striatum. **tegmental n.**, 1. nucleus fastigii. 2. nucleus ruber. **terminal nuclei**, nerve cells on which axons of primary afferent neurons synapse. **triangular n.**, cuneate nucleus. **trophic n.**, macronucleus. **vesicular n.**, one with visible nuclear membrane and chromatin material usually lightly diffused throughout the karyolymph. **n. vestibula'ris**, the four cellular masses in the floor of the fourth ventricle. **Westphal's n.**, a group of small nerve cells in the rostral part of the nucleus of the oculomotor nerve. **yolk**

n., the area of the cytoplasm of an ovum in which the synthetic activities leading to the accumulation of food supplies in the oocyte are initiated. **zygote n.**, fertilization nucleus.

nuclide (nu'klīd) any atomic configuration capable of existing for a measurable lifetime, usually more than 10^{-9} seconds.

nudomania (nu″do-ma'ne-ah) a morbid desire to be nude.

nudophobia (-fo'be-ah) a morbid dread of being nude.

nullipara (nu-lip'ah-rah) a woman who has not produced a viable offspring. adj., **nullip'arous**.

nulliparity (nul″ĭ-par'ĭ-te) the state of being a nullipara.

number (num'ber) a symbol, as a figure or word, expressive of a certain value or a specified quantity. **atomic n.**, a number expressive of the number of protons in an atomic nucleus, or the positive charge of the nucleus expressed in terms of the electronic charge. **Avogadro's n.**, the number of particles of the type specified by the chemical formula of a certain substance in one gram mole of the substance. **mass n.**, the number expressive of the mass of a nucleus, being the total number of nucleons — protons and neutrons — in the nucleus of an atom or nuclide.

nummular (num'u-lar) resembling a pile of coins.

Numorphan (nu-mor'fan) trademark for preparations of oxymorphone hydrochloride.

Nupercaine (nu'per-kān) trademark for preparations of dibucaine.

nurse (ners) 1. a person who makes a profession of caring for the sick, disabled or enfeebled. 2. to care for a sick or disabled person or one unable to provide for his own needs. 3. to nourish at the breast. **community n.**, one maintained by an agency (Community Nursing Service) to provide part-time health services in their homes to residents of the area. **dry n.**, an infant's nurse who does not suckle the babe. **general duty n.**, one who is prepared to do any sort of nursing duty. **graduate n.**, a nurse who is a graduate of a training school offering a diploma or degree entitling the holder to take the examination for registered nurse. **head n.**, one in charge of a nursing unit of a hospital. **hospital n.**, one who serves in a hospital ward. **practical n.**, one who performs simpler nursing duties and has had a shorter course of nursing education. **private n.**, one who attends an individual patient. **probationer n.**, a student during the early months of nurse's training, before acceptance as a full-fledged student nurse. **public health n.**, a graduate nurse employed in a community to safeguard the health of its people by giving care to the sick in their homes, teaching families how to keep well, and assisting in the prevention of disease. **Queen's Nurse**, in the United Kingdom, a district nurse who has been trained at or in accordance with the regulations of the Queen Victoria Jubilee Institute for Nurses. **registered n.**, a graduate nurse registered and licensed to practice by a State Board of Nurse Examiners or other state authority. **school n.,** a trained nurse who supplements the work of the physician in medical inspection of schools. **scrub n.,** a nurse in the operating room, wearing sterile gloves, who passes instruments to the surgeon. **trained n.,** a nurse trained in and graduated from a nurses' training school. **visiting n.,** one who provides essential services on a part-time basis in their homes to patients who do not require full-time nursing care. **wet n.,** a woman who furnishes breast feeding for the infants of others.

nursery (ner'sĕ-re) the department in a hospital where newborn infants are cared for. **day n.,** an institution devoted to the care of young children during the day.

nutation (nu-ta'shun) nodding.

nutatory (nu'tah-tor"e) nodding.

nutrient (nu'tre-ent) 1. nourishing; aiding nutrition. 2. a nourishing substance, or food.

nutriment (nu'trĭ-ment) nourishment; nutritious material.

nutriology (nu"tre-ol'o-je) the study of foods and their use in diet and therapy.

nutrition (nu-trish'un) the assimilation of food.

nutritious (nu-trish'us) affording nourishment.

nutriture (nu'trĭ-tūr) the status of the body in relation to nutrition.

Nuttallia (nŭ-tal'e-ah) a genus of protozoan blood parasites causing a disease of horses.

Nuttalliellidae (nŭ-tal"le-el'ĭ-de) a family of arthropods (suborder Ixodides), including a single species, *Nuttalliella namaqua.*

nuttalliosis (nŭ-tal"e-o'sis) infection with Nuttallia.

nux (nuks) [L.] nut. **n. vom'ica,** the dried ripe seed of *Strychnos nux-vomica;* used as a tincture, extract or fluidextract for its bitter tonic properties.

nyctalgia (nik-tal'je-ah) pain that occurs only in sleep.

nyctalope (nik'tah-lōp) a person affected with nyctalopia.

nyctalopia (nik"tah-lo'pe-ah) night blindness.

nycterine (nik'ter-in) occurring at night.

nyctohemeral (nik"to-hem'er-al) pertaining to both day and night.

nyctophilia (-fil'e-ah) a preference for darkness or for night.

nyctophobia (nik"to-fo'be-ah) morbid dread of darkness.

nyctophonia (-fo'ne-ah) loss of voice during the day.

nyctotyphlosis (-tif-lo'sis) night blindness.

Nydrazid (ni'drah-zid) trademark for preparations of isoniazid.

nylidrin (nil'ĭ-drin) a compound used as a peripheral vasodilator.

nymph (nimf) a newly hatched young of certain insects, which resembles the adult in appearance and habitat.

nympha (nim'fah), pl. *nym'phae* [L.] labium minus.

nymphectomy (nim-fek'to-me) excision of the nymphae.

nymphitis (nim-fi'tis) inflammation of a nympha.

nymphomania (nim"fo-ma'ne-ah) insatiable sexual desire in the female.

nymphoncus (nim-fong'kus) swelling or enlargement of the nymphae.

nymphotomy (nim-fot'o-me) surgical incision of the nymphae or clitoris.

nystagmiform (nis-tag'mĭ-form) resembling nystagmus.

nystagmograph (nis-tag'mo-graf) instrument for recording the movements of the eyeball in nystagmus.

nystagmoid (nis-tag'moid) resembling nystagmus.

nystagmus (nis-tag'mus) continuous rolling movement of eyeball. adj., **nystag'mic. aural n.,** a form due to labyrinthine disturbance. **Cheyne's n.,** a peculiar rhythmical eye movement. **disjunctive n.,** nystagmus in which the eyes move away from each other. **labyrinthine n.,** vestibular nystagmus. **lateral n.,** horizontal movement of the eyes. **miners' n.,** a variety of nystagmus peculiar to miners. **optokinetic n.,** nystagmus induced by looking at a moving object. **rotatory n.,** rotation of eyes about the visual axis. **vertical n.,** up-and-down movement of eyes. **vestibular n.,** nystagmus due to vestibular disease.

nystatin (nis'tah-tin) an antibiotic substance produced by growth of *Streptomyces noursei;* used in treatment of infections due to *Candida albicans.*

nystaxis (nis-tak'sis) nystagmus.

nyxis (nik'sis) puncture or pricking.

O

O chemical symbol, *oxygen.*

O. [L.] oculus *(eye);* [L.] octarius *(pint);* opening.

o- symbol, *ortho-.*

O₂ both eyes.

O₃ chemical symbol, *ozone* (triatomic oxygen).

O.A.R. Office of Aerospace Research.

oath (ōth) a solemn declaration or affirmation. **hippocratic o.,** a statement of principles for

the medical profession, attributed to Hippocrates and subscribed to by physicians on graduation from medical school.

O.B. obstetrics.

ob- (ob) word element [L.], *against; in front of.*

obdormition (ob"dor-mish'un) local numbness from nerve pressure.

obelion (o-be'le-on) junction of the sagittal

suture and a line between the parietal foramina.

obesity (o-bēs'ĭ-te) an excessive accumulation of fat in the body. adj., **obese'**.

obex (o'beks) the thickening of the ependyma at the caudal angle of the roof of the fourth ventricle.

objective (ob-jek'tiv) 1. perceptible by the external senses. 2. a result for whose achievement an effort may be made. 3. the lens or system of lenses of a microscope nearest the object that is being examined. **achromatic o.**, one in which the chromatic aberration is corrected for two colors. **apochromatic o.**, one in which chromatic aberration is corrected for three colors. **semiapochromatic o.**, one in which the chromatic aberration for three colors is almost entirely overcome.

obligate (ob'lĭ-gāt) imposed by necessity; incapable of adaptation to different conditions.

oblique (o-blēk', o-blīk') slanting; inclined.

obliquity (ob-lik'wĭ-te) the state of being oblique or slanting. **Litzmann's o.**, presentation of the posterior parietal bone to the parturient canal. **Nägele's o.**, presentation of the anterior parietal bone to the birth canal, the biparietal diameter being oblique to the brim of the pelvis. **Roederer's o.**, presentation of the occiput to the birth canal.

oblongata (ob-long-gah'tah) medulla oblongata. adj., **oblonga'tal.**

obsession (ob-sesh'un) an unwanted idea or impulse that persistently intrudes into the consciousness. adj., **obses'sional.**

obsessive-compulsive (ob-ses'iv-kom-pul'-siv) characterized by both obsessional thoughts and compulsions.

obstetrician (ob″stē-trish'an) one who practices obstetrics.

obstetrics (ob-stet'riks) the branch of medicine dealing with pregnancy, labor and the puerperium. adj., **obstet'ric, obstet'rical.**

obstipation (ob″stī-pa'shun) intractable constipation.

obstruction (ob-struk'shun) the act of blocking or clogging; state of being clogged. **intestinal o.**, any hindrance to the passage of feces.

obstruent (ob'stroo-ent) 1. causing obstruction. 2. an astringent remedy.

obtund (ob-tund') to dull or blunt.

obtundent (ob-tun'dent) a soothing or demulcent agent.

obturator (ob″tu-ra'tor) a disk or plate that closes an opening.

obtusion (ob-tu'zhun) a deadening or blunting of sensitiveness.

occipitalization (ok-sip″ĭ-tal-i-za'shun) fusion of the first cervical vertebra with the skull (occiput).

occiput (ok'si-put) the back part of the head. adj., **occip'ital.**

occlude (o-klood') to fit close together; to close tight.

occlusion (ŏ-kloo'zhun) 1. the act of closure or state of being closed. 2. the contact of the teeth of both jaws when closed or during those excursive movements of the mandible essential to the function of mastication. adj., **occlu'sal. abnormal o.**, malocclusion. **afunctional o.**, malocclusion which prevents mastication. **anatomic o.**, occlusion in which all the teeth are present and occlude properly. **balanced o.**, occlusion in which the teeth are in harmonious working relation. **capsular o.**, surgical closure of the perinephric capsule for the relief of floating kidney. **central o.**, **centric o.**, occlusion of the teeth with the jaws closed in normal position. **coronary o.**, obstruction to the flow of blood through an artery of the heart. **eccentric o.**, occlusion of the teeth when the lower jaw has moved from the position of rest. **functional o.**, occlusion providing the highest efficiency during all the excursive movements of the jaws essential to the function of mastication without producing trauma. **hyperfunctional o.**, traumatic occlusion. **lateral o.**, occlusion of the teeth when the lower jaw is moved to the right or left of central occlusion. **mesial o.**, position of a tooth too mesial to be normal. **normal o.**, meeting of the teeth in the normal position and relationship. **protrusive o.**, anterocclusion. **retrusive o.**, posterocclusion. **traumatic o.**, occlusion in which the contact relation of the masticatory surfaces of the teeth is directly due to trauma.

occult (ŏ-kult') obscure or hidden from view.

ocellus (o-sel'us) a simple light-sensitive organ; one of the constituents of a compound eye.

Ochrobium (o-kro'be-um) a genus of Schizomycetes (order Pseudomonadales, suborder Pseudomonadineae, family Siderocapsaceae).

ochrodermatosis (o″kro-der″mah-to'sis) a condition marked by yellowness of the skin.

ochrodermia (-der'me-ah) yellowness of the skin.

ochrometer (o-krom'ĕ-ter) an instrument for measuring capillary blood pressure.

ochronosis (o″kro-no'sis) a peculiar discoloration of body tissues caused by deposit of alkapton bodies as the result of a metabolic disorder. **exogenous o.**, ochronosis allegedly due to exposure to a noxious substance. **ocular o.**, brown or gray discoloration of the sclera, sometimes involving also the conjunctivae and eyelids.

octa- (ok'tah) word element [Gr., L.], *eight.*

octad (ok'tad) an element having a valency of eight.

octan (ok'tan) recurring on the eighth day (every seven days).

octapeptide (ok″tah-pep'tĭd) a peptide which on hydrolysis yields eight amino acids.

octaploid (ok'tah-ploid) 1. pertaining to or characterized by octaploidy. 2. an individual or cell having eight sets of chromosomes.

octaploidy (ok'tah-ploi″de) the state of having eight sets of chromosomes (8n).

octavalent (ok″tah-va'lent) having a valency of eight.

Octin (ok'tin) trademark for preparations of isometheptene.

octipara (ok-tip'ah-rah) a woman who has had

eight pregnancies which resulted in viable offspring; para VIII.

ocul(o)- (ok′u-lo) word element [L.], *eye.*

ocular (ok′u-lar) 1. pertaining to the eye. 2. eyepiece.

oculocutaneous (ok″u-lo-ku-ta′ne-us) pertaining to or affecting both the eyes and the skin.

oculofacial (-fa′shal) pertaining to the eyes and face.

oculogyration (-ji-ra′shun) the movement of the eyeball.

oculometroscope (-met′ro-skōp) an instrument for performing skiametry.

oculomotor (-mo′tor) pertaining to eye movements.

oculomotorius (-mo-to′re-us) the oculomotor nerve.

oculonasal (-na′zal) pertaining to the eye and the nose.

oculopupillary (-pu′pĭ-ler″e) pertaining to the pupil of the eye.

oculus (ok′u-lus), pl. *oc′uli* [L.] eye.

O.D. Doctor of Optometry; [L.] *oc′ulus dex′ter* (right eye).

odont(o)- (o-don′to) word element [Gr.], *tooth.*

odontalgia (o″don-tal′je-ah) toothache. **phantom o.,** alveolar neuralgia.

odontectomy (-tek′to-me) excision of a tooth.

odontexesis (-tek′sĕ-sis) cleaning, scraping and polishing of the teeth.

odontiasis (-ti′ah-sis) eruption of the teeth, or any disorder caused thereby.

odontic (o-don′tik) pertaining to the teeth.

odontinoid (o-don′tĭ-noid) a tumor composed of tooth substance.

odontitis (o″don-ti′tis) inflammation of a tooth.

odontoblast (o-don′to-blast) one of the connective tissue cells forming the outer surface of the dental pulp adjacent to the dentin.

odontoblastoma (o-don″to-blas-to′mah) a tumor made up of odontoblasts.

odontoclamis (-kla′mis) the presence of a hood of gingival tissue over an erupted tooth.

odontoclasis (o″don-tok′lah-sis) breaking of a tooth.

odontoclast (o-don′to-klast) a multinucleated giant cell associated with absorption of roots of deciduous teeth.

odontodynia (o-don″to-din′e-ah) odontalgia.

odontogen (o-don′to-jen) the substance which develops into the dentin of the teeth.

odontogenesis (o-don″to-jen′ĕ-sis) the origin and development of the teeth. adj., **odontogenet′ic. o. imperfec′ta,** dentinogenesis imperfecta.

odontogenic (-jen′ik) originating from a tooth or tooth-forming tissue.

odontogeny (o″don-toj′ĕ-ne) odontogenesis.

odontography (-tog′rah-fe) a description of the teeth.

odontoid (o-don′toid) like a tooth.

odontolith (o-don′to-lith) a concretion on a tooth; dental calculus.

odontology (o″don-tol′o-je) scientific study of the teeth.

odontoma (-to′mah) a tumor derived from tissues involved in tooth formation. **amelo-**

blastic o., an odontogenic neoplasm characterized by simultaneous occurrence of ameloblastoma and a composite odontoma. **composite o.,** one consisting of both enamel and dentin in an abnormal pattern. **coronary o.,** one attacking the crown of a tooth. **follicular o.,** a dentigerous cyst. **radicular o.,** one attacking the root of a tooth.

odontopathy (o″don-top′ah-the) any disease of the teeth.

odontoperiosteum (o-don″to-per″e-os′te-um) periodontium.

odontorrhagia (-ra′je-ah) hemorrhage following extraction of a tooth.

odontoscope (o-don′to-skōp) a dental mirror for examining the teeth.

odontosis (o″don-to′sis) formation or eruption of the teeth.

odontotomy (-tot′o-me) incision of a tooth.

odontotrypy (-tot′rĭ-pe) the boring or drilling of a tooth.

odynacusis (o-din″ah-ku′sis) painful hearing.

-odynia (o-din′e-ah) word element [Gr.], *pain.*

odynometer (o″din-om′ĕ-ter) an instrument for measuring pain.

odynophagia (o-din″o-fa′je-ah) painful swallowing of food.

oe- for words beginning thus, see also those beginning *e-.*

oesophagostomiasis (e-sof″ah-go-sto-mi′ah-sis) infection with Œsophagostomum.

Oesophagostomum (-gos′to-mum) a genus of nematode worms found in the intestines of various animals.

Oestrus (es′trus) a genus of flies whose larvae parasitize the nasal cavities and sinuses of ruminants. **O. o′vis,** a widespread species which deposits its larvae on the nostrils of sheep and goats, and which may cause ocular myiasis in man.

Of. official.

official (ŏ-fish′al) authorized by pharmacopeias and recognized formularies.

officinal (o-fis′ĭ-nal) regularly kept for sale in druggists' shops.

OH symbol, *hydroxyl ion.*

ohm (ōm) a unit of electric resistance, being that of a column of mercury 1 sq. mm. in cross section and 106.25 cm. long.

oidiomycosis (o-id″e-o-mi-ko′sis) candidiasis

oil (oil) a generally combustible substance that is not miscible with water, but is soluble in ether. **allspice o.,** pimenta oil. **almond o.,** fixed oil from kernels of varieties of *Prunus amygdalus,* used as an emollient and in the mixing of prescriptions. **anise o.,** volatile oil from dried ripe fruit of *Pimpinella anisum* or *Ilicium verum;* used as a flavoring agent for drugs and as a carminative. **apricot kernel o.,** persic oil. **arachis o.,** peanut oil. **Benne o.,** sesame oil. **betula o., birch o., sweet,** methyl salicylate. **cade o.,** juniper tar. **camphorated o.,** camphor liniment. **caraway o.,** volatile oil from dried ripe fruit of *Carum carvi;* used as a flavoring agent. **cardamom o.,** volatile oil from seed of *Elettaria cardamomum;* used as a flavoring agent. **cassia o.,** cinnamon oil. **castor o.,** a fixed oil obtained from the see-of *Ricinus communis*; used as a cathartic. **castor o., aromatic,** castor oil mixed with cinnamon and clove oils, saccharin, vanillin and alcohol; used as a cathartic. **cedar o.,** a distilled oil from cedar wood, used for preparing specimens for microscopy. **chaulmoogra o.,** a fixed oil from ripe seeds of *Taraktogenos kurzii* or species of Hydnocarpus; formerly used in the treatment of leprosy. **chenopodium o.,** a volatile oil from *Chenopodium ambrosiodes*; an active anthelmintic principle. **chloriodized o.,** an iodine monochloride product of vegetable oil; used as a radiopaque medium in roentgenography of the uterus and uterine tubes and of the bronchi. **cinnamon o.,** a volatile oil from leaves and twigs of *Cinnamonum cassia*; used as a flavoring agent. **citronella o.,** a fragrant oil used as an insect repellent. **clove o.,** a volatile oil from dried flower buds of *Eugenia caryophyllus*; used as a dental analgesic and to relieve nausea and stimulate the appetite. **cod liver o.,** partially destearinated, fixed oil from fresh livers of *Gadus morrhua* and other fish of the family Gadidae; used as a source of vitamins A and D. **cod liver o., nondestearinated,** entire fixed oil from fresh livers of *Gadus morrhua* and other fish of the family Gadidae. **coriander o.,** a volatile oil from dried ripe fruit of *Coriandrum sativum*; used as a flavoring agent. **corn o.,** refined, fixed oil from the embryo of *Zea mays*; used as a solvent for drugs. **cottonseed o.,** refined, fixed oil from seeds of cultivated plants of various species of Gossypium; used as a solvent for drugs. **distilled o.,** volatile oil. **drying o.,** a type of fixed oil which thickens and hardens on exposure to the air. **essential o., ethereal o.,** volatile oil. **eucalyptus o.,** a volatile oil from fresh leaf of species of Eucalyptus; used as a flavoring agent. **expressed o., fatty o.,** fixed oil. **fennel o.,** a volatile oil from dried ripe fruit of *Foeniculum vulgare*; used as a flavoring agent. **fixed o.,** a nonvolatile substance of plant or animal origin, containing mixtures of fatty acids and their esters, and occurring as a solid, semisolid or liquid. **flaxseed o.,** linseed oil. **gaultheria o.,** methyl salicylate. **gingilli o.,** sesame oil. **groundnut o.,** peanut oil. **Haarlem o.,** juniper tar. **halibut liver o.,** a fixed oil from fresh or suitably preserved livers of halibut species; used as a source of vitamin A. **heavy o.,** an oily product obtained by the action of sulfuric acid on alcohol. **hydnocarpus o.,** an oil from species of Hydnocarpus, which resembles chaulmoogra oil. **iodized o.,** a sterile preparation of vegetable oil or oils containing 38-42 per cent of organically combined iodine; used as a contrast medium in hysterosalpingography. **juniper o.,** a volatile oil from dried ripe fruit of *Juniperus communis*. **lavender o.,** a volatile oil from fresh flowering tops of *Lavandula officinalis*; used as a perfuming agent. **lemon o.,** a volatile oil from fresh peel of fruit of *Citrus limon*; used as a flavoring agent. **linseed o.,** a fixed oil

from dried ripe seed of *Linum usitatissimum*. **maize o.,** corn oil. **mineral o.,** a mixture of liquid hydrocarbons from petroleum; used as a softening agent. **myristica o.,** a volatile oil distilled with steam from dried kernels of ripe seeds of *Myristica fragrans*; used as a flavoring agent. **nutmeg o.,** myristica oil. **olive o.,** a fixed oil obtained from ripe fruit of *Olea europaea*; used as an emollient. **orange o.,** a volatile oil from fresh peel of ripe fruit of *Citreus sinensis*; used as a flavoring agent. **orange flower o.,** a volatile oil from fresh flowers of *Citrus aurantium*; used as a flavoring and perfuming agent. **peach kernel o.,** persic oil. **peanut o.,** a refined fixed oil from seed kernels of cultivated varieties of *Arachis hypogaea*; used as a solvent for drugs administered by injection. **peppermint o.,** a volatile oil from fresh overground parts of flowering plant of *Mentha piperita*; used as a flavoring agent. **persic o.,** oil expressed from kernels of varieties of *Prunus armeniaca* or *Prunus persica*; used as a vehicle for dispensing drugs. **pimenta o.,** a volatile oil from the fruit of *Pimenta officinalis*; used as a flavoring agent. **pine o.,** a volatile oil from *Pinus palustris* and other species; used as a deodorant and disinfectant. **pine needle o.,** a volatile oil from fresh leaf of *Pinus mugo*; used as a perfuming and flavoring agent. **ricinus o.,** castor oil. **rose o.,** a volatile oil from fresh flowers of different species of Rosa; used as a perfuming agent. **rosemary o.,** a volatile oil from fresh flowering tops of *Rosmarinus officinalis*; used as a flavoring and perfuming agent. **safflower o.,** an oily liquid from the seeds of the safflower; used as a dietary supplement in the management of hypercholesterolemia. **sassafras o.,** a volatile oil from the root of *Sassafras albidum*; used as a flavoring agent. **sesame o.,** a refined, fixed oil from seeds of cultivated varieties of *Sesamum indicum*; used as a solvent for drugs administered by intramuscular injection. **spearmint o.,** a volatile oil from fresh parts of flowering plants of *Mentha spicata* or *M. cardiaca*; used as a flavoring agent. **sweet o.,** olive oil. **tar o., rectified,** a volatile oil from pine tar rectified by steam distillation. **teel o.,** sesame oil. **theobroma o.,** fat from roasted seed of *Theobroma cacao*; used as a base in suppositories. **thyme o.,** a volatile oil from flowering plant of *Thymus vulgaris or T. zygis*; used as a flavoring agent. **turpentine o.,** a volatile oil from an oleoresin obtained from *Pinus palustris* and other species of Pinus; used as a local irritant. **volatile o.,** a readily evaporating substance of plant origin, containing aromatic hydrocarbons, aldehydes, alcohols, ethers, acids, terpenes or camphors. **wheatgerm o.,** oil derived from the germ of wheat kernels; it is rich in vitamin E. **wintergreen o.,** methyl salicylate.

ointment (oint′ment) a semisolid preparation for external application to the body, official ointments consisting of medicinal substances incorporated in suitable vehicles (bases).

ammoniated mercury o., a preparation of ammoniated mercury, liquid petrolatum and white ointment; used as a local anti-infective. **benzoic and salicylic acid o.,** a preparation of benzoic acid and salicylic acid in a water-soluble base; used topically as an antifungal agent. **calamine o.,** a mixture of calamine, yellow wax, anhydrous lanolin and petrolatum; used as an astringent protectant. **chrysarobin o.,** a preparation of chrysarobin, chloroform and white ointment; used in local treatment of psoriatic lesions. **hydrophilic o.,** an oil-in-water emulsion used as a vehicle for local anti-infectives and antibiotics. **polyethylene glycol o.,** an ointment prepared by combining polyethylene glycol 4000 and polyethylene glycol 400. **undecylenic acid o., compound,** undecylenic acid and zinc undecylanate in polyethylene glycol ointment. **white o.,** a mixture of white wax and white petrolatum; used as a vehicle for medications to be applied to the skin. **yellow o.,** a mixture of yellow wax and petrolatum; used as a vehicle for medications. **zinc o., zinc oxide o.,** a preparation of zinc oxide and liquid petrolatum in white ointment; used topically as an astringent and protective.

-ol word termination indicating an alcohol or a phenol.

oleaginous (o″le-aj′ĭ-nus) oily; greasy.

oleandomycin (o″le-an″do-mi′sin) an antibiotic substance produced by growth of *Streptomyces antibioticus;* used chiefly in treatment of infections by gram-positive organisms.

oleate (o′le-āt) 1. a salt of oleic acid. 2. a solution of a substance in oleic acid.

olecranarthritis (o-lek″ran-ar-thri′tis) inflammation of the elbow joint.

olecranarthrocace (-ar-throk′ah-se) tuberculosis of the elbow joint.

olecranarthropathy (-ar-throp′ah-the) disease of the elbow joint.

olecranoid (o-lek′rah-noid) resembling the olecranon.

olecranon (o-lek′rah-non) bony projection of the ulna at the elbow. adj., **olec′ranal.**

oleoresin (o″le-o-rez′in) an extract containing the resinous and oily constituents of the drug, obtained by evaporating ethereal acetone, or alcoholic percolates.

oleotherapy (-ther′ah-pe) treatment by injections of oil.

oleothorax (-tho′raks) intrapleural injection of oil.

oleovitamin (-vi′tah-min) a preparation of fat-soluble vitamins in fish liver or edible vegetable oil.

oleum (o′le-um), pl. *o′lea* [L.] oil.

olfactie (ol-fak′te) a unit of odor.

olfaction (ol-fak′shun) 1. the act of smelling. 2. the sense of smell.

olfactology (ol″fak-tol′o-je) the science of the sense of smell.

olfactometer (-tom′ĕ-ter) instrument for testing the sense of smell.

olfactory (ol-fak′to-re) pertaining to the sense of smell.

olig(o)- (ol′ĭ-go) word element [Gr.], *few; little; scanty.*

oligemia (ol″ĭ-ge′me-ah) deficiency in volume of the blood. adj., **olige′mic.**

oligidria (ol″ig-id′re-ah) deficiency in sweat secretion.

oligoblast (ol′ĭ-go-blast″) a primitive oligodendrocyte.

oligocardia (ol″ĭ-go-kar′de-ah) bradycardia.

oligocholia (-ko′le-ah) deficiency of bile.

oligochromemia (-kro-me′me-ah) deficiency of hemoglobin in blood.

oligochylia (-ki′le-ah) deficiency of chyle.

oligochymia (-ki′me-ah) deficiency of chyme.

oligocythemia (-si-the′me-ah) scarcity of red corpuscles in the blood.

oligodactylia (-dak-til′e-ah) congenital absence of a digit of a hand or foot.

oligodendria (-den′dre-ah) oligodendroglia.

oligodendrocyte (-den′dro-sīt) a cell of oligodendroglia.

oligodendroglia (-den-drog′le-ah) non-nervous tissue of ectodermal origin forming part of the adventitial structure of the central nervous system.

oligodendroglioma (-den″dro-gli-o′mah) a tumor composed of oligodendroglia.

oligodipsia (-dip′se-ah) abnormally diminished thirst.

oligodontia (-don′she-ah) presence of fewer teeth than normal, due to congenital absence of some.

oligodynamic (-di-nam′ik) active in a small quantity.

oligogalactia (-gah-lak′she-ah) deficient secretion of milk.

oligogenic (-jen′ik) produced by a few genes at most; used in reference to certain hereditary characters.

oligohemia (-he′me-ah) oligemia.

oligohydramnios (-hi-dram′ne-os) deficiency of the liquor amnii in pregnancy.

oligohydruria (-hi-droo′re-ah) abnormally high concentration of urine.

oligolecithal (-les′ĭ-thal) having only a little yolk.

oligomania (-ma′ne-ah) disordered mental activity on a few subjects.

oligomenorrhea (-men″o-re′ah) infrequent or scanty menstrual flow.

oligomorphic (-mor′fik) passing through only a few forms of growth.

oligo-ovulation (-ov″u-la′shun) maturation and discharge of fewer than the normal number of ova from the ovaries.

oligophosphaturia (-fos″fah-tu′re-ah) deficiency of phosphates in the urine.

oligophrenia (-fre′ne-ah) mental deficiency. **phenylpyruvic o., o. phenylpyru′vica,** mental deficiency due to a genetically determined inability to convert phenylalanine to tyrosine, with accumulation of phenylalanine in body fluids and excretion of abnormally large amounts of its metabolites in the urine (phenylketonuria).

oligoplasmia (-plaz′me-ah) deficiency of blood plasma.

oligopnea (ol″ĭ-gop′ne-ah) retarded breathing.

oligoposia (ol″ĭ-go-po′ze-ah) abnormally diminished intake of fluids.

oligoposy (ol″ĭ-gop′o-se) oligoposia.

oligoptyalism (ol″ĭ-go-ti′al-izm) diminished secretion of saliva.

oligoria (ol″ĭ-go′re-ah) abnormal indifference toward persons or objects.

oligosaccharide (ol″ĭ-go-sak′ah-rīd) a carbohydrate that, on acid hydrolysis, yields two to ten monosaccharides.

oligospermia (-sper′me-ah) deficiency of spermatozoa in the semen.

oligotrichia (-trik′e-ah) congenital thinness of growth of the hair.

oligotrophia (-tro′fe-ah) a state of poor (insufficient) nutrition.

oligotrophy (ol″ĭ-got′ro-fe) oligotrophia.

oligozoospermia (ol″ĭ-go-zo″o-sper′me-ah) oligospermia.

oliguria (ol″ĭ-gu′re-ah) diminution of urinary secretion to between 100 and 400 ml. in 24 hours. adj., **oligu′ric.**

oliva (o-li′vah), pl. *oli′vae* [L.] olive.

olivary (ol′ĭ-ver″e) shaped like an olive.

olive (ol′iv) 1. fruit of the tree *Olea europaea.* 2. a rounded elevation lateral to the upper part of each pyramid of the medulla oblongata.

-oma (o′mah) word element [Gr.], *tumor.*

omagra (o-mag′rah) gout in the shoulder.

omalgia (o-mal′je-ah) pain in the shoulder.

omarthritis (o″mar-thri′tis) inflammation of the shoulder joint.

omasitis (o″mah-si′tis) inflammation of the omasum.

omasum (o-ma′sum) the third division of the stomach of a ruminant animal.

omentectomy (o″men-tek′to-me) excision of omentum.

omentitis (-ti′tis) inflammation of the omentum.

omentofixation (o-men″to-fik-sa′shun) omentopexy.

omentopexy (o-men′to-pek″se) fixation of the omentum, to establish collateral circulation in portal obstruction.

omentorrhaphy (o″men-tor′ah-fe) suture of the omentum.

omentum (o-men′tum), pl. *omen′ta* [L.] a fold of peritoneum extending from stomach to adjacent abdominal organs. adj., **omen′tal. gastrocolic o.,** greater omentum. **gastrohepatic o.,** lesser omentum. **greater o., o. ma′jus,** a peritoneal fold attached to the anterior surface of the transverse colon. **lesser o., o. mi′nus,** a peritoneal fold joining the lesser curvature of the stomach and the first part of the duodenum to the porta hepatis.

omitis (o-mi′tis) inflammation of the shoulder.

omocephalus (o″mo-sef′ah-lus) a fetal monster with no arms and incomplete head.

omodynia (-din′e-ah) pain in the shoulder.

omoplata (-plat′ah) the scapula.

omphalectomy (om″fah-lek′to-me) excision of the umbilicus.

omphalic (om-fal′ik) pertaining to the umbilicus.

omphalitis (om″fah-li′tis) inflammation of the umbilicus.

omphalocele (om′fal-o-sēl″) protrusion, at birth, of part of the intestine through a defect in the abdominal wall at the umbilicus.

omphaloncus (om″fah-long′kus) tumor of the umbilicus.

omphalophlebitis (om″fah-lo-fle-bi′tis) inflammation of umbilical veins.

omphaloproptosis (-prop-to′sis) prolapse of the umbilical cord.

omphalorrhagia (-ra′je-ah) hemorrhage from the umbilicus.

omphalorrhea (-re′ah) effusion of lymph at the umbilicus.

omphalorrhexis (-rek′sis) rupture of the umbilicus.

omphalosite (om′fal-o-sīt″) a fetal monster with no heart, which cannot live after the umbilical cord is cut.

omphalotaxis (om″fah-lo-tak′sis) replacement of prolapsed umbilical cord.

omphalotomy (om″fah-lot′o-me) the cutting of the umbilical cord.

omphalotripsy (om-fal′o-trip″se) separation of the umbilical cord by crushing.

onanism (o′nah-nizm) incomplete sexual relations with withdrawal just before emission; sometimes incorrectly used as a synonym for masturbation.

Onchocerca (ong″ko-ser′kah) a genus of nematode parasites of the superfamily Filarioidea. **O. vol′vulus,** a species causing human infection, dwelling in tumors in subcutaneous connective tissue.

onchocerciasis (-ser-ki′ah-sis) infection by nematodes of the genus Onchocerca.

oncogenesis (ong″ko-jen′ĕ-sis) the production of tumors. adj., **oncogenet′ic.**

oncogenic (-jen′ik) causing tumor formation.

oncogenous (ong-koj′ĕ-nus) arising in or originating from a tumor.

oncology (ong-kol′o-je) sum of knowledge regarding tumors.

oncolysis (ong-kol′ĭ-sis) destruction or dissolution of a neoplasm. adj., **oncolyt′ic.**

oncoma (ong-ko′mah) a tumor.

oncometer (ong-kom′ĕ-ter) instrument for measuring variations in size of viscera.

oncosis (ong-ko′sis) the formation of multiple tumors.

oncosphere (ong′ko-sfēr) the larva of a tapeworm in the spherical stage.

oncotherapy (ong″ko-ther′ah-pe) the treatment of tumors.

oncothlipsis (-thlip′sis) pressure caused by a tumor.

oncotic (ong-kot′ik) pertaining to swelling.

oncotomy (ong-kot′o-me) the incision of an abscess or tumor.

oncotropic (ong″ko-trop′ik) having special affinity for tumor cells.

oneiric (o-ni′rik) pertaining to dreams.

oneirism (o-ni′rizm) a waking dream state.

oneiroanalysis (o-ni″ro-ah-nal′ĭ-sis) exploration of conscious and unconscious person-

ality by interpretation of drug-induced dreams.

oneirogenic (o″ni-ro-jen′ik) producing a dreamlike state.

oneirology (o″ni-rol′o-je) the science of dreams.

oneiroscopy (o″ni-ros′ko-pe) analysis of dreams for diagnosis of a patient's mental state.

oniomania (o″ne-o-ma′ne-ah) insane desire to make purchases.

onomatology (on″o-mah-tol′o-je) the science of names and nomenclature.

onomatomania (on″o-mat″o-ma′ne-ah) mental derangement with regard to words or names.

onomatophobia (-fo′be-ah) morbid aversion to a certain word or name.

ontogeny (on-toj′e-ene) the complete developmental history of an individual organism.

onychalgia (on″ī-kal′je-ah) pain in the nails.

onychatrophia (o-nik″ah-tro′fe-ah) atrophy of the nails.

onychectomy (on″ī-kek′to-me) excision of a fingernail or toenail.

onychia (o-nik′e-ah) inflammation of the nail bed, resulting in loss of the nail. **o. latera′lis,** paronychia. **o. malig′na,** onychia with fetid ulceration. **o. parasit′ica,** onychomycosis.

onychitis (on″ī-ki′tis) inflammation of the matrix of a nail.

onychogenic (on″ī-ko-jen′ik) producing nail substance.

onychograph (o-nik′o-graf) instrument for recording variations of blood pressure in capillaries of fingertips.

onychogryposis (on″ī-ko-grī-po′sis) abnormal elongation and twisting of the nails, giving a clawlike appearance.

onychoid (on′ī-koid) resembling a fingernail.

onycholysis (on″ī-kol′ī-sis) loosening or separation of a nail from its bed.

onychomadesis (on″ī-ko-mah-de′sis) complete loss of the nails.

onychomalacia (-mah-la′she-ah) softening of the fingernail.

onychomycosis (-mi-ko′sis) fungus infection of the nails.

onychopathy (on″ī-kop′ah-the) disease of the nails.

onychophagy (-kof′ah-je) biting of the nails.

onychorrhexis (on″ī-ko-rek′sis) spontaneous splitting and brittleness of the nails.

onychoschizia (-skiz′e-ah) loosening of the nail from its bed.

onychosis (on″ī-ko′sis) disease or malformation of the nails.

onychotillomania (on″ī-ko-til″o-ma′ne-ah) neurotic picking or tearing at the nails.

onychotomy (on″ī-kot′o-me) incision into a fingernail or toenail.

onychotrophy (-kot′ro-fe) nutrition of the nails.

onyx (on′iks) 1. a variety of hypopyon. 2. a fingernail or toenail.

onyxitis (on″ik-si′tis) onychitis.

ooblast (o′o-blast) a cell from which an ovum is developed.

oocyst (o′o-sist) the membrane surrounding a zygote after union of the gametes.

oocyte (o′o-sīt) a cell developed from an oogonium in oogenesis. **primary o.,** the original large cell into which an oogonium develops. **secondary o.,** the large cell produced by unequal meiotic division of a primary oocyte.

oogenesis (o″o-jen′ē-sis) the development of mature ova from oogonia.

oogonium (o″o-go′ne-um), pl. *oogo′nia* [Gr.] one of the primitive germ cells in the ovary.

oophor(o)- (o-of′or-o) word element [Gr.], *ovary.*

oophoralgia (o″of-o-ral′je-ah) pain in an ovary.

oophorectomy (-rek′to-me) excision of an ovary.

oophoritis (-ri′tis) inflammation of an ovary. **mumps o.,** involvement of the ovaries in epidemic parotitis.

oophorocystectomy (o-of″o-ro-sis-tek′to-me) excision of an ovarian cyst.

oophorocystosis (-sis-to′sis) formation of an ovarian cyst.

oophorohysterectomy (-his″ter-ek′to-me) excision of ovaries and uterus.

oophoroma (o-of″o-ro′mah) a malignant tumor of the ovary.

oophoron (o-of′o-ron) an ovary.

oophoropexy (o-of′o-ro-pek″se) fixation of an ovary.

oophoroplasty (o-of′o-ro-plas″te) plastic repair of an ovary.

oophororrhaphy (o″of-o-ror′ah-fe) suture of an ovary.

oosperm (o′o-sperm) a fertilized ovum.

ootid (o′o-tid) the cell produced by unequal meiotic division of a secondary oocyte, which develops into the ovum.

oozooid (o″o-zo′oid) an individual developed from an ovum, i.e. as a result of sexual reproduction.

opacity (o-pas′ī-te) 1. the condition of being opaque. 2. an opaque area.

opening (o′pen-ing) an unobstructed area or aperture. **aortic o.,** 1. the aperture of the ventricle into the aorta. 2. the aperture in the diaphragm for passage of the descending aorta. **duodenal o. of stomach,** pylorus. **saphenous o.,** the aperture in the fascia lata for passage of the long saphenous vein. **o. of stomach, anterior,** pylorus.

operate (op′er-āt) 1. to perform an operation. 2. the subject of an experiment which has undergone a specific surgical procedure in contrast to the normal control.

operation (op″er-a′shun) 1. any action performed with instruments or by the hands of a surgeon. 2. the specific effect of a drug. **Albee's o.,** spinal fusion. **Bassini's o.,** plastic repair of inguinal hernia. **Billroth's o.,** gastrectomy. **Brunschwig's o.,** pancreatoduodenectomy. **Caldwell-Luc o.,** radical maxillary sinusotomy. **cosmetic o.,** one for correction of an unsightly defect. **Crosby-Cooney o.,** introduction of flanged glass tube into the peritoneal cavity for drainage of fluid in ascites. **Elliot's o.,** sclerectomy by trephine. **explora-**

tory o., opening of the body for determination of the cause of otherwise unexplainable symptoms. **Fredet-Ramstedt o.,** pyloromyotomy. **Heller's o.,** cardiomyotomy. **Holth's o.,** sclerectomy by punch. **Kelly's o.,** **King's o.,** arytenoidopexy. **Kondoleon's o.,** excision of fascia in treatment of elephantiasis. **Kraske's o.,** proctectomy. **Lagrange's o.,** sclerectomy by scissors. **Le Forte's o.,** partial colpectomy. **McBurney's o.,** radical surgery for the cure of inguinal hernia. **McGill's o.,** suprapubic prostatectomy. **Macewen's o.,** supracondylar section of the femur for genu valgum. **Marshall-Marchetti o.,** surgical correction of stress incontinence. **Partsch o.,** partial removal of a dental cyst. **Phemister o.,** use of an onlay graft of cancellous bone for treatment of a stable but ununited fracture. **Porro's o.,** cesarean hysterectomy. **radical o.,** one by which all diseased or involved tissue is removed, effecting complete cure without effort to preserve body structures. **Ramstedt o.,** pyloromyotomy. **Ransohoff o.,** cruciate incision of thickened scars of the visceral pleura. **Schede's o.,** resection of parietal pleura, ribs and intercostal muscle. **Semb's o.,** extrafascial apicolysis. **Sistrunk o.,** a surgical procedure for removal of thyroglossal cysts and sinuses. **tagliacotian o.,** rhinoplasty. **Talma-Morison o.,** omentopexy. **Taussig's o.,** excision of the central portion of the uterine tube. **Torkildsen's o.,** ventriculocisternostomy. **Wertheim's o.,** radical hysterectomy.

operative (op″er-a′tiv) 1. pertaining to an operation. 2. acting to produce an effect.

operculum (o-per′ku-lum), pl. *oper′cula* [L.] applied to folds from the frontal, parietal and temporal lobes of the cerebrum overlying the insula. adj., **oper′cular. dental o.,** the hood of gingival tissue overlying the crown of an erupting tooth. **trophoblastic o.,** the plug of trophoblast that helps close the gap in the endometrium made by the implanting blastocyst.

operon (op′er-on) a system of hereditary units on a chromosome, one of which, the operator gene, interacts with repressor in the cell and controls activity of the remaining structural genes of the system.

ophiasis (o-fi′ah-sis) baldness in winding streaks.

ophidiophobia (o-fid″e-o-fo′be-ah) morbid dread of snakes.

ophidism (o′fi-dizm) poisoning by snake venom.

ophryon (o′fre-on) middle point of transverse supraorbital line.

Ophthaine (of′thān) trademark for a preparation of proparacaine hydrochloride.

ophthalm(o) word element [Gr.], *eye.*

ophthalmectomy (of″thal-mek′to-me) excision of an eye.

ophthalmia (of-thal′me-ah) severe inflammation or affection of the eye. **Egyptian o.,** trachoma. **o. neonato′rum,** purulent ophthalmia of newborn. **periodic o.,** a recurring inflammation primarily of the iris and ciliary body, a common cause of blindness in horses and mules. **phlyctenular o.,** a form with vesicles on epithelium of cornea or conjunctiva. **sympathetic o.,** inflammation of a sound eye accompanying involvement of the other.

ophthalmic (of-thal′mik) pertaining to the eye.

ophthalmitis (of″thal-mi′tis) inflammation of the eyeball.

ophthalmoblennorrhea (of-thal″mo-blen″ō-re′ah) gonorrheal ophthalmia.

ophthalmocele (of-thal′mo-sēl) exophthalmos.

ophthalmodynamometry (of-thal″mo-di″nah-mom′ē-tre) determination of the blood pressure in the retinal artery.

ophthalmodynia (-din′e-ah) neuralgic pain of the eye.

ophthalmo-eikonometer (-i-ko-nom′ē-ter) an instrument for measuring retinal images.

ophthalmofunduscope (-fun′du-skōp) an instrument for examining the fundus of the eye.

ophthalmography (of″thal-mog′rah-fe) description of the eye and its diseases.

ophthalmogyric (of-thal″mo-ji′rik) causing movements of the eye.

ophthalmolith (of-thal′mo-lith) a lacrimal calculus.

ophthalmologist (of″thal-mol′o-jist) a specialist in ophthalmology.

ophthalmology (-mol′o-je) the study of the eye and its diseases.

ophthalmomalacia (of-thal″mo-mah-la′she-ah) abnormal softness of the eyeball.

ophthalmometer (of″thal-mom′ē-ter) instrument for measuring the refractive power of the eye.

ophthalmometry (-mom′ē-tre) determination of refractive power of eye.

ophthalmomycosis (of-thal″mo-mi-ko′sis) any disease of the eye caused by a fungus.

ophthalmomyotomy (-mi-ot′o-me) division of the muscles of the eyes.

ophthalmonouritis (-nu-ri′tis) inflammation of the optic nerve.

ophthalmopathy (of″thal-mop′ah-the) any disease of the eye.

ophthalmophantom (of-thal″mo-fan′tom) a model of the eye for demonstration purposes.

ophthalmophthisis (of″thal-mof′thi-sis) abnormal softness of the eye; phthisis bulbi.

ophthalmoplasty (of-thal′mo-plas″te) plastic surgery of the eye.

ophthalmoplegia (of-thal″mo-ple′je-ah) paralysis of the eye muscles. **o. exter′na,** paralysis of extraocular muscles. **o. inter′na,** paralysis of the intraocular muscles. **nuclear o.,** that due to a lesion of nuclei of motor nerves of eye. **partial o.,** that affecting some of the eye muscles. **progressive o.,** gradual paralysis of all the eye muscles. **total o.,** paralysis of all the eye muscles, both intraocular and extraocular.

ophthalmoptosis (of-thal″mop-to′sis) exophthalmos.

ophthalmoreaction (of-thal″mo-re-ak′shun) ophthalmic reaction.

ophthalmorrhagia (of-thal"mo-ra'je-ah) hemorrhage from the eye.

ophthalmorrhea (-re'ah) oozing of blood from the eye.

ophthalmorrhexis (-rek'sis) rupture of an eyeball.

ophthalmoscope (of-thal'mo-skōp) an instrument for observing the interior of the eye.

ophthalmoscopy (of"thal-mos'ko-pe) examination of the eye by means of the ophthalmoscope. **direct o.**, observation of an upright or erect mirrored image. **indirect o.**, observation of an inverted image. **medical o.**, that performed for diagnostic purposes. **metric o.**, that performed for measurement of refraction.

ophthalmosteresis (of-thal"mo-stě-re'sis) loss of an eye.

ophthalmosynchysis (-sin'kĭ-sis) effusion into the eye.

ophthalmotomy (of"thal-mot'o-me) incision of the eye.

ophthalmotrope (of-thal'mo-trōp) a mechanical eye that moves like a real eye.

ophthalmoxerosis (of-thal"mo-ze-ro'sis) xerophthalmia.

opian (o'pe-an) noscapine.

opianine (o-pi'ah-nin) noscapine.

opiate (o'pe-āt) 1. a remedy containing opium. 2. any drug that induces sleep and anesthesia.

opiomania (o"pe-o-ma'ne-ah) intense craving for opium.

opisthion (o-pis'the-on) midpoint of lower border of foramen magnum.

opisthorchiasis (o"pis-thor-ki'ah-sis) infection by flukes of the genus Opisthorchis.

Opisthorchis (o"pis-thor'kis) a genus of flukes parasitic in the liver and biliary tract of various birds and mammals, including man. **O. sinen'sis,** a species widely distributed in China, Japan, Korea, Vietnam and parts of India.

opisthotonos (o"pis-thot'o-nos) tetanic spasm which flexes the head and feet backward.

opium (o'pe-um) air-dried milky exudation from incised unripe capsules of *Papaver somniferum,* yielding not less than 9.5 per cent anhydrous morphine. **granulated o.,** opium reduced to a coarse powder. **powdered o.,** opium reduced to a very fine powder.

opiumism (o'pe-u-mizm") habitual misuse of opium, and its consequences.

opocephalus (o"po-sef'ah-lus) a fetal monster with ears fused, one orbit, no mouth and no nose.

opodidymus (-did'ĭ-mus) a fetal monster with two fused heads and sense organs partly fused.

oppilative (op'ĭ-la"tiv) 1. closing the pores. 2. constipating.

opsinogen (op-sin'o-jen) a substance which forms opsonins. adj., **opsinog'enous.**

opsiuria (op"se-u're-ah) excretion of urine more rapidly during fasting than after a meal.

opsogen (op'so-jen) opsinogen.

opsomania (op"so-ma'ne-ah) an abnormal craving for some special food.

opsoniferous (op"so-nif'er-us) bearing opsonin.

opsonification (op-son"ĭ-fĭ-ka'shun) the rendering of bacteria and other cells subject to phagocytosis.

opsonin (op-so'nin) an antibody which renders bacteria and other cells susceptible to phagocytosis. adj., **opson'ic. immune o.**, an antibody which sensitizes a particulate antigen to phagocytosis, after combination with the homologous antigen in vivo or in vitro.

opsonize (op'so-nīz) to treat with opsonins.

opsonocytophagic (op"so-no-si"to-faj'ik) pertaining to the phagocytic activity of blood in the presence of serum opsonins and homologous leukocytes.

opsonoid (op'so-noid) an opsonin in which the active element has been destroyed.

opsonology (op"so-nol'o-je) the study of opsonins and opsonic action.

opsonometry (-nom'ě-tre) measurement of the opsonic index.

opsonophilia (op"so-no-fil'e-ah) affinity for opsonins. adj., **opsonophil'ic.**

opsonotherapy (-ther'ah-pe) treatment by use of bacterial vaccines to increase the opsonic index.

optesthesia (op"tes-the'ze-ah) visual sensibility.

optic (op'tik) pertaining to the eye.

optical (op'tĭ-kal) pertaining to vision.

optician (op-tish'an) a specialist in opticianry.

opticianry (op-tish'an-re) the translation, filling and adapting of ophthalmic prescriptions, products and accessories.

opticist (op'tĭ-sist) a specialist in the science of optics.

opticociliary (op"tĭ-ko-sil'e-er"e) pertaining to optic and ciliary nerves.

opticokinetic (-ki-net'ik) pertaining to movement of the eyes.

opticopupillary (-pu"pĭ-ler"e) pertaining to optic nerve and pupil.

optics (op'tiks) the science of light and vision.

optogram (op'to-gram) visual image formed on the retina.

optometer (op-tom'ě-ter) device for measuring power and range of vision.

optometrist (op-tom'ě-trist) a specialist in optometry.

optometry (op-tom'ě-tre) measurement of the powers of vision and the adaptation of lenses or prisms for the aid thereof, utilizing any means other than drugs.

optostriate (op"to-stri'āt) pertaining to optic thalamus and corpus striatum.

O.R. operating room.

ora (o'rah), pl. *o'rae* [L.] an edge or margin. **o. serra'ta ret'inae,** the zigzag margin of the retina of the eye.

Orabilex (o"rah-bi'leks) trademark for a preparation of bunamiodyl.

orad (o'rad) toward the mouth.

oral (o'ral) pertaining to the mouth.

Oranixon (or"ah-nik'son) trademark for a preparation of mephenesin.

orbicular (or-bik'u-lar) circular; rounded.

orbiculare (or-bik″u-la're) the orbicular bone; an ossicle of the ear.

orbit (or'bit) the bony cavity containing the eyeball. adj., **or'bital.**

orbita (or'bĭ-tah), pl. *or'bitae* [L.] the bony cavity containing the eyeball and its associated muscles, vessels and nerves.

orbitale (or″bĭ-ta'le) the lowest point on the inferior edge of the orbit.

orbitalis (or″bĭ-ta'lis) [L.] pertaining to the orbit.

orbitonometer (or″bĭ-to-nom'ĕ-ter) an instrument for measuring backward displacement of eyeball produced by given pressure on its anterior aspect.

orbitotomy (or″bĭ-tot'o-me) incision into the orbit.

orcein (or-se'in) a brownish-red coloring substance obtained from orcinol.

orchi(o)- (or'ke-o) word element [Gr.], *testis.*

orchialgia (or″ke-al'je-ah) pain in a testis.

orchichorea (-ko-re'ah) twitching or jerking of a testis.

orchidectomy (or″kĭ-dek'to-me) orchiectomy.

orchidic (or-kid'ik) pertaining to a testis.

orchidoptosis (or″kĭ-dop-to'sis) falling or relaxation of the testis.

orchidorrhaphy (or″kĭ-dor'ah-fe) orchiopexy.

orchidotherapy (or″kĭ-do-ther'ah-pe) treatment with testicular extract.

orchidotomy (or″kĭ-dot'o-me) incision and drainage of a testis.

orchiectomy (or″ke-ek'to-me) excision of a testis.

orchiepididymitis (-ep″ĭ-did″ĭ-mi'tis) inflammation of testis and epididymis.

orchiocele (or'ke-o-sēl″) hernial protrusion of a testis.

orchiodynia (or″ke-o-din'e-ah) pain in a testis.

orchiomyeloma (-mi″ĕ-lo'mah) myeloma of a testis.

orchioncus (-ong'kus) tumor of a testis.

orchioneuralgia (-nu-ral'je-ah) pain in a testis.

orchiopathy (or″ke-op'ah-the) any disorder of the testes.

orchiopexy (or'ke-o-pek″se) fixation of an undescended testis in the scrotum.

orchioplasty (or'ke-o-plas″te) plastic surgery of a testis.

orchioscheocele (or″ke-os'ke-o-sēl″) scrotal tumor with scrotal hernia.

orchioscirrhus (or″ke-o-skir'us) hardening of a testis.

orchitis (or-ki'tis) inflammation of a testis. adj., **orchit'ic. mumps o.,** involvement of the testes in epidemic parotitis.

orcinol (or'sĭ-nol) a chemical compound occurring in many species of lichens.

order (or'der) 1. arrangement systematically or in proper sequence. 2. a taxonomic category subordinate to a class and superior to a family (or suborder).

orderly (or'der-le) a male hospital attendant who does general work, attending especially to needs of male patients.

ordinate (or'dĭ-nāt) the vertical line in a graph along which is plotted one of the factors considered in the study, as temperature in a time-temperature study.

O.R.E.F. Orthopedic Research and Education Foundation.

Oretic (o-ret'ik) trademark for a preparation of hydrochlorothiazide.

Oreton (or'e-ton) trademark for preparations of testosterone.

orexigenic (o-rek″sĭ-jen'ik) increasing the appetite.

orf (orf) a contagious pustular dermatitis of sheep, communicable to man.

organ (or'gan) a structural unit of a plant or animal body which serves a specific function or functions. **acoustic o.,** organ of Corti. **cell o.,** a structural part of a cell having some definite function in its life or reproduction, as a nucleus or a centrosome. **cement o.,** the embryonic tissue which develops into the cement layer of the tooth. **o. of Corti,** the terminal acoustic apparatus within the scala media, including the rods of Corti and the auditory cells, with their supporting elements. **enamel o.,** a process of epithelium forming a cap over a dental papilla and developing into the enamel. **o. of Giraldès,** the paradidymis. **Golgi tendon o.,** one of the mechanoreceptors arranged in series with muscle in the tendons of mammalian muscles, being the receptor for stimuli responsible for the lengthening reaction. **gustatory o.,** the organ concerned with the perception of taste. **Jacobson's o.,** a sac in the nasal septum, rudimentary in man except in the fetus. **lateral line o's,** sense organs in the skin of fishes and amphibians, intermediate in type between organs of touch and hearing. **Meyer's o.,** an area of circumvallate papillae on either side of the posterior part of the tongue. **olfactory o.,** the organ concerned with the perception of odors. **primitive fat o.,** interscapular gland. **o. of Rosenmüller,** epoophoron. **segmental o.,** the pronephros, mesonephros and metanephros together. **sense o., sensory o's,** a specialized structure containing receptors which are remarkably sensitive to the appropriate stimulus. **o. of shock,** the organ which reacts in anaphylactic shock. **target o.,** the organ affected by a particular hormone. **terminal o.,** the organ at either end of a reflex neural arc. **vestigial o.,** one which was functional in some earlier animal, but which, through a change in environment or mode of life in the species, has become unnecessary to survival. **vomeronasal o.,** Jacobson's organ, **Weber's o.,** utriculus prostaticus. **o's of Zuckerkandl,** two rounded masses of chromaffin cells about the root of the inferior mesenteric artery, formed before birth and persisting to puberty.

organelle (or″gah-nel′) 1. a specific particle of organized living substance present in practically all cells. 2. a minute structure serving a specific function in the life processes of a cell, e.g. a specific particle of organized living substance contained in the cytoplasm, or a flagellum of a protozoan.

organic (or-gan′ik) 1. pertaining to or having organs. 2. pertaining to carbon compounds produced by living plants or animals, or by synthetic processes.

organicist (or-gan′ĭ-sist) one who believes that the symptoms of disease are due to organic changes.

organism (or′gah-nizm) an individual animal or plant. **pleuropneumonia-like o's,** an apparently homogeneous group of highly pleomorphic, filterable microorganisms, one species of which causes pleuropneumonia in cattle.

organization (or″gah-ni-za′shun) 1. the process of organizing or being organized, especially the conversion of a plastic mass, such as a blood clot or inflammatory exudate, into fibrous tissue. 2. an organism or organized body.

organizer (or′gah-nīz″er) a special region of the embryo which is capable of determining the differentiation of other regions.

organogenesis (or″gah-no-jen′ĕ-sis) the segregation of tissues into different organs in embryonic development.

organogeny (or″gah-noj′ĕ-ne) organogenesis.

organography (-nog′rah-fe) 1. description of organs. 2. roentgen visualization of body organs.

organoleptic (or″gah-no-lep′tik) making an impression on or affecting an organ or the entire organism.

organology (or″gah-nol′o-je) scientific study of the organs of plants and animals.

organon (or′gah-non), pl. *or′gana* [Gr.] organum.

organotherapy (or″gah-no-ther′ah-pe) therapeutic administration of animal organs or their extracts.

organotropism (or-gah-not′ro-pizm) the special affinity of chemical compounds or pathogenic agents for particular tissues or organs of the body. adj., **organotrop′ic.**

organum (or′gah-num), pl. *or′gana* [L.] a somewhat independent part of the body that performs a special function.

orgasm (or′gazm) the crisis or climax of sexual excitement.

orientation (o″re-en-ta′shun) the recognition of one's position in relation to time and space.

orientomycin (o-re-en″to-mi′sin) cycloserine.

orifice (or′ĭ-fis) 1. the entrance or outlet of any body cavity. 2. any foramen, meatus or opening. **canal o.,** root canal orifice. **duodenal o. of stomach,** pylorus. **pilosebaceous o's,** the opening of the hair follicles. **root canal o.,** an opening in the floor of the pulp chamber of a tooth, leading into a root canal.

orificium (or″i-fish′e-um), pl. *orific′ia* [L.] orifice.

origin (or′ĭ-jin) a beginning, as of a nerve or blood vessel, or the end of a skeletal muscle that remains relatively fixed when the muscle contracts.

Orinase (or′ĭ-nās) trademark for a preparation of tolbutamide.

ornithine (or′nĭ-thēn) a naturally occurring amino acid isolated from the urine and excrement of fowls.

Ornithodoros (or″nĭ-thod′o-ros) a genus of arthropods (family Argasidae), including *O. moubata,* a vector of the organism causing relapsing fever, and many other species which transmit pathogenic microorganisms.

ornithosis (or″nĭ-tho′sis) a viral infection of birds that is occasionally transmitted to man, to produce an acute viral pneumonitis; that transmitted by parrots is commonly called psittacosis.

orolingual (o″ro-ling′gwal) pertaining to mouth and tongue.

oronasal (-na′zal) pertaining to mouth and nose.

oropharynx (-phar′inks) part of pharynx behind the mouth and tongue.

orphenadrine (or-fen′ah-drēn) a compound used as an antihistaminic, antitremor and antispasmodic agent for relaxation of skeletal muscle spasm and tremor.

orrhology (or-rol′o-je) scientific study of serums.

orrhomeningitis (or″o-men″in-ji′tis) inflammation of a serous membrane.

orrhoreaction (-re-ak′shun) a serum reaction.

orrhorrhea (-re′ah) a watery or serous discharge.

orrhotherapy (-ther′ah-pe) serum therapy.

O.R.S. Orthopedic Research Society.

orth(o) (or′tho) word element [Gr.], *straight normal; correct.*

orthesis (or-the′sis), pl. *orthe′ses* [Gr.] orthosis.

orthetics (or-thet′iks) orthotics.

orthetist (or′thĕ-tist) orthotist.

orthoarteriotony (or″tho-ar-te″re-ot′o-ne) normal arterial pressure.

orthobiosis (-bi-o′sis) proper and hygienic living.

orthocephalic (-sĕ-fal′ik) having a vertical index of 70.1–75.

orthochorea (-ko-re′ah) choreic movements in the erect posture.

orthochromatic (-kro-mat′ik) staining normally.

orthocrasia (-kra′ze-ah) normal reaction of the body to drugs, proteins, etc.

orthodiagram (-di′ah-gram) an outline of an organ, such as the heart, as visualized on the fluoroscopic screen.

orthodiagraph (-di′ah-graf) an instrument for use in orthodiagraphy.

orthodiagraphy (-di-ag′rah-fe) the recording of outlines of organs as seen by the fluoroscope.

orthodontia (-don′she-ah) orthodontics.

orthodontics (-don′tiks) that branch of dentistry concerned with irregularities of teeth and malocclusion, and associated facial problems. **corrective o.,** that concerned with correction of existing malocclusion and its sequelae. **interceptive o.,** that concerned with elimination of conditions that might lead to malocclusion. **preventive o.,** that concerned with preservation of the integrity of normal occlusion.

orthodontist (or"tho-don'tist) a dentist who specializes in orthodontics.

orthodromic (-drom'ik) traveling or conducting impulses forward or in the normal direction.

orthogenics (-jen'iks) eugenics.

orthoglycemic (-gli-se'mik) having the normal amount of sugar in the blood.

orthognathous (or-thog'nah-thus) having a gnathic index below 98.

orthograde (or'tho-grād) carrying the body upright in walking.

orthometer (or-thom'ĕ-ter) instrument for determining relative protrusion of the eyeballs.

orthopedic (or"tho-pe'dik) pertaining to the correction of deformities or to orthopedics.

orthopedics (-pe'diks) the art and science of prevention, diagnosis and treatment of diseases and abnormalities of the musculoskeletal system.

orthopedist (-pe'dist) a specialist in orthopedics.

orthopercussion (-per-kush'un) percussion with the distal phalanx of the finger held perpendicularly to the body wall.

orthophoria (-fo're-ah) normal equilibrium of the eye muscles, or muscular balance.

orthopnea (or"thop-ne'ah) ability to breathe only in the upright position.

orthopsychiatry (or"tho-si-ki'ah-tre) the study of intrapsychic factors in the development of normal personality in children; preventive psychiatry.

orthoptic (or-thop'tik) pertaining to correction of deviation of the visual axes.

orthoptics (or-thop'tiks) treatment of strabismus by exercise of the ocular muscles.

orthoptoscope (or-thop'to-skōp) an instrument for exercising the ocular muscle in treating strabismus.

orthoroentgenography (or"tho-rent"gen-og'rah-fe) orthodiagraphy.

orthorrhachic (-rak'ik) having a vertebral column showing practically no curvature in the lumbar region.

orthoscope (or'tho-skōp) apparatus which neutralizes the corneal refraction by means of a layer of water; used in ocular examinations.

orthoscopic (or"tho-skop'ik) affording a correct and undistorted view.

orthoscopy (or-thos'ko-pe) examination by means of an orthoscope.

orthosis (or-tho'sis) a brace or other orthopedic device which is applied to a segment of the body for the purpose of protecting the segment or assisting in restoration or improvement of its function.

orthostatic (or"tho-stat'ik) pertaining to the upright position.

orthostatism (or'tho-stat"izm) an erect standing position of the body.

orthotic (or-thot'ik) serving to protect or to restore or improve function; pertaining to the use or application of an orthosis.

orthotics (or-thot'iks) the field of knowledge relating to orthoses and their use.

orthotist (or'tho-tist) a person skilled in orthotics and practicing its application in individual cases.

orthotonos (or-thot'o-nos) tetanic spasm which fixes the head, body and limbs in a rigid straight line.

Orthoxine (or-thok'sēn) trademark for preparations of methoxyphenamine.

orthuria (or-thoo're-ah) normal frequency of urination.

O.S. [L.] *oculus sinister* (left eye).

Os chemical symbol, *osmium.*

os[1] (os), pl. *o'ra* [L.] an opening or mouth.

os[2] (os), pl. *os'sa* [L.] a bone.

O.S.A. Optical Society of America.

osazone (o'sah-zōn) any one of a series of compounds obtained by heating sugars with phenylhydrazine and acetic acid.

osche(o) (os'ke-o) word element [Gr.], *scrotum.*

oscheitis (os"ke-i'tis) inflammation of the scrotum.

oscheocele (os'ke-o-sēl") a swelling or tumor of the scrotum.

oscheoma (os"ke-o'mah) tumor of the scrotum.

oscheoplasty (os'ke-o-plas"te) plastic repair of the scrotum.

oscillogram (ŏ-sil'o-gram) a graphic record made by an oscillograph.

oscillograph (ŏ-sil'o-graf) an instrument for recording electric oscillations.

oscillometer (os"ĭ-lom'ĕ-tcr) an instrument for measuring oscillations.

oscillometry (-lom'ĕ-tre) the measurement of oscillations, as by the string galvanometer.

oscillopsia (-lop'se-ah) a visual sensation that stationary objects are swaying back and forth.

oscilloscope (ŏ-sil'lo-skōp) an instrument for displaying the shape or wave form of transient or recurrent electrical signals.

Oscillospira (os"sil-lo-spi'rah) a genus of Schizomycetes (order Caryophanales, family Oscillospiraceae).

Oscillospiraceae (-spi-ra'se e) a family of Schizomycetes (order Caryophanales) found as nonpathogenic parasites in the intestinal tract of vertebrates.

oscitation (os"ĭ-ta'shun) the act of yawning.

osculum (os'ku-lum) [L.] an aperture or little opening.

-osis (-o'sis) word element [Gr.], *disease, morbid state; abnormal increase.*

osmatic (oz-mat'ik) pertaining to the sense of smell.

osmesthesia (os"mes-the'ze-ah) the sense by which odors are perceived and distinguished.

osmics (oz'miks) the science dealing with the sense of smell.

osmidrosis (oz"mĭ-dro'sis) bromhidrosis.

osmium (oz'me-um) chemical element *(see table),* at. no. 76, symbol Os.

osmolality (os"mo-lal'ĭ-te) the concentration of the solute in a solution per unit of solvent.

osmolarity (-lar'ĭ-te) the concentration of the solute in a solution per unit of total volume of solution.

osmole (os'mōl) the standard unit of osmotic

pressure, being the amount produced by one mole of solute in a liter of water.

osmometer (oz-mom′ĕ-ter) 1. device for testing the sense of smell. 2. instrument for measuring osmotic pressure.

osmophore (oz′mo-for) the group of atoms in a molecule of a compound which is responsible for its odor.

osmoreceptor (oz″mo-re-sep′tor) 1. a specialized sensory nerve ending sensitive to stimulation giving rise to the sensation of odors. 2. a specialized sensory nerve ending which is stimulated by changes in osmotic pressure of the surrounding medium.

osmoregulation (-reg″u-la′shun) adjustment of internal osmotic pressure of a simple organism in relation to that of the surrounding medium.

osmoregulator (-reg′u-la″tor) an instrument for regulating the penetrating power of roentgen rays.

osmoregulatory (-reg′u-lah-to″re) pertaining to or accomplishing adaptation to osmotic pressure of the surrounding medium.

osmose (oz′mōs) to pass through a membrane.

osmosis (oz-mo′sis) diffusion of water or solvent molecules through a semipermeable membrane, passing from the side of lower concentration to that of the higher. adj., **osmot′ic**.

osmosity (oz-mos′ĭ-te) a measure of the osmotic pressure of a solution, expressed numerically by the molarity.

osphresiology (os-fre″ze-ol′o-je) the science of odors and sense of smell.

osphresiometer (os-fre″ze-om′ĕ-ter) instrument for measuring acuteness of the sense of smell.

osphresis (os-fre′sis) the sense of smell. adj., **osphret′ic**.

ossein (os′e-in) the animal matter of bone.

osseous (os′e-us) composed of bone.

ossicle (os′ĭ-kl) a small bone, especially one of those in the middle ear. adj., **ossic′ular. Andernach's o's,** wormian bones. **auditory o's,** the small bones of the middle ear: incus, malleus and stapes.

ossiculectomy (os″ĭ-ku-lek′to-me) excision of one or more of the ossicles of the middle ear.

ossiculum (ŏ-sik′u-lum), pl. *ossic′ula* [L.] ossicle.

ossiferous (ŏ-sif′er-us) producing bone.

ossific (ŏ-sif′ik) forming bone.

ossification (os″ĭ-fĭ-ka′shun) formation of or conversion into bone. **cartilaginous o., endochondral o.,** ossification which occurs in and replaces cartilage. **intramembranous o.,** development of bone in and replacing connective tissue. **perichondral o.,** development of bone peripherally within the perichondrium of a cartilaginous model. **periosteal o.,** development of parallel plates of compact bone on the inner surface of periosteum surrounding centers of ossification in mesenchymal tissue.

ostalgia (os-tal′je-ah) pain in the bones.

oste(o)- (os′te-o) word element [Gr.], *bone.*

osteanagenesis (os″te-an″ah-jen′ĕ-sis) regeneration or reproduction of bone.

ostearthritis (-ar-thri′tis) inflammation of bones and joints.

ostearthrotomy (-ar-throt′o-me) excision of an articular end of a bone.

ostectomy (os-tek′to-me) excision of a bone.

osteectopia (os″te-ek-to′pe-ah) displacement of a bone.

ostein (os′te-in) ossein.

osteitis (os″te-i′tis) inflammation of bone. **o. conden′sans generalisa′ta,** osteopoikilosis. **condensing o.,** osteosclerosis. **o. defor′mans,** a chronic skeletal disease of unknown origin, leading to progressive deformity of bones. **o. fibro′sa cys′tica, o. fibro′sa osteoplas′tica,** rarefying osteitis with fibrous degeneration and formation of cysts and with the presence of fibrous nodules on the affected bones; it is due to hyperfunction of the parathyroid gland. **o. fibro′sa cys′tica generalisa′ta,** a skeletal disorder associated with hyperparathyroidism and characterized by generalized decalcification of the bones. **o. fragil′itans,** osteogenesis imperfecta. **gummatous o.,** chronic form with syphilitic gummata. **parathyroid o.,** osteitis fibrosa cystica generalisata. **rarefying o.,** a bone disease in which the inorganic matter is diminished and the hard bone becomes cancellated. **sclerosing o.,** osteosclerosis. **o. tuberculo′sa cys′tica, o. tuberculo′sa mul′tiplex cystoi′des,** a nonsequestrating spina ventosa with cystlike alteration of the long bones. **vascular o.,** rarefying osteitis in which the spaces formed become occupied by blood vessels.

ostempyesis (os″tem-pi-e′sis) suppuration within a bone.

osteoarthritis (os″te-o-ar-thri′tis) hypertrophic degenerative joint disease of unknown cause. **interphalangeal o.,** arthritis involving the joints of the fingers with intermittent inflammatory episodes leading to deformities and ankylosis.

osteoarthropathy (-ar-throp′ah-the) any disease of the joints and bones. **hypertrophic o.,** osteoarthritis associated with clubbing of fingers and toes and periostosis of shafts of cylindrical bones of the extremities; called also *pulmonary* or *secondary hypertrophic osteoarthropathy.*

osteoarthrotomy (-ar-throt′o-me) ostearthrotomy.

osteoblast (os′te-o-blast″) an immature bone-producing cell.

osteoblastoma (os″te-o-blas-to′mah) a tumor whose cells tend to differentiate into bone cells.

osteocampsia (-kamp′se-ah) curvature of a bone.

osteocarcinoma (-kar″sĭ-no′mah) osteoma combined with carcinoma.

osteochondritis (-kon-dri′tis) inflammation of bone and cartilage. **o. defor′mans juveni′lis,** degeneration of the epiphysis of a bone due to interference with its blood supply. **o. defor′mans juveni′lis dor′si,** osteochondrosis of vertebrae. **o. dis'secans,** a condition in which a fragment of articular cartilage becomes separated from the epiphysis of the parent bone.

osteochondrodystrophia (os″te-o-kon″dro-dis-tro′fe-ah) osteochondrodystrophy.

osteochondrodystrophy (-kon″dro-dis′tro-fe) a disorder of bone and cartilage formation. **familial o.,** a disorder of bone and cartilage appearing between the ages of one and four years, causing shortness of stature, and thought to be transmitted by a recessive gene.

osteochondrofibroma (-kon″dro-fi-bro′mah) a tumor containing osseous, cartilaginous and fibrous elements.

osteochondrolysis (-kon-drol′ĭ-sis) osteochondritis dissecans.

osteochondroma (-kon-dro′mah) a benign bone tumor consisting of projecting adult bone capped by cartilage.

osteochondromatosis (-kon″dro-mah-to′sis) occurrence of multiple osteochondromas. **synovial o.,** a condition in which cartilage bodies are formed in the synovial membrane of the joints, tendon sheaths or bursae, and later undergo secondary calcification and ossification.

osteochondropathy (-kon-drop′ah-the) any morbid condition involving both bone and cartilage, or marked by abnormal enchondral ossification.

osteochondrophyte (kon′dro-fīt) a tumor of cartilage and bone.

osteochondrosarcoma (-kon″dro-sar-ko′mah) an osteosarcoma containing considerable cartilage.

osteochondrosis (-kon-dro′sis) a disorder of a bony epiphysis due to interference with the blood supply; known by various names, depending on the bone involved. **o. defor′mans tib′iae,** tibia vara.

osteoclasis (os″te-ok′lah-sis) surgical fracture of a bone.

osteoclast (os′te-o-klast″) 1. a surgical instrument used for fracturing bone. 2. a large, multinuclear cell frequently associated with resorption of bone.

osteoclastoma (os″te-o-klas-to′mah) giant cell tumor of bone.

osteocope (os′te-o-kōp″) severe pain in a bone. adj., **osteocop′ic.**

osteocranium (os″te-o-kra′ne-um) the fetal skull during the period of ossification, from early in the third month of gestation.

osteocystoma (-sis-to′mah) a cystic tumor in bone.

osteocyte (os′te-o-sīt″) one of the cells lodged in flat, oval cavities in bone, communicating with each other by cytoplasmic processes.

osteodentin (os″te-o-den′tin) dentin that resembles bone.

osteodermia (-der′me-ah) a bony formation in the skin.

osteodynia (-din′e-ah) pain in a bone.

osteodystrophia (-dis-tro′fe-ah) osteodystrophy. **o. juveni′lis,** osteitis fibrosa cystica generalisata.

osteodystrophy (-dis′tro-fe) abnormal devel-

opment of bone. **renal o.,** a condition due to chronic renal disease, and marked by hyperactivity of the parathyroid glands, resulting in deossification of previously normally mineralized bone.

osteo-epiphysis (os″te-o-e-pif′ĭ-sis) a bony epiphysis.

osteofibroma (-fi-bro′mah) tumor of osseous and fibrous tissues.

osteogen (os′te-o-jen″) soft material from which bone is formed.

osteogenesis (-jen′ĕ-sis) the development of the bones. **o. imperfec′ta,** a congenital condition with skeletal deformity due to imperfect formation and mineralization of bone.

osteogenic (os″te-o-jen′ik) 1. forming bone. 2. arising from bone.

osteogeny (os″te-oj′ĕ-ne) osteogenesis.

osteography (-og′rah-fe) description of the bones.

osteohalisteresis (os″te-o-hah-lis″ter-e′sis) deficiency in mineral elements of bone.

osteoid (os′te-oid) resembling bone.

osteolathyrism (os″te-o-lath′ĭ-rizm) a skeletal disorder in animals caused by diets containing the sweet pea (*Lathyrus odoratus*) or its active principle.

osteologia (-lo′je-ah) osteology.

osteologist (os″te-ol′o-jist) a specialist in osteology.

osteology (-ol′o-je) scientific study of the bones.

osteolysis (-ol′ĭ-sis) the decay or soft necrosis of bone. adj., **osteolyt′ic.**

osteoma (os″te-o′mah) a tumor composed of bone. **o. du′rum, o. ebur′neum,** one containing hard bony tissue. **o. medulla′re,** one containing marrow spaces. **osteoid o.,** a benign bone tumor consisting of osteoid tissue surrounded by sclerotic, reactive bone. **o. spongio′sum,** one containing cancellous bone.

osteomalacia (os″te-o-mah-la′she-ah) softening of mature bone due to deficient mineralization of osteoid formed to replace bone lost by normal catabolic lysis. adj., **osteomala′cic. infantile o., juvenile o.,** late rickets. **puerperal o.,** that due to exhaustion of skeletal stores of calcium and phosphorus by repeated pregnancies and lactation. **renal tubular o.,** that due to acidosis and hypercalciuria.

osteomalacosis (-mal″ah-ko′sis) osteomalacia.

osteomatoid (os″te-o′mah-toid) resembling an osteoma.

osteomere (os′te-o-mēr″) one of a series of similar bony structures, such as the vertebrae.

osteometry (os″te-om′ĕ-tre) measurement of the bones.

osteomyelitis (os″te-o-mi″ĕ-li′tis) infection of the substance of bone by pyogenic organisms. **Garré's o.,** sclerosing, nonsuppurative osteomyelitis. **hemorrhagic o.,** osteitis fibrosa cystica.

osteomyelodysplasia (-mi″ĕ-lo-dis-pla′ze-ah) a condition characterized by thinning of the osseous tissue of bones, increase in size of the marrow cavities and associated leukopenia and fever.

osteomyelography (os″te-o-mi″ē-log′rah-fe) roentgen examination of bone marrow.

osteon (os′te-on) the basic unit of structure of compact bone, comprising a haversian canal and its concentrically arranged lamellae.

osteoncus (os″te-ong′kus) tumor of a bone.

osteonecrosis (os″te-o-ne-kro′sis) necrosis of a bone.

osteoneuralgia (-nu-ral′je-ah) neuralgia of a bone.

osteonosus (os″te-on′ō-sus) disease of bone.

osteopath (os′te-o-path″) a practitioner of osteopathy.

osteopathia (os″te-o-path′e-ah) osteopathy (1). **o. conden′sans dissemina′ta,** osteopoikilosis. **o. stria′ta,** an asymptomatic condition characterized radiographically by multiple condensations of cancellous bone tissue, giving a striated appearance.

osteopathology (-pah-thol′o-je) any disease of bone.

osteopathy (os″te-op′ah-the) 1. any disease of a bone. 2. a system of therapy utilizing generally accepted physical, medicinal and surgical methods of diagnosis and therapy, and emphasizing the importance of normal body mechanics and manipulative methods of detecting and correcting faulty structure. adj., **osteopath′ic. disseminated condensing o.,** osteopoikilosis. **hunger o.,** disturbances of the skeletal system observed in famine areas, characterized by a reduction in the amount of normally calcified bone.

osteopecilia (os″te-o-pe-sil′e-ah) osteopoikilosis.

osteopedion (-pe′de-on) lithopedion.

osteoperiosteal (-per″e-os′te-al) pertaining to bone and periosteum.

osteoperiostitis (-per″e-os-ti′tis) inflammation of a bone and its periosteum.

osteopetrosis (-pē-tro′sis) a rare abnormality in bone growth, with extreme hardness and density of bones throughout the skeleton.

osteophage (os′te-o-fāj″) osteoclast.

osteophlebitis (os″te-o-fle-bi′tis) inflammation of the veins of a bone.

osteophyma (-fi′mah) a tumor of a bone.

osteophyte (os′te-o-fīt″) a bony excrescence or outgrowth.

osteoplasty (os′te-o-plas″te) plastic surgery of the bones.

osteopoikilosis (os″te-o-poi″kĭ-lo′sis) a mottled condition of bones, apparent radiographically and due to the presence of multiple sclerotic foci. adj., **osteopoikilot′ic.**

osteoporosis (-po-ro′sis) abnormal rarefaction of bone due to failure of osteoblasts to lay down bone matrix. adj., **osteoporot′ic. adipose o.,** that in which the enlarged spaces are filled with fat. **o. circumscrip′ta,** demineralization occurring in localized areas of bone, especially in the skull.

osteopsathyrosis (os″te-op-sath″ĭ-ro′sis) osteogenesis imperfecta.

osteoradionecrosis (os″te-o-ra″de-o-ne-kro′sis) necrosis of bone as a result of excessive exposure to radiation.

osteorrhagia (os″te-o-ra″je-ah) hemorrhage from bone.

osteorrhaphy (os″te-or′ah-fe) fixation of fragments of bone with sutures or wires.

osteosarcoma (os″te-o-sar-ko′mah) a malignant tumor arising from undifferentiated fibrous tissue of bone. adj., **osteosarco′matous.**

osteosclerosis (-skle-ro′sis) abnormal hardness of bone; osteopetrosis. adj., **osteosclerot′ic. o. congen′ita,** achondroplasia. **o. frag′ilis,** osteopetrosis; so called because of frequency of pathologic fracture of affected bones. **o. frag′ilis generalisa′ta,** osteopoikilosis. **o. myelofibro′sis,** a condition of excessive erythroblastic activity of the bone marrow characterized by fibrotic changes in the blood vessels of the marrow and calcification of the bones.

osteoseptum (-sep′tum) the bony part of the nasal septum.

osteosis (os″te-o′sis) the formation of bony tissue.

osteospongioma (os″te-o-spon″je-o′mah) a spongy tumor of bone.

osteostixis (-stik′sis) surgical puncture of a bone.

osteosuture (-su′tūr) osteorrhaphy.

osteosynovitis (-sin″o-vi′tis) synovitis with osteitis of neighboring bones.

osteosynthesis (-sin′thē-sis) surgical fastening of the ends of a fractured bone.

osteotabes (-ta′bēz) a disease, chiefly of infants, in which bone marrow cells are destroyed and the marrow disappears.

osteothrombophlebitis (-throm″bo-fle-bi′tis) inflammation through intact bone by a progressive thrombophlebitis of small venules.

osteothrombosis (-throm-bo′sis) thrombosis of the veins of a bone.

osteotome (os′te-o-tōm″) a knife or chisel for cutting bone.

osteotomy (os″te-ot′o-me) incision or transection of a bone. **cuneiform o.,** removal of a wedge of bone. **linear o.,** the sawing or simple cutting of a bone. **Macewen's o.,** supracondylar cuneiform section of the femur for genu valgum.

osteotrite (os′te-o-trīt″) an instrument for rasping carious bone.

ostitis (os-ti′tis) osteitis.

ostium (os′te-um), pl. os′*tia* [L.] a mouth or orifice. adj., **os′tial. o. abdomina′le,** fimbriated end of oviduct. **o. inter′num,** uterine end of oviduct. **o. pharyn′geum,** nasopharyngeal end of eustachian tube. **o. pri′mum,** an opening in the lower portion of the membrane dividing the embryonic heart into right and left sides. **o. secun′dum,** a defect in the upper portion of the membrane dividing the embryonic heart into right and left sides, appearing later than the ostium primum. **o. tympan′icum,** tympanic end of eustachian tube. **o. vagi′nae,** external orifice of vagina.

O.S.U.K. Ophthalmological Society of the United Kingdom.

O.T. occupational therapy; old terminology; old tuberculin.

otalgia (o-tal′je-ah) pain in the ear.

OTC over the counter; applied to drugs not required by law to be sold on prescription only.

OTD organ tolerance dose (the amount of radiation tolerated by tissues of a normal organ).

otectomy (o-tek′to-me) excision of tissues of internal and middle ear.

othelcosis (ōt″hel-ko′sis) suppuration of the ear.

othemorrhea (ōt″hem-o-re′ah) flow of blood from the ear.

otiatrics (o″te-at′riks) the science and treatment of ear diseases.

otic (o′tik) pertaining to the ear.

oticodinia (o″ti-ko-din′e-ah) vertigo from ear disease.

otitis (o-ti′tis) inflammation of the ear. adj., **otit′ic**. aviation o., aero-otitis media. **o. exter′na**, inflammation of external ear. **furuncular o.**, formation of furuncles in external meatus. **o. inter′na**, inflammation of the inner ear. **o. labyrin′thica**, inflammation of the labyrinth. **o. mastoi′dea**, inflammation of the mastoid spaces. **o. me′dia**, inflammation of the middle ear. **o. me′dia, secretory**, a painless accumulation of mucoid fluid in the middle ear, due to obstruction of the eustachian tube and causing conduction deafness. **o. parasit′ica**, otitis due to a microorganism. **o. sclerot′ica**, otitis marked by hardening of the ear structures.

otoantritis (o″to an-tri′tis) inflammation of the attic of the tympanum and the mastoid antrum.

Otobius (o-to′be-us) a genus of arthropods (family Argasidae) parasitic in the ears of various animals and known also to bite man.

otoblennorrhea (o″to-blen″o-re′ah) mucous discharge from the ear.

Otocentor (-sen′tor) a genus of ticks, formerly classified as *Dermacentor*.

otocephalus (-sef′ah-lus) a fetal monster lacking lower jaw and having ears united below the face.

otocleisis (-kli′sis) closure of the auditory passages.

otoconia (-ko′ne-ah) a dustlike substance found in the membranous labyrinth of the inner ear.

otocyst (o′to-sist) 1. the auditory vesicle of the embryo. 2. the organ of hearing in invertebrates.

Otodectes (o″to-dek′tēz) a genus of mites which may be parasitic on man.

otodynia (-din′e-ah) pain in the ear; earache.

otoencephalitis (-en-sef″ah-li′tis) inflammation of brain extending from the middle ear.

otoganglion (-gang′gle-on) the otic ganglion.

otography (o-tog′rah-fe) description of the ear.

otolaryngology (o″to-lar″in-gol′o-je) otology and laryngology regarded as a single specialty.

otolith (o′to-lith) a calcareous mass in the inner ear of vertebrates or the otocyst of invertebrates.

otologist (o-tol′o-jist) a specialist in otology.

otology (o-tol′o-je) the branch of medicine dealing with the ear and its diseases.

otomassage (o″to-mah-sahzh′) massage of tympanic cavity and ossicles.

Oto-microscope (-mi′kro-skōp) trademark for an operating microscope devised to improve visualization of the surgical field in operations on the ear.

Otomyces (-mi′sēz) genus of fungi infesting the ear.

otomycosis (-mi-ko′sis) fungus infection of the ear.

otopathy (o-top′ah-the) any disease of the ear.

otoplasty (o′to-plas″te) plastic repair of the ear.

otopolypus (o″to-pol′i-pus) polyp in the ear.

otopyorrhea (-pi″o-re′ah) purulent discharge from ear.

otorhinolaryngology (-ri″no-lar″in-gol′o-je) the branch of medicine dealing with the ear, nose and throat.

otorhinology (-ri-nol′o-je) the branch of medicine dealing with the ear and nose.

otorrhagia (-ra′je-ah) hemorrhage from the ear.

otorrhea (-re′ah) a discharge from the ear.

otosclerosis (-skle-ro′sis) primary focal disease of the capsule of the labyrinth of the ear, with irregularly arranged new bone occurring in and replacing dense bone, and sometimes causing fixation of the stapes to the oval window. adj., **otosclerot′ic**.

otoscope (o′to-skōp) instrument for inspecting the ear.

otoscopy (o-tos′ko-pe) examination of the external auditory canal with a speculum or endoscope.

otosteal (o-tos′te-al) pertaining to the small bones of the ear.

ototomy (o-tot′o-me) dissection of the ear.

ototoxic (o″to-tok′sik) having a deleterious effect upon the eighth nerve or on the organs of hearing and balance.

ototoxicity (-tok-sis′i-te) the property of exerting deleterious effects upon the ear or the sense of hearing.

Otrivin (o′tri-vin) trademark for preparations of xylometazoline hydrochloride.

O.U. 1. [L.] *oculi unitas* (both eyes together). 2. [L.] *oculi uterque* (each eye).

ouabain (wah-ba′in) a white crystalline compound used for its stimulating effect upon the heart.

ounce (owns) a unit of weight in the avoirdupois (437.5 grains, 28.35 grams) or apothecaries′ (480 grains, 31.1 grams) system. **fluid o.**, a unit of liquid measure of the apothecaries′ system, being 8 fluid drams, or the equivalent of 29.57 ml.

outlay (owt′la) a graft applied to the surface of an organ or structure.

outlet (owt′let) a means or route of exit or egress. **pelvic o.**, the inferior opening of the pelvis.

outlimb (owt′lim) the distal part or segment of an extremity.

outpatient (owt-pa′shent) an ambulatory patient who comes to a hospital for treatment.

outpocketing (owt-pok'et-ing) 1. evagination. 2. enclosure of the distal end of a pedicle flap within an opening made in the body tissues.

output (owt'put) the yield or total of anything produced; substance eliminated from the body, usually expressed as quantity per unit of time. **cardiac o.,** the quantity of blood ejected from the heart per unit of time, being the product of stroke volume times the number of beats in the interval. **energy o.,** the energy a body is able to manifest in work or activity. **stroke o.,** the amount of blood ejected by each ventricle at each beat of the heart. **urinary o.,** the amount of urine secreted by the kidneys.

ovalbumin (ov"al-bu'min) albumin from the whites of eggs.

ovalocyte (o'vah-lo-sīt") elliptocyte.

ovalocytosis (o-val"o-si-to'sis) elliptocytosis.

ovarialgia (o-va"re-al'je-ah) pain in an ovary.

ovarian (o-va're-an) pertaining to an ovary.

ovariectomy (o-va"re-ek'to-me) excision of an ovary.

ovariocele (o-va're-o-sēl") hernia of an ovary.

ovariocentesis (o-va"re-o-sen-te'sis) surgical puncture of an ovary.

ovariocyesis (-si-e'sis) ovarian pregnancy.

ovariorrhexis (-rek'sis) rupture of an ovary.

ovariosalpingectomy (-sal"pin-jek'to-me) excision of ovary and oviduct.

ovariostomy (o-va"re-os'to-me) incision of an ovary, with drainage.

ovariotomy (-ot'o-me) surgical removal of an ovary, or removal of an ovarian tumor.

ovariotubal (o-va"re-o-tu'bal) pertaining to ovary and oviduct.

ovaritis (o"vah-ri'tis) inflammation of an ovary.

ovarium (o-va're-um), pl. *ova'ria* [L.] ovary.

ovary (o'var-e) the structure in the female in which the ova develop; the female gonad corresponding to the testis in the male. **polycystic o.,** one containing multiple, small follicular cysts filled with yellow or blood-stained, thin serous fluid.

overbite (o'ver-bīt) extension of incisal ridges of the upper anterior teeth below the incisal ridges of the anterior teeth in the lower jaw when the jaws are closed normally.

overcompensation (o"ver-kom"pen-sa'shun) exaggerated correction of a real or imagined physical or psychologic defect.

overjet (o'ver-jet) extension of the incisal or buccal cusp ridges of the upper teeth labially or buccally to the ridges of the teeth in the lower jaw when the jaws are closed normally.

overlay (o'ver-la) a later component superimposed on a pre-existing state or condition. **psychogenic o.,** an emotionally determined increment to a pre-existing symptom or disability of organic or physically traumatic origin.

overventilation (o"ver-ven"tī-la'shun) hyperventilation.

ovi (o'vi) [L.] genitive of *o'vum.* **o. albu'men,** white of egg. **o. vitel'lus,** yolk of egg.

ovicide (o'vī-sīd) 1. the destruction of ova. 2. an agent destructive to the ova of certain organisms.

oviduct (o'vī-dukt) a tube for the passage of ova; a uterine tube. adj., **ovidu'cal.**

oviferous (o-vif'er-us) producing or conveying ova.

ovigenesis (o"vī-jen'ĕ-sis) oogenesis. adj., **ovigenet'ic.**

ovine (o'vīn) pertaining to or derived from sheep.

oviparous (o-vip'ah-rus) producing eggs in which the embryo develops outside of the maternal body.

ovisac (o'vī-sak) a graafian follicle.

ovist (o'vist) one who believed that the individuals of successive generations are contained, completely formed, within the eggs of the maternal organism.

Ovocylin (o"vo-sil'in) trademark for a preparation of estradiol.

ovoflavin (o"vo-fla'vin) riboflavin derived from eggs.

ovoglobulin (-glob'u-lin) the globulin of white of egg.

ovolytic (-lit'ik) splitting up egg albumin.

ovomucoid (-mu'koid) a mucoid principle from egg albumin.

ovotestis (-tes'tis) a gonad containing both testicular and ovarian tissue.

ovoviviparous (-vi-vip'ah-rus) producing eggs with a definite shell, in which the embryo develops within the maternal body.

ovulation (o"vu-la'shun) the maturation and discharge of the ovum from the ovary. adj., **ov'ulatory.**

ovule (o'vūl) the ovum in the ovary, or any small egglike structure. **primitive o., primordial o.,** a rudimentary ovum in the ovary.

ovulum (ov'u-lum), pl. *ov'ula* [L.] an ovule.

ovum (o'vum), pl. *o'va* [L.] egg; the female reproductive element that may develop into a new organism; sometimes applied to any stage of the fertilized germ cell during cleavage and even until hatching or birth of the new individual. adj., **o'vular. alecithal o.,** one with no or very little food yolk. **blighted o.,** a fertilized ovum in which development has become arrested. **centrolecithal o.,** one with the yolk concentrated at the center of the egg, surrounded by a thin layer of cytoplasm. **holoblastic o.,** one that undergoes total cleavage. **isolecithal o.,** one with a small amount of yolk evenly distributed throughout the cytoplasm. **meroblastic o.,** one that undergoes partial cleavage. **permanent o.,** the mature ovum ready for fertilization. **primitive o., primordial o.,** any egg cell which may eventually become an oocyte within the graafian follicle. **telolecithal o.,** one with a comparatively large amount of yolk massed at one pole.

oxacid (ok-sas'id) an acid containing oxygen.

oxacillin (ok"sah-sil'in) a semisynthetic penicillin which is relatively stable in an acid medium and resistant to inactivation by penicillinase. **sodium o.,** an antibacterial compound for oral administration.

Oxaine (ok'sān) trademark for a preparation of oxethazaine.

oxalate (ok'sah-lāt) a salt of oxalic acid. **po-**

tassium o., colorless, odorless crystals used extensively as a reagent. **sodium o.,** a white, odorless, crystalline powder, formerly used as an anticoagulant in collection of blood for laboratory examination.

oxalemia (ok"sah-le'me-ah) excess of oxalates in the blood.

oxalism (ok'sah-lizm) poisoning by oxalic acid or by an oxalate.

oxalosis (ok"sah-lo'sis) a metabolic disorder with deposits of oxalate crystals in the kidneys and other body tissues.

oxaluria (ok"sah-lu're-ah) oxalic acid or oxalates in the urine.

oxanamide (ok-san'ah-mīd) a compound used as a tranquilizer.

oxethazaine (ok-seth'ah-zān) a compound used as a gastric mucosal anesthetic, antacid and demulcent.

oxidant (ok'sĭ-dant) the electron acceptor in an oxidation-reduction (redox) reaction.

oxidase (ok'sĭ-dās) an enzyme which catalyzes oxidation. **cytochrome o.,** an oxidation-catalyzing enzyme which receives electrons transferred by a cytochrome.

oxidation (ok"sĭ-da'shun) the combination of a substance with oxygen.

oxide (ok'sīd) a compound of oxygen with an element or radical.

oxidize (ok'sĭ-dīz) to cause to combine with oxygen.

oxidoreductase (ok"sĭ-do-re-duk'tās) an enzyme that catalyzes the reversible transfer of electrons from one substance to another.

oxidosis (ok"sĭ-do'sis) acidosis.

oxime (ok'sīm) a compound formed by action of hydroxylamine on an aldehyde or ketone.

oximeter (ok-sim'ĕ-ter) a device for measuring oxygen content.

oxophenarsine (ok"so-fen-ar'sin) a compound used as an antitreponemal agent.

Oxsoralen (ŏk-sŏr'ah len) trademark for preparations of methoxsalen.

oxtriphylline (oks-trif'ĭ-lēn) a compound used as mild diuretic, cardiac stimulant and a vasodilator and bronchodilator.

oxyacid (ok'se-as"ĭd) oxacid.

oxybenzene (ok"sĭ-ben'zēn) phenol.

oxyblepsia (-blep'se-ah) unusual acuity of vision.

Oxycel (ok'sĭ-sel) trademark for preparations of oxidized cellulose.

oxycephalia (-sĕ-fa'le-ah) oxycephaly.

oxycephaly (ok-sĭ-sef'ah-le) a high, pointed condition of the skull, with a vertical index of 77 or more. adj., **oxycephal'ic.**

oxychloride (-klo'rīd) an element or radical combined with oxygen and chlorine.

oxychromatic (-kro-mat'ik) staining with acid dyes.

oxychromatin (-kro'mah-tin) that part of chromatin that stains with acid dyes.

oxycinesia (-si-ne'ze-ah) pain on motion.

oxydoreductase (ok"sĭ-do-re-duk'tās) one of the enzymes of the zymase system of alcoholic fermentation which rearranges aldehydes.

oxyesthesia (ok"se-es-the'ze-ah) abnormal acuteness of the senses.

oxygen (ok'sĭ-jen) chemical element (see table), at. no. 8, symbol O. **o. debt,** deficiency of oxygen occurring in violent exercise. **heavy o.,** an isotope of oxygen of atomic weight 18.

oxygenase (ok'sĭ-jen-ās") an enzyme that transfers oxygen from the air.

oxygenation (ok"sĭ-je-na'shun) saturation with oxygen. **hyperbaric o.,** exposure to oxygen under conditions of greatly increased pressure.

oxygonator (-je-na'tor) an apparatus by which oxygen is introduced into the blood during circulation outside the body, as during open-heart surgery.

oxygeusia (-gu'ze-ah) extreme acuteness of the sense of taste.

oxyhemoglobin (-he"mo-glo'bin) hemoglobin charged with oxygen.

oxyhemoglobinometer (-he"mo-glo"bin-om'ĕ-ter) instrument for measuring oxygen content of the blood.

oxyhemogram (-he'mo-gram) a graphic record of the oxygen saturation of the blood as determined by use of the oxyhemograph.

oxyhemograph (-he'mo-graf) an apparatus for determining oxygen content of the blood.

oxyhydrocephalus (-hi"dro-sef'ah-lus) hydrocephalus with the top of the head pointed.

oxyhyperglycemia (-hi"per-gli-se'me-ah) a condition in which there is slight glycosuria and an oral glucose tolerance curve which rises to about 180-200 mg. per 100 ml., but returns to fasting values 2½ hours after ingestion of the glucose.

oxyiodide (ok"se-i'o-dīd) an element or radical combined with oxygen and iodine.

oxylalia (ok"sĭ-la'le-ah) rapidity of speech.

Oxylone (ok'sĭ-lōn) trademark for a preparation of fluorometholone.

oxymetholone (ok"sĭ-meth'o-lōn) a steroid compound with low androgenic action, but high anabolic activity.

oxymorphone (-mor'fōn) a compound used as a narcotic analgesic.

oxymyoglobin (-mi"o-glo'bin) myoglobin charged with oxygen.

oxyntic (ok-sin'tik) secreting an acid substance.

oxyopia (ok"se-o'pe-ah) abnormal acuteness of sight.

oxyosis (-o'sis) acidosis.

oxyosmia (-oz'me-ah) extreme acuteness of the sense of smell.

oxypathia (ok"sĭ-path'e-ah) 1. acuteness of sensation. 2. oxypathy.

oxypathy (ok-sip'ah-the) inability of the body to eliminate unoxidizable acids.

oxyphenbutazone (ok"sĭ-fen-bu'tah-zōn) a compound used as an anti-inflammatory agent and in treatment of joint diseases.

oxyphencyclimine (-fen-si'klĭ-mēn) a compound used in parasympathetic blockade.

oxyphenisatin (-fĕ-ni'sah-tin) a compound used as an enema for cleansing the colon.

oxyphenonium (-fĕ-no'ne-um) a compound used in parasympathetic blockade.

oxyphil (ok′sĭ-fil) a structure or element readily stainable with an acid dye. adj., **oxyphil′ic, oxyph′ilous.**

oxyphonia (ok″sĭ-fo′ne-ah) an abnormally sharp quality of the voice.

oxypurine (-pu′rēn) a purine containing oxygen.

oxyrhine (ok′sĭ-rīn) having a sharp-pointed nose.

oxysalt (ok′sĭ-sawlt) a salt of an oxacid.

oxytetracycline (ok″sĭ-tet-rah-si′klēn) an antibiotic substance isolated from the elaboration products of *Streptomyces rimosus*, effective against a wide range of microorganisms.

oxytocic (-to′sik) 1. hastening the process of childbirth. 2. an agent that accelerates childbirth.

oxytocin (-to′sin) a principle from the posterior lobe of the pituitary, or prepared synthetically, which stimulates contraction of the uterine muscle.

oxyuriasis (ok″se-u-ri′ah-sis) infection with Oxyuris.

oxyuricide (-u′rĭ-sīd) a drug destructive to Oxyuris.

oxyurid (-u′rid) a seatworm or threadworm; an individual organism of the genus Oxyuris.

oxyurifuge (-u′ri-fūj) an agent that promotes expulsion of worms of the genus Oxyuris.

Oxyuris (-u′ris) a genus of nematode parasites. **O. e′qui,** a species found in horses. **O. vermicula′ris,** *Enterobius vermicularis.*

oz. ounce.

ozena (o-ze′nah) an offensive-smelling discharge from the nose.

ozone (o′zōn) an allotropic form of oxygen, O_3; antiseptic and disinfectant.

ozonometer (o″zo-nom′ĕ-ter) apparatus for measuring ozone in the atmosphere.

ozostomia (-sto′me-ah) foulness of the breath.

P

P chemical symbol, *phosphorus.*

P. Pharmacopeia; position; presbyopia; [L.] proximum*(near)*; pulse, [L.] punctum*(point)*; pupil.

p- symbol, *para-.*

P₁ parental generation.

P₂ pulmonic second sound.

P.A. pulpoaxial.

Pa chemical symbol, *protactinium.*

PAB, PABA para-aminobenzoic acid.

pabulum (pab′u-lum) food or aliment.

Pacatal (pak′ah-tal) trademark for a preparation of mepazine.

pacemaker (pās′māk-er) that which sets the pace at which a phenomenon occurs. **artificial p.,** a device designed to stimulate, by electrical impulses, contraction of the heart muscle at a certain rate; worn by or implanted in the body of the patient. **cardiac p.,** the sinoatrial node, which normally emits the impulses that dominate the rhythm of the heart beat. **wandering p.,** a condition in which occasional isolated beats of the heart are controlled by the atrioventricular node instead of by the sinoatrial node as normally.

pachy- (pak′e) word element [Gr.], *thickened; thickening.*

pachyacria (pak″e-a′kre-ah) acropachydermia.

pachyblepharon (pak″ĭ-blef′ah-ron) thickening of the eyelids.

pachycephalia (-sĕ-fa′le-ah) abnormal thickness of the bones of the skull. adj., **pachycephal′ic.**

pachychromatic (-kro-mat′ik) having the chromatin in thick strands.

pachydactylia (-dak-til′e-ah) enlargement of the fingers and toes.

pachyderma (pak″ĭ-der′mah) abnormal thickening of the skin. adj., **pachyder′matous. p. laryn′gis,** warty thickenings on the vocal cords. **p. ves′icae,** thickening of the mucous membrane of the bladder.

pachydermatocele (-der-mat′o-sēl) cutis laxa.

pachydermatosis (-der″mah-to′sis) chronic pachyderma.

pachydermia (-der′me-ah) pachyderma.

pachydermoperiostosis (-der″mo-per″e-os-to′sis) thickening of the skin associated with periostosis.

pachyglossia (-glos′e-ah) abnormal thickness of the tongue.

pachygyria (-ji′re-ah) a condition in which the cerebral convolutions are broad and flat.

pachyhematous (-hem′ah-tus) having thickened blood.

pachyhemia (-he′me-ah) thickening of the blood.

pachyleptomeningitis (-lep″to-men″in-ji′tis) inflammation of dura mater and pia mater.

pachylosis (-lo′sis) a thickened, dry, scaly state of the skin.

pachymeningitis (-men″in-ji′tis) inflammation of the dura mater.

pachymeningopathy (-men″ing-gop′ah-the) noninflammatory disease of the dura mater.

pachymeninx (-me′ninks) the dura mater.

pachymeter (pah-kim′ĕ-ter) instrument for measuring thickness of objects.

pachynsis (pah-kin′sis) thickening. adj., **pachyn′tic.**

pachyonychia (pak″e-o-nik′e-ah) abnormal thickening of the nails. **p. congen′ita,** a rare congenital disorder characterized by the presence, at birth, of massively thickened, clawlike nails.

pachyostosis (pak″e-os-to′sis) hypertrophy of the bones.

pachyotia (pak″e-o′she-ah) marked thickness of the ears.

pachypelviperitonitis (pak″ĭ-pel″vĭ-per″ĭ-to-ni′tis) pelvic peritonitis with thickening of the peritoneum.

pachyperiostitis (-per″e-os-ti′tis) periostitis of long bones resulting in abnormal thickness of the bones.

pachyperitonitis (-per″ĭ-to-ni′tis) inflammation and thickening of the peritoneum.

pachypleuritis (-ploo-ri′tis) inflammation and thickening of the pleura.

pachypodous (pah-kip′o-dus) having thick feet.

pachysalpingitis (pak″ĭ-sal″pin-ji′tis) salpingitis with thickening.

pachysalpingo-ovaritis (-sal-ping″go-o″var-i′tis) inflammation of ovary and oviduct, with thickening.

pachysomia (-so′me-ah) thickening of parts of the body.

pachyvaginalitis (-vaj″ĭ-nal-i′tis) inflammation and thickening of tunica vaginalis.

pachyvaginitis (-vaj″ĭ-ni′tis) chronic vaginitis with thickening of the vaginal walls.

pack (pak) 1. treatment by wrapping a patient in blankets, wet or dry and either hot or cold; also the blankets in which a patient is wrapped. 2. a dressing which is inserted firmly into a wound or body cavity, as the nose, uterus or vagina, principally for stopping hemorrhage. **periodontal p.,** a mixture consisting of a zinc oxide powder and eugenol liquid, applied to the gingiva around the teeth after surgical peridontal procedures.

packer (pak′er) an instrument for introducing a dressing into the vagina or other body cavity.

packing (pak′ing) 1. the filling of a wound or cavity with gauze, sponge or other material. 2. the substance used for filling a cavity. 3. treatment with the pack.

pad (pad) a cushion-like mass of soft material. **abdominal p.,** a pad for the absorption of discharges from abdominal wounds. **dinner p.,** a pad placed over the stomach before a plaster jacket is applied; the pad is then removed, leaving space under the jacket to take care of expansion of the stomach after eating. **fat p.,** 1. a large pad of fat lying behind and below the patella. 2. sucking pad. **kidney p.,** a pad held in place by a belt for support of movable kidney. **Malgaigne's p's,** adipose pads in the knee joint immediately above the articular surface of the femur and on either side of the upper end of the patella. **Mikulicz's p.,** a pad made of folded gauze, for packing off viscera in surgical procedures. **occlusal p.,** a pad which covers the occlusal surface of a tooth. **retromolar p.,** a cushion-like mass of tissue situated at the distal termination of the mandibular residual ridge. **sucking p., suctorial p.,** a lobulated mass of fat which occupies the space between the masseter and the external surface of the buccinator; it is well developed in infants. **sur-**

gical p., a rubber sheet for the carrying off of fluids in surgical operation.

pae- for words beginning thus, see those beginning with *pe-*.

Pagitane (paj′i-tān) trademark for a preparation of cycrimine.

-pagus (pa′gus) word element [Gr.], *twin fetal monster.*

PAH, PAHA para-aminohippuric acid.

P.A.H.O. Pan American Health Organization.

pain (pān) a feeling of distress, suffering or agony, caused by stimulation of specialized nerve endings. **bearing-down p.,** a variety of pain in childbirth. **boring p.,** a sensation as of being pierced with a gimlet. **false p.,** pains in the latter part of pregnancy which simulate those of labor. **fulgurant p.,** intense shooting pain. **growing p.,** quasirheumatic pain peculiar to youth. **hunger p.,** pain coming on at the time for feeling hunger for a meal; a symptom of gastric disorder. **labor p's,** the rhythmic pains of increasing severity and frequency due to contraction of the uterus at childbirth. **lancinating p.,** sharp darting pain. **lightning p's,** the cutting pains of locomotor ataxia. **osteocopic p.,** pain in bones, peculiar to syphilis. **parenchymatous p.,** pain at the peripheral end of a nerve. **phantom limb p.,** pain felt as if it were in the patient's limb, although the limb has been amputated. **referred p.,** pain in a part other than that in which the cause that produced it is situated. **terebrant p., terebrating p.,** boring pain.

paint (pānt) 1. a substance designed for application to the surface. 2. to apply a substance to a specific area as a remedial or protective measure. **Castellani's p.,** a mixture of basic fuchsin, phenol, boric acid, acetone and resorcinol; used for skin disinfection and in treatment of dermatophytosis, tinea and other infections.

palat(o)- (pal′ah-to) word element [L.], *palate.*

palate (pal′at) roof of the mouth. adj., **pal′a-tal. artificial p.,** a prosthesis to close a cleft palate. **bony p.,** the rigid framework of the hard palate, formed by parts of the maxilla and the palatine bone. **cleft p.,** congenital fissure of median line of palate. **hard p.,** the anterior portion of the palate, separating the oral and nasal cavities, consisting of the bony framework and covering membranes. **soft p.,** the posterior portion of the palate, partially separating the nasopharynx and oropharynx and consisting of muscle fibers and covering mucous membrane.

palatine (pal′ah-tin) pertaining to the palate.

palatitis (pal″ah-ti′tis) inflammation of the palate.

palatognathus (pal″ah-tog′nah-thus) congenital fissure of hard and soft palates.

palatoplasty (pal′ah-to-plas″te) plastic repair of the palate.

palatoplegia (pal″ah-to-ple′je-ah) paralysis of the palate.

palatorrhaphy (pal″ah-tor′ah-fe) suture of the palate.

palatoschisis (pal″ah-tos′kĭ-sis) fissure of the palate.

palatostaphylinus (pal″ah-to-staf″ĭ-li′nus) muscular slip to the uvula.

pale(o)- (pa′le-o) word element [Gr.], *old*.

paleogenesis (pa″le-o-jen′ĕ-sis) palingenesis (2).

paleogenetic (-jĕ-net′ik) originated in the past.

paleokinetic (-ki-net′ik) noting the motor mechanism concerned in automatic associated movements.

paleontology (pa″le-on-tol′o-je) the study of life in the early eras of the earth's history.

paleopathology (pa″le-o-pah-thol′o-je) study of disease in bodies which have been preserved from ancient times.

paleostriatum (-stri-a′tum) the more early formed portion of the corpus striatum, represented by the globus pallidus. adj., **paleostria′tal.**

paleothalamus (-thal′ah-mus) the medial (noncortical) portion of the thalamus.

pali(n)- (pal′in) word element [Gr.], *again; pathologič repetition.*

palikinesia (pal″ĭ-ki-ne′ze-ah) pathologic repetition of movements.

palilalia (-la′le-ah) a disorder of enunciation in which a phrase or word is repeated with increasing rapidity.

palinal (pal′ĭ-nal) directed or moved backward.

palindromia (pal″in-dro′me-ah) a recurrence or relapse. adj., **palindrom′ic.**

palinesthesia (-es-the′ze-ah) the return of sensation after anesthesia or coma.

palingenesis (-jen′ĕ-sis) 1. regeneration or restoration 2. reappearance of ancestral characters; atavism.

palingraphia (-gra′fe-ah) repetition of words or letters in writing.

palinphrasia (-fra′ze-ah) repetition of words or phrases in speaking.

palladium (pah-la′de-um) chemical element (*see table*), at. no. 46, symbol Pd.

pallanesthesia (pal″an-es-the′ze-ah) insensibility of bone to vibrations of a tuning fork.

pallesthesia (pal″es-the′ze-ah) sensibility of bone to vibrations of a tuning fork.

palliative (pal′e-a″tiv) relieving symptoms.

pallidectomy (pal″ĭ-dek′to-me) extirpation of the globus pallidus by surgical means.

pallidofugal (pal″ĭ-dof′u-gal) conducting impulses away from the globus pallidus.

pallidotomy (-dot′o-me) surgical creation of lesions in the globus pallidus.

pallidum (pal′ĭ-dum) the globus pallidus. adj., **pal′lidal.**

pallium (pal′e-um) the gray matter covering the cerebral hemispheres, characterized by a distinctive layering of the cellular elements.

pallor (pal′or) absence of skin coloration.

palm (pahm) the hollow or flexor surface of the hand. adj., **pal′mar.**

palma (pahl′mah), pl. *pal′mae* [L.] palm. adj.,

pal′mae plica′tae, the branching folds of the mucosa of the vagina.

palmaris (pahl-ma′ris) palmar.

palmus (pahl′mus) 1. palpitation. 2. clonic spasm of leg muscles, producing jumping motion.

palpate (pal′pāt) to perform palpation; to feel with the fingers or hand.

palpation (pal-pa′shun) feeling with the fingers or hand, to determine by use of the tactile senses the physical characteristics of tissues or organs.

palpebra (pal′pĕ-brah), pl. *pal′pebrae* [L.] eyelid. adj., **pal′pebral. p. ter′tius,** nictitating membrane.

palpebralis (pal″pĕ-bra′lis) [L.] palpebral.

palpebritis (pal″pĕ-bri′tis) inflammation of the eyelid.

palpitation (pal″pī-ta′shun) rapid beating of the heart.

palsy (pawl′ze) paralysis. **Bell's p.,** neuropathy of facial nerve (facial paralysis) due to pressure. **birth p.,** obstetric paralysis. **bulbar p.,** facial paralysis due to lesion of the facial nerve, resulting in characteristic distortion of the face. **cerebral p.,** persisting qualitative motor disorder appearing before age three, due to nonprogressive damage of the brain. **Erb's p.,** paralysis of the muscles of the arm and chest wall in the newborn, due to injury of the nerve roots of the brachial plexus occurring in delivery. **shaking p.,** paralysis agitans. **wasting p.,** progressive muscular atrophy.

paludal (pal′u-dal) pertaining to, or arising from, marshes.

paludism (pal′u-dizm) malaria.

Paludrine (pal′u-drin) trademark for a preparation of proguanil hydrochloride.

pamaquine naphthoate (pam′ah-kwin naf′-tho-āt) odorless yellow powder; antimalarial.

Pamine (pam′ēn) trademark for preparations of methscopolamine.

Pamisyl (pam′ĭ-sil) trademark for preparations of aminosalicylic acid.

pampiniform (pam-pin′ĭ-form) shaped like a tendril.

pampinocele (pam-pin′o-sēl) varicocele.

pan- (pan) word element [Gr.], *all.*

panacea (pan″ah-se′ah) a remedy for all diseases.

panagglutinin (pan″ah-gloo′tĭ-nin) an agglutinin which agglutinates the corpuscles of all groups.

panangiitis (pan″an-je-i′tis) inflammation involving all the coats of a vessel. **necrotizing p.,** diffuse, extensive inflammation involving both arteries and veins, with cutaneous and visceral manifestations.

panarteritis (pan″ar-tĕ-ri′tis) periarteritis nodosa.

panarthritis (pan″ar-thri′tis) inflammation of all the joints.

panasthenia (pan″as-the′ne-ah) neurasthenia.

panatrophy (pan-at′ro-fe) atrophy of several parts.

pancarditis (pan"kar-di'tis)   general inflammation of the heart.

panchromia (pan-kro'me-ah) the condition of staining with various dyes.

pancolectomy (pan"ko-lek'to-me) excision of the entire colon, with creation of an outlet from the ileum on the body surface.

pancrealgia (pan"kre-al'je-ah) pain in the pancreas.

pancreas (pan'kre-as), pl. *pancrea'ta* [Gr.] a large, elongated, racemose gland behind the stomach and in relation with the spleen and the duodenum. adj., **pancreat'ic. aberrant p.**, an exclave of pancreatic tissue. **annular p.**, one which forms a ring surrounding the duodenum. **lesser p.**, small, partially detached portion of the pancreas lying dorsad of its head. **ventral p.**, an outgrowth on the ventral side of the embryonic intestine.

pancreatalgia (pan"kre-ah-tal'je-ah) pain in the pancreas.

pancreatectomy (-tek'to-me) excision of the pancreas.

pancreatemphraxis (-tem-frak'sis)   congestion of pancreas from stoppage of pancreatic duct.

pancreathelcosis (pan"kre-ath"el-ko'sis) ulceration of the pancreas.

pancreatico- (pan"kre-at'ĭ-ko) word element [Gr.], *pancreatic duct.*

pancreaticoduodenal (pan"kre-at"ĭ-ko-du"o-de'nal) pertaining to pancreas and duodenum.

pancreaticoduodenostomy (-du"o-de-nos'to-me) anastomosis of the pancreatic duct to a different site on the duodenum.

pancreaticogastrostomy (-gas-tros'to-me) anastomosis of the pancreatic duct to the stomach.

pancreaticojejunostomy (-je"joo-nos'to-me) anastomosis of the pancreatic duct to the jejunum.

pancreatin (pan'kre-ah-tin) a substance from the pancreas of the hog or ox containing enzymes, principally pancreatic amylase, trypsin and pancreatic lipase.

pancreatism (pan'kre-ah-tizm") activity of the pancreas.

pancreatitis (pan"kre-ah-ti'tis) inflammation of the pancreas. **acute hemorrhagic p.**, a form due to hemorrhage into the gland. **chronic p.**, fibrosis of the pancreas.

pancreato- (pan'kre-ah-to) word element [Gr.], *pancreas.*

pancreatoduodenectomy (pan"kre-ah-to-du"o-de-nek'to me) resection of the head of the pancreas, part of the common bile duct, pyloric portion of the stomach, and duodenum.

pancreatoenterostomy (-en"ter-os'to-me) anastomosis of the pancreas to the intestinal tract.

pancreatogenous (pan"kre-ah-toj'ĕ-nus) arising in the pancreas.

pancreatography (-tog'rah-fe) roentgenography of the pancreas.

pancreatolithectomy (pan-kre"ah-to-lĭ-thek'-to-me) excision of a calculus from the pancreas.

pancreatolithiasis (pan-kre"ah-to-lĭ-thi'ah-sis) presence of calculi in the ductal system or parenchyma of the pancreas.

pancreatolithotomy (-lĭ-thot'o-me) incision of the pancreas for the removal of calculi.

pancreatolysis (pan"kre-ah-tol'ĭ-sis) destruction of pancreatic tissue. adj., **pancreatolyt'ic.**

pancreatoncus (pan"kre-ah-tong'kus) tumor of the pancreas.

pancreatotomy (-tot'o-me) incision of the pancreas.

pancreatotropic (pan-kre"ah-to-trop'ik) having a special influence on the pancreas.

pancreolithotomy (pan"kre-o-lĭ-thot'o-me) pancreatolithotomy.

pancreoprivic (-priv'ik) deprived of the pancreas.

pancreotherapy (-ther'ah-pe) the therapeutic use of pancreas tissue.

pancytopenia (pan"si-to-pe'ne-ah) abnormal depression of all the cellular elements of the blood.

pandemic (pan-dem'ik)   a widespread epidemic.

panendoscope (-en'do-skōp)   a cystoscope which gives a wide view of the bladder.

panesthesia (pan"es-the'ze-ah) the sum of the sensations experienced. adj., **panesthet'ic.**

pangenesis (pan-jen'ĕ-sis) the doctrine that in reproduction each cell of the parent body is represented by a particle.

panhematopenia (pan"hem-ah-to-pe'ne-ah) abnormal decrease of all the cellular elements of the blood. **primary splenic p.**, a form of hypersplenism with indiscriminate elimination of all circulating elements of the blood.

panhidrosis (pan"hĭ-dro'sis) perspiration of the whole surface of the body.

panhypopituitarism (pan-hi"po-pĭ-tu'ĭ-tar-izm) anterior pituitary insufficiency; Simmonds's disease.

panhysterectomy (pan"his-tĕ-rek'to-me) complete extirpation of the uterus and cervix.

panhystero-oophorectomy (pan"his-ter-o-o"of-o-rek'to-me) excision of the entire uterus and ovaries.

panhysterosalpingectomy (-sal"pin-jek'to-me) excision of the entire uterus and oviducts.

panhysterosalpingo-oophorectomy (-sal ping"go-o"of-o-rek'to-me) excision of the uterus, cervix, oviducts and ovaries.

panic (pan'ik) an episode of acute anxiety, with abandonment of reason.

panimmunity (pan"ĭ-mu'nĭ-te) immunity to several infections.

Panmycin (pan-mi'sin) trademark for preparations of tetracycline.

panmyelophthisis (-mi-ĕ-lof'thĭ-sis) general aplasia of the bone marrow.

panmyelosis (-mi"ĕ-lo'sis) proliferation of all the elements of the bone marrow.

panneuritis (-nu-ri'tis) general or multiple neuritis. **p. epidem'ica,** beriberi.

panniculitis (pah-nik"u-li'tis) inflammation of the panniculus adiposus. **nodular nonsup-**

purative p., a disease marked by painful nodules in the subcutaneous fatty tissue.

panniculus (pah-nik'u-lus), pl. *pannic'uli* [L.] a layer of tissue. **p. adipo'sus,** subcutaneous tissue containing large amounts of fat. **p. carno'sus,** a muscular layer in superficial fascia.

pannus (pan'us) a membrane-like structure, as produced by (*a*) superficial vascularization of the cornea with infiltration of granulation tissue, or (*b*) exudate overlying synovial cells on the inside of a joint capsule.

panophobia (pan"o-fo'be-ah) fear of everything; vague and persistent dread of an unknown evil.

panophthalmitis (pan"of-thal-mi'tis) inflammation of all the eye structures.

panosteitis (pan"os-te-i'tis) inflammation of every part of a bone.

panotitis (pan"o-ti'tis) inflammation of all the parts or structures of the ear.

Panparnit (pan-par'nit) trademark for a preparation of caramiphen hydrochloride.

panphobia (-fo'be-ah) panophobia.

panproctocolectomy (-prok"to-ko-lek'to-me) excision of the entire rectum and colon, with creation of an outlet from the ileum on the body surface.

pansinusitis (pan"si-nu-si'tus) inflammation of all the accessory sinuses of the nose.

Panstrongylus (pan-stron'ji-lus) a genus of arthropods (order Hemiptera), species of which are vectors of trypanosomes.

pantalgia (-tal'je-ah) pain over the whole body.

pantomography (-to-mog'rah-fe) a method of body-section roentgenography used for visualization of curved surfaces at any depth. adj., **pantomograph'ic.**

pantophobia (pan"to-fo'be-ah) panophobia.

pantothenate (pan-to'then-āt) a salt of pantothenic acid.

pantotropic (pan"to-trop'ik) pantropic.

pantropic (pan-trop'ik) having affinity for tissues derived from all three of the germ layers.

panturbinate (-ter'bĭ-nāt) the entire turbinate structure.

panzootic (pan"zo-ot'ik) occurring pandemically among animals.

papain (pah-pa'in, pah-pi'in) a digestant from papaw fruit.

papaverine (pah-pav'er-in) an alkaloid obtained from opium or prepared synthetically. **p. hydrochloride,** a white, crystalline compound used as a smooth muscle relaxant.

paper (pa'per) a substance of various types of fibers, made in thin sheets. **bibulous p.,** paper which absorbs moisture. **litmus p.,** paper prepared with a solution of litmus, a slightly acid solution to produce red paper (used in indicating alkalinity) and a slightly alkaline solution to produce blue paper (used in indicating acidity). **test p.,** paper stained with a compound which changes visibly on occurrence of a chemical reaction.

papilla (pah-pil'ah), pl. *papil'lae* [L.] a small, nipple-shaped projection or elevation. adj., **pap'illary. circumvallate p.,** vallate papilla.

dental p., dentinal p., the small mass of condensed mesenchyme capped by each of the enamel organs. **duodenal p.,** either of the small elevations (major and minor) on the mucosa of the duodenum, the *major* at the entrance of the conjoined pancreatic and common bile ducts, the *minor* at the entrance of the accessory pancreatic duct. **filiform p.,** one of the threadlike elevations covering most of the tongue surface. **foliate p.,** one of the parallel mucosal folds on the tongue margin at the junction of its body and root. **fungiform p.,** one of the knoblike projections of the tongue scattered among the filiform papillae. **gingival p.,** the triangular pad of the gingiva filling the space between the proximal surfaces of two adjacent teeth. **hair p.,** a mass within the corium beneath each hair bulb. **incisive p.,** an elevation at the anterior end of the raphe of the palate. **interdental p.,** gingival papilla. **lacrimal p.,** an elevation on the margin of either eyelid, near the medial angle of the eye. **mammary p.,** the nipple of the mammary gland. **nervous papillae,** papillae of the skin enclosing special nerve terminations. **optic p.,** optic disk. **palatine p.,** incisive papilla. **p. pi'li,** hair papilla. **renal p.,** the blunted apex of a renal pyramid. **p. spira'lis,** the spiral edge formed by Corti's organ. **tactile p.,** a papilla on the true skin inclosing a tactile corpuscle. **urethral p.,** a slight elevation in the vestibule of the vagina at the external orifice of the urethra. **vallate p.,** one of the 8 to 12 large papillae arranged in a v near the base of the tongue. **vascular papillae,** papillae of the corium which contain loops of blood vessels. **p. of Vater, Vater's p.,** major duodenal papilla.

papillectomy (pap"i-lek'to-me) excision of a papilla.

papilledema (pap"il-ĕ-de'mah) edema and hyperemia of the optic disk (choked disk), usually associated with increased intracranial pressure.

papillitis (pap"ĭ-li'tis) inflammation of a papilla, especially of the optic disk.

papillo-adenocystoma (pap"ĭ-lo-ad"ĕ-no-sisto'mah) a tumor containing elements of papilloma, adenoma and cystoma.

papillocarcinoma (-kar"sĭ-no'mah) a malignant papilloma.

papilloma (pap"i-lo'mah) a benign tumor derived from epithelium. **Shope p.,** a virus-induced lesion occurring in rabbits.

papillomatosis (pap"i-lo"mah-to'sis) development of multiple papillomas.

papilloretinitis (pap"ĭ-lo-ret"ĭ-ni'tis) inflammation of optic nerve and disk.

papillosphincterotomy (-sfingk"ter-ot'o-me) partial incision of the sphincter of the majo duodenal papilla.

papulation (pap"u-la'shun) the formation of papules.

papule (pap'ūl) a circumscribed, solid, elevated lesion of the skin, up to 5 mm. in diameter. adj., **pap'ular.**

papyraceous (pap"ĭ-ra'shus) like paper.

par (par) [L.] pair.

para- (par′ah) word element [Gr.], *beside.*

para (par′ah) a woman who has produced one or more viable offspring. **p. I,** primipara. **p. II,** secundipara, etc.

para-agglutinin (par″ah-ah-gloo′tĭ-nin) partial agglutinin.

para-anesthesia (-an″es-the′ze-ah) anesthesia of the lower part of the body.

para-appendicitis (-ah-pen″dĭ-si′tis) appendicitis involving nearby structures.

parabion (-bi′on) parabiont.

parabiont (-bi′ont) one of two organisms living in a condition of parabiosis.

parabiosis (-bi-o′sis) the cooperative association of two distinct organisms, or the anatomic and physiologic union of two animals as created surgically for experimental purposes or as occurs naturally in Siamese twins. adj., **parabiot′ic. dialytic p.,** the separate circulation of the blood of two animals through a dialyzer to eliminate harmful factors from the blood of one and add to it essential factors from the blood of the other.

parablepsia (-blep′se-ah) false or perverted vision.

parabulia (-bu′le-ah) perversion of will.

paracarbinoxamine (-kar″bin-ok′sah-min) carbinoxamine.

paracasein (-ka′se-in) the compound into which casein is converted in the stomach by rennin or pepsin, before undergoing complete digestion.

paracenesthesia (-se″nes-the′ze-ah) any disturbance of the general sense of well-being.

paracentesis (-sen-te′sis) surgical puncture of a cavity for the aspiration of fluid, as of the abdominal (peritoneal) or thoracic (pleural) cavity. adj., **paracentet′ic.**

paracephalus (-sef′ah-lus) a fetus with defective head and imperfect sense organs.

paracetaldehyde (par-as″et-al′dē-hīd) paraldehyde.

paracetamol (par-as″et-am′ol) acetaminophen.

parachloramine (par″ah-klor′ah-mēn) meclizine.

parachlorophenol (-klo″ro-fe′nol) a crystalline compound used as a topical antibacterial agent.

paracholia (-ko′le-ah) disordered bile secretion.

parachordal (-kor′dal) beside the notochord.

parachroma (-kro′mah) skin discoloration.

parachromatin (-kro′mah-tin) the nucleoplasm of the spindle formed in mitosis.

parachromatopsia (-kro″mah-top′se-ah) color blindness.

parachromophoric (-kro″mo-for′ik) secreting coloring matter, but retaining it in the organism.

paracinesia (-si-ne′se-ah) perversion of motor powers.

paracoccidioidomycosis (-kok-sid″e-oi″do-mi-ko′sis) a skin infection due to *Blastomyces* (*Paracoccidioides*) *brasiliensis.*

Paracolobactrum (-ko″lo-bac′trum) a genus of Schizomycetes (order Eubacteriales, family Enterobacteriaceae, tribe Escherichieae) found in the intestinal tract of animals, including man.

Paracort (par′ah-kort) trademark for a preparation of prednisone.

Paracortol (par″ah-kor′tol) trademark for a preparation of prednisolone.

paracusis (-ku′sis) derangement of the hearing. **p. duplica′ta,** diplacusis. **p. lo′ci,** inability to locate correctly the origin of sounds. **p. willisia′na,** ability to hear best in a loud din.

paracyesis (-si-e′sis) extrauterine pregnancy.

paradental (-den′tal) 1. having some connection with or relation to the science or practice of dentistry. 2. periodontal.

paradidymis (-did′ĭ-mis) a small, vestigial structure found occasionally in the adult in the lower part of the spermatic cord.

Paradione (-di′ōn) trademark for preparations of paramethadione.

paradipsia (-dip′se-ah) a perverted appetite for fluids.

paradox (par′ah-doks) a seemingly contradictory occurrence. **Weber's p.,** elongation of a muscle which has been so stretched that it cannot contract.

paraffin (par′ah-fin) purified mixture of solid hydrocarbons obtained from petroleum. **light liquid p.,** light liquid petrolatum. **liquid p.,** liquid petrolatum (mineral oil).

paraffinoma (par″ah-fĭ-no′mah) a swelling forming around a deposit of paraffin in the tissues.

Paraflex (par′ah-fleks) trademark for a preparation of chlorzoxazone.

paragammacism (par″ah-gam′ah-sizm) faulty enunciation of *g, k* and *ch sounds.*

paraganglioma (-gang″gle-o′mah) a tumor of the tissue composing the paraganglia. **medullary p.,** pheochromocytoma. **nonchromaffin p.,** carotid body tumor.

paraganglion (-gang′gle-on), pl. *paragan′glia* [Gr.] a collection of chromaffin cells derived from neural ectoderm, occurring outside the adrenal medulla.

parageusia (-gu′ze-ah) perversion of the sense of taste.

paraglobulin (-glob′u-lin) a globulin from blood serum, blood cells, lymph and various tissues.

paraglossa (-glos′ah) swelling of the tongue.

paragonimiasis (-gon′ĭ-mi′ah-sis) infection with flukes of the genus Paragonimus.

Paragonimus (-gon′ĭ-mus) a genus of trematode parasites. **P. wester man′i,** a species occurring primarily in Asia, but also in Africa and South and Central America; found in the lungs of man and crab-eating mammals.

paragrammatism (-gram′ah-tizm) disorder of speech, with confusion in the use and order of words and grammatical forms.

paragraphia (-graf′e-ah) slight impairment of ability to express thoughts in writing.

parahemophilia (-he″mo-fil′e-ah) a condition resembling hemophilia, but due to lack of a different blood coagulation factor.

parahormone (-hor′mōn) a substance, not a true hormone, which has a hormone-like action in controlling the functioning of some distant organ.

parakeratosis (par″ah-ker″ah-to′sis) 1. any disorder of the horny layer of the skin. 2. retention of the nuclei in the cells of the keratin or horny layer, normally seen in true mucous membrane.

paralalia (-la′le-ah) a disorder of speech, especially the production of a vocal sound different from the one desired, or the substitution in speech of one letter for another.

paralambdacism (-lam′dah-sizm) faulty enunciation of the *l* sound.

paralbumin (par″al-bu′min) an albumin showing characteristics differing from those of the normal compound.

paralbuminemia (-bu″mi-ne′me-ah) presence in the blood of abnormal albumins (paralbumins).

paraldehyde (pah-ral′dĕ-hīd) colorless, transparent liquid; hypnotic and sedative.

paralepsy (par′ah-lep″se) psycholepsy.

paralexia (par″ah-lek′se-ah) slight impairment of ability to comprehend written ·language.

paralgesia (par″al-je′ze-ah) an abnormal and painful sensation.

parallagma (par″ah-lag′mah) displacement of a bone or of the fragments of a broken bone.

parallax (par′ah-laks) an apparent displacement of an object due to change in the observer's position.

parallergy (par-al′er-je) a predisposition to allergy produced by previous sensitization. adj., **paraller′gic.**

paralogia (par″ah-lo′je-ah) derangement of the reasoning faculty.

paralysin (pah-ral′ĭ-sin) agglutinin.

paralysis (pah-ral′ĭ-sis) loss of power of voluntary motion or of sensation due to a lesion of nerve substance. **abducens p.,** lesion of the abducens nerve causing paralysis of the external rectus muscle of the eye. **p. of accommodation,** paralysis of the ciliary muscles of the eye so as to prevent accommodation. **p. ag′itans,** a progressive disease of late life, with masklike facies, tremor, slowing of voluntary movements, festinating gait, peculiar posture and muscle weakness. **ascending p.,** spinal paralysis which progresses cephalad. **birth p.,** that due to injury received at birth. **brachial p.,** paralysis of an arm. **brachiofacial p.,** paralysis of the face and arm. **bulbar p.,** paralysis due to changes in motor centers of the medulla oblongata. **central p.,** paralysis due to a lesion of the brain or spinal cord. **cerebral p.,** paralysis caused by some intracranial lesion. **cerebrospinal p., hereditary,** a hereditary condition which develops usually in early middle life, with gradually developing paralyses in the upper or lower extremities, in the two extremities on one side, or in all four extremities. **creeping p.,** locomotor ataxia. **crossed p.,** affecting one side of face and other side of body. **diver's p.,** decompression sickness. **Duchenne's p.,** progressive bulbar paralysis. **emotional p.,** inaction due to opposing psychic drives of equal strength.

facial p., Bell's palsy. **infantile p.,** acute anterior poliomyelitis. **Landry's p.,** acute ascending myelitis. **obstetric p.,** paralysis of the newborn resulting from injuries received at birth. **pseudobulbar p.,** paralysis simulating bulbar paralysis, but due to a lesion in the cerebrum. **pseudohypertrophic p.,** paralysis with enlargement and fatty degeneration of affected muscles. **spastic p.,** paralysis with rigidity of the muscles and heightened deep muscle reflexes. **spinal p.,** 1. anterior poliomyelitis. 2. paraplegia. **spinal p., spastic,** congenital lateral sclerosis of the spinal cord, producing atrophy and rigidity of the muscles of the extremities. **Weber's p.,** alternating oculomotor hemiplegic paralysis.

paralytic (par″ah-lit′ik) 1. pertaining to paralysis. 2. a person affected with paralysis.

paralytogenic (par″ah-lit″o-jen′ik) causing paralysis.

paralyzant (par′ah-līz″ant) 1. causing paralysis. 2. a drug that causes paralysis.

paramania (par″ah-ma′ne-ah) a condition in which the patient exhibits joy by complaining.

Paramecium (-me′she-um) a genus of ciliate protozoans.

paramecium (-me′she-um) an organism belonging to the genus Paramecium.

paramedical (-med′ĭ-kal) related to the science or practice of medicine.

paramenia (-me′ne-ah) disordered or difficult menstruation.

parameter (pah-ram′ĕ-ter) an arbitrary constant whose values characterize the mathematical expressions into which it enters.

paramethadione (par″ah-meth″ah-di′ŏn) a compound used as an anticonvulsant in petit mal epilepsy.

paramethasone (-meth′ah-sōn) a compound used as a corticosteroid with anti-inflammatory action.

parametric (-met′rik) around the uterus.

parametrismus (-me-triz′mus) painful spasm of muscle in the broad ligament.

parametritis (-me-tri′tis) inflammation of parametrium.

parametrium (-me′tre-um) loose connective tissue and smooth muscle within the broad ligaments and near the uterus.

paramimia (-mim′e-ah) loss of power to make natural gestures and movements.

paramitome (-mi′tōm) hyaloplasm (1).

paramnesia (par″am-ne′ze-ah) an unconsciously false memory.

paramorphia (par″ah-mor′fe-ah) abnormality of form.

paramyoclonus (-mi-ok′lo-nus) a condition characterized by myoclonic contractions of various muscles. **p. mul′tiplex,** a condition characterized by sudden shocklike contractions.

paramyotonia (-mi″o-to′ne-ah) impairment of muscular tonicity. **p. congen′ita,** myotonia congenita.

paranesthesia (par″an-es-the′ze-ah) paraanesthesia.

para-nitrosulfathiazole (par″ah-ni″tro-sul″-fah-thi′ah-zōl) a compound used as an antibacterial.

paranoia (-noi′ah) a mental disorder marked by well systematized delusions of grandeur and persecution.

paranoiac (-noi′ak) a person affected with paranoia.

paranomia (-no′me-ah) aphasia in which the names of objects seen (*visual paranomia*) or touched (*myotactic paranomia*) are not recollected.

paranuclein (-nu′kle-in) nucleoalbumin.

paranucleus (-nu′kle-us) a body sometimes seen in cell protoplasm near the nucleus.

paraphasia (-fa′ze-ah) slight defect in ability to comprehend, elaborate or express speech concepts.

paraphemia (-fe′me-ah) distorted speech.

paraphia (par-a′fe-ah) disorder of the sense of touch.

paraphilia (par″ah-fil′e-ah) expression of the sexual instinct in practices biologically or socially undesirable.

paraphiliac (-fil′e-ak) a person who exhibits paraphilia.

paraphimosis (-fi-mo′sis) retraction of foreskin behind the glans penis.

paraphobia (-fo′be-ah) a mild phobia.

paraphrasia (-fra′ze-ah) disorderly arrangement of spoken words.

paraphrenia (-fre′ne-ah) 1. any one of a group of psychoses including paranoia and dementia precox. 2. paraphrenitis. **p. confab'u-lans**, paraphrenia distinguished by falsifications of memory. **p. expan'siva**, paraphrenia marked by delusions of grandeur, and exalted mood and mild excitement. **p. phantas'tica**, paraphrenia marked by fantastic, changeable and unsystematized delusions. **p. systemat'ica**, paraphrenia marked by gradual development of delusions of persecution, with later delusion of grandeur without deterioration of personality.

paraplasm (par′ah-plazm) 1. any abnormal growth. 2. hyaloplasm (1).

paraplastic (par″ah-plas″tik) having morbid formative power.

paraplectic (par″ah-plek′tik) paraplegic.

paraplegia (-ple′je-ah) paralysis of half of the body, usually referring to paralysis of the lower half, including the legs. adj., **paraple'-gic. superior p., upper p.**, paralysis of the upper half of the body, including the arms, shoulders and usually the upper trunk.

paraplexus (-plek′sus) the choroid plexus of the lateral ventricle.

parapophysis (-pof′i-sis) lower vertebral transverse process.

parapoplexy (par-ap′o-plek″se) slight apoplexy.

parapraxia (par″ah-prak′se-ah) inability to perform movements properly.

paraprotein (-pro′te-in) a protein having unusual physical characteristics.

paraproteinemia (-pro″te-in-e′me-ah) presence in the blood of an abnormal serum globu-lin, such as a cryoglobulin or a macroglobulin.

parapsis (par-ap′sis) perversion of the sense of touch.

parapsoriasis (par″ah-so-ri′ah-sis) a chronic skin eruption resembling psoriasis.

parapsychology (-si-kol′o-je) the study of psychic phenomena, i.e. relations between persons and events which apparently occur without the apparent intervention of the five human senses.

parapsychosis (-si-ko′sis) perversion of the function of thought.

parareflexia (-re-flek′se-ah) any disorder of the reflexes.

pararhotacism (-ro′tah-sizm) faulty enunciation of *r* sound.

pararrhythmia (-rith′me-ah) cardiac arrhythmia with two separate rhythms at one time.

pararthria (par-ar′thre-ah) imperfect utterance of words.

Parasal (par′ah-sal) trademark for preparations of para-aminosalicylic acid.

parasigmatism (par″ah-sig′mah-tizm) faulty enunciation of *s* and *z* sounds.

parasite (par′ah-sit) an individual or species which nourishes itself at the expense of an organism of another species, which it affects adversely, but does not immediately destroy. adj., **parasit'ic. erratic p.**, one that invades an organ of a host in which it is not usually found. **facultative p.**, one that is not entirely dependent on a host for its survival, but can adapt itself to a parasitic way of life. **incidental p.**, an organism that accidentally acquires an unnatural host and survives. **obligatory p.**, one that is entirely dependent upon a host for its survival. **pathogenic p.**, one that causes an almost immediate disease in the host. **periodic p., sporadic p.**, one that intermittently visits a host to obtain some benefit.

parasiticide (par″ah-sit′i-sīd) a substance destructive to parasites.

parasitism (par′ah-si″tizm) the biological association of two individuals or populations of different species, one of which nourishes itself at the expense of the other, which it often affects adversely, but does not rapidly destroy.

parasitogenic (par″ah-si″to-jen′ik) due to parasites.

parasitologist (-si-tol′o-jist) a person skilled in parasitology.

parasitology (-si-tol′o-je) the scientific study of parasites. **medical p.**, that particularly concerned with the study of disease-causing parasites.

parasitophobia (-si″to-fo′be-ah) morbid dread of parasites.

parasitotropic (-trop′ik) having affinity for parasites.

paraspadias (par″ah-spa′de-as) opening of the urethra on one side of the penis.

paraspasm (par′ah-spazm) spasm of the corresponding muscles on both sides of the body.

Paraspirillum (par″ah-spi-ril′um) a genus of Schizomycetes (order Pseudomonadales, suborder Pseudomonadineae, family Spirilla-ceae).

parasteatosis (par″ah-ste″ah-to′sis) disorder of sebaceous secretions.

parasternal (-ster′nal) beside the sternum.

parasthenia (par″as-the′ne-ah) abnormal functioning of organic tissue.

parasympatholytic (par″ah-sim″pah-tho-lit′ik) producing effects resembling those of interruption of the parasympathetic nerve supply of a part; having a destructive effect on the parasympathetic nerve fibers or blocking the transmission of impulses by them.

parasympathomimetic (-mi-met′ik) producing effects resembling those of stimulation of the parasympathetic nerve supply of a part.

parasystole (par″ah-sis′to-le) an abnormally prolonged interval between systole and diastole.

paratenon (-ten′on) the fatty areolar tissue filling the interstices of the fascial compartment in which a tendon is situated.

paratherapeutic (-ther″ah-pu′tik) caused by treatment of some other disease.

parathion (-thi′on) an insecticidal compound, which may cause fatal poisoning in man.

Parathormone (-thor′mōn) trademark for a preparation of parathyroid extract.

parathymia (-thi′me-ah) disordered emotion.

parathyroid (-thi′roid) one of four small glands on the lateral lobes of the thyroid.

parathyroidectomy (-thi″roi-dek′to-me) excision of a parathyroid gland.

parathyroidoma (-thi″roi-do′mah) a tumor composed of tissue resembling the parathyroid gland.

parathyroprivia (-thi″ro-pri′ve-ah) the condition due to absence of functioning parathyroid glands. adj., **parathyropriv′ic.**

paratrachoma (-trah-ko′mah) conjunctivitis resembling trachoma.

paratrichosis (-tri-ko′sis) growth of hair in abnormal situations.

paratrophy (par-at′ro-fe) 1. bacterial nutrition in which the growth energy is obtained from the host. 2. dystrophy.

paratuberculosis (par″ah-tu-ber″ku-lo′sis) a disease of cattle, sometimes occurring in sheep and goats, characterized by persistent diarrhea and rapid loss of weight, and due to *Mycobacterium paratuberculosis.*

paratyphoid (-ti′foid) diseased state associated with typhoid fever.

paravaccinia (-vak-sin′e-ah) an eruption of tubercles sometimes following vaccination.

paravertebral (-ver′tē-bral) near the vertebrae.

paravitaminosis (-vi″tah-mi-no′sis) vitamin deficiency without the usual symptoms.

paraxial (par-ak′se-al) alongside an axis.

Paredrine (par′ah-drēn) trademark for preparations of hydroxyamphetamine.

paregoric (par″ē-gor′ik) a mixture of powdered opium, anise oil, benzoic acid, camphor and glycerin, in diluted alcohol.

parenchyma (pah-reng′ki-mah) the essential or functional elements of an organ, as distinguished from its stroma or framework. adj., **paren′chymal.**

parenchymatitis (par″eng-ki″mah-ti′tis) inflammation of a parenchyma.

Parenogen (par-en′o-gen) trademark for a preparation of fibrinogen.

parenteral (pah-ren′ter-al) otherwise than through the alimentary canal.

parepididymis (par″ep-ĭ-did′ĭ-mis) paradidymis.

parergasia (par″er-ga′ze-ah) a psychic disorder marked by incongruities, mannerisms, etc., as schizophrenia and paranoia.

paresis (pah-re′sis, par′ĕ-sis) paralysis. adj., **paret′ic. syphilitic p.,** dementia paralytica.

paresthesia (par″es-the′ze-ah) an abnormal or perverted sensation due to disorder of the sensory nervous system.

paridrosis (par″ĭ-dro′sis) any disorder of the perspiration.

paries (pa′re-ez), pl. *pari′etes* [L.] a wall, as of an organ or cavity. adj., **pari′etal.**

parietography (pah-ri″ĕ-tog′rah-fe) roentgenographic visualization of the walls of an organ.

parkinsonism (par′kin-sun-izm″) a condition marked by rigidity and tremor characteristic of paralysis agitans.

Parnate (par′nāt) trademark for a preparation of tranylcypromine.

paroccipital (par″ok-sip′ĭ-tal) beside the occipital bone.

paromomycin (par″o-mo-mi″sin) a stable antibiotic derived from a strain of Streptomyces and effective against Entamoeba, Salmonella, Shigella, Proteus, Aerobacter and *Escherichia coli.*

paromphalocele (par″om-fal′o-sēl) hernia near the navel.

paronychia (par″o-nik′e-ah) infection of the soft tissues adjacent to the nail. **p. tendino′sa,** septic inflammation of sheath of tendon of a finger.

paroophoron (par″o-of′o-ron) a small, vestigial structure found between the layers of the mesosalpinx.

parophthalmia (par″of-thal′me-ah) inflammation of the connective tissue around the eye.

paropsis (par-op′sis) a disorder of vision.

parorchidium (par″or-kid′e-um) displacement of a testis.

parorexia (par″o-rek′se-ah) nervous perversion of the appetite, with craving for special articles of food.

parosmia (par-oz′me-ah) perversion of sense of smell.

parostosis (par″os-to′sis) ossification of tissues outside of the periosteum.

parotid (pah-rot′id) near the ear.

parotidectomy (pah-rot″ĭ-dek′to-me) excision of a parotid gland.

parotiditis (-di′tis) parotitis.

parotitis (par″o-ti′tis) inflammation of the parotid gland. **contagious p., epidemic p.,** an acute, communicable viral disease involving chiefly the parotid gland, but frequently affecting other oral glands or the pancreas or gonads.

parovarian (par″o-va′re-an) beside the ovary.

parovarium (-va′re-um) epoophoron.

paroxysm (par'ok-sizm) an episode or occurrence of abrupt onset and termination. adj., **paroxys'mal.**

pars (pars), pl. *par'tes* [L.] part. **p. mastoi'dea,** the mastoid portion of the temporal bone, being the irregular, posterior part. **p. petro'sa,** the petrous portion of the temporal bone, containing the inner ear and wedged in at the base of the skull between the sphenoid and occipital bones. **p. tympan'ica,** the tympanic portion of the temporal bone, the curved plate lying below the squama and in front of the mastoid process.

Parsidol (par'si-dol) trademark for a preparation of ethopropazine.

parthenogenesis (par"thĕ-no-jen'ĕ-sis) development of an ovum not initiated by combination with a male gamete; it may occur as a natural phenomenon or be induced by chemical or mechanical stimulation (*artificial parthenogenesis*).

parthogenesis (par"tho-jen'ĕ-sis) parthenogenesis.

particle (par'tĭ-kl) an extremely small mass or portion of substance or matter. **disperse p's,** the particles of colloid in a colloid system. **elementary p.,** one of the smallest units of which atoms are composed and which are capable of independent existence. **high-velocity p's,** elementary charged particles, such as electrons and protons, given greater speed and energy in an accelerator. **ionizing p.,** one that directly produces ion pairs in its passage through matter.

particulate (par-tik'u-lāt) composed of separate particles.

parturient (par-tu're-ent) giving birth or pertaining to birth; by extension, a woman at childbirth.

parturifacient (par-tu"rĭ-fa'shent) a medicine which facilitates childbirth.

parturiometer (-om'ĕ-ter) device used in measuring expulsive power of uterus.

parturition (par"tu-rish'un) expulsion or delivery of the fetus from the body of the maternal organism.

parulis (pah-roo'lis) abscess of a gingiva.

parumbilical (par"um-bil'ĭ-kal) near the navel.

parvicellular (par"vĭ-sel'u-lar) composed of small cells.

PAS, PASA para-aminosalicylic acid.

passion (pash'un) 1. suffering; pain. 2. strong emotion. **ileac p.,** ileus.

paste (pāst) a semisolid preparation, generally for external use, of a fatty base, a viscous or mucilaginous base, or a mixture of starch and petrolatum.

pastern (pas'tern) the part of a horse's foot occupied by the first and second phalanges.

Pasteurella (pas"tĕ-rel'ah) a genus of Schizomycetes (order Eubacteriales, family Brucellaceae).

pasteurellosis (pas"ter-ĕ-lo'sis) infection with organisms of the genus Pasteurella.

Pasteuria (pas-tu're-ah) a genus of Schizomycetes (order Hyphomicrobiales, family Pasteuriaceae) parasitic on fresh-water crustacea.

Pasteuriaceae (pas-tu"re-a'se-e) a family of Schizomycetes (order Hyphomicrobiales), including the genera Blastocaulis and Pasteuria.

pasteurization (pas"tūr-ĭ-za'shun) exposure to a temperature of 60°C. for 30 minutes, killing pathogenic bacteria and delaying other bacterial development.

patch (pach) a small area differing from the rest of a surface. **Peyer's p's,** whitish patches of lymph follicles in mucous and submucous layers of the small intestine.

patella (pah-tel'ah), pl *patel'lae* [L.] a bone at the knee. adj., **patel'lar.**

patellapexy (-pek"se) surgical fixation of the patella to the lower end of the femur.

patellectomy (pat"ĕ-lek'to-me) excision of the patella.

patelliform (pah-tel'ĭ-form) shaped like the patella.

patellofemoral (pah-tel"o-fem'o-ral) pertaining to patella and femur.

patency (pa'ten-se) the condition of being wide open. adj., **pa'tent.**

path(o)- (path'o) word element [Gr.], *disease; morbid condition.*

pathergasia (path"er-ga'ze-ah) mental malfunction, implying functional or structural damage.

pathergy (path'er-je) 1. a condition in which the application of a stimulus leaves the body abnormally susceptible to subsequent stimuli. 2. a condition of being allergic to several antigens. adj., **pather'gic.**

pathic (path'ik) pertaining to disease.

Pathilon (path'ĭ-lon) trademark for preparations of tridihexethyl.

patho-anatomy (path"o-ah-nat'o-me) pathologic anatomy.

pathobiology (-bi-ol'o-je) pathology.

pathogen (path'o-jen) any disease-producing agent or microorganism. adj., **pathogen'ic.**

pathogenesis (path"o-jen'ĕ-sis) the development of disease or a morbid or pathologic state. adj., **pathogenet'ic.**

pathogenicity (-jĕ-nis'ĭ-te) the quality of producing morbid changes (disease) in an organism or tissue.

pathogeny (pah-thoj'ĕ-ne) pathogenesis.

pathoglycemia (path"o-gli-se'me-ah) sugar in the blood as a result of some disease.

pathognomonic (path"og-no-mon'ik) specifically distinctive or characteristic of a disease or pathologic condition.

pathologic (path"o-loj'ik) pertaining to or caused by disease.

pathologist (path-thol'o-jist) a specialist in pathology. **speech p.,** a specialist in disorders of speech and language.

pathology (pah-thol'o-je) the scientific study of the alterations produced by disease. adj., **patholog'ic. behavior p.,** psychopathology. **cellular p.,** that which considers the morbid changes in body cells. **clinical p.,** pathology applied to the solution of clinical problems. **comparative p.,** that which considers human disease processes in comparison with those of the lower animals. **experimental p.,** the study of artificially induced pathologic processes. **general p.,** that taking cognizance of processes which may occur in various diseases and in different organs. **oral p.,** that treating of conditions causing or resulting from morbid anatomic or functional changes in the structures of the mouth. **pediatric p.,** that dealing especially with diseases of children. **special p.,** that dealing with changes produced by certain diseases or in a specific organ. **surgical p.,** that dealing with conditions requiring surgical treatment.

patholysis (pah-thol'ĭ-sis) dissolution of tissues by disease.

pathomania (path"o-ma'ne-ah) moral insanity.

pathomimesis (-mi-me'sis) malingering.

pathomorphism (-mor'fizm) abnormal morphology.

pathonomy (pah-thon'o-me) science of the laws of disease.

pathophobia (path"o-fo'be-ah) morbid fear of disease.

pathophoresis (-fo-re'sis) the transmission of disease. adj., **pathophor'ic.**

pathophysiology (-fiz"e-ol'o-je) the physiology of disordered function.

pathopleiosis (-pli-o'sis) the tendency to magnify the gravity of one's disease.

pathopsychology (-si-kol'o-je) the psychology of mental disease.

pathosis (pah-tho'sis) a diseased condition.

pathway (path'wa) a course usually followed. **biosynthetic p.,** sequence of enzymic steps in the synthesis of a specific end-product in a living organism.

-pathy (path'e) word element [Gr.], *morbid condition* or *disease*; generally used to designate a noninflammatory condition.

patient (pa'shent) a person who is undergoing treatment for disease.

patroclinous (pat"ro-kli'nus) inheriting or inherited from the father.

patulous (pat'u-lus) spread widely apart.

Paveril (pav'er-il) trademark for preparations of dioxyline.

pavilion (pah-vil'yun) a dilated or flaring expansion at the end of a canal.

pavor (pa'vor) extreme fear reaction; terror. **p. diur'nus,** extreme fear reaction in a child during a daytime nap. **p. noctur'nus,** extreme fear reaction in a child during sleep or at night.

P.B. *Pharmacopoeia Britannica* (British pharmacopoeia).

Pb chemical symbol, *lead* (L. *plumbum*).

P.B.I. protein-bound iodine.

p.c. [L.] *post ci'bum* (after meals).

PCG phonocardiogram.

P.C.M.O. Principal Colonial Medical Officer.

P.C.V. packed cell volume.

Pd chemical symbol, *palladium.*

p.d. potential difference; prism diopter (dioptry).

pearl (perl) 1. a small medicated granule. 2. a glass globule with a single dose of volatile medicine. **epithelial p.,** a form of granule found in epithelioma. **Laennec's p's,** round masses of sputum in bronchial asthma.

pecazine (pe'kah-zēn) mepazine.

peccant (pek'ant) unhealthy; causing ill health.

pectase (pek'tās) an enzyme which catalyzes the demethylation of pectin, thus producing pectic acid.

pecten (pek'ten), pl. *pec'tines* [L.] 1. a narrow zone in the anal canal distal to the line separating rectal mucosa and skin of the canal. 2. anterior border of the superior ramus of the pubis. adj., **pectin'eal. p. os'sis pu'bis,** the sharp anterior border of the os pubis.

pectenitis (pek"tĕ-ni'tis) inflammation of the pecten of the anus.

pectenosis (-no'sis) stenosis of the anal canal due to an inelastic ring of tissue.

pectenotomy (-not'o-me) incision of the constricting band in pectenosis.

pectin (pek'tin) purified carbohydrate product from dilute acid extract of inner portion of the rind of citrus fruits or from apple pulp; used as a plasma substitute or an emulsifying or gelling agent.

pectinase (pek'tĭ-nās) an enzyme in plants which catalyzes the hydrolysis of pectin to sugars and galacturonic acid.

pectinate (pek'tĭ-nāt) comb-shaped.

pectiniform (pek-tin'ĭ-form) shaped like a comb.

pectoral (pek'tor-al) 1. pertaining to the chest or breast. 2. effective in diseases of the chest.

pectoralgia (pek"to-ral'je-ah) pain in the chest.

pectoralis (-ra'lis) pertaining to the chest or breast.

pectoriloquy (-ril'o-kwe) transmission of the sound of spoken words through the chest wall.

pectorophony (-rof'o-ne) exaggeration of vocal resonance heard on auscultation.

pectose (pek'tōs) a principle in unripe fruits which in ripening becomes converted into pectin.

pectus (pek'tus) the breast, chest or thorax. **p. carina'tum,** undue prominence of the sternum. **p. excava'tum,** undue depression of the sternum.

ped- word element, (1) *child*; (2) *foot.*

pedal (ped'al) pertaining to the foot or feet.

pederasty (ped"er-as'te) sexual intercourse per anum; usually applied to that between human males, especially between an adult and a youth.

pediatric (pe"de-at'rik) pertaining to diseases of children.

pediatrician (pe"de-ah-trish'an) a specialist in pediatrics.

pediatrics (pe"de-at'riks) the department of medicine dealing especially with problems and diseases of young children.

pedicellation (ped"ĭ-sel-la'shun) the development of a pedicle.

pedicle (ped'ĭ-kl) a footlike or stemlike part or attaching structure.

pediculation (pĕ-dik"u-la'shun) 1. the process of forming a pedicle. 2. infestation with lice.

pediculicide (pĕ-dik'u-lĭ-sīd) an agent which destroys lice.

Pediculoides (pe-dik"u-loi'dēz) a name formerly given a genus of mites. **P. ventri-co'sus,** *Pyemotes ventricosus.*

pediculophobia (pě-dik″u-lo-fo′be-ah) morbid dread of lice.

pediculosis (-lo′sis) infestation with lice.

Pediculus (pe-dik′u-lus) a genus of lice. **P. huma'nus,** a species which feeds on human blood and is an important vector of relapsing fever, typhus and trench fever; two subspecies were formerly recognized: *P. humanus* var. *capitis,* occurring on the head, and *P. humanus* var. *corporis,* occurring elsewhere on the body. **P. inguina'lis, P. pu'bis,** *Phthirus pubis.*

Pediococcus (pe″de-o-kok′us) a genus of Schizomycetes (order Eubacteriales, family Lactobacillaceae, tribe Streptococceae) found in fermenting fruit juices.

pediophobia (-fo′be-ah) morbid dread of children or dolls.

peditis (pe-di′tis) inflammation of the pedal bone of a horse.

pedodontia (pe″do-don′she-ah) pedodontics.

pedodontics (-don′tiks) the department of dentistry dealing with the teeth and mouth conditions of children.

pedodontist (-don′tist) a dentist who specializes in pedodontics.

pedograph (ped′o-graf) an imprint of the weight-bearing surface of the foot.

pedomorphism (pe″do-mor′fizm) retention in adult organisms of bodily characters that in early evolutionary history were only infantile.

pedophilia (-fil′e-ah) abnormal fondness for children.

peduncle (pe-dung′kl) a stemlike part; applied to collections of nerve fibers coursing between different regions in the central nervous system. adj., **pedun'cular. cere-bellar p's,** three sets of paired bundles of the hindbrain (*superior, middle* and *inferior*) connecting the cerebellum to the midbrain, pons and medulla oblongata, respectively. **cerebral p's,** two massive bundles, one on each side, constituting the ventral portion of the midbrain. **pineal p.,** slender band going forward on either side from pineal body.

pedunculated (pe dung′ku-lāt″ed) having a peduncle.

pedunculotomy (pe-dung″ku-lot′o-me) incision of a peduncle of the brain.

pedunculus (pe-dung′ku-lus) peduncle.

Peganone (peg′ah-nōn) trademark for a preparation of ethotoin.

peladophobia (pel″ah-do-fo′be-ah) morbid fear of baldness.

pelage (pel′ij) the hairy covering of the body.

peliosis (pe″le-o′sis) purpura. **p. hep'atis,** a condition characterized by multiple small cystic, blood-filled spaces in the liver.

pella (pel′ah) cutis.

pellagra (pě-la′grah, pě-lag′rah) a condition due to deficiency of nicotinic acid, marked by anorexia, weakness, malaise and characteristic cutaneous lesions, and sometimes leading to mental depression. adj., **pellag'-rous.**

pellagrin (pě-la′grin, pě-lag′rin) a person affected with pellagra.

pellagroid (pě-lag′roid) resembling pellagra.

pellet (pel′et) a small pill or granule.

pellicle (pel′i-kl) a thin scum forming on the surface of liquids.

pellicula (pě-lik′u-lah) epidermis.

Pelodictyon (pe″lo-dik′te-on) a genus of Schizomycetes (order Pseudomonadales, suborder Rhodobacteriineae, family Chlorobacteriaceae).

Pelonema (pe″lo-ne′mah) a genus of Schizomycetes (order Chlamydobacteriales, family Peloplocaceae).

Peloploca (pe-lo′plo kah) a genus of Schizomycetes (order Chlamydobacteriales, family Peloplocaceae).

Peloplocaceae (pe-lo″plo-ka′se-e) a family of Schizomycetes (order Chlamydobacteriales).

pelta (pel′tah) a crescent-shaped membrane observed in certain flagellates.

pelvicephalometry (pel″vi-sef″ah-lom′ě-tre) measurement of the fetal head in relation to the maternal pelvis.

pelvimeter (pel-vim′ě-ter) instrument for measuring the pelvis.

pelvimetry (pel-vim′ě-tre) measurement of capacity and diameter of pelvis.

pelvioileoneocystostomy (pel″ve-o-il″e-o-ne″o-sis-tos′to-me) interposition of an isolated segment of ileum to provide a new communication between renal pelvis and the urinary bladder.

pelviotomy (pel″ve-ot′o-me) 1. incision or transection of a pelvic bone. 2 pyelotomy.

pelviperitonitis (pel″vi-per″ě-to-ni′tis) inflammation of the pelvic peritoneum.

pelviroentgenography (-rent″gen-og′rah-fe) roentgenography of the organs of the pelvis.

pelvis (pel′vis) 1. the basin formed by the hip bones and lower portion of the vertebral column, constituting the lowest part of the trunk. 2. the expanded, proximal portion of the ureter, usually contained in the substance of the kidney, in which the calices of the kidney open. adj., **pel'vic. android p.,** one with a wedge-shaped inlet and narrow anterior segment typically found in the male. **anthropoid p.,** one whose anteroposterior diameter equals or exceeds the transverse diameter. **assimilation p.,** one in which the ilia articulate with the vertebral column higher (*high assimilation pelvis*) or lower (*low assimilation pelvis*) than normal, the number of lumbar vertebrae being correspondingly decreased or increased. **brachy-pellic p.,** one in which the transverse diameter exceeds the anteroposterior diameter by 1 to 3 cm. **contracted p.,** one showing a decrease of 1.5 to 2 cm. in an important diameter. **dolichopellic p.,** a long, oval pelvis with the anteroposterior diameter greater than the transverse diameter. **false p.,** part of the pelvic cavity above a plane determined by a line on the inner surface of the ilium extending from the sacroiliac joint to the iliopubic eminence anteriorly. **flat p.,** one in which the anteroposterior dimension is abnormally reduced. **frozen p.,** a condition in which the fornices of the uterus are filled with a hardened exudate. **gynecoid p.,** one with a rounded, oval shape, typical of the normal female. **infantile p.**, a generally contracted pelvis with an oval shape, a high sacrum and inclination of the walls. **inverted p.**, split pelvis. **juvenile p.**, infantile pelvis. **kyphotic p.**, one marked by increase of conjugate diameter at brim with decrease of transverse diameter at outlet. **p. major**, false pelvis. **malacosteon p.**, one deformed as a result of rickets. **mesatipellic p.**, one in which the transverse diameter is equal to the anteroposterior diameter or exceeds it by no more than 1 cm. **p. minor**, true pelvis. **Nägele's p.**, one contracted in an oblique diameter, with complete ankylosis of the sacroiliac synchondrosis of one side and imperfect development of the sacrum and coxa on the same side. **platypellic p.**, one in which the transverse diameter exceeds the anteroposterior diameter by 3 cm. or more. **platypelloid p.**, one shortened in the anteroposterior aspect, with a flattened transverse, oval shape. **rachitic p.**, one affected with rickets. **renal p.**, the funnel-shaped expansion of the ureter within the substance of the kidney. **Robert's p.**, one deformed by osteoarthritis, with involvement of both sacroiliac synchondroses. **scoliotic p.**, one tilted as a result of scoliosis. **split p.**, one with a congenital separation at the symphysis pubis. **spondylolisthetic p.**, one deformed by sliding of the body of one of the lower lumbar vertebrae over the first sacral and into the pelvis. **true p.**, the part of the pelvic cavity below a plane determined by a line on the inner surface of the ilium, extending from the sacroiliac joint to the iliopubic eminence anteriorly.

pelvospondylitis (pel"vo-spon"dǐ-li'tis) inflammation of the pelvic portion of the spine. **p. ossif'icans**, rheumatoid spondylitis.

pemphigoid (pem'fĭ-goid) resembling pemphigus.

pemphigus (pem'fĭ-gus) a condition marked by chronic vesiculobullous lesions on the skin. **benign chronic familial p.**, a genetically transmitted condition which resembles pemphigus vulgaris, but heals spontaneously. **Brazilian p.**, a condition resembling pemphigus foliaceus, of unknown origin and endemic in Brazil. **bullous p.**, a chronic, generalized bullous eruption occurring in elderly adults predominantly, and usually not fatal. **p. erythemato'sus**, a condition resembling lupus erythematosus, with lesions limited to the face and chest. **p. folia'ceus**, a condition beginning with insignificant vesicles, with scaling and crusting at the site of the lesions, resembling exfoliative dermatitis. **p. gangreno'sus**, dermatitis gangrenosa infantum. **hemorrhagic p., p. hemorrhag'icus**, a condition characterized by the presence of bullae filled with hemorrhagic fluid. **p. neonato'rum**, neonatal impetigo. **South American p.**, Brazilian pemphigus. **p. veg'etans**, a variant of pemphigus bullosa in which verrucoid hypertrophic vegetative masses replace many of the bullous lesions. **p. vulga'ris**, a rare relapsing disease with tense or flaccid bullae on skin and mucous membranes; sometimes fatal. **wildfire p.**, Brazilian pemphigus.

penetrance (pen'ě-trans) the frequency with which a heritable trait is manifested by individuals carrying the principal gene or genes conditioning it.

penetrometer (pen"ě-trom'ě-ter) 1. an instrument for measuring the penetrating power of x-rays. 2. a device for registering the resistance of semisolid material to penetration.

-penia (pe'ne-ah) word element [Gr.], *scarcity.*

penicillamine (pen"ĭ-sil-am'in) an amino acid obtained from penicillin by treatment with hot mineral acids.

penicillin (pen"ĭ-sil'in) an antibiotic substance extracted from cultures of certain molds of the genus Penicillium that have been grown on special media.

penicillinase (-sil'ĭ-nās) a substance produced by bacteria which inactivates penicillin.

Penicillium (-sil'e-um) a genus of fungi.

penis (pe'nis) the male organ of urination and copulation.

penitis (pe-ni'tis) inflammation of the penis.

penniform (pen'ĭ-form) shaped like a feather.

penta (pen'tah) word element [Gr.], *five.*

pentachlorin (pen"tah-klo'rin) chlorophenothane.

pentad (pen'tad) an element or radical with a valence of five.

pentamethazene (pen"tah-meth'ah-zēn) azamethonium.

pentamethylenediamine (-meth"ĭ-lěn-di-am-ēn) a bacterial decomposition product of proteins, arising from the decarboxylation of lysine.

pentamethylenetetrazol (-tet'rah-zol) pentylenetetrazol.

pentapeptide (pen"tah-pep'tīd) a polypeptide containing five amino acids.

pentaploid (pen'tah-ploid) 1. characterized by pentaploidy. 2. an individual or cell having five sets of chromosomes.

pentaploidy (pen'tah-ploi"de) the state of having five sets of chromosomes (5n).

pentapyrrolidinium (pen"tah-pir-ro"lǐ-din'e-um) pentolinium.

pentavalent (pen"tah-va'lent, pen-tav'ah-lent) having a valence of five.

penthienate (pen-thi'ě-nāt) a compound used in parasympathetic blockade.

Penthrane (pen'thrān) trademark for a preparation of methoxyflurane.

Pentids (pen'tidz) trademark for preparations of potassium penicillin G.

pentobarbital (pen"to-bar'bĭ-tal) a short- to intermediate-acting barbiturate. **sodium p.**, a hypnotic compound.

pentobarbitone (-bar'bĭ-tōn) pentobarbital.

pentolinium (-lin'e-um) a compound used in ganglionic blockade to reduce blood pressure.

pentolysis (pen-tol'ĭ-sis) the disintegration or splitting up of pentose.

pentose (pen'tōs) any sugar or hydrocarbon of formula $C_5H_{10}O_5$.

pentoside (pen'to-sīd) a compound of pentose with another substance.

pentosuria (pen"to-su're-ah) pentose in the urine.

Pentothal (pen'to-thal) trademark for preparations of thiopental.

pentylenetetrazol (pen"tĭ-lēn-tet'rah-zol) a compound used as a central nervous system stimulant.

Pen-vee (pen've) trademark for preparations of penicillin V.

peonin (pe'o-nin) a dye used as an indicator for alkalis and acids.

peppermint (pep'er-mint) the dried leaves and flowering tops of *Mentha piperita*, used as a flavoring vehicle for drugs.

pepsic (pep'sik) peptic.

pepsin (pep'sin) a proteolytic enzyme secreted and stored in inactive form by the chief cells of the stomach wall, and activated by gastric acid; a preparation from the fresh stomach of the hog is used therapeutically. **saccharinated p.**, pepsin triturated with powdered lactose to a uniform fine powder.

pepsinogen (pep-sin'o-jen) the inactive precursor of pepsin, secreted by the chief cells of the stomach and converted to pepsin under the influence of hydrogen ions.

peptic (pep'tik) pertaining to pepsin or to digestion.

peptid (pep'tid) peptide.

peptidase (pep'tĭ-dās) an enzyme which catalyzes the hydrolysis of peptide linkages in polypeptides.

peptide (pep'tīd, pep'tid) a compound of low molecular weight which yields two or more amino acids on hydrolysis; known as di-, tri-, tetra-, etc., peptides, depending on the number of amino acids.

peptidolytic (pep"tĭ-do-lit'ik) splitting up peptides.

Peptococcus (pep"to-kok'us) a genus of Schizomycetes (order Eubacteriales, family Micrococcaceae).

peptogenic (-jen'ik) producing pepsin or peptones.

peptoid (pep'toid) a product of proteolytic digestion which does not give the biuret reaction.

peptolysis (pep-tol'ĭ-sis) the splitting up of pepsin. adj., **peptolyt'ic.**

peptone (pep'tōn) an intermediate product formed in the digestion of protein.

Peptostreptococcus (pep"to-strep"to-kok'us) a genus of Schizomycetes (order Eubacteriales, family Lactobacillaceae, tribe Streptococceae) occurring as parasitic inhabitants of the intestinal tract.

peracidity (per"ah-sid'ĭ-te) excessive acidity.

peracute (per"ah-kūt') very acute.

Perandren (per-an'dren) trademark for a preparation of testosterone.

per anum (per a'num) [L.] by anus.

Perazil (per'ah-zil) trademark for preparations of chlorcyclizine.

percentile (per-sen'tīl, per-sen'til) one of the values establishing the division of a series of

variables into hundredths, or the range of items included in such a segment.

percept (per'sept) the impression registered in the brain as the result of stimulation of a sense organ.

perception (per-sep'shun) recognition and proper interpretation of stimuli received in the brain, especially from the organs of special sense. **depth p.**, the ability to recognize depth or the relative distances to different objects in space. **extrasensory p.**, awareness gained otherwise than through the usual physical senses.

perceptive (per-sep'tiv) related to or important in the function of perception.

perceptivity (per"sep-tiv'ĭ-te) ability to receive sense impressions.

percipient (per-sip'e-ent) 1. pertaining to perception. 2. an individual who perceives or is capable of perception.

percolate (per'ko-lāt) 1. to submit to percolation. 2. any solution obtained by percolation.

percolation (per"ko-la'shun) the extraction of soluble parts of a drug by passing a solvent liquid through it.

percolator (-la'tor) vessel used in percolation.

Percorten (per-kor'ten) trademark for preparations of desoxycorticosterone.

percuss (per-kus') to perform percussion.

percussion (per-kush'un) the act of striking a part to produce vibrations in underlying tissues, the sound of which may provide information on their condition or structure; one of the methods of physical diagnosis. **auscultatory p.**, percussion combined with auscultation. **immediate p.**, that in which the blow is struck directly against the body surface. **instrumental p.**, that in which the blow is delivered by an instrument rather than the examiner's hand or fingers. **mediate p.**, that in which the blow is struck against another object or material placed on the surface of the body.

percussor (per-kus'or) an instrument for performing percussion.

percutaneous (per"ku-ta'ne-us) performed through the skin.

perflation (per-fla'shun) the blowing of air into a space to force secretions out.

perforans (per'fo-rans) [L.] perforating.

perforating (per"fo-rāt'ing) piercing or passing through a part.

perforation (-ra'shun) 1. an act of piercing. 2. a hole through a part.

perfrication (per"frĭ-ka'shun) rubbing with an ointment or embrocation.

perfusion (per-fu'zhun) the act of pouring through or into.

peri- (per'e) word element [Gr.], *around; near.* See also words beginning *para-.*

periacinous (per"e-as'ĭ-nus) around an acinus.

Periactin (-ak'tin) trademark for preparations of cyproheptadine hydrochloride.

periadenitis (-ad"ĕ-ni'tis) inflammation of tissues around a gland.

perianal (per″e-a′nal) around the anus.

periangiocholitis (-an″je-o-ko-li′tis) inflammation of tissues around the bile ducts.

periaortitis (-a″or-ti′tis) inflammation of tissues around the aorta.

periapical (-a′pĭ-kal) surrounding the apex of the root of a tooth.

periappendicitis (-ah-pen″dĭ-si′tis) inflammation of appendix and surrounding tissues.

periarterial (-ar-te′re-al) around an artery.

periarteritis (-ar″tĕ-ri′tis) inflammation of the outer coat of an artery. **p. gummo′sa**, accumulation of gummas in the blood vessels in syphilis. **p. nodo′sa**, an inflammatory disease of the coats of small and medium-sized arteries with inflammatory changes around the vessels and marked by symptoms of systemic infection.

periarthritis (-ar-thri′tis) inflammation around a joint.

periarticular (-ar-tik′u-lar) situated around a joint.

periaxial (-ak′se-al) around an axis.

periaxillary (-ak′sĭ-ler″e) around the axilla.

periblast (per′i-blast) the portion of the blastoderm of telolecithal eggs the cells of which lack complete cell membranes.

peribronchiolitis (per″ĭ-brong″ke-o-li′tis) inflammation around the bronchioles.

peribronchitis (-brong-ki′tis) inflammation of an entire lobe with bronchitis in that portion of the lung and thickening of the peribronchial tissue.

pericardiac (-kar′de-ak) pertaining to the pericardium; around the heart.

pericardicentesis (-kar″dĭ-sen-te′sis) puncture of the pericardial cavity with aspiration of fluid.

pericardiectomy (-kar″de-ek′to-me) excision of the pericardium.

pericardiocentesis (-kar″de-o-sen-te′sis) pericardicentesis.

pericardiolysis (-kar″de-ol′ĭ-sis) the freeing of adhesions between the visceral and parietal pericardium.

pericardiomediastinitis (-kar″de-o-me″de-as″tĭ-ni′tis) inflammation of pericardium and mediastinum.

pericardiophrenic (-fren′ik) pertaining to pericardium and diaphragm.

pericardiopleural (-ploo′ral) pertaining to pericardium and pleura.

pericardiorrhaphy (per″ĭ-kar″de-or′ah-fe) suture of the pericardium.

pericardiostomy (-kar″de-os′to-me) creation of an opening into the pericardial cavity through the chest wall for drainage of effusions.

pericardiosymphysis (-kar″de-o-sim″fĭ-sis) adhesion between visceral and parietal pericardium.

pericardiotomy (-kar″de-ot′o-me) incision of pericardium.

pericarditis (-kar-di′tis) inflammation of the pericardium. adj., **pericardit′ic**. **constrictive p.**, inflammatory thickening and calcification of the pericardium, constricting the heart and restricting its pulsation. **dry p.**, pericarditis not attended with effusion. **p. with effusion**, pericarditis with collection of a serous or purulent exudate in the pericardial cavity. **fibrinous p.**, **fibrous p.**, chronic pericarditis with formation of fibrous bands causing adhesion of the layers.

pericardium (per″ĭ-kar′de-um) the fibroserous sac enclosing the heart. adj., **pericar′dial**. **adherent p.**, one abnormally connected with the heart by dense fibrous tissue. **fibrous p.**, the external layer of the pericardium, consisting of dense fibrous tissue. **parietal p.**, the parietal layer of the serous pericardium, which is in contact with the fibrous pericardium. **serous p.**, the inner, serous portion of pericardium, consisting of two layers, visceral and parietal, enclosing a potential space, the pericardial cavity. **visceral p.**, the inner layer of the serous pericardium, which is in contact with the heart.

pericardosis (-kar-do′sis) disease of the pericardium.

pericecal (-se′kal) around the cecum.

pericecitis (-se-si′tis) inflammation around the cecum.

pericementitis (-se″men-ti′tis) periodontitis.

pericementoclasia (-se-men″to-kla′ze-ah) disintegration of the periodontal membrane and alveolar bone without loss of the overlying gingival tissue.

pericementum (-se-men′tum) the tissue between the root of a tooth and the alveolus of the jaw.

pericholecystic (-ko″le-sis′tik) around the gallbladder.

pericholecystitis (-ko″le-sis-ti′tis) inflammation of tissues around the gallbladder. **gaseous p.**, emphysematous cholecystitis.

perichondritis (-kon-dri′tis) inflammation of perichondrium.

perichondrium (-kon′dre-um) the membrane covering the surface of a cartilage.

perichondroma (-kon-dro′mah) a tumor of the perichondrium.

perichordal (-kor′dal) surrounding the notochord.

perichoroidal (-ko-roi′dal) surrounding the choriad.

Periclor (per′i-klor) trademark for a preparation of petrichloral.

pericolic (per″ĭ-ko′lik) around the colon.

pericolitis (-ko-li′tis) inflammation around the colon.

pericolonitis (-ko″lon-i′tis) inflammation around the colon.

pericolpitis (-kol-pi′tis) inflammation of tissues around the vagina.

periconchal (-kong′kal) around the concha.

pericorneal (-kor′ne-al) around the cornea.

pericoronal (-kŏ-ro′nal) around the crown of a tooth.

pericranitis (-kra-ni′tis) inflammation of pericranium.

pericranium (-kra′ne-um) the periosteum of the skull.

pericystitis (-sis-ti′tis) inflammation of tissues about the bladder.

pericyte (per'ĭ-sīt) a peculiar elongated cell found wrapped around capillaries.

pericytial (per"ĭ-si'shal) around a cell.

peridens (per"ĭ-dens) a supernumerary tooth elsewhere than in the midline of the dental arch.

peridesmitis (-dez-mi'tis) inflammation of the peridesmium.

peridesmium (-dez'me-um) the membrane investing a ligament.

perididymis (-did'ĭ-mis) the tunica vaginalis testis.

perididymitis (-did"ĭ-mi'tis) inflammation of tunica vaginalis testis.

peridiverticulitis (-di"ver-tik"u-li'tis) inflammation around an intestinal diverticulum.

periductal (-duk'tal) around a duct.

periduodenitis (-du"o-dē-ni'tis) inflammation around the duodenum.

periencephalitis (per"e-en-sef"ah-li'tis) inflammation of the surface of the brain.

periencephalomeningitis (-en-sef"ah-lo-men"-in-ji'tis) inflammation of cerebral cortex and meninges.

perienteritis (-en"ter-i'tis) inflammation of peritoneal coat of intestines.

periepithelioma (-ep"ĭ-the"le-o'mah) a tumor of the adrenal gland.

periesophagitis (-e-sof"ah-ji'tis) inflammation of tissues around the esophagus.

perifascicular (per"ĭ-fah-sik'u-lar) surrounding a fasciculus of nerve or muscle fibers.

perifistular (-fis'tu-lar) around a fistula.

perifolliculitis (-fŏ-lik"u-li'tis) inflammation around the hair follicles.

perigangliitis (-gang"gle-i'tis) inflammation around a ganglion.

perigastric (-gas'trik) around the stomach.

perigastritis (-gas-tri'tis) inflammation of peritoneal coat of stomach.

perihepatitis (-hep"ah-ti'tis) inflammation around the liver.

perijejunitis (-je"ju-ni'tis) inflammation around the jejunum.

perilabyrinthitis (-lab"ĭ-rin-thi'tis) inflammation of tissues around the labyrinth.

perilaryngitis (-lar"in-ji'tis) inflammation of tissues around the larynx.

perilymph (per'ĭ-limf) fluid in the space separating the membranous and osseous labyrinth.

perilymphadenitis (per"ĭ-lim"fad-ē-ni'tis) inflammation of tissues around a lymph node.

perilymphangitis (-lim"fan-ji'tis) inflammation around a lymphatic vessel.

perimeningitis (-men"in-ji'tis) pachymeningitis.

perimeter (pĕ-rim'ĕ-ter) 1. the boundary of a plane figure. 2. an apparatus for determining the extent of the peripheral visual field.

perimetrium (per"i-me'tre-um) the serous membrane enveloping the uterus.

perimetry (pĕ-rim'ĕ-tre) measurement of the visual field.

perimyelitis (per"ĭ-mi"ĕ-li'tis) inflammation of the pia of the spinal cord.

perimyelography (-mi"ĕ-log'rah-fe) roentgenography of the spine after injection of a

contrast medium into the subarachnoid space.

perimyositis (per"ĭ-mi"o-si'tis) inflammation of connective tissue around a muscle.

perimysiitis (-mis"e-i'tis) inflammation of the perimysium.

perimysium (-mis'e-um) connective tissue binding together the fasciculi of striated muscle.

perinatal (-na'tal) relating to the period shortly before and after birth; from the twenty-ninth week or gestation to one to four weeks after birth.

perineal (-ne'al) pertaining to the perineum.

perineocele (-ne'o-sēl) a hernia between the rectum and the prostate or between the rectum and the vagina.

perineoplasty (-ne'o-plas"te) plastic repair of the perineum.

perineorrhaphy (-ne-or'ah-fe) suture of the perineum.

perineotomy (-ne-ot'o-me) incision of the perineum.

perinephric (-nef'rik) around the kidney.

perinephritis (-nē-fri'tis) inflammation of peritoneal envelope of kidney.

perinephrium (-nef're-um) the membrane surrounding the kidney.

perineum (-ne'um) the lower surface of the trunk, or floor of the pelvis, bounded anteriorly by the pubic symphysis, laterally by the ischial tuberosities and posteriorly by the coccyx.

perineuritis (-nu-ri'tis) inflammation of perineurium.

perineurium (-nu're-um) the sheath of a nerve or of a bundle of nerve fibers.

periocular (per"e-ok'u-lar) around the eye.

period (pe're-od) an interval or division of time. **childbearing p.,** the duration of the reproductive ability in the human female, roughly from puberty to menopause. **gestational p.,** the duration of pregnancy, in the human female about 266 days. **incubation p.,** the interval required for development; especially the time between invasion of the body by a pathogenic organism and appearance of the first symptoms of disease. **intersystolic p.,** the atriocarotid interval. **isoelectric p.,** the moment in muscular contraction when no deflection of the galvanometer is produced. **latency p.,** 1. the period between the ages of five and twelve, separating the periods of pregenital and genital sexuality. 2. latent period. **latent p.,** the period between application of a stimulus and manifestation of its results. **menstrual p., monthly p.,** menstruation. **postsphygmic p.,** a short period (0.08 second) of ventricular diastole, after the sphygmic period, and lasting until opening of the atrioventricular valves. **presphygmic p.,** a short period (0.04–0.06 second) early in ventricular systole when both the atrioventricular and semilunar valves are closed. **refractory p.,** a short period succeeding entrance into a condition of functional activity during which the nerve or muscle does not respond to a second stimulus. **safe p.**, the period during the menstrual cycle when conception is considered least likely to occur. **sphygmic p.**, the second phase of ventricular systole (0.21–0.30 second), between the opening and closing of the semilunar valves, while the blood is entering the aorta and pulmonary artery.

periodic (pe″re-od′ik) repeated or recurring at intervals; applied to disease, designating a condition occurring at intervals, separated by periods of freedom from symptoms.

periodicity (pe″re-o-dis′ĭ-te) the recurrence of certain phenomena at approximately regular intervals.

periodontal (per″e-o-don′tal) around a tooth.

periodontics (-don′tiks) the branch of dentistry dealing with periodontal tissue and its diseases.

periodontist (-don′tist) a dentist who specializes in periodontics.

periodontitis (-don-ti′tis) inflammation of periodontium.

periodontium (-don′she-um) the tissues investing and supporting the teeth.

periodontoclasia (-don″to-kla′ze-ah) a degenerative or destructive disease of the periodontium.

periodontology (-don-tol′o-je) the science and study of the periodontium and its diseases.

periodontopathy (-don-top′ah-the) a noninflammatory disorder of the periodontium.

periodontosis (-don-to′sis) noninflammatory disease of the periodontium, with migration of teeth.

periomphalic (per″e-om-fal′ik) situated around the umbilicus.

perionychium (per″e-o-nik′e-um) the epidermis bordering a nail.

perionyxis (-nik′sis) inflammation of the skin around a nail.

perioophoritis (-o″of-o-ri′tis) inflammation of tissues around the ovary.

perioophorosalpingitis (-o-of″o-ro-sal″pin-ji′tis) inflammation of tissues around ovary and oviduct.

periople (per′e-o″pl) the smooth, shiny layer on the outer surface of the hoofs of animals.

perioptometry (per″e-op-tom′ĕ-tre) measurement of acuity of peripheral vision or of limits of the visual field.

periorbita (per″e-or′bĭ-tah) periosteum of the eye socket.

periorbital (-or′bĭ-tal) around the eye socket.

periorbitis (-or-bi′tis) inflammation of the periorbita.

periorchitis (-or-ki′tis) inflammation of the tunica vaginalis testis.

periosteitis (-os″te-i′tis) periostitis.

periosteo-edema (-os″te-o-ĕ-de′mah) edema of the periosteum.

periosteomyelitis (-mi″ĕ-li′tis) inflammation of the entire bone, including periosteum and marrow.

periosteophyte (per″e-os′te-o-fīt″) bony growth on periosteum.

periosteorrhaphy (-os″te-or′ah-fe) suture of the periosteum.

periosteotomy (per″e-os″te-ot′o-me) incision of the periosteum.

periosteum (-os′te-um) a specialized connective tissue covering all bones and having bone-forming potentialities. adj., **perios′teal.**

periostitis (-os-ti′tis) inflammation of periosteum. **dental p.**, periodontitis. **diffuse p.**, widespread periostitis of the long bones.

periostoma (-os-to′mah) a bony growth around bone.

periostosis (-os-to′sis) abnormal deposition of periosteal bone.

periotic (-ot′ik) situated around the ear.

peripachymeningitis (per″ĭ-pak″ĭ-men″in-ji′tis) inflammation of tissue between the dura mater and its bony covering.

peripancreatitis (-pan″kre-ah-ti′tis) inflammation of tissues about the pancreas.

peripericarditis (-per″ĭ-kar-di′tis) inflammation of tissues around the pericardium.

periphacitis (-fah-si′tis) inflammation of the capsule of the eye lens.

peripherad (pĕ-rif′er-ad) toward the periphery.

peripheroceptor (pĕ-rif″er-o-sep′tor) any one of the receptors at the peripheral ends of the sensory peripheral neuron which receives the stimulus.

periphery (pĕ-rif′er-e) an outward part or surface. adj., **periph′eral.**

periphlebitis (per″ĭ-fle-bi′tis) inflammation of external coat of vein.

periphoria (-fo′re-ah) cyclophoria.

periphrenitis (-fre-ni′tis) inflammation of diaphragm and adjoining structures.

periplast (per′ĭ-plast) protoplasm of a cell outside the nucleus.

peripleural (per″ĭ-ploo′ral) surrounding the pleura.

peripleuritis (-ploo-ri′tis) inflammation of tissue about the pleura.

peripneumonia (-nu-mo′ne-ah) 1. pneumonia. 2. pleuropneumonia.

periproctitis (-prok-ti′tis) inflammation of tissues around the rectum and anus.

periprostatic (-pros-tat′ik) around the prostate.

periprostatitis (-pros″tah-ti′tis) inflammation of substance around the prostate.

peripylephlebitis (-pi″le-fle-bi′tis) inflammation of tissues around the portal vein.

peripylic (-pi′lik) around the portal vein.

peripyloric (-pi-lo′rik) around the pylorus.

perirectal (-rek′tal) around the rectum.

perirectitis (-rek-ti′tis) periproctitis.

perirenal (-re′nal) around the kidney.

perirhinal (-ri′nal) around the nose.

perisalpingitis (-sal″pin-ji′tis) inflammation of tissues around the uterine tube.

periscopic (-skop′ik) affording a wide range of vision.

perisigmoiditis (-sig″moi-di′tis) inflammation of peritoneum of sigmoid flexure.

perisinusitis (-si″nu-si′tis) inflammation of substance about a sinus.

perispermatitis (-sper″mah-ti′tis) inflammation of tissues about the spermatic cord.

perisplanchnic (per″ĭ-splangk′nik) around a viscus or the viscera.

perisplanchnitis (-splangk-ni′tis) inflammation of tissues around the viscera.

perisplenic (-splen′ik) around the spleen.

perisplenitis (-sple-ni′tis) inflammation of peritoneal surface of the spleen.

perispondylitis (-spon″dĭ-li′tis) inflammation of tissues around a vertebra.

perissad (pĕ-ris′ad) any element or radical with an odd-numbered valence.

peristalsis (per″ĭ-stal′sis) an aboral, wave-like progression of alternate contraction and relaxation of the muscle fibers of the esophagus and intestines, by which contents are propelled along the alimentary tract. adj., **peristal′tic. reversed p.,** that which impels the contents of the intestine cephalad.

peristaphyline (-staf′ĭ-līn) situated around the uvula.

peristole (pĕ-ris′to-le) the capacity of the walls of the digestive tract to surround or grasp its contents after the ingestion of food.

perisynovial (per″ĭ-sĭ-no′ve-al) around a synovial structure.

peritectomy (-tek′to-me) excision of a ring of conjunctiva around the cornea in treatment of pannus.

peritendineum (-ten-din′e um) connective tissue investing larger tendons and extending between fibers composing them.

peritendinitis (-ten″di-ni′tis) inflammation of the sheath of a tendon.

peritenontitis (-ten″on-ti′tis) peritendinitis.

perithelioma (-the″le-o′mah) a tumor of the perithelium.

perithelium (-the′le-um) fibrous layer around the capillaries.

perithyroiditis (-thi″roi-di′tis) inflammation of capsule of the thyroid.

peritomy (pĕ rit′o-me) peritectomy.

peritonealgia (per″ĭ-to″ne al′je-ah) pain in the peritoneum.

peritoneocentesis (-to″ne-o-sen-te′sis) paracentesis of the abdominal (peritoneal) cavity.

peritoneoclysis (per″ĭ-to″ne-ok′lĭ-sis) injection of fluid into the peritoneal cavity.

peritoneopathy (-op′ah-the) any disease of the peritoneum.

peritoneoscope (per″ĭ-to′ne-o-skōp″) an endoscope for use in peritoneoscopy.

peritoneoscopy (-to″ne-os′ko-pe) visual examination of the organs of the abdominal (peritoneal) cavity with a peritoneoscope.

peritoneotomy (-ot′o-me) incision into the peritoneum.

peritoneum (per″ĭ-to-ne′um) serous membrane lining the walls of the abdominal and pelvic cavities (*parietal peritoneum*) and investing contained viscera (*visceral peritoneum*), the two layers enclosing a potential space, the peritoneal cavity. adj., **peritone′al.**

peritonism (per′ĭ-to-nizm) a condition of shock simulating peritonitis.

peritonitis (per″ĭ-to-ni′tis) inflammation of the peritoneum.

peritonsillar (per″ĭ-ton′sĭ-lar) around a tonsil.

peritonsillitis (-ton″sĭ-li′tis) inflammation of peritonsillar tissues.

peritrichous (pĕ-rit′rĭ-kus) having flagella distributed over the whole surface.

perityphlitis (per″ĭ-tif-li′tis) inflammation of tissues around the cecum.

periureteral (-u-re′ter-al) around the ureter.

periureteritis (-u-re″tĕ-ri′tis) inflammation of tissues around the ureter.

periurethral (-u-re′thral) around the urethra.

periuterine (-u′ter-īn) around the uterus.

perivaginal (-vaj′ĭ-nal) around the vagina.

perivaginitis (-vaj″ĭ-ni′tis) inflammation of tissues around the vagina.

perivascular (-vas′ku-lar) around a vessel.

perivasculitis (-vas″ku-li′tis) inflammation of a perivascular sheath.

perivesical (-ves′ĭ-kal) around the bladder.

perivesiculitis (-ve-sik″u-li′tis) inflammation of tissues around the seminal vesicles.

perlèche (per-lesh′) a form of oral moniliasis at the labial commissures in children.

permanganate (per-man′gah-nāt) a salt of permanganic acid.

permeability (per″me-ah-bil′ĭ-te) the rate at which a substance moves through a permeable layer under a given force.

permeable (per′me-ah-bl) not impassable; pervious.

permease (per′me-ās) a stereospecific membrane transport system.

pernicious (per-nish′us) tending to a fatal issue.

pernio (per′ne-o) chilblain.

perniosis (per″ne-o′sis) chilblain affecting several areas of the body.

pero (pe′ro) the external layer of the olfactory lobe of the brain.

pero- (pe′ro) word element [Gr.], *deformity.*

perobrachius (pe″ro-bra′ke-us) fetus with deformed feet and arms.

perocephalus (-sef′ah-lus) fetus with a deformed head.

perochirus (-ki′rus) fetus with deformed hands.

peromelia (-me′le-ah) congenital deformity of the limbs.

peromelus (pe rom′ĕ-lus) fetus with deformed limbs.

peroneal (per″o-ne′al) pertaining to the fibula.

peropus (pe′ro-pus) fetus with malformed legs and feet.

peroral (per-o′ral) performed or administered through the mouth.

per os (per os) [L.] by mouth.

peroxidase (pĕ-rok′sĭ-dās) an enzyme which catalyzes the decomposition of peroxides.

peroxide (pĕ-rok′sīd) an oxide with more than the normal proportion of oxygen.

perphenazine (per-fen′ah-zēn) a phenothiazine compound used as a tranquilizer and antiemetic.

per primam intentionem (per pri′mam in-ten″she-o′nem) [L.] by first intention.

per rectum (per rek′tum) [L.] through the rectum.

persalt (per′sawlt) any salt which contains a

greater amount of the acid radical than a protosalt.

per saltum (per sal′tum) [L.] at a leap.

Persantin (per-san′tin) trademark for preparations of dipyridamole.

per secundam intentionem (per se-kun′dam in-ten″she-o′nem) [L.] by second intention.

perseveration (per-sev″er-a′shun) persistence of one reply or one idea in response to various questions; continuance of activity after cessation of the causative stimulus.

persona (per-so′nah) Jung's term for the personality "mask" or facade presented by a person to the outside world.

personality (per″sŏ-nal′ĭ-te) the total social, emotional and intellectual attributes of an individual. **alternating p.,** dual personality. **disordered p.,** a condition in which the patient thinks that he is someone other than himself. **double p., dual p.,** a state of disordered consciousness in which the subject leads two lives, alternately, with amnesia for the other. **multiple p.,** a state of disordered consciousness in which the subject leads three or more lives, alternatively, with amnesia for those not lived at the moment. **psychopathic p.,** a constitutional tendency to mental disorder; a type of personality marked by lessened voluntary control and increased emotional response to stimuli.

perspiration (per″spĭ-ra′shun) 1. the excretion of moisture through the pores of the skin. 2. the material excreted through the pores of the skin. **insensible p.,** the constant excretion of the skin, of such small amount as to be imperceptible. **sensible p.,** the noticeable excretion of the sweat glands, which appears as moisture upon the skin.

persulfate (per-sul′fāt) a sulfate which contains more sulfuric acid than the ordinary sulfate.

per tertiam intentionem (per ter′she-am in-ten″she-o′nem) [L.] by third intention.

per tubam (per tu′bam) [L.] through a tube.

pertussis (per-tus′is) an infectious disease due to *Bordetella pertussis*, and characterized by coryza, bronchitis and typical explosive cough ending in crowing inspiration.

pertussoid (per-tus′oid) 1. resembling whooping cough. 2. an influenzal cough resembling that of whooping cough.

per vaginam (per vah-ji′nam) [L.] through the vagina.

perversion (per-ver′zhun) deviation from the normal course. **sexual p.,** paraphilia.

pervert (per′vert) a person who deviates from a normal course, especially a paraphiliac.

pes (pes), pl. *pe′des* [L.] foot; the terminal organ of the leg, or lower limb; any footlike part. **p. abduc′tus,** a deformity in which the anterior part of the foot is displaced and lies laterally to the vertical axis of the leg. **p. adduc′tus,** a deformity in which the anterior part of the foot is displaced and lies medially to the vertical axis of the leg. **p. ca′vus,** a foot with an abnormally high longitudinal arch. **p. corvi′nus,** wrinkles radiating from the lateral canthus of the eye. **p. gi′gas,** mac-

ropodia. **p. pla′nus,** flatfoot; one with an abnormally low longitudinal arch. **p. supina′tus,** a deformity in which the inner border of the anterior part of the foot is higher than the outer border. **p. val′gus,** flatfoot.

pessary (pes′ah-re) 1. an instrument placed in the vagina to support the uterus or rectum. 2. a medicated vaginal suppository.

pesticide (pes′tĭ-sīd) a poison used to destroy pests of any sort.

pestiferous (pes-tif′er-us) causing a pestilence.

pestilence (pes′tĭ-lens) 1. a virulent epidemic contagious disease. 2. an epidemic of a virulent contagious disease. adj., **pestilen′tial.**

pestle (pes′el) an instrument with rounded end, used in a mortar to reduce a solid to a powder or produce a homogeneous mixture of solids.

-petal word element [L.], *directed* or *moving toward.*

petechia (pe-te′ke-ah), pl. *pete′chiae* [L.] a minute red spot due to escape of a small amount of blood. adj., **pete′chial.**

pethidine (peth′ĭ-dēn) a compound having less analgesic effect than morphine, but not causing nausea.

petit mal (pĕ-te′ mahl′) an epileptic seizure with a brief blackout of consciousness and only minor rhythmic movements.

petrichloral (pet″rĭ-klo′ral) a derivative of chloral used as a hypnotic and sedative.

pétrissage (pa-trĭ-sahzh′) [Fr.] kneading action in massage.

petrolatum (pet″ro-la′tum) a purified mixture of semisolid hydrocarbons obtained from petroleum. **hydrophilic p.,** a mixture of cholesterol, stearyl, alcohol, white wax and white petrolatum. **liquid p.,** a mixture of liquid hydrocarbons from petroleum, used as a lubricant and laxative. **liquid p., heavy,** liquid petrolatum. **liquid p., light,** a mixture of liquid hydrocarbons from petroleum, used as a laxative. **white p.,** a decolorized, purified mixture of semisolid hydrocarbons from petroleum, used as an ointment base.

petroleum (pĕ-tro′le-um) the liquid mixture of organic compounds obtained from the upper strata of the earth, consisting chiefly of paraffinic, alicyclic or aromatic hydrocarbons, in varying proportions.

petrolization (pet″rol-i-za′shun) spreading of petroleum on bodies of water to destroy mosquito larvae.

petromastoid (pet″ro-mas′toid) 1. the periotic bone. 2. pertaining to petrous and mastoid bones.

petrosal (pĕ-tro′sal) pertaining to the petrous bone.

petrosalpingostaphylinus (pet″ro-sal-ping″-go-staf′ĭ-li′nus) the levator veli palatini muscle.

petrosectomy (-sek′to-me) excision of the cells of the apex of the petrous portion of the temporal bone.

petrositis (-si′tis) inflammation of the petrous part of the temporal bone.

petrous (pet′rus) resembling rock or stone.

pexis (pek′sis) the fixation of a substance or chemical compound in a tissue. adj., **pex′ic.**

-pexy (pek′se) word element [Gr.], *surgical fixation.* adj., **-pec′tic.**

peyote (pa-o′te) a drug obtained from the Mexican cactus, Anhalonium; sometimes used to produce an intoxication marked by feelings of ecstasy.

pfropfhebephrenia (propf″he-be-fre′ne-ah) schizophrenia in a person already mentally defective.

pg. picogram.

PGA pteroylglutamic (folic) acid.

pH symbol, *hydrogen ion concentration.*

phac(o)- (fak′o) word element [Gr.], *lens.* See also words beginning *phako-.*

phacitis (fah-si′tis) inflammation of the eye lens.

phacoanaphylaxis (fak″o-an″ah-fi-lak′sis) anaphylaxis to protein of the eye lens.

phacocele (fak′o-sēl) hernia of the eye lens.

phacocystectomy (fak″o-sis-tek′to-me) excision of part of lens capsule for cataract.

phacocystitis (-sis-ti′tis) inflammation of capsule of eye lens.

phacoerysis (-er′ĭ-sis) removal of the eye lens in cataract by suction.

phacoglaucoma (-glaw-ko′mah) glaucoma affecting the lens.

phacohymenitis (-hi″men-i′tis) inflammation of the capsule of the eye lens.

phacoid (fak′oid) shaped like a lens.

phacoiditis (fak″oi-di′tis) inflammation of the eye lens.

phacoidoscope (fah-koi′do-skōp) phacoscope.

phacolysis (fah-kol′ĭ-sis) dissolution of the crystalline lens by operation or by medical means. adj., **phacolyt′ic.**

phacomalacia (fak″o-mah-la′she-ah) soft cataract.

phacometachoresis (-met″ah-ko-re′sis) displacement of the eye lens.

phacosclerosis (-skle-ro′sis) hardening of the eye lens.

phacoscope (fak′o-skōp) instrument for viewing accommodative changes of the eye lens.

phacotoxic (fak″o-tok′sik) exerting a deleterious effect upon the crystalline lens.

phacozymase (-zi′mās) an enzyme from extract of the crystalline lens.

phag(o)- (fag′o) word element [Gr.], *eating; ingestion.*

phage (fāj) bacteriophage.

phagedena (faj″ĕ-de′nah) rapidly spreading and sloughing ulcer. adj., **phageden′ic.**

phagocyte (fag′o-sīt) any cell that destroys microorganisms or harmful cells.

phagocytin (fag″o-si′tin) a bactericidal substance from neutrophilic leukocytes.

phagocytoblast (-si′to-blast) a cell giving rise to phagocytes.

phagocytolysis (-si-tol′ĭ-sis) destruction of phagocytes. adj., **phagocytolyt′ic.**

phagocytose (-si′tōs) to envelope and destroy bacteria and other foreign material.

phagocytosis (-si-to′sis) the uptake or envelopment of solid particles by living cells.

phagodynamometer (fag″o-di″nah-mom′ĕ-ter) apparatus for measuring the force exerted in chewing food.

phagokaryosis (-kar″e-o′sis) phagocytosis allegedly effected by the cell nucleus.

phagomania (-ma′ne-ah) an insatiable craving for food or an obsessive preoccupation with the subject of eating.

phagotherapy (-ther′ah-pe) treatment by feeding.

phakoma (fah-ko′mah) a lenslike mass or tumor.

phakomatosis (fak″o-mah-to′sis) a heredofamilial tumorous state, with formation of lenslike masses.

phalangeal (fah-lan′je-al) pertaining to a phalanx.

phalangectomy (fal″an-jek′to-me) excision of a phalanx.

phalangitis (-ji′tis) inflammation of one or more phalanges.

phalangosis (-go′sis) a condition in which the eyelashes grow in rows.

phalanx (fa′lanks), pl. *phalan′ges* [Gr.] any bone of a finger or toe. adj., **phalan′geal.**

phallectomy (fal-ek′to-me) amputation of the penis.

phallitis (fal-li′tis) inflammation of the penis.

phallocampsis (fal″o-kamp′sis) curvature of penis during erection.

phallodynia (-din′e-ah) pain in the penis.

phallotomy (fal-ot′o-me) incision of the penis.

phallus (fal′us) the penis. adj., **phal′lic.**

phaneromania (fan″er-o-ma′ne-ah) abnormal attention to some external growth, as picking at a wart, etc.

phanerosis (fan″er-o′sis) the process of becoming visible.

phanic (fan′ik) visible; apparent.

Phanodorn (fan′o-dorn) trademark for a preparation of cyclobarbital.

phantasm (fan′tazm) an optical illusion or hallucination.

phantom (fan′tom) 1. a shadowy image or impression. 2. a model of the body or of a specific part, used for demonstration or other purposes; in nuclear medicine, a device which simulates conditions encountered in vivo, to permit accurate determination of radiation received from a radioactive source. **anatomic p.,** one used in nuclear medicine which corresponds as closely as possible to the configuration of the organ it represents. **basic p.,** one used in nuclear medicine, constructed in a geometric configuration, with little resemblance to the organ it represents. **intermediate p.,** one used in nuclear medicine which has a strong geometric flavor, but bears some resemblance to the organ it represents.

Phar. pharmacopeia.

pharm. pharmaceutical; pharmacy.

pharmacal (far′mah-kal) pertaining to pharmacy.

pharmaceutical (far″mah-su′tĭ-kal) 1. pertaining to pharmacy or drugs. 2. a medicinal drug.

pharmaceutics (-su′tiks) the apothecary's art.

pharmacist (far'mah-sist) a person licensed to compound or dispense drugs.

pharmacodiagnosis (far"mah-ko-di"ag-no'sis) use of drugs in diagnosis.

pharmacodynamics (-di-nam'iks) the study of the action of drugs.

pharmacogenetics (-jĕ-net'iks) study of the effects of genetic factors on the individual organism's response to drugs.

pharmacognosy (far"mah-kog'no-se) the study of crude medicines.

pharmacology (-kol'o-je) the study of drugs, their sources, preparations and therapeutic uses.

pharmacomania (far"mah-ko-ma'ne-ah) abnormal fondness for taking or administering medicines.

pharmacopeia (-pe'ah) an authoritative treatise on drugs and their preparations.

pharmacophobia (-fo'be-ah) morbid dread of medicines.

pharmacophore (far'mah-ko-for") the group of atoms in the molecule of a drug which causes the therapeutic effect.

pharmacopoeia (far"mah-ko-pe'ah) pharmacopeia.

pharmacopsychosis (-si-ko'sis) a mental disease due to alcohol, drugs or poisons.

pharmacoradiography (-ra"de-og'rah-fe) roentgen examination of a body or organ under influence of a drug which best facilitates such examination.

pharmacotherapy (-ther'ah-pe) treatment of disease with medicines.

pharmacy (far'mah-se) 1. the art of preparing and compounding medicines. 2. a shop for the compounding and dispensing of drugs and medical supplies. **galenical p.**, that related to crude drugs only.

pharyng(o)- (fah-ring'go) word element [Gr.], *pharynx.*

pharyngalgia (far"ing-gal'je-ah) pain in the pharynx.

pharyngeal (fah-rin'je-al) pertaining to the pharynx.

pharyngectomy (far"in-jek'to-me) excision of part of the pharynx.

pharyngemphraxis (-jem-frak'sis) obstruction of the pharynx.

pharyngismus (-jiz'mus) muscular spasm of the pharynx.

pharyngitis (-ji'tis) inflammation of the pharynx. **p. sic'ca**, pharyngitis with atrophy of the submucous tissue and absence of normal secretion of the glands in the lining of the mucosa.

pharyngocele (fah-ring'go-sēl) herniation of the pharynx.

pharyngoconjunctivitis (fah-ring"go-kon-junk"ti-vi'tis) inflammation involving the pharynx and conjunctiva, the result of a virus infection.

pharyngodynia (-din'e-ah) pain in the pharynx.

pharyngoesophageal (-e-sof"ah-je'al) pertaining to pharynx and esophagus.

pharyngolaryngitis (-lar"in-ji'tis) inflammation of pharynx and larynx.

pharyngology (far"ing-gol'o-je) scientific study of the pharynx.

pharyngomycosis (fah-ring"go-mi-ko'sis) fungus disease of the pharynx.

pharyngoparalysis (-pah-ral'ĭ-sis) paralysis of the pharyngeal muscles.

pharyngopathy (far"ing-gop'ah-the) disease of the pharynx.

pharyngoperistole (fah-ring"go-pĕ-ris'to-le) narrowing of the pharynx.

pharyngoplasty (fah-ring'go-plas"te) plastic repair of the pharynx.

pharyngoplegia (fah-ring"go-ple'je-ah) paralysis of pharyngeal muscles.

pharyngorhinitis (-ri-ni'tis) inflammation of the nasopharynx.

pharyngoscope (fah-ring'go-skōp) instrument for inspecting the pharynx.

pharyngoscopy (far"ing-gos'ko-pe) examination of the pharynx.

pharyngospasm (fah-ring'go-spazm) spasm of pharyngeal muscles.

pharyngostenosis (fah-ring"go-ste-no'sis) narrowing of the pharynx.

pharyngotomy (far"ing-got'o-me) incision of the pharynx.

pharynx (far'ingks) the musculomembranous cavity behind the nasal cavities, mouth and larynx, communicating with them and with the esophagus.

phase (fāz) 1. one of the aspects or stages through which a varying entity may pass. 2. in a heterogeneous system, a component which is homogeneous of itself, bounded by an interface, and mechanically separable from other phases of the system. **continuous p.**, in a heterogeneous system, the component in which the disperse phase is distributed, corresponding to the solvent in a true solution. **disperse p.**, the discontinuous portion of a heterogeneous system, corresponding to the solute in a true solution.

phatnorrhagia (fat"no-ra'je-ah) hemorrhage from a tooth socket.

Phe-mer-nite (fe'mer-nīt) trademark for preparations of phenylmercuric nitrate.

Phemerol (fe'mer-ol) trademark for preparations of benzethonium.

phemitone (fem'ĭ-tōn) mephobarbital.

phenacaine (fen'ah-kān) a compound used as a local anesthetic.

phenacemide (fĕ-nas'e-mīd) phenacetylurea, used as an anticonvulsant in psychomotor and grand mal epilepsy.

phenadone (fen'ah-dōn) methadone.

phenaglycodol (fen"ah-gli'ko-dol) a compound used as a tranquilizer.

phenanthrene (fe-nan'thrēn) a colorless, crystalline hydrocarbon.

phenate (fe'nāt) a salt formed by union of a base with phenic acid.

phenazocine (fĕ-naz'o-sēn) a compound used as an analgesic.

phenelzine (fen'el-zēn) a compound used as an antidepressant.

Phenergan (fen'er-gan) trademark for preparations of promethazine hydrochloride.

phenethicillin (fĕ-neth″ĭ-sil′in) phenoxymethyl penicillin.

phenformin (fen-for′min) a compound used orally as a hypoglycemic agent.

phenindamine (fĕ-nin′dah-min) a compound used as an antihistaminic.

phenindione (fen-in′dĭ-ōn) a compound used as an anticoagulant.

pheniramine (fe-nir′ah-min) a compound used as an antihistaminic.

phenmetrazine (fen-met′rah-zēn) a compound used to reduce the appetite.

phenobarbital (fe″no-bar′bĭ-tal) a barbituric acid compound used as a hypnotic and sedative. **sodium p.**, a hypnotic, sedative compound for parenteral administration.

phenocopy (fe′no-kop″e) 1. an individual whose phenotype mimics that of another genotype, but whose character is determined by environment and is not hereditary. 2. the simulated trait in a phenocopy individual.

phenol (fe′nol) 1. an extremely poisonous compound; a pharmaceutic aid as a bacteriostatic agent. 2. a type of organic compound containing one or more hydroxyl groups attached to an aromatic or carbon ring. **liquefied p.**, phenol maintained in liquid state by the presence of 10 per cent of water; used in diluted form in preparations for use on skin. **p. red**, phenolsulfonphthalein. **p. salicylate**, phenyl salicylate.

phenolphthalein (fe″nol-tha′lēn) a white or faintly yellowish-white crystalline powder used as a cathartic.

phenolsulfonphthalein (fe″nol-sul″fōn-tha′-lēn) a reddish crystalline powder used in tests of renal function.

phenomenon (fe-nom′ĕ-non) an unusual or distinctive event whose occurrence is considered indicative of a certain quality or condition. **"fall-and-rise" p.**, initial decrease in the number of tubercle bacilli observed in sputum after initiation of chemotherapy, with subsequent increase in number indicative of multiplication of resistant organisms **Fick's p.**, fogging of vision, with appearance of halos around lights, occurring in persons wearing contact lenses. **Huebner-Thomsen-Friedenreich p.**, the susceptibility of red cells to agglutination by all normal human serums after activation by a bacterial enzyme of a latent "T" receptor common to all erythrocytes. **L.E. p.**, production of L.E. cells on incubation of normal neutrophils with the serum of affected patients, as a diagnostic test for lupus erythematosus. **Raynaud's p.**, episodic, symmetrical constriction of small arteries of the extremities, resulting in cyanosis or pallor of the part, followed by hyperemia, producing a red color. **rebound p.**, an opposite reaction occurring on the withdrawal of a stimulus. **second set p.**, occurrence in a recipient of a more severe immunologic reaction to a second graft of tissue from the same donor.

phenopropazine (fe″no-pro′pah-zēn) ethopropazine.

phenothiazine (-thi′ah-zēn) a compound originally used as an anthelmintic, urinary antiseptic and insecticide.

phenotype (fe′no-tīp) the outward, visible expression of the hereditary constitution of an organism. adj., **phenotyp′ic.**

Phenoxene (fen-ok′sēn) trademark for a preparation of chlorphenoxamine.

phenoxybenzamine (fĕ-nok″se-ben′zah-mēn) a compound used in adrenergic blockade to reduce blood pressure and as a vasodilator.

phenozygous (fe″no-zi′gus) having the calvaria narrower than the face, so that the zygomatic arches are visible when the head is viewed from above.

phenprocoumon (fen-pro′koo-mon) an anticoagulant of the coumarin type.

phensuximide (fen-suk′sĭ-mīd) a whitish crystalline powder used as an anticonvulsant in petit mal epilepsy.

phentolamine (fen-tol′ah-mēn) a compound used as an adrenolytic agent for the diagnosis of pheochromocytoma.

Phenurone (fen′u-rōn) trademark for a preparation of phenacemide.

phenyl (fen′il, fe′nil) the monovalent radical, C_6H_5. adj., **phenyl′ic. p. salicylate**, a compound used as an enteric coating for tablets.

phenylalanine (fen″il-al′ah-nīn) a naturally occurring amino acid essential for optimal growth in infants and for nitrogen equilibrium in human adults.

phenylbutazone (-bu′tah-zōn) a compound used as an analgesic and antipyretic.

phenylephrine (-ef′rin) a compound with sympathomimetic action used mainly as a nasal decongestant, mydriatic, a local vasoconstrictor or a pressor agent in hypotensive states.

phenylketonuria (-ke″to-nu′re-ah) excretion in the urine of abnormally large amounts of phenylpyruvic acid and other metabolites of phenylalanine as a result of a genetically determined metabolic disorder, and associated with mental retardation (phenylpyruvic oligophrenia). adj., **phenylketonu′ric.**

phenylmercuric (-mer-ku′rik) denoting a compound containing the radical C_6H_5Hg-, some of which have bacteriostatic and bactericidal properties. **p. nitrate**, a compound of phenol, mercury and nitric acid; used as a local antibacterial.

phenylpropylmethylamine (-pro″pil-meth″il-am′ēn) a compound used as a nasal decongestant.

phenylthiocarbamide (-thi″o-kar-bam′īd) a compound used in genetics research.

phenyltoloxamine (-tol-ok′sah-mēn) a compound used as an antihistaminic.

phenylurea (-u-re′ah) a hypnotic compound prepared from urea and aniline.

phenyramidol (fen″ĭ-ram′ĭ-dol) a benzyl alcohol compound suggested as an analgesic.

phenytoin (fen′ĭ-to-in) diphenylhydantoin.

pheochrome (fe′o-krōm) staining dark with chromium salts.

pheochromoblast (fe″o-kro′mo-blast) an embryonic structure which develops into pheochromocytes.

pheochromocyte (fe"o-kro'mo-sīt) a chromaffin cell.

pheochromocytoma (-kro"mo-si-to'mah) a tumor of chromaffin tissue of the adrenal medulla or sympathetic paraganglia.

Ph.G. Graduate in Pharmacy.

-phil(e) word element [Gr.], *entity* (person or thing); *having affinity for or morbid fondness for something.* adj., **-phil'ic.**

-philia (fil'e-ah) word element [Gr.], *affinity for; morbid fondness of.* adj., **-phil'ic.**

philtrum (fil'trum) the vertical groove in the median portion of the upper lip.

phimosis (fi-mo'sis) tightness of the foreskin, which cannot be drawn back from the glans.

pHisoHex (fi'so-heks) trademark for an emulsion containing hexachlorophene.

phleb(o)- (fleb'o) word element [Gr.], *vein.*

phlebangioma (fleb"an-je-o'mah) a venous aneurysm.

phlebarteriectasia (fleb"ar-te"re-ek-ta'ze-ah) dilatation of veins and arteries.

phlebectasia (fleb"ek-ta'ze-ah) dilatation of a vein or veins.

phlebectomy (fle-bek'to-me) excision of a vein.

phlebemphraxis (fleb"em-frak'sis) stoppage of a vein.

phlebismus (fle-biz'mus) obstruction and turgescence of veins.

phlebitis (flē-bi'tis) inflammation of a vein. **sinus p.,** inflammation of a cerebral sinus.

phleboclysis (flē-bok'lī-sis) introduction of a solution into a vein.

phlebogram (fleb'o-gram) 1. a sphygmographic tracing of a venous pulse. 2. a film obtained at phlebography.

phlebography (fle-bog'rah-fe) radiography of the veins after introduction of a contrast medium.

phlebolith (fleb'o-lith) a venous calculus or concretion.

phlebology (fle-bol'o-je) a treatise on veins.

phlebomanometer (fleb"o-mah-nom'ē-ter) an instrument for the direct measurement of venous blood pressure.

phlebophlebostomy (fleb"o-fle-bost'to-me) anastomosis of two veins, as of the portal vein and inferior vena cava.

phleboplasty (fleb'o-plas"te) plastic repair of a vein.

phleborrhaphy (flē-bor'ah-fe) suture of a vein.

phleborrhexis (fleb"o-rek'sis) rupture of a vein.

phlebosclerosis (-skle-ro'sis) abnormal thickening and hardening of the walls of veins.

phlebostasis (fle-bos'tah-sis) 1. retardation of blood flow in veins. 2. temporary abstraction of a portion of blood from the general circulation by compressing the veins of an extremity.

phlebothrombosis (fleb"o-throm-bo'sis) the development of venous thrombi in the absence of antecedent inflammation of the vessel wall.

phlebotome (fleb'o-tōm) a lancet for venesection.

Phlebotomus (fle-bot'o-mus) a genus of flies, called sandflies, the females of which have piercing-sucking mouth parts and are hematophagous; various species are vectors of various disease-producing organisms. **P. papatas'ii,** the sandfly, an insect of India and the Mediterranean countries, believed to convey the causative organism of sandfly fever.

phlebotomy (flē-bot'o-me) incision of a vein.

phlegm (flem) 1. mucus. 2. an old name for a supposed bodily humor.

phlegmasia (fleg-ma'ze-ah) inflammation with fever. **p. al'ba do'lens,** phlebitis of the femoral vein. **p. al'ba do'lens puerpera'rum,** phlebitis of the femoral vein in puerperal women. **p. ceru'lea do'lens,** acute fulminating form of deep venous thrombosis, with pronounced edema and severe cyanosis of the extremity.

phlegmatic (fleg-mat'ik) of dull and sluggish temperament.

phlegmon (fleg'mon) cellulitis. adj., **phleg'-monous. bronze p.,** cellulitis with bronze-colored spots along the incision line after a kidney operation. **diffuse p.,** diffuse cellulitis with septic symptoms. **gas p.,** cellulitis in which gas is formed. **ligneous p., woody p.,** inflammation causing induration of the involved tissues.

phlog(o)- (flo"go) word element [Gr.], *inflammation.*

phlogistic (flo-jis'tik) inflammatory.

phlogogenic (flo"go-jen'ik) producing inflammation.

phlogotic (flo-got'ik) inflammatory.

phlorhizin (flo-ri'zin) a bitter glycoside which causes glycosuria by blocking the tubular reabsorption of glucose.

P.H.L.S. Public Health Laboratory Service (British).

phlyctena (flik-te'nah) a vesicle containing a thin ichor or lymph.

phlyctenoid (flik'tē-noid) resembling a phlyctena.

phlyctenosis (flik"tē-no'sis) any pustular disease or lesion.

phlyctenule (flik'ten-ūl) a minute vesicle; an ulcerated nodule of cornea or conjunctiva. adj., **phlycten'ular.**

phlyctenulosis (flik-ten"u-lo'sis) a condition marked by formation of phlyctenules.

-phobe (fōb) word element [Gr.], *entity* (person or thing); *having antipathy toward or morbid fear of something.*

phobia (fo'be-ah) a persistent abnormal dread or fear; combined with other word elements to designate fear of the thing indicated, e.g. claustrophobia, agoraphobia. adj., **pho'bic.**

phobophobia (fo"bo-fo'be-ah) morbid fear of one's own fears.

phocomelus (fo-kom'ē-lus) fetus with hands and feet, but no legs or arms.

phonal (fo'nal) pertaining to the voice.

phonarteriogram (fōn"ar-te"re-o-gram") a tracing or graphic record of arterial sounds obtained in phonarteriography.

phonarteriography (fōn"ar-te"re-og'rah-fe)

the recording of arterial sounds by means of a phonocardiograph.

phonasthenia (fo″nas-the′ne-ah) weakness of the voice from fatigue.

phonation (fo-na′shun) the utterance of vocal sounds.

phone (fōn) the smallest unit of sound.

phoneme (fo′nēm) 1. an objective auditory sensation occurring in the absence of the stimuli usually responsible for its production. 2. the smallest distinguishable unit of sound.

phonendoscope (fo-nen′do-skōp) a stethoscope that intensifies auscultatory sounds.

phonetics (fo-net′iks) science of vocal sounds.

phonic (fon′ik, fo′nik) pertaining to the voice.

phonism (fo′nizm) a sensation of hearing produced by the effect of something seen, felt, tasted, smelled or thought of.

phonocardiogram (fo″no-kar′de-o-gram) the record produced by phonocardiography.

phonocardiography (-kar″de-og′rah-fe) graphic recording of the sounds produced by the action of the heart. adj., **phonocardiograph′ic. intracardiac p.,** recording of sounds transmitted by a phonocatheter passed into a chamber of the heart.

phonocatheter (-kath′ĕ-ter) a catheter with a device in its tip for picking up and transmitting sound.

phonocatheterization (-kath″ĕ-ter-i-za′shun) use of a phonocatheter for detection of sounds produced in the circulatory system. **intracardiac p.,** detection of sounds by means of a phonocatheter passed into the heart as an aid in the diagnosis of cardiac defects.

phonogram (fo′no-gram) a graphic record of a sound.

phonology (fo-nol′o-je) phonetics.

phonomassage (fo″no-mah-sahzh′) massage of the middle ear.

phonometer (fo-nom′ĕ-ter) device for measuring intensity of vocal sounds.

phonomyogram (fo″no-mi′o-gram) a record produced by phonomyography.

phonomyography (-mi-og′rah-fe) the recording of sounds produced by muscle contraction.

phonopathy (fo-nop′ah-the) disease of organs of speech.

phonophobia (fo″no-fo′be-ah) morbid dread of sounds or of speaking aloud

phonophore (fo′no-for) a form of stethoscope.

phonophotography (fo″no-fo-tog′rah-fe) photographic recording of sound waves.

phonopneumomassage (-nu″mo-mah-sahzh′) air massage of the middle ear.

phonopsia (fo-nop′se-ah) a visual sensation caused by the hearing of sounds.

phonoreception (fo″no-re-sep′shun) the reception of stimuli perceived as sound.

phonoreceptor (-re-sep′tor) a receptor for sound stimuli.

phonorenogram (-re′no-gram) record of sounds produced by pulsation of the renal artery obtained by a phonocatheter passed through a ureter into the kidney pelvis.

-phore (for) word element [Gr.], *a carrier.*

phoresis (fo-re′sis) introduction of chemical ions into the tissues by passage of an electric current.

phoria (fo′re-ah) tendency of the visual axis of one eye to deviate when the other eye is covered and fusion is prevented.

phorology (fo-rol′o-je) study of disease carriers and the transmission of disease.

phorometer (fo-rom′ĕ-ter) an instrument for measuring heterophoria.

phose (fōz) a subjective light sensation.

phosgene (fos′jēn) a toxic gas, $COCl_2$.

phosphagen (fos′fah-jen) a compound, such as phosphocreatine and phosphoarginine, present in tissue which yields high-energy phosphate.

Phosphaljel (fos′fal jel) trademark for a preparation of aluminum phosphate gel.

phosphatase (fos′fah-tās) one of a group of enzymes capable of catalyzing the hydrolysis of esterified phosphoric acid. **acid p.,** a type showing optimal activity at a pH between 3.4 and 6. **alkaline p.,** a type showing optimal activity at a pH between 8.6 and 9.4.

phosphate (fos′fāt) a salt of phosphoric acid containing the trivalent PO_4 radical. adj., **phosphat′ic. acid p.,** a salt of phosphoric acid in which only one or two of the hydrogen atoms have been replaced. **ammoniomagnesium p.,** double salt of magnesium, ammonium and orthophosphoric acid. **arginine p.,** phosphoarginine. **calcium p.,** a compound containing calcium and the phosphate radical (PO_4). **creatine p.,** phosphocreatine. **earthy p.,** any phosphate of an alkaline earth. **ferric p.,** a yellowish-white powder insoluble in water or acetic acid. **ferric p., soluble,** ferric phosphate rendered soluble by the presence of sodium citrate; used as a hematinic. **magnesium p.,** a salt of phosphoric acid used as a laxative or antacid. **normal p.,** a phosphate in which all the hydrogen atoms of the acid have been replaced.

phosphatemia (fos″fah-te′me-ah) phosphates in the blood.

phosphatide (fos′fah-tīd) a fatty acid ester of a phosphorylated polyvalent alcohol. **prothromboplastic p′s,** substances that are believed to function as parts of both thromboplastin and antithromboplastin.

phosphaturia (fos″fah-tu′re-ah) excess of phosphates in the urine.

phosphene (fos′fēn) an objective visual sensation that occurs with the eyes closed, and in the absence of retinal stimulation by visible light.

phosphide (fos′fīd) a binary compound of phosphorus.

phosphite (fos′fīt) a salt of phosphorous acid.

phosphoarginine (fos″fo-ar′ji-nin) an arginine phosphoric acid compound found in invertebrate muscles.

phosphocreatine (-kre′ah-tin) a creatine-phosphoric acid compound occurring in muscle, being the most important storage form of high-energy phosphate.

phosphoguanidine (-gwan′i-dēn) a guanidine—phosphoric acid compound which on hydrolysis yields low-energy phosphate.

phospholipid (fos″fo-lip′id) a compound of an alcohol, fatty acids and phosphoric acid.

phospholipin (-lip′in) phospholipid.

phosphonecrosis (-ne-kro′sis) necrosis of the jaw in phosphorus poisoning.

phosphopenia (-pe′ne-ah) deficiency of phosphorus in the body.

phosphoprotein (-pro′te-in) a protein containing phosphoric acid as a prosthetic group.

phosphorated (fos′fo-rāt″ed) charged with phosphorus.

phosphorescence (fos″fo-res′ens) emission of light without heat.

phosphorhidrosis (fos″for-hǐ-dro′sis) secretion of phosphorescent or luminous sweat.

phosphorism (fos′fo-rizm) poisoning by phosphorus.

phosphorolysis (fos″fo-rol′ĭ-sis) the reversible combination and separation of sugar and phosphoric acid in carbohydrate metabolism.

phosphoruria (fos″for-u′re-ah) phosphorus in the urine.

phosphorus (fos′fo-rus) chemical element (*see table*), at. no. 15, symbol P. **amorphous p.**, phosphorus in a dark red powder, not poisonous. **metallic p.**, an allotropic form produced by heating ordinary phosphorus. **ordinary p.**, a waxy solid, exceedingly poisonous. **P³²**, **radioactive p.**, the radioactive isotope with an atomic weight of 32; used in treating leukemia and allied disorders. **red p.**, amorphous phosphorus. **rhombohedral p.**, metallic phosphorus.

phosphorylase (fos-for′ĭ-lās) an enzyme which catalyzes the conversion of glycogen into glucose-1-phosphate.

phosphotransacetylase (fos″fo-trans″ah-set′ĭ-lās) an enzyme which catalyzes the transfer of an acetyl group between acetylphosphate and acetyl coenzyme A.

phosphotransferase (-trans′fer-ās) an enzyme which catalyzes the transfer of a phosphate group.

phosphuresis (fos″fu-re′sis) the urinary excretion of phosphorus (phosphates). adj., **phosphuret′ic.**

phot(o)- (fo′to) word element [Gr.], *light.*

photalgia (fo-tal′je-ah) pain, as in the eye, caused by light.

phote (fōt) a unit of illumination, being 1 lumen per square centimeter.

photechy (fo′tek-e) the production of radioactivity in a nonactive substance by exposure to radiation.

photic (fo′tik) pertaining to light.

photism (fo′tizm) a visual sensation produced by the effect of something heard, felt, tasted, smelled or thought of.

photoallergy (fo″to-al′er-je) allergic sensitiveness to light. adj., **photoaller′gic.**

Photobacterium (-bak-te′re-um) a genus of Schizomycetes (order Pseudomonadales, suborder Pseudomonadineae, family Pseudomonadaceae) found on dead fish and other salt-water animals and in sea water.

photobiology (-bi-ol′o-je) the branch of biology dealing with the effect of light on organisms.

photobiotic (-bi-ot′ik) living only in the light.

photocatalysis (fo″to-kah-tal′ĭ-sis) promotion or stimulation of a reaction by light. adj., **photocatalyt′ic.**

photochemistry (-kem′is-tre) science of chemical action of light rays.

photochromogen (-kro′mo-jen) a microorganism whose pigmentation develops as a result of exposure to light. adj., **photochromogen′ic.**

photocoagulation (-ko-àg″u-la′shun) condensation of protein material by controlled use of light rays, as in treatment of pathologic conditions of the eye.

photodermatitis (-der″mah-ti′tis) an abnormal state of the skin in which light is an important causative factor.

photodynamics (-di-nam′iks) the science of the activating effects of light. adj., **photodynam′ic.**

photodynesis (-di-ne′sis) initiation of cyclosis under the influence of light.

photodynia (-din′e-ah) photalgia.

photofluorography (-floo″or-og′rah-fe) the photographic recording of fluoroscopic images on small films, using a fast lens.

photogene (fo′to-jēn) after-image.

photogenic (fo″to-jen′ik) produced by light, or producing light.

photokinetic (-ki-net′ik) moving in response to the stimulus of light.

photolysis (fo-tol′ĭ-sis) decomposition by light. adj., **photolyt′ic.**

photolyte (fo′to-līt) a substance decomposed by light.

photomania (fo″to-ma′ne-ah) mania developed under the influence of light.

photometer (fo-tom′ĕ-ter) a device for measuring intensity of light.

photometry (fo-tom′ĕ-tre) measurement of the intensity of light.

photomicrograph (fo″to-mi′kro-graf) a photograph of an object as seen through an ordinary light microscope.

photon (fo′ton) a párticle (quantum) of electromagnetic radiation.

photonosus (fo-ton′o-sus) disease due to too much sunlight.

photoperceptive (fo″to-per-sep′tiv) able to perceive light.

photoperiodicity (-pe″re-o-dis′ĭ-te) regularly recurrent alteration in relation of light and darkness noted in annual passage of the earth about the sun; applied also to the rhythm of certain biological phenomena as determined by that alteration.

photophilic (-fil′ik) fond of or thriving in light.

photophobia (-fo′be-ah) abnormal intolerance of light.

photophthalmia (fo″tof-thal′me-ah) a morbid condition of the eyes caused by excessive exposure to radiant energy (ultraviolet rays).

photopia (fo-to′pe-ah) the adjustment of the eye for light.

photopsy (fo′top-se) appearance as of sparks or flashes, in retinal disease.

photoptarmosis (fo″to-tar-mo′sis) sneezing caused by the influence of light.

photoptometer (fo"top-tom'ĕ-ter) device for measuring sensitiveness to light.

photoreception (fo"to-re-sep'shun) the process of detecting radiant energy, usually of wavelengths between 3900 and 7700 angstroms, being the range of visible light.

photoreceptive (-re-sep'tiv) able to perceive light.

photoreceptor (-re-sep'tor) a receptor organ which responds to stimulation of light rays.

photoscan (fo'to-skan) a two-dimensional representation of gamma rays emitted by a radioactive isotope in body tissue, produced by a printout mechanism utilizing a light source to expose a photographic film.

photosensitive (fo"to-sen'sĭ-tiv) sensitive to light.

photostable (fo'to-sta"bl) unchanged by the influence of light.

photosynthesis (fo"to-sin'thĕ-sis) the formation of carbohydrates from carbon dioxide and water under the influence of light. adj., **photosynthet'ic.**

phototaxis (-tak'sis) movement of a freely motile organism in response to the stimulation of light. adj., **phototac'tic.**

phototherapy (-ther'ah-pe) treatment of disease by light rays.

phototoxic (-tok'sik) having a toxic effect triggered by exposure to light.

phototrophic (-trof'ik) utilizing light in metabolism.

phototropism (fo-tot'ro-pizm) a growth curvature occurring in response to the stimulation of light. adj., **phototrop'ic.**

photuria (fo-tu're-ah) phosphorescence of the urine.

Phragmidiothrix (frag-mid'e-o-thriks") a genus of Schizomycetes (order Chlamydobacteriales, family Crenotrichaceae).

phren (fren). 1. the mind or heart. 2. the diaphragm.

phrenalgia (fre-nal'je-ah) 1. pain in the diaphragm. 2. melancholia.

phrenemphraxis (fren"em-frak'sis) phrenicotripsy.

phrenetic (frĕ-net'ik) maniacal.

phrenic (fren'ik) pertaining to the diaphragm or to the mind.

phrenicectomy (fren"ĭ-sek'to-me) resection of the phrenic nerve.

phrenicoexeresis (-ko-ek-ser'ĕ-sis) avulsion of the phrenic nerve.

phrenicotomy (-kot'o-me) cutting of the phrenic nerve.

phrenicotripsy (fren"ĭ-ko-trip'se) surgical crushing of the phrenic nerve.

phrenitis (frĕ-ni'tis) delirium or frenzy.

phrenocardia (fren"o-kar'de-ah) a psychic condition marked by cardiac symptoms.

phrenocolic (-kol'ik) pertaining to diaphragm and colon.

phrenodynia (-din'e-ah) pain in the diaphragm.

phrenology (frĕ-nol'o-je) study of the faculties and qualities of mind from the shape of the skull.

phrenopathy (-nop'ah-the) any mental disease.

phrenoplegia (fren"o-ple'je-ah) a sudden attack of mental disorder.

phrenosin (fren'o-sin) a cerebroside containing cerebronic acid attached to the sphingosine.

phrenotropic (fren"o-trop'ik) exerting its principal effect upon the mind.

phrynoderma (frin"o-der'mah) a dry dermatosis, probably due to deficiency of vitamin A.

phthalein (thal'e-in) any one of a series of coloring matters formed by the condensation of phthalic anhydride with the phenols.

phthalylsulfacetamide (thal"il-sul"fah-set'ah-mĭd) white or creamy white crystalline compound used as an intestinal anti-infective.

phthalylsulfathiazole (-thi'ah-zōl) a white or yellowish-white, crystalline powder used as an intestinal antibacterial.

phthalylsulfonazole (thal"il-sul-fon'ah-zōl) phthalylsulfacetamide.

phthiriasis (thi-ri'ah-sis) infestation with lice of the species *Phthirus pubis.*

Phthirus (thir'us) a genus of lice. **P. pu'bis,** a species of louse which infests the pubic hair, and sometimes the eyebrows.

phthisiology (tiz"e-ol'o-je) the scientific study of tuberculosis.

phthisiophobia (tiz"e-o-fo'be-ah) morbid fear of tuberculosis.

phthisis (thi'sis) 1. a wasting of the body. 2. tuberculosis. **p. bul'bi,** shrinkage of eyeball. **miner's p.,** anthracosis. **pulmonary p.,** tuberculosis of the lungs. **p. ventric'uli,** atrophy of the mucous membrane of stomach and alimentary canal.

phycochrome (fi'ko-krōm) a pigment derived from algae.

phycocyanin (fi"ko-si'ah-nin) a blue photosynthetic pigment contained in the blue-green algae.

phycocyanogen (-si-an'o-jen) a blue pigment derived from blue-green algae.

phycoerythrin (-er'ĭ-thrin) a red pigment derived from red algae.

phylaxin (fi-lak'sin) any defensive proteid in an animal which has become immune against a disease.

phylaxis (fi-lak'sis) the bodily defense against infection. adj., **phylac'tic.**

phylloquinone (fil"o-kwin'ōn) phytonadione.

phylogeny (fi-loj'ĕ-ne) the complete developmental history of a race or group of organisms. adj., **phylogen'ic.**

phylum (fi'lum) a primary division of the plant or animal kingdom, including organisms which are assumed to have a common ancestry.

phyma (fi'mah) a skin tumor.

phymatosis (fi"mah-to'sis) a disease characterized by the presence of skin tumors.

physiatrics (fiz"e-at'riks) that branch of medicine using physical agents, such as light, heat, water and electricity, and mechanical apparatus, in the diagnosis, prevention and treatment of bodily disorders.

physiatrist (fiz"e-at'rist) a specialist in physiatrics.

physic (fiz'ik) 1. the art of medicine and of

therapeutics. 2. a medicine, especially a cathartic.

physical (fiz'ĭ-kal) pertaining to nature or to the body.

physician (fĭ-zish'un) an authorized practitioner of medicine. **attending p.**, one who attends a hospital at stated times to visit the patients and give directions as to their treatment. **resident p.**, a graduate and licensed physician resident in a hospital.

physicochemical (fiz"ĭ-ko-kem'ĭ-kal) pertaining to both physics and chemistry.

physics (fiz'iks) the study of the laws and phenomena of nature, especially of forces and general properties of matter.

physinosis (fiz"ĭ-no'sis) a disease due to physical agents.

physio- (fiz'e-o) word element [Gr.], *nature; physiology.*

physiochemical (fiz"e-o-kem'ĭ-kal) pertaining to both physiology and chemistry.

physiognomy (fiz"e-og'no-me) 1. determination of mental or moral character and qualities by the face. 2. the face.

physiology (-ol'o-je) the science dealing with the function of various parts and organs of living organisms. **cell p.**, scientific study of phenomena involved in cell growth and maintenance, self-regulation and division of cells, interactions between nucleus and cytoplasm, and general behavior of protoplasm. **comparative p.**, that concerned with many different types of organisms. **general p.**, that concerned with establishment of the general principles of functional mechanisms underlying life processes of all organisms. **morbid p., pathologic p.**, the study of disordered function or of function in diseased tissues. **special p.**, that concerned with a specific group of animals, e.g. mammals or insects.

physiometry (-om'ĕ-tre) measurement of physiologic functions by physiologic or serologic methods.

physiotherapist (fiz"-e-o-ther'ah-pist) physical therapist.

physiotherapy (-ther'ah-pe) physical therapy.

physique (fĭ-zēk') the body organization, development and structure.

physis (fi'sis) the segment of tubular bone concerned mainly with growth.

physohematometra (fi"so-hem"ah-to-me'trah) gas and blood in the uterine cavity.

physohydrometra (-hi"dro-me'trah) gas and serum in the uterine cavity.

physometra (-me'trah) gas in the uterine cavity.

physopyosalpinx (-pi"o-sal'pinks) gas and pus in the oviduct.

physostigmine (-stig'min) an alkaloid usually obtained from dried ripe seed of *Physostigma venenosum.* **p. salicylate, p. sulfate,** salts of physostigmine used topically in the conjunctival sac to produce miosis.

phyt(o)- (fi'to) word element [Gr.], *plant; an organism of the vegetable kingdom.*

phytalbumin (fi"tal-bu'min) albumin of vegetable origin.

phytalbumose (fi-tal'bu-mōs) albumose of vegetable origin.

phytobezoar (fi"to-be'zōr) a bezoar composed of vegetable fibers.

phytochemistry (-kem'is-tre) study of chemical processes occurring in plants, the nature of plant chemicals and various applications of such chemicals to science and industry.

phytodetritus (-de-tri'tus) detritus produced by disintegration and decomposition of vegetable organisms or tissue.

phytogenous (fi-toj'ĕ-nus) derived from plants.

phytoglobulin (fi"to-glob'u-lin) a plant globulin.

phytohemagglutinin (-hem"ah-gloo'tĭ-nin) a hemagglutinin of plant origin.

phytohormone (-hōr'mōn) a plant hormone.

phytoid (fi'toid) resembling a plant.

phytomelin (fi"to-mel'in) rutin.

phytomenadione (-men"ah-di'ōn) phytonadione.

phytomitogen (-mi'to-jen) a substance of plant origin which induces mitosis in human cells.

phytonadione (-nah-di'ōn) a vitamin K preparation used as a prothrombogenic agent.

phytoparasite (-par"ah-sīt) a parasitic vegetable organism.

phytopathology (-pah-thol'o-je) 1. the pathology of plants. 2. pathology of diseases caused by schizomycetes.

phytophotodermatitis (-fo"to-der"mah-ti'tis) a morbid condition of the skin due to contact with certain plants and subsequent exposure to light.

phytoplankton (-plank'ton) minute plant organisms, mostly algae, found floating free in practically all natural waters.

phytoplasm (fi'to-plazm) protoplasm of plants.

phytosis (fi-to'sis) any disease caused by a phytoparasite.

phytosterol (fi"to-ste'rol) one of a group of compounds which are closely related to cholesterol, found in plants.

phytotoxin (-tok'sin) an exotoxin produced by certain species of higher plants.

pia (pi'ah) [L.] soft; tender. **p. ma'ter,** the innermost of the three membranes covering the brain and spinal cord.

pia-arachnitis (pi"ah-ar"ak-ni'tis) leptomeningitis.

pia-arachnoid (-ah-rak'noid) the pia and arachnoid considered together.

piarachnitis (pi"ar-ak-ni'tis) pia-arachnitis.

piarachnoid (pi"ar-ak'noid) pia-arachnoid.

piarrhemia (pi"ah-re'me-ah) lipemia.

pica (pi'kah) craving for unnatural articles as food.

piceous (pi'se-us) of the nature of pitch.

pico- (pi'ko) word element used to designate an amount 10^{-12} (one trillionth) the size of the unit to which it is joined, e.g. picocurie.

picocurie (pi"ko-ku're) a unit of radioactivity, 10^{-12} curie or 10^{-6} microcurie.

picogram (pi'ko-gram) a unit of mass, 10^{-12} gram or 10^{-6} microgram.

picornavirus (pi-kor″nah-vi′rus) an extremely small, ether-resistant ribonucleic acid virus, one of the group comprising the enteroviruses and the coryzaviruses.

picounit (pi″ko-u′nit) one trillionth part of a unit (10⁻¹²).

picrate (pik′rāt) a salt of picric acid.

picrotoxin (pik″ro-tok′sin) an active principle from the seed of *Anamirta cocculus*, used as a central nervous system stimulant and as an antidote in barbiturate poisoning.

piedra (pe-a′drah) hair disease in which nodules form on the shafts.

piesesthesia (pi-e″zes-the′ze-ah) the sense by which pressure stimuli are felt.

piesimeter (pi″e-sim′ē-ter) instrument for testing the sensitiveness of the skin to pressure.

-piesis (pi-e′sis) word element [Gr.], *pressure*. adj., **-pies′ic.**

piezocardiogram (pi-e″zo-kar′de-o-gram″) a graphic tracing of the changes in pressure caused by pulsation of the heart against the esophageal wall, recorded through the esophagus.

pigment (pig′ment) a coloring matter or dyestuff. adj., **pig′mentary.** **bile p's,** substances formed by the degradation of heme and removed from the blood by the liver. **respiratory p.,** a substance in the blood or body fluid of animals which carries oxygen to the various tissues of the body for use in the oxidative processes of the cells, such as the hemoglobin of human blood.

pigmentation (pig″men-ta′shun) the deposit of coloring matter; the coloration or discoloration of a part by a pigment. **hematogenous p.,** pigmentation produced by accumulation of hemoglobin derivatives, such as hematoidin or hemosiderin. **malarial p.,** pigmentation due to accumulation, especially in spleen and liver, of dark brown pigment liberated from red blood cells which are destroyed by malarial parasites. **vagabonds' p.,** pigmentation of the skin due to lice.

pigmented (pig′ment-ed) containing pigment.

pigmentogenic (pig″men-to-jen′ik) inducing formation or deposit of pigment.

pigmentolysin (pig″men-tol′ĭ-sin) a lysin which destroys pigment.

pigmentolysis (tol′ĭ-sis) destruction of pigment.

piitis (pi-i′tis) inflammation of pia mater.

pilary (pil′ar-e) pertaining to the hair.

pile (pīl) 1. hemorrhoid. 2. in nucleonics, a chain-reaction fission device for producing slow neutrons and radioactive isotopes. **sentinel p.,** an edematous tag of skin, usually in the midline and posteriorly, marking the outer limit of a fissure in the wall of the anus.

pileous (pil′e-us) hairy.

pileus (pil′e-us) 1. one of the cerebellar hemispheres. 2. a membrane which sometimes covers a child's head at birth.

pill (pil) a plastic mass made up of a medicated powder incorporated in a gummy or syrupy material, fashioned into convenient size for oral administration. **aloe p.,** a pill containing finely powdered aloe and hard soap, mixed with distilled water. **asafetida p.,** a pill composed of asafetida, hard soap and distilled water. **Blaud's p.,** ferrous carbonate pill. **cathartic p., compound,** compound mild mercurous chloride pill. **chalybeate p.,** ferrous carbonate pill. **colocynth and jalap p., compound,** a pill containing compound colocynth extract, hyoscyamus extract, jalap resin, leptandra extract and podophyllum resin. **enteric-coated p.,** one enclosed in a substance that dissolves only when it has reached the intestines. **ferrous carbonate p.,** ferrous sulfate, potassium carbonate, sucrose, tragacanth, althea, glycerin, distilled water. **hexylresorcinol p.,** one containing hexylresorcinol, with a rupture-resistant coating which disintegrates in the digestive tract. **Hinkle's p.,** aloin, belladonna, cascara and podophyllum pill. **mercurous chloride, mild p., compound,** pill containing compound colocynth extract, mild mercurous chloride, jalap resin, and gamboge. **vegetable cathartic p.,** compound colocynth and jalap pill.

pillar (pil-ar) a supporting structure. **p's of the fauces,** folds of mucous membrane at sides of fauces.

pilleus (pil′e-us) pileus.

pillion (pil′yon) a temporary artificial leg.

pilocarpine (pi″lo-kar′pin) an alkaloid from leaflets of *Pilocarpus jaborandi* and *P. microphyllus*. **p. hydrochloride, p. nitrate,** salts of pilocarpine used to produce constriction of the pupil.

pilocystic (-sis′tik) cystic and containing hair.

pilo-erection (-e-rek′shun) erection of the hair.

pilojection (-jek′shun) introduction of one or more hairs into an aneurysmal sac, to promote formation of a blood clot.

pilology (pi-lol′o-je) the study of the hair.

pilomotor (pi″lo-mo′tor) causing movements of the hairs.

pilonidal (-ni′dal) having a nidus of hairs.

pilose (pi′lōs) hairy; covered with hair.

pilosebaceous (pi″lo-se-ba′shus) pertaining to hair and sebaceous glands.

pilus (pi′lus), pl. **pi′li** [L.] hair. **p. annula′tus** (pl. **pi′li annula′ti**), ringed hair. **p. cunicula′tus** (pl. **pi′li cunicula′ti**), burrowing hair. **p. incarna′tus** (pl. **pi′li incarna′ti**), ingrown hair. **pi′li multigem′ini,** the growth of several hairs from the same follicle. **p. tor′tus** (pl. **pi′li tor′ti**), twisted hair.

piminodine (pi-min′o-dēn) a compound used as a narcotic analgesic.

pin (pin) a slender, elongated piece of metal used for securing fixation of parts. **Steinmann p.,** a pin driven through the distal part of a fractured bone as a means of applying traction, or used to immobilize the fragments of a fractured bone.

pincement (pans-maw′) [Fr.] pinching of the flesh in massage.

pineal (pin′e-al) 1. like a pine cone. 2. the pineal gland.

pinealectomy (pin″e-al-ek′to-me)   excision of the pineal gland.

pinealism (pin″e-al-izm) derangement of secretion of the pineal gland.

pinealoma (pin″e-ah-lo′mah)   a tumor of the pineal gland.

pinealopathy (-lop′ah-the)   a disease of the pineal gland.

pinguecula (pin-gwek′u-lah) pinguicula.

pinguicula (pin-gwik′u-lah), pl. *pinguic′ulae* [L.]   a small, yellowish spot on the cornea.

piniform (pin′ĭ-form) shaped like a pine cone.

pink-eye (pink′i)   epidemic, contagious conjunctivitis.

pinna (pin′ah)   the part of the ear outside the cranial bones.

pinocyte (pin′o-sīt)   a cell which absorbs and digests tissue fluids.

pinocytosis (pi″no-si-to′sis) the uptake of fluid material by a living cell. adj., **pinocytot′ic.**

pinosome (pi′no-sōm)   a small, fluid-filled vacuole occurring in the cytoplasm of a cell after the breakdown of the canal-like intrusions formed during pinocytosis.

pint (pīnt)   a unit of liquid measure in the apothecaries' system, 16 fluidounces or equivalent to 473.17 milliliters.

pinta (pin′tah)   a treponemal infection characterized by bizarre pigmentary changes, occurring in Cuba and hot lowlands of the American continent.

pinworm (pin′werm)   a name applied to various nematode parasites, especially to individuals of the species *Enterobius vermicularis*, but also to those parasitic in animals other than man.

pionemia (pi″o-ne′me-ah)   fat in the blood.

pipamazine (pi-pam′ah-zēn)   a phenothiazine compound used as an antiemetic.

Pipanol (pip′ah-nol)   trademark for a preparation of trihexyphenidyl.

pipenzolate (pi-pen′zo-lāt)   a compound used in parasympathetic blockade.

piperazine (pi-per′ah-zēn)   a compound, various salts of which are used as anthelmintics.

piperidione (pi″per-ĭ-di′ōn) dihyprylone.

piperidolate (pi″per-id′o-lāt) a compound used in parasympathetic blockade.

piperocaine (pi′per-o-kān″) a compound used as a local anesthetic.

pipet (pi-pet′)   1. a heavy-walled glass tube of small bore, with a slightly beveled end, used to draw up by suction small quantities of liquid.   2. to draw into and discharge from a pipet.   **diluting p.,** one incorporating a bulbous expansion in which the liquid under study can be diluted with the appropriate solution.   **measuring p.,** one with a graduated scale, permitting accurate measurement of a quantity of liquid.   **transfer p.,** one used to convey a small quantity of liquid from one container to another.

pipethanate (pi-peth′ah-nāt)   a compound used in parasympathetic blockade.

pipette (pi-pet′) pipet.

Pipizan (pi′pĭ-zan)   trademark for a preparation of piperazine.

pipradrol (pi′prah-drol)   a compound used as a central nervous system stimulant.

Piptal (pip′tal)   trademark for preparations of pipenzolate methylbromide.

Piroplasma (pi″ro-plaz′mah)   former genus name for Babesia.

piroplasmosis (-plaz-mo′sis) babesiosis.

pit (pit)   a depressed area or hollow. **anal p.,** proctodeum. **auditory p.,** a cuplike depression in an auditory placode, a stage in development of the auditory vesicle. **ear p.,** a slight depression in front of the helix, and above the tragus, sometimes leading to a congenital preauricular cyst or fistula. **nasal p.,** olfactory p., a depression appearing in the olfactory placodes in the early stages of development of the nose.

pitch (pich)   a black substance derived from tar. **black p.,** inflammable solid prepared by boiling tar. **Burgundy p.,** an aromatic, oily resin much used in plasters. **Canada p.,** a resin useful in plasters, etc. **mineral p.,** bitumen. **naval p.,** black pitch. **Trinidad p.,** asphalt from Trinidad, West Indies.

pithecoid (pith′ē-koid) apelike.

pithing (pith′ing)   piercing of the brain or spinal cord in experimental animals.

Pitocin (pi-to′sin)   trademark for a solution of oxytocin for injection.

Pitressin (pi-tres′in)   trademark for a solution of vasopressin for injection.

pitting (pit′ing)   the formation of depressions or hollows.

pituita (pi-tu′ĭ-tah)   glutinous mucus or phlegm.

pituitarigenic (pi-tu″ĭ-tar″ĭ-jen′ik)   produced by secretions of the pituitary gland.

pituitarism (pi-tu′ĭ-tar-izm″)   disorder of pituitary function.

pituitary (pi-tu′ĭ-tār″e)   1. pertaining to mucus or phlegm.   2. the hypophysis cerebri. **anterior p.,** the pars anterior of the hypophysis cerebri, or a pharmaceutic preparation thereof. **posterior p.,** 1. the posterior lobe of the hypophysis cerebri.   2. powder prepared from clean, dried posterior lobe of pituitary body of domesticated animals used for food by man.

Pituitrin (pi-tu′ĭ-trin)   trademark for a preparation of posterior pituitary injection.

pityriasis (pit″ĭ-ri′ah-sis)   a skin condition with formation of branny scales. **p. al′ba,** a chronic condition with patchy scaling and hypopigmentation of the skin of the face. **p. ro′sea,** a dermatosis due to a virus and marked by a rash and mild to moderate pruritus. **p. ru′bra,** a condition marked by scarlatiniform patches beginning on the forearms and spreading to the entire body, with scaling of the skin and shedding of hair. **p. versi-co′lor,** tinea versicolor.

pityroid (pit′ĭ-roid)   like bran; branny.

pix (piks) [L.] pitch.

PKU phenylketonuria.

placebo (plah-se′bo)   an inactive substance resembling a medication that may be given experimentally or for its psychologic effects.

placenta (plah-sen′tah)   an organ developed in

the uterus by the fertilized ovum, which subserves the anabolic and catabolic needs of the developing fetus. adj., **placen'tal**. **p. accre'ta**, one abnormally adherent to the uterine wall, with partial or complete absence of the decidua basalis. **battledore p.**, one with the umbilical cord inserted at the edge. **p. circumvalla'ta**, one encircled with a raised white nodular ring, the attached membranes being doubled back over the edge of the placenta. **p. fenestra'ta**, one which has spots where placental tissue is lacking. **p. incre'ta**, one abnormally adherent and penetrating the uterine wall. **p. membrana'cea**, one spread over an unusually large area of the uterine wall. **p. nappifor'mis**, placenta circumvallata. **p. percre'ta**, one abnormally adherent with invasion of the uterine wall to the serosal layer. **p. prae'via**, one located in the lower uterine segment, partially or entirely covering the internal os. **p. reflex'a**, one in which the margin is thickened, appearing to turn back on itself. **p. spu'ria**, an accessory portion without blood vessels connecting it with the placenta. **p. succenturia'ta**, an accessory portion with blood vessels connecting it with the placenta.

placentation (plas″en-ta'shun) the series of events following implantation of the embryo and leading to development of the placenta.

placentitis (-ti'tis) bacterial infection of the placenta.

placentography (-tog'rah-fe) radiography of the pregnant uterus to determine the position of the placenta.

placentoid (plah-sen'toid) resembling the placenta.

placentologist (plas″en-tol'o-jist) a specialist in placentology.

placentology (-tol'o-je) scientific study of the development, structure and functioning of the placenta.

placentolysin (-tol'ĭ-sin) an antibody capable of destroying placental cells.

placentoma (-to'mah) a neoplasm derived from retained placenta.

Placidyl (plas'ĭ-dil) trademark for a preparation of ethchlorvynol.

placode (plak'od) a platelike structure, especially a thickening of the ectoderm marking the site of future development in the early embryo of an organ of special sense, e.g. the *auditory placode* (ear), *lens placode* (eye) and *olfactory placode* (nose).

pladaroma (plad″ah-ro'mah) a soft tumor on the eyelid.

plagiocephaly (pla″je-o-sef'ah-le) bizarre distortion of the shape of the skull. adj., **plagiocephal'ic**.

plague (plāg) an acute febrile, infectious, highly fatal disease due to *Pasteurella pestis* and characterized by inflammation of the lymphatics, septicemia, and petechial and diffuse hemorrhages into the skin, subcutaneous tissues and viscera. **bubonic p.**, plague in which the nodes along lymphatic vessels draining the site of infection become edematous, congested and hemorrhagic and often

necrotic. **cattle p.**, contagious typhus in cattle. **hemorrhagic p.**, a severe form with hemorrhages into the mucous membrane and skin. **murine p.**, infection in domestic rodents due to *Pasteurella pestis*. **pneumonic p.**, that in which the air passages are intensely congested, with hemorrhagic exudate in the alveoli and bronchi, but with little or no fibrin formation; the bronchial and hilar lymph nodes are also involved. **rodent p.**, a plague which affects rodents. **septicemic p.**, that occurring with *Pasteurella pestis* in the blood stream, with death before the appearance of buboes or of pulmonic manifestations. **swine p.**, an epidemic, infectious disease of swine, affecting the respiratory and alimentary tracts. **sylvatic p.**, plague in wild rodents, such as the ground squirrel, which serve as a reservoir from which man may be infected.

plane (plān) a flat surface. **axial p.**, one parallel with the long axis of a solid body, such as a tooth. **axiobuccolingual p.**, a plane parallel with the long axis of a tooth and passing through the buccal and lingual surfaces. **axiolabiolingual p.**, a plane parallel with the long axis of a tooth and cutting its labial and lingual surfaces. **axiomesiodistal p.**, a plane parallel with the long axis of a tooth and cutting its mesial and distal surfaces. **base p.**, an imaginary plane upon which is estimated the retention of an artificial denture. **coronal p.**, frontal plane. **datum p.**, a given horizontal plane from which craniometric measurements are made. **equatorial p.**, one perpendicular to the longitudinal axis of a spherical body, dividing it into two approximately equal parts. **frontal p.**, one which includes the anterior-posterior and the left-right axis, but is at right angles to the dorsoventral axis. **horizontal p.**, one passing through the body at right angles to the median and frontal planes, and dividing the body into upper and lower parts. **median p.**, one passing longitudinally through the body from front to back and dividing it into right and left halves. **nuchal p.**, the outer surface of the occipital bone between the foramen magnum and the superior curved line. **occipital p.**, the outer surface of the occipital bone above the superior curved line. **orbital p.**, 1. the orbital surface of the maxilla. 2. the plane that passes through the visual axis of each eye. **sagittal p.**, a vertical plane through the body parallel to the median plane and dividing the body into left and right portions. **sternal p.**, the anterior surface of the sternum. **temporal p.**, the depressed area on the side of the skull below the inferior temporal line. **transverse p.**, one passing horizontally through the body, at right angles to the sagittal and frontal planes, and dividing the body into upper and lower portions. **visual p.**, orbital plane (2).

planigraphy (plah-nig'rah-fe) a method of body-section roentgenography with the x-ray tube moved in many directions, usually through circles or spirals. adj., **planigraph'ic**.

plankton (plangk'ton) the minute, free-floating organisms living in practically all natural waters.

planocellular (pla″no-sel′u-lar) composed of flat cells.

planoconcave (-kon′kāv) flat on one side and concave on the other.

planoconvex (-kon′veks) flat on one side and convex on the other.

planocyte (plan′o-sīt) a wandering cell.

planography (plah-nog′rah-fe) a special technique of body-section roentgenography.

plant (plant) a living organism without sense organs and incapable of voluntary motion.

planta (plan′tah) the sole of the foot.

plantalgia (plan-tal′je-ah) pain in the sole of the foot.

plantar (plan′tar) pertaining to the sole of the foot.

plantaris (plan-ta′ris) [L.] plantar.

plantation (-ta′shun) insertion or application of material into or on the human body.

plantigrade (plan′tĭ-grād) walking or running flat on the lower surface of the foot; characteristic of man and of such quadrupeds as the bear.

planula (plan′u-lah) the embryo in the stage when it consists of two primary layers.

planum (pla′num), pl. *pla′na* [L.] plane.

plaque (plak) a flat, platelike body. **bacterial p.,** a collection of bacteria growing in a deposit of material on the surface of a tooth. **blood p.,** a blood platelet. **dental p.,** a deposit of material on the surface of a tooth.

Plaquenil (pla′kwĕ-nil) trademark for a preparation of hydroxychloroquine.

plasm (plazm) 1. plasma. 2. formative substance (cytoplasm, hyaloplasm, etc.). **germ p.,** the line of cells which by successive divisions give rise to the gametes.

plasma (plaz′mah) the fluid portion of whole blood, obtained by centrifuging or sedimentation. adj., **plasmat′ic. antihemophilic human p.,** normal human plasma which has been processed promptly to preserve the antihemophilic properties, being frozen within six hours and dispensed in frozen or dried state. **normal human p.,** plasma derived from pooled blood of eight or more adult humans, considered free of disease, which is treated with ultraviolet irradiation to remove possible contamination; it may transmit the virus which causes homologous serum jaundice.

plasmacyte (plaz′mah-sīt) plasma cell.

plasmacytoma (plaz″mah-si-to′mah) a primary tumor of lymph nodes, composed of mature, well differentiated or more anaplastic plasma cells.

plasmacytosis (-si-to′sis) the presence of plasma cells in the blood.

plasmagene (plaz′mah-jēn) a self-reproducing copy of a nuclear gene persisting in the cytoplasm of a cell.

plasmalogen (plaz-mal′o-jen) a term applied to a member of a group of phospholipids present in platelets which liberate higher fatty aldehydes on hydrolysis.

plasmapheresis (plaz″mah-fĕ-re′sis) removal of blood, separation of the corpuscles by centrifugation, replacement of the plasma by Locke's solution, and reinjection of the cells into the body.

plasmasome (plaz′mah-sōm) a leukocyte granule.

plasmatocyte (plaz-mat′o-sīt) monocyte.

plasmatorrhexis (plaz″mah-to-rek′sis) bursting of a cell from internal pressure.

plasmic (plaz′mik) plasmatic.

plasmin (plaz′min) a proteolytic enzyme with a high specificity for fibrin and the particular ability to dissolve formed fibrin clots.

plasminogen (plaz-min′o-jen) the inactive precursor of plasmin, occurring in the beta globulin fraction of the plasma.

Plasmochin naphthoate (plaz″mo-kin naf′tho-āt) trademark for a preparation of pamaquine naphthoate.

plasmocyte (plaz′mo-sīt) a cell of the plasmocytic series with chromatin aggregated into large, sharply demarcated clumps, without nucleoli.

plasmodicidal (plaz-mo″dī-si′dal) destructive to plasmodia.

Plasmodium (plaz-mo′de-um) a multispecies genus of sporozoa parasitic in the red blood cells of various animals; four species, *P. fal-cip′arum*, *P. mala′riae*, *P. ova′le* and *P. vi′vax*, cause the four specific types of malaria in man.

plasmodium (plaz-mo′de-um), pl. *plasmo′dia* [Gr.] an organism of the genus Plasmodium.

plasmogen (plaz′mo-jen) bioplasm.

plasmology (plaz-mol′o-je) the science of the minute particles of living matter.

plasmolysis (-mol′ĭ-sis) contraction of cell protoplasm due to loss of water by osmosis.

plasmorrhexis (plaz″mo-rek′sis) erythrocytorrhexis.

plasmoschisis (plaz-mos′kĭ-sis) the splitting up of cell protoplasm.

plasmosome (plaz′mo-sōm) the true nucleolus of a cell.

plasmotropism (plaz-mot′ro-pizm) the property of spleen and bone marrow of attracting and destroying red blood cells.

plasmozyme (plaz′mo-zīm) thrombogen.

plasome (pla′sōm) hypothetical unit of living protoplasm.

plaster (plas′ter) an adhesive substance spread on fabric or other suitable backing material, for application to the skin, often containing some medication, such as an anodyne or rubefacient. **adhesive p.,** fabric spread with pressure-sensitive adhesive mixture, for application to the skin. **dental p.,** a gypsum preparation used for the making of impressions of structures of the mouth. **p. of Paris,** calcium sulfate.

plastic (plas′tik) 1. tending to build up tissues. 2. capable of being molded. 3. a substance produced by chemical condensation or by polymerization.

plasticity (plas-tis′ĭ-te) the quality of being plastic.

plastid (plas′tid) any cell or constructive unit.

-plasty (plas'te) word element [Gr.], *formation or plastic repair of.*

plate (plāt) a flattened process, chiefly of bone. **approximation p.**, a disk of bone, or the like, used in intestinal surgery. **auditory p.**, bony roof of auditory meatus. **axial p.**, the primitive streak of embryo. **bite p.**, a plate of rigid material used to support a bite-rim. **collecting p's**, the electronegative element of a galvanic battery. **cribriform p.**, the upper perforated plate of the ethmoid bone. **deck p.**, roof plate. **dental p.**, a plate of acrylic resin, metal or other material which is fitted to the shape of the mouth, and serves for the support of artificial teeth. **dorsal p.**, lengthwise ridge on either side on the dorsum of embryo. **floor p.**, the unpaired ventral longitudinal zone of the neural tube. **foot p.**, flat portion of stapes. **generating p.**, the plate in an electric cell which is chemically acted on. **growth p.**, the area between the epiphysis and diaphysis of long bones within which growth in length occurs. **medullary p.**, neural plate. **muscle p.**, myotome. **neural p.**, a thickened band of ectoderm in the midbody region of the developing embryo, which develops into the nervous system. **roof p.**, the unpaired dorsal longitudinal zone of the neural tube. **sole p.**, a mass of protoplasm in which a motor nerve ending is embedded. **tarsal p.**, the quasicartilaginous substance which gives firmness to the eyelid. **tympanic p.**, bony plate forming floor and sides of meatus auditorius. **ventral p.**, floor plate.

platelet (plāt'let) a small disk or platelike structure. **blood p.**, a microscopic circular or oval disk found in the blood of all mammals, which is concerned in coagulation of the blood and contraction of the clot.

platinectomy (plat"ĭ-nek'to-me) excision of the footplate in surgical mobilization of the stapes, in treatment of hearing loss.

platinode (plat'ĭ-nōd) collecting plate of an electric battery.

platinum (plat'ĭ-num) chemical element (*see table*), at. no. 78, symbol Pt.

platy- (plat'e) word element [Gr.], *flat.*

platybasia (plat"ĭ-ba'ze-ah) malformation of the base of the skull, with upward displacement of the upper cervical vertebrae.

platycelous (-se'lus) having one surface flat and the other concave.

platycephalous (-sef'ah-lus) having a wide, flat head.

platycoria (-ko're-ah) a dilated condition of the pupil of the eye.

platycrania (-kra'ne-ah) flattening of the skull.

Platyhelminthes (-hel-min'thēz) a phylum of acoelomate, dorsoventrally flattened, bilaterally symmetrical animals, commonly known as flatworms.

platyhieric (-hi-er'ik) having a sacral index above 100.

platypellic (-pel'ik) having a pelvic index below 90.

platypodia (-po'de-ah) flatness of the sole of the foot.

Platyrrhina (plat"ĭ-ri'nah) a superfamily of the order Primates (suborder Anthropoidea), characterized by a broad nasal septum and often a prehensile tail, and including the New World monkeys.

platyrrhine (plat'ĭ-rīn) having a nasal index above 53.

platysma (plah-tiz'mah) a muscle of the neck.

pledge (plej) a solemn statement of intention. **Nightingale p.**, a statement of principles for the nursing profession, formulated by a committee in 1893 and subscribed to by student nurses at the time of the capping ceremonies.

pledget (plej'et) a small compress or tuft.

pleiotropy (pli-ot'ro-pe) 1. the quality of having affinity for tissues derived from the different germ layers. 2. ability of a gene to manifest itself in many ways. adj., **pleiotrop'ic.**

pleochromatic (ple"o-kro-mat'ik) showing various colors under varying circumstances.

pleochromocytoma (-kro"mo-si-to'mah) a tumor composed of tissues of varying colors.

pleocytosis (-si-to'sis) presence of a greater than normal number of cells, as of more than the normal number of lymphocytes in cerebrospinal fluid.

pleomastia (-mas'te-ah) the presence of supernumerary mammary glands.

pleomorphic (-mor'fik) occurring in various distinct forms.

pleomorphism (-mor'fizm) quality of being pleomorphic.

pleonasm (ple'o-nazm) an excess of parts.

pleonemia (ple"o-ne'me-ah) increased volume of blood in a part. adj., **pleone'mic.**

pleonexia (-nek'se-ah) morbid greediness.

pleoptics (ple-op'tiks) a technique of eye exercises designed to develop fuller vision of an amblyopic eye and assure proper binocular cooperation.

plessesthesia (ples"es-the'ze-ah) palpatory percussion.

plessimeter (ple-sim'ĕ-ter) pleximeter

plessor (ples'or) plexor.

plethora (pleth'o-rah) vascular turgescence, excess of blood, and fullness of habit. adj., **plethor'ic.**

plethysmograph (plĕ-thiz'mo-graf) instrument for recording variations in volume of parts.

plethysmography (pleth"iz-mog'rah-fe) the determination of changes in volume by means of a plethysmograph.

pleur(o)- (ploor'o) word element [Gr.], *pleura; rib; side.*

pleura (ploo'rah), pl. *pleu'rae* [Gr.] serous membrane investing the lungs (*pulmonary pleura*) and lining the walls of the thoracic cavity (*parietal pleura*), the two layers enclosing a potential space, the pleural cavity. adj., **pleu'ral.**

pleuracotomy (ploo"rah-kot'o-me) thoracotomy.

pleuralgia (ploo-ral'je-ah) pain in the pleura or in the side.

pleurapophysis (ploo"rah-pof'ĭ-sis) a rib or its homologue.

pleurectomy (ploo-rek'to-me)   excision of a portion of the pleura.

pleurisy (ploo'ri-se)   inflammation of the pleura. adj., **pleurit'ic. adhesive p.**, dry pleurisy. **diaphragmatic p.**, pleurisy limited to a spot near the diaphragm. **dry p.**, a variety with dry fibrinous exudate. **fibrinous p.**, pleurisy with a fibrinous exudate. **plastic p.**, pleurisy characterized by deposition of a soft, semisolid exudate. **purulent p.**, empyema. **serous p.**, pleurisy characterized by free exudation of serum. **wet p.**, **p. with effusion**, pleurisy marked by serous exudation.

pleuritis (ploo-ri'tis)   pleurisy.

pleurocele (ploo'ro-sēl)   hernia of lung tissue or of pleura.

pleurocentesis (ploo″ro-sen-te'sis)   paracentesis of the thoracic (pleural) cavity.

pleurocentrum (-sen'trum)   the lateral element of the vertebral column.

pleurocholecystitis (-ko″le-sis-ti'tis)   inflammation of the pleura and gallbladder.

pleuroclysis (ploo-rok'li-sis)   injection of fluids into the pleural cavity.

pleurodesis (ploo-rod'ĕ-sis)   production of adhesions between the parietal and the visceral pleura.

pleurodont (ploor'o-dont)   having teeth attached by one side on the inner surface of the jaw elements.

pleurodynia (ploo″ro-din'e-ah)   pain of intercostal muscles or of the pleural nerves. **epidemic p., epidemic diaphragmatic p.**, an epidemic disease marked by a sudden attack of pain in the chest, fever, and a tendency to recrudescence on the third day.

pleurogenic (-jen'ik)   originating in the pleura.

pleurography (ploo-rog'rah-fe)   radiography of the lungs.

pleurohepatitis (ploo″ro-hep″ah-ti'tis)   hepatitis with inflammation of pleura near the liver.

pleurolith (ploo'ro-lith)   a concretion in the pleura.

pleurolysis (ploo-rol'i-sis)   surgical separation of the pleura from its attachments.

pleuroparietopexy (ploo″ro-pah-ri'ĕ-to-pek″se)   fixation of lung to chest wall by adhesion of the visceral and parietal pleura.

pleuropericarditis (-per″i-kar-di'tis)   inflammation involving the pleura and the pericardium.

pleuropexy (-pek'se)   surgical induction of fusion between the visceral and parietal pleura.

pleuropneumonia (-nu-mo'ne-ah)   1. pneumonia accompanied by pleurisy. 2. a highly contagious disease of cattle, due to a filterable microorganism and occurring in many parts of the world.

pleuropneumonolysis (-nu″mo-nol'i-sis)   collapse of a tuberculous lung by removal of ribs from one side.

pleurorrhea (-re'ah)   a pleural effusion.

pleuroscopy (ploo-ros'ko-pe)   direct examination of the pleural cavity by incision of the chest wall.

pleurosomia (ploo″ro-so'me-ah)   developmental anomaly with imperfect development of the arm and protrusion of the intestine on one side.

pleurosomus (ploo″ro-so'mus)   a fetal monster exhibiting pleurosomia.

pleurothotonos (-thot'o-nus)   tetanic bending of the body to one side.

pleurotomy (ploo-rot'o-me)   incision of the pleura.

pleurovisceral (ploo″ro-vis'er-al)   pertaining to pleura and viscera.

plexiform (plek's i-form)   resembling a plexus.

pleximeter (plek-sim'ĕ-ter)   1. a plate to be struck in mediate percussion. 2. a glass plate used to show condition of the skin under pressure.

plexitis (plek-si'tis)   inflammation of a nerve plexus.

plexor (plek'sor)   hammer used in diagnostic percussion.

plexus (plek'sus), pl. *plex'us, plex'uses* [L.]   a network or tangle, chiefly of veins or nerves. adj., **plex'al. celiac p.**, solar plexus. **choroid p.**, the ependyma lining the ventricles of the brain with the vascular fringes of the pia mater invaginating them; concerned with formation of cerebrospinal fluid. **cystic p.**, a nerve plexus near the gallbladder. **Exner's p.**, a mesh of medullated fibers in the cerebral cortex. **Heller's p.**, an arterial network in the submucosa of the intestine. **Meissner's p.**, a network of nerve fibers beneath intestinal mucosa. **molecular p.**, Exner's plexus. **nerve p.**, a distinct network formed by fibers from several adjacent spinal nerves. **solar p.**, a network of ganglia and nerves supplying the abdominal viscera. **tympanic p.**, a network of nerve fibers supplying the mucous lining of the tympanum, mastoid air cells and pharyngotympanic tube.

plica (pli'kah), pl. *pli'cae* [L.]   a plait or fold. **pli'cae gas'tricae**, the series of folds in the mucous membrane of the stomach. **p. muco'sa**, a fold of mucous membrane. **pli'cae palma'tae**, folds of the arbor vitae uterinus. **p. polon'ica**, a matting of the hair with crusts and vermin. **p. semiluna'ris**, fold of mucous membrane on inner canthus of the eye.

plicate (pli'kāt)   plaited or folded.

plication (pli-ka'shun)   the process of taking a fold or plait, for shortening or decreasing the size of an organ or structure.

plicotomy (pli-kot'o-me)   myringotomy.

plombage (plom-bahzh') [Fr.]   the filling of a space or cavity in the body with inert material.

plug (plug)   an obstructing mass. **copulation p.**, vaginal plug. **Dittrich's p's**, obstructing masses in the bronchial tubes in gangrene of the lungs. **epithelial p.**, a mass of ectodermal cells that temporarily closes the external naris of the fetus. **mucous p.**, a plug formed by secretions of the mucous glands of the cervix uteri and closing the cervical canal during pregnancy. **vaginal p.**, one consisting of a mass of coagulated sperm which forms in the vagina of animals after coitus.

plugger (plug'er)   an instrument for compacting filling material in a tooth cavity.

plumbic (plum'bik) pertaining to lead.

plumbism (plum'bizm) a chronic form of poisoning caused by absorption of lead or lead salts.

plumbum (plum'bum) [L.] lead (symbol Pb).

pluri- (ploor'e) word element [L.], *many*.

pluriglandular (ploor"ĭ-glan'du-lar) pertaining to, derived from or affecting several glands.

plurigravida (-grav'ĭ-dah) multigravida.

plurilocular (-lok'u-lar) multilocular.

plurimenorrhea (-men"o-re'ah) increased frequency of menstrual periods.

pluriorificial (-or"ĭ-fish'al) pertaining to or affecting several body orifices.

pluripara (ploo-rip'ah-rah) multipara.

pluriparity (ploor"ĭ-par'ĭ-te) multiparity.

pluripotentiality (-po-ten"she-al'ĭ-te) ability to develop or act in any one of several different ways.

plutonium (ploo-to'ne-um) chemical element (*see table*), at. no. 94, symbol Pu.

Pm chemical symbol, *promethium*.

P.M.I. point of maximal impulse (of the heart).

-pnea (ne'ah) word element [Gr.], *respiration; breathing*. adj., **-pneic**.

pneodynamics (ne"o-di-nam'iks) dynamics of respiration.

pneograph (ne'o-graf) device for registering respiratory movements.

pneometer (ne-om'ĕ-ter) spirometer.

pneoscope (ne'o-skōp) pneumograph.

pneum(o) (nu'mo) word element [Gr.], *air or gas; lung*.

pneumarthrogram (nu-mar'thro-gram) a film obtained by pneumarthrography.

pneumarthrography (nu"mar-throg'rah-fe) radiography of a joint after injection into it of oxygen or other gas.

pneumarthrosis (-thro'sis) gas or air in a joint.

pneumat(o)- (nu'mah-to) word element [Gr.], *air or gas; lung*.

pneumatic (nu-mat'ik) pertaining to air or respiration.

pneumatocele (nu-mat'o-sēl) 1. hernia of lung tissue. 2. a swelling containing a gas.

pneumatodyspnea (nu"mah-to-disp'ne-ah) dyspnea from emphysema.

pneumatogram (nu-mat'o gram) a tracing made by a pneumatograph.

pneumatograph (nu-mat'o-graf) device for registering movements of chest wall.

pneumatology (nu"mah-tol'o-je) science of gases and air and of their therapeutic use.

pneumatometer (-tom'ĕ-ter) spirometer.

pneumatometry (-tom'ĕ-tre) measurement of respiratory movements.

pneumatorrhachis (-tor'ah-kis) presence of gas in vertebral canal.

pneumatosis (-to'sis) air or gas in an abnormal location in the body. **p. cystoi'des intestina'lis, p. cystoi'des intestino'rum,** a condition characterized by the presence of thin-walled, gas-containing cysts in the wall of the intestines.

pneumatotherapy (nu"mah-to-ther'ah-pe) treatment by rarefied or compressed air. **cerebral p.,** injection of pure oxygen into subarachnoid space, in treatment of psychoses.

pneumaturia (-tu're-ah) gas or air in urine.

pneumoamnios (nu"mo-am'ne-os) gas in the amniotic fluid.

pneumoangiogram (-an'je-o-gram") a composite of radiographs obtained by pneumoencephalography and cerebral angiography.

pneumoarthrography (-ar-throg'rah-fe) radiography of a joint after injection of air or gas into the articular capsule.

pneumocephalus (-sef'ah-lus) air in the cerebral ventricles.

pneumococcemia (-kok-se'me-ah) pneumococci in the blood.

pneumococcidal (-kok-si'dal) destroying pneumococci.

pneumococcosis (-kok-o'sis) infection with pneumococci.

pneumococcosuria (-kok"o-su're-ah) pneumococci in the urine.

pneumococcus (-kok'us) pl. *pneumococ'ci*, the organism, *Diplococcus pneumoniae*, which causes lobar pneumonia; it is a small, slightly elongated coccus, one end of which is pointed or lance-shaped, and commonly occurs in pairs; 33 serologic strains or types have been described. adj., **pneumococ'cal**.

pneumoconiosis (-ko"ne-o'sis) a lung disease due to inhalation of inorganic dust.

pneumocranium (-kra'ne-um) air under the dura mater.

pneumocystography (-sis-tog'rah-fe) radiography of the urinary bladder after injection of air or gas.

pneumocystotomography (-sis"to-to-mog'rah-fe) body section roentgenography after inflation of the bladder with air.

pneumoderma (-der'mah) subcutaneous emphysema.

pneumoencephalogram (-en-sef'ah-lo-gram") the film produced by pneumoencephalography.

pneumoencephalography (-en-sef"ah-log'rah-fe) radiography of the intracranial contents after injection of air or gas into the subarachnoid space, usually by spinal puncture.

pneumoencephalomyelogram (-en-sef"ah-lo-mi'el-o-gram") the roentgenogram obtained by pneumoencephalomyelography.

pneumoencephalomyelography (-en-sef"ah-lo-mi"ĕ-log'rah-fe) the making of x-ray films of the brain and spinal cord after injection of air or gas into the subarachnoid space.

pneumography (nu-mog'rah-fe) 1. description of lungs. 2. radiography after injection of air or other gas as a contrast medium.

pneumohemopericardium (nu"mo-he"mo-per"ĭ-kar'de-um) air and blood in the pericardium.

pneumohemothorax (-tho'raks) gas or air and blood in pleural cavity.

pneumohydrometra (nu"mo-hi"dro-me'trah) gas and fluid in the uterus.

pneumohydropericardium (-per"ĭ-kar'de-um)

air or gas with effused serum in the pericardium.

pneumohydrothorax (nu″mo-hi″dro-tho′raks) air or gas with effused fluid in the thoracic cavity.

pneumohypoderma (-hi″po-der′mah) air in the subcutaneous tissues.

pneumolith (nu′mo-lith) a pulmonary concretion.

pneumolithiasis (nu″mo-lĭ-thi′ah-sis) the presence of concretions in the lungs.

pneumology (nu-mol′o-je) the study of diseases of the air passages.

pneumomediastinogram (nu″mo-me″de-as-ti′no-gram) the film produced by pneumomediastinography.

pneumomediastinography (-me″de-as″tĭ-nog′rah-fe) radiography of the mediastinum after injection of air or gas.

pneumomediastinum (-me″de-as-ti′num) presence of air or gas in tissues of the mediastinum, occurring pathologically or introduced intentionally.

pneumometer (nu-mom′ĕ-ter) spirometer.

pneumomyelography (nu″mo-mi″ĕ-log′rah-fe) roentgenography of the spinal canal after injection of air or gas.

pneumonectasis (-nek′tah-sis) emphysema of lungs.

pneumonectomy (-nek′to-me) resection of long tissue: of an entire lung (*total pneumonectomy*) or less (*partial pneumonectomy*), or of a single lobe (*lobectomy*).

pneumonemia (-ne′me-ah) pulmonary congestion.

pneumonia (nu-mo′ne-ah) an acute inflammatory condition of the lung marked by formation of an exudate in the interstitial and cellular portions of the lung. **aspiration p.**, pneumonia due to aspiration of foreign material into the lungs. **atypical p.**, virus pneumonia. **bronchial p.**, bronchopneumonia. **congenital aspiration p.**, idiopathic respiratory distress of newborn. **double p.**, pneumonia affecting both lungs. **Friedländer's p.**, **Friedländer's bacillus p.**, a form characterized by massive mucoid inflammatory exudates in a lobe of the lung, and due to *Klebsiella pneumoniae*. **hypostatic p.**, pneumonia due to dorsal decubitus in weak or aged persons. **inhalation p.**, aspiration pneumonia. **interstitial p.**, a chronic form with increase of the interstitial tissue and decrease of the proper lung tissue, with induration. **lipid p.**, **lipoid p.**, patchy or diffuse consolidation of lung tissue caused by the aspiration of oil. **lobar p.**, an acute infectious disease due to the pneumococcus and marked by inflammation of one or more lobes of the lungs followed by consolidation. **lobular p.**, bronchopneumonia. **primary atypical p.**, **virus p.**, any one of several atypical forms of pneumonia in which no bacteria have been found, especially a peculiar form of bronchopneumonia; generally attributed to an unknown virus.

pneumonic (nu-mon′ik) pertaining to the lung or to pneumonia.

pneumonitis (nu″mo-ni′tis) inflammation of lung tissue.

pneumono- (nu-mo′no) word element [Gr.], *lung*. See also words beginning *pneumato-*, *pneumo-*.

pneumonocentesis (nu-mo″no-sen-te′sis) puncture of a lung for drainage of a cyst or abscess.

pneumonocirrhosis (-sĭ-ro′sis) cirrhosis of the lung.

pneumonoconiosis (-ko″ne-o′sis) pneumoconiosis.

pneumonograph (nu-mon′o-graf) a radiogram of the lungs.

pneumonography (nu″mo-nog′rah-fe) radiography of the lungs.

pneumonolysis (-nol′ĭ-sis) division of tissues attaching the lung to the wall of the chest cavity, to permit collapse of the lung. **extraperiosteal p.**, that in which the separation is between the inner surface of the ribs and the periosteum, which, with the intercostal muscle bundles, remains attached to the parietal pleura. **extrapleural p.**, pneumonolysis in which the separation is between the parietal pleura and the chest wall. **intrapleural p.**, that in which the separation is between the visceral and the parietal pleura.

pneumonometer (-nom′ĕ-ter) spirometer.

pneumonomycosis (nu-mo″no-mi-ko′sis) fungus disease of the lungs.

pneumonopathy (nu″mo-nop′ah-the) any lung disease.

pneumonopexy (nu-mo′no-pek″se) fixation of the lung to the thoracic wall.

pneumonophthisis (nu″mon-of-thi′sis) pulmonary tuberculosis.

pneumonorrhaphy (nu″mon-or′ah-fe) suture of the lung.

pneumonosis (nu″mo-no′sis) any lung disease.

pneumonotomy (-not′o-me) incision of the lung.

pneumopericardium (-per″ĭ-kar′de-um) the presence of air or gas in the pericardial cavity.

pneumoperitoneum (-per″ĭ-to-ne′um) the presence of air or gas in the peritoneal cavity, occurring pathologically or introduced intentionally.

pneumoperitonitis (-ni′tis) peritonitis with formation of gas.

pneumophone (nu′mo-fōn) an instrument for measuring pressure in the middle ear.

pneumopleuritis (nu″mo-ploo-ri′tis) inflammation of lungs and pleura.

pneumopyelography (-pi″ĕ-log′rah-fe) radiography after injection of oxygen into the kidney pelvis.

pneumopyopericardium (-pi″o-per″ĭ-kar′de-um) air or gas and pus in the pericardium.

pneumopyothorax (-tho′raks) air or gas and pus in the pleural cavity.

pneumoradiography (nu″mo-ra″de-og′rah-fe) radiography of a part after injection of oxygen or other gas as contrast material.

pneumoresection (nu″mo-re-sek′shun) removal of a portion of the lung.

pneumoretroperitoneum (-ret″ro-per″ĭ-to-ne′um) presence of air or gas in the retroperitoneal space.

pneumorrhagia (-ra′je-ah) hemorrhage from the lungs.

pneumosilicosis (-sil″ĭ-ko′sis) the deposit of silica particles in the lungs.

pneumotherapy (-ther′ah-pe) 1. treatment of disease of lungs. 2. pneumatotherapy.

pneumothorax (-tho′raks) the presence of air or gas in the pleural cavity or between the pleura and the chest wall, occurring spontaneously or introduced by accident or intent (*artificial pneumothorax*). **extrapleural p.,** injection of air or gas between the chest wall and parietal pleura, to collapse the lung. **spontaneous p.,** entrance of air into the pleural cavity without operation or causative disease.

pneumotomography (-to-mog′rah-fe) body-section radiography after injection of air or other gas into the region or organ being visualized roentgenographically.

pneumotomy (nu-mot′o-me) pneumonotomy.

pneumotoxin (nu″mo-tok′sin) a toxin produced by the bacteria of pneumonia.

pneumotropic (-trop′ik) 1. having a special affinity for lung tissue. 2. having a selective affinity for pneumococci.

pneumotropism (nu-mot′ro-pizm) predilection of an agent or organism for lung tissue.

pneumoventriculography (nu″mo-ven-trik″u-log′rah-fe) pneumoencephalography.

Po chemical symbol, *polonium.*

pock (pok) a pustule, especially of smallpox.

podagra (po-dag′rah) gouty pain in the great toe.

podalgia (po-dal′je-ah) pain in the feet.

podalic (po-dal′ik) accomplished by means of the feet, as podalic version.

Podangium (po-dan′je-um) a genus of Schizomycetes (order Myxobacterales, family Polyangiaceae).

podarthritis (pod″ar-thri′tis) inflammation of the joints of the feet.

podencephalus (pod″en-sef′ah-lus) fetal monster without a cranium, the brain hanging by a pedicle.

podiatrist (po-di′ah-trist) a specialist in podiatry.

podiatry (po-di′ah-tre) the scientific study and care of the feet.

podium (po′de-um) a footlike part, such as an extension of the protoplasm of a cell.

podobromidrosis (pod″o-brom″ĭ-dro′sis) fetid perspiration of the feet.

pododynamometer (-di″nah-mom′ĕ-ter) a device for determining strength of the leg muscles.

pododynia (-din′e-ah) pain in the feet.

podology (po-dol′o-je) study of the foot.

podophyllin (pod″o-fil′in) the yellow purgative resin of Podophyllum.

podophyllum (-fil′um) the dried rhizome and roots of *Podophyllum peltatum;* formerly used as a cathartic.

poe- for words beginning thus, see those beginning *pe-.*

pogoniasis (po″go-ni′ah-sis) excessive or abnormal growth of the beard.

pogonion (po-go′ne-on) the anterior midpoint of the chin.

-poiesis (-poi-e′sis) word element [Gr.], *formation.* adj., **-poiet′ic.**

poikilionia (poi″kil-e-o′ne-ah) variation in the ionic content of the blood.

poikiloblast (poi′kĭ-lo-blast″) a large, nucleated red blood corpuscle.

poikilocyte (poi′kĭ-lo-sīt″) a malformed blood corpuscle.

poikilocytosis (poi″kĭ-lo-si-to′sis) presence of poikilocytes in the blood.

poikiloderma (-der′mah) a condition characterized by pigmentary and atrophic changes in the skin, giving it a mottled appearance.

poikiloplastocyte (-plas′to-sīt) an irregularly shaped blood platelet.

poikiloploid (poi′kĭ-lo-ploid″) 1. pertaining to or characterized by poikiloploidy. 2. an individual having different cells with different numbers of chromosomes.

poikiloploidy (poi′kĭ-lo-ploi′de) the state of having different numbers of chromosomes in different cells.

poikilosmosis (poi″kil-oz-mo′sis) adjustment by a cell, tissue, organ or organism of the tonicity of its fluid milieu to the tonicity of the surrounding medium. adj., **poikilosmot′ic.**

poikilotherm (poi′kĭ-lo-therm″) an organism whose temperature varies with that of the external environment.

poikilothermal (poi″kĭ-lo-ther′mal) poikilothermic.

poikilothermy (-ther′me) the state of having body temperature which varies with that of the environment. adj., **poikilother′mic.**

point (point) a spot having a definite location, but not extending in space. **auricular p.,** the center of the opening of the external auditory meatus. **boiling p.,** the temperature at which a liquid will boil: at sea level, 100°C., or 212°F. **boiling p., normal,** the temperature at which a liquid boils at one atmosphere pressure. **cardinal p′s,** the points on the different refracting media of the eye which determine the direction of the entering or emerging light rays. **cardinal p′s of Capuron,** the ilopectineal eminences and the sacroiliac joints of the pelvis. **craniometric p′s,** the established points of reference for measurement of the skull. **dew p.,** the temperature at which dew is deposited. **disparate p′s,** points on the two retinas on which incident light rays do not produce the same impression. **p′s douloureux,** tender points along certain nerves in neuralgia. **far p.,** the remotest point at which an object is clearly seen when the eye is at rest. **fixation p.,** the point for which accommodation of the eye is momentarily adjusted and where vision is clearest. **freezing p.,** the temperature at which a liquid begins to freeze; for water, 0°C., or 32°F. **ice p.,** the temperature of equilibrium between ice and air-saturated water under one atmosphere pressure. **identical p's,** corresponding points on the retinas of the two eyes. **isoelectric p.,** the pH of a solution at which a dipolar ion does not migrate in an electric field. **isoionic p.,** the pH of a solution at which the number of cations equals the number of anions, solutes other than water and other ions being absent. **lacrimal p.,** a small aperture situated on a slight elevation at the medial end of the lid margin at the junction of its ciliary and lacrimal portions. **McBurney's p.,** a point of special tenderness in appendicitis, on a line connecting the umbilicus and anterior superior spine of the right ilium, about 2 inches from the latter. **melting p.,** the temperature to which a solid must be raised to become liquid. **near p.,** the nearest point of clear vision, the *absolute near point* being that for either eye alone, and the *relative near point* being that for the two eyes together. **nodal p's,** two points on the axis of an optical system situated so that a ray falling on one will produce a parallel ray emerging through the other. **subnasal p.,** the central point at the base of the nasal spine.

pointillage (pwahn-til-yahzh′) [Fr.] massage with the points of the fingers.

poise (poiz) the unit of absolute viscosity, being that of a fluid which would require a shearing force of one dyne to move a square centimeter area of a layer of fluid 1 cm. per second relative to a parallel layer of fluid 1 cm. distant, the space between the layers being filled with the fluid.

poison (poi′zun) a substance which, on ingestion, inhalation, absorption, application, injection or development within the body, in relatively small amounts, produces injury to the body by its chemical action. **corrosive p.,** a poison which acts by directly destroying tissue.

poisoning (poi′zu-ning) the morbid condition produced by a poison. **blood p.,** septicemia. **food p.,** acute illness caused by food which is inherently poisonous or contaminated by certain bacteria. **forage p.,** a disease produced in animals, especially horses, as a result of eating moldy or fermented food. **ivy p.,** dermatitis produced by contact with *Rhus toxicodendron,* or poison ivy. **loco p.,** locoism. **meat p.,** acute gastroenteritis caused by bacterial toxins present in meat. **sausage p.,** botulism. **trinitrotoluene p.,** a toxic condition produced in workers with the chemical, marked by gastritis, abdominal pain, etc.

Polaramine (po-lar′ah-mēn) trademark for preparations of dexchlorpheniramine maleate.

polarimeter (po″lah-rim′ĕ-ter) device for measuring the rotation of polarized light.

polarimetry (-rim′ĕ-tre) measurement of the rotation of polarized light.

polariscope (po-lar′i-skōp) instrument for the study of polarization.

polarity (po-lar′i-te) condition of having poles or of exhibiting opposite effects at the two extremities.

polarization (po″lar-i-za′shun) the production

of that condition in light in which its vibrations are parallel to each other in one plane, or in circles and ellipses.

polarizer (po′lah-rīz-er) an appliance for polarizing light.

poldine (pol′dēn) a compound used in parasympathetic blockade and to reduce acid formation in the stomach.

pole (pōl) 1. either extremity of any axis, as of the fetal ellipse or eye lens. 2. either one of two points which have opposite physical qualities (electric or other). adj., **po′lar. animal p.,** that pole at which the cytoplasm is concentrated in a telolecithal ovum. **anterior p.,** the front or facial end of the anteroposterior axis of the eye. **antigerminal p.,** vegetative pole. **cephalic p.,** the end of the fetal ellipse at which the head of the fetus is situated. **frontal p.,** the most prominent part of the anterior end of each hemisphere of the brain. **germinal p.,** animal pole. **negative p.,** the terminal of an electric cell which has the lower potential, and toward which the current flows. **nutritive p.,** vegetative pole. **occipital p.,** the posterior end of the occipital lobe of the brain. **pelvic p.,** the end of the fetal ellipse at which the breech of the fetus is situated. **placental p.,** the pole of the chorion at which a dome-shaped placenta is located. **positive p.,** the terminal of an electric cell which has the higher potential, and from which the current flows. **posterior p.,** the retinal end of the anteroposterior axis of the eye, usually between the macula lutea and the optic papilla. **temporal p.,** the prominent anterior end of the temporal lobe of the brain. **twin p.,** that part of a spiral-fibered nerve cell from which both the straight and the spiral fibers arise. **vegetal p., vegetative p., vitelline p.,** that pole at the end of an ovum at which the yolk is massed.

poli(o)- (po′le-o) word element [Gr.], *gray substance.*

policeman (po-lēs′man) a tool, usually with a long handle and a stiff or flexible blade or other device at the end, for cleaning laboratory equipment or brushing down precipitates.

policlinic (pol″ĭ-klin′ik) a city hospital or infirmary.

poliencephalitis (po″le-en-sef″ah-li′tis) polioencephalitis.

poliencephalomyelitis (-en-sef″ah-lo-mi″ĕ-li′tis) inflammatory disease of the gray matter of the brain and spinal cord.

polioclastic (po″le-o-klas′tik) destroying gray matter of the nervous system.

polioencephalitis (-en-sef″ah-li′tis) inflammatory disease of the gray substance of the brain. **inferior p.,** bulbar paralysis.

polioencephalomeningomyelitis (-en-sef″ah-lo-mĕ-ning″go-mi″ĕ-li′tis) inflammation of the gray substance of the brain and spinal cord and of the meninges.

polioencephalomyelitis (-mi″ĕ-li′tis) inflammation of the gray substance of the brain and spinal cord.

polioencephalopathy (-en-sef″ah-lop′ah-the)

disease of the gray substance of the brain.

poliomyelencephalitis (po"le-o-mi"el-en-sef"-ah-li'tis) polioencephalomyelitis.

poliomyelitis (-mi"ĕ-li'tis) inflammation of gray substance of spinal cord. **acute anterior p.,** an acute infectious virus disease usually marked by fever, paralysis and muscular atrophy. **ascending p.,** poliomyelitis with a cephalad progression. **bulbar p.,** inflammation affecting the substance of the medulla oblongata.

poliomyelopathy (-mi"ĕ-lop'ah-the) disease of the gray substance of the spinal cord.

polioplasm (po'le-o-plazm") protoplasm.

poliosis (po"le-o'sis) premature grayness of the hair.

poliovirus (-o-vi'rus) the causative agent of poliomyelitis, separable, on the basis of specificity of neutralizing antibody, into three serotypes designated types 1, 2 and 3.

politzerization (pol"it-zer-i-za'shun) inflation of the middle ear by means of a Politzer bag.

pollen (pol'en) the male fertilizing element of flowering plants.

pollenogenic (pol"ĕ-no-jen'ik) caused by the pollen of plants.

pollenosis (-no'sis) pollinosis.

pollex (pol'eks) [L.] thumb. **p. pe'dis,** great toe; hallux.

pollinosis (pol"ĭ-no'sis) an allergic reaction to pollen; hay fever.

polocyte (po'lo-sit) a polar body.

polonium (po-lo'ne-um) chemical element *(see table),* at. no. 84, symbol Po.

poloxalkol (pol-ok'sal-kol) a pharmacologically inert oxyalkylene polymer used as a fecal softener.

polus (po'lus), pl. *po'li* [L.] pole.

poly- (pol'e) word element [Gr.], *many.*

polyadenia (pol"e-ah-de'ne-ah) pseudoleukemia.

polyadenomatosis (-ad"ĕ-no"mah-to'sis) multiple adenomas in a part.

polyadenous (-ad'ĕ-nus) having many glands.

polyagglutinability (-ah gloo"ti-nah-bil'ĭ-te) susceptibility to agglutination by a number of agents.

polyandry (-an'dre) 1. concurrent marriage of a woman to more than one man. 2. union of two or more male pronuclei with a female pronucleus, resulting in polyploidy of the zygote.

Polyangiaceae (-an"je-a'se-e) a family of Schizomycetes (order Myxobacterales) found in soil and decaying organic matter.

polyangiitis (-an"je-i'tis) inflammation involving multiple blood or lymph vessels.

Polyangium (-an'je-um) a genus of Schizomycetes (order Myxobacterales, family Polyangiaceae).

polyarteritis (-ar"tĕ-ri'tis) inflammation of several arteries. **p. nodo'sa,** periarteritis nodosa.

polyarthric (-ar'thrik) polyarticular.

polyarthritis (-ar-thri'tis) inflammation of several joints. **p. rheumat'ica,** rheumatic fever.

polyarticular (pol"e-ar-tik'u-lar) affecting many joints.

polyatomic (-ah-tom'ik) made up of several atoms.

polyauxotroph (-awk'so-trōf) an organism, especially a mutant, requiring multiple growth factors. adj., **polyauxotroph'ic.**

polybasic (-ba'sik) having several replaceable hydrogen atoms.

polyblast (pol'e-blast) any cell in new-formed connective tissue which is neither a leukocyte nor a fibroblast.

Polybrene (pol'e-brēn) trademark for a preparation of hexadimethrine bromide.

polyceptor (pol"e-sep'tor) an amboceptor capable of binding several different complements.

polychemotherapy (-ke"mo-ther'ah-pe) simultaneous administration of several chemotherapeutic agents.

polycholia (-ko'le-ah) excessive secretion of bile.

polychondritis (-kon-dri'tis) inflammation of many cartilages of the body. **chronic atrophic p., p. chron'ica atro'phicans, relapsing p.,** an acquired disease of unknown origin, chiefly involving various cartilages and showing both chronicity and a tendency to recurrence.

polychondropathy (-kon-drop'ah-the) relapsing polychondritis.

polychrest (pol'e-krest) 1. useful in many conditions. 2. a remedy useful in many diseases.

polychromatic (pol"e-kro-mat'ik) many-colored.

polychromatophil (-kro-mat'o fil) an element stainable with many kinds of stain.

polychromatophilia (-kro-mat"o-fil'e-ah) 1. the property of being stainable with various stains. 2. excess of polychromatophilic cells in the blood. adj., **polychromatophil'ic.**

polychromemia (-kro-me'me-ah) increase in coloring matter of the blood.

polychromia (-kro'me-ah) increased color formation.

polyclinic (-klin'ik) hospital or infirmary treating patients with many kinds of diseases.

polyclonia (-klo'ne-ah) a disease marked by many clonic spasms.

polycoria (-ko're-ah) the presence of more than one pupil.

polycrotism (po-lik'ro-tizm) the quality of having several secondary waves to each beat of the pulse. adj., **polycrot'ic.**

Polycycline (pol"e-si'klēn) trademark for preparations of tetracycline hydrochloride.

polycyesis (-si-e'sis) multiple pregnancy.

polycystic (-sis'tik) containing many cysts or cavities.

polycyte (pol'e-sit) a hypersegmented polymorphonuclear leukocyte of normal size.

polycythemia (pol"e-si-the'me-ah) abnormal increase in the erythrocytes in the circulating blood. **p. hyperton'ica,** polycythemia with hypertrophy of the heart and hypertension. **myelopathic p., primary p.,** polycythemia vera. **relative p.,** apparent increase in erythrocytes due to decrease in the fluid portion of the blood. **p. ru'bra,** polycythemia vera. **secondary p.,** any absolute increase in the total red cell mass other than polycythemia vera. **splenomegalic p.,** polycythemia vera. **stress p.,** stress erythrocytosis. **p. ve'ra,** a familial disease of unknown origin, marked by an absolute increase in the red cell mass and total blood volume, with splenomegaly, leukocytosis, thrombocytosis and signs of bone marrow hyperactivity.

polycytosis (pol"e-si-to'sis) excess of cells in the blood.

polydactylia (-dak-til'e-ah) the presence of supernumerary digits on hands or feet.

polydentia (-den'she-ah) polyodontia.

polydipsia (-dip'se-ah) excessive thirst.

polydysspondylism (-dis-spon'dĭ-lizm) malformation of several vertebrae and the sella turcica, with dwarfed stature and low intelligence.

polyembryony (-em-bri'o-ne) the production of two or more embryos from a single ovum.

polyemia (-e'me-ah) excessive blood in the body. **p. hyperalbumino'sa,** excess of albumin in blood plasma. **p. polycythem'ica,** an increase in red corpuscles of blood. **p. sero'sa,** increase in amount of blood serum.

polyesthesia (-es-the'ze-ah) a sensation as if several points were touched on application of a stimulus to a single point.

polyesthetic (-es-thet'ik) affecting several senses.

polyethylene (-eth'ĭ-lēn) a compound formed by polymerization of ethylene. **p. glycol,** a polymer of ethylene oxide and water, available in liquid form (polyethylene glycol 300 or 400) or as waxy solids (polyethylene glycol 1540 or 4000), used in various pharmaceutical preparations.

polygalactia (-gah-lak'she-ah) excessive secretion of milk.

polygenic (-jen'ik) pertaining to or influenced by several different genes.

polyglandular (-glan'du-lar) affecting many glands.

polygnathus (po-lig'nah-thus) double fetal monster united by the jaws.

polygram (pol'e-gram) a tracing made by a polygraph.

polygraph (pol'e-graf) an apparatus for simultaneously recording blood pressure, pulse and respiration, and variations in electrical resistance of the skin; popularly known as a lie-detector.

polygyny (po-lij'ĭ-ne) 1. concurrent marriage of a man to more than one woman. 2. union of two or more female pronuclei with one male pronucleus, resulting in polyploidy of the zygote.

polygyria (pol"e-ji're-ah) excess of cerebral gyri.

polyhedral (-he'dral) having many sides or surfaces.

polyhydramnios (-hi-dram'ne-os) excess of liquor amnii in pregnancy.

polyhydrosis (-hi-dro'sis) excessive secretion of sweat.

polyhydruria (pol"e-hi-droo're-ah) abnormal dilution of the urine.

polyidrosis (-ĭ-dro'sis) polyhydrosis.

polyinfection (-in-fek'shun) infection with more than one organism.

polykaryocyte (-kar'e-o-sīt") a giant cell containing several nuclei.

Polykol (pol'e-kol) trademark for preparations of poloxalkol.

polyleptic (pol"e-lep'tik) having many remissions and exacerbations.

polymastia (-mas'te-ah) presence of supernumerary mammary glands.

polymelus (po-lim'ē-lus) fetus with supernumerary limbs.

polymenia (pol"e-me'ne-ah) polymenorrhea.

polymenorrhea (-men"o-re'ah) abnormally frequent menstruation.

polymer (pol'ĭ-mer) a compound, usually of high molecular weight, formed by combination of simpler molecules. **addition p.,** one formed by repeated combination of the smaller molecules (monomers) without formation of any other product. **condensation p.,** one formed by repeated combination of the smaller molecules, with simultaneous elimination of water or other simple compound.

polymeria (pol"ĭ-me're-ah) presence of supernumerary parts of the body.

polymeric (-mer'ik) characterized by polymerism.

polymerism (po-lim'ē-rizm, pol'ĭ-mĕ-rizm") the state of being a polymer.

polymerization (po-lim"er-i-za'shun, -mer"i-za'shun) the formation of a compound, usually of high molecular weight, by the combination of several identical molecules (monomers).

polymicrobic (pol"e-mi-kro'bik) pertaining to or caused by several varieties of pathogenic microorganisms.

polymorphism (-mor'fizm) the quality of existing in several different forms. adj., **polymor'phous.**

polymorphocellular (-mor"fo-sel'u-lar) having cells of many forms.

polymorphonuclear (-nu'kle-ar) having a nucleus so deeply lobed or so divided as to appear to be multiple.

polymyalgia (pol"e-mi-al'je-ah) pain involving many muscles.

polymyoclonus (-mi-ok'lo-nus) 1. a minute muscular tremor. 2. polyclonia.

polymyopathy (-mi-op'ah-the) disease affecting several muscles simultaneously.

polymyositis (-mi"o-si'tis) inflammation of many muscles.

polymyxin (-mik'sin) an antibiotic substance derived from culture of various strains of *Bacillus polymyxa,* several closely related compounds being designated by letters. **p. B,** a compound effective against gram-negative bacteria.

polynesic (pol"ĭ-ne'sik) affecting many separate locations.

polyneural (-nu'ral) pertaining to many nerves.

polyneuralgia (pol"e-nu-ral'je-ah) neuralgia of several nerves.

polyneuritis (-nu-ri'tis) inflammation involving many peripheral nerves.

polyneuromyositis (-nu"ro-mi-o-si'tis) inflammation involving several muscles, with loss of reflexes, sensory loss and paresthesias.

polyneuropathy (-nu-rop'ah-the) a disease involving several nerves.

polyneuroradiculitis (-nu"ro-rah-dik"u-li'tis) inflammation of spinal ganglia, nerve roots and peripheral nerves.

polynuclear (-nu"kle-ar) 1. polynucleate. 2. polymorphonuclear.

polynucleate (-nu'kle-āt) having many nuclei.

polyodontia (-o-don'she-ah) presence of supernumerary teeth.

polyonychia (-o-nik'e-ah) presence of supernumerary nails.

polyopia (-o'pe-ah) visual perception of several images of a single object.

polyorchidism (-or'ki-dizm) the presence of more than two testes.

polyorchis (-or'kis) a person exhibiting polyorchidism.

polyorchism (-or'kizm) polyorchidism.

polyorrhymenitis (-or"hi-mē-ni'tis) malignant inflammation of serous membranes.

polyostotic (-os-tot'ik) affecting several bones.

polyotia (-o'she-ah) presence of more than two ears.

polyovulatory (-ov'u-lah-tor"e) normally discharging several ova in one ovarian cycle.

polyp (pol'ip) a morbid excrescence from a mucous membrane. **adenomatous p.,** one that has undergone malignant degeneration. **fibrinous p.,** intrauterine polyp made up of fibrin from retained blood.

polyparesis (pol"e-par'ē-sis) general paresis.

polypathia (-path'e-ah) the presence of several diseases at one time.

polypectomy (-pek'to-me) surgical excision of a polyp.

polypeptidase (-pep'tī-dās) an enzyme which catalyzes the hydrolysis of polypeptides.

polypeptide (-pep'tīd) a compound containing two or more amino acids linked by a peptide bond; called dipeptide, tripeptide, etc., depending on the number of amino acids present.

polyperiostitis (-per"e-os-ti'tis) inflammation of the periosteum of several bones. **p. hyperesthet'ica,** a chronic disease of the periosteum with extreme tenderness of the skin and soft parts.

polyphagia (-fa'je-ah) excessive ingestion of food.

polyphalangism (-fah-lan'jizm) excess of phalanges in a finger or toe.

polypharmacy (-far'mah-se) the simultaneous administration of several therapeutic agents in combination or separately.

polyphasic (-fa'zik) having or existing in many phases; having unlike particles in the disperse phase.

polyphobia (-fo'be-ah) abnormal fear of many things.

polyphrasia (-fra'ze-ah) morbid volubility.

polyplastic (pol"e-plas'tik) 1. composed of many cells. 2. passing through many changes of form.

polyplegia (-ple'je-ah) paralysis of several muscles.

polyploid (pol'e-ploid) 1. characterized by polyploidy. 2. an individual or cell characterized by polyploidy.

polyploidy (pol'e-ploi"de) the state of having more than two sets of homologous chromosomes.

polypnea (pol"ip-ne'ah) rapid or panting respiration.

polypodia (pol"e-po'de-ah) the presence of supernumerary feet.

polypoid (pol'ĭ-poid) resembling a polyp.

polyposia (pol"ĭ-po'ze-ah) ingestion of abnormally increased amounts of fluids for long periods of time.

polyposis (-po'sis) the formation of numerous polyps. **familial p.,** the appearance in childhood of innumerable adenomatous polyps in the lower bowel, tending to occur in several members of the same family.

polypus (pol'ĭ-pus), pl. *pol'ypi* [L.] polyp.

polyradiculitis (pol"e-rah-dik"u-li'tis) inflammation of the nerve roots.

polyradiculoneuritis (-rah-dik"u-lo-nu-ri'tis) acute infectious polyneuritis which involves the peripheral nerves, the spinal nerve roots and the spinal cord.

polyribosome (-ri'bo-sōm) a cluster of ribosomes in the cytoplasm of a cell.

polysaccharide (-sak'ah-rīd) a carbohydrate which, on acid hydrolysis, yields 10 or more monosaccharides.

polysarcous (-sar'kus) corpulent; too fleshy.

polyscelia (-se'le-ah) presence of more than two legs.

polysensitivity (-sen"sĭ-tiv'ĭ-te) sensitivity to a number of different stimuli.

polyserositis (-se"ro-si'tis) general inflammation of serous membranes.

polysinusectomy (-si"nu-sek'to-me) excision of diseased mucous membrane of several paranasal sinuses.

polysinusitis (-si"nu-si'tis) inflammation of several sinuses.

polysome (pol'e-sōm) polyribosome.

polysomia (pol"e-so'me-ah) developmental anomaly with doubling or tripling of the body.

polysomus (-so'mus) a fetal monster exhibiting polysomia.

polysomy (-so'me) an excess of a particular chromosome.

polysorbate 80 (-sor'bāt) an oleate ester of sorbitol and its anhydride condensed with polymers of ethylene oxide, consisting of approximately 20 oxyethylene units; used as a surfactant agent.

polyspermia (-sper'me-ah) 1. excessive secretion of semen. 2. polyspermy.

polyspermy (-sper'me) fertilization of an ovum by more than one spermatozoon; occurring normally in certain species (*physiologic polyspermy*) and sometimes abnormally in others (*pathologic polyspermy*).

polystichia (pol″e-stik′e-ah) two or more rows of eyelashes on a lid.

polystyrene (-sti′rēn) the resin produced by polymerization of styrene, a clear resin of the thermoplastic type, used in the construction of denture bases.

polytene (pol′e-tēn) composed of or containing many strands of chromatin (chromonemata).

polyteny (pol″e-te′ne) reduplication of chromonemata in the chromosome without separation into distinct daughter chromosomes.

polythelia (-the′le-ah) presence of supernumerary nipples.

polytocous (po-lit′ŏ-kus) giving birth to several offspring at one time.

polytrichia (pol″e-trik′e-ah) hypertrichiasis.

polytrophia (-tro′fe-ah) overnutrition.

polytropic (-trop′ik) affecting many kinds of bacteria or several kinds of tissue.

polyunguia (-ung′gwe-ah) presence of supernumerary nails on fingers or toes.

polyuria (-u′re-ah) excessive secretion of urine.

polyvalent (-va′lent) multivalent.

polyvinylpyrrolidine (-vi″nil-pi-rol′ĭ-dēn) a polymer of formaldehyde, used extensively as a plasma substitute.

pompholyx (pom′fo-liks) a skin disease with small, deep-seated vesicles on the palms and soles and between the digits.

pomphus (pom′fus) a wheal.

pomum (po′mum), pl. *po′ma* [L.] apple. **p. ada′mi,** the prominence on the throat caused by thyroid cartilage.

ponophobia (po″no-fo′be-ah) abnormal fear of pain or fatigue.

ponos (po′nos) infantile kala-azar.

pons (ponz) that part of the hindbrain lying above the medulla oblongata and, with the cerebellum and middle part of the fourth ventricle, constituting the metencephalon. **p. hep′atis,** a projection partially bridging the longitudinal fissure of the liver. **p. tari′ni,** the floor of the posterior perforated space. **p. varo′lii,** the organ connecting the cerebrum, cerebellum and oblongata.

pontic (pon′tik) the portion of a bridge which substitutes for an absent tooth.

ponticulus (pon-tik′u-lus), pl. *pontic′uli* [L.] propons. adj., **pontic′ular.**

pontine (pon′tin) pertaining to the pons varolii.

Pontocaine (pon′to-kān) trademark for preparations of tetracaine.

pontocerebellar (pon″to-ser″ĕ-bel′ar) pertaining to pons varolii and cerebellum.

popliteal (pop″lĭ-te′al) pertaining to the area behind the knee.

population (pop″u-la′shun) the collection of individuals constituting a certain class, or occupying a certain area. **C₃ p.,** those individuals who are mentally or physically defective.

poradenitis (pōr″ad-ĕ-ni′tis) suppurative inflammation of lymph nodes with formation of draining fistulas. **p. nos′tras,** lymphogranuloma venereum.

porcelain (pōr′sĕ-lin) a fused mixture of kaolin, felspar, quartz and other substances, used in the making of artificial teeth, jacket crowns, facings and veneers.

pore (pōr) a small opening or empty space.

porencephalia (po″ren-se-fa′le-ah) porencephaly.

porencephalitis (-sef″ah-li′tis) porencephaly with inflammation of brain.

porencephalous (-sef″ah-lus) characterized by porencephaly.

porencephaly (-sef′ah-le) development or presence of abnormal cavities in the brain tissue.

porocele (po′ro-sēl) scrotal hernia with thickening of the coverings.

porocephaliasis (po″ro-sef″ah-li′ah-sis) infection with parasites of the genus Porocephalus.

Porocephalus (-sef′ah-lus) a genus of wormlike animals, including the species *P. crotalus,* parasitic in rattlesnakes and water moccasins.

porokeratosis (-ker″ah-to′sis) hypertrophy of the stratum corneum, followed by its atrophy.

porosis (po-ro′sis) formation of callus at the ends of fractured bones.

porosity (po-ros′ĭ-te) the condition of being porous.

porotomy (po-rot′o-me) meatotomy.

porphin (por′fin) the fundamental ring structure of four linked pyrrole nuclei around which porphyrins, hemin and chlorophyll are built.

porphobilinogen (por″fo-bi-lin′o-jen) an intermediary product in the biosynthesis of heme.

porphobilinogenuria (-bi-lin″o-jen-u′re-ah) excretion of porphobilinogen in the urine.

porphyria (por-fēr′e-ah) a disturbance of porphyrin metabolism characterized by increase in formation and excretion of porphyrins or their precursors. **p. cuta′nea tar′da heredita′ria,** a familial or genetic abnormality of porphyrin metabolism in which cutaneous manifestations are in the foreground of the clinical picture. **p. cuta′nea tar′da symptomat′ica,** a cutaneous form of porphyria which is not believed to be hereditary. **p. erythropoiet′ica,** a form of porphyria in which the excessive porphyrin formation takes place in bone marrow normoblasts.

porphyrin (por′fĭ-rin) one of a group of complex cyclic compounds which are important components of hemoglobin, myoglobin, cytochrome and catalase.

porphyrinogen (por″fĭ-rin′o-jen) a colorless, fully hydrogenated compound giving rise to the corresponding porphyrin by oxidation.

porphyrinopathy (por″fir-in-op′ah-the) a disorder of porphyrin metabolism.

porphyrinuria (por″fĭ-rĭ-nu′re-ah) excretion of an abnormal type or quantity of porphyrin in the urine.

porrigo (por′ĭ-go) ringworm or other disease of the scalp. **p. decal′vans,** alopecia areata. **p. favo′sa,** favus. **p. larva′lis,** eczema with impetigo of scalp.

porta (por′tah), pl. *por′tae* [L.] an entrance or

gateway. **p. hep'atis,** the transverse fissure of the liver.

portacaval (por"tah-ka'val) pertaining to portal vein and inferior vena cava.

portal (por'tal) 1. an avenue of entrance. 2. pertaining to an entrance. **p. of entry,** the pathway by which bacteria or other pathogenic agents gain entry to the body.

porte-polisher (port-pol'ish-er) a hand instrument for holding a wooden point to be used in a dental engine for applying polishing paste and burnishing teeth.

portio (por'she-o), pl. *portio'nes* [L.] a part or division; used in names of parts of various structures of the body. **p. du'ra,** the facial nerve. **p. interme'dia,** a fasciculus which joins the facial and acoustic nerves. **p. mol'lis,** acoustic nerve. **p. vagina'lis,** portion of uterus which projects into the vagina.

portogram (por'to-gram) the film obtained by portography.

portography (por-tog'rah-fe) radiography of the portal vein after injection of opaque material. **portal p.,** portography after injection of opaque material into the superior mesenteric vein or one of its branches, the abdomen being opened. **splenic p.,** portography after percutaneous injection of opaque material into the substance of the spleen.

porus (po'rus), pl. *po'ri* [L.] an opening; used in names of various openings in the body. **p. acus'ticus exter'nus,** outer end of external auditory meatus. **p. acus'ticus inter'nus,** opening of internal auditory canal into cranial cavity. **p. op'ticus,** the opening in the sclera for passage of the optic nerve.

-posia (po'ze-ah) word element [Gr.], *drinking; intake of fluids.*

position (po-zish'un) attitude or placement of the body, especially the relation of the body of the fetus to the maternal pelvis at the beginning of parturition (see table of *Various Fetal Positions in Utero*). **anatomic p.,** that of the human body, standing erect and arms with palms facing forward, used as the position of reference in designating the site or direction of structures of the body. **decubitus p.,** that of the body lying on a horizontal surface, designated according to the aspect of the body touching the surface as *dorsal decubitus, left* or *right lateral decubitus* and *ventral decubitus position.* **Fowler's p.,** that in which the head of the patient's bed is raised 18–20 inches above the level. **genucubital p.,** knee-chest position. **genupectoral p.,** the patient resting on his knees and chest, arms crossed above his head. **knee-chest p.,** the patient on his knees and elbows, his head on his hands. **lithotomy p.,** the patient on his back, legs flexed on his thighs, thighs flexed on his abdomen and abducted. **Sims's p.,** patient on left side and chest, right knee and thigh drawn up, left arm along the back. **Trendelenburg's p.,** patient on back, on a plane inclined 45 degrees, legs and feet hanging down over end of table.

positive (poz'i-tiv) having a value greater than

VARIOUS FETAL POSITIONS IN UTERO

IN CEPHALIC PRESENTATION

Vertex — occiput the point of direction
  Left occiput anterior (L.O.A.)
  Left occiput transverse (L.O.T.)
  Right occiput posterior (R.O.P.)
  Right occiput transverse (R.O.T.)
  Right occiput anterior (R.O.A.)
  Left occiput posterior (L.O.P.)
Face — chin the point of direction
  Right mentoposterior (R.M.P.)
  Left mento-anterior (L.M.A.)
  Right mentotransverse (R.M.T.)
  Right mento-anterior (R.M.A.)
  Left mentotransverse (L.M.T.)
  Left mentoposterior (L.M.P.)
Brow — the point of direction
  Right frontoposterior (R.F.P.)
  Left fronto-anterior (L.F.A.)
  Right frontotransverse (R.F.T.)
  Right fronto-anterior (R.F.A.)
  Left frontotransverse (L.F.T.)
  Left frontoposterior (L.F.P.)

IN BREECH PRESENTATION

Complete breech — sacrum, the point of direction (feet crossed and thighs flexed on abdomen)
  Left sacro-anterior (L.S.A.)
  Left sacrotransverse (L.S.T.)
  Right sacroposterior (R.S.P.)
  Right sacro-anterior (R.S.A.)
  Right sacrotransverse (R.S.T.)
  Left sacroposterior (L.S.P.)
Incomplete breech — sacrum the point of direction. Same designations as above, adding the qualifications footling, knee, etc.

IN TRANSVERSE PRESENTATION

Shoulder — scapula the point of direction

Left scapulo-anterior (L. Sc. A.)	Back anterior positions
Right scapulo-anterior (R. Sc. A.)	
Right scapuloposterior (R. Sc. P.)	Back posterior positions
Left scapuloposterior (L. Sc. P.)	

zero; indicating the existence or presence, as chromatin-positive; characterized by affirmation or cooperation.

positron (poz'i-tron) a positively charged electron.

posology (po-sol'o-je) science or system of dosage.

post (post) [L.] preposition, *after;* used also as a prefix, *after, behind* (in time or space).

postalbumin (post"al-bu'min) a serum protein which has an electrophoretic mobility between albumin and alpha-globulin at pH 8.6.

postaurale (post"aw-ra'le) an anthropometric landmark, the most posterior point on the helix of the ear.

postaxial (post-ak'se-al) behind an axis.

postcardiotomy (-kar"de-ot'o-me) occurring after or as a consequence of open-heart surgery.

postcava (pōst-ka'vah) the inferior vena cava. adj., **postca'val.**

postcibal (-si'bal) after eating.

postclavicular (pōst"klah-vik'u-lar) behind the clavicle.

postclimacteric (pōst"kli-mak'ter"ik) after the climacteric.

postcommissure (pōst-kom'ĭ-shūr) the posterior commissure of the brain.

postcornu (-kor'nu) the posterior horn of the lateral ventricle.

postcyclodialysis (-si"klo-di-al'ĭ-sis) occuring after or as a consequence of cyclodialysis.

postdiastolic (-di"as-tol'ik) after diastole.

postdicrotic (pōst"di-krot'ik) after the dicrotic elevation of the sphygmogram.

postencephalitis (pōst"en-sef"ah-li'tis) a condition sometimes remaining after recovery from epidemic encephalitis.

postepileptic (pōst"ep-ĭ-lep'tik) following an epileptic attack.

posterior (pos-tēr'e-or) directed toward or situated at the back; opposite of anterior.

postero- (pos'ter-o) word element [L.], *the back; posterior to.*

posteroanterior (pos"ter-o-an-te're-or) directed from the back toward the front.

posteroclusion (-kloo'zhun) malrelation of dental arches with the mandibular arch posterior to the maxillary arch.

postero-external (-ek-ster'nal) situated on the outside of a posterior aspect.

posterolateral (-lat'er-al) situated on the side and toward the posterior aspect.

posteromedian (-me'de-an) situated on the middle of a posterior aspect.

posterosuperior (-su-pēr'e-or) situated behind and above.

postesophageal (pōst"e-sof"ah-ge'al) behind the esophagus.

postethmoid (pōst-eth'moid) behind the ethmoid bone.

postglomerular (pōst"glo-mer'u-lar) distal to a ganglion.

postgeminum (pōst-jem'ĭ-num) the posterior corpora quadrigemina.

postgeniculatum (pōst"jē-nik"u-la'tum) the internal geniculate body.

postglomerular (pōst"glo-mer'u-lar) distal to a glomerulus.

posthepatitic (post"hep-ah-tit'ik) occurring after or as a consequence of hepatitis.

posthioplasty (pos'the-o-plas"te) plastic repair of the prepuce.

posthitis (pos-thi'tis) inflammation of the prepuce.

postligation (pōst"li-ga'shun) occurring after or as a consequence of ligation of a blood vessel.

postmaturity (pōst"mah-tū'rĭ-te) the quality of exceeding the period of maturity, used of a fetus not born at the end of the usual period of gestation.

postmedian (pōst-me'de-an) behind a median line or plane.

postmeiotic (post"mi-ot'ik) occurring after or pertaining to time following meiosis.

postminimus (pōst-min'ĭ-mus) an appendage

attached to the proximal phalanx of the fifth finger or toe.

postmitotic (post"mi-tot'ik) occurring after or pertaining to time following mitosis.

post mortem (pōst mor'tem) after death.

postmortem (pōst-mor'tem) performed or occurring after death.

postnatal (-na'tal) occurring after birth.

postoblongata (pōst"ob-long-gah'tah) part of oblongata below the pons.

postoperative (pōst-op'er-a"tiv) after a surgical operation.

postoral (-o'ral) in the back part of the mouth.

postpallium (-pal'e-um) the cerebral cortex behind the fissure of Rolando.

postparalytic (pōst"par-ah-lit'ik) following an attack of paralysis.

post partum (pōst par'tum) after parturition.

postpartum (pōst-par'tum) occurring after childbirth or delivery.

postpontile (-pon'til) behind the pons varolii.

postprandial (-pran'de-al) after a meal.

postpubescent (pōst"pu-bes'ent) after puberty.

postsynaptic (post"sĭ-nap'tik) situated distal to a synapse, or occurring after the synapse is crossed.

postulate (pos'tu-lāt) anything assumed or taken for granted. **Koch's p's,** a statement of the kind of experimental evidence required to establish the causative relation of a given microorganism to a given disease.

posture (pos'tūr) an attitude of the body. adj., **pos'tural.**

postuterine (pōst-u'ter-īn) behind the uterus.

postvaccinal (-vak'sĭ-nal) occurring after vaccinia or after inoculation of vaccinia virus.

postvermis (-ver'mis) the lower surface of the vermis of the cerebellum.

postvital (-vi'tal) following cessation of life.

postzygotic (post"zi-got'ik) occurring after or pertaining to the time following the union of the gametes (formation of the zygote).

potable (po'tah-bl) fit to drink.

potamophobia (po"tah-mo-fo'be-ah) a dread of large bodies of water.

potash (pot'ash) impure potassium carbonate. **caustic p.,** potassium hydroxide. **sulfurated p.,** a mixture of potassium polysulfides and potassium thiosulfate; antiparasitic, local stimulant.

potassa (po-tas'ah) potassium hydroxide.

potassemia (pot"ah-se'me-ah) excess of potassium in the blood.

potassic (po-tas'ik) containing potassium.

potassium (po-tas'e-um) chemical element *(see table),* at. no. 19, symbol K. **p. acetate,** a compound used as a systemic and urinary alkalizer. **p. bicarbonate,** a transparent, crystalline salt used as a gastric antacid and to replenish electrolytes in the body. **p. bismuth tartrate,** bismuth potassium tartrate. **p. bitartrate,** a white, crystalline salt used as a diuretic, cathartic and refrigerant. **p. bromide,** a colorless, crystalline body used as a sedative and antiepileptic. **p. carbonate,** white, crystalline or granular salt, used chiefly in pharmaceutical and chemical manufacturing procedures. **p. chlorate,** a highly toxic compound used as an oxidizing germicide and for hemorrhoids and proctitis. **p. chloride,** a white, crystalline compound used orally or intravenously as an electrolyte replenisher. **p. citrate,** a white, granular powder used as a diuretic, expectorant, sudorific and systemic alkalizer. **p. guaiacolsulfonate,** a white, crystalline compound used as an expectorant. **p. hydroxide,** a white, crystalline compound with alkaline and caustic properties. **p. iodide,** a colorless, transparent body used as an expectorant and in prophylaxis of goiter. **p. mercuric oxide,** a complex used as a germicide and as an ingredient of various reagents. **p. nitrate,** a white, crystalline salt used as a diuretic. **p. nitrite,** a compound sometimes used in place of sodium nitrite. **p. permanganate,** a dark purple, crystalline salt used as an oxidant and local anti-infective. **p. phosphate,** a salt used as a mild laxative and diuretic. **p. sodium tartrate,** a compound used as a saline cathartic and also in combination with sodium bicarbonate and tartaric acid (Seidlitz powders). **p. sulfate,** a compound having an extremely irritant action on stomach and intestines. **p. sulfite,** a white, crystalline salt used as a mild laxative and diuretic. **p. sulfocyanate,** potassium thiocyanate. **p. tartrate,** a compound used as a diuretic, diaphoretic and cathartic. **p. thiocyanate,** a colorless, crystalline salt used as a reagent and a vasodilator.

potency (po'ten-se) power or ability; sexual adequacy, especially in the male. **prospective p.,** the total developmental possibilities of an embryonic part.

potential (po-ten'shal) 1. existing and ready for action, but not active. 2. electric tension or pressure. **action p.,** the temporary change in potential between stimulated and resting portions of a cell. **biotic p.,** the inherent power of a population to increase in numbers when the age ratio is stable and all environmental conditions are optimal. **injury p.,** the potential measured between electrodes placed on the intact and on the injured portion of a cell. **resting p.,** the potential present within the resting cell.

potentiation (po-ten″she-a'shun) enhancement of one agent by another so that the combined effect is greater than the sum of the effects of each one alone.

potion (po'shun) a large dose of liquid medicine.

pouch (powch) a pocket-like space, cavity or sac, e.g. one formed by reflection of the peritoneum on the surfaces of adjoining organs. **abdominovesical p.,** the pouchlike reflection of the peritoneum from the abdominal wall to the anterior surface of the bladder. **Rathke's p.,** a diverticulum from the embryonic buccal cavity from which the anterior lobe of the hypophysis cerebri is developed.

poudrage (poo-drahzh') [Fr.]. application of a powder (e.g. talc or asbestos) to a surface, as

done to promote fusion of serous membranes (e.g. two layers of pericardium or pleura).

poultice (pōl'tis) a soft, pultaceous mass to be placed hot upon the skin.

pound (pownd) a unit of weight in the avoirdupois (453.6 grams, or 16 ounces) or apothecaries' (373.2 grams, or 12 ounces) system.

povidone-iodine (po'vĭ-dōn-i'o-dīn) a complex produced by reacting iodine with the polymer polyvinylpyrrolidone; used as a mild anti-infective agent.

powder (pow'der) aggregation of particles obtained by grinding or triturating a solid. **aromatic p.,** powder of cinnamon, ginger, cardamon seed and myristica. **Dover's p.,** powder of ipecac and opium. **dusting p.,** an absorbent, antiseptic, astringent or soothing powder for external use. **effervescent p., compound,** (1) a mixture of sodium bicarbonate and potassium tartrate and (2) tartaric acid, each to be dissolved in water and the solutions mixed as the effervescence subsides; aperient. **Seidlitz p's,** a mixture of sodium bicarbonate, potassium sodium tartrate and tartaric acid; used as a cathartic.

power (pow'er) the ability to accomplish an act. **candle p.,** the luminous intensity of a light source, expressed in international candles. **carbon dioxide-combining p.,** ability of the blood plasma to combine with carbon dioxide. **defining p.,** the ability of a lens to make an object clearly visible. **penetrating p.,** focal length.

pox (poks) an eruptive disease.

poxvirus (poks-vi'rus) one of a group of morphologically similar and immunologically related agents, including the viruses of vaccinia and variola.

P.P.D. purified protein derivative.

ppg. picopicogram.

PPLO pleuropneumonia-like organisms.

p.p.m. parts per million.

Pr chemical symbol, *praseodymium.*

practice (prak'tis) the putting of knowledge into use; the use of knowledge and skill in a particular endeavor. **dental p.,** the occupation of a dentist in caring for the dental conditions of patients. **family p.,** a specialized area of medicine in which the physician assumes responsibility for physical and mental care of all members of the basic family unit to prevent and to treat illness or accident. **general p.,** the provision of comprehensive medical care as a continuing responsibility regardless of age of the patient or of the condition that may temporarily require the services of a specialist. **medical p.,** the occupation of a physician in caring for the medical conditions of patients.

practitioner (prak-tish'un-er) one who uses his knowledge and skills to a specific purpose. **general p.,** a legally qualified doctor of medicine whose practice is not limited to a particular field of medicine or surgery. **nurse p.,** any person prepared and authorized by law to practice nursing, and therefore deemed competent to render safe nursing care.

prae- for words beginning thus, see those beginning *prae-*.

pragmatagnosia (prag″mat-ag-no′ze-ah) loss of ability to recognize objects.

pragmatamnesia (prag″mat-am-ne′ze-ah) loss of power of remembering appearance of objects.

pramoxine (pram-ok′sēn) a compound used as a local anesthetic.

prandial (pran′de-al) pertaining to a meal.

Pranone (pra′nōn) trademark for a preparation of ethisterone.

Prantal (pran′tal) trademark for preparations of diphemanil.

praseodymium (pra″ze-o-dim′e-um) chemical element *(see table)*, at. no. 59, symbol Pr.

praxiology (prak″se-ol′o-je) the science of conduct.

pre- (pre) [L.] preposition, *before;* used also as a prefix, *before* (in time or space).

preagonal (pre-ag′o-nal) immediately before the death agony.

prealbumin (pre″al-bu′min) one of a group of serum proteins which have an electrophoretic mobility slightly faster than albumin at pH 8.6.

preanesthetic (pre″an-es-thet′ik) before anesthesia.

preantiseptic (pre″an-tī-sep′tik) before the days of antiseptic surgery.

preaurale (pre″aw-ra′le) a cephalometric landmark, the point at which a straight line from the postaurale, perpendicular to the long axis of the auricle, meets the base of the auricle.

preaxial (pre-ak′se-al) in front of the axis of the body.

precancerous (-kan′ser-us) preceding development of a cancer.

precava (-ka′vah) the superior vena cava. adj., **preca′val.**

preceptor (pre′sep-tor) a practicing physician whom a student accompanies, observes and assists, as one facet of his education in medicine.

prechordal (pre-kor′dal) in front of the notochord.

precipitant (-sip′ĭ-tant) a substance that causes precipitation.

precipitate (-sip′ĭ-tāt) 1. to cause settling in solid particles of substance in solution. 2. a deposit of solid particles settled out of a solution. **red p.,** red mercuric oxide. **white p.,** ammoniated mercury. **yellow p.,** yellow mercuric oxide.

precipitation (-sip″ĭ-ta′shun) act or process of precipitating.

precipitin (-sip′ĭ-tin) an antibody produced by artificial immunization and able to precipitate from solution the proteid producing it.

precipitinogen (-sip″ĭ-tin′o-jen) a soluble antigen which stimulates the formation of a precipitin.

precipitinoid (-sip′ĭ-tin-oid) a precipitin whose activity has been destroyed by heat.

precipitophore (-sip′ĭ-to-fōr″) the group in a precipitin which is the active cause of precipitation.

preclinical (pre-klin′ĭ-kal) 1. before the appearance or development of disease. 2. preceding the study of diseases in living patients.

preclival (-kli′val) in front of the clivus.

precocity (-kos′ĭ-te) unusually early development of mental or physical traits.

precognition (pre″kog-nish′un) the extrasensory perception of a future event.

precommissure (pre-kom′ĭ-shūr) the anterior commissure.

preconscious (-kon′shus) not present in consciousness, but readily recalled into it.

preconvulsive (pre″kon-vul′siv) preceding convulsions.

precordia (pre-kor′de-ah) epigastrium. adj., **precor′dial.**

precordium (-kor′de-um) epigastrium.

precornu (-kor′nu) anterior cornu of lateral ventricle.

precuneus (-ku′ne-us), pl. *precu′nei* [L.] a small convolution on the medial surface of the parietal lobe of the cerebrum.

precursor (-ker′sor) something that normally precedes or may develop into another, as a premalignant lesion or an intermediate compound in a metabolic or synthetic process.

predation (-da′shun) the biological association of two individuals or populations of different species, one of which feeds upon the other, which it rapidly destroys.

predator (pred′ah-tor) an individual or species that feeds upon and destroys organisms of another species, on which it is dependent for survival.

predentin (pre-den′tin) the soft, primitive dentin.

prediabetes (-di″ah-be′tēz) a state of latent impairment of carbohydrate metabolism in which the criteria for diabetes mellitus are not all satisfied.

predicrotic (pre″dĭ-krot′ik) occurring before the dicrotic wave of the sphygmogram.

predigestion (-di-jes′chun) partial artificial digestion of food before its ingestion into the body.

predisposition (pre-dis″po-zish′un) a special tendency toward some disease.

prednisolone (pred-nis′o-lōn) a compound used as an adrenocortical steroid of glucogenic type.

prednisone (pred′nĭ-sōn) a compound used as an adrenocortical steroid of glucogenic type.

preeclampsia (pre″e-klamp′se-ah) a toxemia of late pregnancy, characterized by hypertension, albuminuria and edema.

preflagellate (pre-flaj′ĕ-lāt) preceding the flagellate stage.

prefrontal (-frun′tal) the central part of the ethmoid bone.

preganglionic (pre″gang-gle-on′ik) proximal to a ganglion.

pregeniculatum (pre″jĕ-nik″u-la′tum) the external geniculate body.

pregenital (pre-jen′ĭ-tal) antedating the emergence of genital interests.

preglomerular (pre″glo-mer′u-lar) proximal to a glomerulus.

pregnancy (preg′nan-se) the state of being

pregnant; the development of the fertilized ovum with the maternal body. **abdominal p.,** development of the fetus in the abdominal cavity. **ectopic p., extrauterine p.,** development of the fetus outside the cavity of the uterus. **false p.,** development of all the signs of pregnancy without the presence of an embryo. **hydatid p.,** pregnancy with formation of hydatid mole. **interstitial p.,** development of the fetus in that part of the oviduct within the wall of the uterus. **molar p.,** conversion of ovum into a mole. **multiple p.,** presence of more than one fetus in the uterus at the same time. **mural p.,** interstitial pregnancy. **ovarian p.,** pregnancy occurring in an ovary. **oviducal p.,** tubal pregnancy. **phantom p.,** false pregnancy. **tubal p.,** development of the embryo within an oviduct. **tuboabdominal p.,** development of the products of conception partly in the fimbriated end of the oviduct and partly in the abdominal cavity.

pregnane (preg'nān) a crystalline saturated steroid hydrocarbon related to cholone.

pregnanediol (preg-nān'de-ol) a crystalline, biologically inactive dihydroxy derivative of pregnane, formed by reduction of progesterone and found especially in urine of pregnant women.

pregnant (preg'nant) having a developing ovum within the uterus.

pregnene (preg'nēn) a compound which forms the chemical nucleus of progesterone.

pregneninolone (preg"nēn-in'o-lōn) ethisterone.

pregnenolone (preg nēn'o-lōn) a compound used as an antiarthritic.

pregravidic (pre"grah-vid'ik) preceding pregnancy.

prehallux (pre-hal'uks) a supernumerary bone of the foot growing from the inner border of the navicular.

prehemiplegic (pre"hem-ī-ple'jik) preceding hemiplegia.

prehensile (pre-hen'sil) capable of grasping or seizing.

prehension (-hen'shun) the act of grasping.

prehyoid (-hi'oid) in front of the hyoid bone.

prehypophysis (pre"hi-pof'ĭ-sis) the anterior lobe of the hypophysis cerebri.

preictal (pre-ik'tal) occurring before a stroke, seizure or attack.

pre-immunization (pre"im-u-ni-za'shun) artificial immunization produced in very young infants.

preinsula (pre-in'su-lah) the cephalic portion of the insula.

preinvasive (pre"in-va'siv) not yet invading tissues outside the site of origin.

prelimbic (pre-lim'bik) in front of a limbus.

Preludin (-lu'din) trademark for preparations of phenmetrazine hydrochloride.

premalignant (pre"mah-lig'nant) preceding malignancy.

premature (pre"mah-tūr') born or interrupted before the state of maturity.

prematurity (-tūr'ĭ-te) the quality of not reaching the state of maturity, used of a fetus

weighing less than 2500 gm. (5.5 pounds) at birth, regardless of the period of gestation.

premaxillary (pre-mak'sī-ler"e) in front of the maxilla.

premedication (pre"med-ĭ-ka'shun) administration of drugs to produce basal narcosis before giving a general anesthetic.

premeiotic (pre"mi-ot'ik) occurring before or pertaining to time preceding meiosis.

premenarchal (pre"mĕ-nar'kal) occurring before establishment of menstruation.

premenstrual (pre-men'stroo-al) preceding menstruation.

premenstruum (-men'stroo-um) the period before menstruation.

premitotic (pre"mi-tot'ik) occurring before or pertaining to the time preceding mitosis.

premolar (pre-mo'lar) in front of the molar teeth.

premonocyte (-mon'o-sīt) promonocyte.

premorbid (-mor'bid) occurring before development of disease.

premortal (-mor'tal) occurring before death.

premunition (pre"mu-nish'un) resistance to hyperinfection by the same organism sometimes stimulated by and existing during the presence of a specific parasite in the host. adj., **premu'nitive.**

premyeloblast (pre-mi'ĕ-lo-blast") an early precursor of a myelocyte.

premyelocyte (-mi'ĕ-lo-sīt") promyelocyte.

prenarcosis (pre"nar-ko'sis) narcosis induced preliminary to general or local anesthesia.

prenasale (pre"na sa'le) a cephalometric landmark, the most projecting point, in the midsagittal plane, at the tip of the nose.

prenatal (pre-na'tal) preceding birth.

preneoplastic (pre"ne-o-plas'tik) before the formation of a tumor.

preoperative (pre-op'er-a"tiv) preceding an operation.

preoptic (-op'tik) in front of the optic lobes.

preoral (-o'ral) in front of the mouth.

preoxygenation (-ok"sĭ-jē-na'shun) prolonged breathing of oxygen before exposure to low atmospheric pressure, to prevent decompression sickness.

prepallium (-pal'e-um) the brain cortex in front of the fissure of Rolando.

preparalytic (pre"par-ah-lit'ik) preceding paralysis.

prepatellar (pre"pah-tel'ar) in front of the patella.

preprandial (pre-pran'de-al) before meals.

prepuce (pre'pūs) a cutaneous fold over the glans penis or glans clitoridis. adj., **preputial.**

preputiotomy (pre-pu"she-ot'o-me) incision of the prepuce of the penis to relieve phimosis.

preputium (-pu'she-um) prepuce.

presacral (-sa'kral) anterior to the sacrum.

presby- (pres'be) word element [Gr.], *old age.*

presbyatry (pres"be-ah'tre) treatment of the diseases of old age.

presbycardia (pres"bī-kar'de-ah) impairment of cardiac function with advancing years, with senescent changes in the body and no evidence of other cause of heart disease.

presbycusis (pres″be-ku′sis) impairment of hearing due to old age.

presbyesophagus (-e-sof′ah-gus) a condition characterized by alteration in motor function of the esophagus as a result of degenerative changes occurring with advancing age.

presbyophrenia (-o-fre′ne-ah) disorientation and confabulation occurring in old age.

presbyopia (-o′pe-ah) impairment of eyesight due to old age.

prescription (pre-skrip′shun) a written directive, as for the compounding or dispensing and administration of drugs, or for other service to a particular patient. **compounded p., extemporaneous p.,** a written directive to a pharmacist giving names and quantities of ingredients to be combined and dispensed for use by a particular patient. **magistral p.,** extemporaneous prescription. **ophthalmic p.,** directions for the grinding of lenses to be worn by a person to correct visual defects. **precompounded p.,** a written directive to a pharmacist calling for an agent that is supplied by a pharmaceutical manufacturer and dispensed without alteration.

presentation (prez″en-ta′shun) the particular part of the body of the fetus appearing at the os uteri or bounded by the girdle of resistance at birth. **breech p.,** presentation of the fetal buttock in labor. **cephalic p.,** presentation of any part of the fetal head in labor, whether the vertex, face or brow. **compound p.,** prolapse of an extremity of the fetus alongside the head in cephalic presentation or of one or both arms alongside a presenting breech at the beginning of labor. **placental p.,** placenta praevia. **transverse p.,** presentation of any portion of the side of the fetal body at the os uteri in labor.

presomite (pre-so′mīt) referring to embryos before the appearance of somites.

presphenoid (-sfe′noid) anterior portion of the body of the sphenoid bone.

presphygmic (-sfig′mik) preceding the pulse wave.

prespinal (-spi′nal) in front of the spine.

pressor (pres′or) increasing blood pressure and vasomotor activity.

pressoreceptive (pres″o-re-sep′tiv) sensitive to stimuli due to vasomotor activity.

pressoreceptor (-re-sep′tor) a receptor or nerve ending sensitive to stimuli of vasomotor activity.

pressosensitive (-sen′sĭ-tiv) pressoreceptive.

pressure (presh′ur) stress or strain, by compression, expansion, pull, thrust or shear. **arterial p.,** the blood pressure in the arteries. **atmospheric p.,** the pressure exerted by the atmosphere, about 15 pounds to the square inch at sea level. **blood p.,** the tension in the walls of blood vessels derived from the blood current. **capillary p.,** blood pressure in the capillaries. **diastolic p.,** arterial pressure during diastole. **intracranial p.,** pressure of the subarachnoidal fluid. **intraocular p.,** the pressure exerted against the outer coats by the contents of the eyeball. **negative p.,** pressure less than that of the atmosphere.

oncotic p., the osmotic pressure of a colloid system. **osmotic p.,** pressure which brings about diffusion between solutions of different concentration or between a solute and the fluid in which it is dissolved. **partial p.,** pressure exerted by each of the constituents of a mixture of gases. **positive p.,** pressure greater than that of the atmosphere. **pulse p.,** the difference between systolic and diastolic pressures. **systolic p.,** arterial pressure during systole. **venous p.,** blood pressure in the veins.

presternum (pre-ster′num) manubrium.

presubiculum (pre″su-bik′u-lum) the portion of the hippocampal gyrus between the olfactory portion and the subiculum.

presuppurative (pre-sup′u-ra″tiv) preceding suppuration.

presynaptic (pre″sī-nap′tik) situated proximal to a synapse, or occurring before the synapse is crossed.

presystole (pre-sis′to-le) interval just before systole.

presystolic (pre″sis-tol′ik) preceding systole.

pretarsal (pre-tar′sal) in front of the tarsus.

pretibial (-tib′e-al) in front of the tibia.

prevalence (prev′ah-lens) the number of cases of a specific disease in existence in a given population at a certain time.

preventive (pre-ven′tiv) prophylactic.

prevertebral (-ver′tĕ-bral) in front of a vertebra.

prevesical (-ves′ĭ-kal) anterior to the bladder.

previable (-vi′ah-bl) not yet viable; said of a fetus incapable of extrauterine existence.

previtamin (-vi″tah-min) a precursor of a vitamin.

prezygotic (pre″zi-got′ik) occurring before or pertaining to the time preceding union of the gametes (formation of the zygote).

prezymogen (pre-zi′mo-jen) a substance in the cell which is converted into zymogen.

priapism (pri′ah-pizm) persistent abnormal erection of penis.

primaquine (pri′mah-kwin) a compound used as an antimalarial agent.

primate (pri′māt) an individual belonging to the highest order of mammals.

Primates (pri-ma′tēz) the highest order of mammals, containing man and the apes, monkeys, etc.

primer (prīm′er) a substance which prepares for or facilitates the action of another.

primidone (pri′mĭ-dōn) a compound used as an anticonvulsant.

primigravida (pri″mĭ-grav′ĭ-dah) a woman pregnant for the first time; gravida I.

primipara (pri-mip′ah-rah) a woman who has had one pregnancy which resulted in a viable offspring; para I. adj., **primip′arous.**

primiparity (pri″mĭ-par′ĭ-te) the state of being a primipara.

primordium (pri-mor′de-um) the first beginnings of an organ or part in the developing embryo.

Prinadol (prin′ah-dol) trademark for a preparation of phenazocine.

princeps (prin′seps) a principal artery.

principle (prin'sĭ-pl) 1. a chemical component. 2. a substance on which certain of the properties of a drug depend. 3. a law of conduct. **active p.**, any constituent of a drug which helps to confer upon it a medicinal property. **antianemia p.**, the constituent in liver and certain other tissues that produces the hematopoietic effect in pernicious anemia. **pleasure p.**, the automatic instinct or tendency to avoid pain and secure pleasure. **proximate p.**, any one of the definite compounds into which a substance may be directly or readily resolved. **reality p.**, the mental activity which develops to control the pleasure principle under the pressure of necessity or the demands of reality.

Priodax (pri'o-daks) trademark for a preparation of iodoalphionic acid.

Priscoline (pris'ko-lēn) trademark for preparations of tolazoline.

prism (prizm) a solid with a triangular or polygonal cross section. **enamel p.**, any one of the columns which make up the enamel of teeth. **Nicol p.**, one composed of two slabs of Iceland spar, for polarizing light.

prismosphere (priz'mo-sfēr) a prism combined with a spherical lens.

Privine (pri'vēn) trademark for preparations of naphazoline.

p.r.n. [L.] *pro re na'ta* (according to circumstances).

pro- (pro) word element [L., Gr.], *before; in front of; favoring.*

proaccelerin (pro"ak-sel'er-in) factor V.

proactivator (pro-ak"tĭ-va'tor) a precursor of an activator; a factor which reacts with an enzyme to form an activator.

proamnion (-am'ne-on) that part of the embryonal area at front and sides of head which remains without mesoderm for some time.

proarrhythmic (pro"ah-rith'mik) 1. tending to produce cardiac arrhythmia. 2. an agent which tends to produce cardiac arrhythmia.

proazamine (pro-az'ah-mēn) promethazine.

proband (pro'band) propositus.

probang (pro'bang) a flexible rod with a ball, tuft or sponge at the end; used in diseases of the esophagus or larynx.

Pro-banthine (pro-ban-thīn') trademark for preparations of propantheline bromide.

probarbital (-bar'bĭ-tal) a barbiturate compound used as a sedative and hypnotic.

probe (prōb) a long, slender instrument for exploring wounds or body cavities or passages. **pocket p.**, a dental instrument having a tapered, rodlike blade with a blunt, rounded tip, used to measure the depth and determine the outline of a periodontal pocket.

probenecid (pro-ben'ĕ-sid) a white, crystalline compound, used in the treatment of gout to promote excretion of uric acid.

procainamide (-kăn'ah-mĭd) a compound used in the treatment of cardiac arrhythmia.

procaine (pro'kān) a compound used to produce local anesthesia. **p. butyrate**, an effective compound for infiltration anesthesia, used especially for surface anesthesia for eyes and mucous membrane. **p. hydrochloride,** white crystalline powder used for infiltration and spinal anesthesia, and nerve block.

procarboxypeptidase (pro"kar-bok"se-pep'tĭ-dās) the inactive precursor of carboxypeptidase, which is converted to the active enzyme by the action of trypsin.

procelous (pro-se'lus) having the anterior surface concave; said of vertebrae.

procephalic (pro"sĕ-fal'ik) pertaining to the anterior part of the head.

procercoid (pro-ser'koid) a larval stage of fish tapeworms.

process (pros'es) 1. a prominence or projection, as from a bone. 2. a series of operations or events leading to achievement of a specific result. **axis-cylinder p.**, axon. **basilar p.**, a forward projection of the occipital bone, articulating with the sphenoid bone. **capitular p.**, the articular process on a vertebra for the head of a rib. **caudate p.**, the portion connecting the right lobe and caudate lobe of the liver. **ciliary p's,** fringelike processes encircling the margin of the eye lens. **coracoid p.**, projection from anterior and upper edge of scapula. **coronoid p.**, 1. a projection on the ulna which articulates in the coronoid fossa of the humerus. 2. a process of the mandible. **Deiters' p.**, axon. **dendritic p.**, the branched process of a nerve cell. **ensiform p.**, xiphoid process. **epiphyseal p.**, epiphysis. **ethmoid p.**, projection from upper border of inferior turbinated bone. **falciform p.**, 1. process of fascia lata around the saphenous opening. 2. the falx cerebri. **falciform p.**, flocculus. **frontonasal p.**, an expansive facial process in the embryo which develops into the forehead and bridge of the nose. **funicular p.**, the portion of the tunica vaginalis surrounding the spermatic cord. **lacrimal p.**, process of inferior turbinate which joins with the lacrimal bone. **malar p.**, eminence by which the superior maxilla articulates with the zygoma. **mammillary p.**, a tubercle on each superior articular process of a lumbar vertebra. **mandibular p.**, one of the processes formed by bifurcation of the first branchial arch in the embryo, which unites ventrally with its fellow to form the base of the lower jaw. **mastoid p.**, conical projection at base of mastoid portion of temporal bone. **maxillary p.**, one of the processes formed by bifurcation of the first branchial arch in the embryo, which joins with the ipsilateral median nasal process in the formation of the upper jaw. **odontoid p.**, toothlike projection of axis which articulates with atlas. **pterygoid p.**, one of the wing-shaped processes of the sphenoid. **spinous p.**, a slender, more or less sharp-pointed projection. **xiphoid p.**, the lowest segment of the sternum. **zygomatic p.**, a projection from the frontal or temporal bone, or from the maxilla, by which they articulate with the zygoma.

processus (pro-ses'us), pl. *proces'sus* [L.] process; used in official names of various anatomic structures.

procheilon (pro-ki′lon) central prominence of the mucocutaneous margin of the upper lip.

prochlorpemazine (pro″klor-pem′ah-zēn) prochlorperazine.

prochlorperazine (-per′ah-zēn) a phenothiazine derivative used as a tranquilizer and antiemetic.

procidentia (pro″sī-den′she-ah) a falling down, or state of prolapse.

proconceptive (pro″kon-sep′tiv) aiding or promoting conception.

proconvertin (-ver′tin) factor VII.

procreation (pro″kre-a′shun) the act of begetting or generating.

proctagra (prok-tag′rah) proctalgia.

proctalgia (-tal′je-ah) pain in the rectum.

proctatresia (prok″tah-tre′ze-ah) imperforation of the anus.

proctectasia (prok″tek-ta′ze-ah) dilatation of the rectum or anus.

proctectomy (prok-tek′-to-me) excision of the rectum.

procteurynter (-tu-rin′ter) an instrument for dilating the anus.

proctitis (-ti′tis) inflammation of the rectum.

proctocele (prok′to-sēl) hernial protrusion of part of the rectum.

proctoclysis (prok-tok′lī-sis) slow injection of liquid into the rectum.

proctocolectomy (prok″to-ko-lek′to-me) excision of the rectum and colon.

proctocolonoscopy (-ko″lon-os′ko-pe) inspection of interior of rectum and lower colon.

proctocolpoplasty (-kol′po-plas″te) repair of a rectovaginal fistula.

proctocystoplasty (-sis′to-plas″te) repair of a rectovesical fistula.

proctocystotomy (-sis-tot′o-me) removal of vesical stone through rectum.

proctodeum (-de′um) the ectodermal depression of the caudal end of the embryo, which becomes the anal canal.

proctodynia (-din′e-ah) pain in the rectum.

proctogenic (-jen′ik) derived from anus or rectum.

proctology (prok-tol′o-je) branch of medicine treating of the rectum and its diseases.

proctoparalysis (prok″to-pah-ral′ĭ-sis) paralysis of the anal sphincter.

proctoperineoplasty (-per″ĭ-ne′o-plas″te) plastic repair of rectum and perineum.

proctoperineorrhaphy (-per″ĭ-ne-or′ah-fe) suture of rectum and perineum.

proctopexy (prok′to-pek″se) surgical fixation of the rectum.

proctophobia (prok″to-fo′be-ah) mental apprehension in patients with rectal disease.

proctoplasty (prok′to-plas″te) plastic repair of the rectum and anus.

proctoplegia (prok″to-ple′je-ah) proctoparalysis.

proctoptosis (prok″top-to′sis) prolapse of the rectum.

proctorrhaphy (prok-tor′ah-fe) suture of the rectum.

proctorrhea (prok″to-re′ah) a discharge from the anus.

proctoscope (prok′to-skōp) an endoscope specially designed for passage through the anus to permit inspection of the lower part of the intestine.

proctoscopy (prok-tos′ko-pe) inspection of the lower part of the intestine with a proctoscope.

proctosigmoid (prok″to-sig′moid) the rectum and sigmoid colon.

proctosigmoidectomy (-sig″moi-dek′to-me) excision of rectum and sigmoid.

proctosigmoiditis (-sig″moi-di′tis) inflammation of rectum and sigmoid.

proctosigmoidopexy (-sig-moid′o-pek″se) surgical fixation of the rectum and sigmoid colon.

proctosigmoidoscopy (-sig″moi-dos′ko-pe) direct visual examination of the rectum and sigmoid.

proctospasm (prok′to-spazm) spasm of the rectum.

proctostat (prok′to-stat) a radium-containing tube for insertion into the rectum.

proctostenosis (prok″to-ste-no′sis) stricture of the rectum.

proctostomy (prok-tos′to-me) creation of a new opening of the rectum on the body surface.

proctotomy (-tot′o-me) incision of the rectum.

proctovalvotomy (prok″to-val-vot′o-me) incision of the rectal valves.

procumbent (pro-kum′bent) prone; lying on the face.

procursive (-ker′siv) tending to run forward.

procyclidine (-si′klī-dēn) tricyclamol.

prodrome (pro′drōm) a premonitory symptom.

product (prod′ukt) something produced. **cleavage p.**, a substance formed by splitting of a compound molecule into a simpler one. **contact activation p.**, a product of the interaction of blood coagulation factors XII and XI, which functions to activate factor IX during the formation of intrinsic thromboplastin. **fission p.**, an isotope, usually radioactive, of an element in the middle of the periodic table, produced by fission with a heavy element under bombardment with high-energy particles. **intermediate p.**, one which is formed as a step in a definite sequence of events. **spallation p's**, the isotopes of many different chemical elements produced in small amounts in nuclear fission. **substitution p.**, a substance formed by substitution of a different element or radical in a molecule.

proencephalus (pro″en-sef′ah-lus) a fetus with a protrusion of the brain through a frontal fissure.

proenzyme (pro-en′zīm) zymogen; an inactive precursor of an enzyme.

proerythroblast (pro″ĕ-rith′ro-blast) an early precursor of an erythrocyte.

profenamine (pro-fen′ah-mēn) ethopropazine.

profibrillatory (-fib″rĭ-lah-to′re) tending to produce cardiac fibrillation.

profibrinolysin (-fi″brĭ-no-li′sin) plasminogen.

proflavine (-fla′vin) a reddish-brown, crystalline powder used in the treatment of infected wounds.

profundus (-fun′dus) [L.] deep.

progeria (pro-je're-ah) premature development of the characteristics usually associated with old age.

progestational (pro"jes-ta'shun-al) preceding gestation; referring to changes in the endometrium preparatory to implantation of the developing ovum should fertilization occur.

progesteroid (pro-jes'tĕ-roid) a progesterone-like compound.

progesterone (-jes'tĕ-rōn) a steroid with progestational activity, isolated from human ovaries, adrenal cortex and placenta.

progestin (-jes'tin) a substance having the biological activity of the specific hormone of the corpus luteum, preparing the endometrium for implantation of the fertilized ovum.

progestogen (-jes'to-jen) a substance which induces changes in the uterus similar to those (progestational changes) occurring after ovulation.

proglossis (-glos'is) the tip of the tongue.

proglottid (-glot'id) one of the segments making up the body of a tapeworm (strobila).

proglottis (-glot'is) proglottid.

prognathism (prog'nah-thizm) abnormal protrusion of the lower jaw. adj., **prognath'ic.**

prognathous (prog'nah-thus, prog-na'thus) having a gnathic index above 103.

prognosis (prog-no'sis) the probable outcome of an attack of a disease. adj., **prognos'tic.**

progoitrin (pro-goi'trin) an inactive compound found in the seeds of most plants belonging to the genus Brassica, which liberates goitrin through specific enzymatic hydrolysis.

progranulocyte (-gran'u-lo-sīt") a cell of the granulocytic series which has a coarse nuclear structure and no discernible specific granules.

proguanil (-gwan'il) a compound used as an antimalarial.

Progynon (-jin'on) trademark for preparations of estradiol.

proiosystole (pro"e-o-sis'to-le) a contraction of the heart occurring before its normal time; a premature heart beat.

proiosystolia (-sis-to'le-ah) occurrence of proiosystoles.

proiotia (pro"e-o'she-ah) sexual or genital precocity.

projection (pro-jek'shun) 1. a throwing forward, especially the reference of impressions made on the sense organs to their proper source. 2. the act of extending or jutting out, or a part that juts out. 3. a mental mechanism by which a repressed complex is regarded as belonging to someone else; the attribution to others of one's own ideas.

prokaryocyte (-kar'e-o-sīt") an immature erythrocyte intermediate between a karyoblast and a karyocyte.

prokaryosis (pro"kar-e-o'sis) the state of not having a true nucleus, the nuclear material being scattered in the protoplasm of the cell. adj., **prokaryot'ic.**

prolabium (pro-la'be-um) the prominent central part of the upper lip.

prolactin (-lak'tin) a hormone secreted by the anterior pituitary, which stimulates milk secretion.

prolamine (pro-lam'in) one of a class of simple proteins insoluble in water and absolute alcohol, but soluble in 70–80 per cent ethyl alcohol; obtained principally from cereal seeds.

prolan (pro'lan) gonadotropic hormone.

prolapse (pro'laps) the falling down, or downward displacement, of a part or viscus. **p. of cord,** protrusion of the umbilical cord ahead of the presenting part of the fetus in labor. **frank p.,** prolapse of the uterus in which the vagina is inverted and hangs from the vulva. **p. of the iris,** protrusion of the iris through a wound in the cornea. **Morgagni's p.,** chronic inflammatory hyperplasia of the mucosa and submucosa of the sacculus laryngis. **rectal p., p. of rectum,** protrusion of the rectal mucous membrane through the anus. **p. of uterus,** protrusion of the uterus through the vaginal orifice.

prolapsus (pro-lap'sus) [L.] prolapse.

prolepsis (-lep'sis) recurrence of a paroxysm before the expected time. adj., **prolep'tic.**

proleukemia (pro"lu-ke'me-ah) leukanemia.

proliferation (pro-lif"ĕ-ra'shun) the reproduction or multiplication of similar forms, especially of cells and morbid cysts. adj., **prolif'erous.**

proligerous (-lij'er-us) producing offspring.

proline (pro'lēn) a naturally occurring amino acid discovered in 1901.

Prolixin (pro-lik'sin) trademark for preparations of fluphenazine.

Proluton (pro-lu'ton) trademark for preparations of progesterone.

prolymphocyte (-lim'fo-sīt) a cell of the lymphocytic series intermediate between the lymphoblast and lymphocyte.

promazine (pro'mah-zēn) a phenothiazine derivative used as a tranquilizer.

promegakaryocyte (pro"meg-ah-kar'e-o-sīt") a cell of the thrombocytic series having a coarse chromatin structure and nucleoli in the nucleus.

promegaloblast (pro-meg'ah-lo-blast") a cell developing from a lymphoidocyte into a megaloblast.

promethazine (-meth'ah-zēn) a phenothiazine derivative used as an antihistaminic.

promethestrol (-meth'es-trol) a compound used as an estrogenic substance.

promethium (-me'the-um) chemical element (*see table*), at. no. 61, symbol Pm.

Promin (pro'min) trademark for a preparation of glucosulfone sodium.

promine (pro'mēn) a substance widely distributed in animal cells which is characterized by its ability to promote cell division and growth.

prominence (prom'ĭ-nens) a conspicuously elevated area.

promonocyte (pro-mon'o-sīt) a cell of the monocytic series intermediate between the monoblast and monocyte, with coarse chromatin structure and one or two nucleoli.

promontory (prom'on-tor"e) a projecting

process or eminence. **p. of the sacrum,** the upper, projecting part of the sacrum.

promoxolane (pro-mok′so-lān) a compound used as a tranquilizer.

promyelocyte (-mi′ĕ-lo-sīt″) a cell intermediate between myeloblast and myelocyte, containing a few undifferentiated cytoplasmic granules.

pronate (pro′nāt) to place in or assume a prone position.

pronation (pro-na′shun) the act of assuming the prone position; placing or lying face downward; applied to the foot, a combination of eversion and abduction, resulting in lowering of the longitudinal arch.

prone (prōn) 1. lying face downward, or on the ventral surface. 2. especially susceptible or liable. **accident-p.,** especially likely to be involved in accidents.

pronephros (pro-nef′ros), pl. *proneph′roi* [Gr.] the earliest and simplest excretory organ in the embryo; although it serves no purpose in many vertebrates, its development precedes that of a mesonephros.

Pronestyl (-nes′til) trademark for preparations of procainamide hydrochloride.

pronograde (pro′no-grād) carrying the body in a horizontal position when walking.

pronormoblast (pro-nor′mo-blast) a name given early forms of the erythrocytic series.

pronucleus (-nu′kle-us) the nucleus of an ovum or spermatozoon before their fusion in the fertilized ovum. **female p.,** the nucleus of an ovum before it unites with that of the spermatozoon that has penetrated its cytoplasm. **male p.,** the nucleus of the spermatozoon after it has penetrated the cytoplasm of an ovum.

prootic (-ot′ik) in front of the ear.

Propadrine (pro′pah-drēn) trademark for a preparation of synthetic alkaloid, resembling ephedrine in composition and action.

propagation (prop″ah-ga′shun) reproduction. adj., **prop′agative.**

propalinal (pro-pal′ĭ-nal) having a backward and forward motion or direction.

propane (pro′pān) a hydrocarbon from petroleum.

propanolide (pro-pan′o-līd) betapropiolactone.

propantheline (-pan′thĕ-lēn) a compound used in parasympathetic blockade.

proparacaine (-par′ah-kān) a compound used as a local anesthetic.

propedeutics (pro″pĕ-du′tiks) the introduction to an art or science.

propepsin (pro-pep′sin) pepsinogen.

propeptone (-pep′tōn) hemialbumose.

properdin (-pār′din) a euglobulin isolated from normal serum which is capable of destroying bacteria and viruses.

prophase (pro′fāz) the first stage of division of the nucleus of a cell in either meiosis or mitosis.

prophenpyridamine (pro″fen-pi-rid′ah-mēn) pheniramine.

prophylactic (pro″fĭ-lak′tik) tending to ward off disease.

prophylactodontics (pro″fĭ-lak″to-don′tiks)

the branch of dentistry concerned with prevention of dental and oral diseases.

prophylactodontist (pro″fĭ-lak″to-don′tist) a specialist in prophylactodontics.

prophylaxis (pro″fĭ-lak′sis) prevention of disease.

propiodal (pro-pi′o-dal) an iodide compound used as source of iodine.

propiolactone (pro″pe-o-lak′tōn) betapropiolactone.

propiomazine (-ma′zēn) a phenothiazine derivative used to potentiate the sedative action of barbiturates and as an adjunct to ether anesthesia.

Propionibacteriaceae (pro″pe-on″e-bak-te″re-a′se-e) a family of Schizomycetes (order Eubacteriales).

Propionibacterium (-bak-te′re-um) a genus of Schizomycetes (order Eubacteriales, family Propionibacteriaceae) found as saprophytes in dairy products.

proplasmocyte (pro-plaz′mo-sīt) a cell of the plasmocytic series with a coarse nuclear structure and one or more nucleoli.

proplexus (-plek′sus) the choroid plexus of the lateral ventricle.

propons (pro′pons) delicate plates of white matter passing across the anterior end of the pyramid and just below the pons varolii.

propositus (pro-poz′ĭ-tus), pl. *propos′iti* [L.] the original person presenting a mental or physical disorder who serves as the basis for a hereditary or genetic study.

propoxycaine (-pok′se-kān) a compound used as a local anesthetic.

propoxyphene (-pok′se-fēn) dextropropoxyphene.

proprietary (-pri′ĕ-ter″e) manufactured and sold exclusively by a single person or organization.

proprioceptive (pro″pre-o-sep′tiv) receiving stimuli within the body.

proprioceptor (-sep′tor) one of the specialized nerve endings in muscles, tendons and joints which are sensitive to changes in tension of muscle or tendon.

proptometer (pro-tom′ĕ-ter) an instrument for measuring exophthalmos.

proptosis (prop-to′sis) downward or forward displacement of an organ or part.

propulsion (pro-pul′shun) 1. a tendency to fall forward. 2. festination.

propylene glycol (pro′pĭ-lēn gli′kol) a colorless, viscous liquid, used as a substitute for glycerin.

propylhexedrine (pro″pil-hek′se-drēn) a compound used as an inhalant to decongest nasal mucosa.

propyliodone (-i′o-dōn) a compound used as a radiopaque medium in bronchography.

propylparaben (-par′ah-ben) a compound used as an antifungal preservative.

propylthiouracil (-thi″o-u′rah-sil) a compound used as a thyroid inhibitor.

pro re nata (pro ra nah′tah) [L.] according to circumstances.

prorennin (pro-ren′in) a precursor of rennin.

prorrhaphy (pro′rah-fe) advancement.

prorubricyte (pro-roo′brĭ-sīt) proerythroblast.

prosecretin (pro″se-kre′tin) the precursor of secretin.

prosection (pro-sek′shun) carefully programmed dissection for demonstration of anatomic structure.

prosector (-sek′tor) a person skilled in the performance of prosection.

prosencephalon (pros″en-sef′ah-lon) the forebrain, comprised of the cerebral hemispheres, diencephalon, hypothalamus and thalamencephalon.

prosodemic (pros″o-dem′ĭk) passing from one person to another.

prosogaster (-gas′ter) foregut.

prosopagnosia (-pag-no′se-ah) inability to recognize the faces of other people or one's own features in a mirror.

prosopalgia (-pal′je-ah) neuralgia of the trigeminal nerve.

prosopantritis (-pan-tri′tis) inflammation of the frontal sinuses.

prosopectasia (-pek-ta′ze-ah) oversize of the face.

prosoplasia (-pla′ze-ah) development into a higher state of organization.

prosopodiplegia (-po-di-ple′je-ah) paralysis of the face and one lower extremity.

prosoponeuralgia (-nu-ral′je-ah) facial neuralgia.

prosopoplegia (-ple′je-ah) facial paralysis. adj., **prosopople′gic.**

prosoposchisis (pros″o-pos′kĭ-sis) congenital fissure of the face.

prosopospasm (pros′o-po-spazm″) spasm of the face.

prosoposternodymia (pros″o-po-ster″no-dim′e-ah) double fetal monster joined from face to sternum.

prosopothoracopagus (-tho″rah-kop′ah-gus) twin fetuses joined in the thorax, face and neck.

prosopotocia (-to′she-ah) face presentation in labor.

prostatalgia (pros″tah-tal′je-ah) pain in the prostate.

prostate (pros′tāt) a gland surrounding the neck of the bladder and urethra in the male. adj., **prostat′ic.**

prostatectomy (pros″tah-tek′to-me) excision of the prostate.

prostaticovesiculectomy (pros-tat″ĭ-ko-ve-sik″u-lek′to-me) excision of the prostate gland and seminal vesicles.

prostatism (pros′tah-tizm) a morbid state due to prostatic disease.

prostatitis (pros″tah-ti′tis) inflammation of the prostate.

prostatocystitis (pros″tah-to-sis-ti′tis) inflammation of the prostate and the bladder.

prostatocystotomy (-sis-tot′o-me) incision of bladder and prostate.

prostatodynia (-din′e-ah) pain in the prostate.

prostatolith (pros-tat′o-lith) a calculus in the prostate.

prostatolithotomy (pros″tah-to-lĭ-thot′o-me) incision of prostate for removal of calculus.

prostatomegaly (pros″tah-to-meg′ah-le) hypertrophy of the prostate.

prostatomyomectomy (-mi″o-mek′to-me) excision of a prostatic myoma.

prostatorrhea (-re′ah) catarrhal discharge from the prostate.

prostatotomy (pros″tah-tot′o-me) surgical incision of the prostate.

prostatovesiculectomy (pros″tah-to-ve-sik″u-lek′to-me) excision of the prostate and seminal vesicles.

prostatovesiculitis (-ve-sik″u-li′tis) inflammation of prostate and seminal vesicles.

prosthesis (pros-the′sis), pl. *prosthe′ses* [Gr.] an artificial substitute for a missing body part, as an arm or leg, eye or tooth, used for either functional or cosmetic reasons, or both. **cleft palate p.,** an appliance used to restore the integrity of the roof of the mouth in patients with cleft palate. **dental p.,** artificial substitutes for missing teeth or parts of teeth. **internal p.,** a substitute for a diseased or nonfunctioning internal structure of the body, as the head of the femur or a valve of the heart. **maxillofacial p.,** a replacement for parts of the upper jaw or the face missing because of disease or injury.

prosthetic (-thet′ik) serving as a substitute; pertaining to the use or application of prostheses.

prosthetics (-thet′iks) the field of knowledge relating to prostheses and their use.

prosthetist (pros′thĕ-tist) a person skilled in prosthetics and practicing its application in individual cases.

prosthion (pros′the-on) the lowest anterior point on the gum between the maxillary central incisors.

prosthodontics (pros″tho-don′tiks) the branch of dental art and science concerned with construction of artificial appliances to replace missing teeth, and sometimes other parts of the oral cavity and face.

prosthodontist (-don′tist) a specialist in prosthodontics.

Prostigmin (pro-stig′min) trademark for preparations of neostigmine.

prostration (pros-tra′shun) extreme exhaustion or lack of energy or power.

protactinium (pro″tak-tin′e-um) chemical element (*see table*), at. no. 91, symbol Pa.

Protalba (pro-tal′bah) trademark for preparations of protoveratrine A.

protamine (pro′tah-min) one of a class of simple proteins, soluble in water, not coagulated by heat, and precipitated from aqueous solution by addition of alcohol; found combined with nucleic acids in ripe fish sperm.

Protaminobacter (-mi″no-bak′ter) a genus of Schizomycetes (order Pseudomonadales, suborder Pseudomonadineae, family Pseudomonadaceae) found in soil or water.

protandrous (pro-tan′drus) functioning first as a male and later as a female.

protanopia (pro″tah-no′pe-ah) blindness to red and green.

protean (pro′te-an) changing form or assuming different shapes.

protease (pro'te-ās) peptidase.

protectant (pro-tek'tant) a preparation which affords protection against a noxious agent or influence.

Proteeae (-te'e-e) a tribe of Schizomycetes (order Eubacteriales, family Enterobacteriaceae).

proteid (pro'te-id) protein.

protein (pro'te-in) a compound containing carbon, hydrogen, oxygen, nitrogen, and usually sulfur and phosphorus, the characteristic element being nitrogen. adj., **protein'ic.** **Bence Jones p.,** a low-molecular weight, heat-sensitive urinary protein found in multiple myeloma, which coagulates when heated to 45–55°C. and redissolves partially or wholly on boiling. **compound p.,** a protein which on hydrolysis yields a simple protein and a nonprotein matter. **defensive p.,** any protein formed within the body and serving as a protection against disease. **immune p's,** proteins formed by the combination of albuminous matters of the body with the enzymes of pathogenic bacteria. **native p.,** an unchanged, naturally occurring animal or vegetable protein. **protective p.,** defensive protein. **serum p.,** any protein found in the serum of the blood.

proteinase (pro'te-ĭ-nās") an enzyme which splits protein.

proteinemia (pro"te-ĭ-ne'me-ah) excess of protein in the blood.

proteinivorous (pro"te-ĭ-niv'o-rus) feeding on protein.

proteinogram (pro"te-in'o-gram) a graphic representation of proteins present in a solution, such as blood serum.

proteinosis (pro"te-in-o'sis) the accumulation of protein in the tissues. **lipid p.,** a disturbance of lipid metabolism marked by yellowish deposits of a lipid-protein mixture on the inner surface of the lips, under the tongue, on the fauces. **tissue p.,** amyloidosis.

proteinuria (-u're-ah) protein in the urine.

proteoclastic (pro"te-o-klas'tik) splitting up proteins.

proteolipid (-lip'id) a combination of a protein and a lipid, having the solubility characteristics of a lipid.

proteolipin (-lip'in) proteolipid.

proteolysin (pro"te-ol'ĭ-sin) a specific substance causing proteolysis.

proteolysis (-ol'ĭ-sis) the breaking down of proteins into simpler compounds. adj., **proteolyt'ic.**

proteometabolism (pro"te-o-mĕ-tab'o-lizm) the metabolism of protein.

proteopeptic (-pep'tik) digesting protein.

proteopexy (pro'te-o-pek"se) the fixation of protein within the organism. adj., **proteopex'ic.**

proteose (pro'te-ōs) any albumose or other substance intermediate between a protein and a peptone.

proteosuria (pro"te-o-su're-ah) presence of proteose in urine.

proteotoxin (pro"te-o-tok'sin) anaphylatoxin.

proteuria (pro"te-u're-ah) proteinuria.

Proteus (pro'te-us) a genus of Schizomycetes (order Eubacteriales, family Enterobacteriaceae, tribe Proteeae) usually found in fecal and other putrefying material.

prothipendyl (pro-thi'pen-dil) a compound used as a tranquilizer.

prothrombin (-throm'bin) a glycoprotein in plasma which is the precursor of thrombin.

prothrombinase (-throm'bin-ās) thromboplastin.

prothrombinogen (pro"throm-bin'o-gen) factor VII.

prothrombinogenic (pro-throm"bī-no-jen'ik) promoting the production of prothrombin.

prothrombinokinase (-ki'nās) factor VII.

prothrombinopenia (-pe'ne-ah) deficiency of prothrombin in the blood.

protistologist (pro"tis-tol'o-jist) a microbiologist.

protistology (-tol'o-je) microbiology.

proto- (pro'to) word element [Gr.], *first.*

proto-albumose (pro"to-al'bu-mōs) a primary albumose.

protobiology (-bi-ol'o-je) scientific study of the simplest forms of living organisms.

protoblast (pro'to-blast) a cell with no cell wall; an embryonic cell. adj., **protoblas'tic.**

protochloride (pro"to-klo'rīd) that one of a series of chlorides of the same element which contains the least chlorine.

protochrome (pro'to-krōm) a substance derived from proteins giving reactions identical with urochrome.

protocol (pro'to-kol) a written statement of the history and treatment of any particular patient, especially one made for a medicolegal purpose.

protocooperation (pro"to-ko-op"er-a'shun) the interaction between coexisting populations of different species, each of which is benefited, but is able to survive in the absence of the other.

protoduodenum (-du"o-de'num) the first portion of the duodenum, developed from the embryonic foregut.

proto-elastose (-e-las'tōs) a product of the digestion of elastin.

protofibril (-fi'bril) the first elongated unit appearing in formation of any type of fiber.

protogaster (-gas'ter) foregut.

protoglobulose (-glob'u-lōs) an albumose produced in the digestion of globulin.

protogynous (pro-toj'ĭ-nus) functioning first as a female and later as a male.

protokylol (pro"to-ki'lol) a compound used as a sympathomimetic agent and as a bronchodilator.

protomerite (-mer'īt) the anterior portion of certain gregarine protozoa.

protomyosinose (-mi-o'sĭ-nōs) an albumose formed in the digestion of myosin.

proton (pro'ton) an elementary particle of mass number 1, with a positive charge equal to the negative charge of the electron; a constituent particle of every nucleus, the number of protons in the nucleus of each atom of a chemical element being indicated by its atomic number.

protonephros (pro″to-nef′ros), pl. *protoneph′-roi* [Gr.] pronephros.

protoneuron (-nu′ron) the first neuron in a peripheral reflex arc.

Protophyta (pro-tof′i-tah) the lowest division of the vegetable kingdom, made up of unicellular organisms and including the algae, bacteria and viruses.

protophyte (pro′to-fīt) a unicellular plant or vegetable organ; an individual belonging to the Protophyta.

protophytology (pro″to-fi-tol′o-je) scientific study of the simplest forms of plants (protophytes).

protoplasm (pro′to-plazm) the viscid, translucent colloid material, the essential constituent of the living cell. adj., **protoplas′mic.**

protoplast (pro′to-plast) a bacterial or plant cell deprived of its rigid wall and dependent for its integrity on an isotonic or hypertonic medium.

protoporphyria (pro″to-por-fēr′e-ah) porphyria in which protoporphyrin is the compound present. **erythropoietic p.,** a form in which excessive amounts of free protoporphyrin are found in red blood cells, plasma and bone marrow, with sensitivity of skin to sunlight and sometimes liver damage.

protoporphyrin (-por′fī-rin) the porphyrin, $C_{34}H_{34}N_4O_4$, whose iron complex united with protein occurs in hemoglobin and other respiratory pigments.

protoporphyrinuria (-por″fī-rī-nu′re-ah) protoporphyrin in the urine.

protosalt (pro′to-sawlt) that one of a series of salts of the same base which contains the smallest amount of the combining substance.

protospasm (pro′to-spazm) a spasm which begins in a limited area and extends to other parts.

prototoxin (pro″to-tok′sin) the most virulent of a series of toxins.

prototroph (pro′to-trōf) an organism, especially a mutant, which does not require a growth factor. adj., **prototroph′ic.**

protoveratrine (pro″to-ver′ah-trēn) an antihypertensive alkaloid isolated from *Veratrum album.*

protovertebra (-ver′tĕ-brah) somite.

protoxide (pro-tok′sid) that one of a series of oxides of the same element which contains the least amount of oxygen.

Protozoa (pro″to-zo′ah) a phylum of the animal kingdom, comprising the lowest forms and made up of microscopic, unicellular organisms. adj., **protozo′an.**

protozoacide (-zo′ah-sīd) destructive to protozoa.

protozoiasis (-zo-i′ah-sis) infestation with protozoa.

protozoology (-zo-ol′o-je) scientific study of the simplest forms of animals (protozoa).

protozoon (-zo′on), pl. *protozo′a* [Gr.] a unicellular animal organism; an individual belonging to the Protozoa.

protozoophage (pro″to-zo′o-fāj) a phagocyte which consumes protozoa.

protraction (pro-trak′shun) a forward extension in space or time. **mandibular p.,** a facial anomaly in which the gnathion is anterior to the orbital plane. **maxillary p.,** a facial anomaly in which the subnasion is anterior to the orbital plane.

protractor (-trak′tor) instrument for drawing foreign bodies from wounds.

protrusion (-troo′zhun) extension beyond the usual limits, or above a plane surface.

protuberance (-tu′ber-ans) a projecting part, or prominence.

protuberantia (-tu″ber an′she-ah), pl. *protuberan′tiae* [L.] protuberance.

Provell (pro-vel′) trademark for a preparation of protoveratrines A and B.

Provera (-ver′ah) trademark for preparations of medroxyprogesterone acetate.

provertebra (-ver′tĕ-brah) somite.

provirus (-vi′rus) a latent stage of an animal virus, equivalent to prophage.

provitamin (-vi′tah-min) the precursor of a vitamin.

provocative (-vok′ah-tiv) stimulating the appearance of a sign, reflex, reaction or therapeutic effect.

proximad (prok′sī-mad) in a proximal direction.

proximal (prok′sī-mal) nearest to a point of reference, as to a center or median line or to the point of attachment or origin.

proximalis (prok″sī-ma′lis) [L.] proximal.

proximate (prok′sī-mit) nearest; nearest.

proximo-ataxia (prok″sī-mo-ah-tak′se-ah) ataxia of the proximal part of an extremity.

prozymogen (pro-zi′mo-jen) prezymogen.

pruriginous (proo-rij′ī-nus) of the nature of prurigo.

prurigo (proo-ri′go) a chronic skin disease marked by small, pale papules and intense itching. **p. estiva′lis,** a form occurring during warm weather. **p. fe′rox,** prurigo of a severe type. **p. mi′tis,** prurigo of a mild type. **p. nodula′ris,** a form marked by intense itching and formation of discrete, firm, erythematous nodules. **p. sim′plex,** a mild form with crops of papules tending to recur in cycles. **summer p.,** prurigo estivalis. **p. universa′lis,** prurigo covering the entire body.

pruritogenic (proo″rī-to-jen′ik) causing pruritus, or itching.

pruritus (proo-ri′tus) itching. adj., **prurit′ic. p. a′ni,** itching in the anal region. **essential p.,** that occurring without known cause. **p. seni′lis,** itching in the aged, due to degeneration of the skin. **symptomatic p.,** that which occurs secondarily to another condition. **p. vul′vae,** itching of the external genitalia in the female.

prussiate (proo′she-āt) cyanide.

p.s. per second.

psalis (sal′is) fornix.

psalterium (sal-te′re-um) lyra.

psammoma (sah-mo′mah) a tumor (of brain or ovary) containing granular material.

psammosarcoma (sam″o-sar-ko′mah) a sarcoma containing granular material.

pseud(o)- (su′do) word element [Gr.], *false*.

pseudacousma (su″dah-koōz′mah) an auditory defect with sounds seemingly altered in quality or pitch.

pseudarthritis (su″dar-thri′tis) a hysterical joint affection.

pseudarthrosis (su″dar-thro′sis) a pathologic condition in which failure of callus formation following pathologic fracture through an area of deossification in a weight-bearing long bone results in formation of a false joint.

pseudencephalus (su″den-sef′ah-lus) a fetus with tumor in place of brain.

pseudesthesia (su″des-the′ze-ah) a subjective sensation occurring in the absence of the appropriate stimuli.

pseudoacromegaly (su″do-ak″ro-meg′ah-le) acropachyderma.

pseudoagraphia (-ah-graf′e-ah) a condition in which the patient can copy writing, but cannot write except in a meaningless and illegible manner.

pseudoallele (-ah-lēl′) one of two or more genes which are seemingly allelic, but which can be shown to have distinctive loci on the chromosome. adj., **pseudoallel′ic.**

pseudoanemia (-ah-ne′me-ah) a condition marked by paleness without true anemia.

pseudoaneurysm (-an′u-rizm) an appearance resembling an aneurysm, but due to enlargement and tortuosity of a vessel.

pseudoangina (-an-ji′nah) nervous disorder resembling angina.

pseudoangioma (-an″je-o′mah) a venous thrombus that has become canalized.

pseudoapoplexy (-ap′o-plek″se) condition like apoplexy, but without hemorrhage.

pseudoataxia (-ah-tak′se-ah) general incoordination resembling ataxia.

pseudoatheroma (-ath″er-o′mah) a sebaceous cyst.

pseudoblepsis (-blep′sis) perversion of vision, objects appearing different from what they really are.

pseudocartilaginous (-kar″ti-laj′ĭ-nus) resembling cartilage.

pseudocast (su′do-kast) an accidental formation of urinary sediment resembling a true cast.

pseudocele (su′do-sēl) the fifth ventricle of the brain.

pseudocholesteatoma (su″do-ko″les-te″ah-to′-mah) a horny mass of epithelial cells in the tympanic cavity, resembling cholesteatoma.

pseudochorea (-ko-re′ah) a state of general incoordination resembling chorea.

pseudochromesthesia (-krō″mes-the′ze-ah) a sensation of color experienced on hearing sounds.

pseudochromhidrosis (-krōm″hĭ-dro′sis) discoloration of sweat by surface contaminants, such as pigment-producing bacteria or chemical substances on the skin.

pseudocide (su′do-sīd) the deliberate taking of measures to harm one's self without wishing to die.

pseudocirrhosis (su″do-sĭ-ro′sis) apparent cirrhosis of liver, due to pericarditis.

pseudocoarctation (-ko″ark-ta′shun) a condition resembling coarctation, without narrowing of the lumen. **p. of the aorta,** a congenital anomaly similar to coarctation, but without occlusion of the vessel.

pseudocoele (su′do-sēl) the fifth ventricle.

pseudocoloboma (su″do-kol″o-bo′mah) a scar on the iris resembling a coloboma.

pseudocopulation (-kop″u-la′shun) the fertilization of animal ova by the spermatozoa of the male without sexual union.

pseudocrisis (-kri′sis) a false crisis.

pseudocroup (su′do-kroōp) laryngismus stridulus.

pseudocyesis (su″do-si-e′sis) false pregnancy.

pseudocyst (su′do-sist) a dilated space resembling a cyst. **pancreatic p.,** an accumulation of pancreatic juice in the retroperitoneal space as a result of necrosis and rupture of a pancreatic duct.

pseudodementia (su″do-de-men′she-ah) state of general apathy resembling dementia.

pseudodiphtheria (-dif-the′re-ah) a condition resembling diphtheria, but not due to *Mycobacterium diphtheriae.*

pseudodipsia (-dip′se-ah) false thirst.

pseudoedema (-ĕ-de′mah) a puffy state resembling edema.

pseudoemphysema (-em″fĭ-ze′mah) a condition resembling emphysema, but due to obstruction of the bronchi.

pseudoephedrine (-ĕ-fed′rin) one of the optical isomers of ephedrine; used as a nasal decongestant.

pseudoerysipelas (-er″ĭ-sip′ĕ-las) an inflammatory subcutaneous disease resembling erysipelas.

pseudoganglion (-gang′gle-on) an enlargement on a nerve resembling a ganglion.

pseudogeusesthesia (-gūs″es-the′ze-ah) a false sensation of taste associated with a sensation of another modality.

pseudogeusia (-gu′ze-ah) a sensation of taste occurring in the absence of a stimulus or inappropriate to the exciting stimulus.

pseudoglioma (-gli-o′mah) an exudate in the vitreous simulating glioma.

pseudoglottis (-glot′is) the space between the false vocal cords.

pseudogout (su′do-gowt) a condition resembling gout, but with calcium salt rather than urate crystals in the synovial fluid.

pseudographia (su″do-graf′e-ah) the production of meaningless written symbols.

pseudohaustration (-haw-stra′shun) a false appearance of normal sacculation of the wall of the colon.

pseudohemophilia (-he″mo-fil′e-ah) thrombopenic purpura.

pseudohemoptysis (-he-mop′tĭ-sis) spitting of blood which comes from some source other than the lungs.

pseudohereditary (-hĕ-red′ĭ-tār″e) occurring

in successive generations because of imposition of the same environmental factors and not because of genetic transmission.

pseudohermaphrodite (su″do-her-maf′ro-dīt) an individual exhibiting pseudohermaphroditism. **female p.,** one whose gonads are ovaries. **male p.,** one whose gonads are testes.

pseudohermaphroditism (-her-maf′ro-dit-izm″) a state in which the gonads are of one sex, but the morphologic criteria of sex are ambiguous or contradictory.

pseudohernia (-her′ne-ah) an inflamed sac or gland simulating strangulated hernia.

pseudohydrocephalus (-hi″dro-sef′ah-lus) abnormally large appearance of a normal sized head, due to smallness of the face and body.

pseudohydrophobia (-hi″dro-fo′be-ah) hydrophobophobia.

pseudohypertrichosis (-hi″per-trī-ko′sis) persistence after birth of fine hair present during fetal life, due to inability of the skin to throw it off.

pseudohypertrophy (-hi-per′tro-fe) increase of size with loss of function.

pseudohypoparathyroidism (-hi″po-par″ah-thi′roi-dizm) a condition clinically resembling hypoparathyroidism, but caused by failure of response to rather than deficiency of parathyroid hormone.

pseudoleukemia (-lu-ke′me-ah) a condition clinically resembling leukemia, but without its characteristic blood findings.

pseudologia (-lo′je-ah) the writing of anonymous letters to people of prominence, to one's self, etc. **p. fantas′tica,** a tendency to tell extravagant and fantastic falsehoods centered about one's self.

pseudomania (-ma′ne-ah) 1. false or pretended mental disorder. 2. pathologic lying.

pseudomelanosis (-mel″ah-no′sis) pigmentation of tissues after death.

pseudomelia (-me′le-ah) phantom limb. **p. parœsthet′ica,** the perception of morbid or perverted sensations as occurring in an absent or paralyzed limb.

pseudomembrane (-mem′brān) a tough layer of gray-white exudate, resembling a true membrane formed on the mucosa in certain diseases. adj., **pseudomem′branous.**

Pseudomonadaceae (-mo″nah-da′se-e) a family of Schizomycetes (order Pseudomonadales, suborder Pseudomonadineae) found in soil and fresh or salt water.

Pseudomonadales (-mo″nah-da′lez) an order of Schizomycetes, including suborders Rhodobacteriineae and Pseudomonadineae.

Pseudomonadineae (-mo″nah-di′ne-e) a suborder of Schizomycetes (order Pseudomonadales).

Pseudomonas (-mo′nas) a genus of Schizomycetes (order Pseudomonadales, suborder Pseudomonadineae, family Pseudomonadaceae).

pseudomucin (-mu′sin) a variety of mucin from ovarian cysts.

pseudo-obstruction (-ob-struk′shun) a condition simulating obstruction. **intestinal p.,** a

condition characterized by constipation, colicky pain and vomiting, but without evidence of organic obstruction at laparotomy.

pseudopapilledema (su″do-pap″ĭ-lĕ-de′mah) anomalous elevation of the optic disk.

pseudoparalysis (-pah-ral′ĭ-sis) loss of muscular power without real paralysis.

pseudoparaphrasia (-par″ah-fra′ze-ah) complete general incoherence in which the patient calls everything by a wrong name.

pseudoparaplegia (-par″ah-ple′je-ah) paralysis of the lower limbs, but with normal reflexes.

pseudoparasite (-par′ah-sīt) a facultative parasite.

pseudoparesis (-par′ĕ-sis) a hysterical condition simulating paresis.

pseudopelade (-pe′lād) alopecia with formation of small white cicatrices.

pseudophakia (-fa′ke-ah) failure of development of the crystalline lens, its place being occupied by tissue of abnormal type.

pseudophthisis (su″dof-thi′sis) a wasting not due to tuberculosis.

pseudoplegia (su″do-ple′je-ah) hysterical paralysis.

pseudopodium (-po′de-um) a temporary protrusion of the protoplasm of an ameba, serving for purposes of locomotion or to engulf food.

pseudopolyp (-pol′ip) a hypertrophied tab of mucous membrane resembling a polyp.

pseudopolyposis (-pol″ĭ-po′sis) numerous pseudopolyps in the colon and rectum, due to long standing inflammation.

pseudopregnancy (-preg′nan-se) false pregnancy.

pseudo-pseudohypoparathyroidism (-su″do-hi″po-par″ah-thi′roi-dizm) a condition resembling pseudohypoparathyroidism, but with normal levels of calcium and phosphorus in the blood serum.

pseudopsia (su-dop′se-ah) pseudoblepsis.

pseudopterygium (su″do-ter-ij′e-um) a fold of conjunctiva attached to any part of the cornea, following ulceration of the cornea.

pseudoptosis (-to′sis) decrease in the size of the palpebral aperture.

pseudorabies (-ra′be-ēz) a highly contagious viral disease of cattle, sometimes present as an unrecognized infection of swine, and communicable also to dogs and cats.

pseudorickets (-rik′ets) renal osteodystrophy.

pseudoscarlatina (-skar″lah-te′nah) a septic condition with fever and eruption resembling scarlet fever.

pseudosclerosis (-skle-ro′sis) hepaticolenticular degeneration, with tremors, rigidity, emotional disturbance and optic atrophy.

pseudoscrotum (-skro′tum) a solid partition with a median raphe, resembling the scrotum in the male, obliterating the opening into the vagina in female pseudohermaphroditism.

pseudosmia (su-doz′me-ah) a sensation of odor without the appropriate stimulus.

pseudostoma (su-dos′to-mah) an apparent communication between stained endothelial cells.

pseudosyphilis (su″do-sif′ĭ-lis) a condition resembling syphilis, but not caused by *Treponema pallidum*.

pseudotabes (-ta′bēz) a disease simulating locomotor ataxia.

pseudotetanus (-tet′ah-nus) persistent muscular contractions not associated with *Clostridium tetani*.

pseudotuberculosis (-tu-ber″ku-lo′sis) condition like tuberculosis, but not caused by *Mycobacterium tuberculosis*.

pseudotyphoid (-ti′foid) spurious typhoid fever.

P.S.G.B.I. Pathological Society of Great Britian and Ireland.

p.s.i. pounds per square inch.

psilocin (si′lo-sin) a hallucinogenic substance closely related to psilocybin.

psilocybin (si″lo-si′bin) a hallucinogenic crystalline compound isolated from a species of mushrooms.

psilosis (si-lo′sis) 1. sprue. 2. falling out of the hair.

psittacosis (sit″ah-ko′sis) a viral disease first observed in parrots and known to be transmitted by them to man, later discovered in other birds and domestic fowl.

psodymus (sod′ĭ-mus) a fetal monster with two heads and two trunks, but united below.

psoitis (so-i′tis) inflammation of a psoas muscle or its sheath.

psora (so′rah) 1. scabies. 2. psoriasis.

psorelcosis (sor″el-ko′sis) ulceration due to scabies.

psoriasis (so-ri′ah-sis) a chronic, recurrent papulosquamous dermatosis with silvery gray scaling papules or plaques.

psorous (so′rus) affected with itch.

P.S.P. phenolsulfonphthalein.

psych(o) (si′ko) word element [Gr.], *mind*.

psychalgia (si-kal′je-ah) pain experienced in the mind and due to psychic causes, e.g. anxiety or depression. adj., **psychal′gic**.

psychalia (si-ka′le-ah) a morbid state in which voices seem to be heard and images to be seen.

psychanalysis (si″kah-nal′ĭ-sis) psychoanalysis.

psychanopsia (-nop′se-ah) psychic blindness.

psychasthenia (si″kas-the′ne-ah) a functional neurosis marked by anxiety, pathologic fears and obsessions.

psychataxia (si″kah-tak′se-ah) disordered mental state with confusion, agitation and inability to fix the attention.

psyche (si′ke) the human faculty for thought, judgment and emotion; the mental life, including both conscious and unconscious processes.

psycheclampsia (si″ke-klamp′se-ah) acute mania.

psychedelic (si″kĕ-del′ik) pertaining to freedom from anxiety and, by relaxation, enjoyable perceptional changes and highly creative thought patterns; by extension, applied to a type of drug which produces these effects.

psychiatrist (si-ki′ah-trist) a specialist in psychiatry.

psychiatry (si-ki′ah-tre) the branch of medicine devoted to study of the genesis, diagnosis, prevention and treatment of emotional illness and mental disorders. adj., **psychiat′ric**. **descriptive p.**, that based on observation and study of external factors that can be seen, heard or felt. **dynamic p.**, the study of emotional processes, their origins and the mental mechanisms underlying them.

psychic (si′kik) pertaining to the mind.

psychics (si′kiks) psychology.

psycho-allergy (si″ko-al′er-je) a condition of sensitization to certain words, ideas, people and other symbols of emotional patterns.

psychoanaleptic (-an″ah-lep′tik) stimulating the mind.

psychoanalysis (-ah-nal′ĭ-sis) a method of diagnosing and treating mental and emotional disorders through ascertaining and analyzing the facts of the patient's mental life.

psychobiology (-bi-ol′o-je) study of the interrelations of body and mind in the formation and functioning of personality. adj., **psychobiolog′ical**.

psychocoma (-ko′mah) melancholic stupor.

psychocutaneous (-ku-ta′ne-us) pertaining to the relations between mental or emotional factors and skin disorders.

psychodelic (-del′ik) psychedelic.

psychodiagnosis (-di″ag-no′sis) the use of psychologic testing in the diagnosis of disease.

psychodrama (-drah′mah) the psychiatric technique of having a patient act out conflicting situations of his daily life.

psychodynamics (-di-nam′iks) the science of human behavior and motivation.

psychodysleptic (-dis-lep′tik) inducing a delusional state of mind.

psychogalvanometer (-gal″vah-nom′ĕ-ter) a galvanometer for recording the electrical agitation produced by emotional stresses.

psychogenesis (-jen′ĕ-sis) mental development.

psychogenic (-jen′ik) originating in the mind.

psychogeriatrics (-jer″e-at′riks) psychologic and psychiatric treatment of the aged.

psychognosis (si″kog-no′sis) study of mental activity.

psychogram (si′ko-gram) a tabulation of personality traits.

psychokinesis (si″ko-ki-ne′sis) the influence of mind on matter without the intermediation of physical force.

psycholepsy (-lep′se) a mild and temporary attack of confusion, tachycardia and blindness occurring in nervous or hysterical persons.

psycholeptic (-lep′tik) exerting a relaxing effect on the mind.

psychology (si-kol′o-je) the scientific study of mental processes and behavior. adj., **psycholog′ic**. **abnormal p.**, the study of derangements or deviations of mental functions. **analytic p.**, psychology by introspective methods. **animal p.**, the study of the mental activity of animals **child p.**, the study of the development of the mind of the child. **clinical p.**, the use of psychologic knowledge and techniques in the treatment of persons with emotional difficulties. **criminal p.**, the study of the mental action of criminals. **depth p.**, that dealing with intrapsychic phenomena rather than the more superficial, behavioral phenomena. **dynamic p.**, a school of psychology which stresses the element of energy in mental processes. **experimental p.**, the study of the mind and mental operations by the use of experimental methods. **genetic p.**, that branch of psychology which deals with the development of mind in the individual and with its evolution in the race. **gestalt p.**, gestaltism. **physiologic p.**, that branch of psychology which applies the facts taught in neurology to show the relation between the mental and the neural. **social p.**, that branch of psychology which treats of the social aspects of mental life.

psychotrician (si"ko-mĕ-trish'an) a person skilled in psychometry.

psychometrics (-met'riks) the testing and measuring of mental and psychologic ability, efficiency, potentials and functioning.

psychometry (si-kom'ĕ-tre) measurement of work done and of time consumed in mental operations.

psychomotor (si"ko-mo'tor) pertaining to motor effects of cerebral or psychic activity.

psychoneurosis (-nu-ro'sis) neurosis. adj., **psychoneurot'ic.**

psychonomy (si-kon'o-me) the science of the laws of mental activity.

psychopath (si'ko-path) a person who has a psychopathic personality. **sexual p.**, one whose sexual behavior is manifestly antisocial and criminal.

psychopathic (si"ko-path'ik) pertaining to mental disease.

psychopathology (-pah-thol'o-je) the study of abnormal behavior, its manifestations, development and causation.

psychopathy (si-kop'ah-the) any disease of the mind.

psychopharmacology (si"ko-fahr"mah-kol'o je) the study of the action of drugs on the mind. adj., **psychopharmacolog'ic.**

psychophylaxis (-fi-lak'sis) mental hygiene.

psychophysics (-fiz'iks) scientific study of quantitative relations between characteristics or patterns of physical stimuli and the sensations induced by them.

psychophysiology (-fiz"e-ol'o-je) scientific study of interaction and interrelations of psychic and physiologic factors. adj., **psychophysiolog'ic.**

psychoplegic (-ple'jik) an agent lessening cerebral excitability.

psychoprophylaxis (-pro"fi-lak'sis) , psychophysical training aimed at suppression of painful sensation associated with normal childbirth. adj., **psychoprophylac'tic.**

psychorrhea (-re'ah) an incoherent stream of thought.

psychorrhythmia (-rith'me-ah) involuntary repetition of various mental actions.

psychosensory (si"ko-sen'sor-e) perceiving and interpreting sensory stimuli.

psychosexual (-seks'u-al) pertaining to the psychic or emotional portion of the sex instinct.

psychosis (si-ko'sis), pl. *psycho'ses* Gr.] a major emotional disorder with derangement of the personality and loss of contact with reality, often with delusions, hallucinations or illusions. adj., **psychot'ic. affective p.**, one marked by severe disorder of mood or emotional feeling. **alcoholic p.**, mental disorder caused by excessive use of alcohol. **depressive p.**, one characterized by mental depression, melancholy, despondency, inadequacy and feelings of guilt. **drug p.**, a toxic psychosis due to the ingestion of drugs. **exhaustion p.**, a psychosis due to some exhausting or depressing occurrence, as an operation. **functional p.**, a psychosis not caused by organic disease or dysfunction. **gestational p.**, a psychosis developing during pregnancy. **involutional p.**, psychosis occurring in late middle life, marked by severe depression and sometimes by paranoid thinking. **Korsakoff's p.**, a syndrome marked by amnesia, confabulation and peripheral neuritis, usually associated with alcoholism and vitamin deficiencies. **manic p.**, one characterized by emotional instability. **manic-depressive p.**, an essentially benign affective psychosis, chiefly marked by emotional instability, striking mood swings and a tendency to recurrence; seen in the manic, depressed, circular, mixed, perplexed and stuporous types. **organic p.**, a psychosis due to a lesion of the central nervous system, such as general paresis. **paranoiac p., paranoid p.**, one in which the patient has delusions that others are plotting to injure him. **periodic p.**, a condition in which intermittent periods of depression or hypomania recur regularly in a seemingly mentally healthy or nearly healthy person. **polyneuritic p.**, Korsakoff's psychosis. **senile p.**, mental deterioration of old age, with tendency to confabulation, loss of memory of recent events, irritability and assaultiveness. **situational p.**, psychosis caused by an unbearable situation over which the patient has no control.

psychosolytic (si"ko-so-lit'ik) relieving or abolishing psychotic symptoms.

psychosomatic (-mat'ik) pertaining to the interrelations of mind and body.

psychosomimetic (si-ko"so-mi-met'ik) psychotomimetic.

psychosurgery (si"ko-ser'jer-e) the performance of operations on the brain as a means of treating emotional or mental disorder.

psychotherapy (-ther'ah-pe) treatment designed to produce a response by mental rather than by physical effects.

psychotogenic (si-kot"o-jen'ik) producing a psychosis.

psychotomimetic (-mi-met'ik) characterized by or producing symptoms similar to those of a psychosis.

psychotonic (si″ko-ton′ik) elevating or stimulating the mind.

psychotropic (-trop′ik) exerting an effect upon the mind.

psychr(o)- (si′kro) word element [Gr.], *cold.*

psychralgia (si-kral′je-ah) a painful sensation of cold.

psychrometer (si-krom′ĕ-ter) an instrument for measuring the moisture of the atmosphere.

psychrophile (si′kro-fīl) an organism growing best at 15–20°C. adj., **psychrophil′ic.**

psychrophobia (-fo′be-ah) morbid dread of cold.

psychrotherapy (-ther′ah-pe) treatment of disease by applying cold.

Pt. chemical symbol, *platinum.*

pt. pint.

PTA plasma thromboplastin antecedent.

ptarmic (tar′mik) causing sneezing.

ptarmus (tar′mus) spasmodic sneezing.

PTC plasma thromboplastin component.

pterin (ter′in) a colorless or yellow compound found in the wings of butterflies and wasps, characterized by fluorescence in neutral solution.

pterion (te′re-on) point of junction of frontal, parietal, temporal and sphenoid bones.

pterygium (tĕ-rij′e-um) a winglike structure, especially a patch of thickened conjunctiva extending over part of the cornea, or an abnormal extension and adherence of the cuticle over the proximal portion of the nail plate. **p. col′li,** a band of tissue from the mastoid region to the region of the sternum.

pterygoid (ter′ĭ-goid) shaped like a wing.

pterygomaxillary (ter″ĭ-go-mak′sĭ-ler″e) pertaining to a pterygoid process and the maxilla.

pterygopalatine (-pal′ah-tīn) pertaining to a pterygoid process and the palate bone.

ptilosis (ti-lo′sis) falling out of the eyelashes.

ptomaine (to′mān, to-mān′) a basic substance derived from putrefying tissues.

ptosis (to′sis) abnormal downward displacement of an organ or body structure, especially paralytic drooping of the upper eyelid. adj., **ptot′ic.**

-ptosis (to′sis) word element [Gr.], *downward displacement.* adj., **-ptot′ic.**

PTT partial thromboplastin time.

ptyalagogue (ti-al′ah-gog) sialagogue.

ptyalectasis (ti″ah-lek′tah-sis) 1. a state of dilatation of a salivary duct. 2. surgical dilation of a salivary duct.

ptyalin (ti′ah-lin) an enzyme found in saliva.

ptyalinogen (ti″ah-lin′o-jen) the precursor of ptyalin.

ptyalism (ti′al-izm) excessive secretion of saliva.

ptyalocele (ti-al′o-sēl) ranula.

ptyalogenic (ti″ah-lo-jen′ik) formed from saliva.

ptyaloreaction (-re-ak′shun) a reaction occurring in or performed on the saliva.

ptyalorrhea (-re′ah) ptyalism.

Pu chemical symbol, *plutonium.*

pubarche (pu-bar′ke) the first appearance of pubic hair.

puberty (pu′ber-te) the period marked by the beginning development of secondary sex characteristics. adj., **pu′beral, pu′bertal.**

pubes (pu′bēz) 1. the hair on the external genitalia, or the region covered with it. 2. plural of *pubis.* adj., **pu′bic.**

pubescence (pu-bes′ens) 1. puberty. 2. lanugo.

pubescent (pu-bes′ent) 1. arriving at the age of puberty. 2. covered with down or lanugo.

pubiotomy (pu″be-ot′o-me) transection of the symphysis pubis.

pubis (pu′bis), pl. *pu′bes* [L.] the anterior portion of the pelvic bone, a distinct bone in early life.

pubofemoral (pu″bo-fem′o-ral) pertaining to pubis and femur.

puboprostatic (-pros-tat′ik) pertaining to pubis and prostate.

pubovesical (-ves′ĭ-kal) pertaining to pubis and bladder.

pudendum (pu-den′dum), pl. *puden′da* [L.] external structures of the reproductive system in the female, including the mons pubis and the labia majora and minora. adj., **puden′dal, pu′dic.**

puericulture (pu′er-ĭ-kul″tūr) art of rearing children.

puerile (pu′er-il) pertaining to a child or to childhood.

puerilism (pu′er-il-izm″) reversion of the mind to the state of childhood.

puerpera (pu-er′per-ah) a woman who has just given birth to a child.

puerperal (pu-er′per-al) pertaining to a puerpera or to the puerperium.

puerperalism (pu-er′per-al-izm″) morbid condition incident to childbirth.

puerperium (pu″er-pe′re-um) the period or state of confinement after childbirth.

Pulex (pu′leks) a genus of fleas, several species of which transmit the microorganism causing plague. **P. ir′ritans,** a widely distributed species, known as the human flea, which infests domestic animals as well as man.

pulicicide (pu-lis′ĭ-sīd) an agent destructive to fleas.

pulicosis (pu″lĭ-ko′sis) irritation of the skin caused by flea bites.

pullulation (pul″u-la′shun) development by sprouting or budding.

pulmin (pul′min) a substance which inhibits plasmin and trypsin, found in lung tissue of the ox, but not of other animals.

pulmo-aortic (pul″mo-a-or′tik) pertaining to lungs and aorta.

pulmometer (pul-mom′ĕ-ter) an apparatus for measuring lung capacity.

pulmometry (-mom′ĕ-tre) measurement of lung capacity.

pulmonary (pul′mo-ner″e) pertaining to the lungs.

pulmonectomy (pul″mo-nek′to-me) pneumonectomy.

pulmonic (pul-mon′ik) pulmonary.

pulmonitis (pul″mo-ni′tis) inflammation of the lung.

pulmonohepatic (pul-mo″no-hě-pat′ik) pertaining to lung and liver.

pulmonologist (pul″mo-nol′o-jist) a person skilled in pulmonology.

pulmonology (-nol′o-je) the science concerned with the anatomy, physiology and pathology of the lungs.

pulmonoperitoneal (pul-mo″no-per″ĭ-to-ne′al) pertaining to lung and peritoneum.

pulmotor (pul′mo-tor) apparatus for forcing oxygen into the lungs.

pulp (pulp) soft, juicy animal or vegetable tissue. adj., **pul′pal. coronal p.**, the part of the dental pulp contained in the crown portion of the pulp cavity. **dental p.**, richly vascularized and innervated connective tissue inside a tooth. **digital p.**, a cushion of soft tissue on the palmar or plantar surface of the distal phalanx of a finger or toe. **tooth p.**, dental pulp. **white p.**, sheaths of lymphatic tissue surrounding the arteries of the spleen.

pulpa (pul′pah), pl. *pul′pae* [L.] pulp.

pulpalgia (-pal′je-ah) pain in the dental pulp.

pulpectomy (-pek′to-me) removal of dental pulp.

pulpefaction (pul″pě-fak′shun) conversion into pulp.

pulpitis (pul-pi′tis), pl. *pulpit′ides* [L.] inflammation of dental pulp.

pulpoaxial (pul″po-ak′se-al) pertaining to pulpal and axial walls of a tooth cavity.

pulpobuccoaxial (-buk″o-ak′se-al) pertaining to pulpal, buccal and axial walls of a tooth cavity.

pulpodistal (-dis′tal) pertaining to pulpal and distal walls of a tooth cavity.

pulpodontics (-don′tiks) the branch of dentistry concerned with diagnosis and treatment of diseases of the dental pulp.

pulpolabial (-la′be-al) pertaining to pulpal and labial walls of a tooth cavity.

pulpolingual (-ling′gwal) pertaining to pulpal and lingual walls of a tooth cavity.

pulpolinguoaxial (-ling″gwo-ak′se-al) pertaining to pulpal, lingual and axial walls of a tooth cavity.

pulpomesial (-mc′ze-al) pertaining to pulpal and mesial walls of a tooth cavity.

pulpotomy (pul-pot′o-me) incision into the pulp cavity of a tooth.

pulpy (pul′pe) soft; of the consistency of pulp.

pulsatile (pul′sah-til) characterized by a rhythmic pulsation.

pulsation (pul-sa′shun) a throb, or rhythmic beat, as of the heart.

pulse (puls) the impact felt in a vessel caused by blood forced out by contraction of the heart. **abdominal p.**, that in the abdominal aorta. **abrupt p.**, one which strikes the finger rapidly. **anacrotic p.**, one which makes a break in the ascending limb of the sphygmogram. **ardent p.**, one which appears to strike the finger at a single point. **bigeminal p.**, one in which two beats occur in rapid succession, the groups of two being separated by a longer interval. **catacrotic p.**, one which makes a break in the descending limb of the sphygmogram. **cordy p.**, a tense, firm pulse. **Corrigan's p.**, jerky pulse with full expansion and sudden collapse. **dicrotic p.**, one with exaggerated recoil wave. **full p.**, one with copious volume of blood. **hard p.**, one characterized by high tension. **hyperdicrotic p.**, one showing an aortic notch below the base line of the sphygmogram; a sign of extreme exhaustion. **jerky p.**, one in which the artery is suddenly and markedly distended. **paradoxical p.**, one that is weaker during inspiration, as in some cases of adherent pericardium. **quick p.**, one which strikes the finger smartly and leaves it quickly. **Quincke's p.**, reddening of the nail bed with each systole; seen in aortic insufficiency. **radial p.**, that felt over the radial artery. **Riegel's p.**, one which is smaller during respiration. **thready p.**, one that is very fine and scarcely perceptible. **tricrotic p.**, one showing three sphygmographic waves to the pulse beat. **undulating p.**, one giving the sensation of successive waves. **unequal p.**, one in which some beats are strong and others weak. **vagus p.**, a slow pulse caused by influence of the vagus nerve on the heart. **water-hammer p.**, Corrigan's pulse. **wiry p.**, a small, tense pulse.

pulsimeter (pul-sim′ě-ter) apparatus for measuring force of pulse.

pulsus (pul′sus) [L.] pulse. **p. bigem′inus**, bigeminal pulse. **p. ce′ler**, a swift, abrupt pulse. **p. dif′ferens**, inequality of the pulse observable at corresponding sites on either side of the body. **p. paradox′us**, paradoxical pulse. **p. ra′rus**, a slow pulse due to prolongation of the heart beat. **p. tar′dus**, an abnormally slow pulse.

pultaceous (pul-ta′shus) like a poultice; pulpy.

pulverulent (pul-ver′u-lent) powdery; dusty.

pulvinar (pul vi′nar) the posterior inner part of the optic thalamus.

pumice (pum′is) a substance consisting of silicates of aluminum, potassium and sodium; used in dentistry as an abrasive or polishing agent.

pump (pump) apparatus for drawing and removing liquid. **air p.**, one for exhausting or forcing in air. **blood p.**, a machine used to propel blood through the tubing of extracorporeal circulation devices. **breast p.**, pump for taking milk from the breast. **dental p.**, device for removing saliva during dental operations. **stomach p.**, pump for removing contents from the stomach.

punctate (pungk′tāt) spotted; marked with points or punctures.

punctiform (pungk′tĭ-form) like a point.

punctum (pungk′tum), pl. *punc′ta* [L.] point. **p. cae′cum**, blind spot. **punc′ta doloro′sa**, painful spots along a nerve. **p. lacrima′le** (pl. *punc′ta lacrima′lia*), an opening of a lacrimal canal on the edge of the eyelid. **p. lu′teum**, macula lutea. **p. ossificatio′nis,**

center of ossification. **p. prox'imum,** near point. **p. remo'tum,** far point. **punc'ta vasculo'sa,** minute red spots which mark the cut surface of white substance of the brain.

puncture (pungk'tŭr) 1. the piercing of an organ or other body structure with a long hollow needle for the withdrawal of fluid or the removal of tissue for microscopic study. 2. a wound made by a pointed instrument. **cisternal p.,** puncture of the cisterna magna through the atlanto-occipital ligament. **lumbar p.,** puncture of the spinal canal in the region of the lumbar vertebrae. **spinal p.,** puncture of the spinal canal. **sternal p.,** removal of bone marrow from the manubrium of the sternum through a spinal puncture needle.

P.U.O. pyrexia of unknown origin.

pupil (pu'pil) the opening in the center of the iris. adj., **pu'pillary. Argyll Robertson p.,** one which is miotic and responds to accommodative effort, but not to light. **Hutchinson's p.,** one which is dilated while the other is not.

pupilla (pu-pil'ah) [L.] pupil.

pupillatonia (pu″pil-ah-to'ne-ah) failure of the pupil to react to light.

pupillometry (-lom'ĕ-tre) measurement of the diameter or width of the pupil of the eye.

pupilloplegia (pu″pī-lo-ple'je-ah) pupillatonia.

pupilloscopy (pu″pī-los'ko-pe) skiascopy.

pupillostatometer (pu″pī-lo-stah-tom'ĕ-ter) instrument for measuring distance between the pupils.

pupillotonia (-to'ne-ah) abnormal tonic reaction of the pupil, as in Adie's syndrome.

purgation (per-ga'shun) catharsis; purging effected by a cathartic medicine.

purgative (per'gah-tiv) 1. effecting purgation; cathartic. 2. a medicine which causes purgation.

purge (perj) 1. a purgative medicine or dose. 2. to cause free evacuation of feces.

purine (pu'rēn) the cystalline compound $C_5H_4N_4$, or one of a group of compounds of which it is the base, such as uric acid, adenine, xanthine, guanidine, hypoxanthine and theobromine.

Purinethol (pu'rēn-thol) trademark for a preparation of mercaptopurine.

Purodigin (pu″ro-dī'jin) trademark for a preparation of crystalline digitoxin.

purpura (per'pu-rah) a condition characterized by confluent petechiae or ecchymoses over any area of the body. adj., **purpu'ric. allergic p., anaphylactic p.,** a form of unknown origin, associated with increased capillary permeability and one or more allergic symptoms. **p. annula'ris telangiecto'des,** a rare form in which punctate erythematous lesions coalesce to form an annular or serpiginous pattern. **p. ful'minans,** a nonthrombocytopenic purpura observed mainly in children, usually following an infectious disease, and often associated with extensive extravascular thromboses and gangrene. **p. hemorrha'gica,** idiopathic thrombocytopenic purpura. **Henoch's p.,**

nonthrombocytopenic purpura with acute visceral symptoms such as vomiting, diarrhea, hematuria and renal colic. **p. hyperglobuline'mica,** purpura with an increase in gamma globulins; no longer considered a specific entity. **malignant p.,** cerebrospinal fever. **nonthrombocytopenic p.,** purpura without any decrease in the platelet count of the blood. **Schönlein-Henoch p.,** idiopathic purpura in which there may be concomitant articular symptoms (Schönlein's disease) and intestinal symptoms with onset of abdominal pain. **thrombocytopenic p.,** purpura associated with a decrease in the number of platelets in the blood, occurring as a primary disease *(idiopathic thrombocytopenic purpura)* or as a consequence of another disorder *(secondary thrombocytopenic purpura).* **thrombotic thrombocytopenic p.,** thrombocytopenic purpura associated with thrombosis in terminal arterioles and capillaries.

purpureaglycoside (per-pu″re-ah-gli'ko-sīd) a cardiac glycoside from the leaves of *Digitalis purpurea.* **p.,** deslanoside.

purpurin (per'pu-rin) a red coloring matter of the urine.

purulence (pu'roo-lens) the formation or presence of pus.

purulent (pur'roo-lent) containing or consisting of pus.

puruloid (pu'roo-loid) resembling pus.

pus (pus) a thick fluid composed of viable and necrotic polymorphonuclear leukocytes, with necrotic tissue debris partially liquefied by enzymes liberated from the dead leukocytes, and other tissue breakdown products, characteristically produced in infections due to certain bacteria.

pustula (pus'tu-lah), pl. *pus'tulae* [L.] pustule.

pustulant (pus'tu-lant) causing pustulation.

pustulation (pus″tu-la'shun) the formation of pustules.

pustule (pus'tūl) a circumscribed, pus-containing lesion of the skin, up to 5 mm. in diameter. adj., **pus'tular. malignant p.,** anthrax.

pustulosis (pus″tu-lo'sis) a condition marked by an eruption of pustules.

putamen (pū-ta'men) the darker and outer part of the lenticular nucleus.

putrefaction (pū″trĕ-fak'shun) decomposition of animal or vegetable matter effected largely by action of microorganisms. adj., **putrefac'tive.**

putrescent (pū-tres'ent) undergoing putrefaction.

putrescine (pū-tres'in) tetramethylene-diamine.

PVP polyvinylpyrrolidine.

pyarthrosis (pi″ar-thro'sis) suppurative inflammation of a joint; suppurative arthritis.

pyc- for words beginning thus, see those beginning *pyk-.*

pyel(o) (pi'ĕ-lo) word element [Gr.], *renal pelvis.*

pyelectasis (pi″ĕ-lek′tah-sis) dilatation of the kidney pelvis.

pyelephlebitis (pi″ĕ-lĕ-fle-bi′tis) pylephlebitis.

pyelitis (-li′tis) inflammation of the kidney pelvis. adj., **pyelit′ic. p. cys′tica,** chronic pyelitis with cyst formation.

pyelocaliectasis (pi″ĕ-lo-kal″e-ek′tah-sis) dilatation of the kidney pelvis and calyces.

pyelocystitis (-sis-ti′tis) inflammation of renal pelvis and bladder.

pyelogram (pi′ĕ-lo-gram″) the film produced by pyclography.

pyelography (pi″e-log′rah-fe) radiography of the kidney and ureter after injection of contrast material. **ascending p.,** retrograde pyelography. **p. by elimination,** intravenous pyelography. **excretion p.,** radiography of the kidney with opacification achieved by contrast material injected into the blood stream and excreted by the kidney. **intravenous p.,** pyelography after intravenous injection of a contrast medium which is excreted in the urine. **retrograde p.,** radiography of the kidney after introduction of contrast material into the ureter.

pyeloileocutaneous (pi″e-lo-il″e-o-ku-ta′ne-us) pertaining to the kidney pelvis, ileum and skin.

pyelolithotomy (-li-thot′o-me) incision of the renal pelvis for removal of calculi.

pyelometer (pi″ĕ-lom′ĕ-ter) a pelvimeter.

pyelometry (-lom′ĕ-tre) 1. measurement of the renal pelvis. 2. pelvimetry.

pyelonephritis (pi″ĕ-lo-nĕ-fri′tis) inflammation of kidney and renal pelvis. **p. bacillo′sa bo′vum,** purulent inflammation of the renal pelvis in cows.

pyelonephrosis (-nĕ-fro′sis) any disease of the kidney and its pelvis.

pyelopathy (pi″ĕ-lop′ah-the) any disease of the renal pelvis.

pyelophlebitis (pi″e-lo-fle-bi′tis) inflammation of the veins of the renal pelvis.

pyeloplasty (pi′ĕ-lo-plas″te) plastic repair of the renal pelvis.

pyelostomy (pi″e-los′to-me) fistulization of the renal pelvis.

pyolotomy (-lot′o-me) incision of the renal pelvis.

pyemesis (pi-em′e-sis) the vomiting of pus

pyemia (pi-e′me-ah) the presence of pus cells in the circulating blood. adj., **pye′mic.**

pyemotes (pi″ĕ-mo′tēz) a genus of mites. **P. ventrico′sus,** a species parasitic on various insect pests which occasionally causes a dermatitis in man (straw itch).

pyencephalus (pi″en-sef′ah-lus) abscess of the brain.

pygal (pi′gal) pertaining to the buttocks.

pygalgia (pi-gal′je-ah) pain in the buttocks.

pygodidymus (pi″go-did′ĭ-mus) a fetal monster with double hips and pelvis.

pygomelus (pi-gom′ĕ-lus) a fetal monster with extra limbs on the buttocks.

pygopagus (pi-gop′ah-gus) a twin fetal monster joined at the buttocks.

ykn(o)- (pik′no) word element [Gr.], *thick; compact; frequent.*

pyknemia (pik-ne′me-ah) thickening of the blood.

pyknic (pik′nik) having a short, thick, stocky build.

pyknolepsy (pik′no-lep″se) a form of idiopathic epilepsy in which momentary lapses of consciousness may occur as frequently as hundreds of times daily.

pyknometer (pik-nom′ĕ-ter) 1. instrument for measuring thickness of parts. 2. instrument for determining specific gravity of urine.

pyknomorphous (pik″no-mor′fus) having the stained portions of the cell body compactly arranged.

pyknophrasia (-fra′ze-ah) thickness of speech.

pyknosis (pik-no′sis) thickening and shrinkage of the nucleus after death of a cell. adj., **pyknot′ic.**

pylemphraxis (pi″lem-frak′sis) obstruction of the portal vein.

pylephlebectasis (pi″le-fle-bek′tah-sis) dilatation of the portal vein.

pylephlebitis (-fle-bi′tis) inflammation of the portal vein.

pylethrombophlebitis (-throm″bo-fle-bi′tis) thrombosis and inflammation of the portal vein.

pylethrombosis (-throm-bo′sis) thrombosis of the portal vein.

pyloralgia (pi″lo-ral′je-ah) pain and spasm of the pylorus.

pylorectomy (-rek′to-me) excision of the pylorus.

pyloroduodenitis (pi-lor″o-du″o-de-ni′tis) inflammation of pyloric and duodenal mucosa.

pyloromyotomy (-mi-ot′o-me) incision of muscles of the pylorus.

pyloroplasty (pi-lor′o-plas″te) plastic surgery of the pylorus.

pyloroscopy (pi″lor-os′ko-pe) inspection of the pylorus.

pylorospasm (pi-lor′o-spazm) functional obstruction of the orifice between stomach and duodenum. **congenital p.,** spasm of the pylorus in infants from birth. **reflex p.,** pylorospasm due to extragastric conditions.

pylorostenosis (pi-lor″o-ste-no′sis) stenosis of the pylorus.

pylorostomy (pi″lor-os′to-me) formation of an opening into the pylorus through the abdominal wall.

pylorotomy (-ot′o-me) 1. gastrotomy. 2. pyloromyotomy.

pylorus (pi-lo′rus) the distal aperture of the stomach, opening into the duodenum. adj., **pylor′ic.**

pyo- (pi′o) word element [Gr.], *pus.*

pyocalix (pi″o-ka′liks) pus in the calix of the kidney pelvis.

pyocele (pi′o-sēl) collection of pus about the testis.

pyocelia (pi″o-se′le-ah) pus in the abdominal cavity.

pyocephalus (-sef′ah-lus) abscess in the brain.

pyochezia (-ke′ze-ah) presence of pus corpuscles in the feces.

pyococcus (pi″o-kok′us) a micrococcus which causes suppuration.

pyocolpos (-kol′pos) pus in the vagina.

pyocyanase (-si′ah-nās) an antibacterial substance from cultures of *Pseudomonas aeruginosa* (*pyocyanea*).

pyocyanin (-si′ah-nin) a pigment, $C_{14}H_{14}NO_2$, from blue pus.

pyocyst (pi′o-sist) a cyst containing pus.

pyoderma (pi″o-der′mah) a purulent skin disease. **p. gangreno′sum,** a cutaneous ulcer originating in an operative or traumatic wound, with undermining of the border.

pyodermatitis (-der″mah-ti′tis) dermatitis from pyogenic infection.

pyodermatosis (-der″mah-to′sis) any skin disease of pyogenic origin.

pyodermia (-der′me-ah) pyoderma.

pyofecia (-fe′se-ah) pus in the feces.

pyogenesis (-jen′ĕ-sis) the formation of pus.

pyogenic (-jen′ik) producing suppuration.

pyohemia (-he′me-ah) pyemia.

pyohemothorax (-he″mo-tho′raks) pus and blood in the pleural cavity.

pyoid (pi′oid) resembling or like pus.

pyolabyrinthitis (pi″o-lab″ĭ-rin-thi′tis) inflammation of the labyrinth of the ear, with suppuration.

pyometra (-me′trah) accumulation of pus within the uterus.

pyometritis (-me-tri′tis) purulent inflammation of the uterus.

pyonephritis (-nĕ-fri′tis) purulent inflammation of the kidney.

pyonephrolithiasis (-nef″ro-lĭ-thi′ah-sis) pus and stones in the kidney.

pyonephrosis (-nĕ-fro′sis) suppurative destruction of the renal parenchyma, with total or almost complete loss of kidney function.

pyonychia (-nik′e-ah) bacterial infection of the fold surrounding a nail.

pyo-ovarium (-o-va′re-um) an abscess of the ovary.

pyopericarditis (-per″ĭ-kar-di′tis) purulent pericarditis.

pyopericardium (-per″ĭ-kar′de-um) pus in the pericardium.

pyoperitoneum (-per″ĭ-to-ne′um) pus in the peritoneal cavity.

pyoperitonitis (-per″ĭ-to-ni′tis) purulent inflammation of the peritoneum.

pyophthalmitis (pi″of-thal-mi′tis) purulent inflammation of the eye.

pyophysometra (pi″o-fi″so-me′trah) pus and gas in the uterus.

pyoplania (-pla′ne-ah) wandering of pus from one place to another.

pyopneumocholecystitis (-nu″mo-ko″le-sis-ti′tis) inflammation of the gallbladder, with presence of pus and gas.

pyopneumohepatitis (-hep″ah-ti′tis) abscess of the liver with pus and gas in the abscess cavity.

pyopneumopericardium (-per″ĭ-kar′de-um) pus and gas in the pericardium.

pyopneumoperitonitis (-per″ĭ-to-ni′tis) peritonitis with presence of pus and gas.

pyopneumothorax (pi″o-nu″mo-tho′raks) the presence of both purulent exudates and air or gas within the pleural cavity.

pyopoiesis (-poi-e′sis) pyogenesis.

pyoptysis (pi-op′tĭ-sis) expectoration of purulent matter.

pyopyelectasis (pi″o-pi″ĕ-lek′tah-sis) dilatation of the renal pelvis with pus.

pyorrhea (-re′ah) a copious discharge of pus. **p. alveola′ris,** a purulent inflammation of the dental periosteum, with progressive necrosis of the alveoli and looseness of the teeth.

pyosalpingitis (-sal″pin-ji′tis) inflammation of the uterine tube with formation of pus.

pyosalpingo-oophoritis (-sal-ping″go-o″of-o-ri′tis) purulent inflammation of the uterine tube and ovary.

pyosalpinx (-sal′pinks) accumulation of pus in a uterine tube.

pyosis (pi-o′sis) suppuration.

pyospermia (pi″o-sper′me-ah) pus in the semen.

pyostatic (-stat′ik) arresting suppuration.

pyostomatitis (-sto″mah-ti′tis) inflammation of the mucous membrane of the mouth, with suppuration.

pyothorax (-tho′raks) an accumulation of pus in the thorax; empyema.

pyourachus (-u′rah-kus) pus in the urachus.

pyoureter (-u-re′ter) pus in the ureter.

pyovesiculosis (-vĕ-sik″u-lo′sis) pus in the seminal vesicles.

pyoxanthine (-zan′thēn) brownish pigment from oxidation of pyocyanine.

pyoxanthose (-zan′thōs) a yellow pigment from pus.

pyramid (pir′ah-mid) a pointed or cone-shaped structure or part. adj., **pyram′idal. p. of the cerebellum,** the central portion of the inferior vermiform process. **p. of Ferrein,** one of the intracortical prolongations of the malpighian pyramid. **Lalouette's p.,** pyramid of the thyroid. **p. of light,** a triangular reflection seen upon the tympanic membrane. **malpighian p.,** one of the conical masses of the medulla of the kidney. **p's of the medulla,** two anterior and two posterior columns within the oblongata. **petrous p.,** pars petrosa. **renal p.,** one of the wedge-shaped masses constituting the medulla of the kidney, the base toward the cortex and culminating at the summit in the renal papilla. **p. of the thyroid,** the third lobe of the thyroid body. **p. of tympanum,** the elevation in the middle ear which contains the stapedius. **Wistar's p's,** the sphenoturbinal bones.

pyramis (pir′ah-mis), pl. *pyram′ides* [Gr.] pyramid.

pyranisamine (pi″rah-nis′ah-mēn) pyrilamine.

pyrathiazine (-thi′ah-zēn) a phenothiazine compound used as an antihistaminic.

pyrazinamide (-zin′ah-mīd) pyrazinoic acid amide; used as a tuberculostatic agent.

pyrectic (pi-rek′tik) pertaining to fever; feverish.

pyrethrum (pi-re′thrum) dried flowerhead of various species of Chrysanthemum; insecticide.

pyretic (pi-ret′ik) pertaining to fever.

pyretogenesis (pi-re″to-jen′ĕ-sis) the origination of fever.

pyretogenous (pi″rĕ-toj′ĕ-nus) producing fever.

pyretolysis (-tol′ĭ-sis) reduction of fever.

pyretotherapy (pi-re″to-ther′ah-pe) treatment by artificially increasing the patient's body temperature.

pyrexia (pi-rek′se-ah) fever; elevated body temperature. adj., **pyrex′ial.**

pyrexiogenic (pi-rek″se-o-jen′ik) pyrogenic.

Pyribenzamine (pir″ĭ-ben′zah-mēn) trademark for preparations of tripelennamine.

pyridine (pir′ĭ-din) a compound, C_5H_5N, originally isolated from bone oil and coal tar.

pyridostigmine (pir″ĭ-do-stig′mēn) a compound used as a cholinesterase inhibitor in the treatment of myasthenia gravis.

pyridoxine (pir″ĭ-dok′sēn) a component of the vitamin B complex, sometimes used in the treatment of nausea and vomiting of pregnancy and in irradiation sickness.

pyridoxol (-dok′sol) pyridoxine.

pyrilamine (pi-ril′ah-mēn) a compound used as an antihistaminic.

pyrimethamine (pi″rĭ-meth′ah-mēn) a compound used as an antimalarial.

pyrimidine (pi-rim′ĭ-dēn) an organic compound which is the fundamental form of the pyrimidine bases.

pyroborate (pi″ro-bo′rāt) a salt of pyroboric acid.

pyrogen (pi″ro-jen) an agent which causes fever. adj., **pyrogen′ic. bacterial p.,** a fever-producing agent of bacterial origin.

pyroglobulin (pi″ro-glob′u-lin) a blood globulin which precipitates from serum on heating.

pyroglobulinemia (-glob″u-lin-e′me-ah) presence in the blood of an abnormal globulin constituent which is precipitated by heat.

pyroligneous (pi″ro-lig′ne-us) obtained by destructive distillation of wood.

pyrolysis (pi-rol′ĭ-sis) the decomposition of a substance at high temperatures in the absence of oxygen.

pyromania (pi″ro-ma′ne-ah) a morbid compulsion to start fires.

pyrometer (pi-rom′ĕ-ter) a device for measuring high degrees of heat.

Pyronil (pi′ro-nil) trademark for a preparation of pyrrobutamine.

pyronine (pi′ro-nin) a red aniline histologic stain.

pyrophobia (pi″ro-fo′be-ah) morbid dread of fire.

pyrophosphate (-fos′fāt) a salt of pyrophosphoric acid.

pyrosis (pi-ro′sis) burning sensation in the esophagus and stomach, with sour eructation.

pyrotic (pi-rot′ik) caustic.

pyrotoxin (pi″ro-tok′sin) a toxin developed during a fever.

pyroxylin (pi-rok′sĭ-lin) a product of the action of a mixture of nitric and sulfuric acids on cotton, consisting chiefly of cellulose tetranitrate.

pyrrobutamine (pir″ro-bu′tah-min) a compound used as an antihistaminic.

pyrrole (pir′ōl) a compound, found in coal tar and tars, obtained by distillation of waste animal matter.

pyrrolidine (pĭ-rol′ĭ-din) a simple base, tetramethylene imine, which may be obtained from tobacco or prepared from pyrrole.

pyruvate (pi′roo-vāt) a salt or ester of pyruvic acid.

pyrvinium (pir-vin′e-um) a compound used as an anthelminthic.

pyuria (pi-u′re-ah) excretion of urine containing pus corpuscles.

PZI protamine zinc insulin.

Q

Q. quadrant; electric quantity.

q.d. [L.] *qua′que di′e* (every day).

q.h. *qua′que ho′ra* (every hour).

q.i.d. [L.] *qua′ter in di′e* (four times a day).

Q.N.S. Queen's Nursing Sister (of Queen's Institute of District Nursing).

q.q.h. [L.] *qua′que quar′ta ho′ra* (every four hours).

q.s. [L.] *quan′tum sa′tis* (a sufficient amount).

qt. quart.

quack (kwak) one who misrepresents his ability and experience in diagnosis and treatment of disease or effects to be achieved by his treatment.

quackery (kwak′er-e) misrepresentation of one's ability to diagnose and treat disease.

quadr(i)- (kwod′re) word element [L.], *four.*

quadrangular (kwod-rang′gu-lar) having four angles.

quadrant (kwod′rant) 1. one fourth of the circumference of a circle. 2. one of four corresponding parts, or quarters, as of the surface of the abdomen or of the field of vision.

quadrantanopia (kwod″ran-tah-no′pe-ah) loss of vision in one fourth of the visual field.

quadrate (kwod′rāt) square or squared.

quadriceps (kwod′rĭ-seps) having four heads.

quadrigemina (kwod″rĭ-jem′ĭ-nah) the corpora quadrigemina.

quadrigeminal (-jem′ĭ-nal) fourfold; in four parts.

quadrilateral (-lat′er-al) having four sides.

quadrilocular (-lok′u-lar) having four cavities.

quadripara (kwod-rip'ah-rah) A woman who has had four pregnancies which resulted in viable offspring; para IV.

quadripartite (kwod″rī-par'tīt) divided into four.

quadriplegia (-ple'je-ah) tetraplegia.

quadrisect (kwod'rī-sekt) to cut into four parts.

quadritubercular (kwod″rī-tu-ber'ku-lar) having four tubercles or cusps.

quadrivalent (kwod″rī-va'lent, kwod-riv'ah-lent) having a valence of four.

quadruplet (kwod'roo-plet) one of four offspring produced at one birth.

qualimeter (kwah-lim'ĕ-ter) an instrument for measuring the penetrating power of roentgen rays.

quantimeter (kwon-tim'ĕ-ter) an instrument for measuring quantity of roentgen rays generated by a tube.

quantity (kwon'tī-te) 1. a characteristic, as of energy or mass, susceptible of precise physical measurement. 2. a measurable amount. **scalar q.,** a quantity that is expressed only in terms of magnitude. **vector q.,** a quantity that is expressed in terms of magnitude and direction.

quantivalence (kwon-tiv'ah-lens) chemical valence.

quantum (kwon'tum) an elemental unit of energy; the amount emitted or absorbed at each step when energy is emitted or absorbed by atoms or molecules.

quarantine (kwor'an-tēn) 1. place or period of detention of ships coming from infected or suspected ports. 2. restrictions placed on entering or leaving premises where a case of communicable disease exists. **land q.,** quarantine against persons by land from an infected region.

quartan (kwor'tan) recurring in four-day cycles (every third day).

quarter (kwor'ter) the part of a horse's hoof between the heel and the toe. **black q.,** blackleg. **false q.,** a cleft in a horse's hoof from the top to the bottom.

quartile (kwor'tīl, kwor'til) one of the values establishing the division of a series of variables into fourths, or the range of items included in such a segment.

quartipara (kwor-tip'ah-rah) quadripara.

quaternary (kwah'ter-ner″e, kwah-ter'nar-e) 1. fourth in a series. 2. made up of four elements or radicals.

Quelicin (kwel'ī-sin) trademark for a preparation of succinylcholine.

quercetin (kwer'cĕ-tin) the aglucon of rutin and other glycosides, used to reduce abnormal capillary fragility.

Quiactin (kwi-ak'tin) trademark for a preparation of oxanamide.

quickening (kwik'en-ing) the first perceptible movement of the fetus in the uterus.

quinacrine (kwin'ah-krin) a compound used as an antimalarial and anthelminthic.

quinalbarbitone (kwin″al-bar'bī-tōn) secobarbital.

quinidine (kwin'ī-din) an isomer of quinine, used in treatment of cardiac arrhythmias.

quinine (kwi'nīn) white, bitter alkaloid usually obtained from cinchona; tonic, antiperiodic. **q. sulfate,** $(C_{20}H_{24}N_2O_2)_2.H_2SO_4.2H_2O.$ **q. and urea hydrochloride,** double salt of quinine and urea hydrochlorides; sclerosing agent for internal hemorrhoids. **q. and urethan injection,** sterile solution containing quinine hydrochloride and urethan; sclerosing agent for varicose veins.

quininism (kwin'ī-nizm) cinchonism.

quinone (kwi-non', kwin'ōn) a principle, $C_6H_4O_2$, obtained by oxidizing quinic acid.

quinquevalent (kwing″kwē-va'lent, kwing-kwev'ah-lent) pentavalent.

quinsy (kwin'ze) acute suppurative inflammation of the tonsil and 'the surrounding tissue.

quint- (kwint) word element [L.], *five.*

quintan (kwin'tan) recurring every five days (every fourth day).

quintipara (kwin-tip'ah-rah) a woman who has had five pregnancies which resulted in viable offspring; para V.

quintuplet (kwin'tu-plet) one of five offspring produced at one birth.

Quotane (kwo'tān) trademark for preparations of dimethisoquin hydrochloride.

quotid [L.] *quoti'die* (every day).

quotidian (kwo-tid'e-an) recurring every day.

quotient (kwo'shent) a number obtained by division. **achievement q.,** the achievement age divided by the mental age, indicating the progress in learning. **caloric q.,** the heat evolved (in calories) divided by the oxygen consumed (in milligrams) in a metabolic process. **intelligence q.,** see under *intelligence.* **respiratory q.,** an expression of the ratio of the carbon dioxide produced to the oxygen consumed by an organism.

R

R 1. symbol for *roentgen.* 2. a symbol used in general chemical formulas to represent an organic radical.

R. Réaumur; rectal; L. remo'tum *(far);* respiration; right; ohmic resistance.

℞. symbol, L. *rec'ipe* (take).

Ra chemical symbol, *radium.*

rabiate (ra'be-āt) affected with rabies.

rabid (rab'id) affected with hydrophobia or rabies.

rabies (ra'be-ēz) an acute infectious virus disease communicated to man by the bite of an infected animal, usually a dog, and marked by spasm of the muscles of deglutition and respiration, fever, delirium, coma and death. adj., **ra'bic.**

racemic (ra-se'mik) optically inactive, being composed of equal amounts of dextrorotatory and levorotatory isomers.

racemization (ras"e-mī-za'shun) the conversion of a compound having optical activity in either direction into a mixture of compounds having activity in each direction.

racemose (ras'e-mōs) shaped like a bunch of grapes.

racephedrine (ra-sef'e-drin) the racemic mixture of ephedrine; used as a sympathomimetic.

-rachia (ra'ke-ah) word element [Gr.], *state of the spinal fluid;* also sometimes spelled *-rrachia.*

rachialgia (ra"ke-al'je-ah) pain in the vertebral column.

rachianesthesia (-an"es-the'ze-ah) loss of sensation produced by injection of an anesthetic into the spinal canal.

rachicentesis (ra"kī-sen-te'sis) puncture of the subarachnoid space for aspiration of fluid.

rachidian (rah-kid'e-an) pertaining to the spine.

rachilysis (rah-kil'ī-sis) correction of lateral curvature of the spine by combined traction and pressure.

rachiocampsis (ra"ke-o-kamp'sis) spinal curvature.

rachiometer (ra"ke-om'e-ter) apparatus for measuring spinal curvature.

rachiomyelitis (ra"ke-o-mi"e-li'tis) myelitis.

rachioplegia (-ple'je-ah) spinal paralysis.

rachiotomy (ra"ke-ot'o-me) incision of the vertebral column.

rachis (ra'kis) the vertebral column.

rachischisis (rah-kis'kī-sis) congenital fissure of the vertebral column. **r. poste'rior,** spina bifida.

rachitic (rah-kit'ik) pertaining to rickets.

rachitis (rah-ki'tis) rickets.

rachitogenic (rah-kit"o-jen'ik) causing rickets.

rad. [L.] *ra'dix* (root).

rad (rad) a unit of radiation equal to the absorption of 100 ergs per gram of tissue.

radectomy (rah-dek'to-me) excision of the root of a tooth.

radiability (ra"de-ah-bil'ī-te) the state of being susceptible to treatment by radiant energy (as x-rays or gamma rays).

radiad (ra'de-ad) toward the radial side or aspect.

radial (ra'de-al) pertaining to the radius.

radialis (ra"de-a'lis) [L.] radial.

radiant (ra'de-ant) diverging from a center.

radiatio (ra"de-a'she-o), pl. *radiatio'nes* [L.] a structure made up of diverging elements; radiation.

radiation (-a'shun) 1. divergence from a common center. 2. a structure made up of diverging elements, especially a tract of the central nervous system made up of diverging fibers. 3. energy transmitted through space, as electromagnetic or corpuscular radiation. **acoustic r.,** a fiber tract arising in the medial geniculate nucleus and passing laterally to terminate in the transverse temporal gyri of

the temporal lobe. **r. of corpus callosum,** the fibers of the corpus callosum radiating to all parts of the neopallium. **corpuscular r.,** particles emitted in nuclear disintegration, including alpha and beta particles, protons, neutrons, positrons and deuterons. **electromagnetic r.,** energy, unassociated with matter, which is transmitted through space by means of waves (electromagnetic waves) traveling in all instances at 3×10^{10} cm., or 186,284 miles per second, but ranging in length from 10^{11} cm. (electrical waves) to 10^{-12} cm. (cosmic rays) and including radio waves, infra-red, visible light and ultraviolet, x-rays, and gamma rays. **r. illness,** an acute, self-limiting organic disorder due to exposure to x-rays or gamma rays or other dangerous forms of radiation. **infra-red r.,** the portion of the spectrum of electromagnetic radiation of wavelengths ranging between 7700 and 120,000 angstroms. **interstitial r.,** energy emitted by radium or radon inserted directly into the tissue. **ionizing r.,** corpuscular or electromagnetic radiation which is capable of producing ions, directly or indirectly, in its passage through matter. **optic r.,** a fiber tract starting at the lateral geniculate body, passing through the pars retrolentiformis of the internal capsule, and terminating in the striate area on the medial surface of the occipital lobe, on either side of the calcarine sulcus. **pyramidal r.,** fibers extending from the pyramidal tract to the cortex. **r. striothalam'ica,** a fiber system joining the thalamus and the hypothalamic region. **tegmental r.,** fibers radiating laterally from the red nucleus. **thalamic r.,** fibers streaming out through the lateral surface of the thalamus, through the internal capsule to the cerebral cortex. **ultraviolet r.,** the portion of the spectrum of electromagnetic radiation of wavelengths ranging between 1800 and 3900 angstroms.

radical (rad'i-kal) 1. designed to eliminate all possible extensions of a morbid process. 2. a group of atoms which enters and goes out of chemical combination without undergoing change in its configuration.

radiole (rad'i-kal) one of the smallest branches of a vessel or nerve.

radicotomy (rad"ī-kot'o-me) rhizotomy.

radiculalgia (rah-dik"u-lal'je-ah) neuralgia of the nerve roots.

radicular (rah-dik'u-lar) pertaining to a root or radicle.

radiculitis (rah-dik"u-li'tis) inflammation of spinal nerve roots.

radiculoganglionitis (rah-dik"u-lo-gang"gle-o-ni'tis) inflammation of posterior spinal nerve roots and their ganglia.

radiculomedullary (-med'u-lar"e) affecting nerve roots and spinal cord.

radiculomeningomyelitis (-me-ning"go-mi"e-li'tis) inflammation of nerve roots, meninges and spinal cord.

radiculomyelopathy (-mi"e-lop'ah-the) disease of nerve roots and spinal cord.

radiculoneuropathy (-nu-rop'ah-the) disease of the nerve roots and spinal nerves.

radiculopathy (rah-dik″u-lop′ah-the) disease of nerve roots.

radiectomy (ra″de-ek′to-me) excision of the root of a tooth.

radio- (ra′de-o) word element [L.], *radiation; radium; radius*; affixed to the name of a chemical element to designate a radioactive isotope of that element.

radioactinium (ra″de-o-ak-tin′e-um) a substance formed by the disintegration of actinium.

radioactive (-ak′tiv) characterized by radioactivity.

radioactivity (-ak-tiv′ĭ-te) emission of corpuscular or electromagnetic radiations consequent to nuclear disintegration, a natural property of all chemical elements of atomic number above 83 and possible of induction in all other known elements. **artificial r., induced r.,** that produced by bombarding an element with high-velocity particles.

radioautogram (-aw′to-gram) autoradiogram.

radioautography (-aw-tog′rah-fe) autoradiography.

radiobicipital (-bi-sip′ĭ-tal) pertaining to radius and biceps muscle.

radiobiologist (-bi-ol′o-jist) an expert in radiobiology.

radiobiology (-bi-ol′o-je) the branch of science concerned with effects of light and of ultraviolet and ionizing radiations on living tissue or organisms.

radiocalcium (-kal′se-um) a radioactive isotope of calcium, Ca^{45}, with a half-life of 180 days; used as a tracer in the study of calcium metabolism.

radiocarbon (-kar′bon) a radioactive isotope of carbon; the isotope of mass 14 (C^{14}) is used in many diagnostic procedures and physiologic investigations; with a half-life of 5568 years, it has provided a means of determining the age of many ancient substances and articles.

radiocarcinogenesis (-kar″sĭ-no-jen′ĕ-sis) cancer formation due to exposure to radiation.

radiocardiogram (-kar′de-o-gram) the graphic record produced by radiocardiography.

radiocardiography (-kar″de-og′rah-fe) graphic recording of variation with time of the concentration, in a selected chamber of the heart, of a radioactive isotope, usually injected intravenously.

radiocarpal (-kar′pal) pertaining to radius and carpus.

radiochemistry (-kem′is-tre) chemistry dealing with radionuclides and their properties and uses.

radiocurable (-kūr′ah-bl) curable by radiation.

radiode (ra′de-ōd) an apparatus for therapeutic application of radioactive substance.

radiodermatitis (ra″de-o-der″mah-ti′tis) cutaneous reaction to exposure to excessive quantities of ionizing or corpuscular radiation.

radiodiagnosis (-di″ag-no′sis) diagnosis by means of x-rays or gamma rays.

radiodontics (-don′tiks) the branch of dentistry dealing with the making and interpretation of radiographs of teeth and associated oral structures.

radiodontist (ra″de-o-don′tist) a specialist in radiodontics.

radioecology (-e-kol′o-je) the science dealing with the effects of radiation on species of plants and animals in natural communities or ecosystems.

radioelectrocardiogram (-e-lek″tro-kar′de-o-gram) the tracing obtained by radioelectrocardiography.

radioelectrocardiograph (-kar′de-o-graf″) the apparatus used in radioelectrocardiography.

radioelectrocardiography (-kar″de-og′rah-fe) electrocardiography with impulses beamed by radio waves from the subject to the recording device.

radio-element (ra″de-o-el′ĕ-ment) a radioactive element.

radioencephalogram (-en-sef′ah-lo-gram″) 1. a tracing showing the variation with time of the concentration of a radioactive isotope injected in the cerebral circulation. 2. the record obtained by radioencephalography.

radioencephalography (-en-sef″ah-log′rah-fe) electroencephalography with impulses beamed by radio waves from the subject to the recording device.

radiogram (ra′de-o-gram″) a picture of internal structures of the body produced by the action of x-rays or gamma rays on a specially sensitized film.

radiograph (ra′de-o-graf″) the film produced by radiography.

radiography (ra″de-og′rah-fe) the taking of pictures (radiograms) of internal structures of the body by exposure of specially sensitized film to x-rays or gamma rays.

radiohumeral (ra″de-o-hu′mer-al) pertaining to radius and humerus.

radio-immunity (-ĭ-mu′nĭ-te) a condition of decreased sensitivity to radiation sometimes produced by repeated irradiation.

radio-iodine (-i′o-dīn) a radioactive isotope of iodine; I^{131} is frequently used in thyroid investigation and in treatment of toxic goiter.

radioisotope (-i′so-tōp) a radioactive isotope; one that disintegrates with emission of corpuscular or electromagnetic radiations.

radiologist (ra″de-ol′o-jist) a specialist in radiology.

radiology (-ol′o-je) the branch of medical science dealing with use of radiant energy in diagnosis and treatment of disease.

radiolucency (ra″de-o-lu′scn-se) the quality or property of permitting the passage of radiant energy, such as x-rays (roentgenolucency) or gamma rays. adj., **radiolu′cent.**

radiometer (ra″de-om′ĕ-ter) instrument for measuring the penetrating power of radiant energy.

radiomimetic (ra″de-o-mi-met′ik) producing effects similar to those of ionizing radiations.

radion (ra′de-on) a particle given off by radioactive matter.

radionecrosis (ra″de-o-ne-kro′sis) necrosis from exposure to radiant energy.

radioneuritis (-nu-ri′tis) neuritis from exposure to radiant energy.

radionuclide (-nu′klīd) a radioactive nuclide;

one that disintegrates with the emission of corpuscular or electromagnetic radiations.

radiopacity (ra″de-o-pas′ĭ-te) the quality or property of obstructing the passage of radiant energy, such as x-rays (roentgenopacity) or gamma rays. adj., **radiopaque′**.

radioparent (-par′ent) offering no obstruction to the passage of radiant energy.

radiopathology (-pah-thol′o-je) the pathology of radiation effects on tissues.

radiopelvimetry (-pel-vim′ĕ-tre) measurement of the pelvis by radiography.

radiophosphorus (-fos′fo-rus) a radioactive isotope of phosphorus; P^{32} has been used in treatment of skin cancer, hyperkeratoses and other skin conditions, and in various tests of red cell volume or circulatory efficiency.

radioreceptor (-re-sep′tor) a receptor which is stimulated by radiant energy.

radioscopy (ra″de-os′ko-pe) fluoroscopy.

radiosensibility (ra″de-o-sen″sĭ-bil′ĭ-te) sensibility to irradiation.

radiosensitive (-sen′sĭ-tiv) sensitive to irradiation.

radiosodium (-so′de-um) a radioactive isotope of sodium; Na^{24} has been used in studies of circulation time and measurement of extracellular fluid.

radiosurgery (-ser′jer-e) surgical treatment by the use of radium.

radiotelemetry (-tel-em′ĕ-tre) measurement based on data transmitted by radio waves from the subject to the recording apparatus.

radiotherapy (-ther′ah-pe) treatment by means of irradiation. **interstitial r.,** that administered with the radioactive element contained in devices (e.g. needles) inserted directly into the tissues. **intracavitary r.,** that in which the radioactive element is introduced into a natural body cavity.

radiotoxemia (-tok-se′me ah) toxemia produced by radiant energy.

radiotransparent (-trans-pār′ent) offering no obstruction to transmission of radiant energy, such as x-rays.

radiotropic (-trop′ik) influenced by radiation.

radio-ulnar (-ul′nar) pertaining to radius and ulna.

radium (ra′de-um) chemical element (see table), at. no. 88, symbol Ra.

radius (ra′de-us), pl. **ra′dii** [L.] a line from the center of a circle to a point on its circumference. **r. fix′us,** straight line from hormion to inion.

radix (ra′diks), pl. **rad′ices** [L.] root.

radon (ra′don) chemical element (see table), at. no. 86, symbol Rn.

raffinase (raf′ĭ-nās) an enzyme which splits up raffinose.

raffinose (raf′ĭ-nōs) a sugar, melitose, occurring in cotton seed and in beet molasses.

rage (rāj) a violently aggressive emotional state. **sham r.,** a state resembling rage occurring in decorticated animals or in certain pathologic conditions in man.

rale (rahl) an abnormal respiratory sound heard in auscultation. **amphoric r.,** a musical, tinkling sound. **clicking r.,** a small, sticky sound, heard in early pulmonary tuberculosis. **dry r.,** a whistling, musical or squeaky sound, heard in asthma and bronchitis. **moist r.,** a sound produced by fluid in the bronchial tubes.

R.A.M.C. Royal Army Medical Corps.

Ramibacterium (ra″me-bak-te′re-um) a genus of Schizomycetes (order Eubacteriales, family Lactobacillaceae, tribe Lactobacilleae) found in the intestinal tract and occasionally associated with purulent infections.

ramification (ram″ĭ-fĭ-ka′shun) distribution in branches.

ramify (ram′ĭ-fi) to branch; to diverge in different directions.

ramisectomy (ram″ĭ-sek′to-me) rhizotomy.

ramitis (rah-mi′tis) inflammation of a nerve root.

ramose (ra′mos) branching; having many branches.

ramus (ra′mus), pl. **ra′mi** [L.] a branch, as of a nerve, vein or artery. **r. commu′nicans** (pl. *ra′mi communican′tes*), a branch of a spinal nerve given off mesially to the autonomic ganglion. **dorsal r.,** a branch given off by a spinal nerve, just beyond the union of its dorsal and ventral roots. **ventral r.,** the continuation of a spinal nerve after the branching off of the dorsal ramus and the ramus communicans, dividing ultimately into the lateral and ventral divisions.

range (rānj) the difference between the maximum and minimum of a series of variables, or between the extremes of a varying quantity or ability. **r. of accommodation,** difference in diopters between accommodation of eye at its near and at its far point.

ranine (ra′nīn) pertaining to a ranula, or to the lower surface of the tongue.

ranula (ran′u-lah) a cystic tumor beneath the tongue.

raphe (ra′fe) the line of union of the halves of a symmetrical organ or part as of the palate or pharynx, medulla oblongata or pons.

rapport (rah-port′) a relation of harmony and accord between patient and physician.

rarefaction (rar″ĕ-fak′shun) condition of being or becoming less dense.

rash (rash) an outbreak of lesions on the skin; a skin eruption. **diaper r.,** dermatitis occurring in infants on the areas covered by the diaper. **drug r.,** one due to a drug to which the patient is sensitive. **heat r.,** miliaria rubra. **mulberry r.,** peculiar eruption of typhus fever, looking like the eruption of measles. **nettle r.,** urticaria. **serum r.,** a rash following the injection of antitoxic sera. **tooth r.,** strophulus. **vaccine r.,** erythema following vaccination. **wildfire r.,** strophulus.

rate (rāt) the speed or frequency with which an event or circumstance occurs per unit of time, population or other standard of comparison. **attack r.,** the rate at which new cases of a specific disease occur. **basal metabolic r.,** an expression of the rate at which oxygen is utilized in a fasting subject at complete rest as a percentage of a value established as normal for such a subject. **birth r.,** the number of births during one year for the total population (*crude birth rate*), for the female population (*refined birth rate*) or for the female population of childbearing age (*true birth rate*). **case r.**, morbidity rate. **case fatality r.**, the number of deaths due to a specific disease. **death r.**, the number of deaths per stated number of persons (1,000 or 10,000 or 100,000) in a certain region in a certain year. **dose r.**, the amount of any therapeutic agent administered per unit of time. **erythrocyte sedimentation r.**, an expression of the extent of settling of erythrocytes in a vertical column of blood per unit of time. **fatality r.**, the number of deaths caused by a specific circumstance or disease, expressed as the absolute or relative number among individuals encountering the circumstance or having the disease. **growth r.**, an expression of the increase in size of an organic object per unit of time. **heart r.**, the number of contractions of the cardiac ventricles per unit of time. **metabolic r.**, an expression of the amount of oxygen consumed by the body cells. **morbidity r.**, the number of cases of a given disease occurring in a specified period per unit of population. **mortality r.**, death rate. **pulse r.**, the number of pulsations noted in a peripheral artery per unit of time; normally 72–80 per minute in an adult. **respiration r.**, the number of movements of the chest wall per unit of time, indicative of inspiration and expiration; normally 16–20 per minute in an adult. **sedimentation r.**, erythrocyte sedimentation rate.

ratio (ra'she-o) a numerical expression of the quantitative relations between different factors or elements. **arm r.**, a figure expressing the relation of the length of the longer arm of a mitotic chromosome to that of the shorter arm. **cardiothoracic r.**, the ratio of the transverse diameter of the heart to the internal diameter of the chest at its widest point just above the dome of the diaphragm. **sex r.**, the number of females in a population per number of males, usually stated as the number of females per 1000 males.

rational (rash'un-al) accordant with reason.

rationalization (rash"un-al-i-za'shun) justification by the conscious mind of attitudes and behavior determined by unacceptable unconscious emotions and motives.

Rau-sed (row'sed) trademark for a preparation of reserpine.

Rauwiloid (row'wĭ-loid) trademark for preparations of alseroxylon.

Rauwolfia (raw-wul'fe-ah) a genus of climbing shrubs indigenous to Asia, including over 100 species and providing numerous alkaloids of medical interest.

rauwolfia (raw-wul'fe-ah) an alkaloid derived from shrubs of the genus Rauwolfia. **r. serpenti'na**, the dried root of *Rauwolfia serpentina*, sometimes with fragments of rhizome and other parts, used chiefly as a hypotensive.

ray (ra) a line of light, heat or other form of radiant energy, emanating from an object or substance. **actinic r.**, a light ray which produces chemical changes. **alpha r's**, high-speed helium nuclei ejected from radioactive substances. **Becquerel's r's**, emanations given off by radium, uranium and other radioactive substances. **beta r's**, emanations with moderate velocity and power. **border r's**, grenz rays. **cathode r.**, a ray resembling roentgen rays, but carrying negative electricity and capable of being deflected by the magnet. **cosmic r's**, penetrating radiations which apparently move through interplanetary space in every direction. **delta r's**, secondary beta rays produced in a gas by the passage of alpha particles. **digital r.**, a digit of the hand or foot and corresponding metacarpal or metatarsal bone, regarded as a continuous unit. **gamma r's**, electromagnetic radiation of wavelengths between 0.02 and 0.1 angstrom. **grenz r's**, electromagnetic radiation of wavelengths of 1–5 angstroms. **hertzian r's**, electromagnetic waves with a greater wavelength than a light wave, used in wireless transmission of signals, speech, etc. **infra red r's**, rays beyond the red end of the visible spectrum, of 7700–120,000 angstroms wavelength. **medullary r.**, a cortical extension of a bundle of tubules from a malpighian pyramid of the kidney. **Millikan r's**, cosmic rays. **roentgen r's**, x-rays. **transition r's**, grenz rays. **ultraviolet r's**, radiant energy beyond the violet end of the visible spectrum, of 3900–1800 angstroms wavelength. **x-r's**, electromagnetic radiation of wavelengths ranging between 0.05 and 5 angstroms (including grenz rays). **x-r's, diagnostic**, x-rays of wavelengths of 0.12–0.30 angstrom. **x-r's, therapeutic**, x-rays of wavelength of 0.05–0.12 angstrom.

Rb chemical symbol, *rubidium*.

RBC red blood cells; red blood (cell) count.

R.B.E. relative biological effectiveness; effectiveness of other types of radiation compared with that of 1 R of gamma or roentgen rays.

R.C.M. Royal College of Midwives.

R.C.N. Royal College of Nursing.

R.C.O.G. Royal College of Obstetricians and Gynaecologists.

R.C.P. Royal College of Physicians.

R.C.S. Royal College of Surgeons.

R.D.S. respiratory distress syndrome.

Re chemical symbol, *rhenium*.

reaction (re-ak'shun) 1. opposite action or counteraction. 2. a phenomenon caused by chemical action of substances on each other. **Abderhalden's r.**, production by the body of enzymes capable of digesting foreign proteins which gain entrance to the blood stream. **adjustment r.**, one elicited by a change in situation or environment, sometimes evidenced as a transient personality disorder. **alarm r.**, the first and defensive stage of the stress reaction. **anxiety r.**, a neurotic reaction characterized by abnormal apprehension or uneasiness. **biuret r.**, biuret dissolved in water and heated with Fehling's solution gives a violet reaction. **Calmette's r.**, ophthalmic reaction. **Cannizzaro's r.**, decomposition of aldehyde on contact with animal tissue, one molecule being reduced to the corresponding alcohol and another being oxidized to the corresponding acid. **Casoni's**

r., formation of a white papule on the skin after injection of fluid from a hydatid cyst. **chain r.,** one which is self-propagating; a chemical process in which each time a free radical is destroyed a new one is formed. **citochol r.,** a quick flocculation test in which concentrated cholesterolized extract of heart muscle is used as the antigen. **conversion r.,** a loss or alteration of a sensory or motor function as an expression of anxiety. **cross r.,** one between an antigen and an antibody of closely related but not identical species. **defense r.,** a mental reaction which shuts out from consciousness ideas not acceptable to the ego. **r. of degeneration,** loss of response to a faradic stimulation in a muscle, and to galvanic and faradic stimulation in a nerve. **delayed-blanch r.,** pallor instead of erythema appearing 5 to 10 minutes after intradermal injection of acetylcholine or methacholine and persisting for 15–30 minutes; associated with atopic disease. **depressive r.,** a response to an environmental loss or stress characterized by morbid sadness or melancholy. **dissociative r.,** a neurotic reaction in which amnesia, fugue, somnambulism or splitting of the personality occurs. **dyssocial r.,** disregard by a person of the normal codes of social behavior. **Ehrlich's diazo r.,** deep red color in urine produced by the diazo reagent in certain diseases. **Herxheimer r., Jarisch-Herxheimer r.,** accentuation of symptoms after antisyphilitic therapy. **immunologic r.,** response of an organism to elements recognized as non-self, with production of plasma cells, lymphocytes and antigens, leading to ultimate rejection of the foreign material. **involutional psychotic r.,** a reaction occurring in late middle life, with severe depression and sometimes with paranoid thinking. **lengthening r.,** reflex elongation of extensor muscles which permits flexion of a limb. **luetin r.,** Noguchi's reaction (2). **Moro's r.,** a red eruption on the skin after rubbing in tuberculin ointment. **Much-Holzmann r.,** inhibition of the hemolytic action of cobra venom on the red corpuscles, seen in dementia precox and manic-depressive insanity. **near-point r.,** constriction of the pupil when the gaze is fixed on a near point. **Neufeld r.,** swelling of the capsules of pneumococci, seen under the microscope, on mixture with specific antiserum. **Noguchi's r.,** 1. a modification of the Wassermann reaction for syphilis. 2. in syphilis, on the injection of a drop of luetin a distinct papule is formed. **ophthalmic r.,** local reaction of the conjunctiva after instillation into the eye of toxins of organisms causing typhoid fever and tuberculosis. **pancreatic r.,** a test for recognizing pancreatic disease. **Pirquet's r.,** appearance of a papule with a red areola 24–48 hours after introduction of two small drops of old tuberculin by slight scarification of the skin. **Prausnitz-Küstner r.,** local hypersensitiveness produced by intradermal injection of the serum of an allergic person. **psychotic depressive r.,** severe, nonrecurrent depression of psychotic intensity. **Schultz-Charlton r.,** disappearance of scarlet fever rash around the site of an injection of scarlet fever antitoxin. **serum r.,** seroreaction. **stress r.,** a disturbance of balance and regulation of functioning in response to stress. **Weil-Felix r.,** agglutination by blood serum of typhus patients of a bacillus of the proteus group from the urine and feces. **Wernicke's r.,** a peculiar reaction of the pupil in hemianopia when exposed to light. **Wildbolz r.,** intradermal injection of a few drops of the patient's urine produces a local reaction if the patient is tuberculous. **Wolff-Eisner r.,** ophthalmic reaction. **xanthoproteic r.,** orange color produced by heating proteins with nitric acid.

Reactrol (re-ak'trol) trademark for a preparation of clemizole hydrochloride.

reagent (re-a'jent) substance used to produce chemical reaction. **diazo r., Ehrlich's diazo r.,** a mixture of aqueous solutions of sodium nitrite and of sulfanilic and hydrochloric acids. **Millon's r.,** aqueous solution of mercury dissolved in fuming nitric acid. **Nessler's r.,** mercuric chloride, potassium iodide, and potash, dissolved in water; used in estimating small amounts of ammonia.

reagin (re'ah-jin) an antibody or substance behaving like an antibody in complement fixation and similar reactions.

reamer (re'mer) an instrument used in dentistry for enlarging root canals.

recapitulation (re"kah-pit"u-la'shun) repetition in the development and growth of an individual of the evolutionary stages through which the species evolved.

receiver (re-sēv'er) a vessel for collecting a gas or distillate.

receptaculum (re"sep-tak'u-lum), pl. *receptac'ula* [L.] a vessel or receptacle. **r. chy'li,** expansion at lower end of thoracic duct.

receptor (re-sep'tor) a sensory nerve terminal which responds to stimulation by transmitting impulses to the central nervous system.

recess (re'ses) a small, empty space or cavity.

recessive (re-ses'iv) tending to recede; in genetics, incapable of expression unless carried by both members of a set of homologous chromosomes.

recessus (re-ses'us), pl. *reces'sus* [L.] a recess.

recidivation (re-sid"i-va'shun) 1. the relapse or recurrence of a disease. 2. the repetition of an offense or crime.

recidivism (re-sid'i-vizm) a tendency to relapse, especially the tendency to return to a life of crime.

recidivist (re-sid'i-vist) a person who tends to relapse, especially one who tends to return to criminal habits after treatment or punishment.

recipe (res'i-pe) a document giving quantities and directions for combining ingredients for a specific preparation.

reciprocation (re-sip"ro-ka'shun) the complementary interaction of two distinct entities; in dentistry, applied to the means whereby one part of an appliance is made to counter the effect created by another part.

recompression (re″kom-presh′un) return to normal environmental pressure after exposure to greatly diminished pressure.

recon (re′kon) a hereditary unit indivisible by genetic recombination.

recrement (rek′rē-ment) saliva, or other secretion, which is reabsorbed into the blood. adj., **recrementi′tious.**

recrudescence (re″kroo-des′ens) recurrence of symptoms after temporary abatement. adj., **recrudes′cent.**

rect(o)- (rek′to) word element [L.], *rectum*. See also words beginning *proct(o)-.*

rectalgia (rek-tal′je-ah) proctalgia.

rectectomy (rek-tek′to-me) excision of the rectum.

rectification (rek″tĭ-fĭ-ka′shun) the process of purifying or correcting.

rectified (rek′tĭ-fīd) brought to an established standard of purity.

rectitis (rek-ti′tis) proctitis.

rectocele (rek′to-sēl) herniation of the rectum into the vagina.

rectocolitis (rek″to-co-li′tis) inflammation of rectum and colon.

rectolabial (-la′be-al) pertaining to or communicating with the rectum and a labium majus.

rectopexy (rek′to-pek″se) proctopexy.

rectoplasty (rek′to-plas″te) proctoplasty.

rectoscope (rek′to-skōp) proctoscope.

rectosigmoid (rek″to-sig′moid) the terminal portion of the sigmoid colon and the proximal portion of the rectum.

rectosigmoidectomy (-sig″moi-dek′to-me) excision of the rectosigmoid colon.

rectostomy (rek-tos′to-me) proctostomy.

rectourethral (rek″to-u-re′thral) pertaining to rectum and urethra.

rectouterine (-u′ter-in) pertaining to rectum and uterus.

rectovaginal (-vaj′ĭ-nal) pertaining to rectum and vagina.

rectovesical (-ves′ĭ-kal) pertaining to rectum and bladder.

rectovestibular (-ves-tib′u-lar) pertaining to or communicating with the rectum and the vestibule of the vagina.

rectovulvar (-vul′var) pertaining to or communicating with the rectum and vulva.

rectum (rek′tum) distal portion of large intestine. adj., **rec′tal.**

rectus (rek′tus) [L.], straight.

recumbent (re-kum′bent) lying down.

recurrence (re-ker′ens) the return of symptoms after a temporary absence.

recurrent (re-ker′ent) returning after a remission; reappearing.

red (red) 1. one of the primary colors produced by the longest waves of the visible spectrum. 2. a dye of the color of blood. **cholera r.**, a red pigment derived from *Vibrio comma*. **Congo r.**, a dark red or brownish powder; a medicinal dye. **phenol r.**, phenolsulfonphthalein. **scarlet r.**, an azo dye which stimulates wound healing.

redia (re′de-ah), pl. *re′diae* [L.] the second or third larval stage of certain trematode parasites, which develops in the body of a snail host.

redintegration (red″in-tĕ-gra′shun) restitution of a part.

Redisol (red′ĭ-sol) trademark for a preparation of crystalline vitamin B_{12}.

redox (red′oks) oxidation-reduction.

reduce (re-dūs′) 1. to replace in normal position. 2. to decrease in size. 3. to deprive of oxygen.

reductant (re-duk′tant) the electron donor in an oxidation-reduction (redox) reaction.

reductase (re-duk′tās) an enzyme that has a reducing action on chemicals.

reduction (re-duk′shun) 1. restoration of the normal relation of parts, as in fracture, luxation or hernia. 2. the subtraction of oxygen from, or the addition of hydrogen to, a substance; the loss of positive charges or the gain of negative charges. **closed r.**, restoration of the proper position of the fragments of a fractured bone by external manipulation, and application of a cast to maintain immobilization. **open r.**, restoration of the proper position of the fragments of a fractured bone under direct visualization at operation, with some form of internal or external fixation.

reduplication (re-du″plĭ-ka′shun) a developmental anomaly resulting in the doubling of an organ or part, with a connection between them at some point and the excess part usually a mirror image of the other.

refection (re-fek′shun) recovery; repair.

refine (re-fīn′) to purify or free from foreign matter.

reflection (re-flek′shun) a turning or bending back.

reflector (re-flek′tor) a device for reflecting light or sound waves.

reflex (re′fleks) 1. directed backward; produced by deflection of a nervous impulse which does not penetrate the level of consciousness. 2. a reflection. 3. an automatic response to a given stimulus, depending only on the anatomic relations of the neurons involved. **abdominal r.**, contraction of recti muscles and deviation of linea alba on stroking of the abdominal skin. **accommodation r.**, adjustment of direction of visual axis, size of pupil and convexity of lens when an individual fixes his eyes on a point at a different distance. **Achilles r.**, triceps surae reflex. **anal r.**, momentary contraction of sphincter muscles when skin around the anus is touched. **ankle r.**, triceps surae reflex. **Babinski r.**, Babinski toe sign. **biceps r.**, tensing of the tendon of the biceps muscle felt on percussion over the tendon with the arm and forearm relaxed. **carotid sinus r.**, slowing of the heart beat on pressure on the carotid artery at the level of the cricoid cartilage. **ciliospinal r.**, dilation of ipsilateral pupil on scratching or pinching of skin at side of neck. **clasp-knife r.**, lengthening reaction. **conditioned r.**, one which is acquired as the result of experience. **convergency r.**, convergence of the visual axes with fixation on a near point. **corneal r.**, blinking of the ipsilateral eyelids (*direct corneal reflex*) or of the eyelids of the opposite eye (*consensual corneal reflex*) when the cornea is touched lightly. **cremasteric r.**, contraction of the ipsilateral cremasteric muscle, drawing the testis upward, when the upper inner aspect of the thigh is stroked longitudinally. **deep r.**, one elicited by stimulation of a deep body structure, as a tendon or the periosteum of a bone. **embrace r.**, Moro reflex. **gag r.**, elevation of the soft palate and retching elicited by touching the back of the tongue or the wall of the pharynx. **gastrocolic r.**, stimulation of emptying of the colon resulting from filling of the stomach. **gastroileac r.**, relaxation of the ileocecal valve in response to the stimulus of food in the stomach. **grasp r.**, flexion or clenching of the fingers or toes on stimulation of the palm of the hand or sole of the foot. **Hoffmann's r.**, Hoffmann's sign (2). **knee r.**, quadriceps reflex. **light r.**, constriction of the pupil when a light is shown into the same (*direct light reflex*) or the opposite eye (*indirect* or *consensual light reflex*). **Mayer's r.**, adduction of the thumb on downward pressure of the index finger. **Magnus-DeKleijn r.**, tonic neck reflex. **Mendel-Bechterew r.**, plantar flexion of the toes when the dorsum of the foot is struck on its outer part. **Moro r.**, flexion of an infant's thighs and knees, fanning and then clenching of fingers, with arms first thrown outward and then brought together as though embracing something. **myotactic r.**, stretch reflex. **Oppenheim r.**, Oppenheim's sign. **patellar r.**, quadriceps reflex. **perianal r.**, anal reflex. **pharyngeal r.**, gag reflex. **pilomotor r.**, contraction of the arrectores pilorum on stroking of the nape of the neck or the axillary region. **plantar r.**, plantar flexion of the foot when the ankle is grasped firmly and the lateral border of the sole is stroked or scratched from the heel toward the toes. **pupillary r.**, a change in size of the pupil in response to various stimuli (change in illumination or point of fixation, or emotional stimulation). **quadriceps r.**, contraction of the quadriceps and extension of the leg when the quadriceps tendon is tapped between the patella and the tibial tubercle. **quadrupedal extensor r.**, extension of a hemiplegic flexed arm on assumption of the quadrupedal position. **red r.**, the usually bright red appearance of the pupil when viewed through the ophthalmoscope at a distance of a foot or less. **righting r.**, the ability to assume an optimal position when there has been a departure from it. **spinal r.**, any reflex action mediated through a center of a spinal cord. **startle r.**, Moro reflex. **stretch r.**, reflex contraction of a muscle in response to passive longitudinal stretching. **sucking r.**, sucking movements of the lips of an infant elicited by touching the lips or the skin near the mouth. **superficial r.**, one elicited by stimulation of superficial nerve endings, as in the skin. **tendon r.**, contraction of a muscle caused by percussion of its tendon. **tonic neck r.**, extension of the

arm and sometimes of the leg on the side to which the head is forcibly turned, with flexion of the contralateral limbs. **triceps r.**, contraction of the belly of the triceps muscle and slight extension of the arm when the tendon of the muscle is tapped directly, with the arm flexed and fully supported and relaxed. **triceps surae r.**, plantar extension of the foot elicited by a tap on the Achilles tendon, preferably while the patient kneels on a bed or chair, the feet hanging free over the edge.

reflexogenic (re-flek″so-jen′ik) producing reflex action.

reflexograph (re-flek′so-graf) an instrument for recording a reflex.

reflexometer (re″flek-som′ĕ-ter) instrument for measuring force required to produce myotatic contraction.

reflux (re′fluks) a return flow.

refract (re-frakt′) to ascertain errors of ocular refraction.

refraction (re-frak′shun) 1. the deviation of light in traversing obliquely a medium of differing density. 2. determination of the distortion of vision caused by defect of any of the refractive media of the eye. adj., **refrac′tive. double r.**, refraction in which incident rays are divided into two refracted rays. **dynamic r.**, refraction of the eye when at rest. **static r.**, refraction of the eye when its accommodation is paralyzed.

refractionist (re-frak′shun-ist) one skilled in determining errors of refraction of the eye.

refractometer (re″frak-tom′ĕ-ter) apparatus for measuring defects of vision.

refractory (re-frak′to-re) not readily yielding to treatment.

refrangible (re-fran′ji-bl) susceptible of being refracted.

refresh (re-fresh′) to make raw again.

refrigerant (re-frij′er-ant) relieving fever and thirst.

refrigeration (re-frij″er-a′shun) therapeutic application of low temperature.

refusion (re-fu′zhun) the temporary removal and subsequent return of blood to the circulation.

regeneration (re-jen″ĕ-ra′shun) the natural replacement of a lost or injured organ or part.

regimen (rej′ĭ-men) a methodical system of diet and habits.

regio (re′je-o), pl. *regio′nes* [L.] region.

region (re′jun) a particular part of the body. adj., **re′gional. abdominal r's**, the areas into which the anterior surface of the abdomen is divided, including the *epigastric*, *hypochondriac* (right and left), *inguinal* (right and left), *lateral* (right and left), *pubic* and *umbilical*. **basilar r.**, the base of the skull. **ecphylactic r.**, a region of infection that cannot be protected by the defensive agencies of the body, owing to the virulence of the infecting agent. **extrapolar r.**, that part of the body which is outside the influence of the poles in electrotherapy. **facial r's**, the areas into which the face is divided, including the *buccal* (side of oral cavity), *infraorbital* (below the eye), *mental* (chin), *nasal* (nose), *oral* (lips), *orbital* (eye), *parotideomasseter* (angle of the jaw) and *zygomatic* (cheek bone). **motor r.**, the ascending frontal and parietal convolutions of the cerebrum. **parietotemporal r.**, sensory region. **pectoral r's,** the areas into which the anterior surface of the chest is divided, including the *axillary*, *infraclavicular* and *mammary.* **perineal r.,** the inferior surface of the trunk, including the anal and urogenital regions. **precordial r.,** a part of the anterior surface of the body covering the heart and the pit of the stomach. **prefrontal r.,** the part of the frontal lobe of the cerebrum in front of the precentral fissures. **sensory r.,** a part of the cerebral cortex on either side of the motor region.

registrant (rej'is-trant) a nurse listed on the books of a registry as available for duty.

registrar (rej'is-trar) 1. an official keeper of records. 2. in British hospitals, a resident specialist who acts as assistant to the chief or attending specialist.

registration (rej"is-tra'shun) the act of recording; in dentistry, the making of a record of the jaw relations present or desired, in order to transfer them to an articulator to facilitate proper construction of a dental prosthesis.

registry (rej'is-tre) an office in which official lists or records are kept. **nurse's r.,** an office with lists of nurses available for duty.

Regitine (rej'ĭ-tēn) trademark for a preparation of phentolamine.

regression (re-gresh'un) 1. return to an earlier or primitive state. 2. subsidence of symptoms or of a disease process. 3. in biology, the tendency in successive generations toward mediocrity. 4. defensive retreat to an earlier pattern of behavior or stage of development. **atavistic r.,** a process by which the mind ceases to function at a logical critical level and reverts to a biologically more primitive mode of functioning. adj., **regres'sive.**

regurgitant (re-ger'jĭ-tant) flowing back.

regurgitation (re-ger"jĭ-ta'shun) abnormal backward progression of fluids or other vessel contents, as the return of undigested food from the stomach to the oral cavity, or of blood through valves of the heart. **aortic r.,** reverse passage of blood from the aorta into the left ventricle in insufficiency of the valve guarding its entrance.

rehabilitation (re"hah-bil"ĭ-ta'shun) restoration to useful activity of persons with physical or other disability.

rehabilitee (re"hah-bil'ĭ-te) the subject of rehabilitation.

rehalation (re"hah-la'shun) rebreathing.

rehydration (re"hi-dra'shun) the restoration of water or fluid content to a body or to a substance which has become dehydrated.

reimplantation (re"im-plan-ta'shun) replacement of a structure in a site from which it was dislodged.

reinfection (re"in-fek'shun) a second infection by the same agent.

reinforcement (re"in-fors'ment) the increas-

ing of force or strength. **r. of reflex,** strengthening of a reflex response by the patient's performance of some action during elicitation of the reflex.

reinnervation (re"in-er-va'shun) restoration of nerve supply of an organ by anastomosis with a living nerve.

relapse (re-laps') a recurrence, or an exacerbation in the course of an illness.

relaxant (re-lak'sant) 1. causing relaxation. 2. an agent which causes relaxation.

relaxation (re"lak-sa'shun) a lessening of tension.

relaxin (re-lak'sin) a hormone occurring in pregnant mammals which promotes relaxation of the symphysis pubis and sacroiliac joints.

Releasin (re-le'sin) trademark for a preparation of relaxin.

reline (re-līn') to resurface the tissue side of a denture with new base material in order to achieve a more accurate fit.

rem (rem) the amount of any ionizing radiation which has the same biological effectiveness of 1 rad of x (roentgen) rays.

remedy (rem'ĕ-de) an agent which alleviates or banishes disease. adj., **reme'dial. specific r.,** one that is invariably effective in treatment of a certain condition.

remission (re-mish'un) improvement or abatement of the symptoms of a disease.

remittent (re-mit'ent) having periods of abatement and of exacerbation.

ren (ren), pl. *re'nes* [L.] kidney. **r. mo'bilis,** wandering kidney.

renal (re'nal) pertaining to the kidney.

reniform (ren'ĭ-form) kidney-shaped.

renin (re'nin) an enzyme elicited by ischemia of the kidneys or by diminished pulse pressure, which converts hypertensinogen to hypertensin.

renipelvic (ren"ĭ-pel'vik) pertaining to the pelvis of the kidney.

reniportal (-por'tal) pertaining to the portal system of the kidney.

renipuncture (-pungk'tūr) surgical incision of capsule of kidney.

rennet (ren'et) preparation of calf's stomach which coagulates milk.

rennin (ren'in) an enzyme of gastric juice which catalyzes the conversion of casein from a soluble to an insoluble form; a preparation from the stomach of the calf is used to coagulate milk protein to facilitate its digestion.

renninogen (rĕ-nin'o-jen) the proenzyme in the gastric glands which is converted into rennin.

renogastric (re"no-gas'trik) pertaining to kidney and stomach.

renography (re-nog'rah-fe) roentgen study of the kidney.

reno-intestinal (re"no-in-tes'tĭ-nal) pertaining to kidney and intestine.

renopathy (re-nop'ah-the) any disease of the kidneys.

renoprival (re"no-pri'val) pertaining to or caused by lack of kidney function.

reovirus (re"o-vi'rus) one of a subgroup of enteric cytopathogenic human orphan (ECHO) viruses.

rep (rep) roentgen-equivalent-physical, a unit of radiation equivalent to the absorption of 93 ergs per gram of tissue.

repair (re-pār') the physical or mechanical restoration of damaged tissues, especially the replacement of dead or damaged cells in a body tissue or organ by healthy new cells. **plastic r.**, restoration of anatomic structure by means of tissue transferred from other sites or derived from other individuals, or by other substance.

repellent (re-pel'ent) 1. capable of dispersing a swelling. 2. capable of driving away, as insects or mosquitoes. 3. a substance which repels insects or mosquitoes.

repercussion (re″per-kush′un) 1. the driving in of an eruption, or scattering of a swelling. 2. ballottement.

replantation (re″plan-ta′shun) restoration of an organ or other body structure to its original site.

replication (rĕ″pli-ka′shun) 1. a turning back of a part so as to form a duplication. 2. repetition of an experiment to ensure accuracy.

repolarization (re-po″lar-i-za′shun) the re-establishment of polarity, or the restoration of the exhibition of opposite effects at the two extremities.

repositor (re poz′ĭ-tor) instrument for replacing displaced parts.

repression (re-presh′un) a forcing back, as banishment from consciousness of unacceptable ideas or impulses, or diminution of the concentration of one (*enzyme repression*) or several (*coordinate repression*) enzymes involved in a metabolic pathway.

repressor (re-pres′sor) a compound which represses the formation of a specific enzyme; the term has been used to refer both to a small molecule (corepressor) which can be added exogenously and to the postulated active repressor (corepressor plus aporepressor).

reproduction (re″pro-duk′shun) the production by a living entity or organism of a new individual of the same kind. **asexual r.**, reproduction without the fusion of sexual cells. **cytogenic r.**, production of a new individual from a single germ cell or zygote. **sexual r.**, reproduction by the fusion of a female sexual cell with a male sexual cell or by the development of an unfertilized egg. **somatic r.**, production of a new individual from a multicellular fragment by fission or budding.

reproductive (-duk′tiv) serving purposes of reproduction.

rescinnamine (re-sin′ah-min) an alkaloid from various species of Rauwolfia; used as an antihypertensive and tranquilizer.

resection (re-sek′shun) surgical removal of a considerable portion of an organ or body part. **gastric r.**, partial gastrectomy. **root r.**, apicoectomy. **submucous r.**, excision of a portion of a deflected nasal septum after first laying back a flap of mucous membrane. **transurethral r.**, removal of the prostate by means of an instrument passed through the urethra. **wedge r.**, removal of a triangular mass of tissue, as from the ovary. **window r.**, submucous resection.

resectoscope (re-sek′to-skōp) an instrument for transurethral prostatic resection.

resectoscopy (re″sek-tos′ko-pe) transurethral resection of the prostate.

reserpine (res′er-pēn) an active alkaloid from *Rauwolfia serpentina*, used as an antihypertensive and tranquilizer.

reserve (re-zerv′) 1. to hold back for future use. 2. a supply, beyond that ordinarily used, which may be utilized in emergency. **alkali r.**, **alkaline r.**, the buffer compounds in the blood capable of neutralizing acidity **cardiac r.**, potential ability of the heart to perform work beyond that necessary under basal conditions.

reservoir (rez′er-vwar) a storage space. **biological r.**, the animals capable of harboring, without injury to themselves, pathogenic microorganisms which may at any time be transmitted to man and produce disease. **r. of infection**, a source of pathogenic organisms in permanent hosts or healthy carriers, from which they spread to cause disease. **r. of Pecquet**, receptaculum chyli. **r. of virus**, the alternate host or passive carrier of a virus, from which it passes to a person who shows clinical signs of infection.

resident (rez′ĭ-dent) a graduate and licensed physician resident in a hospital.

residuum (re-zid′u-um) a residue or remainder. **r. ova′rii**, the dried, powdered ovary of cattle, sheep or swine, with corpus luteum removed.

resin (rez′in) 1. a naturally occurring solid, brittle, amorphous substance, as an exudate from plants and trees. 2. a precipitate obtained by mixing an alcohol solution with water. adj., **res′inous. acrylic r′s,** products of the polymerization of acrylic or methacrylic acid or their derivatives, used in fabrication of medical prostheses and dental restorations and appliances. **activated r., autopolymer r.**, self-curing resin. **heat-curing r.**, one which requires the use of heat to effect its polymerization. **ion-exchange r.**, a high-molecular weight insoluble polymer of simple organic compounds capable of exchanging its attached ions for other ions in the surrounding medium; classified as *cation* or *anion exchange resin*, depending on the charge of the ion exchanged. **podophyllum r.**, an amorphous powder obtained by percolation of podophyllum with alcohol; used in treatment of venereal warts. **quick-cure r., self-curing r.**, any resin which can be polymerized by addition of an activator and a catalyst without the use of external heat. **synthetic r.**, an amorphous, organic solid or semisolid substance produced by polymerization of simple compounds.

Resinat (rez′ĭ-nat) trademark for preparations of polyamine-methylene resin.

resistance (re-zis′tans) opposition, or counteracting force, as opposition of a conductor to passage of electricity or other energy or substance, or ability of an organism to withstand a noxious influence; in studies of respiration, an expression of the opposition to flow of air produced by tissues of air passages, in terms of pressure per amount of air per unit of time. **age r.**, a condition of apparently decreased susceptibility to infection by various agents sometimes observed in older persons. **environmental r.**, the sum of physical and biotic factors which prevent the reproduction of a species at its maximum rate. **essential r.**, resistance to conductivity with an electric battery. **peripheral r.**, the resistance to the passage of the blood through the small blood vessels, especially the capillaries.

resolution (rez″o-lu′shun) 1. subsidence of a pathologic state. 2. perception as separate of two adjacent points; in microscopy, the smallest distance at which two adjacent objects can be distinguished as separate.

resolvent (re-zol′vent) promoting resolution.

resonance (rez′o-nans) 1. a rich quality of sound. 2. a fairly sustained note of moderate pitch elicited by percussion. **skodaic r.**, resonance of a paradoxical tympanic quality over the upper part of the thorax when the lower portion of a lung is entirely compressed by pleuritic effusion and the upper portion is reduced in volume. **tympanic r.**, drumlike reverberation of a cavity filled with air. **tympanitic r.**, peculiar sound elicited by percussing a tympanitic abdomen. **vesicular r.**, normal pulmonary resonance. **vocal r.**, the sound of ordinary speech as heard through the chest wall.

resonant (rez′o-nant) giving an intense, rich sound on percussion.

resonator (rez′o-na″tor) 1. an instrument used to intensify sounds. 2. an electric circuit in which oscillations of a certain frequency are set up by oscillations of the same frequency in another circuit.

resorcin (rĕ-zor′sin) resorcinol.

resorcinism (rĕ-zor′sĭ-nizm) chronic poisoning by resorcinol.

resorcinol (rĕ-zor′sĭ-nol) a compound used as a local anti-infective. **r. monoacetate**, a viscous, pale yellow or amber liquid; used as a local irritant and antibacterial and antifungal agent.

resorcinolphthalein (rĕ-zor″sĭ-nol-thal′e-in) fluorescein.

resorption (re-sorp′shun) removal by absorption of something already secreted or formed in the body, as reabsorption in the kidney of certain elements from the urine, or destruction of bone or of cementum or dentin of teeth.

respirable (rĕ-spīr′ah-bl) suitable for respiration.

respiration (res″pǐ-ra′shun) the exchange of oxygen and carbon dioxide in the body (1) in the lungs, (2) between the cell and its environment, and (3) in the metabolism of the cell. adj., **respir′atory. abdominal r.**, the inspiration and expiration of air by the lungs accomplished mainly by the abdominal muscles and diaphragm. **artificial r.**, that which is maintained by force applied to the body, such as *Eve's method* (patient face down on a stretcher placed on a trestle, the ends being alternately lowered and raised); *Schafer's method* (pressure alternately applied and relaxed over the lower ribs, the patient lying face downward); or *Silvester's method* (patient supine, arms pulled firmly over head, raising ribs, until air no longer enters chest); stimulation of the phrenic nerve by application of electric current; or *mouth-to-mouth method* (resuscitation of an apneic victim by direct application of the mouth to his, regularly taking a deep breath and blowing into the victim's lungs). **Biot's r.**, rapid, short breathing, with pauses of several seconds. **Cheyne-Stokes r.**, breathing characterized by rhythmic alterations in intensity. **cogwheel r.**, breathing with jerky inspiration. **cutaneous r.**, normal passage of gases and vapors through the skin. **electrophrenic r.**, induction of respiration by electric stimulation of the phrenic nerve. **external r.**, the exchange of carbon dioxide and oxygen by diffusion between the external environment and the blood stream. **internal r.**, the exchange of oxygen and carbon dioxide between the blood stream and the cells of the body. **paradoxical r.**, that in which a lung, or a portion of a lung, is deflated during inspiration and inflated during expiration. **tissue r.**, internal respiration.

respirator (res′pǐ-ra″tor) 1. an apparatus to modify the quality of the air which is inhaled. 2. a device for maintaining artificial respiration. **cuirass r.**, an apparatus which is applied only to the chest, either completely surrounding the trunk or applied only to the front of the chest and abdomen. **Drinker r.**, an apparatus for maintaining artificial respiration for long periods of time, popularly called "iron lung."

respirometer (res″pǐ-rom′ĕ-ter) instrument for determining the nature of the respiration.

response (re-spons′) any action or change of condition evoked by a stimulus. **reticulocyte r.**, increase in the formation of reticulocytes in response to a bone marrow stimulus.

rest (rest) 1. a period of cessation of activity. 2. a fragment of undifferentiated tissue retained within the adult organism. 3. an extension which helps support a dental appliance. **adrenal r.**, an accessory adrenal gland. **incisal r., lingual r., occlusal r.**, a metallic extension from a removable partial denture to aid in supporting the appliance. **suprarenal r.**, adrenal rest. **Walthard cell r's**, rests of squamous epithelium in the ovary.

restenosis (re″stĕ-no′sis) recurrent stenosis, especially of a cardiac valve after surgical correction of the primary condition. **false r.**, stenosis recurring after failure to divide either commissure of the cardiac valve beyond the area of incision of the papillary muscles.

restibrachium (res″tǐ-bra′ke-um) inferior peduncle of cerebellum.

restiform (res′tǐ-form) shaped like a rope.

restim (res′tim) a biologically derived nonpyrogenic, nontoxic lipid material which has a stimulating effect on the reticuloendothelial system.

restis (res'tis) the restiform body.

restoration (res"to-ra'shun) 1. induction of a return to a previous state, as a return to health or replacement of a part to normal position. 2. partial or complete reconstruction of a body part, or the device used in its place.

restorative (re-stŏr'ah-tiv) 1. promoting a return of health. 2. a remedy that aids in restoring health.

restraint (re-strānt') forcible control. **chemical r.,** control of the behavior of a disturbed psychotic patient by means of sedatives. **mechanical r.,** control of the behavior of a disturbed psychotic patient by mechanical means.

resuscitation (re-sus"ĭ-ta'shun) restoration to life of one apparently dead.

resuscitator (re-sus'ĭ-ta"tor) an apparatus for initiating respiration in persons whose breathing has stopped.

retainer (re-tān'er) an appliance or device that keeps a tooth or partial denture in proper position.

retardate (re-tar'dāt) a mentally retarded person.

retardation (re"tar-da'shun) hindrance or delay in any process, as in mental or physical development.

retching (rech'ing) strong involuntary effort to vomit.

rete (re'te), pl. re'tia [L.] a network; usually applied to an anastomosing network of small arteries or veins or of other channels. **r. malpig'hii,** rete mucosum. **r. mirab'ile,** a network of small anastomosing blood vessels, chiefly from a single trunk. **r. muco'sum,** the innermost stratum of epidermis. **r. tes'tis,** the network formed in the mediastinum of the testis by the vasa recta.

retention (re-ten'shun) the process of holding back or keeping in position, as persistence in the body of material normally excreted, or maintenance of a dental prosthesis in proper position in the mouth.

reticular (re-tik'u-lar) resembling a network.

reticulated (re-tik'u-lāt"ed) reticular.

reticulation (re-tik"u-la'shun) the formation of a network.

reticulemia (-le'me-ah) presence in the blood of increased numbers of immature red blood cells.

reticulin (re-tik'u-lin) a scleroprotein present in connective tissue, closely related to collagen in composition.

reticulitis (re-tik"u-li'tis) inflammation of the reticulum of a ruminant animal.

reticulocyte (re-tik'u-lo-sīt) a non-nucleated cell of the erythrocytic series, grossly indistinguishable from an erythrocyte, but, on special staining, showing granules or a diffuse network of fibrils.

reticulocytogenic (re-tik"u-lo-si"to-jen'ik) causing the formation of reticulocytes.

reticulocytopenia (-si"to-pe'ne-ah) deficiency of reticulocytes in the blood.

reticulocytosis (re-tik"u-lo-si-to'sis) excess of reticulocytes in the blood.

reticuloendothelioma (-en"do-the"le-o'mah) a tumor of the reticuloendothelial system.

reticuloendotheliosis (-en"do-the"le-o'sis) hyperplasia of reticuloendothelial tissue.

reticuloendothelium (-en"do-the'le-um) the tissue of the reticuloendothelial system.

reticuloma (re-tik"u-lo'mah) a tumor composed of cells of reticuloendothelial origin (monocytes).

reticulopenia (re-tik"u-lo-pe'ne-ah) reticulocytopenia.

reticulopodium (-po'de-um) a threadlike, branching pseudopod.

reticulosarcoma (-sar-ko'mah) a sarcoma composed of reticulum cells.

reticulosis (re-tik"u-lo'sis) reticulocytosis.

reticulum (re-tik'u-lum), pl. retic'ula [L.] 1. a small network. 2. the second stomach of a ruminant animal. **endoplasmic r.,** a system of membrane-bounded cavities in the cytoplasm of a cell, occurring in two types, granular, or rough-surfaced, and agranular, or smooth-surfaced. **sarcoplasmic r.,** a network of smooth-surfaced tubules surrounding the myofibrils of striated muscle fibers. **stellate r.,** the soft, middle part of the enamel organ of a developing tooth.

retiform (re'tĭ-form, ret'ĭ-form) reticular.

retina (ret'ĭ-nah) the innermost tunic of the eyeball, containing the nervous elements for reception and transmission of visual stimuli. adj., **ret'inal.**

retinaculum (ret"ĭ-nak'u-lum), pl. retinac'ula [L.] a structure or device for holding a thing in place, as an anatomic structure or a surgical instrument. **r. morgag'ni,** ridge formed by the coming together of segments of ileocecal valve. **r. peroneo'rum infe'rius,** band across peroneal tendons on outside of calcaneum. **r. peroneo'rum supe'rius,** external annular ligament of ankle. **r. ten'dinum,** a tendinous restraining structure, such as an annular ligament. **Weitbrecht's r.,** retinacular fibers attached to the neck of the femur.

retine (ret'ēn) a substance widely distributed in animal cells, capable of inhibiting cell division and growth.

retinene (ret'ĭ-nen) a pigment which is transformed into rhodopsin under the influence of light.

retinitis (ret"ĭ-ni'tis) inflammation of the retina. **r. circina'ta, circinate r.,** retinitis with brilliant white spots surrounding the macula or disk like a wreath. **r. discifor'mis,** retinitis with formation of a yellowish mass in the macular region. **r. exudati'va, exudative r.,** retinitis with areas of exudation beneath the retinal vessels. **r. pigmento'sa,** retinitis with pigmentation, atrophy and sclerosis. **r. prolif'erans,** retinitis with connective tissue bands formed in the vitreous.

retinoblastoma (ret"ĭ-no-blas-to'mah) glioma of the retina.

retinochoroiditis (-ko"roi-di'tis) inflammation of retina and choroid.

retinoid (ret'ĭ-noid) resembling the retina.

retinomalacia (ret″ĭ-no-mah-la'she-ah) softening of the retina.

retinopapillitis (-pap″ĭ-li'tis) inflammation of retina and optic papilla.

retinopathy (ret″ĭ-nop'ah-the) any noninflammatory disease of the retina.

retinoschisis (-nos'kĭ-sis) 1. a congenital cleft of the retina. 2. cleavage of retinal layers with formation of holes, due to degenerative changes occurring with age.

retinoscope (ret'ĭ-no-skōp″) skiascope.

retinoscopy (ret″ĭ-nos'ko-pe) skiametry.

retinosis (-no'sis) any degenerative condition of the retina.

retinotoxic (ret″ĭ-no-tok'sik) having a deleterious effect the retina.

retisolution (ret″ĭ-so-lu'shun) dissolution of the Golgi apparatus.

retort (re-tort') a globular, long-necked vessel used in distillation.

retothelioma (re″to-the″le-o'mah) a tumor composed of reticuloendothelium.

retothelium (-the'le-um) reticuloendothelium.

retractile (re-trak'til) susceptible of being drawn back.

retraction (re-trak'shun) the act of drawing back, or condition of being drawn back.

retractor (re-trak'tor) instrument for holding open the lips of a wound.

retribution (rĕ-trĭ-bū'shun) the unconscious granting or inflicting of one's desserts as requital for good or evil.

retro- (ret'ro, re'tro) word element [L.], *behind; posterior to.*

retroaction (ret″ro-ak'shun) action in a reversed direction.

retroauricular (-aw-rik'u-lar) behind the auricle.

retrobulbar (-bul'bar) behind the eyeball.

retrocecal (-se'kal) behind the cecum.

retrocedent (-se'dent) going back; coming back or returning.

retrocervical (-ser'vĭ-kal) behind the cervix uteri.

retrocession (-sesh'un) a going back, or return.

retrocolic (-ko'lik) behind the colon.

retrocollic (-kol'ik) pertaining to the back of the neck.

retrocollis (-kol'is) spasmodic wryneck in which the head is drawn back.

retrocursive (-ker'siv) marked by stepping backward.

retrodeviation (-de″ve-a'shun) a bending backward.

retrodisplacement (-dis-plās'ment) backward displacement.

retro-esophageal (-e-sof″ah-je'al) behind the esophagus.

retroflexion (-flek'shun) the bending of an organ so that its top is thrust backward.

retrogasserian (-gas-se're-an) pertaining to the posterior root of the gasserian ganglion.

retrognathia (-nath'e-ah) position of the jaws behind the frontal plane of the forehead.

retrognathic (ret″ro-nath'ik) having a receding lower jaw.

retrograde (ret'ro-grād) going backward; retracing a former course.

retrography (re-trog'rah-fe) mirror writing.

retroinfection (ret″ro-in-fek'shun) infection of a mother by the fetus in utero.

retroinsular (-in'su-lar) behind the island of Reil.

retrolabyrinthine (-lab″ĭ-rin'thin) behind the labyrinth of the ear.

retrolental (-len'tal) behind the lens of the eye.

retrolingual (-ling'gwal) behind the tongue.

retromammary (-mam'ar-e) behind the mammary gland.

retromandibular (-man-dib'u-lar) behind the lower jaw.

retromastoid (-mas'toid) behind the mastoid process.

retromorphosis (-mor-fo'sis) reversion to an earlier or more primitive form; catabolism.

retronasal (-na'zal) pertaining to the back part of the nose.

retro-ocular (-ok'u-lar) behind the eye.

retroparotid (-pah-rot'id) behind the parotid gland.

retropatellar (-pah-tel'ar) behind the patella.

retroperitoneal (-per″ĭ-to-ne'al) behind the peritoneum.

retroperitoneum (-per″ĭ-to-ne'um) the retroperitoneal space.

retroperitonitis (-per″ĭ-to-ni'tis) inflammation in the space behind the peritoneum.

retropharyngeal (-fah-rin'je-al) behind the pharynx.

retropharyngitis (-far″in-ji'tis) inflammation of posterior part of the pharynx.

retroplasia (-pla'ze-ah) change of a cell to an earlier type.

retroposed (-pōsd') displaced backward.

retroposition (-po-zish'un) backward displacement.

retropulsion (-pul'shun) 1. a driving back, as of the fetal head in labor. 2. tendency to walk backward, as in some cases of tabes dorsalis.

retrotarsal (-tar'sal) behind tarsus of the eye.

retro-uterine (-u'ter-in) behind the uterus.

retroversion (-ver'zhun) the tipping backward of an entire organ.

reversal (re-ver'sal) a turning or change in the opposite direction. **sex r.,** a change in characteristics from those typical of one sex to those typical of the other.

revulsant (re-vul'sant) 1. causing revulsion. 2. an agent causing revulsion.

revulsion (re-vul'shun) derivation of blood from a diseased part to another part.

revulsive (re-vul'siv) 1. causing revulsion. 2. an agent causing revulsion.

Rezipas (rez'ĭ-pas) trademark for a preparation of para-aminosalicylic acid.

R.F.A. right fronto-anterior (position of the fetus).

R.F.N. Registered Fever Nurse (England).

R.F.P. right frontoposterior (position of the fetus).

R.G.N. Registered General Nurse (Scotland).

Rh chemical symbol, *rhodium.*

rhabd(o) (rab'do) word element [Gr.], *rod; rod-shaped.*

Rhabditis (rab-di'tis)   a genus of parasitic nematode worms.

rhabdium (rab'de-um)   a voluntary muscle fiber.

rhabdocyte (rab'do-sīt) metamyelocele.

rhabdoid (rab'doid)   resembling a rod; rod-shaped.

Rhabdomonas (rab″do-mo'nas)   a genus of Schizomycetes (order Pseudomonadales, suborder Rhodobacteriineae, family Thiorhodaceae).

rhabdomyoblastoma (-mi″o-blas-to'mah)   a tumor whose cells tend to differentiate into striated muscle cells.

rhabdomyolysis (-mi-ol'ĭ-sis) disintegration of striated muscle fibers with excretion of myoglobin in the urine.

rhabdomyoma (-mi-o'mah)   a tumor containing striated muscle fibers.

Rhabdonema (-ne'mah) rhabditis.

rhabdosarcoma (-sar-ko'mah) a sarcoma containing striated muscle fibers.

rhachi- (rak'e) for words beginning thus, see those beginning *rachi-*.

rhacoma (rah-ko'mah)   1. excoriation.   2. a pendulous scrotum.

rhagades (rag'ah-dēz)   painful fissures in the skin.

rhaphe (ra'fe) raphe.

rhenium (re'ne-um)   chemical element *(see table)*, at. no. 75, symbol Re.

rheo- (re'o) word element [Gr.], *flow.*

rheobase (re'o-bās)   the minimum potential of electric current necessary to produce stimulation.

rheocardiogram (re″o-kar'de-o-gram″)   the graphic record obtained by rheocardiography.

rheocardiography (-kar″de-og'rah-fe)   a recording of the variation occurring during the cardiac cycle in the total resistance to the flow of an alternating current sent through the body.

rheochord (re'o-kord) rheostat.

rheometer (re-om'ē-ter)   1. galvanometer.   2. instrument for measuring rapidity of the blood current.

rheonome (re'o-nōm)   apparatus for determining the effect of irritation on a nerve.

rheophore (re'o-fōr) electrode.

rheoscope (re'o-skōp)   device indicating the presence of an electric current.

rheostat (re'o-stat)   apparatus for regulating resistance in an electric circuit.

rheostosis (re″os-to'sis) melorheostosis.

rheotaxis (re″o-tak'sis)   orientation of a longitudinal body in a stream of liquid, with its long axis parallel with the direction of flow, designated *negative* (moving in the same direction) or *positive* (moving in the opposite direction).

rheotome (re'o-tōm)   a device for breaking an electric circuit.

rheotrope (re'o-trōp)   an instrument for reversing a current.

rheum (rōm)   a watery discharge from the nose, eyes or sores.

rheumarthritis (roo″mar-thri'tis)   rheumatism of the joints.

rheumatalgia (roo″mah-tal'je-ah)   rheumatic pain.

rheumatid (roo'mah-tid)   a skin lesion occurring in rheumatism.

rheumatism (roo'mah-tizm)   a disease marked by pain in joints or muscles, usually recurrent, and often due to exposure. adj., **rheumat'ic. acute articular r.,** inflammatory r., rheumatic fever. **muscular r.,** rheumatism of voluntary muscles and their fibrous structures. **palindromic r.,** repeated attacks of arthritis and periarthritis without fever.

rheumatoid (roo'mah-toid)   resembling rheumatism.

rheumatologist (roo″mah-tol'o-jist)   a specialist in rheumatology.

rheumatology (-tol'o-je)   the study of rheumatic conditions.

rheumatosis (-to'sis)   any disorder of rheumatic origin.

rheumic (roo'mik)   pertaining to a rheum or flux.

rhexis (rek'sis)   the rupture of a blood vessel or of an organ.

rhigosis (ri-go'sis)   the perception of cold.

rhin(o)- (ri'no)   word element [Gr.], *nose; nose-like structure.*

rhinal (ri'nal)   pertaining to the nose.

rhinalgia (ri-nal'je-ah)   pain in the nose.

rhinencephalon (ri″nen-sef'ah-lon)   the portion of the brain concerned with the sense of smell, consisting of the olfactory lobe, the anterior perforated substance, the subcallosal gyrus and the parolfactory area.

rhinesthesia (ri″nes-the'ze-ah)   the sense of smell.

rhineurynter (ri″nu-rin'ter)   dilatable bag for plugging a nostril.

rhinion (rin'e-on)   lower end of the suture between nasal bones.

rhinitis (ri-ni'tis)   inflammation of nasal mucous membrane. **allergic r., anaphylactic r.,** hay fever. **atrophic r.,** rhinitis with wasting of mucous membrane and glands. **r. caseo'sa,** rhinitis with caseous, fetid discharge. **fibrinous r.,** rhinitis with development of false membrane. **hypertrophic r.,** rhinitis with hypertrophy of mucous membrane. **membranous r.,** chronic rhinitis with a fibrinous exudate. **purulent r.,** chronic rhinitis with formation of pus. **vasomotor r.,** hay fever.

rhinoantritis (ri″no-an-tri'tis)   inflammation of mucous membrane of the nose and antrum of Highmore.

rhinocanthectomy (-kan-thek'to-me)   rhinomectomy.

rhinocele (ri'no-sēl)   the ventricle of the olfactory lobe of the brain.

rhinocephalus (ri″no-sef'ah-lus)   a fetal monster with a nose like a proboscis.

rhinocleisis (-kli'sis)   obstruction of the nasal passage.

rhinodacryolith (-dak're-o-lith″)   lacrimal concretion in the nasal duct.

rhinodynia (ri″no-din'e-ah) pain in the nose.

rhinogenous (ri-noj'e-nus) arising in the nose.

rhinolalia (ri″no-la'le-ah) nasal quality of speech from defect or disease of the nasal passages. **r. aper′ta,** due to too great opening of the nasal passages. **r. clau′sa,** due to too great closure of the nasal passages.

rhinolaryngitis (-lar″in-ji'tis) inflammation of mucous membrane of nose and larynx.

rhinolith (ri'no-lith) a nasal calculus.

rhinolithiasis (ri″no-li-thi'ah-sis) the formation of nasal calculi.

rhinologist (ri-nol'o-jist) a specialist in rhinology.

rhinology (ri-nol'o-je) the sum of knowledge about the nose and its diseases.

rhinometer (ri-nom'e-ter) apparatus for measuring the nose.

rhinomycosis (ri″no-mi-ko'sis) fungus infection of the nose.

rhinonecrosis (-ne-kro'sis) necrosis of the nasal bones.

rhinopathy (ri-nop'ah-the) any disease of the nose.

rhinopharyngitis (ri″no-far″in-ji'tis) inflammation of nasopharynx.

rhinopharyngocele (-fah-ring'go-sēl) a tumor of the nasopharynx.

rhinophonia (-fo'ne-ah) nasal twang or quality of voice.

rhinophore (ri'no-fōr) a nasal cannula to facilitate breathing.

rhinophyma (ri″no-fi'mah) nodular congestion and enlargement of the nose.

rhinoplasty (ri'no-plas″te) plastic reconstruction of the nose.

rhinopolypus (ri″no-pol'ĭ-pus) a nasal polyp.

rhinorrhagia (-ra'je-ah) copious hemorrhage from nose.

rhinorrhea (-re'ah) copious mucous discharge from the nose.

rhinosalpingitis (-sal″pin-ji'tis) inflammation of the mucosa of the nose and eustachian tube.

rhinoscleroma (-skle-ro'mah) respiratory scleroma involving the nose.

rhinoscope (ri'no-skōp) speculum for nasal examination.

rhinoscopy (ri-nos'ko-pe) specular examination of the nose.

rhinostegnosis (ri″no-steg-no'sis) obstruction of the nasal passages.

rhinotomy (ri-not'o-me) incision into the nose.

rhinovirus (ri″no-vi'rus) one of a group of viral agents found associated with the common cold.

Rhipicephalus (ri″pĭ-sef'ah-lus) a genus of arthropods (family Ixodidae), comprising some 46 species and including *R. distinctus* and *R. sanguineus.*

Rhizobiaceae (ri-zo″be-a'se-e) a family of Schizomycetes (order Eubacteriales).

Rhizobium (ri-zo'be-um) a genus of Schizomycetes (order Eubacteriales, family Rhizobiaceae).

rhizoblast (ri'zo-blast) a delicate fibril connecting the basal granule and nucleus of a protozoan.

rhizode (ri'zōd) a rootlike structure, such as a projection from a colony of microorganisms into the medium on which it is grown.

rhizodontropy (ri″zo-don'tro-pe) fixing an artificial crown to a root of a tooth.

rhizodontrypy (-don'trĭ-pe) perforation of the root of a tooth for the escape of morbid matter.

rhizoid (ri'zoid) resembling a root.

rhizome (ri'zōm) the subterranean root stem of a plant.

rhizomelic (ri″zo-mel'ik) pertaining to the hips and shoulders (the roots of the limbs).

rhizomeningomyelitis (-mĕ-ning″go-mi″ĕ-li'tis) radiculomeningomyelitis.

rhizoneure (ri'zo-nūr) a nerve cell forming a nerve root.

Rhizopoda (ri-zop'o-dah) a division of protozoa which includes the amebae.

rhizopodium (ri″zo-po'de-um), pl. *rhizopo′dia* [Gr.] a filamentous pseudopodium, finer than filopodia, and characterized by branching and anastomosis of the branches.

rhizotomy (ri-zot'o-me) division or transection of a nerve root.

rhod(o)- (ro'do) word element [Gr.], *red.*

rhodium (ro'de-um) chemical element *(see table),* at. no. 45, symbol Rh.

Rhodnius (rod'ne-us) a genus of arthropods (order Hemiptera), species of which are naturally infected with trypanosomes.

Rhodobacteriineae (ro″do-bak-te″re-in'e-e) a suborder of Schizomycetes (order Pseudomonadales), including the families Athiorhodaceae, Chlorobacteriaceae and Thiorhodaceae.

rhodocyte (ro'do-sīt) erythrocyte.

rhodogenesis (ro″do-jen'e-sis) regeneration of rhodopsin after its bleaching by the light.

Rhodomicrobium (-mi-kro'be-um) a genus of Schizomycetes (order Hyphomicrobiales, family Hyphomicrobiaceae).

rhodophane (ro'do-fān) a red pigment from retinal cones.

rhodophylaxis (ro″do-fi-lak'sis) the supposed property of the retinal epithelium of protecting and increasing the power of the retinal purple to regain its color after bleaching.

rhodoporphyrin (-por'fi-rin) a porphyrin derived from chlorophyll.

Rhodopseudomonas (-su″do-mo'nas) a genus of Schizomycetes (order Pseudomonadales, suborder Rhodobacteriineae, family Athiorhodaceae).

rhodopsin (ro-dop'sin) the purple-red pigment of outer segment of retinal rods.

Rhodospirillum (ro″do-spi-ril'lum) a genus of Schizomycetes (order Pseudomonadales, suborder Rhodobacteriineae, family Athiorhodaceae).

Rhodothece (-the'se) a genus of Schizomycetes (order Pseudomonadales, suborder Rhodobacteriineae, family Thiorhodaceae).

rhombencephalon (romb″en-sef'ah-lon) the hindbrain, including the medulla oblongata, pons and cerebellum.

rhombocele (rom'bo-sēl) the terminal expansion of the canal of the spinal cord.

rhomboid (rom'boid) shaped like a rhomb or kite. **Michaelis' r.**, a diamond-shaped area over the posterior aspect of the pelvis.

rhomboideus (rom-boi'de-us) [L.] rhomboid.

rhonchus (rong'kus) a coarse dry rale in the bronchial tubes. adj., **rhon'chal, rhon'chial.**

rhotacism (ro'tah-sizm) faulty enunciation of r sounds.

rhubarb (roo'barb) the dried rhizome and root of *Rheum officinale;* used in fluidextract or aromatic tincture as a cathartic.

Rhus (rus) a name formerly given a genus of trees and shrubs, many of them poisonous, and most of which are now classified in the genus Toxicodendron. **R. diversilo'ba,** poison oak. **R. toxicoden'dron,** poison ivy, a plant which causes a severe dermatitis in susceptible persons. **R. venena'ta,** poison sumac, another species capable of causing severe dermatitis.

rhypophagy (ri-pof'ah-je) the eating of filth.

rhypophobia (ri″po-fo'be-ah) morbid fear of filth.

rhythm (rithm) regularity of occurrence, as of variation of energy, electrical discharge, muscular contraction or other phenomenon. **biological r.**, the established regularity with which certain phenomena recur in living organisms. **cantering r.**, gallop rhythm. **circadian r.**, the regular recurrence in cycles of approximately 24 hours from one stated point to another, e.g. certain biological activities that occur at that interval regardless of constant darkness or other conditions of illumination. **coupled r.**, an abnormal relation between pulse and heart beat, every other beat of the heart producing no pulse at the wrist. **gallop r.**, a cardiac cycle with an accentuated extra sound, creating an auscultatory effect like the sound of a galloping horse. **sinus r.**, the normal heart rhythm originating in the sinoatrial node. **ventricular r.**, the ventricular contractions occurring in complete heart block.

rhythmicity (rith-mis'i-te) a state of rhythmical contraction.

rhytidoplasty (rit'i do-plas″te) plastic surgery for the elimination of wrinkles from the skin.

rhytidosis (rit″i-do'sis) a wrinkling, as of the cornea.

rib (rib) any one of the paired bones, 12 on either side, extending from the thoracic vertebrae toward the median line on the ventral aspect of the trunk. **abdominal r's, asternal r's,** false ribs. **cervical r.**, a supernumerary rib arising from a cervical vertebra. **false r's,** the five lower ribs on either side, not attached directly to the sternum. **floating r's,** the two lower false ribs on either side, attached only to the vertebra. **slipping r.**, one whose attaching cartilage is repeatedly dislocated. **true r's,** the seven upper ribs on either side, attached to both vertebrae and sternum. **vertebral r's,** floating ribs. **vertebrocostal r's,** the three upper false ribs on either side, attached to vertebrae and costal cartilages. **vertebrosternal r's,** true ribs.

riboflavin (ri″bo-fla'vin) a water-soluble vitamin, one of the components of the B complex.

ribonuclease (ri″bo-nu'kle-ās) an enzyme which catalyzes the depolymerization of ribonucleic acid.

ribose (ri'bōs) an aldopentose found in and characteristic of yeast nucleic acid (ribose nucleic acid).

ribosome (ri'bo-sōm) a submicroscopic ribonucleic acid-containing particle in the cytoplasm of a cell, sometimes closely associated with endoplasmic reticulum.

R.I.C. Royal Institute of Chemistry.

rice (rīs) the grain of *Oryza sativa,* the common cultivated rice. **r. polishings,** fine yellowish powder from certain parts of rice; used in vitamin B deficiency.

ricinism (ri'sī-nizm) intoxication due to inhalation or ingestion of a poisonous principle (ricin) of castor bean.

Ricinus (ris'i-nus) a genus of euphorbiaceous plants. **R. commu'nis,** the plant whose seeds afford castor oil.

rickets (rik'ets) a deficiency disease of infancy and childhood with disturbance of the normal process of ossification, the bones becoming crooked and deformed. **fetal r.**, achondroplasia. **renal r.**, renal osteodystrophy. **tardy r.**, a disease resembling rickets, occurring in an adult.

Rickettsia (ri-ket'se-ah) a genus of Microtatobiotes (order Rickettsiales, family Rickettsiaceae, tribe Rickettsieae) transmitted by lice, fleas, ticks and mice to man and other animals, causing various diseases.

rickettsia (ri-ket'se-ah), pl. *rickett'siae,* an individual organism of the genus Rickettsiae.

Rickettsiaceae (ri-ket″se-a'se-e) a family of Microtatobiotes (order Rickettsiales), including the tribes Ehrlichieae, Rickettsieae and Wolbachieae.

rickettsial (ri-ket'se-al) pertaining to or caused by rickettsiae.

Rickettsiales (ri-ket″se-a'lez) an order of Microtatobiotes, parasitic in both vertebrates and invertebrates.

rickettsialpox (rik-et'se-al-poks″) a febrile disease with vesiculopapular eruption, caused by rickettsiae.

rickettsicidal (rik-et″sī-si'dal) destructive to rickettsiae.

Rickettsieae (rik″et-si'e-e) a tribe of Microtatobiotes (order Rickettsiales, family Rickettsiaceae).

Rickettsiella (ri-ket″se-el'lah) a genus of Microtatobiotes (order Rickettsiales, family Rickettsiaceae, tribe Wolbachieae).

rickettsiosis (rik-et″se-o'sis) infection with rickettsiae.

Ricolesia (rik″o-le'ze-ah) a genus of Microtatobiotes (order Rickettsiales, family Chlamydiaceae).

ridge (rij) a linear projection or elevation, as on a bone, or a linear thickening of other tissue, as in the embryo. **dental r.**, any linear elevation on the crown of a tooth. **germ r.**, epithelial ridge on the embryonic mesonephros, giving rise to the sexual elements.

mammary r., an ectodermal thickening in early embryos, along which the mammary glands subsequently develop. **oblique r.**, a variable linear elevation obliquely crossing the occlusive surface of a maxillary molar tooth.

ridgling (rij'ling) an animal with one testis removed.

R.I.F. right iliac fossa.

rigidity (rĭ-jid'ĭ-te) inflexibility or stiffness. **clasp-knife r.**, increased tension in the extensors of a joint when it is passively flexed, giving way suddenly on exertion of further pressure. **cogwheel r.**, tension in a muscle which gives way in little jerks when the muscle is passively stretched. **decerebrate r.**, abnormal stiffness and inflexibility in experimental animals caused by transection of the brain stem.

rigor (rig'or, ri'gor) a chill; rigidity. **r. mor'tis**, rigidity of skeletal muscles, developing six to ten hours after death and persisting for three or four days.

rim (rim) a border or edge. **bite r.**, occlusion r., **record r.**, a border constructed on temporary or permanent denture bases in order to record the maxillomandibular relation and for positioning of the teeth.

rima (ri'mah), pl. *ri'mae* [L.] a linear opening between two more or less parallel borders. **r. glot'tidis**, the opening between the vocal cords. **r. o'ris**, the opening of the mouth. **r. palpebra'rum**, the slit between the eyelids. **r. puden'di**, the space between the labia minora.

Rimifon (rim'ĭ-fon) trademark for a preparation of isoniazid.

rimula (rim'u-lah), pl. *rim'ulae* [L.] a minute fissure.

rinderpest (rin'der-pest) cattle plague.

ring (ring) a circular or continuous structure, as one surrounding an opening in an organ or in the body wall. **abdominal r., external,** opening in aponeurosis of external oblique for spermatic cord or round ligament. **abdominal r., internal,** aperture in transverse fascia for spermatic cord or round ligament. **Bandl's r.**, pathologic retraction ring. **benzene r.**, the hexagon representing the arrangement of carbon atoms in a molecule of benzene, different compounds being derived by replacement of the hydrogen atoms by different elements. **constriction r.**, a thickened area of myometrium during labor, over a point of depression in the fetal body or at a point just below it. **retraction r., pathologic,** a complication of prolonged labor marked by failure of relaxation of the circular fibers at the internal os of the cervix, obstructing delivery of the infant. **retraction r., physiologic,** the demarcation between the upper, contracting portion of the uterus in labor and the lower, dilating part. **tympanic r.**, the bony ring forming part of the temporal bone at birth and developing into the tympanic plate. **umbilical r.**, the orifice in the abdominal wall of the fetus for transmission of the umbilical vein and arteries. **vascular r.**, a congenital anomaly of the aortic arch and its tributaries, the vessels forming a ring about the trachea and esophagus and causing varying degrees of compression.

ring-bone (ring'bōn) enlargement of some part of the pastern bone in horses.

ringworm (ring'werm) a skin disease marked by characteristic ring-shaped patches, due to various fungi (dermatophytes). **honeycomb r.**, favus. **Tokelau r.**, tinea imbricata.

R.I.P.H.H. Royal Institute of Public Health and Hygiene.

Risa (ri'sah) trademark for a preparation of radio-iodinated serum albumin.

ristocetin (ris"to-se'tin) an antibiotic substance derived from culture of *Nocardia lurida*; used in treatment of infections by gram-positive cocci.

risus (ri'sus) [L.] laughter. **r. sardon'icus,** grinning expression produced by spasm of facial muscles.

Ritalin (rit'ah-lin) trademark for preparations of methylphenidate.

riziform (riz'ĭ-form) resembling grains of rice.

R.L.L. right lower lobe.

R.M.A. right mento-anterior (position of the fetus).

R.M.N. Registered Mental Nurse (England).

R.M.P. right mentoposterior (position of the fetus).

R.M.P.A. Royal Medico-Psychological Association.

R.N. Registered Nurse.

Rn chemical symbol. *radon.*

RNA (ribonucleic acid) a nucleic acid found in all living cells which on hydrolysis yields adenine, guanine, cytosine, uracil, ribose and phosphoric acid, the material taking part in the protein synthesis in the cell. **messenger RNA,** an RNA fraction of intermediate molecular weight which transmits genetic information from DNA to the protein-forming system of the cell. **ribosomal RNA,** nonspecific RNA present in ribosomes with almost equal proportions of protein. **soluble RNA, transfer RNA,** a fraction of low molecular weight which transfers a specific amino acid from an activating enzyme to a ribosome to facilitate synthesis of a specific polypeptide.

R.N.M.S. Registered Nurse for the Mentally Subnormal.

R.O.A. right occipito-anterior (position of the fetus).

roaring (rōr'ing) a condition in the horse marked by a rough sound on inspiration and sometimes on expiration.

Robalate (ro'bah-lāt) trademark for preparations of dihydroxyaluminum aminoacetate.

Robaxin (ro-bak'sin) trademark for preparations of methocarbamol.

Roccal (Ro'kal) trademark for a preparation of benzalkonium chloride.

rod (rod) a straight, slim mass of substance, specifically one of the rodlike bodies of the retina, which contain rhodopsin. **Corti's r's,** stiff, pillar-like structures forming two rows in the organ of Corti. **enamel r.**, one of the rodlike structures forming the enamel of the teeth. **Heidenhain's r's,** rodlike epithelial striations in the tubules of the kidney.

rodenticide (ro-den'tĭ-sīd) an agent destructive to rodents.

rodonalgia (ro″do-nal'je-ah) erythromelalgia.

roentgen (rent'gen) a special unit (l e.s.u. per 0.001293 gm., or 2.58 × 10⁻⁴ coulomb per kilogram of air) used in expressing the amount of exposure to x-rays or gamma rays; abbreviated R.

roentgenism (rent'gen-izm) disease due to excessive exposure to x-rays.

roentgenkymogram (rent″gen-ki'mo-gram) the film obtained by roentgenkymography.

roentgenkymograph (-ki'mo-graf) the apparatus used in roentgenkymography.

roentgenkymography (-ki-mog'rah-fe) a technique of graphically recording the movements of an organ by means of x-rays.

roentgenogram (rent'gen-o-gram″) radiogram.

roentgenography (rent″gĕ-nog'rah-fe) the taking of pictures (roentgenograms) of internal structures of the body by passage of x-rays through the body to act on specially sensitized film. **body-section r.,** x-ray visualization of structures lying in a particular plane of the body by various techniques which cause blurring of the images of structures in other places. **mass r.,** the rapid taking of radiograms of large numbers of people. **miniature r.,** the taking of radiograms on small films, to screen for certain diseases. **mucosal relief r.,** a technique permitting visualization of the intestinal mucosa, and revealing any defect in its continuity. **serial r.,** the making of several exposures of a particular area at arbitrary intervals. **spot film r.,** the recording on film of any desired area at any time during fluoroscopic examination.

roentgenologist (-nol'o-jist) a specialist in roentgenology.

roentgenology (-nol'o-je) the scientific study of the diagnostic and therapeutic use of roentgen (x) rays.

roentgenolucent (rent″gen-o-lu'sent) permitting the passage of x-rays.

roentgenometry (rent″gĕ-nom'ĕ-tre) measurement of roentgen (x) rays.

roentgenopaque (rent″gen-o-pak′) not permitting the passage of x-rays.

roentgenoscopy (rent″gĕ-nos'ko-pe) fluoroscopy.

roentgenotherapy (rent″gen-o-ther'ah-pe) treatment by roentgen (x) rays.

Rolicton (ro-lik'ton) trademark for a preparation of amisometradine.

rolitetracycline (ro″le-tet″rah-si'klēn) a tetracycline compound used for intravenous or intramuscular injection.

rombergism (rom'berg-izm) tendency of a patient to sway when he stands still with feet close together and eyes closed.

Romilar (ro'mil-ar) trademark for preparations of dextromethorphan hydrobromide.

rongeur (ron-zher′) [Fr.] gouge forceps or nippers.

room (room) a place in a building, enclosed and set apart for occupancy, or equipped for a special purpose. **delivery r.,** one in which infants are delivered. **labor r.,** one in which the obstetrical patient is observed during the first stage of labor. **operating r.,** one especially equipped for the performance of surgical operations. **recovery r.,** a hospital unit adjoining operating or delivery rooms, with special equipment and personnel for care of patients immediately after operation or childbirth.

root (root) 1. the descending and subterranean part of a plant. 2. that portion of an organ, such as a tooth, hair or nail, that is buried in the tissues, or by which it arises from another structure. **nerve r., anterior,** the structure composed of efferent (motor) fibers emerging from the anterior aspect of the spinal cord and, with the fibers of the posterior root, forming the spinal nerve; called also *motor root* and *ventral root.* **nerve r., posterior,** the structure composed of afferent (sensory) fibers emerging from a spinal nerve and entering the dorsolateral aspect of the spinal cord; called also *dorsal root* and *sensory root.*

R.O.P. right occipitoposterior (position of the fetus).

rosacea (ro-za'she-ah) a disease of the nose and cheeks marked by acnelike lesions, dilatation of the capillaries and sometimes leading to hypertrophy of the nose (rhinophyma).

rosaniline (ro-zan'ĭ-lin) a substance from coal tar, the basis of various dyes and stains.

rosary (ro'zah-re) a structure resembling a string of beads. **rachitic r.,** a succession of beadlike prominences along the costal cartilages, in rickets.

roseola (ro-ze'o-lah) a rose-colored rash. **r. choler'ica,** eruption sometimes seen in cholera. **epidemic r.,** rubeola. **r. infan'tum,** exanthem subitum. **syphilitic r.,** eruption of rose-colored spots in early secondary syphilis. **r. typho'sa,** the eruption of typhoid or typhus fever. **r. vacci'nia,** a rash sometimes occurring after vaccination.

rosette (ro-zet′) any structure or formation resembling a rose.

rosin (roz'in) solid resin obtained from species of Pinus; used in preparation of ointments and plasters.

Rossiella (ros″e-el'ah) a genus of protozoan organisms parasitic in the blood of certain animals.

rostellum (ros-tel'um) the hook-bearing part of the head of worms.

rostral (ros'tral) 1. resembling a rostrum. 2. directed toward the front end of the body.

rostrate (ros'trāt) beaked.

rostrum (ros'trum), pl. *ros'tra* [L.] a beak-shaped process.

rot (rot) 1. decay. 2. a disease of sheep.

rotation (ro-ta'shun) process of turning around an axis.

rotenone (ro'tĕ-nōn) a poisonous compound from derris root and other roots; used as an insecticide and as a scabicide.

rotula (rot′u-lah) 1. the patella. 2. a lozenge or troche.

rotular (rot′u-lar) pertaining to the patella.

rotz (rotz) glanders in horses.

roughage (ruf′ij) coarse material, such as bran, cereals, fruit and vegetable fibers, which acts as an irritant to stimulate intestinal evacuation.

rouleau (roo-lo′), pl. *rouleaux′* [Fr.] a roll of red blood corpuscles resembling a pile of coins.

roundworm (rownd′werm) a parasite of the genus Ascaris.

roup (roop) an infectious disease of fowls.

R.P.F. renal plasma flow.

rpm. revolutions per minute.

R.Q. respiratory quotient.

-rrhachia word element [Gr.], *state of the spinal fluid;* also spelled **-rachia.**

-rrhachis word element [Gr.], *spinal cord.*

-rrhage, -rrhagia (rāj, ra′je-ah) word element [Gr.], *excessive flow.* adj., **-rrhagic.**

-rrhaphy (rah-fe) word element [Gr.], *stitching; suture.* adj., **-rrhaphic.**

-rrhea (re′ah) word element [Gr.], *profuse flow.* adj., **-rrheic.**

-rrhexis (rek′sis) word element [Gr.], *rupture; bursting.* adj., **-rrhec′tic.**

R.R.L. Registered Record Librarian.

R.S.A. right sacro-anterior (position of the fetus).

R.Sc.A. right scapulo-anterior (position of the fetus).

R.S.C.N. Registered Sick Children's Nurse.

R.Sc.P. right scapuloposterior (position of the fetus).

R.S.M. Royal Society of Medicine.

R.S.N.A. Radiological Society of North America.

R.S.P. right sacroposterior (position of the fetus).

R.S.T. right sacrotransverse (position of the fetus).

R.S.T.M.H. Royal Society of Tropical Medicine and Hygiene.

R.U. rat unit.

Ru chemical symbol, *ruthenium.*

rubber-dam (rub′er-dam) a sheet of thin latex rubber used by dentists to isolate a tooth from the fluids of the mouth during dental treatment.

rubedo (roo-be′do) redness of the skin.

rubefacient (roo″bĕ-fa′shent) 1. reddening the skin. 2. an agent that reddens the skin.

rubella (roo-bel′ah) an extremely mild constitutional disease, caused by a virus and characterized by fever and a transient eruption resembling the exanthem of measles; occurring in early pregnancy, it may cause serious anomalies in the developing fetus. **r. scarlatino′sa,** a disease attended with eruption, sore throat and desquamation, somewhat resembling scarlet fever, but much milder.

rubeola (roo-be′o-lah, ru″be-o′lah) measles.

rubeosis (roo″be-o′sis) redness. **r. i′ridis,** a condition characterized by a new formation of vessels and connective tissue on the surface of the iris, frequently seen in diabetics.

rubescent (roo-bes′ent) growing red.

rubidium (roo-bid′e-um) chemical element *(see table),* at. no. 37, symbol Rb.

rubor (roo′bor) redness, one of the cardinal signs of inflammation.

Rubramin (roo′brah-min) trademark for preparations of vitamin B_{12} activity concentrate.

rubriblast (roo′brī-blast) a cell of the erythrocytic series having fine chromatin structure in the nucleus, and usually discernible nucleoli.

rubricyte (roo′brī-sīt) a cell of the erythrocytic series having a definite chromatin structure in the nucleus, but no discernible nucleoli.

rubrospinal (roo″bro-spi′nal) pertaining to the red nucleus and the spinal cord.

rubrum (roo′brum) [L.] red. **r. scarlati′num,** scarlet red.

rudiment (roo′dĭ-ment) 1. a vestigial organ. 2. primordium.

rudimentary (roo″dĭ-men′ter-e) incompletely developed.

ruga (roo′gah), pl. *ru′gae* [L.] a ridge or fold.

rugose (roo′gōs) marked by ridges; wrinkled.

rugosity (roo-gos′ĭ-te) 1. condition of being rugose. 2. a ridge or ruga.

R.U.L. right upper lobe.

rule (rool) a statement of conditions commonly observed in a given situation, or of a prescribed procedure to obtain a given result. **Arey's r.,** a formula correlating the length of the embryo and the conception age. **Bastedo's r.,** the dose of a drug for a child is obtained by multiplying the adult dose by the child's age in years, adding 3 to the product, and dividing the sum by 30. **Clark's r.,** the dose of a drug for a child is obtained by multiplying the adult dose by the child's weight in pounds and dividing the result by 150. **Fried's r.,** the dose of a drug for an infant less than two years old is obtained by multiplying the child's age in months by the adult dose and dividing the result by 150. **Nägele's r.,** (for predicting day of labor) subtract three months from the first day of the last menstruation and add seven days. **Young's r.,** the dose of a drug for a child is obtained by multiplying the adult dose by the child's age in years and dividing the result by the sum of the child's age plus 12.

rumen (roo′men) the first stomach of a ruminant.

rumenitis (roo″mĕ-ni′tis) inflammation of the rumen.

ruminant (roo′mī-nant) an animal which has a stomach with four complete cavities: rumen, reticulum, omasum and abomasum, which characteristically regurgitates undigested food from the rumen and masticates it when at rest.

rumination (roo″mī-na′shun) 1. merycism. 2. persistent meditation on a certain subject.

rump (rump) the buttock or gluteal region.

rupia (roo′pe-ah) an eruption in tertiary syphilis, with formation of bullae.

rupture (rup′tūr) 1. to break apart or disrupt. 2. the bursting or breaking of a part. 3. hernia.

rush (rush) a rapid movement. **peristaltic r's,**

vigorous peristaltic movements, propelling intestinal contents 20 to 50 cm. before dying out.

rut (rut) the period of testicular activity in the males of certain species of animals, coinciding with the period of sexual excitement (estrus) in the females.

ruthenium (roo-the'ne-um) chemical element *(see table)*, at. no. 44, symbol Ru.

rutherford (ruth'er-ford) a unit of radioactive disintegration, representing one million disintegrations per second.

rutin (roo'tin) tasteless, greenish-yellow powder from buckwheat and other sources; used to decrease capillary fragility.

rutoside (roo'to-sīd) rutin.

rye (ri) the cereal plant *Secale cereale,* and its nutritious seed. **ergotized r., spurred r.,** rye affected with fungus, *Claviceps purpurea,* from which ergot is derived.

S

S chemical symbol, *sulfur.*

S. [L.] se'mis *(half);* sight; [L.] sig'na *(sign);* [L.] sin'ister *(left);* south; spherical (lens).

S.A.B. Society of American Bacteriologists.

sabulous (sab'u-lus) gritty or sandy.

saburra (sah-bur'ah) sordes or foulness of the mouth or stomach.

saburral (sah-bur'al) 1. pertaining to saburra. 2. gritty; gravelly.

sac (sak) a pouchlike cavity. **air s.,** an alveolus of the lung. **amnionic s.,** the sac enclosing the fetus suspended in the amniotic fluid. **conjunctival s.,** the space between the bulbar and palpebral conjunctivae. **dental s.,** the dense fibrous layer of mesenchyme surrounding the enamel organ and dental papilla. **enamel s.,** the enamel organ when its outer layer forms a sac enclosing the whole dental germ. **heart s.,** the pericardium. **hernial s.,** peritoneal pouch which encloses protruding intestine. **Hilton's s.,** laryngeal pouch. **lacrimal s.,** a membranous reservoir into which the lacrimal canaliculi drain and which is continuous with the nasolacrimal duct. **yolk s.,** a membranous structure formed in early embryonic development, connected with the midgut.

saccate (sak'āt) 1. shaped like a sac. 2. contained in a sac.

saccharase (sak'ah-rās) invertase.

saccharate (sak'ah-rāt) a salt of saccharic acid.

saccharated (sak'ah-rāt"ed) sugary; charged with sugar.

saccharide (sak'ah-rīd) one of a series of carbohydrates, including the sugars.

sacchariferous (sak"ah-rif'er-us) containing sugar.

saccharin (sak'ah-rin) a white, crystalline compound several hundred times sweeter than sucrose; used as a noncaloric sweetening agent. **calcium s.,** an artificial sweetening agent.

saccharogalactorrhea (sak"ah-ro-gah-lak"to-re'ah) secretion of milk containing an excess of sugar.

saccharolytic (-lit'ik) capable of splitting up sugar.

saccharometabolic (-met"ah-bol'ik) pertaining to metabolism of sugar.

saccharometabolism (sak"ah-ro-mě-tab'o-lizm) metabolism of sugar.

saccharometer (sak"ah-rom'ě-ter) apparatus for measuring proportion of sugar in a solution.

Saccharomyces (sak"ah-ro-mi'sēz) a genus of protophytes, the yeast fungi.

saccharomycosis (-mi-ko'sis) 1. any disease due to yeast fungi. 2. a skin disease marked by presence of nodules containing Saccharomyces.

saccharorrhea (re'ah) glycosuria.

saccharose (sak'ah-rōs) ordinary cane or beet sugar.

saccharosuria (sak"ah-ro-su're-ah) saccharose in urine.

saccharum (sak'ah-rum) [L.] sugar. **s. lac'tis,** lactose.

sacciform (sak'sī-form) shaped like a bag or sac.

saccular (sak'u-lar) pertaining to or resembling a sac.

sacculated (sak'u-lāt"ed) containing saccules.

sacculo (sak'ūl) a little bag or sac; a small, pouchlike cavity.

sacculus (sak'u-lus), pl. *sac'culi* [L.] a saccule. **s. laryn'gis,** fovea on outside of either false vocal cord.

saccus (sak'us), pl. *sac'ci* [L.] a sac. **s. endolymphat'icus,** sac of dura in the aqueduct of the vestibule. **s. lacrima'lis,** lacrimal sac.

sacrad (sa'krad) toward the sacrum.

sacral (sa'kral) pertaining to the sacrum.

sacralgia (sa-kral'je-ah) pain in the sacrum.

sacralization (sa"kral-i-za'shun) fusion of the fifth lumbar vertebra with the sacrum.

sacrectomy (sa-krek'to-me) excision or resection of the sacrum.

sacrococcygeal (sa"kro-kok-sij'e-al) pertaining to sacrum and coccyx.

sacrocoxalgia (-kok-sal'je-ah) pain in the sacroiliac joint.

sacrocoxitis (-kok-si'tis) inflammation of the sacroiliac joint.

sacrodynia (-din'e-ah) pain in the sacral region.

sacroiliac (-il'e-ak) pertaining to the sacrum and ilium, or to their articulation.

sacroiliitis (-il"e-i'tis) inflammation of the sacroiliac joint.

sacrolumbar (sa″kro-lum′bar) pertaining to sacrum and loins.

sacrosciatic (-si-at′ik) pertaining to sacrum and ischium.

sacrospinal (-spi′nal) pertaining to sacrum and vertebral column.

sacrouterine (-u′ter-in) pertaining to sacrum and uterus.

sacrovertebral (-ver′tē-bral) pertaining to sacrum and vertebrae.

sadism (sad′izm) 1. the derivation of sexual gratification through the infliction of pain on another. 2. the needless infliction of pain on another. adj., **sadis′tic.**

sadist (sad′ist) a person exhibiting or characterized by sadism.

sadomasochism (sad″o-mas′o-kizm) a state characterized by both sadistic and masochistic tendencies. adj., **sadomasochis′tic.**

sadomasochist (-mas′o-kist) a person exhibiting sadomasochism.

Saff (saf) trademark for a preparation of safflower oil.

Safflor (saf′flor) trademark for a preparation of safflower oil.

sagittal (saj′ĭ-tal) 1. shaped like an arrow. 2. situated in the direction of the sagittal suture; said of an anteroposterior plane or section coinciding with (median sagittal plane) or parallel to the long axis of the body.

sagittalis (saj″i-ta′lis) [L.] sagittal.

sago (sa′go) starch from pith of various palm trees.

sal (sal) [L.] salt. **s. ammo′niac,** ammonium chloride. **s. so′da,** sodium carbonate. **s. volat′ile,** ammonium carbonate.

salamander (sal″ah-man′der) a lizard-like animal used in various physiologic experiments.

salicylamide (sal″ĭ-sil-am′īd) a white, crystalline powder used as an analgesic.

salicylanilide (-an′ĭ-līd) a white or slightly pink crystalline compound used as an antifungal agent.

salicylate (sal′ĭ-sil″āt, sah-lis′ĭ-lāt) a salt of salicylic acid.

salicylated (sal′ĭ-sil-āt″ed) impregnated or charged with salicylic acid.

salicylazosulfapyridine (sal″ĭ-sil″ah-zo-sul″-fah-pir′ĭ-dēn) a salicylic acid compound used in treatment of chronic ulcerative colitis.

salicylide (sal′ĭ-sil″īd) an anhydride of salicylic acid.

salicylism (sal′ĭ-sil″izm) toxic symptoms caused by salicylic acid.

salicyltherapy (sal″ĭ-sil-ther′ah-pe) treatment with salicylic acid and the salicylates.

salifiable (sal″ĭ-fi′ah-bl) capable of combining with an acid to form a salt.

salimeter (sah-lim′ē-ter) an instrument for determining the strength of saline solutions.

saline (sa′līn) salty; of the nature of a salt.

saliva (sah-li′vah) the enzyme-containing secretion of the salivary glands. adj., **sal′ivary.**

salivant (sal′ĭ-vant) causing an excessive flow of saliva.

salivation (sal″ĭ-va′shun) 1. the secretion of saliva. 2. ptyalism.

sallenders (sal′en-derz) eczema at the bend of the hock in the hind leg of a horse.

salmiac (sal′me-ak) ammonium chloride.

Salmonella (sal″mo-nel′ah) a genus of Schizomycetes (order Eubacteriales, family Enterobacteriaceae, tribe Salmonelleae), including the typhoid-paratyphoid bacilli and bacteria usually pathogenic for lower animals which are often transmitted to man.

salmonella (-nel′ah) an individual organism of the genus Salmonella.

Salmonelleae (-nel′e-e) a tribe of Schizomycetes (order Eubacteriales, family Enterobacteriaceae).

salmonellosis (-nel-lo′sis) infection with Salmonella.

salping(o)- (sal-ping′go) word element [Gr.], *tube (eustachian tube* or *uterine tube).*

salpingectomy (sal″pin-jek′to-me) excision of a uterine tube.

salpingemphraxis (-jem-frak′sis) 1. obstruction of a uterine tube. 2. obstruction of a eustachian tube.

salpingian (sal-pin′je-an) pertaining to the auditory or the uterine tube.

salpingion (sal-pin′je-on) a point at the apex of the petrous bone on the lower surface.

salpingitis (sal″pin-ji′tis) 1. inflammation of a uterine tube. 2. inflammation of the eustachian tube.

salpingocele (sal-ping′go-sēl) hernial protrusion of a uterine tube.

salpingocyesis (sal-ping″go-si-e′sis) pregnancy in a uterine tube.

salpingography (sal″ping-gog′rah-fe) roentgenologic visualization of the uterine tubes after intrauterine injection of a radiopaque medium.

salpingolithiasis (sal-ping″go-lĭ-thi′ah-sis) the presence of calcareous deposits in the wall of the uterine tubes.

salpingolysis (sal″ping-gol′ĭ-sis) surgical separation of adhesions involving the uterine tubes.

salpingo-oophorectomy (sal-ping″go-o″of-o-rek′to-me) excision of a uterine tube and ovary.

salpingo-oophoritis (-o″of-o-ri′tis) inflammation of a uterine tube and ovary.

salpingo-oophorocele (-o-of″o-ro-sēl″) hernia of a uterine tube and ovary.

salpingo-ovariotripsy (-o-va″re-o-trip″se) ablation of uterine tube, ovary and adnexa.

salpingopexy (-pek′se) fixation of a uterine tube.

salpingoplasty (sal-ping′go-plas″te) plastic repair of a uterine tube.

salpingoscope (sal-ping′go-skōp) an instrument for examination of nasopharynx and eustachian tube.

salpingostaphylinus (sal-ping″go-staf″ĭ-li′i-nus) the tensor veli palatini muscle.

salpingostomy (sal″ping-gos′to-me) restoration of the patency of a uterine tube.

salpingotomy (-got′o-me) surgical incision of a uterine tube.

salpinx (sal′pinks) 1. a uterine tube. 2. a eustachian tube.

salt (sawlt) 1. sodium chloride. 2. a compound

of a metal with an acid radical. 3. (plural: salts) a saline purgative. **acid s.**, a salt in which some of the replaceable hydrogen atoms remain in the molecule, giving it the properties of an acid. **baker's s.**, ammonium carbonate. **basic s.**, a salt with OH groups in the molecule, giving it the properties of a base. **bile s's**, compounds formed in the liver which aid in digestion and absorption of fats and absorption of fat-soluble vitamins. **buffer s.**, a salt in the blood which is able to absorb slight excesses of acid or alkali. **common s.**, sodium chloride. **double s.**, a salt in which the hydrogen atoms of the acid have been replaced by two metals. **Epsom s.**, magnesium sulfate. **Glauber's s.**, sodium sulfate. **haloid s.**, a binary compound of a halogen— i.e. of chlorine, iodine, bromine, fluorine. **neutral s., normal s.**, a salt in which all the hydrogen of the acid has been replaced by a metal. **Rochelle s.**, potassium sodium tartrate. **smelling s.**, aromatic ammonium carbonate.

saltation (sal-ta'shun) 1. leaping or dancing as in chorea. 2. in genetics, an abrupt variation in species; a mutation.

salubrious (sah-lu'bre-us) conducive to health; wholesome.

saluresis (sal"u-re'sis) excretion of sodium and chloride in the urine. adj., **saluret'ic.**

salutary (sal'u-tār"e) healthful.

salvarsan (sal'var-san) arsphenamine.

salve (sav) ointment.

Salyrgan (sal'er-gan) trademark for a preparation of mersalyl.

S.A.M.A. Student American Medical Association.

samarium (sah-ma're-um) chemical element (see table), at. no. 62, symbol Sm.

S.A.N.A. Society of Alienists and Neurologists of America.

sanative (san'ah-tiv) curative; healing.

sanatorium (san"ah-to're-um) an institution for treatment of sick persons, especially a private hospital for convalescents or patients who are not extremely ill.

sanatory (san'ah-tor"e) conducive to health.

sand (sand) substance composed of fine gritty particles. **brain s.**, acervulus cerebri.

Sandril (san'dril) trademark for preparations of reserpine.

sane (sān) sound in mind.

sangui- (sang'gwe) word element [L.], blood.

sanguicolous (sang-gwik'o-lus) living in the blood.

sanguifacient (sang"gwī-fa'shent) forming blood.

sanguimotor (-mo'tor) pertaining to circulation of the blood.

sanguinaria (-na're-ah) dried rhizome of San-guinaria canadensis; local irritant and sternutatory.

sanguine (sang'gwin) 1. abounding in blood. 2. ardent; hopeful.

sanguineous (sang-gwin'e-us) bloody; abounding in blood.

sanguinolent (sang-gwin'o-lent) of a bloody tinge.

sanguirenal (sang"gwī-re'nal) pertaining to blood and kidneys.

sanguis (sang'gwis) [L.] blood.

sanguivorous (sang-gwiv'o-rus) subsisting on blood.

sanies (sa'ne-ēz) a fetid ichorous discharge containing serum, pus and blood. adj., **sa'nious.**

saniopurulent (sa"ne-o-pu'roo-lent) purulent, with serum and blood.

sanioserous (-se'rus) serous, with pus and blood.

sanitarium (san"ī-ta're-um) an institution for the promotion of health.

sanitary (san'ī-tār"e) promoting or pertaining to health.

sanitation (san"ī-ta'shun) the establishment of conditions favorable to health.

sanitization (-ti-za'shun) the process of making or the quality of being made sanitary.

sanitize (san'ī-tīz) to clean and sterilize.

sanity (san"ī-te) soundness, especially soundness of mind.

santonin (san'to-nin) a lactone from the unexpanded flower heads of Artemisia cina; used as an anthelmintic.

sap (sap) the natural fluid substance of animal or vegetable tissue. **cell s.**, hyaloplasm. **nuclear s.**, karyolymph.

sapid (sap'id) having taste or flavor.

sapo (sa'po) [L.] soap. **s. du'rus**, hard soap. **s. mol'lis**, soft soap. **s. mol'lis medicina'lis**, medicinal soft soap.

saponaceous (sa"po-na'shus) soapy; of soaplike feel or quality.

saponification (sah-pon"ī-fi-ka'shun) conversion of an oil or fat into a soap by combination with an alkali.

saponin (sap'o-nin) a glycosidal principle from various plants which characteristically foams when shaken with water.

sapophore (sap'o-for) the group of atoms in the molecule of a compound which gives the substance its characteristic taste.

sapphism (saf'izm) homosexual behavior in the female; lesbianism.

sapr(o)- (sap'ro) word element [Gr.], rotten; putrid; decay; decayed material.

sapremia (sah-pre'me-ah) the presence of septic material in the blood.

saprogen (sap'ro-jen) an agent which causes putrefaction.

saprogenic (sap"ro-jen'ik) causing putrefaction.

saprogenous (sap-roj'ĕ-nus) arising or resulting from putrefaction.

saprophilous (sah-prof'ī-lus) living on dead matter.

saprophyte (sap'ro-fīt) a plant organism, such as yeasts, molds and most bacteria, that absorbs required nutrients directly through the cell membrane, from decomposing animal or plant bodies or from masses of plant and animal by-products. adj., **saprophyt'ic.**

Saprospira (sap"ro-spi'rah) a genus of Schizomycetes (order Spirochaetales, family Spirochaetaceae).

saprozoic (-zo'ik) living in decayed organic

matter; said of animals, especially protozoa.

sarc(o)- (sar'ko) word element [Gr.], *flesh.*

Sarcina (sar-si'nah) a genus of Schizomycetes (order Eubacteriales, family Micrococcaceae) found in soil and water as saprophytes and rarely observed in disease processes.

sarcitis (sar-si'tis) inflammation of muscle tissue.

sarcoadenoma (sar″ko-ad″ĕ-no'mah) adenosarcoma.

sarcoblast (sar'ko-blast) a primitive cell which develops into a muscle cell.

sarcocarcinoma (sar″ko-kar″si-no'mah) carcinosarcoma.

sarcocele (sar'ko-sēl) a fleshy swelling of the testis.

Sarcocystis (sar″ko-sis'tis) a genus name applied to parasitic organisms of uncertain taxonomic status found in muscle tissue of various animals.

sarcocyte (sar'ko-sīt) the middle layer of the ectoplasm of protozoans.

sarcode (sar'kōd) protoplasm.

Sarcodina (sar″ko-di'nah) a subphylum of Protozoa, including all the amebas, characterized by an extremely flexible plasmalemma covering the body surface, permitting body cytoplasm to flow in all directions, with constant alteration in the outline of the body.

sarcogenic (-jen'ik) forming flesh.

sarcoid (sar'koid) 1. resembling flesh; fleshy. 2. a sarcoma-like tumor. **Boeck's s.,** sarcoidosis. **Darier-Roussy s.,** a condition occurring most often in women, with firm, nonulcerating nodules deep to the skin, usually on the extremities. **multiple benign s.,** a condition marked by the presence of nodules on the skin, caused by proliferation of connective tissue surrounding the blood vessels, the lesions being of a tuberculous nature. **Schaumann's s.,** a form called benign lymphogranulomatosis by Schaumann. **Spiegler-Fendt s.,** a sarcoid in the subcutaneous tissue in the form of a circumscribed cellular mass containing reticulated cells and lymphocytes; probably a solitary lymphocytoma.

sarcoidosis (sar″koi-do'sis) a disorder involving many organs, with formation of epithelioid cell tubercles in affected tissues.

sarcolemma (sar″ko-lem'ah) the membrane covering a striated muscle fiber.

sarcoleukemia (-lu-ke'me-ah) lymphosarcoma cell leukemia.

sarcology (sar-kol'o-je) scientific study of the soft tissues of the body.

sarcolysis (-kol'ĭ-sis) disintegration of the soft tissues. adj., **sarcolyt'ic.**

sarcolyte (sar'ko-lit) a cell concerned in disintegration of soft tissues.

sarcoma (sar-ko'mah) a tumor of mesenchymal derivation, often highly malignant. **Abernethy's s.,** a circumscribed fatty tumor occurring on the trunk. **alveolar s.,** one with sarcoma cells enclosed in alveolar spaces. **ameloblastic s.,** the malignant counterpart of ameloblastic fibroma. **botryoid s., s. botryoi'des,** a vaginal sarcoma. **osteogenic s.,** one occurring in bone and arising from bone cells of osteogenic tissue. **reticulocytic s., reticuloendothelial s., reticulum cell s.,** a form of malignant lymphoma in which the predominant cell is the primitive mesenchymal element, or one which has differentiated into the identifiable reticulum cell. **Rous s.,** a virus-induced sarcoma of chickens.

sarcomagenesis (sar-ko″mah-jen'ĕ-sis) the production of sarcoma.

sarcomatoid (sar-ko'mah-toid) resembling a sarcoma.

sarcomatosis (sar-ko″mah-to'sis) condition characterized by development of many sarcomas.

sarcomatous (sar-ko'mah-tus) of the nature of a sarcoma.

sarcomere (sar'ko-mēr) the unit of length of a myofibril, between two Z bands.

sarcomphalocele (sar″kom-fal'o-sēl) fleshy tumor of the umbilicus.

sarcoplasm (sar'ko-plazm) the cytoplasm of a striated muscle fiber, filling the spaces between myofibrils.

sarcopoietic (sar″ko-poi-et'ik) forming muscle.

Sarcoptes (sar-kop'tēz) a widely distributed genus of mites, including the species *S. scabiei;* the cause of scabies in man; different varieties of the organism cause mange in different animals.

sarcosis (sar-ko'sis) 1. the presence of multiple fleshy tumors. 2. abnormal increase of flesh.

sarcosome (sar'ko-sōm) the darker contractile part of a muscle fibril.

Sarcosporidia (sar″ko-spo-rid'e-ah) an order of sporozoan parasites found in the muscles of cattle, sheep and other animals.

sarcosporidiosis (-spo-rid″e-o'sis) infection with organisms of the order Sarcosporidia.

sarcostosis (sar″kos-to'sis) ossification of fleshy tissue.

sarcostyle (sar'ko-stīl) a fibrilla of an elementary muscle fiber.

sarcous (sar'kus) pertaining to flesh or muscle tissue.

sat. saturated.

satellite (sat'ĕ-līt) in genetics, a knob of chromatin connected by a stalk to the short arm of certain chromosomes.

satellitosis (sat″ĕ-li-to'sis) a gathering of free cell nuclei around the ganglion cells of the brain cortex in general paresis.

saturated (sat'u-rāt″ed) 1. having all affinities of its elements satisfied (saturated compound). 2. holding all of a solute which can be held in solution by the solvent (saturated solution).

saturation (sat″u-ra'shun) the state of a solvent which holds in solution all of a substance it can possibly contain.

saturnine (sat'ur-nīn) pertaining to lead.

saturnism (sat'urn-izm) lead poisoning.

satyriasis (sat″ĭ-ri'ah-sis) insatiable sexual desire in the male.

satyromania (sat″ĭ-ro-ma'ne-ah) satyriasis.

saucerization (saw″ser-i-za′shun) the formation of a shallow depression, as by excavation or injury.

sauriderma (saw″rĭ-der′mah) a variety of ichthyosis.

sauriosis (saw″re-o′sis) keratitis follicularis.

saw (saw) a cutting instrument with a toothed or serrated edge, used in bone surgery.

saxitoxin (sak″sĭ-tok′sin) a toxic substance obtained from poisonous mussels, clams and plankton.

Sb chemical symbol, *antimony* (L. *stibium*).

S.B.P. Society of Biological Psychiatry.

Sc chemical symbol, *scandium*.

scab (skab) 1. the crust of a superficial sore. 2. to become covered with a crust or scab.

scabicide (ska′bĭ-sid) an agent used in treating scabies.

scabies (ska′be-ēz) a communicable skin disease due to the itch mite, *Sarcoptes scabiei*.

scabieticide (ska″be-et′ĭ-sid) scabicide.

scabiophobia (-o-fo′be-ah) morbid dread of scabies.

scabrities (ska-brish′e-ēz) scabby or rough state.

scala (ska′lah), pl. *sca′lae* [L.] a ladder-like structure. **s. me′dia,** space in ear between membrane of Reissner and membrana basilaris. **s. tym′pani,** part of cochlea below the lamina spiralis. **s. vestib′uli,** part of cochlea above the lamina spiralis.

scale (skāl) 1. a thin flake or compacted platelike body, as of epithelial cells. 2. a scheme or device by which some property may be measured (as hardness, weight, linear dimension). 3. to remove incrustations or other material from a surface, as from the enamel of teeth. **absolute s.,** a temperature scale with zero at the absolute zero of temperature. **Baumé s.,** a graduated scale for indicating the density of a liquid. **Celsius s.,** a temperature scale with zero at the ice point of water and the normal boiling point of water at 100 degrees. **centigrade s.,** one with 100 gradations or steps between two fixed points, as the Celsius scale. **Fahrenheit s.,** a temperature scale with the ice point at 32 and the normal boiling point of water at 212 degrees. **French s.,** one used for denoting size of catheters, sounds and other tubular instruments, each unit being roughly equivalent to 0.33 mm. in diameter; i.e. 18 French indicates a diameter of 6 mm. **Kelvin s.,** an absolute scale on which the unit of measurement corresponds with that of the Celsius scale and the ice point of water is at 273.15 degrees. **Rankin s.,** an absolute scale on which the unit of measurement corresponds with that of the Fahrenheit scale and the ice point of water is at 459.67 degrees. **Réaumur s.,** a temperature scale on which zero represents the ice point and 80 the boiling point of water. **temperature s.,** one used for expressing the temperature, with zero established at absolute zero or with values arbitrarily assigned to the ice point and boiling point of water, and the range between them divided into identical units.

(See also *Table of Temperature Equivalents*, p. 610).

scalenectomy (ska″le-nek′to-me) resection of the scalenus muscle.

scalenotomy (-not′o-me) division of the scalenus muscle.

scaler (skāl′er) a dental instrument for removal of calculus from the teeth.

scall (skawl) a crusty disease, as of the scalp.

scalp (skalp) that area of the head (exclusive of the face) which is usually covered by a growth of hair. **gyrate s.,** cutis verticis gyrata.

scalpel (skal′pel) a straight knife with convex edge.

scalpriform (skal′prĭ-form) shaped like a chisel.

scaly (skāl′e) characterized by scales.

scan (skan) scintiscan.

scandium (skan′de-um) chemical element (*see table*), at. no. 21, symbol Sc.

scanning (skan′ning) 1. close visual examination of a small area or of different isolated areas. 2. a manner of utterance characterized by somewhat regularly recurring pauses. **radioisotope s.,** production of a two-dimensional record of the emissions of a radioactive isotope concentrated in a specific organ or tissue of the body, as brain, kidney or thyroid gland.

scapha (ska′fah), pl. *sca′phae* [L.] the curved depression separating the helix and anthelix.

scaphocephalia (skaf″o-sē-fa′le-ah) scaphocephaly.

scaphocephaly (-sef′ah-le) abnormal length and narrowness of the skull, usually accompanied by mental retardation. adj., **scaphocephal′ic.**

scaphoid (skaf′oid) shaped like a boat.

scaphoiditis (skaf″oi-di′tis) inflammation of the scaphoid bone.

scapulalgia (skap″u-lal′je-ah) pain in the scapula.

scapular (skap′u-lar) pertaining to the scapula.

scapulectomy (skap″u-lek′to-me) excision of the scapula.

scapuloclavicular (skap″u-lo-klah-vik′u-ler) pertaining to scapula and clavicle.

scapulopexy (skap″u-lo-pek″se) surgical fixation of the scapula.

scapulothoracic (skap″u-lo-tho-ras′ik) pertaining to scapula and thorax.

scar (skar) a mark remaining after the healing of a wound or other morbid process; by extension applied to other visible manifestations of an earlier event.

scarification (skar″i-fĭ-ka′shun) production in the skin of many small superficial scratches or punctures, as for introduction of vaccine.

scarificator (-fĭ-ka′tor) an instrument for scarifying.

scarifier (-fi′er) an instrument with many sharp points, used in scarification.

scarlatina (skar″lah-te′nah) scarlet fever. adj., **scarlat′inal. s. angino′sa,** scarlatina with severe throat symptoms. **s. haemorrha′gica,** a form in which there is extravasation of blood into the skin and mucous membranes. **s. malig'na,** a variety with severe symptoms and great prostration.

scarlatinella (skar-lat″ĭ-nel′ah) mild scarlet fever without fever.

scarlatiniform (skar″lah-tin′ĭ-form) resembling scarlet fever.

SCAT sheep cell agglutination test.

scatacratia (skat″ah-kra′she-ah) incontinence of feces.

scatemia (skah-te′me-ah) intestinal toxemia.

scatology (skah-tol′o-je) study and analysis of feces or obscenity.

scatophagy (skah-tof′ah-je) the eating of dung.

scatoscopy (skah-tos′ko-pe) examination of the feces.

scatter (skat′er) the diffusion or deviation of x-rays produced by a medium through which the rays pass. **back s.,** backward diffusion of x-rays.

scattergram (skat′er-gram) a graph in which the values found in a statistical study are represented by disconnected, individual symbols.

Sc.D. Doctor of Science.

schema (ske′mah) a plan, outline or arrangement.

schindylesis (skin″dĭ-le′sis) an articulation in which one bone is received into a cleft in another.

schist(o)- (skis′to) word element [Gr.], *cleft; split.*

schistasis (skis′tah-sis) a splitting; specifically, any congenital split condition of the body.

schistocelia (skis″to-se′le-ah) congenital fissure of the abdomen.

schistocephalus (-sef′ah-lus) a fetal monster with a cleft head.

schistocormus (-kor′mus) a fetal monster with a cleft trunk.

schistocyte (skis′to-sīt) a fragment of a red blood corpuscle, commonly observed in the blood in hemolytic anemia.

schistocytosis (skis″to-si-to′sis) excess of schistocytes in the blood.

schistoglossia (-glos′e-ah) cleft tongue.

schistomelus (skis-tom′ĕ-lus) a fetal monster with a cleft limb.

schistoprosopus (skis″to-pros′o-pus) a fetal monster with a cleft face.

Schistosoma (-so′mah) a genus of trematodes, including several species parasitic in the blood of man and domestic animals. **S. haemato′bium,** a species endemic in north, central and west Africa and the Near East; found in the liver and in the vesical, prostatic and uterine venous plexuses. **S. japon′icum,** a species geographically confined to the Far East, and found chiefly in the superior mesenteric vein, but also in inferior mesenterics and the caval system. **S. manso′ni,** a species widely distributed in Africa and parts of South America; found in the host's portal blood, chiefly in the inferior mesenteric veins.

schistosomiasis (-so-mi′ah-sis) infection with flukes of the genus Schistosoma.

schistosomus (-so′mus) a fetal monster with a cleft abdomen.

schistothorax (skis″to-tho′raks) developmental anomaly with fissure of the chest or sternum.

schiz(o)- (skiz′o) word element [Gr.], *divided; division.* See also words beginning *schist(o)-.*

schizaxon (skiz-ak′son) an axon which divides into two nearly equal branches.

schizogenesis (skiz″o-jen′ĕ-sis) reproduction by fission.

schizogony (skĭ-zog′o-ne) the asexual reproduction of a sporozoan parasite (sporozoite) by multiple fission within the body of the host, giving rise to merozoites. adj., **schizogon′ic.**

schizogyria (skiz″o-ji′re-ah) a condition in which the cerebral convolutions have wedge-shaped cracks.

schizoid (skiz′oid) resembling schizophrenia: a term applied to a shut-in, unsocial, introspective personality.

schizomycete (skiz″o-mi-sēt′) an organism of the class Schizomycetes.

Schizomycetes (-mi-se′tēz) a class of vegetable organisms (division Protophyta), including organisms which usually contain no photosynthetic pigments and usually reproduce by fission.

schizomycosis (-mi-ko′sis) any disease due to Schizomycetes.

schizont (skiz′ont) the stage in the development of the malarial parasite following the trophozoite whose nucleus divides into many smaller nuclei.

schizonychia (skiz″o-nik′e-ah) splitting of the nails.

schizophasia (-fa′ze-ah) incomprehensible, disordered speech.

schizophrenia (-fre′ne-ah) a chronic mental disorder characterized by loosening of associations, autism, ambivalence and inappropriate affect, as well as by hallucinations and delusions; variously classified, according to predominant symptoms or time at onset, as adolescent type (hebephrenic), catatonic, childhood type or paranoid. adj., **schizophren′ic. catatonic s.,** a psychotic reaction in which motor disturbances, especially stupor or excitement, are conspicuous. **hebephrenic s.,** a psychotic state developing during adolescence and characterized by inappropriate affect, unpredictive giggling, silly behavior and mannerisms, and profound regression. **paranoid s.,** a psychotic state marked by illogical and relatively fragmentary delusions, usually accompanied by auditory hallucinations. **simple s.,** schizophrenia marked by apathy, lack of initiative, and withdrawal.

schizophrenosis (-fre-no′sis) any disease of the dementia praecox group.

Schizophyceae (-fi′se-e) a class of vegetable organisms (division Protophyta), including organisms that have both chlorophyll and phycocyanin; known as the blue-green algae, they closely resemble bacteria.

schizotrichia (-trik′e-ah) splitting of the hairs at the ends.

schwannoglioma (shwan″o-gli-o′mah) schwannoma.

schwannoma (shwan-o'mah) a tumor arising from the sheath of Schwann.

sciage (se-ahzh') [Fr.] a sawing movement in massage.

sciatic (si-at'ik) pertaining to the ischium.

sciatica (si-at'ĭ-kah) neuralgia and neuritis of the sciatic nerve.

science (si'ens) an accumulating body of knowledge seeking to establish general laws governing the occurrence of certain observable phenomena. adj., **scientif'ic. applied s.,** search for knowledge for promotion of a specific effect. **pure s.,** search for knowledge without regard for its immediate economic application.

scientist (si'en-tist) an investigator who seeks to establish general laws governing certain observable phenomena.

scieropia (si"er-o'pe-ah) defect of vision in which objects appear in a shadow.

scintigram (sin'tĭ-gram) a graphic record of the particles registered by a scintiscanner, after administration of a radioactive isotope.

scintillascope (sin-til'ah-skōp) spinthariscope.

scintillation (sin"tĭ-la'shun) 1. the emission of charged particles. 2. the sensation of sparks before the eyes.

scintiscan (sin'tĭ-skan) a two-dimensional representation of the gamma rays emitted by a radioactive isotope, revealing its concentration in a specific organ or tissue.

scintiscanner (sin"tĭ-skan'er) an apparatus for recording the concentration of a gamma-emitting isotope in tissue.

scirrhoid (skir'oid) resembling scirrhus.

scirrhoma (skir-ro'mah) scirrhus.

scirrhosarca (skir"o-sar'kah) scleroderma.

scirrhous (skir'us) of the nature of scirrhus.

scirrhus (skir'us) hard cancer with predominance of connective tissue.

scler(o)- (skle'ro) word element [Gr.], *hard; sclera of the eye.*

sclera (skle'rah) the tough, white covering of approximately the posterior five sixths of the eyeball, continuous anteriorly with the cornea and posteriorly with the external sheath of the optic nerve. adj., **scle'ral. blue s.,** abnormal blueness of the sclera, occurring as a hereditary condition transmitted by a dominant gene, and sometimes associated with brittleness of the bones and deafness.

scleradenitis (sklēr"ad-ē-ni'tis) inflammation and hardening of a gland.

sclerectasia (sklēr"ek-ta'ze-ah) a bulging state of the sclera.

sclerectomy (skle-rek'to-me) excision of part of the sclera.

scleredema (skler"ē-de'mah) edematous hardening of the skin. **s. adulto'rum, Buschke's s.,** hardening of the skin and subcutaneous tissues, affecting chiefly the head, neck and trunk, rarely the extremities. **s. neonato'rum,** sclerema neonatorum.

sclerema (skle-re'mah) scleredema. **s. adipo'sum, s. neonato'rum,** a condition characterized by diffuse, rapidly spreading, nonedematous, tallow-like hardening of subcutaneous tissues in the first few weeks of life.

scleriasis (skle-ri'ah-sis) scleroderma.

scleriritomy (skle"rī-rit'o-me) incision of sclera and iris in anterior staphyloma.

scleritis (skle-ri'tis) inflammation of the sclera.

scleroblastema (skle"ro-blas-te'mah) the embryonic tissue from which bone is formed. adj., **scleroblastem'ic.**

sclerochoroiditis (-ko"roi-di'tis) inflammation of the sclera and choroid.

sclerocornea (-kor'ne-ah) the sclera and choroid regarded as one.

sclerodactylia (-dak-til'e-ah) scleroderma of the fingers and toes.

scleroderma (-der'mah) an insidious chronic disorder characterized by progressive collagenous fibrosis of many organs and systems, usually beginning with the skin. **circumscribed s.,** that affecting only localized areas of the skin, with no apparent visceral involvement. **s. neonato'rum,** sclerema neonatorum.

sclerodermitis (-der-mi'tis) inflammation and hardening of the skin.

sclerogenous (skle-roj'ĕ-nus) producing a hard tissue or material.

scleroiritis (skle"ro-i-ri'tis) inflammation of sclera and iris.

sclerokeratitis (-ker"ah-ti'tis) inflammation of sclera and cornea.

sclerokeratoiritis (-ker"ah-to-i-ri'tis) inflammation of sclera, cornea and iris.

scleroma (skle-ro'mah) a hardened patch or induration, especially of the nasal or laryngeal tissues. **respiratory s.,** presence of bluish-red granulomas on the mucosa of the upper respiratory tract, the involved parts enlarging slowly and becoming hard as ivory.

scleromere (skle'ro-mēr) a segment of the skeletal system.

scleromyxedema (skle"ro-mik"sē-de'mah) a variant of lichen myxedematosus characterized by a generalized eruption of the nodules and diffuse thickening of the skin.

scleronyxis (nik'sis) puncture of the sclera.

sclero-oophoritis (-o"of o-rī'tis) sclerosing inflammation of the ovary.

sclerophthalmia (skle"rof-thal'me-ah) encroachment of the sclera upon the cornea, so that only a portion of the latter remains clear.

scleroplasty (skle'ro-plas"te) plastic repair of the sclera.

scleroprotein (skle"ro-pro'te-in) a protein having structural and protective functions in the organism and insoluble in the usual solvents of proteins.

sclerosarcoma (-sar-ko'mah) a firm, fleshy variety of epulis.

sclerose (skle'rōs) to become, or cause to become, hardened.

sclerosis (sklĕ-ro'sis) an induration or hardening, especially from inflammation. adj., **sclerot'ic. amyotrophic lateral s.,** sclerosis of lateral columns and anterior gray matter of cord. **dentinal s.,** regressive alteration in tooth substance with calcification of the dentinal tubules, producing translucent zones (transparent dentin). **disseminated s.,** multiple sclerosis. **dorsal s.,** sclerosis involving the dorsal columns of the spinal cord. **lateral**

s., sclerosis affecting especially the crossed pyramidal tracts. **Mönckeberg's s.,** Mönckeberg's arteriosclerosis. **multiple s.,** sclerosis of brain and cord occurring in scattered patches. **tuberous s.,** a familial disease with tumors on the surfaces of the lateral ventricles of the brain and sclerotic patches on its surface, and marked by mental deterioration and epileptic attacks.

scleroskeleton (skle″ro-skel′ĕ-ton) part of bony skeleton formed by ossification in ligaments, fasciae and tendons.

sclerostenosis (-ste-no′sis) hardening with contraction.

sclerostomy (skle-ros′to-me) incision of the sclera with drainage.

sclerotherapy (skle″ro-ther′ah-pe) injection of sclerosing solutions in the treatment of hemorrhoids or other varicose veins.

sclerothrix (skle′ro-thriks) abnormal hardness and dryness of the hair.

sclerotic (sklĕ-rot′ik) 1. hard or hardening; affected with sclerosis. 2. sclera.

sclerotica (skle-rot′ĭ-kah) sclera.

scleroticopuncture (skle-rot″ĭ-ko-pungk′tūr) puncture of the sclera.

sclerotitis (skle″ro-ti′tis) scleritis.

sclerotium (skle-ro′she-um) hard mass formed by certain fungi, as ergot.

sclerotome (skle′ro-tōm) 1. one of the masses of diffuse cells formed by the breaking down of the ventromesial wall of each somite, which ultimately become the primordia of the vertebrae. 2. a knife for incising the sclera.

sclerotomy (sklĕ-rot′o-me) incision of the sclera.

S.C.M. State Certified Midwife.

scolecology (sko″le-kol′o-je) helminthology.

scolex (sko′leks), pl. *sco′lices* [Gr.] the attachment organ of a tapeworm, generally considered the anterior, or cephalic, end.

scoli(o)- (sko′le-o) word element [Gr.], *crooked; twisted.*

scoliokyphosis (sko″le-o-ki-fo′sis) combined lateral and posterior curvature of the spine.

scoliorachitic (-rah-kit′ik) both scoliotic and rachitic.

scoliosiometry (-se-om′ĕ-tre) measurement of spinal curvature.

scoliosis (sko″le-o′sis) lateral curvature of vertebral column. adj., **scoliot′ic.**

scolopsia (sko-lop′se-ah) a suture between two bones that allows motion of one upon the other.

scopolamine (sko-pol′ah-mēn) an alkaloid derived from various plants, used in parasympathetic blockade and as a central nervous system depressant.

scopophilia (sko-po-fil′e-ah) 1. the derivation of sexual pleasure from looking at genital organs. 2. a morbid desire to be seen.

scopophobia (sko″po-fo′be-ah) morbid dread of being seen.

-scopy (skop′e) word element [Gr.], *examination of.*

scoracratia (sko″rah-kra′she-ah) fecal incontinence.

scorbutic (skor-bū′tik) pertaining to scurvy.

scorbutigenic (skor-bū″tĭ-jen′ik) causing scurvy.

scorbutus (skor-bū′tus) [L.] scurvy.

scordinemia (skor″dĭ-ne′me-ah) yawning and stretching.

score (skōr) a rating, usually expressed numerically, based on specific achievement or the degree to which certain qualities are manifest. **Apgar s.,** a numerical expression of an infant's condition 60 seconds after birth, based on heart rate, respiratory effort, muscle tone, reflex irritability and color.

scotochromogen (sko″to-kro′mo-jen) a microorganism whose pigmentation develops in the dark as well as in the light. adj., **scotochromogen′ic.**

scotodinia (sko″to-din′e-ah) vertigo with headache and dimness of vision.

scotogram, scotograph (sko′to-gram, sko′to-graf) 1. skiagraph. 2. the effect produced upon a photographic plate in the dark by certain substances.

scotoma (sko-to′mah) an isolated area of loss of vision within an otherwise apparently normal peripheral field. adj., **scoto′matous. absolute s.,** an area within the visual field in which perception of light is entirely lost. **annular s.,** a circular area of depressed vision surrounding the point of fixation. **arcuate s.,** an arc-shaped defect of vision arising in an area near the blind spot and extending toward it. **central s.,** an area of depressed vision corresponding with the point of fixation and interfering with central vision. **color s.,** an isolated area of depressed or defective vision for color. **motile s's,** positive scotomas due to opacities in the vitreous, and changing with their movement. **negative s.,** one which appears as a blank spot or hiatus in the visual field. **peripheral s.,** an area of depressed vision distant from the point of fixation, toward the periphery of the visual field. **physiologic s.,** that area of the visual field corresponding with the optic disk, in which the photosensitive receptors are absent. **positive s.,** one which appears as a dark spot in the visual field. **relative s.,** an area of the visual field in which perception of light is only diminished, or loss is restricted to light of certain wavelengths. **ring s.,** annular scotoma. **scintillating s.,** blurring of vision with sensation of luminous appearance before the eyes, with zigzag, wall-like outlines.

scotomagraph (sko-to′mah-graf) instrument for recording a scotoma.

scotometer (sko-tom′ĕ-ter) instrument for measuring scotomas.

scotometry (sko-tom′ĕ-tre) the measurement of scotomas.

scotomization (sko″to-mĭ-za′shun) development of scotomas, or blind spots, especially of mental "blind spots."

scotophilia (-fil′e-ah) love of darkness.

scotophobia (-fo′be-ah) morbid fear of darkness.

scotopia (sko-to′pe-ah) the adjustment of the eye for darkness. adj., **scotop′ic.**

scours (skowrz) diarrhea in newborn animals.

black s., acute dysentery in animals. **white s.**, diarrhea in calves shortly after birth.

scr. scruple.

scratches (skrach'ez) eczematous inflammation of the feet of a horse.

screatus (skre-a'tus) paroxysmal attacks of hawking.

screen (skrēn) 1. a framework used as a shield or protector. 2. to examine. **Bjerrum s.**, a large square of black cloth with a central mark for fixation; used with a campimeter in mapping the field of vision. **fluorescent s.**, a plate in the fluoroscope coated with crystals of calcium tungstate, permitting visualization of internal body structures by roentgen ray. **tangent s.**, Bjerrum screen.

screening (skrēn'ing) examination of a large number of individuals to disclose certain characteristics, or a certain disease, as tuberculosis or diabetes. **multiphasic s.**, multiple s., simultaneous examination of a population for several different diseases.

scrobiculate (skro-bik'u-lāt) marked with pits.

scrobiculus (skro-bik'u-lus) [L.] pit. **s. cor'dis**, pit of the stomach; the precordial depression.

scrofula (skrof'u-lah) tuberculous disease of lymphatic nodes and of bone, with slowly suppurating abscesses. adj., **scrof'ulous.**

scrofuloderma (skrof"u-lo-der'mah) a skin disease of scrofulous nature.

scrofulosis (skrof"u-lo'sis) the scrofulous diathesis.

scrotectomy (skro-tek'to-me) excision of part of the scrotum.

scrotitis (skro-ti'tis) inflammation of the scrotum.

scrotocele (skro'to-sēl) scrotal hernia.

scrotoplasty (skro'to-plas"te) plastic reconstruction of the scrotum.

scrotum (skro'tum) the pouch containing the testes. adj., **scro'tal. lymph s.**, dilatation of the lymph vessels of the scrotum; seen in filariasis.

scruple (skroo'pl) twenty grains apothecaries' weight; symbol ℈.

S.C.S. Society of Clinical Surgery.

scurf (skerf) branny substance of epidermic origin.

scurvy (sker've) a disease due to deficiency of ascorbic acid, marked by weakness, anemia, spongy gums and mucocutaneous hemorrhages. **land s.**, thrombocytopenic purpura.

scute (skūt) bony plate separating upper tympanic cavity and mastoid cells.

scutiform (skū'tĭ-form) shaped like a shield.

scutulum (sku'tu-lum), pl. **scu'tula** [L.] favus crust.

scutum (skū'tum) a protective covering or shield, e.g. a chitinous plate in the exoskeleton of an arthropod.

scybalous (sib'ah-lus) of the nature of a scybalum.

scybalum (sib'ah-lum), pl. **scyb'ala** [Gr.] a hard mass of fecal matter.

scyphoid (si'foid) shaped like a cup or goblet.

scytoblastema (si"to-blas-te'mah) the rudimentary skin.

SD streptodornase.

S.D. skin dose; standard deviation.

S.E. standard error.

Se chemical symbol, *selenium*.

searcher (serch'er) an instrument used in examining the bladder for calculi.

seasickness (se'sik-nes) motion sickness occasioned by ship travel.

seatworm (sēt'werm) an individual of the species *Enterobius vermicularis*.

sebaceous (se-ba'shus) pertaining to sebum.

sebiferous (se-bif'er-us) sebiparous.

sebiparous (se-bip'ah-rus) secreting or producing sebum.

S.E.B.M. Society for Experimental Biology and Medicine.

sebolith (seb'o-lith) calculus in a sebaceous gland.

seborrhagia (seb"o-ra'je-ah) seborrhea.

seborrhea (seb"o-re'ah) excessive discharge from the sebaceous glands, forming greasy scales on the skin. adj., **seborrhe'ic. s. capil-lit'ii,** seborrhea of the scalp. **s. ni'gricans,** seborrhea with dark-colored crusts. **s. sic'ca,** commonest form of seborrhea, characterized by formation of brownish-gray scales.

seborrheid (seb"o-re'id) a seborrheic eruption.

sebum (se'bum) the oily secretion of the sebaceous glands, whose ducts open into the hair follicles.

secale (se-ka'le) [L.] rye. **s. cornu'tum,** ergot.

secobarbital (sek"o-bar'bĭ-tal) a short- to intermediate-acting barbiturate. **sodium s.,** a hypnotic compound for oral or parenteral use.

Seconal (sek'ŏ-nal) trademark for preparations of secobarbital.

secreta (se-kre'tah) [L., pl.] the secretions.

secretagogue (se-krēt'ah-gog) causing a flow of secretion.

secretin (se-kre'tin) a hormone secreted by duodenal mucosa, which stimulates secretion of pancreatic juice and bile.

secretion (se-kre'shun) 1. the expulsion of materials which have been chemically modified by a cell, to serve a purpose elsewhere in some body process. 2. the substance thus expelled by the cell or organ. **antilytic s.,** saliva secreted by the submaxillary gland with nerves intact, as distinguished from that secreted when the nerve is divided. **external s.,** a secretion discharged by a duct on an external or internal surface of the body. **internal s.,** a secretion not discharged by a duct from the secreting tissue, but given off into the blood and lymph. **paralytic s.,** secretion from a gland after paralysis or division of its nerve.

secreto-inhibitory (se-kre"to-in-hib'ĭ-tor"e) inhibiting secretion.

secretomotory (-mo'tor-e) stimulating secretion.

secretor (se-kre'tor) a person having A or B type blood whose saliva and other secretions contain the particular (A or B) substance.

secretory (se-kre"to-re) pertaining to secretion.

sectio (sek'she-o), pl. **sectio'nes** [L.] section.

section (sek'shun) 1. an act of cutting. 2. a cut surface. **abdominal s.,** laparotomy. **cesarean s.,** delivery of a fetus by incision through the abdominal wall and uterus. **frontal s.**, a section through the body passing from left to right at right angles to the median plane. **frozen s.**, a specimen cut by microtome from tissue that has been frozen. **perineal s.**, external urethrotomy. **Pitres' s's**, a series of six vertical sections made transversely at certain specified locations of the brain. **Saemisch's s.**, a surgical operation for the relief of corneal complications. **sagittal s.**, a section through the body coinciding or parallel with the sagittal suture. **serial s's**, histologic sections made in consecutive order and so arranged for the purpose of microscopic examination. **sigaultian s.**, symphysiotomy. **vaginal s.**, incision through the vaginal wall into the abdominal cavity.

sectioning (sek'shun-ing) the cutting of thin sections of tissue for study under the microscope.

sector (sek'tor) the area of a circle included between an arc and the radii bounding it.

sectorial (sek-to're-al) cutting.

secundigravida (se-kun″di-grav'i-dah) a woman pregnant the second time; gravida II.

secundines (se-kun'dinz) afterbirth.

secundipara (se″kun-dip'ah-rah) a woman who has had two pregnancies which resulted in viable offspring; para II.

S.E.D. skin erythema dose.

Sedamyl (sed'ah-mil) trademark for a preparation of acetylcarbromal.

sedation (se-da'shun) the production of a sedative effect.

sedative (sed'ah-tiv) 1. allaying activity and excitement. 2. a remedy that allays excitement. **cardiac s.**, a drug that decreases the force of the heart. **nerve s.**, a hypnotic.

sediment (sed'i-ment) a precipitate, especially that formed spontaneously.

sedimentation (sed″i-men-ta'shun) the settling out of sediment.

seed (sēd) 1. semen. 2. the small body produced by flowering plants containing the embryo of the new individual. **cardamom s.**, dried ripe seed of *Elettaria cardamomum;* used as a flavoring agent. **plantago s.**, cleaned, dried ripe seed of species of Plantago; used as a cathartic. **plantain s., psyllium s.**, plantago seed. **radon s.**, a small sealed container for radon, for insertion into the tissues of the body in radiation therapy.

segment (seg'ment) a demarcated portion of a whole. adj., **segmen'tal. bronchopulmonary s.**, one of the smaller subdivisions of the lobe of a lung, separated from others by a connective tissue septum and supplied by its own branch of the bronchus leading to the particular lobe.

segmentation (seg″men-ta'shun) division into similar parts.

seismesthesia (sīz″mes-the'ze-ah) tactile perception of vibrations in a liquid or aerial medium.

seismocardiogram (sīz″mo-kar'de-o-gram″) the record obtained by seismocardiography.

seismocardiography (-kar″de-og'rah-fe) the selective recording of cardiac vibrations and beats, giving curves of frequencies between 4

and 5, and between 34 and 40 cycles per second.

seismotherapy (sīz″mo-ther'ah-pe) treatment of disease by mechanical vibration.

seizure (se'zhur) a sudden attack, as of a disease. **psychomotor s.**, an episode of mental confusion with apparently purposeful but coarse and poorly coordinated muscular movements.

selenium (sĕ-le'ne-um) chemical element (*see table*), at. no. 34, symbol Se. **s. sulfide,** a bright orange, insoluble powder; used topically in solution in the treatment of seborrheic dermatosis.

Selenomonas (se-le″no-mo'nas) a genus of Schizomycetes (order Pseudomonadales, suborder Pseudomonadineae, family Spirillaceae).

self (self) a name given to constituents native to an organism, which do not stimulate formation of antibodies against them.

selfing (self'ing) continuous cross-fertilization between different proglottids of the same tapeworm.

self-suspension (self″sus-pen'shun) suspension of the body by head and axillae for purpose of stretching the vertebral column.

selfwise (self'wiz) developing in accordance with the region from which it was transplanted; characteristic of tissue transplanted from an amphibian gastrula of a late stage of development.

sella (sel'ah) pl. *sel'lae* [L.] a saddle-shaped depression. adj., **sel'lar. s. tur'cica,** a depression on the upper surface of the sphenoid bone, lodging the pituitary gland.

semantics (se-man'tiks) study of the meanings of words and the rules of their use; study of the relation between language and significance.

semeiography (se″mi-og'rah-fe) symptomatology.

semeiotic (-ot'ik) 1. pertaining to symptoms. 2. pathognomonic.

semeiotics (-ot'iks) symptomatology.

semel (sem'el) [L.] once.

semelincident (sem″el-in'si-dent) affecting a person only once.

semelparity (-par'i-te) the state, in an individual organism, of reproducing only once in a lifetime.

semen (se'men) fluid discharged at ejaculation in the male, consisting of secretion of glands associated with the urogenital tract and containing spermatozoa. adj., **sem'inal.**

semenuria (se″men-u're-ah) discharge of semen in the urine.

semi (sem'e) word element [L.], *half.*

semicanal (sem″i-kah-nal') a trench or furrow open at one side.

semiflexion (-flek'shun) position of a limb midway between flexion and extension.

Semikon (sem'i-kon) trademark for preparations of methapyrilene.

semilunar (sem″i-lu'nar) shaped like a halfmoon.

semimicroanalysis (-mi″kro-ah-nal'i-sis) chemical analysis based on 0.01 to 0.02 gm. of the substance under study.

semination (sem″ĭ-na′shun) insemination.

seminiferous (-nif′er-us) producing or carrying semen.

seminologist (-nol′o-jist) a specialist in the study of semen and spermatozoa.

seminology (-nol′o-je) scientific study of semen and spermatozoa.

seminoma (-no′mah) a dysgerminoma of the testis. **ovarian s.**, a dysgerminoma of the ovary.

semipermeable (-per′me-ah-bl) permitting passage only of certain molecules.

semis (se′mis) [L.] half; abbreviated ss.

semisulcus (sem′ĭ-sul′kus) a depression which, with an adjoining one, forms a sulcus.

semisupination (-su″pĭ-na′shun) a position halfway toward supination.

semisynthetic (-sin-thet′ik) produced partially by natural processes and partially by artificial manipulation.

Semoxydrine (sem-ok′sĭ-drin) trademark for a preparation of methamphetamine.

senescence (se-nes′ens) the process of growing old.

senile (se′nil) pertaining to old age.

senilism (se′nil-izm) premature old age.

senility (sĕ-nil′ĭ-te) feebleness of body and mind incident to old age.

senna (sen′ah) the dried leaflets of *Cassia acutiflora;* used in a syrup, fluidextract or compound powder as a cathartic.

senopia (se-no′pe-ah) improvement of the visual power in old people.

sensation (sen-sa′shun) an impression produced by impulses conveyed by an afferent nerve to the sensorium. **concomitant s.**, secondary sensation. **cutaneous s.**, sensation perceived at or on the skin, as touch, temperature, etc. **girdle s.**, zonesthesia. **gnostic s's**, sensations perceived by the more recently developed senses, such as those of light touch and the epicritic sensibility to muscle, joint and tendon vibrations. **primary s.**, that resulting immediately and directly from application of a stimulus. **reflex s., referred s.**, one felt elsewhere than at the site of application of a stimulus. **secondary s.**, one developed, without special stimulation, along with a primary sensation. **subjective s.**, one originating within the organism and not occurring in response to an external stimulus.

sense (sens) a faculty by which the conditions or properties of things are perceived. **color s.**, the faculty by which colors are perceived and distinguished. **kinesthetic s.**, the muscular sense. **light s.**, the faculty by which degrees of brilliancy are distinguished. **muscle s., muscular s.**, the faculty by which muscular movements are perceived. **posture s.**, a variety of muscular sense by which the position or attitude of the body or its parts is perceived. **pressure s.**, the faculty by which pressure upon the surface of the body is perceived. **sixth s.**, the general feeling of consciousness of the entire body. **space s.**, the faculty by which relative positions and relations of objects in space are perceived. **special s.**, one of the five senses of seeing, feeling, hearing, taste and smell. **stereog-**

nostic s., the sense by which form and solidity are perceived. **temperature s.**, the faculty by which differences of temperature are appreciated.

sensibility (sen″sĭ-bil′ĭ-te) 1. capacity for perception or feeling. 2. sensitivity. **epicritic s.**, the sensibility to gentle stimulations permitting fine discriminations of touch and temperature, localized in the skin. **protopathic s.**, the sensibility to strong stimulations of pain and temperature, which is low in degree and poorly localized, existing in the skin and in the viscera, and acting as a defensive agency against pathologic changes in the tissues. **somesthetic s.**, the sensibility to stimuli received by the somatic sensory receptors. **splanchnesthetic s.**, the sensibility to stimuli received by the splanchnic receptors.

sensibilization (-bil″ĭ-za′shun) 1. the act of making more sensitive. 2. sensitization.

sensibilizer (sen′sĭ-bil-iz″er) amboceptor.

sensible (sen′sĭ-bl) appreciable by the senses.

sensitinogen (sen″sĭ-tin′o-jen) a general term for an antigen having a sensitizing effect on the body.

sensitive (sen′sĭ-tiv) 1. able to receive or transmit a sensation; capable of responding to a stimulus. 2. unusually susceptible to stimulation; showing an exaggerated response, as to painful stimuli.

sensitivity (sen″sĭ-tiv′ĭ-te) the state or quality of being sensitive.

sensitization (-ti-za′shun) the process of becoming sensitive, as the rendering of a cell sensitive to the action of a complement by the action of an amboceptor.

sensitized (sen′sĭ-tizd) rendered sensitive.

sensomobile (sen″so-mo′bēl) moving in response to a stimulus.

sensomotor (-mo′tor) sensorimotor.

sensoparalysis (-pah-ral′ĭ-sis) paralysis of the sensory nerves of a part.

sensorimotor (-re-mo′tor) both sensory and motor.

sensorium (sen-so′re-um) 1. a sensory nerve center. 2. the state of an individual as regards consciousness or mental awareness. adj., **senso′rial. s. commu′ne**, part of cerebral cortex that receives and coordinates all the impulses sent to individual nerve centers.

sensory (sen′so-re) pertaining to sensation.

sentient (sen′she-ent) able to feel; sensitive.

sepsis (sep′sis) a morbid condition resulting from the presence of pathogenic bacteria and their products. adj., **sep′tic.**

septa (sep′tah) word element [L.], *seven.*

septan (sep′tan) recurring every seven days (every sixth day).

septate (sep′tāt) divided by a septum.

septectomy (sep-tek′to-me) excision of part of the nasal septum.

septicemia (sep″tĭ-se′me-ah) a morbid condition due to presence and reproduction of pathogenic bacteria in the blood. adj., **septice′mic. Bruce's s.**, brucellosis. **cryptogenic s.**, a septicemia in which the focus of infection is not evident during life. **fowl s.**, a disease of fowls, marked by diarrhea, hyperemia of the alimentary canal, and the presence of a blood-tinged, yellowish liquid in the small intestine. **hemorrhagic s.,** an infectious disease of animals caused by species of Pasteurella. **puerperal s.,** that in which the focus of infection is a lesion of the mucous membrane received during childbirth.

septicopyemia (sep″tĭ-ko-pi-e′me-ah) septicemia with pyemia.

septipara (sep-tip′ah-rah) a woman who has had seven pregnancies which resulted in living offspring; para VII.

septivalent (sep″tĭ-va′lent) having a valence of seven.

septotomy (sep-tot′o-me) incision of the nasal septum.

septulum (sep′tu-lum), pl. *sep′tula* [L.] a small separating wall or partition.

septum (sep′tum), pl. *sep′ta* [L.] a dividing wall or partition. adj., **sep′tal. atrioventricular s.,** part of the membranous portion of the interventricular septum, intervening between the left ventricle and the right atrium. **Bigelow's s.,** a layer of hard, bony tissue in the neck of the femur. **crural s.,** the layer closing the femoral ring. **enamel s.,** enamel cord. **interalveolar s.,** one of the thin plates of bone separating the alveoli of the different teeth in the mandible and maxilla. **interatrial s.,** the partition separating the right and left atria of the heart. **interdental s.,** interalveolar septum. **interventricular s.,** the partition separating the right and left ventricles of the heart. **s. lu′cidum,** 1. partition between the lateral ventricles of the brain. 2. the stratum corneum of the epidermis. **nasal s.,** the partition between the two nasal cavities. **s. pectinifor′me,** the wall separating the corpora cavernosa. **placental s.,** trophoblastic tissue which divides the placenta into cotyledons. **rectovaginal s.,** tissues between rectum and vagina. **s. scro′ti,** the partition between the two chambers of the scrotum.

septuplet (sep′tu-plet) one of seven offspring produced at one birth.

sequela (se-kwe′lah), pl. *seque′lae* [L.] a morbid condition following or occurring as a consequence of another condition or event.

sequester (se-kwes′ter) to detach or separate abnormally a small portion from the whole.

sequestration (se″kwes-tra′shun) 1. abnormal separation of a part from a whole, as a portion of a bone by a pathologic process, or a portion of the circulating blood in a specific part occurring naturally or produced by application of a tourniquet. 2. isolation of a patient. **pulmonary s.,** loss of connection of lung tissue with the bronchial tree and the pulmonary veins.

sequestrectomy (-trek′to-me) excision of a sequestrum.

sequestrum (se-kwes′trum), pl. *seques′tra* [L.] piece of dead bone separated from the sound bone in necrosis.

serapheresis (se″rah-fĕ-re′sis) the production of serum by permitting the clotting of plasma derived by plasmapheresis.

Serenium (sĕ-re′ne-um) trademark for a preparation of ethoxazene.

Serfin (ser′fin) trademark for a preparation of reserpine.

sericeps (ser′ĭ-seps) a silken bag used in making traction on the fetal head.

series (se′rēz) a group or succession of events, objects or substances arranged in regular order or forming a kind of chain; in electricity, parts of a circuit connected successively end to end to form a single path for the current. adj., **se′rial. aliphatic s.,** the open chain or fatty series of chemical compounds. **aromatic s.,** the compounds derived from benzene. **erythrocytic s.,** the succession of developing cells which ultimately culminates in the erythrocyte. **fatty s.,** methane and its derivatives and the homologous hydrocarbons. **homologous s.,** a series of compounds each member of which differs from the one preceding it by the radical CH_2. **leukocytic s.,** the succession of developing cells which ultimately culminates in the leukocyte.

serine (ser′ēn) a naturally occurring amino acid.

serocolitis (se″ro-ko-li′tis) inflammation of serous coat of the colon.

seroculture (-kul′tūr) a bacterial culture on blood serum.

serodiagnosis (-di″ag-no′sis) diagnosis of disease from the serum reactions.

sero-enteritis (-en″tĕ-ri′tis) inflammation of serous coat of intestine.

sero-enzyme (-en′zīm) an enzyme in blood serum.

serofibrinous (-fi′brĭ-nus) marked by both a serous exudate and precipitation of fibrin.

seroglobulin (-glob′u-lin) the globulin of blood serum.

serohemorrhagic (-hem″o-raj′ik) characterized by serum and blood.

serohepatitis (-hep″ah-ti′tis) inflammation of the peritoneum of the liver.

sero-immunity (-i-mu′ni-te) immunity produced by an antiserum.

serolactescent (-lak-tes′ent) resembling serum and milk.

serolemma (-lem′ah) membrane whence the serosa or chorion is developed.

serolipase (-li′pās) a lipase from blood serum.

serologist (se-rol′o-jist) a specialist in serology.

serology (se-rol′o-je) the study of antigen-antibody reactions in vitro. adj., **serolog′ic.**

serolysin (se-rol′ĭ-sin) a lysin of the blood serum.

seroma (se-ro′mah) a collection of serosanguineous fluid in the body, producing a tumorlike mass.

seromembranous (se″ro-mem′brah-nus) both serous and membranous.

seromucous (-mu′kus) both serous and mucous.

seromuscular (-mus′ku-lar) pertaining to serous and muscular coats of the intestine.

Seromycin (ser′o-mi″sin) trademark for preparations of cycloserine.

seronegativity (se″ro-neg″ah-tiv′ĭ-te) the state of showing negative results on serologic examination.

seroperitoneum (se″ro-per″ĭ-to-ne′um) fluid in the peritoneal cavity.

serophyte (se′ro-fīt) an organism which grows in the body fluids.

seroplastic (se″ro-plas′tik) serofibrinous.

seropneumothorax (-nu″mo-tho′raks) serous effusion and air or gas in the pleural cavity.

seropositivity (-poz″ĭ-tiv′ĭ-te) the state of showing positive results on serologic examination.

seroprognosis (-prog-no′sis) prognosis of disease from the serum reactions.

seroprophylaxis (-pro″fĭ-lak′sis) the prophylactic use of serums.

seropurulent (-pu′roo-lent) both serous and purulent.

seropus (se″ro-pus′) serum mingled with pus.

seroreaction (se″ro-re-ak′shun) 1. any reaction taking place in serum. 2. serum sickness.

serosa (se-ro′sah) any serous membrane.

serosamucin (se-ro″sah-mu′sin) a protein from inflammatory serous exudates.

serosanguineous (se″ro-sang-gwin′e-us) composed of serum and blood.

seroscopy (se-ros′ko-pe) diagnostic examination of serum.

seroserous (se″ro-se′rus) pertaining to two serous surfaces.

serositis (-si′tis) inflammation of a serous membrane.

serosity (se-ros′ĭ-te) the quality of serous fluids.

serosynovitis (se″ro-sin″o-vi′tis) synovitis with effusion of serum.

serotherapy (-ther′ah-pe) the therapeutic use of serums.

serothorax (-tho′raks) hydrothorax.

serotonin (-to′nin) a potent vasoconstrictor substance secreted by argentaffin cells of the small intestine, absorbed by blood platelets and circulated in the blood.

serotoxin (-tok′sin) a toxin existing in the blood serum.

serotype (se′ro-tīp) the type of a microorganism determined by its constituent antigens, or a taxonomic subdivision based thereon.

serous (se′rus) pertaining to serum; thin and watery, like serum.

Serpasil (ser″pah-sil) trademark for preparations of reserpine.

serpiginous (ser-pij′ĭ-nus) creeping from part to part.

serpigo (ser-pi′go) any creeping eruption.

serrated (ser′āt-ed) having a sawlike edge or border.

Serratia (se-ra′she-ah) a genus of Schizomycetes (order Eubacteriales, family Enterobacteriaceae, tribe Serratieae).

Serratieae (ser″ah-ti′e-e) a tribe of Schizomycetes (order Eubacteriales, family Enterobacteriaceae) saprophytic on decaying plant or animal materials.

serration (sĕ-ra′shun) a notch like that between two saw teeth.

serrulate (ser′u-lāt) characterized by minute serrations.

serum (se′rum) pl. *se′ra, serums* [L.] the liquid left after clotting of blood, fibrinogen having been removed. **Foshay's s.,** a serum for treatment of tularemia. **muscle s.,** muscle plasma deprived of myosin.

sesamoid (ses′ah-moid) shaped like a sesame seed.

sesamoiditis (ses″ah-moi-di′tis) inflammation of sesamoid bones of a horse's foot.

sesqui- (ses′kwe) word element [L.], *one and one-half.*

sesquioxide (ses″kwe-ok′sīd) a compound of three parts of oxygen with two of another element.

sesquisalt (ses′kwĭ-sawlt) a salt containing three parts of an acid with two of a base.

sessile (ses′il) not pedunculated; having a broad base.

setaceous (se-ta′shus) bristle-like.

sex (seks) a distinctive character of most animals and plants, based on the type of gametes produced by the gonads, ova (macrogametes) being typical of the female, and sperm (microgametes) of the male, or the category in which the individual is placed on such basis. adj., **sex′ual. chromosomal s., genetic s.,** the category (male or female) in which an individual is placed, depending on the presence or absence of the Y chromosome in the spermatozoon by which the ovum was fertilized. **gonadal s.,** the category in which an individual is placed on the basis of gonadal tissue present (ovarian or testicular). **morphologic s.,** that determined on the basis of the external genital organs. **nuclear s.,** that determined on the basis of the presence or absence of sex chromatin in somatic cells. **psychologic s.,** that determined by the gender role assigned to and played by the growing individual.

sex-linked (seks-linkt′) transmitted by a gene located on a sex (X or Y) chromosome.

sexology (sek-sol′o-je) the scientific study of sex and sexual relations from the biological point of view.

sexopathy (-sop′ah-the) abnormality of sexual expression.

sextan (seks′tan) recurring in six-day cycles (every five days).

sextipara (seks-tip′ah-rah) a woman who has had six pregnancies that resulted in viable offspring; para VI.

sextuplet (seks′tu-plet) any one of six offspring produced at the same birth.

sexuality (seks″u-al′ĭ-te) 1. the characteristic of the male and female reproductive elements. 2. the constitution of an individual in relation to sexual attitudes and behavior.

S.G.O. Surgeon-General's Office.

SGOT serum glutamic oxaloacetic transaminase.

SGPT serum glutamic pyruvic transaminase.

shadow-casting (shad″o-kast′ing) application of a coating of gold, chromium or other metal to ultramicroscopic structures to increase their visibility under the microscope.

shaft (shaft) the mass of a simple elongate structure, as a long bone or a hair, between the extremities.

shank (shangk) the tibia or shin.

sheath (shēth) a tubular case or envelope. **arachnoid s.**, delicate membrane between pial sheath and dural sheath of optic nerve. **crural s.**, femoral sheath. **dentinal s.**, the layer of dentin immediately adjacent to a dentinal tubule. **dural s.**, external investment of the optic nerve. **femoral s.**, fascial sheath of the femoral vessels. **Henle's s.**, a sheath enveloping an isolated nerve fiber exterior to the neurilemma. **Hertwig's s.**, a layer of epithelial cells around an unerupted tooth. **lamellar s.**, the perineurium. **Mauthner's s.**, axilemma. **medullary s., myelin s.**, the sheath surrounding the axon of some nerve fibers, consisting of myelin alternating with the spirally wrapped neurolemma. **perivascular s.**, wide lymphatic tube around the smallest blood vessels. **pial s.**, extension of pia partly intersecting the optic nerve. **root s.**, the epidermic layer of a hair follicle. **s. of Schwann,** neurilemma. **synovial s.**, synovial membrane lining the cavity of a bone through which a tendon moves.

sheet (shēt) an oblong piece of cotton or linen for a bed covering. **draw s.**, one folded and placed under a patient's body so it may be removed with minimal disturbance of the patient.

shield (shēld) a protecting tube or structure. **Buller's s.**, a shield to cover and protect the eye. **embryonic s.**, the dark circular field due to cell proliferation within the area pellucida, in which the primitive streak appears. **nipple s.**, a device to protect the nipple of the mammary gland. **phallic s.**, a device for protecting male genitals during surgical operations.

shift (shift) a change or deviation. **chloride s.**, the exchange of chloride and carbonate between the plasma and the red blood corpuscles which takes place in order to re-establish the equilibrium between carbonate and chloride ions in the plasma and cells. **s. to the left,** a change in the blood picture, with a preponderance of young neutrophils. **s. to the right,** a change in the blood picture, with a preponderance of older neutrophils.

Shigella (shĭ-gel'ah) a genus of Schizomycetes (order Eubacteriales, family Enterobacteriaceae, tribe Salmonelleae) which cause dysentery.

shigella (shĭ-gel'ah), pl. *shigel'lae*, an individual organism of the genus Shigella.

shigellosis (shi"gel-lo'sis) infection with Shigella.

shin (shin) the prominent anterior edge of tibia and leg. **saber s.**, marked anterior convexity of the tibia, seen in congenital syphilis.

shingles (shing'gelz) herpes zoster.

shiver (shiv'er) 1. a slight tremor. 2. to tremble slightly, as from cold.

shivering (shiv'er-ing) 1. involuntary shaking of the body, as with cold. 2. chorea of the muscles of the hip and thigh of a horse.

shock (shok) depression of body function, usually associated with lowered blood volume, but produced also by other conditions, and sometimes leading to death, characterized basically by reduction in the effectively circulating blood and in blood pressure. **allergic s., anaphylactic s.**, a violent attack of symptoms produced by a second injection of serum or protein and due to anaphylaxis. **insulin s.**, circulatory insufficiency resulting from overdosage with insulin, which causes too sudden reduction of blood sugar; marked by tremor, sweating, vertigo, diplopia, convulsions and collapse. **irreversible s.**, a condition in which the changes produced cannot be corrected by treatment, and death is inevitable. **serum s.**, anaphylactic shock. **shell s.**, loss of nervous control, with psychic symptoms, produced by battle conditions.

shoulder (shōl'der) the junction of clavicle and scapula, where the arm joins the trunk. **frozen s.**, limited abduction and rotation of the arm, due to fibrositis.

show (sho) appearance of blood forerunning labor or menstruation.

shunt (shunt) 1. to turn to one side; to divert. 2. an anomalous or artificially created passage connecting two main channels, and diverting (blood) flow from one to the other. 3. a conductor connecting two points in an electric circuit, so as to receive a portion of the current of the main circuit. **left-to-right s.**, diversion of blood from the systemic to the pulmonary circulation. **portacaval s.**, diversion of circulation by anastomosis of portal vein and inferior vena cava or by splenectomy and anastomosis of the splenic and left renal veins. **right-to-left s.**, diversion of blood from the pulmonary to the systemic circulation.

Si chemical symbol, *silicon.*

siagonagra (si"ah-go-nag'rah) pain in the maxilla.

sial(o)- (si"ah-lo) word element [Gr.], *saliva; salivary glands.*

sialadenitis (si"al-ad"ĕ-ni'tis) inflammation of a salivary gland.

sialadenoncus (-nong'kus) a tumor of a salivary gland.

sialagogue (si-al'ah-gog) an agent which stimulates the flow of saliva. adj., **sialagog'ic.**

sialectasia (si"al-ek-ta'ze-ah) dilatation of a salivary duct.

sialine (si'ah-lĭn) pertaining to the saliva.

sialismus (si"ah-liz'mus) ptyalism.

sialoadenectomy (si"ah-lo-ad"ĕ-nek'to-me) excision of a salivary gland.

sialoadenitis (-ad"ĕ-ni'tis) inflammation of a salivary gland.

sialoadenotomy (-ad'ĕ-not'o-me) incision of a salivary gland.

sialoaerophagy (-a"er-of'ah-je) the swallowing of saliva and air.

sialoangiectasis (-an"je-ek'tah-sis) dilatation of a salivary duct.

sialoangiitis (-an"je-i'tis) inflammation of a salivary duct.

sialoangiography (-an"je-og'rah-fe) radiography of the ducts of the salivary glands after injection of radiopaque material.

sialocele (si'ah-lo-sēl") ranula.

sialodochitis (si"ah-lo-do-ki'tis) inflammation of a salivary duct.

sialodochoplasty (-do'ko-plas"te) plastic repair of a salivary duct.

sialoductitis (-duk-ti'tis) inflammation of Stensen's duct.

sialogenous (si"ah-loj'ĕ-nus) producing saliva.

sialogogue (si-al'o-gog) sialagogue.

sialography (si"ah-log'rah-fe) roentgenography of salivary ducts and glands.

sialolith (si-al'o-lith) a salivary calculus.

sialolithiasis (si"ah-lo-li-thi'ah-sis) the formation of salivary calculi.

sialolithotomy (-li-thot'o-me) excision of a salivary calculus.

sialology (si"ah-lol'o-je) the study of the saliva.

sialoma (si"ah-lo'mah) a tumor of the salivary gland.

sialorrhea (si"ah-lo-re'ah) ptyalism.

sialoschesis (si"ah-los'kĕ-sis) suppression of secretion of saliva.

sialosis (si"ah-lo'sis) the flow of saliva. adj., **sialot'ic.**

sialostenosis (si"ah-lo-ste-no'sis) stenosis of a salivary duct.

sialosyrinx (-si'rinks) 1. salivary fistula. 2. a syringe.

sib (sib) a blood relative; one of a group of persons all descended from a common ancestor.

sibilant (sib'i-lant) shrill, whistling or hissing.

sibling (sib'ling) an individual born of the same parents as the person of reference. **half s.,** an individual one of whose parents was also a parent of the person of reference.

sibship (sib'ship) a group of individuals born of the same parents.

siccative (sik'ah-tiv) 1. drying; removing moisture. 2. an agent which produces drying.

sicklemia (sik-le'me-ah) sickle cell anemia.

sickling (sik'ling) the development of sickle cells in the blood.

sickness (sik'nes) a condition of deviation from the normal healthy state. **African sleeping s.,** African trypanosomiasis. **air s.,** 1. motion sickness due to travel by airplane. 2. altitude sickness. **altitude s.,** a condition due to low oxygen pressure, as at high altitudes. **aviation s.,** air sickness. **caisson s.,** decompression sickness. **car s.,** motion sickness due to automobile or other vehicular travel. **decompression s.,** a complex of symptoms due to sudden relative reduction of atmospheric pressure, with bubbles of nitrogen in the tissues and blood stream. **falling s.,** epilepsy. **green s.,** chlorosis. **milk s.,** poisoning in animals caused by white snakeroot, transmitted to man through milk, producing vomiting, constipation and muscular tremors. **monthly s.,** menstruation. **morning s.,** nausea of early pregnancy. **motion s.,** nausea and malaise due to unaccustomed motion, such as may be experienced in various modes of travel, as by airplane, automobile, steamship or train. **mountain s.,** nausea and dyspnea at high altitudes. **radiation s.,** a syndrome of headache, anorexia, nausea, vomiting and diarrhea, sometimes occurring during radiation therapy. **serum s.,** an acute, self-limited disease caused by allergic reaction to some injected foreign protein or allergen, which usually subsides promptly with or without therapy. **sleeping s.,** a disease characterized by increasing drowsiness and lethargy, and due to a protozoan or microbial infection. **sweating s.,** miliary fever.

S.I.D. Society for Investigative Dermatology.

sidebone (sīd'bōn) hardness of the lateral cartilages of horses above the heels, from deposit of lime salts.

side-effect (sīd'ef-fekt") a consequence other than that for which an agent is used, especially an adverse effect on another organ system.

Siderobacter (sid'er-o-bak'ter) a genus of Schizomycetes (order Pseudomonadales, suborder Pseudomonadineae, family Siderocapsaceae).

Siderocapsa (-kap'sah) a genus of Schizomycetes (order Pseudomonadales, suborder Pseudomonadineae, family Siderocapsaceae).

Siderocapsaceae (-kap-sa'se-e) a family of Schizomycetes (order Pseudomonadales, suborder Pseudomonadineae).

Siderococcus (-kok'us) a genus of Schizomycetes (order Pseudomonadales, suborder Pseudomonadineae, family Siderocapsaceae).

siderocyte (sid'er-o-sīt") a red blood corpuscle containing nonhemoglobin iron.

sideroderma (sid"er-o-der'mah) bronzed coloration of the skin from disordered iron metabolism.

siderodromophobia (-dro"mo-fo'be-ah) morbid dread of railway travel.

siderofibrosis (-fi-bro'sis) fibrosis combined with deposits of iron.

siderogenous (sid"er-oj'e-nus) forming iron.

Sideromonas (sid"er-o-mo'nas) a genus of Schizomycetes (order Pseudomonadales, suborder Pseudomonadineae, family Siderocapsaceae).

Sideronema (-ne'mah) a genus of Schizomycetes (order Pseudomonadales, suborder Pseudomonadineae, family Siderocapsaceae).

sideropenia (-pe'ne-ah) deficiency of iron in the body or blood. adj., **siderope'nic.**

Siderophacus (-fa'kus) a genus of Schizomycetes (order Pseudomonadales, suborder Pseudomonadineae, family Caulobacteraceae).

siderophilin (sid"er-of'i-lin) transferrin.

siderophilous (-of'i-lus) tending to absorb iron.

siderophore (sid'er-o-fōr") a macrophage containing hemosiderin.

siderosis (sid"er-o'sis) abnormal deposit of iron or iron pigments.

Siderosphaera (sid"er-o-sfe'rah) a genus of Schizomycetes (order Pseudomonadales, suborder Pseudomonadineae, family Siderocapsaceae).

sigmatism (sig'mah-tizm) faulty enunciation of s sounds.

sigmoid (sig'moid) 1. shaped like the letter C or S. 2. the distal part of the colon, from the level of the iliac crest to the rectum.

sigmoidectomy (sig″moi-dek'to-me) excision of part of the sigmoid colon.

sigmoiditis (-di'tis) inflammation of the sigmoid colon.

sigmoidopexy (sig-moi'do-pek″se) fixation of the sigmoid colon.

sigmoidoproctostomy (sig-moi″do-prok-tos'to-me) anastomosis of the sigmoid colon to the rectum.

sigmoidorectostomy (-rek-tos'to-me) sigmoidoproctostomy.

sigmoidoscope (sig-moi'do-skōp) an endoscope for use in sigmoidoscopy.

sigmoidoscopy (sig″moi-dos'ko-pe) direct examination of the interior of the sigmoid colon.

sigmoidosigmoidostomy (sig-moi″do-sig″moi-dos'to-me) anastomosis of two previously remote portions of the sigmoid colon.

sigmoidostomy (sig″moi-dos'to-me) fistulization of the sigmoid colon.

sigmoidotomy (-dot'o-me) incision of the sigmoid colon.

sigmoidovesical (sig-moi″do-ves'ĭ-kal) pertaining to or communicating with the sigmoid flexure and the urinary bladder.

sign (sīn) an observable physical phenomenon so frequently associated with a given condition as to be considered indicative of its presence. **Abadie's s.**, loss of deep pain from pressure on the Achilles tendon. **Babinski platysma s.**, failure of the platysma to contract when the mouth is opened wide. **Babinski toe s.**, dorsiflexion of the big toe and fanning of the other toes when the foot is grasped firmly and the sole is stroked upward and medially along the lateral margin. **Babinski trunk-thigh s.**, raising of the limb on the hypertonic, paretic side when the patient raises himself from a recumbent position with arms folded on the chest. **Beevor's s.**, apparent upward excursion of the umbilicus when an attempt is made to contract the abdominal muscles. **Biernacki's s.**, loss of deep pain from pressure in the ulnar region. **Blumberg's s.**, pain on abrupt release of steady pressure over the site of a suspected abdominal lesion, indicative of peritonitis. **Branham's s.**, reduction of pulse rate and cessation of murmur on pressure over an arteriovenous fistula. **Braunwald s.**, occurrence of a weak pulse instead of a strong one immediately after a ventricular premature contraction. **Broadbent's s.**, retraction of the left eleventh and twelfth ribs and interspaces posteriorly, attributed to adhesions between the heart and diaphragm. **Brudzinski's s.**, flexion of the hips and knees on passive flexion of the neck. **Cardarelli's s.**, pulsation of the laryngotracheal tube synchronous with the pulse, visible and palpable when the larynx is displaced to the left by pressure on the thyroid cartilage; observed in aortic aneurysm. **Chaddock's s.**, dorsiflexion of the big toe when the foot is stroked around the lateral malleolus and

along the dorsum laterally. **Chadwick's s.**, bluish discoloration of the vestibule and vaginal wall, due to venous congestion, and sometimes a sign of pregnancy. **Chilaiditi s.**, interposition of a loop of bowel between the liver and the diaphragm. **Chvostek's s.**, contraction of the homolateral facial muscles elicited by tapping the cheek along the course of the facial nerve. **Cullen's s.**, bluish discoloration around the umbilicus sometimes occurring in intraperitoneal hemorrhage, as following rupture of the uterine tube in ectopic pregnancy. **Dalrymple's s.**, visibility of the sclera above the iris when the subject's gaze is fixed straight ahead; indicative of thyrotoxicosis (exophthalmos). **Delbet's s.**, maintenance of nutrition of a part distal to an aneurysm of a peripheral artery, despite absence of pulsation; indicates adequacy of the collateral circulation. **de Musset's s.**, rhythmic oscillation of the head caused by pulsations of the carotid arteries; a sign of aortic insufficiency. **Erb's s.**, increased electrical excitability of peripheral nerves associated with hypercalcemia. **Ewart's s.**, dullness over the involved area caused by compression of the left lung in pericarditis with effusion. **flag s.**, variation in color of the hair, seen in children recovering from kwashiorkor, when the color is changing from orange-black to black. **Friedreich's s.**, diastolic collapse of the cervical veins due to adhesion of the pericardium. **Graefe's s.**, delay or absence of downward movement of the upper eyelids when the gaze is directed downward; noted in thyrotoxicosis. **halo s.**, a halo effect produced in the roentgenogram of the fetal head between the subcutaneous fat and the cranium; said to be indicative of intrauterine death of the fetus. **harlequin s.**, reddening of the lower half of the laterally recumbent body and blanching of the upper half, due to temporary vasomotor disturbance in newborn infants. **Hegar's s.**, compressibility of the cervix, owing to softening of the isthmus of the uterus in early pregnancy. **Hoffman's s.**, flexion and adduction of the thumb and index finger when the distal phalanx of the middle finger is fully flexed by the examiner and suddenly released. **Homans's s.**, pain in the calf due to sharp dorsiflexion of the foot when the patient is supine with the knee raised several inches and the leg flexed. **Hoover's s.**, 1. accentuation of downward pressure of the heel on the healthy side on attempting to raise the paretic leg while in the supine position. 2. diminished expansion of the chest due to interference with movements of the diaphragm caused by pericardial effusion. **Joffroy's s.**, absence of or only slight wrinkling of the forehead when the gaze is directed upward; considered an ocular sign of thyrotoxicosis. **Kernig's s.**, limitation of extension of the leg at the knee when the patient is supine and the thigh has been raised to a vertical position with the knee flexed. **Klippel-Feil s.**, adduction and flexion of the thumb when abnormally flexed fingers are extended by the examiner. **Lasègue's s.**, aggravation of pain in the back and leg elicited by passive raising of the heel from the bed with the knee straight. **Leri's s.**, absence of normal flexion of the elbow on passive flexion of the hand at the wrist. **Lhermitte's s.**, paresthesias in the arms, trunk and legs elicited by flexion of the neck. **Litten's s.**, a linear shadow on the lower side of the chest, traveling downward over several intercostal spaces with deep inspiration and expiration with expiration. **Macewen's s.**, a more than normal resonant note on percussion of the skull behind the junction of the frontal, temporal and parietal bones; noted in internal hydrocephalus and cerebral abscess. **Moebius' s.**, insufficiency of ocular convergence; an ocular sign of thyrotoxicosis. **Musset's s.**, jerking of the head with each heartbeat, due to throbbing of the carotid arteries in aortic insufficiency. **Naunyn's s.**, deep tenderness beneath the costal arch on the right side at the end of full inspiration. **Nikolsky's s.**, a condition in which the outer layer of the skin is easily rubbed off by slight injury. **Oliver's s.**, palpable pulsation felt with gentle upward pressure on the cricoid cartilage with the patient erect, mouth closed and chin elevated; transmitted through the trachea when dilatation or aneurysm of the aorta exists. **Oppenheim's s.**, dorsiflexion of the big toe elicited by stroking forcefully down the leg over the anterior margin of the tibia. **Patrick's s.**, limitation by pain of lateral deviation of the knee with the patient supine, hip and knee flexed, and the foot with the lateral malleolus resting as high as possible on the opposite leg, preferably above the patella. **Romberg's s.**, swaying elicited or increased by shutting the eyes and tilting the head back while standing with the feet close together. **Rossolimo's s.**, flexion of the digits (fingers or toes) elicited by tapping their under (palmar or plantar) surface. **setting-sun s.**, downward deviation of the eyes so that each iris appears to "set" beneath the lower lid, with white sclera exposed between it and the upper lid; indicative of intracranial pressure or irritation of the brain stem. **Stellwag's s.**, infrequent or incomplete blinking; considered one of the ocular signs of thyrotoxicosis. **string s.**, 1. a thin linear shadow observed roentgenographically in pyloric stenosis or regional ileitis, permitting passage of only a thin stream of barium. 2. stringing out of tubules observed on teasing tissues of the intact testis or testicular tissue in which there is active spermatogenesis. **Struempell pronation s.**, pronation occurring when the forearm is passively flexed. **Struempell radialis s.**, dorsiflexion of the hand on making a fist. **Struempell tibialis s.**, dorsiflexion of the toes and adduction of the foot on flexion at the knee and hip against resistance. **Throckmorton's s.**, dorsiflexion of the big toe elicited by scratching it on the side adjacent to the second toe. **Tinel's s.**, elicitation of tingling by percussion along the course of an injured nerve; thought to indicate the point to which fibers have regenerated. **Troisier's s.**, presence of a firm node (sentinel node) just above the left clavicle; indicative of visceral carcinoma. **Trousseau's s.**, induction of tetanic spasm in the hand when circulation is reduced by compression of the arm; associated with hypocalcemia. **Turner's s.**, discoloration of the abdominal wall in acute pancreatitis. **Wartenberg's s.**, 1. assumption by the little finger of a position of abduction. 2. reduction or absence of pendulum movements of the arm while walking. **water-silk s.**, the sensation of silken surfaces sliding over one another when the middle finger is moved back and forth across the inguinal canal, discernible when hernia is present.

signature (sig'nah-tūr) the last chief part of a drug prescription, comprising directions to be followed by the patient in its use.

silica (sil'ĭ-kah) silicon dioxide.

silicate (sil'ĭ-kāt) any compound of silicic acid with a base.

silicatosis (sil″ĭ-kah-to'sis) pulmonary disease due to inhalation of silicate dust.

silicon (sil'ĭ-kon) chemical element (see table), at. no. 14, symbol Si. **s. carbide**, a compound of silicon and carbon used in dentistry as an abrasive agent.

silicosis (sil″ĭ-ko'sis) a lung disease due to inhalation of fine particles of silica. adj., **silicot'ic**.

Silicote (sil'ĭ-kot) trademark for preparations of dimethicone.

silicotuberculosis (sil″ĭ-ko-tu-ber″ku-lo'sis) tuberculous infection of the silicotic lung.

silkosis (sil-ko'sis) a complication sometimes following use of silk sutures, with formation of sinuses.

silver (sil'ver) chemical element (see table), at. no. 47, symbol Ag. **colloidal s.**, a silver preparation in which the silver exists as free ions to only a small extent. **s. iodide**, a yellowish, powdery compound; useful in syphilis and in nervous diseases, and also applied locally in conjunctivitis. **s. nitrate**, colorless or white crystals, used as a caustic and local antiinfective. **s. nitrate, toughened**, a mixture of silver nitrate and silver chloride. **s. protein**, silver made colloidal by the presence of, or combination with, protein; an active germicide with a local irritant and astringent effect.

Simonsiella (si″mon se-el'ah) a genus of Schizomycetes (order Caryophadales, family Caryophanaceae).

simul (sim'ul) [L.] at the same time as.

Simulium (sĭ-mu'le-um) a genus of biting gnats.

Sinaxar (sin'ak-sar) trademark for a preparation of styramate.

sinciput (sin'sĭ-put) the upper and front part of the head. adj., **sincip'ital**.

sinew (sin'ū) a tendon or fibrous cord. **weeping s.**, cystoma on a tendon or aponeurosis.

Singoserp (sing'go-serp) trademark for preparations of syrosingopine.

singultus (sing-gul′tus) hiccup.

sinister (sin′is-ter) [L.] left; on the left side.

sinistr(o) (sin′is-tro) word element [L.], *left; left side.*

sinistrad (sin′is-trad) to or toward the left.

sinistral (sin′is-tral) pertaining to the left side.

sinistrality (sin″is-tral′ĭ-te) dominance of the left member of paired organs.

sinistraural (sin″is-traw′ral) hearing better with the left ear.

sinistrocardia (sin″is-tro-kar′de-ah) displacement of the heart to the left.

sinistrocerebral (-ser′ĕ-bral) situated in the left hemisphere of the brain.

sinistrocular (sin″is-trok′u-lar) having the left eye dominant.

sinistrocularity (-trok″u-lar′ĭ-te) dominance of the left eye.

sinistrogyration (sin″is-tro-ji-ra′shun) a turning to the left.

sinistromanual (-man′u-al) left-handed.

sinistropedal (sin″is-trop′ĕ-dal) using the left foot in preference.

sinistrotorsion (sin″is-tro-tor′shun) a twisting toward the left.

sinoatrial (si″no-a′tre-al) pertaining to the sinus venosus and the atrium of the heart.

sinoauricular (-aw-rik′u-lar) sinoatrial.

sinobronchitis (-brong-ki′tis) chronic paranasal sinusitis with recurrent episodes of bronchitis or collapse.

Sintrom (sin′trom) trademark for a preparation of acenocoumarol.

sinuitis (sin″u-i′tis) sinusitis.

sinuous (sin′u-us) bending in and out; winding.

sinus (si′nus) 1. a recess, cavity or space, as (*a*) one in bone or (*b*) a dilated channel for venous blood. 2. an abnormal channel or fistula, permitting escape of pus. adj., **si′-nusal. accessory s's of nose,** paranasal sinuses. **air s.,** an air-containing space within a bone. **anal s's,** furrows, with pouchlike recesses at the distal end, in the mucous lining of the anal canal. **aortic s's,** pouchike dilatations at the root of the aorta, one opposite each segment of the valve at its opening from the left ventricle. **branchial s.,** a branchial fistula opening on the surface of the body. **carotid s.,** a dilatation of the proximal portion of the internal carotid or distal portion of the common carotid artery, containing in its wall pressoreceptors which are stimulated by changes in blood pressure. **cavernous s.,** an irregularly shaped venous channel between the layers of dura mater of the brain, one on either side of the body of the sphenoid bone and communicating across the midline. **cerebral s.,** one of the ventricles of the brain. **circular s.,** the venous channel encircling the hypophysis cerebri, formed by the two cavernous sinuses and the anterior and posterior intercavernous sinuses. **coccygeal s.,** a sinus or fistula just over or close to the tip of the coccyx. **coronary s.,** the dilated terminal portion of the great cardiac vein, receiving blood from other veins draining the heart muscle and ending in the right atrium. **dermal s.,** a congenital sinus tract extending from the surface of the body, between the bodies of two adjacent lumbar vertebrae, to the spinal canal. **ethmoidal s.,** the collection of cavities (4 to 17 on each side) in the ethmoid bone, communicating with the middle and the superior and highest meatuses of the nasal cavity. **frontal s.,** one of the paired paranasal sinuses in the frontal bone, each communicating with the middle meatus of the ipsilateral nasal cavity. **intercavernous s's,** channels connecting the two cavernous sinuses, one passing anterior and the other posterior to the infundibulum of the hypophysis. **lacteal s's, lactiferous s's,** enlargements of the lactiferous ducts just before they open on the mammary papilla. **lymphatic s's,** irregular, tortuous spaces within lymphatic tissue. **marginal s.,** the discontinuous expansions of the intervillous space at the periphery of the placenta. **maxillary s.,** one of the paired paranasal sinuses in the body of the maxilla on either side, and opening into the middle meatus of the ipsilateral nasal cavity. **occipital s.,** a venous sinus between the layers of dura mater, passing upward along the midline of the cerebellum. **oral s.,** stomodeum. **paranasal s's,** mucosa-lined air cavities in bones of the skull, communicating with the nasal cavity and including ethmoidal, frontal, maxillary and sphenoidal sinuses. **petrosal s., inferior,** a venous channel arising from the cavernous sinus and draining into the internal jugular vein. **petrosal s., superior,** one arising from the cavernous sinus and draining into the transverse sinus. **pilonidal s.,** a suppurating sinus containing hair, occurring chiefly in the coccygeal region. **s. pocula′ris,** prostatic utricle. **prostatic s.,** the posterolateral recess between the seminal colliculus and the wall of the urethra. **s's of pulmonary trunk,** spaces between the wall of the pulmonary trunk and cusps of the valve at its opening from the right ventricle. **renal s.,** a recess in the substance of the kidney, lined by a continuation of the fibrous capsule and occupied by the renal vessels and expanded upper end of the ureter. **sacrococcygeal s.,** pilonidal sinus. **sagittal s., inferior,** a small venous sinus of the dura mater, opening into the straight sinus. **sagittal s., superior,** a venous sinus of the dura mater which ends in the confluence of sinuses. **sigmoid s.,** a venous sinus of the dura mater on either side, continuous with the straight sinus and draining into the internal jugular vein of the same side. **sphenoidal s.,** one of the paired paranasal sinuses in the body of the sphenoid bone and opening into the highest meatus of the ipsilateral nasal cavity. **sphenoparietal s.,** one of the venous sinuses of the dura mater. **s's of spleen,** dilated venous channels in the substance of the spleen. **straight s.,** a venous sinus of the dura mater formed by junction of the great cerebral vein and inferior sagittal sinus, and ending in the confluence of sinuses. **tarsal s.**, a space between the calcaneus and talus. **tentorial s.**, straight sinus. **terminal s.**, a vein which encircles the vascular area in the blastoderm. **transverse s. of dura mater**, a large venous sinus on either side of the skull. **transverse s. of pericardium**, a passage within the pericardial sac, behind the aorta and pulmonary trunk and in front of the left atrium and superior vena cava. **tympanic s.**, a deep recess on the medial wall of the tympanic cavity. **urogenital s.**, a space made by division of the cloaca in the early embryo which ultimately forms most of the vestibule in the female, and of the urethra in the male. **uterine s's**, venous channels in the wall of the uterus in pregnancy. **uteroplacental s's**, blood spaces between the placenta and uterine sinuses. **s. of venae cavae**, the posterior portion of the right atrium into which the inferior and the superior vena cava open. **s. venosus**, the common venous receptacle in the early embryo attached to the posterior wall of the primitive atrium. **venous s's of dura mater**, large channels for venous blood forming an anastomosing system between the layers of the dura mater of the brain, receiving blood from the brain and draining into the veins of the scalp or deep veins at the base of the skull. **venous s. of sclera**, a circular channel at the junction of the sclera and cornea, into which aqueous humor filters from the anterior chamber of the eye.

sinusitis (si"nu-si'tis)   inflammation of a sinus.

sinusoid (si'nu-soid)   a small, irregularly shaped, thin-walled space forming the beginning of the venous system in certain organs, as spleen, liver, bone marrow and various glands.

sinusotomy (si"nu-sot'o-me)   incision of a sinus.

siphon (si'fon)   1. a bent tube with arms of unequal length, for drawing liquid from one receptacle to another. 2. to draw liquid from one receptacle to another by means of a bent tube with arms of unequal length.

siqua (si'kwah)   the square of the sitting height.

sirenomelus (si"ren-om'e-lus)   a fetal monster with fused legs and no feet.

-sis (sis)   word element [Gr.], *state; condition.*

sister (sis'ter)   the nurse in charge of a hospital ward (Great Britain).

sitieirgia (sit"e-ir'je-ah)   hysterical anorexia.

sitiology (-ol'o-je)   sitology.

sitology (si-tol'o-je)   the science of food and nourishment.

sitomania (si"to-ma'ne-ah)   1. excessive hunger, or morbid craving for food.   2. periodic bulimia.

sitophobia (-fo'be-ah)   morbid dread of taking food.

sitosterol (si-tos'ter-ol)   one of a group of closely related plant sterols, designated by different Greek letters and sometimes subscript numerals; a preparation of beta-sitoste-

rol and certain saturated sterols is used as an anticholesterolemic agent.

sitotherapy (si"to-ther'ah-pe)   treatment by food; dietotherapy.

sitotropism (si-tot'ro-pizm)   tropism in response to the influence of food.

situs (si'tus), pl. *si'tus* [L.]   site or position.

situs inversus viscerum (si'tus in-ver'sus vis'er-um) [L.]   lateral transposition of the viscera of the thorax and pelvis.

SK   streptokinase.

skatole (skat'ōl)   a compound formed in the putrefaction of proteins which contributes to the characteristic odor of the feces.

skatoxyl (skah-tok'sil)   oxidation product of skatole found in urine in certain diseases of the large intestine.

skein (skān)   the threadlike figure seen in the earlier stages of mitosis.

skelalgia (ske-lal'je-ah)   pain in the leg.

skeletization (skel"e-ti-za'shun)   1. extreme emaciation. 2. removal of soft parts from the skeleton.

skeletogenous (skel"e-toj'e-nus)   producing skeletal structures or tissues.

skeletology (-tol'o-je)   sum of knowledge regarding the skeleton.

skeleton (skel'e-ton)   1. the hardened tissues forming the supporting framework of an animal body. 2. the assemblage of bones of a vertebrate animal. adj., **skel'etal. appendicular s.**, the bones of the limbs and the supporting thoracic (pectoral) and pelvic girdles. **axial s.**, the bones of the body axis, including the skull, vertebral column, ribs and sternum. **dermal s.**, superficial bony structures developed in skin and not preformed in cartilage. **somatic s.**, that composed of the appendicular and axial skeletons. **visceral s.**, hardened elements in viscera or soft organs of certain animals.

skenitis (ske-ni'tis)   inflammation of Skene's glands.

skeocytosis (ske"o-si-to'sis)   presence of immature forms of white cells in the blood.

skeptophylaxis (skep"to-fi-lak'sis)   production of temporary immunity to a toxic substance by administration of a minute quantity of it.

skia- (ski'ah)   word element [Gr.], *shadow* (especially as produced by roentgen rays).

skiameter (ski-am'e-ter)   instrument for measuring intensity of roentgen rays.

skiametry (ski-am'e-tre)   observation of the pupil under a beam of light projected into the eye, as a means of determining refractive errors of the eye.

skiascope (ski'ah-skōp)   1. a fluoroscope. 2. instrument used in skiametry.

skiascopy (ski-as'ko-pe)   skiametry.

skin (skin)   a covering layer; the outer protective covering of the body. **elastic s.**, cutis hyperelastica. **false s.**, epidermis. **lax s.**, cutis laxa. **marble s.**, cutis marmorata. **sailor's s.**, atrophic changes in the skin due to excessive exposure to the sun. **true s.**, corium.

Skiodan (ski'o-dan)   trademark for preparations of methiodal.

skler(o)- for words beginning thus, see those beginning *scler(o)-*.

skot(o)- for words beginning thus, see those beginning *scot(o)-*.

skull (skul) the bony framework of the head, including ethmoid, frontal, hyoid, lacrimal, nasal, occipital, palatine, parietal, sphenoid, temporal and zygomatic bones, and inferior nasal concha, mandible, maxilla and vomer. **steeple s., tower s.,** oxycephaly.

S.L.E. systemic lupus erythematosus.

sleep (slēp) a natural or artificially induced state of suspension of sensory and motor activity. **frozen s.,** suspension of sensory and motor activity produced by extremely low temperature. **twilight s.,** a state of light anesthesia produced by morphine and scopolamine.

slide (slīd) a piece of glass or other transparent substance on which material is placed for examination under the microscope.

sling (sling) a bandage or suspensory for supporting a part.

slough (sluf) a mass of dead tissue in, or cast out from, living tissue.

slows (slōz) milk sickness.

sludge (sluj) a suspension of solid or semisolid particles in a fluid which itself may or may not be a truly viscous fluid. **activated s.,** sludge from well aerated sewage, which, being well supplied with oxidizing bacteria, ensures continuing oxidation of subsequently added material. **dewatered s.,** sludge from which the water has been removed by drying or pressing.

sludging (sluj'ing) settling out of solid particles from solution. **s. of blood,** intravascular agglutination of erythrocytes into irregular masses, interfering with circulation of blood.

Sm chemical symbol, *samarium.*

smallpox (smawl'poks) an acute, highly communicable, febrile viral disease, characterized by sustained high fever and appearance first of macules and later of papules on the skin and mucous membranes. **black s., hemorrhagic s.,** a fulminant form with hemorrhage occurring locally into the lesions and diffusely into the corium. **malignant s.,** a severe type with a high fatality rate. **modified s.,** varioloid.

smear (smēr) a preparation for microscopic study, the material being spread thinly and unevenly across the slide with a swab or loop, or with the edge of another slide.

smegma (smeg'mah) thickened, ill-smelling secretion, consisting principally of desquamated epithelial cells, found chiefly about the external genitalia.

smog (smog) a mixture of smoke and fog.

S.M.P. Society of Medical Psychoanalysts.

Sn chemical symbol, *tin* (L. *stannum*).

snap (snap) a short, sharp sound. **opening s.,** a short, sharp sound occurring just after the beginning of the second heart sound.

snare (snār) a wire loop for removing polyps and other pedunculated growths.

snow (sno) a freezing or frozen mixture consisting of discrete particles or crystals.

carbon dioxide s., the substance formed by rapid evaporation of liquid carbon dioxide; used locally in various skin conditions.

snowblindness (sno'blīnd-nes) temporary loss of sight due to injury to superficial cells of the cornea caused by ultraviolet rays of the sun reinforced by those reflected by snow.

S.N.S. Society of Neurological Surgeons.

snuffles (snuf'elz) catarrhal discharge from the nasal mucous membrane in congenital syphilis in infants.

soap (sōp) a solid or liquid material produced by treatment of oil or fat with an alkali and used with water for the removal of oil or dirt. **green s.,** a soft, unctuous mass produced by saponification of a suitable vegetable oil, excluding coconut and palm kernel oils, with potassium hydroxide, without removal of glycerin and with addition of oleic acid, glycerin and water. **hard s.,** a soda soap occurring as a white or whitish solid or as a fine white or yellowish-white powder. **medicinal soft s.,** a preparation of vegetable oil, oleic acid, potassium hydroxide, glycerin and water; used as a skin cleaner. **soft s.,** a potassium soap occurring as a soft, unctuous mass.

sociologist (so"se-ol'o-jist) a specialist in sociology.

sociology (-ol'o-je) the scientific study of social relationships and phenomena.

sociometry (-om'ē-tre) the branch of sociology concerned with the measurement of human behavior.

sociopathy (-op'ah-the) a disorder of social behavior.

socket (sok'et) a hollow into which a corresponding part fits. **dry s.,** a condition sometimes occurring after tooth extraction, with exposure of bone, inflammation of an alveolar crypt, and severe pain. **tooth s's,** dental alveoli; the cavities in the maxilla and mandible in which the teeth are embedded.

soda (so'dah) sodium carbonate, **baking s.,** sodium bicarbonate. **caustic s.,** sodium hydroxide. **s. lime,** calcium hydroxide with sodium or potassium hydroxide, or both; used as adsorbent of carbon dioxide in equipment for metabolism tests, inhalant anesthesia or oxygen therapy.

sodic (so'dik) containing sodium.

sodium (so'de-um) chemical element (*see table*), at. no. 11, symbol Na; the chief cation of extracellular body fluids. **s. acetate,** a systemic and urinary alkalizer. **s. acetrizoate,** a substance used as contrast medium in angiocardiography and in x-ray visualization of the urinary and biliary tracts. **s. acid phosphate,** sodium biphosphate. **s. alginate,** a product derived from brown seaweeds, used in formulating various pharmaceutical preparations. **s. aminosalicylate,** an antibacterial compound used in tuberculosis. **s. ascorbate,** an antiscorbutic vitamin for parenteral administration. **s. benzoate,** a white, odorless granular or crystalline powder, used chiefly as a test of liver function. **s. bicarbonate,** an antacid compound. **s. biphosphate,** a colorless or white crystalline compound, used as a urinary acidifier. **s. bisulfite,** an antioxidant compound. **s. borate,** a crystalline compound used in pharmaceutical preparations. **s. bromide,** a central nervous system depressant. **s. caprylate,** the sodium salt of caprylic acid; used in treatment of fungal infections of the skin. **s. carboxymethyl cellulose,** sodium salt of a carboxymethyl ether of cellulose, used as a bulk-forming cathartic. **s. chloride,** common salt, a white crystalline compound, a necessary constituent of the body and therefore of the diet; sometimes used parenterally in solution to replenish electrolytes in the body. **s. citrate,** a crystalline compound, largely used as an anticoagulant in blood for transfusion. **s. colistimethate,** an antibacterial compound usually administered intramuscularly. **s. cyclamate,** a compound used as a sweetening agent. **s. fluoride,** a white, odorless powder added to drinking water or applied locally to teeth, in 1 to 2 per cent solution, to reduce the incidence of dental caries. **s. folate,** a compound used in various anemias and in control of diarrhea in sprue. **s. glucosulfone,** a compound used in treatment of leprosy and tuberculosis. **s. glutamate,** the monosodium salt of L-glutamic acid; used in treatment of encephalopathies associated with liver diseases. **s. hydrate, s. hydroxide,** a compound used chiefly in various chemical and pharmaceutical manipulations. **s. hypochlorite,** a compound used in solution as a germicide, deodorant and bleach. **s. indigotindisulfonate,** a compound used in measurement of kidney function and as a test solution. **s. iodate,** a salt used as an alterative, especially in diseases of the mucous surfaces. **s. iodide,** a compound used as a source of iodine. **s. iodipamide,** a water-soluble organic iodine compound used in roentgenography of the biliary tract. **s. iodohippurate,** a compound used as a contrast medium in roentgenography of the urinary tract. **s. iodomethamate,** a white, odorless powder used as a contrast medium in radiography of the urinary tract. **s. lactate,** a compound used in solution to replenish body fluids and electrolytes. **s. lauryl sulfate,** a surface-active agent used as an ingredient in tooth pastes. **s. liothyronine,** the sodium salt of L-3,3',5-triiodothyronine; used in the treatment of hypothyroidism, metabolic insufficiency and certain gynecologic disorders. **s. methicillin,** a semisynthetic penicillin salt for parenteral administration. **s. morrhuate,** sodium salts of the fatty acids of cod liver oil; used as a sclerosing agent in treatment of varicose veins. **s. nitrate,** a compound used as a reagent and in certain industrial processes. **s. nitrite,** a compound used as an antidote in cyanide poisoning. **s. oxacillin,** a semisynthetic penicillin salt for oral administration. **s. para-aminohippurate,** a compound used in studies for measurement of effective renal plasma flow and determination of the functional capacity of the tubular excretory mechanism. **s. para-amino-**

salicylate, sodium aminosalicylate. **s. perborate,** a compound used as an oxidant and local anti-infective. **s. peroxide,** a white powder soluble in water; used as a dental bleach and in ointment form in acne and rosacea pustulosa. **s. phosphate,** a colorless or white granular salt, used as a cathartic. **s. polystyrene sulfonate,** an ion-exchange resin used for removal of potassium ions. **s. propionate,** a compound used in fungal infections. **s. psylliate,** the sodium salt of the liquid fatty acids; used as a sclerosing agent. **s. salicylate,** an analgesic compound. **s. sulfanilate,** a salt used in acute nasal catarrh. **s. sulfate,** a salt used as a saline cathartic. **s. sulfocyanate,** sodium thiocyanate. **s. sulfoxone,** a compound used in treatment of leprosy. **s. tetradecyl sulfate,** a white, waxy, odorless solid; used in solution as a sclerosing agent. **s. thiocyanate,** white or colorless, odorless crystals with a cooling, salty taste; used as a reagent and as a vasodilator. **s. thiosulfate,** a compound used intravenously as an antidote for cyanide poisoning.

sodoku (so'do-koo)   a relapsing type of infection due to *Spirillum minus,* an organism transmitted by the bite of an infected rat.

sodomy (sod'-o-me)   sexual connection between man and a lower animal; sometimes applied to that between human males.

softening (sof'en-ing)   a change of consistency, with loss of firmness or hardness. **red s.,** a form of degeneration of brain and spinal cord. **white s.,** fatty degeneration of brain substance, the affected area becoming anemic and white.

sol (sol)   a liquid colloidal solution. **solid s.,** a colloidal system in which both dispersed phase and dispersion medium are solids.

sol.   solution.

solarization (so"lar-i-za'shun)   exposure to sunlight and the effects produced thereby.

solation (so-la'shun)   the liquefaction of a gel.

solenoid (so'le-noid)   a coil of wire spaced equally between turns; passage of electric current causes it to act like a magnet.

solenonychia (so"le-no-nik'e-ah) a longitudinal tubular deformation of the nail plate.

Solganal (sol'gah-nal)   trademark for a preparation of aurothioglucose.

solid (sol'id)   1. not fluid or gaseous; not hollow.   2. a substance or tissue not fluid or gaseous.

solubility (sol"u-bil'ĭ-te)   quality of being soluble.

solum (so'lum), pl. *so'la* [L.]   the bottom or lowest part.

solute (sol'ūt)   the substance which is dissolved in a liquid (solvent) to form a solution.

solution (so-loo'shun)   1. a liquid preparation of one or more soluble chemical substances usually dissolved in water.   2. the process of dissolving or disrupting. **aluminum acetate s.,** a preparation of aluminum subacetate and glacial acetic acid; used for its antiseptic and astringent action on the skin. **aluminum subacetate s.,** a solution of aluminum oxide and acetic acid used topically on the skin as an antiseptic and astringent. **ammonia s.**, a colorless, transparent liquid of alkaline reaction. **ammoniacal silver nitrate s.**, a mixture of silver nitrate, purified water and strong ammonia solution; used as a dental protective. **ammonium hydroxide s.**, ammonia solution. **anisotonic s.**, one having an osmotic pressure differing from that of the standard of reference. **antiseptic s.**, a preparation of boric acid, thymol, chlorothymol, menthol, eucalyptol, methyl salicylate, thyme oil and alcohol in purified water; used as an antibacterial. **aqueous s.**, one in which water is used as the solvent. **buffer s.**, one which resists appreciable change in its hydrogen ion concentration when acid or alkali is added to it. **Burrow's s.**, aluminum acetate solution. **calcium hydroxide s.**, aqueous solution of $Ca(OH)_2$; used in infant formulas and in treatment of gastric disturbances. **carbolfuchsin s.**, a mixture of basic fuchsin, boric acid, phenol, resorcinol, acetone and alcohol in purified water; used as an antifungal agent. **colloid s., colloidal s.**, a preparation consisting of minute particles of matter suspended in a solvent. **s. of contiguity**, separation of previously contiguous structures, as dislocation, luxation or displacement. **s. of continuity**, disruption of a previously continuous structure, as fracture or rupture of bone or other tissue. **contrast s.**, a solution of a substance opaque to the roentgen ray, used to facilitate x-ray visualization of some organ or structure in the body. **Dakin's s.**, an aqueous solution of chlorine compounds of sodium; germicide. **dilute s.**, one containing only a small proportion of solute. **Dobell's s.**, a solution containing sodium borate, sodium bicarbonate, glycerin and phenol; a nonirritant wash for mucous membranes. **Donovan's s.**, a solution of arsenic and mercuric iodides. **Fehling's s.**, (1) 34.66 gm. cupric sulfate in water to make 500 cc.; (2) 173 gm. crystallized potassium and sodium tartrate and 50 gm. sodium hydroxide in water to make 500 cc.; mix equal volumes of (1) and (2) at time of use. **formaldehyde s.**, a solution containing not less than 37 per cent of formaldehyde with methanol added to prevent polymerization; used as a disinfectant. **Fowler's s.**, a clear colorless liquid, each 100 cc. containing 0.95 – 1.05 gm. As_2O_3; antiperiodic. **gold Au-198 s.**, a sterile, pyrogen-free colloidal solution of radioactive gold of mass number 198; used for suppression of neoplasms. **Hartmann's s.**, a solution containing sodium chloride, sodium lactate and phosphates of calcium and potassium; used parenterally in acidosis and alkalosis. **hyperbaric s.**, one having a greater specific gravity than a standard of reference. **hyperosmotic s., hypertonic s.**, one having an osmotic pressure greater than that of a standard of reference. **hypobaric s.**, one having a specific gravity less than that of a standard of reference. **hyposmotic s., hypotonic s.**, one having an osmotic pressure less than that of a standard of reference. **iodine**

s., a solution prepared with purified water, each 100 ml. containing 1.8-2.2 gm. of iodine and 2.1-2.6 gm. of sodium iodide. **iodine s., strong**, a solution containing, in each 100 ml., 4.5-5.5 gm. of iodine and 9.5-10.5 gm. of potassium iodide. **isobaric s.**, a solution having the same specific gravity as a standard of reference. **isotonic s.**, one having an osmotic pressure the same as that of a standard of reference. **lead subacetate s.**, a solution of lead acetate and lead monoxide in distilled water; astringent and locally sedative. **Locke's s.**, solution of sodium chloride, calcium chloride, potassium chloride, sodium bicarbonate and dextrose. **Lugol's s.**, iodine solution, strong. **magnesium citrate s.**, a preparation of magnesium carbonate, anhydrous citric acid, with syrup, talc, lemon oil and potassium bicarbonate in purified water; used as a cathartic. **molar s.**, a solution each liter of which contains 1 gram-molecule of the active substance. **ophthalmic s.**, a sterile solution, free from foreign particles, for instillation into the eye. **physiologic salt s., physiologic sodium chloride s.**, an aqueous solution of sodium chloride and other components, having an isosmotic pressure identical to that of blood serum. **Ringer's s.**, a solution of sodium chloride, potassium chloride and calcium chloride in purified water, a physiologic salt solution for topical use. **saline s., salt s.**, a solution of sodium chloride, or common salt, in purified water. **saponated cresol s.**, a mixture of cresol, vegetable oil (excluding coconut and palm kernel oil), alcohol, potassium hydroxide and purified water; used as a disinfectant. **saturated s.**, one containing all of the solute which can be held in solution by the solvent. **sclerosing s.**, one containing an irritant substance which will cause obliteration of a space, as the lumen of a varicose vein or the cavity of a hernial sac. **sodium hypochlorite s.**, a solution containing 4-6 per cent by weight of sodium hypochlorite; used as a disinfectant. **sodium phosphate P-32 s.**, a solution containing radioactive phosphorus as sodium phosphate; used orally or intravenously as a diagnostic aid or neoplastic or antipolycythemic agent. **standard s.**, one containing a fixed amount of solute. **supersaturated s.**, one containing a greater quantity of the solute than the solvent can hold in solution under ordinary conditions. **sulfurated lime s.**, a solution of lime and sublimed sulfur in water; used as a scabicide. **test s.**, any standard solution used in making tests. **Vleminckx's s.**, a clear orange solution of sulfurated lime; used in various skin conditions. **volumetric s.**, one which contains a specific quantity of solvent per stated unit of volume.

solvent (sol'vent) 1. capable of dissolving other material. 2. the liquid in which another substance (the solute) is dissolved to form a solution.

Soma (so'mah) trademark for preparations of carisoprodol.

soma (so'mah)   the body. adj., **so'mal, somat'ic.**

somasthenia (so"mas-the'ne-ah)   bodily weakness with poor appetite and poor sleep.

somat(o)- (so'mah-to)   word element [Gr.], *body.*

somatalgia (so"mah-tal'je-ah) bodily pain.

somatesthesia (so"mat-es-the'ze-ah)   body consciousness or awareness.

somatization (so"mah-ti za'shun)   the conversion of mental experiences or states into bodily symptoms.

somatoblast (so-mat'o-blast)   a cytoblast occurring in the protoplasm of the cell outside the nucleus.

somatochrome (so-mat'o-krōm)   a nerve cell whose cell body stains readily.

somatoderm (so-mat'o-derm)   the somatic layer of mesoderm.

somatodidymus (so"mah-to-did'ĭ-mus)   a double fetal monster with fused trunks.

somatogenic (-jen'ik)   originating in the body.

somatology (so"mah-tol'o-je)   the sum of what is known about the body.

somatome (so'mah-tōm)   1. an appliance for cutting the body of a fetus. 2. a somite.

somatometry (so"mah-tom'ĕ-tre)   measurement of the dimensions of the entire body.

somatopagus (-top'ah-gus)   a double fetal monster united at the trunks.

somatopathic (so"mah-to-path'ik)   disordered in body.

somatoplasm (so-mat'o-plazm)   the body substance.

somatopleure (so-mat'o-plŏor)   the ectoderm and somatic mesoderm.

somatopsychic (so"mah-to-si'kik)   pertaining to both mind and body.

somatopsychosis (-si-ko'sis)   any mental disease symptomatic of bodily disease.

somatoschisis (so"mah-tos'kĭ-sis)   splitting of the bodies of the vertebrae.

somatoscopy (-tos'ko-pe)   examination of the body.

somatosexual (so"mah-to-seks'u-al)   pertaining to both body and sex characteristics.

somatotherapy (-ther'ah-pe)   treatment aimed at relieving or curing ills of the body.

somatotonia (-to'ne-ah)   a group of traits characterized by dominance of muscular activity and vigorous body assertiveness; considered typical of a mesomorph.

somatotopic (-top'ik)   related to particular areas of the body; describing organization of motor area of the brain, control of the movement of different parts of the body being centered in specific regions of the cortex.

somatotrophin (-tro'fin)   growth hormone. adj., **somatotro'phic.**

somatotropin (-tro'pin)   growth hormone. adj., **somatotro'pic.**

somatotype (so-mat'o-tīp)   a particular type of body build.

somatotyping (so-mat"o-tīp'ing)   objective classification of individuals according to type of body build.

Sombulex (som'bu-leks)   trademark for a preparation of hexobarbital.

somesthesia (so"mes-the'ze-ah)   sensibility to bodily sensations. adj., **somesthet'ic.**

somite (so'mīt)   one of the paired segments along the spinal cord of a vertebrate embryo, formed by transverse subdivision of the thickened mesoderm next the midplane.

somnambule (som-nam'būl)   one who sleepwalks.

somnambulism (som-nam'bu-lizm)   walking in one's sleep.

somnifacient (som"nĭ-fa'shent) causing sleep.

somniferous (som-nif'er-us) producing sleep.

somniloquism (som-nil'o-kwizm)   habitual talking in one's sleep

somnipathy (som-nip'ah-the)   any disorder of sleep.

somnolence (som'no-lens) sleepiness.

somnolentia (som"no-len'she-ah)   1. incomplete sleep; drowsiness. 2. drunken sleep.

Somnos (som'nos)   trademark for preparations of chloral hydrate.

sonarography (so"nar-og'rah-fe)   ultrasonic scanning that provides a two-dimensional image corresponding to clear sections of acoustic interfaces in tissues.

sonitus (son'ĭ-tus) tinnitus.

sonometer (so-nom'ĕ-ter)   an apparatus for testing acuteness of hearing.

sophistication (so-fis"tĭ-ka'shun)   adulteration of food or medicine.

sophoretin (sof'o-re'tin) quercetin.

sophorin (sof'o-rin) rutin.

sopor (so'por)   coma or deep sleep.

soporific (sop'ŏ-rif'ik, so"pō-rif'ik)   producing deep sleep.

soporose (sop'ŏ-rōs, so'pō-ros)   associated with coma or deep sleep.

Sorangiaceae (so-ran"je-a'se-e)   a family of Schizomycetes (order Myxobacterales).

Sorangium (so-ran'je-um)   a genus of Schizomycetes (order Myxobacterales, family Sorangiaceae).

sorbefacient (sōr"bĕ-fa'shent)   1. promoting absorption. 2. an agent that promotes absorption.

sorbitol (sor'bĭ-tol)   a crystalline, hexahydric alcohol from the tree *Sorbus aucuparia.*

sordes (sōr'dēz)   foul matter collected on lips and teeth in low fevers. **s. gas'tricae,** food lying undigested in the stomach.

sore (sōr)   an abraded or painful area on the body. **cold s.,** a lesion of herpes simplex on the lip. **Delhi s., Natal s., oriental s.,** cutaneous leishmaniasis. **pressure s.,** decubitus ulcer.

sororiation (so-ro"re-a'shun)   development of the breasts at puberty.

sorption (sorp'shun)   1. incorporation of water in a colloid.   2. processes involved in net movement of components of adjoining substances across a boundary separating them, as various membranes of the body.

S.O.S. [L.]   *si o'pus sit* (if necessary).

soteria (so-tēr'e-ah)   derivation of a sense of security and protection, out of proportion to the stimulus, from an external object.

souffle (soo'fel)   a soft, blowing auscultatory sound. **cardiac s.,** any heart murmur of a blowing quality. **fetal s.,** murmur sometimes heard over pregnant uterus, supposed to be due to compression of umbilical cord. **funic s.**, **funicular s.**, hissing souffle synchronous with fetal heart sounds, probably from umbilical cord. **mammary s.**, a murmur sometimes heard in the second, third or fourth intercostal space during pregnancy and the puerperium, attributed to a change of dynamics in blood flow through the internal mammary artery. **placental s.**, the sound supposed to be produced by the blood current in the placenta. **uterine s.**, a sound made by the blood within the arteries of the gravid uterus.

sound (sownd) 1. percept resulting from stimulation of the ear by mechanical radiant energy of frequency between 20 and 20,000 cycles per second; tones and notes resulting from such energy produced by activity of various organs or elicited by the action of the examiner are observed in detection of abnormal states. 2. a slender instrument to be introduced into body passages or cavities, especially for the dilation of strictures or detection of foreign bodies. **entotic s.**, one originating within the ear, as tinnitus. **friction s.**, one produced by rubbing of two surfaces. **heart s's**, the sounds produced by the functioning of the heart, the first, a dull, prolonged sound, occurring with ventricular systole, and the second, a sharp, short sound, occurring with closure of the semilunar valves. **hippocratic s.**, a splashing succussion sound. **percussion s.**, any sound obtained by percussion. **physiologic s's**, those heard when the auditory canals are plugged, caused by the rush of blood through blood vessels in or near the inner ear and by adjacent muscles in continuous low-frequency vibration. **respiratory s.**, any sound heard on auscultation over the respiratory tract. **succussion s's**, splashing sounds heard on succussion over a distended stomach or in hydropneumothorax. **to-and-fro s.**, peculiar friction sound heard in pericarditis and pleuritis. **urethral s.**, a long, slender instrument for exploring and dilating the urethra. **white s.**, that produced by a mixture of all frequencies of mechanical vibration perceptible as sound.

space (spās) 1. a delimited area. 2. an actual or potential cavity of the body. 3. the areas of the universe beyond the earth and its atmosphere. **apical s.**, the region between the wall of the alveolus and the apex of the root of a tooth. **axillary s.**, the axilla. **bregmatic s.**, the anterior fontanel. **cardiac s.**, the space on the surface of the chest which overlies the heart. **cartilage s's**, the spaces in hyaline cartilage which contain the cartilage cells. **cell s's**, the spaces in the ground substance of connective tissue enclosing the connective tissue corpuscles. **corneal s's**, the spaces between the lamellae of the substantia propria of the cornea which contain corneal cells and interstitial lymph. **cupola s.**, the attic of the tympanum. **Czernak's s's**, interglobular spaces. **dead s.**, 1. space remaining in tissues as a result of failure of proper closure of surgical or other wounds, permitting accumulation of blood or serum. 2. the portions of the respiratory tract (passages and space in the alveoli) occupied by gas not concurrently participating in oxygen-carbon dioxide exchange. **epidural s.**, the space between the dura mater and the lining of the vertebral canal. **escapement s's**, spaces which permit the escape of material being comminuted between the occlusal surfaces of the teeth. **haversian s.**, haversian canal. **intercostal s.**, the space between two adjacent ribs. **interglobular s's**, irregular spaces within the dentin. **interpeduncular s.**, the space bounded by the crura cerebri and optic tracts. **interpleural s.**, mediastinum. **intervillous s.**, the cavernous space of the placenta into which the chorionic villi project and through which the maternal blood circulates. **Kiernan's s's**, dilated triangular spaces in fissures between liver lobules, containing the larger interlobular branches of the portal vein, hepatic artery and hepatic duct. **Larrey's s's**, spaces between parts of the diaphragm attached to the sternum and parts attached to the ribs. **lymph s's**, open spaces filled with lymph in connective or other tissue, especially in the brain and meninges. **Meckel's s.**, a recess in the dura mater which lodges the gasserian ganglion. **mediastinal s.**, mediastinum. **medullary s.**, the central cavity and the intervals between the trabeculae of bone which contain the marrow. **palmar s.**, a large fascial space in the hand, divided by a fibrous septum into a midpalmar and a thenar space. **parasinoidal s's**, spaces in the dura mater along the superior longitudinal sinus which receive the venous blood. **perineal s's**, spaces on either side of the inferior fascia of the urogenital diaphragm, the *deep* between it and the superior fascia, the *superficial* between it and the superficial perineal fascia. **perivascular s.**, a lymph space within the walls of an artery. **plantar s.**, a fascial space on the sole of the foot, divided by septa into the lateral, middle and median plantar spaces. **pneumatic s.**, a portion of bone occupied by air-containing cells. **Poiseuille's s.**, that part of the lumen of a tube, at its periphery, where no flow of liquid occurs. **retrobulbar s.**, the space behind the fascia of the bulb of the eye, containing the eye muscles and the ocular vessels and nerves. **retroperitoneal s.**, the space between the peritoneum and the posterior abdominal wall. **retropharyngeal s.**, the space behind the pharynx, containing areolar tissue. **Retzius' s.**, the areolar space bounded by reflection of peritoneum, symphysis pubis and bladder. **subarachnoid s.**, the space between the arachnoid and the pia mater. **subdural s.**, the space between the dura mater and the arachnoid. **subgingival s.**, the space between the gingiva and the tooth surface it overlies. **submaxillary s.**, submaxillary triangle. **subphrenic s.**, the space between the diaphragm and subjacent organs. **subumbilical s.**, somewhat triangular space in the body cavity beneath the umbilicus. **Tenon's s.**, a lymph space between the sclera and Tenon's capsule. **thiocyanate s.**, a quantitative expression of the space occupied by extracellular fluid, computed after intravenous injection of sodium thiocyanate. **web s's**, areas of loose connective tissue between the creases of the fingers.

span (span) reach or extent; the greatest distance from fingertip to fingertip when the arms are widely outstretched.

span(o)- (span'o) word element [Gr.], *scanty; scarce; scarcity.*

spanemia (spah-ne'me-ah) poverty or thinness of the blood.

spanogyny (span'o-jin"e) scarcity of women; decrease in female births.

spanomenorrhea (span"o-men"o-re'ah) scanty menstruation.

spanopnea (span"op-ne'ah) nervous affection with slow, deep breathing and subjective feeling of dyspnea.

sparganosis (spar"gah-no'sis) infection with spargana.

sparganum (spar-ga'num), pl. *sparga'na* [Gr.] a migrating larva of a tapeworm.

spargosis (spar go'sis) 1. distention of a mammary gland with milk. 2. elephantiasis.

Sparine (spar'ēn) trademark for preparations of promazine.

spasm (spazm) a sudden, violent, involuntary muscular contraction. **carpopedal s.**, spasm of the hand or foot, or of the thumbs and great toes, seen in calcium tetany, rickets and laryngismus stridulus. **clonic s.**, spasm with rigidity followed immediately by relaxation. **cynic s.**, risus sardonicus. **habit s.**, spasm acquired by habit. **intention s.**, muscular spasm on attempting voluntary movement. **massive s.**, a seizure marked by contraction of most of the body musculature. **mimic s.**, involuntary contraction of the facial muscles. **mixed s.**, a seizure marked by both extensor and flexor movements. **myopathic s.**, spasm accompanying disease of the muscles. **nodding s.**, chronic spasm of the sternocleidomastoid muscles, causing a nodding motion of the head. **saltatory s.**, clonic spasm of the muscles of the legs, producing a peculiar jumping or springing motion. **tetanic s.**, persistent spasm occurring in tetanus. **tonic s.**, spasm with rigidity persisting for a long period. **toxic s.**, spasm caused by a toxin.

spasmodic (spaz-mod'ik) of the nature of a spasm; occurring in spasms.

spasmolysis (spaz-mol'ĭ-sis) the arrest of spasm. adj., **spasmolyt'ic.**

spasmophemia (spaz"mo-fe'me-ah) stuttering.

spasmophilia (-fil'e-ah) abnormal tendency to convulsions.

spasmotoxin (-tok'sin) a poisonous ptomaine from *Clostridium tetani.*

spasmus (spaz'mus) [L.] spasm. **s. nu'tans,** nodding spasm.

spastic (spas'tik) pertaining to or marked by spasms.

spasticity (spas-tis'ĭ-te) continuous resistance to stretching by a muscle due to abnormally increased tension.

spatium (spa'she-um) pl. *spa'tia* [L.] space.

spatula (spat'u-lah) a wide, flat, blunt, usually flexible instrument of little thickness, used for spreading material on a smooth surface.

spatulation (spat"u-la'shun) the combining of materials into a homogeneous mixture by continuously heaping together and smoothing out on a smooth surface with a spatula.

spay (spa) to deprive of the ovaries.

SPCA serum prothrombin conversion accelerator.

specialist (spesh'ah-list) one who is particularly skilled; a legally qualified doctor of medicine whose practice is limited to diagnosis and treatment of diseases of a certain type or of a specific organ or body system.

specialty (spesh'al-te) a restricted field in which a person is particularly skilled.

species (spe'shēz) a taxonomic category subordinate to a genus (or subgenus) and superior to a subspecies or variety. **type s.**, the original species from which the description of the genus is formulated.

specific (spē-sif'ik) 1. pertaining to a species. 2. having a particular foreordained effect.

specificity (spes"ĭ-fis'ĭ-te) the quality of having a certain action, as of affecting only certain organisms or tissues, or reacting only with certain substances, as antibodies with certain antigens (*antigenic specificity*). **host s.**, the natural adaptability of a particular parasite to a certain species or group of hosts.

specimen (spes'ĭ-men) a small sample or part taken to show the nature of the whole, as a small quantity of urine for urinalysis, or a small fragment of tissue for microscopic study. **corrosion s.**, one showing particular structures, such as blood vessels which have been injected with a permanent substance, after which the surrounding tissues have been destroyed by chemical digestion.

spectacles (spek'tĕ-kuls) pair of lenses in a frame to assist vision.

spectrocolorimeter (spek"tro-kul"ĕ-rim'ĕ-ter) an instrument for detecting color blindness.

spectrometry (spek-trom'ĕ tre) determination of the place of lines in a spectrum.

spectrophobia (spek"tro-fo'be-ah) morbid dread of mirrors or of seeing one's reflection in a mirror.

spectrophotometer (-fo-tom'ĕ-ter) 1. apparatus for measuring light sense by means of a spectrum. 2. apparatus for determining quantity of coloring matter in solution by measurement of transmitted light.

spectrophotometry (-fo-tom'ĕ-tre) the use of the spectrophotometer.

spectroscope (spek'tro-skōp) instrument for developing and analyzing the spectrum of a body.

spectroscopy (spek-tros'ko-pe) examination by means of a spectroscope.

spectrum (spek'trum) a representation of a range of distribution, as of activity of a given antibiotic, or of intensity of a given type of radiation as a function of its various characteristics, such as wavelength, frequency, energy. **absorption s.,** one obtained by passing radiation with a continuous spectrum through a selectively absorbing medium, showing spaces or dark lines for wavelengths for which the spectrum of the medium itself would be bright. **antibacterial s.,** the range of microorganisms against which an antibiotic substance is effective. **chromatic s.,** that portion of the electromagnetic spectrum including wavelengths of 7700 to 3900 angstroms, giving rise to the perception of color by the normal eye. **electromagnetic s.,** the range of electromagnetic energy from cosmic rays to electric waves, including gamma, x- and ultraviolet light, visible light and infrared and radiowaves, with a range of wavelengths from 10^{11} to 10^{-12} cm. **fortification s.,** scintillating scotoma. **prismatic s.,** one produced by the passage of light through a prism. **solar s.,** that portion of the electromagnetic spectrum including vibrations emanating from the sun.

speculum (spek'u-lum) an instrument for opening or distending a body orifice or cavity to permit visual inspection. **bivalve s.,** one having two valves or parts. **Sims's s.,** a form of bivalve speculum for examining the vagina and cervix.

speech (spēch) the expression of thoughts and ideas by vocal sounds. **esophageal s.,** a form of communication possible after laryngectomy, sounds being produced by vibration of a column of air in the esophagus against the contracting inferior constrictor muscle of the pharynx. **explosive s.,** sudden and forcible utterance of words. **mirror s.,** defective expression, the words being spoken backward or in reverse order. **scanning s., staccato s.,** speech in which syllables of words are separated by noticeable pauses.

sperm (sperm) the male reproductive cell which unites with an ovum in sexual reproduction to produce a new individual.

spermaceti (sper″mah-set'e) a waxy substance obtained from the head of the sperm whale; an emollient used in cold cream.

spermacrasia (-kra'ze-ah) a weak state of the semen.

spermatemphraxis (sper″mat-em-frak'sis) obstruction to the discharge of semen.

spermatic (sper-mat'ik) pertaining to the spermatozoa or to semen.

spermatid (sper'mah-tid) a spherical cell produced by meiotic division of a secondary spermatocyte, which develops into the spermatozoon.

spermatitis (sper″mah-ti'tis) inflammation of a vas deferens.

spermato-, spermo (sper'mah-to, sper'mo) word elements [Gr.], *seed;* specifically used to refer to the male germinative element.

spermatoblast (sper-mat'o-blast) spermatid.

spermatocele (sper-mat'o-sēl) a cystic accumulation of semen in the tunica vaginalis.

spermatocelectomy (sper″mah-to-se-lek'to-me) excision of a spermatocele.

supermatocidal (sper″mah-to-si'dal) destructive to spermatozoa.

spermatocyst (sper-mat'o-sist) a seminal vesicle.

spermatocystectomy (sper″mah-to-sis-tek'to-me) excision of a seminal vesicle.

spermatocystitis (-sis-ti'tis) inflammation of a seminal vesicle.

spermatocystotomy (-sis-tot'o-me) incision of a seminal vesicle.

spermatocyte (sper-mat'o-sīt) a cell developed from a spermatogonium in spermatogenesis. **primary s.,** the original large cell into which a spermatogonium develops. **secondary s.,** a cell produced by meiotic division of the primary spermatocyte.

spermatogenesis (sper″mah-to-jen'ĕ-sis) the development of mature spermatozoa from spermatogonia.

spermatogonium (-go'ne-um), pl. *spermatogo'nia* [Gr.] one of the primitive, unspecialized germ cells which line the sperm tubules of the testis.

spermatoid (sper'mah-toid) resembling semen.

spermatolysin (sper″mah-tol'ĭ-sin) a lysin destructive to spermatozoa.

spermatolysis (-tol'ĭ-sis) dissolution of spermatozoa. adj., **spermatolyt'ic.**

spermatopathia (sper″mah-to-path'e-ah) abnormality of the semen.

spermatorrhea (-re'ah) involuntary escape of semen.

spermatoschesis (sper″mah-tos'kĕ-sis) suppression of the semen.

spermatospore (sper-mat'o-spōr) a spermatogonum.

spermatoxin (sper″mah-tok'sin) a toxin which destroys spermatozoa.

spermatozoicide (sper″mah-to-zo'ĭ-sīd) an agent which destroys spermatozoa.

spermatozoon (-zo'on), pl. *spermatozo'a* [Gr.] the male reproductive cell which develops in the testis and is discharged in the semen. adj., **spermatozo'al.**

spermaturia (sper″mah-tu're-ah) semen in the urine.

spermectomy (sper-mek'to-me) excision of the spermatic cord.

spermiation (sper″me-a'shun) the release of mature spermatozoa from the Sertoli cells of the testis, analogous to ovulation in the female.

spermicide (sper'mĭ-sīd) an agent destructive to spermatozoa. adj., **spermici'dal.**

spermiduct (sper'mĭ-dukt) the ejaculatory duct and vas deferens together.

spermine (sper'min) a leukomaine from semen and other animal substances.

spermiocyte (sper'me-o-sīt″) a primary spermatocyte.

spermiogenesis (sper″me-o-jen'ĕ-sis) the second stage in the formation of spermatozoa, in which the spermatids transform into spermatozoa.

spermiogram (sper'me-o-gram″) a diagram or chart of various cells formed in development of the spermatozoon, or of the cells present in a specimen of semen.

spermioteleosis (sper"me-o-te"le-o'sis) progressive development of spermatogonium through various stages to the mature spermatozoon. adj., **spermioteleot'ic.**

spermist (sper'mist) one who believed that the individuals of successive generations are contained, completely formed, within the sperm of the fathers.

spermoblast (sper'mo-blast) spermatid.

spermolith (sper'mo-lith) a stone in the spermatic duct.

spermoneuralgia (sper"mo-nu-ral'je-ah) neuralgic pain in the spermatic cord.

spermophlebectasia (fle"bek-ta'ze-ah) varicose state of the spermatic veins.

spermoplasm (sper'mo-plazm) the protoplasm of the spermatids.

SPF specific-pathogen-free; a term applied to gnotobiotic animals known to be free of specific pathogenic microorganisms.

sp.gr. specific gravity.

sphacelate (sfas'ĕ-lāt) to become gangrenous.

sphacelation (sfas"ĕ-la'shun) mortification or gangrene.

sphacelism (sfas'ĕ-lizm) gangrenous state or process.

sphaceloderma (sfas"ĕ-lo-der'mah) gangrene of the skin.

sphacelous (sfas'ĕ-lus) gangrenous; sloughing.

sphacelus (sfas'ĕ-lus) a slough; a mass of gangrenous tissue.

Sphaerophorus (sfe-rof'o-rus) a genus of Schizomycetes (order Eubacteriales, family Bacteroidaceae) found in necrotic tissues as a secondary invader.

Sphaerotilus (sfe-ro'tī-lus) a genus of Schizomycetes (order Chlamydobacteriales, family Chlamydobacteriaceae).

sphenion (sfe'ne-on) the point at the sphenoid angle of the parietal bone.

spheno- (sfe'no) word element [Gr.], *wedge-shaped, sphenoid bone.*

sphenocephalus (sfe"no-sef'ah-lus) a monster fetus with wedgelike head.

sphenoid (sfe'noid) wedge-shaped.

sphenoiditis (sfe"noi-di'tis) inflammation of the sphenoid sinus.

sphenoidotomy (-dot'o-me) incision of a sphenoid sinus.

sphenomaxillary (-mak"sĭ-lār"e) pertaining to sphenoid and maxilla.

sphenopalatine (-pal'ah-tīn) pertaining to sphenoid and palatine bones.

sphenotresia (-tre'ze-ah) breaking up of the base of the fetal skull.

sphenotribe (sfe'no-trīb) an instrument used in sphenotresia.

sphere (sfēr) a ball or globe. **attraction s.,** centrosome. **segmentation s.,** 1. morula. 2. a blastomere.

sphero- (sfe'ro) word element [Gr.], *round; a sphere.*

spherocyte (sfe'ro-sīt) a small, globular, completely hemoglobinated erythrocyte without the usual central pallor. adj., **spherocyt'ic.**

spherocytosis (sfe"ro-si-to'sis) a hereditary form of hemolytic anemia with presence in the blood of spheroidal red blood cells.

spheroid (sfe'roid) a spherelike body.

spheroidal (sfe-roi'dal) resembling a sphere.

spheroma (sfe-ro'mah) a spherelike tumor.

spherometer (sfe-rom'ĕ-ter) apparatus for measuring the curvature of a surface.

spheroplast (sfer'o-plast) a spherical form of a bacterium, produced in a hypertonic medium under conditions which cause partial or complete absence of the cell wall.

sphincter (sfingk'ter) a ringlike muscle which closes a natural orifice. **cardiac s.,** muscle fibers about the opening of the esophagus into the stomach. **Henle's s.,** a ring of muscular fibers surrounding the prostatic urethra. **O'Beirne's s.,** a band of muscle at the junction of the sigmoid colon and rectum. **Oddi's s.,** the sheath of muscle fibers investing the associated bile and pancreatic passages as they traverse the wall of the duodenum. **pyloric s.,** a thickening of the muscular wall of the stomach around the opening into the duodenum.

sphincteralgia (sfingk"ter-al'je-ah) pain in a sphincter muscle.

sphincterismus (-iz'mus) spasm of a sphincter.

sphincteritis (-i'tis) inflammation of a sphincter.

sphincterolysis (-ol'ĭ-sis) separation of the iris from the cornea in anterior synechia.

sphincteroplasty (sfingk'ter-o-plas"te) plastic reconstruction of a sphincter.

sphincterotomy (sfingk"ter-ot'o-me) incision of a sphincter.

sphingoin (sfing'go-in) a leukomaine from brain substance.

sphingolipid (sfing"go-lip'id) a phospholipid containing sphingosine, occurring in high concentrations in the brain and other nerve tissue.

sphingolipidosis (-lip"ĭ-do'sis), pl. *sphingolipido'ses* [Gr.] a condition characterized by abnormal storage of sphingolipids.

sphingomyelin (-mi'ĕ-lin) a group of phospholipids which on hydrolysis yield phosphoric acid, choline, sphingosine and a fatty acid.

sphingosine (sfing'go-sin) a basic amino alcohol present in sphingomyelin.

sphygmic (sfig'mik) pertaining to the pulse.

sphygmobolometer (sfig"mo-bo-lom'ĕ-ter) an instrument for recording blood pressure.

sphygmochronograph (-kro'no-graf) a self-registering sphygmograph.

sphygmodynamometer (-di"nah-mom'ĕ-ter) an instrument for measuring the force of the pulse.

sphygmogram (sfig'mo-gram) record or tracing made by a sphygmograph.

sphygmograph (sfig'mo-graf) apparatus for registering the movements of the arterial pulse.

sphygmoid (sfig'moid) resembling the pulse.

sphygmology (sfig-mol'o-je) sum of what is known about the pulse.

sphygmomanometer (sfig"mo-mah-nom'ĕ-ter) instrument for measuring arterial blood pressure.

sphygmometer (sfig-mom'ĕ-ter) an instrument for measuring the pulse.

sphygmoplethysmograph (sfĭg″mo-ple-thiz′-mo-graf) an instrument which traces the record of the pulse, together with the curve of fluctuation of volume.

sphygmoscope (sfĭg′mo-skōp) device for rendering the pulse beat visible.

sphygmotonometer (sfĭg″mo-to-nom′ĕ-ter) an instrument for measuring elasticity of arterial walls.

sphyrectomy (sfĭ-rek′to-me) excision of the malleus.

sphyrotomy (sfĭ-rot′o-me) division of the malleus.

spica (spi′kah) a figure-of-8 bandage, with turns crossing each other.

spiculum (spik′u-lum), pl. *spic′ula* [L.] a sharp, needle-like body or spike.

spider (spi′der) 1. an arthropod of the class Arachnida. 2. a spider-like nevus. **black widow s.**, a spider, *Latrodectus mactans*, whose bite causes severe poisoning.

spignet (spĭg′net) aralia.

spiloma (spi-lo′mah) a nevus.

spiloplaxia (spi″lo-plak′se-ah) a red spot occurring in leprosy.

spina (spi′nah), pl. *spi′nae* [L.] spine; used in anatomic nomenclature to designate a slender, thornlike process such as occurs on many bones. **s. bif′ida**, a defect of the vertebral column due to imperfect union of the paired vertebral arches at the midline; it may be so extensive *(spi′na bif′ida aper′ta)* as to allow herniation of the spinal cord and meninges, or covered by intact skin *(spi′na bif′ida occul′ta)* and evident only on radiologic examination. **s. vento′sa**, tuberculous infection of the bones of hands or feet, occurring mostly in infants and children, with enlargement of digits, caseation, sequestration and sinus formation.

spinal (spi′nal) pertaining to a spine or to the vertebral column.

spinalgia (spi-nal′je-ah) pain in the spinal region.

spinate (spi′nāt) shaped like a thorn.

spindle (spin′del) an elongated structure wider in the middle and tapering at each end, such as the figure formed by protoplasmic fibers extending between either centriole and the equator of a dividing cell. **achromatic s.**, a spindle-shaped figure of achromatin formed in the cell nucleus during mitosis. **Krukenberg's s.**, a spindle-shaped, brownish-red opacity of the cornea. **muscle s.**, one of the mechanoreceptors arranged in parallel between the fibers of skeletal muscle, being the receptor of impulses responsible for the stretch reflex. **nuclear s.**, achromatic spindle. **tendon s.**, Golgi tendon organ. **tigroid s's**, Nissl bodies.

spine (spīn) 1. a slender, thornlike process of bone. 2. the vertebral column. **alar s.**, **angular s.**, the spinous process of the sphenoid bone. **bamboo s.**, the ankylosed spine produced by rheumatoid spondylitis. **bifid s.**, **cleft s.**, **cloven s.**, spina bifida. **deltoid s.**, the deltoid tubercle. **mental s.**, genial tubercle. **nasal s.**, **anterior**, a projection from either side of the maxilla at the lower margin of the anterior aperture of the nose. **nasal s.**, **posterior**, a projection at the median plane of the adjacent palatine bones, for attachment of the muscle of the uvula. **neural s.**, the spinous process of a vertebra. **palatine s.**, one of the ridges on the lower surface of the palatal process of the maxilla. **poker s.**, the inflexible vertebral column resulting from rheumatoid arthritis of the spine. **s. of the pubis**, the outer projecting end of the crest of the pubis. **rigid s.**, poker spine. **s. of the scapula**, the projecting ridge on the posterior surface of the scapula. **sciatic s.**, the spine of the ischium. **s. of the sphenoid**, the pointed backward projection of the lower angle of the great wing of the sphenoid. **s. of the tibia**, the upward-projecting eminence on the head of the tibia. **trochlear s.**, a depression on the orbital surface of the frontal bone for attachment of the trochlea of the superior oblique muscle.

spinifugal (spi-nif′u-gal) conducting or moving away from the spinal cord.

spinipetal (spi-nip′ĕ-tal) conducting or moving toward the spinal cord.

spinitis (spi-ni′tis) myelitis.

spinobulbar (spi″no-bul′bar) pertaining to spinal cord and medulla oblongata.

spinocellular (-sel′u-lar) pertaining to prickle cells.

spinocerebellar (-ser″ĕ-bel′ar) pertaining to spinal cord and cerebellum.

spinocortical (-kor′tĭ-kal) corticospinal.

spinoneural (-nu′ral) pertaining to the spinal cord and the peripheral nerves.

spinous (spi′nus) pertaining to or like a spine.

spinthariscope (spin-thar′ĭ-skōp) an instrument for observing the radiations of radium.

spiradenitis (spi″rad-ĕ-ni′tis) inflammation of the sweat glands.

spiradenoma (spi″rad-ĕ-no′mah) adenoma of the sweat glands.

spiral (spi′ral) 1. winding like the thread of a screw. 2. a structure curving around a central point or axis. **Curschmann's s's**, coiled fibrils of mucin found in the sputum of patients with asthma.

spireme (spi′rēm) wreath of chromatin fibrils formed in mitosis.

Spirillaceae (spi″ril-la′se-e) a family of Schizomycetes (order Pseudomonadales, suborder Pseudomonadineae).

spirillicidal (spi-ril″ĭ-si′dal) destroying spirilla.

spirillicide (spi-ril′ĭ-sīd) an agent which destroys spirilla.

spirilliform (spi-ril′ĭ-form) shaped like a spirillum, or the turn of a screw.

spirillolysis (spi″rĭ-lol′ĭ-sis) the breaking up of spirilla.

spirillosis (-lo′sis) a disease caused by presence of spirilla.

spirillotropism (-lot′ro-pizm) the property of having an affinity for spirilla. adj., **spirillotrop′ic.**

Spirillum (spi-ril′um) a genus of Schizomycetes (order Pseudomonadales, suborder Pseudomonadineae, family Spirillaceae).

spirillum (spi-ril'um), pl. *spiril'la* [L.] 1. a relatively rigid, spiral-shaped bacterium. 2. or organism of the genus Spirillum.

spirit (spir'it) 1. a volatile or distilled liquid. 2. a solution of a volatile material in alcohol. **proof s.,** a product containing 50 per cent by volume of C_2H_5OH. **rectified s.,** alcohol.

Spirochaeta (spi"ro-ke'tah) a genus of Schizomycetes (order Spirochaetales, family Spirochaetaceae) found in fresh-water or sea-water slime.

Spirochaetaceae (-ke-ta'se-e) a family of Schizomycetes (order Spirochaetales) found in the intestinal tracts of bivalve mollusks and in stagnant fresh or salt water.

Spirochaetales (-ke-ta'lēz) an order of Schizomycetes.

spirochete (spi'ro-kēt) 1. a highly coiled bacterium; a general term applied to any organism of the order Spirochaetales. 2. an organism of the genus Spirochaeta. adj., **spiroche'tal.**

spirocheticide (spi"ro-ke'tĭ-sīd) an agent which destroys spirochetes. adj., **spirochetici'dal.**

spirochetolysis (-ke-tol'ĭ-sis) the destruction of spirochetes by lysis.

spirochetosis (-ke-to'sis) infection with spirochetes.

spirogram (spi'ro-gram) a graph of respiratory movements.

spirograph (spi'ro-graf) apparatus for recording respiratory movements.

spiroid (spi'roid) resembling a spiral.

spirolactone (spi"ro-lak'tōn) one of a class of chemical compounds that oppose the action of aldosterone.

spirometer (spi-rom'ē-ter) an instrument for measuring air taken into and expelled from the lungs.

spirometry (spi-rom'ē-tre) measurement of breathing capacity of lungs.

spironolactone (spi-ro"no-lak'tōn) one of the spirolactones which is highly effective when given by mouth; used as a diuretic.

spissated (spis'āt-ed) inspissated.

splanchn(o)- (splank'no) word element [Gr.], *viscus* (*viscera*); *splanchnic nerve.*

splanchnapophysis (splangk"nah-pof'ĭ-sis) a skeletal element, such as the lower jaw, connected with the alimentary canal.

splanchnectopia (-nek-to'pe-ah) misplacement of a viscus or of the viscera.

splanchnemphraxis (-nem-frak'sis) obstruction of a viscus, particularly of the intestine.

splanchnesthesia (-nes-the'ze-ah) visceral sensation. adj., **splanchnesthet'ic.**

splanchnic (splangk'nik) pertaining to the viscera.

splanchnicectomy (splangk"nĭ-sek'to-me) excision of part of the splanchnic nerve.

splanchnicotomy (-kot'o-me) transection of the splanchnic nerve.

splanchnoblast (splangk'no-blast) a rudiment of a viscus.

splanchnocele (splangk'no-sēl) hernial protrusion of a viscus.

splanchnocoele (splangk'no-sēl) portion of the coelom from which the visceral cavities are formed.

splanchnodiastasis (splangk"no-di-as'tah-sis) displacement of a viscus.

splanchnodynia (-din'e-ah) pain in an abdominal organ.

splanchnography (splangk-nog'rah-fe) descriptive anatomy of the viscera.

splanchnolith (splangk'no-lith) intestinal calculus.

splanchnologia (splangk"no-lo'je-ah) splanchnology.

splanchnology (splangk-nol'o-je) scientific study or description of the organs of the body, as of the digestive, respiratory and urogenital systems.

splanchnomegaly (splangk"no-meg'ah-le) enlargement of the viscus.

splanchnopathy (splangk-nop'ah-the) disease of the viscera.

splanchnopleure (splangk'no-plōōr) the entoderm and splanchnic mesoderm.

splanchnoptosis (splangk"nop-to'sis) prolapse or downward displacement of the viscera.

splanchnosclerosis (splangk"no-skle-ro'sis) hardening of the viscera.

splanchnoskeleton (-skel'ē-ton) skeletal structures connected with viscera.

splanchnotomy (splangk-not'o-me) anatomy or dissection of the viscera.

splanchnotribe (splangk'no-trīb) an instrument for crushing the intestine to obliterate its lumen.

splayfoot (spla'foot) flatfoot; talipes valgus.

spleen (splēn) a large, glandlike organ situated in the upper part of the abdominal cavity on the left side, lateral to the cardiac end of the stomach. adj., **splen'ic. accessory s.,** a small mass of tissue elsewhere in the body, histologically and functionally identical with that composing the normal spleen. **sago s.,** one with amyloid degeneration, the malpighian corpuscles looking like grains of sand.

splen(o)- word element [Gr.], *spleen.*

splenadenoma (splēn"ad-e-no'mah) hyperplasia of the spleen pulp.

splenalgia (sple-nal'je-ah) pain in the spleen.

splenculus (splen'ku-lus) an accessory spleen.

splenectasis (sple-nek'tah-sis) enlargement of the spleen.

splenectomy (sple-nek'to-me) excision of the spleen.

splenectopy (sple-nek'to-pe) displacement of the spleen.

splenelcosis (sple"nel-ko'sis) ulceration of the spleen.

splenemia (sple-ne'me-ah) congestion of the spleen with blood.

splenicterus (splen-ik'ter-us) inflammation of spleen with jaundice.

splenitis (sple-ni'tis) inflammation of the spleen.

splenium (sple'ne-um) a compress or bandage. **s. cor'poris callo'si,** the posterior, rounded end of the callosum.

splenization (splen"i-za'shun) the conversion of a tissue, as of the lung, into tissue resembling that of the spleen.

splenoblast (sple'no-blast) the cell from which a splenocyte develops.

splenocolic (sple"no-kol'ik) pertaining to spleen and colon.

splenocyte (splen'o-sīt) the monocyte characteristic of splenic tissue.

splenodynia (sple"no-din'e-ah) pain in the spleen.

splenogenous (sple-noj'ĕ-nus) arising in the spleen.

splenography (sple-nog'rah-fe) 1. roentgenography of the spleen. 2. a description of the spleen.

splenohepatomegaly (sple"no-hep"ah-to-meg'ah-le) enlargement of spleen and liver.

splenoid (sple'noid) resembling the spleen.

splenolysin (sple-nol'ĭ-sin) a lysin which destroys spleen tissue.

splenolysis (sple-nol'ĭ-sis) destruction of splenic tissue by a lysin.

splenoma (sple-no'mah) a splenic tumor.

splenomalacia (sple"no-mah-la'she-ah) abnormal softness of the spleen.

splenomegaly (-meg'ah-le) enlargement of the spleen. **congestive s.,** enlargement of the spleen and liver with ascites, recurrent hematemesis, and fatigability. **hemolytic s.,** hemolytic jaundice. **siderotic s.,** splenomegaly with deposit of iron and calcium.

splenometry (sple-nom'ĕ-tre) determination of the size of the spleen.

splenomyelogenous (sple"no-mi"ĕ-loj'e-nus) formed in spleen and bone marrow.

splenomyelomalacia (-mi"ĕ-lo-mah-la'she-ah) softening of spleen and bone marrow.

splenoncus (sple-nong'kus) splenoma.

splenonephroptosis (sple"no-nef"rop-to'sis) downward displacement of spleen and kidney.

splenopancreatic (-pan"kre-at'ik) pertaining to spleen and pancreas.

splenopathy (sple-nop'ah-the) any disease of the spleen.

splenopexy (sple'no-pek"se) surgical fixation of the spleen.

splenoptosis (sple"nop-to'sis) downward displacement of the spleen.

splenorenal (sple"no-re'nal) pertaining to spleen and kidney, or to splenic and renal veins.

splenorrhagia (-ra'je-ah) hemorrhage from the spleen.

splenorrhaphy (sple-nor'ah-fe) suture of the spleen.

splenosis (sple-no'sis) the presence of numerous implants of splenic tissue as the result of autotransplantation. **pericardial s.,** development between the heart and pericardium of splenic tissue deliberately introduced into the pericardial cavity as a means of increasing the blood supply to the heart muscle.

splenotomy (sple-not'o-me) incision of spleen.

splint (splint) 1. a rigid or flexible appliance for fixation of displaced or movable parts. 2. a small tumor along the metacarpal bone of horses, producing lameness. **Agnew's s.,** one for fracture of the patella or of the metacarpus. **airplane s.,** one which holds the splinted limb suspended in the air. **anchor s.,** one for fracture of the jaw, with metal loops fitting over the teeth and held together by a rod. **Angle's s.,** one for fastening the lower teeth to the upper ones in fracture of the mandible, the wires being held in place by bands cemented to the teeth. **Balkan s.** Balkan frame. **coaptation s's,** small splints adjusted about a fractured limb for the purpose of producing coaptation of fragments. **Denis Browne s.,** one for the correction of clubfoot, consisting of two metal foot plates connected by a cross bar. **dynamic s.,** a supportive or protective apparatus which aids in initiation and performance of motion by the supported or adjacent parts. **Fredjka s.,** one used for securing abduction of the heads of the femurs in congenital dislocation of the hip. **functional s.,** dynamic splint. **Taylor s.,** a horizontal pelvic band and long lateral posterior bars; used with a windlass to apply traction to the lower extremity. **Thomas s.,** two round iron rods joined at the upper end by an oval iron ring, or half ring, and bent at the lower end to form the letter **W**; used to give support to the lower extremity.

splinting (splint'ing) 1. application of a splint, or treatment by use of a splint. 2. in dentistry, the application of a fixed restoration to join two or more teeth into a single rigid unit. 3. rigidity of muscles occurring as a means of avoiding pain caused by movement of the part.

spodo- (spo'do) word element [Gr.], *waste material.*

spodogenous (spo-doj'ĕ-nus) caused by accumulation of waste material in an organ.

spodogram (spod'o-gram) the design of the ash formed on microincineration of tissue or other substance.

spodophagous (spo-dof'ah-gus) consuming waste material of the body.

spondyl(o)- (spon'dĭ-lo) word element [Gr.], *vertebra; vertebral column.*

spondylalgia (spon"dĭ-lal'je-ah) pain in the vertebrae.

spondylarthritis (spon"dil-ar-thri'tis) inflammation of one or more vertebral joints.

spondylexarthrosis (-ek"sar-thro'sis) dislocation of a vertebra.

spondylitis (spon"dĭ-li'tis) inflammation of vertebrae. **s. ankylopoiet'ica, ankylosing s., s. defor'mans,** rheumatoid spondylitis. **s. infectio'sa,** inflammation of the vertebrae of infectious origin. **Kümmell's s.,** a form of unknown origin or occurring at a great interval after the injury causing it, with collapse of the vertebra and thinning of the intervertebral disks. **Marie-Strümpell s.,** rheumatoid spondylitis. **muscular s.,** a morbid condition of the spine due to muscular weakness and not a true inflammation. **posttraumatic s.,** Kümmell's spondylitis. **rheumatoid s.,** a condition of insidious onset, occurring mostly in males aged 20 to 40, with pain and impairment of movement of the sacroiliac, intervertebral and costovertebral joints. **traumatic s.,** spondylitis due to injury. **s. tuberculo'sa,** tuberculous disease of the vertebral joints. **s. typho'sa,** a painful condition of the spine following typhoid fever.

spondylizema (spon"di-li-ze'mah) downward displacement of a vertebra because of destruction of the one below it.

spondylocace (-lok'ah-se) tuberculosis of the vertebrae.

spondylodymus (-lod'i-mus) a twin fetal monster united by the vertebrae.

spondylodynia (spon"di-lo-din'e-ah) pain in a vertebra.

spondylolisthesis (-lis-the'sis) forward displacement of a vertebra over a lower segment, usually of the fourth or fifth lumbar.

spondylolysis (spon"di-lol'i-sis) the breaking down of a vertebra.

spondylopathy (-lop'ah-the) any disease of the vertebrae.

spondyloptosis (spon"di-lo-to'sis) spondylolisthesis.

spondylopyosis (-pi-o'sis) suppuration of a vertebra.

spondyloschisis (spon"di-los'ki-sis) congenital fissure of a vertebral arch; spina bifida.

spondylosis (spon"di-lo'sis) a condition marked by narrowing of the intervertebral spaces and lipping of the vertebral bodies, impinging on the nerve roots. **rhizomelic s.,** spondylitis deformans affecting the movements of the hips and shoulders.

spondylosyndesis (spon"di-lo-sin'de-sis) surgical creation of ankylosis between contiguous vertebrae.

sponge (spunj) a porous, absorbent mass, as a pad of gauze or cotton surrounded by gauze, or the elastic fibrous skeleton of certain species of marine animals. **gelatin s., absorbable,** a sterile, absorbable, water-insoluble, gelatin-base material used in the control of capillary bleeding.

spongi(o) (spun'je-o) word element [L., Gr.], *sponge; spongelike.*

spongiform (spun'ji-form) resembling a sponge.

spongioblast (spun'je-o-blast") an embryonic cell whose processes form the network from which neuroglia is formed.

spongioblastoma (spun"je-o-blas-to'mah) a tumor containing spongioblasts.

spongiocyte (spun'je-o-sit") a neuroglia cell.

spongioid (spun'je-oid) resembling a sponge.

spongioplasm (spun'je-o-plazm") network of fibrils pervading the cell substance.

spongy (spun'je) of spongelike appearance or texture.

Spontin (spon'tin) trademark for a lyophilized preparation of ristocetins A and B.

sporadin (spo'rah-din) trophozoite.

sporangium (spo-ran'je-um), pl. *sporan'gia* [Gr.], a round vesicle containing conidia spores; seen in certain mold fungi.

spore (spor) a reproductive cell of a protozoan or cryptogamic plant.

sporicide (spo'ri-sid) an agent which kills spores. adj., **sporici'dal.**

sporidium (spo-rid'e-um), pl. *sporid'ia* [L.] a protozoan organism in one of the spore stages of its development.

sporiferous (spo-rif'er-us) bearing spores.

sporoblast (spo'ro-blast) one of the bodies formed by cell division in a coccidium.

sporocyst (spo'ro-sist) 1. any cyst or sac containing spores or reproductive cells. 2. the envelope formed about a sporoblast in its development into a spore.

Sporocytophaga (spo"ro-si-to'fah-gah) a genus of Schizomycetes (order Myxobacterales, family Myxococcaceae).

sporogenic (spo"ro-jen'ik) producing spores.

sporogony (spo-rog'o-ne) the third phase of the life cycle of a sporozoan parasite, with development of the zygote into one or several haploid spores, each containing a distinctive number of sporozoites. adj., **sporogon'ic.**

sporont (spo'ront) a mature protozoan in its sexual cycle.

sporophore (spo'ro-for) the spore-bearing part of an organism.

sporoplasm (spo'ro-plazm) protoplasm of reproductive cells.

sporotrichosis (spo"ro-tri-ko'sis) infection with Sporotrichum.

Sporotrichum (spo-rot'ri-kum) a genus of fungi.

Sporozoa (spo"ro-zo'ah) a subphylum of Protozoa, made up exclusively of parasitic forms, which are unable to ingest particulate food or bacteria and depend on the availability of soluble cellular constituents in their environment.

sporozoan (-zo'an) 1. pertaining to sporozoa. 2. a sporozoon.

sporozoite (-zo'it) the infective form of a sporozoan parasite, which undergoes asexual reproduction (schizogony) in the body of the host.

sporozoon (-zo'on), pl. *sporozo'a* [Gr.] an individual organ or species of the subphylum Sporozoa.

sport (sport) an individual deviating beyond the normal range of variation in manifestation of characteristics not found in either of the parents.

sporulation (spor"u-la'shun) formation of spores.

sporule (spor'ul) a small spore.

spot (spot) a circumscribed area or a small blemish. **blind s.,** the area marking the site of entrance of the optic nerve on the retina. **cold s.,** any of the temperature spots where cold is normally perceived, but not heat. **focal s.,** the area of the target of an x-ray tube from which the x-rays are emitted. **germinal s.,** the nucleolus of the fertilized ovum. **hot s.,** any one of the temperature spots where heat is normally perceived, but not cold. **hypnogenetic s's,** superficial areas, stimulation of which brings on sleep. **Koplik's s's,** irregular, bright red spots on the buccal and lingual mucosa, with tiny bluish-white specks in the center of each, pathognomonic of beginning measles. **Mariotte's s.,** blind spot. **pain s's,** spots on the skin where alone the sense of pain can be produced by a stimulus. **Roth's s's,** round or oval white spots sometimes seen in the retina early in the course of subacute bacterial endocarditis. **Soemmerring's s.**, macula lutea. **Tardieu's s's**, spots of ecchymosis under the pleura after death by suffocation. **yellow s.**, macula lutea.

sprain (sprān) wrenching of a joint, with partial rupture of its ligaments.

spray (spra) a liquid minutely divided, as by a jet of air or steam.

sprue (sproo) 1. thrush. 2. a chronic disease marked by sore mouth, indigestion, diarrhea with frothy stools, loss of weight, and anemia.

spur (sper) a projecting piece of bone. **calcaneal s.**, a bone excrescence on the lower surface of the os calcis which frequently causes pain on walking.

sputum (spū'tum) material discharged from throat and respiratory passages and ejected from the mouth. **s. cruen'tum,** bloody sputum. **moss-agate s.**, a grayish, opalescent, gelatinous, mottled sputum, in a more or less globular form. **nummular s.**, sputum in rounded disks, shaped somewhat like coins. **rusty s.**, sputum stained with blood or blood pigments.

SQ subcutaneous.

squalene (skwa'lēn) a compound making up the greater part of liver oil of certain species of sharks of the family Squalidae.

squama (squa'mah), pl. *squa'mae* [L.] a scale, or thin, platelike structure.

squame (skwām) a scale or scalelike mass.

squamoparietal (skwa"mo-pah-ri'ĕ-tal) pertaining to the squamous portion of the temporal bone and the parietal bone.

squamous (skwa'mus) scaly or platelike.

squatting (skwot'ing) a position with hips and knees flexed, the buttocks resting on the heels; sometimes adopted by the parturient at delivery or by children with certain types of cardiac defects.

squill (skwil) the fleshy inner scales of the bulb of the white variety of *Urginea maritima* or *Urginea indica*; used for its effects on the heart.

squint (skwint) strabismus.

S.R. sedimentation rate; sigmoid reaction.

Sr chemical symbol, *strontium*.

S.R.N. State Registered Nurse (England and Wales).

sRNA transfer RNA (soluble RNA).

ss. [L.] *se'mis (one half).*

S. T. 37 (es"te ther"te-sev'en) trademark for a solution of hexylresorcinol.

STA serum thrombotic accelerator.

stability (stah-bil'ĭ-te) the quality of maintaining a constant character despite forces that threaten to disturb it.

stabilization (sta"bĭ-li-za'shun) the process of making firm and steady.

stable (sta'bel) not readily subject to change.

stactometer (stak-tom'ĕ-ter) device for measuring drops.

stadium (sta'de-um), pl. *sta'dia* [L.] stage. **s. decremen'ti,** the stage of defervescence. **s. incremen'ti,** the stage of increase of fever.

staff (staf) 1. an instrument introduced into the urethra as a guide in cutting. 2. the corps of physicians and surgeons attached to a hospital. **s. of Æsculapius,** the rod or staff with entwining snake, symbolic of the god of healing, official insignia of the American Medical Association. **attending s.**, the physicians and surgeons commonly concerned with the care of patients admitted to a hospital. **consulting s.**, specialists associated with a hospital and acting in an advisory capacity to the attending staff. **s. of Wrisberg,** an appearance seen in the normal larynx during laryngoscopic observation.

stage (stāj) 1. a definite period or distinct phase, as of development of a disease or of an organism. 2. the platform of a microscope on which the slide containing the object to be studied is placed. **algid s.**, a period marked by flickering pulse, subnormal temperature and varied nervous symptoms. **amphibolic s.**, the period between the acme and decline of an attack. **cold s.**, the period of chill or rigor in a malarial paroxysm. **eruptive s.**, the period during which an exanthem is appearing. **expulsive s.**, second stage. **first s.** (of labor), the time during which the fetal head is being molded and the cervix is becoming dilated. **fourth s.** (of labor), the period between expulsion of the placenta and occurrence of a satisfactory reaction of the mother to delivery. **hot s.**, period of pyrexia in a malarial paroxysm. **pre-eruptive s.**, the period following infection and preceding appearance of the exanthem of an exanthematous disease. **pyrogenetic s.**, stage of invasion of a febrile attack. **second s.** (of labor), the period during which the fetus is being expelled from the uterus. **third s.** (of labor), the period during which the placenta is being expelled from the uterus.

stain (stān) a substance used to impart color to tissues or cells, to facilitate microscopic study and identification. **acid s.**, one in which the color is carried by an acid and which has an affinity for basic elements in the specimen. **basic s.**, one in which the color is carried by a base and which has an affinity for the acidic elements in the specimen. **contrast s.**, a second stain used in preparation of a specimen, which colors other elements than those colored by the first, increasing the contrast between them. **differential s.**, one which facilitates differentiation of various elements in a specimen. **Gram's s.**, crystal violet solution and iodine solution, successively applied, followed by washing with ethyl alcohol. **metachromatic s.**, one which produces in certain elements colors different from that of the stain itself. **neutral s.**, one which is neither acid nor basic. **nuclear s.**, one which selectively stains cell nuclei, generally a basic stain. **port-wine s.**, nevus flammeus. **protoplasmic s.**, one which selectively stains cell protoplasm, generally an acid stain. **tumor s.**, an area of increased density in a radiograph, due to collection of contrast material in distorted and abnormal vessels, prominent in the capillary and venous phase of arteriography, and presumed to indicate neoplasm.

staining (stān'ing) artificial coloration of a substance to facilitate examination of tissues, microorganisms or other cells under the microscope. **intravital s.**, vital staining. **supravital s.**, staining of living tissue removed from the body. **vital s.**, staining of a tissue by a dye introduced into a living organism.

stalagmometer (stal″ag-mom′ĕ-ter) an instrument for measuring surface tension by determining the exact number of drops in a given quantity of a liquid.

stammering (stam′er-ing) stuttering.

standstill (stand′stil) cessation of motion, as of the heart *(cardiac standstill)* or chest *(respiratory standstill).*

stannum (stan′um) [L.] tin (symbol Sn).

stanolone (stan′o-lōn) a compound used as an androgenic substance.

stanozolol (stan′o-zo-lol″) a steroid compound used to improve appetite and promote gain in weight.

stapedectomy (sta″pe-dek′to-me) excision of the stapes.

stapedial (stah-pe′de-al) pertaining to the stapes.

stapediolysis (stah-pe″de-ol′ĭ-sis) mobilization of the stapes in the surgical treatment of otosclerosis.

stapedioplasty (stah-pe′de-o-plas″te) replacement of the stapes with other material which conducts vibrations from the incus to the oval window.

stapediotenotomy (stah-pe″de-o-tĕ-not′o-me) cutting of the tendon of the stapedius muscle.

stapediovestibular (-ves-tib′u-lar) pertaining to stapes and vestibule.

Staphcillin (staf-sil′in) trademark for a preparation of dimethoxyphenyl penicillin sodium.

staphyl(o)- (staf′i-lo) word element [Gr.], *uvula; like a bunch of grapes.*

staphylectomy (staf″i-lek′to-me) uvulectomy.

staphyledema (staf″il-ĕ-de′mah) edema of the uvula.

staphylin (staf′ĭ-lin) a lysogenic substance produced by active strains of staphylococci which prevents the growth of *Corynebacterium diphtheriae.*

staphyline (staf′ĭ-līn) 1. pertaining to the uvula. 2. shaped like a bunch of grapes.

staphylion (stah-fil′e-on) point at midline of posterior edge of hard palate.

staphylitis (staf″ĭ-li′tis) inflammation of the uvula.

staphyloangina (staf″ĭ-lo-an′jĭ-nah) mild sore throat with pseudomembrane, due to staphylococcus.

staphylocide (staf′ĭ-lo-sīd″) 1. destructive to staphylococci. 2. an agent destructive to staphylococci.

staphylococcemia (staf″ĭ-lo-kok-se′me-ah) staphylococci in the blood.

staphylococcosis (-kok-o′sis) infection caused by staphylococci.

Staphylococcus (-kok′us) a genus of Schizomycetes (order Eubacteriales, family Micrococcaceae).

staphylococcus (-kok′us), pl. *staphylococ′ci* [Gr.], a spherical microorganism which occurs in irregular clumps resembling bunches

of grapes. adj., **staphyloc′cal, staphylococ′cic.**

staphylodialysis (staf″ĭ-lo-di-al′ĭ-sis) relaxation of the uvula.

staphylokinase (-ki′nās) a bacterial kinase produced by certain strains of staphylococci.

staphylolysin (staf″ĭ-lol′ĭ-sin) a substance produced by staphylococci which causes hemolysis.

staphyloma (staf″ĭ-lo′mah) protrusion of the sclera or cornea. **anterior s.**, keratoglobus. **s. cor′neae,** bulging and thinning of the cornea. **posterior s., s. posti′cum,** backward bulging of the sclera at the posterior pole of the eye.

staphyloncus (staf″ĭ-long′kus) tumor of the uvula.

staphyloptosis (staf″ĭ-lop-to′sis) relaxation of the uvula.

staphyloschisis (staf″ĭ-los′kĭ-sis) fissure of the uvula and soft palate.

staphylotomy (-lot′o-me) excision or incision of the uvula or of a staphyloma.

star (star) a structure resembling the five-pointed figure representing the stars in the sky. **daughter s.**, amphiaster. **mother s.**, monaster. **s's of Verheyen,** stellate veins.

starch (starch) 1. the form in which carbohydrate is stored in plants. 2. granular material separated from mature grain of *Zea mays;* used as a dusting powder and pharmaceutic aid. **animal s.**, glycogen. **s. glycerite,** a preparation of starch, benzoic acid, purified water and glycerin, used topically as an emollient. **hydroxyethyl s.**, a starch product which has been suggested as a plasma substitute in man. **iodized s.**, starch that has been treated with iodine.

starvation (star-va′shun) long-continued deprival of food and its morbid effects.

stasibasiphobia (sta″si-ba″si-fo′be-ah) morbid distrust of one's ability to stand or walk.

stasiphobia (sta″si-fo′be-ah) morbid dread of standing erect.

stasis (sta′sis) a stoppage of flow, as of blood or other body fluid, or of intestinal contents. **urinary s.**, stoppage of the flow of urine, at any level of the urinary tract.

-stasis (sta′sis) word element [Gr.], *maintenance of (or maintaining) a constant level; preventing increase or multiplication.* adj., **-stat′ic.**

stat. [L.] *sta′tim* (at once).

state (stāt) condition or situation. **dream s.**, a state of defective consciousness in which the environment is imperfectly perceived. **excited s.**, the condition of a nucleus, atom or molecule produced by the addition of energy to the system as the result of absorption of photons or of inelastic collisions with other particles or systems. **ground s.**, the condition of lowest energy of a nucleus, atom or molecule. **metastable s.**, the condition of a system (nucleus, atom or molecule) capable of undergoing quantum transition to a state of lower energy. **refractory s.**, a condition of subnormal excitability of muscle and nerve following excitation. **resting s.**, the physiologic condition achieved by complete bed rest for at least one hour. **stable s.**, the condition of a system in which it does not readily undergo change. **steady s.**, dynamic equilibrium.

static (stat′ik) not in motion; at rest.

statics (stat′iks) that phase of mechanics which deals with the action of forces and systems of forces on bodies at rest.

statim (sta′tim) [L.] at once.

station (sta′shun) 1. the manner of standing. 2. a fixed place.

statistics (stah-tis′tiks) 1. numerical facts pertaining to a particular subject or body of objects. 2. the science dealing with the collection and tabulation of numerical facts. **vital s.**, numerical facts pertaining to human natality, morbidity and mortality.

statoconia (stat″o-ko′ne-ah), sing. *statoco′-nium* [Gr.] minute calcareous particles in the gelatinous membrane surmounting the macula in the inner ear.

statocyst (stat′o-sist) one of the sacs of the labyrinth to which is attributed an influence in the maintenance of static equilibrium.

statolith (stat′o-lith) a solid or semisolid body occurring in the statocyst of animals.

statometer (stah-tom′ĕ-ter) apparatus for measuring degree of exophthalmos.

status (sta′tus) [L.] condition or state. **s. asthmat′icus**, asthmatic crisis; asthmatic shock. **s. epilep′ticus**, rapid succession of epileptic spasms. **s. lymphat′icus**, a condition marked by enlarged thymus and spleen, hyperplasia of the lymphatic tissues and lowered bodily vitality. **s. thymicolymphat′icus**, a condition resembling status lymphaticus, with enlargement of lymphadenoid tissue and of the thymus. **s. verruco′sus**, a wartlike appearance of the cerebral cortex, produced by disorderly arrangement of the neuroblasts so that the formation of fissures and sulci is irregular and unpredictable.

staurion (staw′re-on) intersection of the median and transverse palatine sutures.

stauroplegia (staw″ro-ple′je-ah) crossed hemiplegia.

steapsin (ste-ap′sin) lipase.

stear(o)- (ste′ah-ro) word element [Gr.], *fat.*

stearate (ste′ah-rāt) any compound of stearic acid.

stearin (ste′ah-rin) a white, solid crystalline substance, $C_3H_5(C_{15}H_{35}COO)_3$, from fat.

stearodermia (ste″ah-ro-der′me-ah) disease of the skin involving the sebaceous glands.

stearopten (ste″ah-rop′ten) the solid constituent of a volatile oil.

steat(o)- (ste′ah-to) word element [Gr.], *fat; oil.*

steatadenoma (ste″at-ad″ĕ-no′mah) adenoma of the sebaceous glands.

steatitis (ste″ah-ti′tis) inflammation of adipose tissue.

steatocele (ste-at′o-sēl) fatty swelling of the scrotum.

steatocryptosis (ste″ah-to-krip-to′sis) disorder of function of sebaceous glands.

steatogenous (ste″ah-toj′ĕ-nus) producing fat.

steatolysis (-tol′ĭ-sis) the emulsification of fats preparatory to absorption. adj., **steatolyt′ic.**

steatoma (ste″ah-to′mah) 1. lipoma. 2. a fatty mass retained within a sebaceous gland.

steatomatosis (ste″ah-to″mah-to′sis) the presence of numerous sebaceous cysts.

steatonecrosis (-ne-kro′sis) fatty necrosis.

steatopathy (ste″ah-top′ah-the) disease of the sebaceous glands.

steatopygia (ste″ah-to-pij′e-ah) excessive fatness of the buttocks.

steatorrhea (-re′ah) excess fat in feces.

steatosis (ste″ah-to′sis) 1. disease of sebaceous glands. 2. fatty degeneration.

stechiology (stek″e-ol′o-je) stoichiology.

stechiometry (-om′ĕ-tre) stoichiometry.

Steclin (stek′lin) trademark for preparations of tetracycline hydrochloride.

stegnosis (steg-no′sis) 1. stoppage of a secretion. 2. stenosis. adj., **stegnot′ic.**

Stegomyia (steg″o-mi′yah) a genus of mosquitoes.

Stelangium (ste-lan′je-um) a genus of Schizomycetes (order Myxobacterales, family Archangiaceae).

Stelazine (stel′ah-zēn) trademark for preparations of trifluoperazine.

stella (stel′ah), pl. *stel′lae* [L.] star.

stellate (stel′āt) star-shaped; arranged in rosettes.

stellectomy (stel-lek′to-me) excision of a portion of the stellate ganglion.

stellula (stel′ú-lah), pl. *stel′lulae* [L.] a little starlike mass or figure. **stel′lulae of Verheyen,** stellate veins.

Stenediol (sten′di-ol) trademark for preparations of methandriol.

steno- (sten′o) word element [Gr.], *narrow; contracted; constriction.*

stenocardia (sten″o-kar′de-ah) angina pectoris.

stenocephaly (-sef′ah-le) narrowness of the head or cranium.

stenochoria (-ko′re-ah) stenosis.

stenocoriasis (-ko-ri′ah-sis) contraction of the pupil.

stenopeic (-pe′ik) having a narrow opening or slit.

stenosed (stĕ-nōst′, stĕ-nōzd′) narrowed; constricted.

stenosis (stĕ-no′sis) narrowing or contraction of a body passage or opening. **aortic s.**, obstruction to the outflow of blood from the left ventricle into the aorta at the subvalvular, valvular or supravalvular level, with a pressure gradient across the site of obstruction. **mitral s.**, a narrowing of the left atrioventricular orifice. **pulmonic s.**, obstruction to the outflow of blood from the right ventricle, with systolic pressure considerably higher in the ventricle than in the pulmonary trunk. **pyloric s.**, hypertrophic obstruction of the pyloric orifice of the stomach. **tricuspid s.**, narrowing or stricture of the tricuspid orifice of the heart.

stenostomia (sten″o-sto′me-ah) narrowing of the mouth.

stenothermal (-ther′mal) stenothermic.

stenothermic (-ther′mik) pertaining to or characterized by tolerance of only a narrow range of temperature.

stenothorax (-tho′raks) an abnormally straight, short or narrow thorax.

stenotic (stĕ-not'ik) marked by abnormal narrowing or constriction.

stent (stent) an impression or mold made of Stent's mass; improperly used as a verb to indicate making such an impression or supporting with such a mold.

stephanion (ste-fa'ne-on), pl. *stepha'nia* [Gr.] intersection of temporal ridge and coronal suture.

Sterane (ster'ān) trademark for preparations of prednisolone.

sterco- (ster'ko) word element [L.], *feces*.

stercobilin (ster″ko-bi'lin) hydrobilirubin from fecal matter.

stercoraceous (-ra'shus) consisting of feces.

stercorolith (ster′ko-ro-lith″) fecalith.

stercoroma (ster″ko-ro'mah) a tumor-like mass of fecal matter in the rectum.

stercus (ster'kus) [L.] dung or feces. adj., **ster′coral, stercorous**.

stereo- (ste're-o) word element [Gr.], *solid; having 3 dimensions; firmly established*.

stereoarthrolysis (ste″re-o-ar-throl'ĭ-sis) formation of a movable new joint in cases of bony ankylosis.

stereoauscultation (-aus″kul-ta'shun) auscultation with two stethoscopes, on different parts of the chest.

stereochemistry (-kem'is-tre) the branch of chemistry treating of the space relations of atoms in molecules. adj., **stereochem'ical**.

stereocinefluorography (-sin″e-floo″or-og'rah-fe) photographic recording by motion picture camera of images observed by stereoscopic fluoroscopy.

stereoencephalotome (-en-sef'ah-lo-tōm″) a guiding instrument used in stereoencephalotomy.

stereoencephalotomy (-en-sef″ah-lot'o-me) the production of sharply circumscribed lesions in subcortical ganglia or pathways by means of accurately placed electrodes.

stereognosis (ste″re-og-no'sis) the sense by which form of objects is perceived

stereoisomer (ste″re-o-i'so-mer) a compound showing stereoisomerism.

stereoisomerism (-i-som'er-izm) isomerism in which the compounds have the same structural formulas, but the atoms are distributed differently in space.

Stereo-orthopter (-or-thop'ter) a proprietary mirror-reflecting instrument for correcting strabismus.

stereoplasm (ste're-o-plazm″) the more solid portion of protoplasm.

stereoroentgenography (ste″re-o-rent″gen-og'rah-fe) the making of a stereoscopic roentgenogram.

stereoscopic (-skop'ik) three-dimensional; having depth, as well as height and width.

stereospecific (-spĕ-sif'ik) exhibiting structural specificity in interacting with a substrate or a limited class of substrates.

stereotaxic (-tak'sik) pertaining to or characterized by precise positioning in space.

stereotaxis (-tak'sis) taxis in response to the stimulus of contact with a solid. adj., **stereotac'tic**.

stereotropism (ste″re-ot'ro-pizm) tropism in

response to contact with a solid or rigid surface.

stereotypy (ste're-o-ti″pe) persistent repetition of senseless acts or words.

sterile (ster'il) 1. free from pathogenic microorganisms. 2. unable to produce offspring.

sterility (stĕ-ril'ĭ-te) 1. freedom from pathogenic microorganisms. 2. inability to produce offspring.

sterilization (ster″il-i-za'shun) 1. the process of rendering an individual incapable of reproduction. 2. the process of destroying all microorganisms and their pathogenic products.

sterilizer (ster'ĭ-līz′er) an apparatus used in ridding instruments, dressings, etc., of all microorganisms and their pathogenic products.

Sterisil (ster'ĭ-sil) trademark for a preparation of hexetidine.

stern(o)- (ster'no) word element, *sternum*.

sternalgia (ster-nal'je-ah) pain in the sternum.

sternebra (ster'ne-brah), pl. *ster'nebrae* [L.] one of the segments forming the sternum in certain animals.

sternoclavicular (ster″no-klah-vik'u-lar) pertaining to sternum and clavicle.

sternoclavicularis (-klah-vik″u-la'ris) [L.] sternoclavicular.

sternocleidomastoid (-kli″do-mas'toid) pertaining to sternum, clavicle and mastoid process.

sternocostal (-kos'tal) pertaining to sternum and ribs.

sternodymia (-dim'e-ah) union of two fetuses by the anterior chest wall.

sternodymus (ster-nod'ĭ-mus) conjoined twins united at the anterior chest wall.

sternohyoid (ster″no-hi'oid) pertaining to the sternum and hyoid bone.

sternoid (ster'noid) resembling the sternum.

sternomastoid (ster″no-mas'toid) sternocleidomastoid.

sternopagus (ster-nop'ah-gus) sternodymus.

sternopericardial (ster″no-per″ĭ-kar'de-al) pertaining to sternum and pericardium.

sternotomy (ster-not'o-me) incision of the sternum.

sternothyroid (ster″no-thy'roid) pertaining to the sternum and thyroid.

sternum (ster'num) a plate of bone forming the middle of the anterior wall of the thorax. adj., **ster'nal**.

sternutatory (ster-nu'tah-tor″e) 1. causing sneezing. 2. an agent that causes sneezing.

steroid (ste'roid) a complex molecule containing carbon atoms in four interlocking rings, three of which contain six carbon atoms each and the fourth of which contains five.

steroidogenesis (ste-roi″do-jen'ĕ-sis) production of steroids, as by the adrenal glands.

sterol (ste'rol) a solid alcohol of animal or vegetable origin, having properties like the fats.

sterolytic (ste″ro-lit'ik) capable of dissolving sterols.

Sterosan (ster'o-san) trademark for preparations of chlorquinaldol.

stertor (ster'tor) snoring; sonorous respiration. adj., **ster'torous**.

steth(o)- (steth'o) word element [Gr.], *chest.*
stethalgia (steth-al'je-ah) pain in the chest or chest wall.
stethogoniometer (steth″o-go″ne-om'ĕ-ter) apparatus for measuring curvature of the chest.
stethoscope (steth'o-skōp) instrument for performing mediate auscultation.
stethoscopy (steth-os'ko-pe) examination with the stethoscope.
stethospasm (steth'o-spazm) spasm of the chest muscles.
STH somatotropic hormone.
sthenic (sthen'ik) characterized by overaction; strong.
sthenophotic (sthen″o-fo'tik) able to see in a strong light.
stibamine (stib'ah-min) sodium amino-phenylstibinate; used in treatment of kala-azar.
stibialism (stib'e-al-izm″) antimonial poisoning.
stibium (stib'e-um) [L.] antimony (symbol Sb).
stigma (stig'mah), pl. *stig'mas, stig'mata* [Gr.] 1. a characteristic abnormality, or an indication of an abnormal or morbid condition. 2. a spot or impression on the skin. adj., **stigmat'ic. stigmata of degeneracy,** bodily abnormalities found in considerable number in degenerate persons. **Giuffrida-Ruggieri s.,** abnormal shallowness of the glenoid fossa. **hysterical stigmata,** bodily marks or signs characteristic of hysteria. **malpighian stigmata,** the points where the smaller veins enter into the larger veins of the spleen. **stigmata may'dis,** zea.
stigmasterol (stig-mas'tĕ-rol) a sterol isolated from soya and calabar beans, which has been converted into progesterone and desoxycorticosterone.
stigmatization (stig″mah-tĭ-za'shun) the formation of stigmas.
stigmatosis (-to'sis) a skin disease marked by ulcerated spots.
stilalgin (stil-al'jin) mephenesin.
stilbestrol (stil-bes'trol) diethylstilbestrol.
Stilbetin (stil-be'tin) trademark for a preparation of diethylstilbestrol.
stilet (sti'let) 1. a delicate probe. 2. a wire used to stiffen or clear a catheter.
stillbirth (stil'berth) birth of a dead child.
stillborn (stil'born) born dead.
stimulant (stim'u-lant) 1. producing stimulation. 2. an agent which stimulates. **alcoholic s.,** one with ethyl alcohol as its basis. **cardiac s.,** one which increases the heart's action. **cerebral s.,** one which exalts action of the brain. **diffusible s.,** one which acts promptly, but transiently. **general s.,** one which acts upon the whole body. **hepatic s.,** one which arouses the functions of the liver. **spinal s.,** one which acts upon or through the spinal cord. **vascular s.,** one which excites vasomotor nerves.
stimulate (stim'u-lāt) to excite functional activity in a part.
stimulation (stim″u-la'shun) the act or process of stimulating; the condition of being stimulated. **audio-visual-tactile s.,** the simultaneous rhythmic excitation of the receptors for the senses of hearing, sight and touch.

stimulon (stim'u-lon) a protein factor produced by interaction of two viruses that favors virus multiplication.
stimulus (stim'u-lus) any agent, act or influence which produces functional or trophic reaction in a receptor or an irritable tissue. **adequate s.,** a stimulus of the specific form of energy to which a given receptor is sensitive. **chemical s.,** one that acts by a chemical process. **electric s.,** application of electricity. **heterologous s.,** one that acts upon all the nerve elements of the sensory apparatus. **homologous s.,** adequate stimulus. **mechanical s.,** one which acts by mechanical means. **thermal s.,** a stimulant application of heat. **threshold s.,** one of such strength that it may or may not be effective.
sting (sting) injury due to a biotoxin introduced into an individual or with which he comes in contact, together with mechanical trauma incident to its introduction.
stippling (stip'pling) a spotted condition or appearance, such as an appearance of the retina as if dotted with light and dark points, or the spotted appearance of red blood corpuscles in basophilia.
stirrup (stir'up) stapes.
stitch (stich) 1. a sudden cutting pain. 2. a loop made in sewing or suturing.
stochastic (sto-kas'tik) arrived at by skillful conjecturing.
stoichiology (stoi″ke-ol'o-je) the science of elements, especially the physiology of the cellular elements of tissues. adj., **stoichiolog'ic.**
stoichiometry (-om'ĕ-tre) the science of the numerical relations of chemical elements and compounds and the mathematical laws of chemical changes. adj., **stoichiomet'ric.**
stoke (stōk) a unit of kinematic viscosity, being that of fluid with a viscosity of one poise and a density of one gram per cubic centimeter.
stoma (sto'mah), pl. *sto'mas, sto'mata* [Gr.] a mouthlike opening, particularly an incised opening which is kept open for drainage or other purposes. adj., **sto'mal.**
stomach (stum'ak) the musculomembranous digestive pouch between the esophagus and duodenum. **hourglass s.,** one shaped somewhat like an hourglass. **leather-bottle s.,** one with severe hypertrophy of the stomach wall, usually leading to contraction of the cavity. **powdered s.,** dried and powdered defatted wall of the stomach of the hog; used in treatment of pernicious anemia.
stomachal (stum'ah-kal) stomachic.
stomachalgia (stum″ah-kal'je-ah) pain in the stomach.
stomachic (sto-mak'ik) a gastric stimulant.
stomat(o)- (sto'mah-to) word element [Gr.], *mouth.*
stomatalgia (sto″mah-tal'je-ah) pain in the mouth.
stomatitis (-ti'tis) generalized inflammation of the oral mucosa. **aphthous s.,** inflammation of the oral mucosa, with vesicle formation. **gangrenous s.,** inflammation of the oral mucosa, with destruction of tissue. **herpetic s.,** an acute infection of the oral mucosa, due to the virus of herpes simplex.

mercurial s., stomatitis arising from mercury poisoning. **mycotic s.**, stomatitis due to a fungus. **ulcerative s.**, stomatitis with shallow ulcers. **ulceromembranous s.**, Vincent's s., Vincent's angina.

stomatodynia (sto″mah-to-din′e-ah) pain in the mouth.

stomatogastric (-gas′trik) pertaining to stomach and mouth.

stomatography (sto″mah-tog′rah-fe) a description of the mouth.

stomatology (-tol′o-je) sum of what is known about the mouth.

stomatomalacia (sto″mah-to-mah-la′she-ah) softening of the structures of the mouth.

stomatomycosis (-mi-ko′sis) a fungus disease of the mouth.

stomatonecrosis (-ne-kro′sis) noma.

stomatopathy (sto″mah-top′ah-the) any disorder of the mouth.

stomatoplasty (sto′mah-to-plas″te) plastic reconstruction of the mouth.

stomatorrhagia (sto″mah-to-ra′je-ah) hemorrhage from the mouth.

stomocephalus (sto″mo-sef′ah-lus) fetus with rudimentary jaws and mouth.

stomodeum (-de′um) the ectodermal depression at the head end of the embryo, which becomes the front part of the mouth.

-stomy (sto′me) word element [Gr.], *creation of an opening into* or *a communication between.*

stone (stōn) 1. a calculus. 2. a unit of weight, equivalent in the English system to 14 pounds avoirdupois.

stool (stōōl) the fecal discharge from the bowels. **lienteric s.**, feces containing much undigested food. **rice water s.**, the watery stool flecked with fragments of necrotic mucosal epithelium, characteristic of cholera.

storax (sto′raks) a balsam obtained from the trunk of trees of the genus Liquidambar; used locally in scabies.

stosstherapy (stos″ther′ah-pe) treatment of a disease by a single massive dose of a therapeutic agent or by short-term administration of unphysiologically large doses.

strabismometer (strah-biz-mom′e-ter) apparatus for measuring strabismus.

strabismus (strah-biz′mus) absence of normal relations of the visual axes in the primary position or failure of the eyes to follow one another normally in any conjunctive or disjunctive movement. adj., **strabis′mic. comitant s.**, that in which the angle of deviation of the visual axis of the squinting eye is always the same, no matter what the direction of gaze. **convergent s.**, esotropia. **divergent s.**, exotropia. **horizontal s.**, that in which the visual axis of the squinting eye deviates in the horizontal plane (esotropia or exotropia). **noncomitant s.**, that in which the angle of deviation does not remain the same in the various positions of gaze. **vertical s.**, that in which the visual axis of the squinting eye deviates in the vertical plane (hypertropia or hypotropia).

strabotomy (strah-bot′o-me) section of an ocular tendon in treatment of strabismus.

strain (strān) 1. to overexercise. 2. to filter. 3. an overstretching or overexertion of some part of the musculature. 4. excessive effort. 5. a group of organisms within a species or variety, characterized by some particular quality, as rough or smooth strains of bacteria. **rough s., r s.**, a type of microorganisms resulting from microbic dissociation, producing colonies with a dull, uneven surface and irregular border; the growth in fluid media tends to flake out, no capsules are seen, and the culture tends to be less virulent. **smooth s., s s.**, a type of microorganisms resulting from microbic dissociation, producing colonies with a smooth surface and unbroken border; the culture tends to be more virulent. **Vi s.**, a strain of *Eberthella typhi* which is encapsulated and virulent.

strait (strāt) a narrow passage. **s's of the pelvis,** the openings of the true pelvis, distinguished as superior and inferior.

stramonium (strah-mo′ne-um) dried leaves and flowering or fruiting tops of *Datura stramonium;* used in parasympathetic blockade.

strangles (strang′gelz) infectious disease of horses with mucopurulent inflammation of the respiratory mucous membrane.

strangulation (strang″gu-la′shun) 1. arrest of respiration by occlusion of the air passages. 2. impairment of the blood supply to a part by mechanical constriction of the vessels.

strangury (strang′gu-re) slow and painful discharge of urine.

strap (strap) to bind with overlapping strips of adhesive plaster.

stratiform (strat′ĭ-form) occurring in layers.

stratigraphy (strah-tig′rah-fe) a method of body-section roentgenography with the x-ray tube moved in only one direction, usually an arc. adj., **stratigraph′ic.**

stratosphere (strat′o-sfēr) the outermost layer of the earth's atmosphere, extending between the altitudes of 8 to 10 miles.

stratum (stra′tum), pl. *stra′ta* [L.] a sheetlike mass of tissue of fairly uniform thickness; used in anatomic nomenclature to designate distinct layers making up various tissues or organs, as of the skin, brain, retina. **s. cor′neum,** outer, horny layer of the epidermis. **s. granulo′sum,** 1. the layer of epidermis next to the stratum corneum. 2. one of the layers of the retina. 3. a layer of the cortex of the cerebellum. 4. the cellular layer of the wall of an ovarian follicle. **s. lu′cidum,** stratum corneum. **s. malpig′hii, s. muco′sum, s. spino′sum,** rete mucosum. **zonal s.,** a layer of white fibers on the surface of the thalamus.

streak (strēk) a line or stripe. **angioid s's,** pigmented streaks appearing in the retina after hemorrhage. **meningeal s.,** tache cérébrale. **primitive s.,** a thickened axial band appearing caudally on the surface of the embryonic disk.

strephosymbolia (stref″o-sim-bo′le-ah) reading difficulty with confusion between similar but opposite letters (b-d, p-q), and a tendency to read backward.

strepogenin (strep″o-jen′in) a factor in casein

and certain other proteins which is essential to optimal growth of animals.

strepto- (strep'to) word element [Gr.], *twisted.*

Streptobacillus (strep''to-bah-sil'lus) a genus of Schizomycetes (order Eubacteriales, family Bacteroidaceae).

streptobacillus (-bah-sil'lus) an organism of the genus Streptobacillus.

Streptococceae (-kok'se-e) a tribe of Schizomycetes (order Eubacteriales, family Lactobacillaceae).

streptococcemia (-kok-se'me-ah) occurrence of streptococci in the blood.

streptococcolysin (-kok-ol'ĭ-sin) streptolysin.

streptococcosis (-kok-o'sis) infection caused by streptococci.

Streptococcus (-kok'us) a genus of Schizomycetes (order Eubacteriales, family Lactobacillaceae, tribe Streptococceae).

streptococcus (-kok'us), pl. *streptococ'ci* [Gr.] an organism of the genus Streptococcus.

streptocyte (strep'to-sīt) an amebiform body from vesicles of foot-and-mouth disease.

streptodermatitis (strep''to-der''mah-ti'tis) dermatitis produced by streptococci.

streptodornase (-dor'nās) a substance produced by hemolytic streptococci which catalyzes the depolymerization of deoxyribonucleic acid (DNA).

streptokinase (-ki'nās) an enzyme produced by streptococci which catalyzes the conversion of plasminogen to plasmin. **s.-streptodornase,** a mixture of enzymes elaborated by hemolytic streptococci; used as a proteolytic and fibrinolytic agent.

streptoleukocidin (-lu''ko-si'din) a toxin from streptococci which is destructive to leukocytes.

streptolysin (strep-tol'ĭ-sin) the hemolysin of hemolytic streptococci.

Streptomyces (strep''to-mi'sēz) a genus of Schizomycetes (order Actinomycetales, family Streptomycetaceae), usually soil forms, but occasionally parasitic on plants and animals, and notable as the source of various antibiotics, e.g. the tetracyclines.

Streptomycetaceae (-mi''se-ta'se-e) a family of Schizomycetes (order Actinomycetales), primarily soil forms and some parasitic species.

streptomycin (-mi'sin) an antibiotic substance produced by a species of Streptomyces.

streptonivicin (-ni'vĭ-sin) novobiocin.

Streptosporangium (-spo-ran'je-um) a genus of Schizomycetes (order Actinomycetales, family Actinoplanaceae) found in soil and water.

streptothricin (-thri'sin) an antibiotic substance active against gram-negative and gram-positive bacteria.

stress (stres) 1. forcibly exerted influence; pressure. 2. the sum of all nonspecific biological phenomena elicited by adverse external influences, including damage and defense.

stretcher (strech'er) a contrivance for carrying sick or wounded.

stria (stri'ah), pl. *stri'ae* [L.] 1. a streak or line. 2. a narrow, bandlike structure; used in anatomic nomenclature to designate longitudinal collections of nerve fibers in the brain. **stri'ae acus'ticae,** striae medullares. **atrophic striae, stri'ae atroph'icae,** abnormal lines on the skin after subsidence of distention, as by a pregnant uterus or a tumor, or occurring in adrenal cortical hyperactivity or idiopathically. **stri'ae gravida'rum,** striae atrophicae occurring in pregnancy. **striae longitudina'les latera'les,** two white lines across upper surface of the callosum. **striae medulla'res,** white lines across the floor of fourth ventricle. **s. pinea'lis,** the anterior peduncle of the pineal gland.

striate (stri'āt) having streaks or striae.

striation (stri-a'shun) 1. quality of being streaked. 2. a streak or scratch, or a series of streaks.

Striatran (stri'ah-tran) trademark for a preparation of emylcamate.

stricture (strik'tūr) abnormal narrowing of a duct or passage.

stricturotome (strik'tu-ro-tōm'') instrument for cutting strictures.

stricturotomy (strik''tu-rot'o-me) incision of a stricture.

stridor (stri'dor) a shrill, harsh sound. adj., **strid'ulous. s. den'tium,** grinding of the teeth, especially during sleep.

striocerebellar (stri''o-ser''ĕ-bel'ar) pertaining to corpus striatum and cerebellum.

strobila (stro-bi'lah) the entire adult tapeworm, including the scolex, neck and proglottids.

stroboscope (stro'bo-skōp) an apparatus for exhibiting the successive phases of animal movements.

stroke (strōk) a sudden, severe attack; a popular term for rupture of a cerebral blood vessel, causing symptoms of varying severity. **apoplectic s.,** apoplexy. **heat s.,** a condition caused by exposure to excessive heat. **little s.,** a slight extravasation of blood from a cerebral blood vessel, often causing only slight or no symptoms.

stroma (stro'mah), pl. *stro'mata* [Gr.] the tissue forming the ground substance, framework or matrix of an organ. adj., **stro'mal, stromat'ic.**

stromuhr (strōm'oor) an instrument for measuring the velocity of blood flow.

Strongyloides (stron''jĭ-loi'dēz) a genus of nematode parasites. **S. stercora'lis,** a species found in the intestine of man and other mammals, primarily in the tropics and subtropics.

strongyloidiasis (stron''jĭ-loi-di'ah-sis) infection with organisms of the genus Strongyloides.

strongyloidosis (-do'sis) strongyloidiasis.

strongylosis (stron''jĭ-lo'sis) infection with Strongylus.

Strongylus (stron'jĭ-lus) a genus of nematode parasites.

strontium (stron'she-um) chemical element (*see table*), at. no. 38, symbol Sr. **s. bromide,** odorless, bitter, crystalline substance, suggested as a substitute for potassium bromide.

s. salicylate, odorless, sweet and salty crystalline powder, used in salicylic acid therapy.

strontiuresis (stron″she-u-re′sis) elimination of strontium from the body through the kidneys. adj., **strontiuret′ic.**

strophulus (strof′u-lus) a papular eruption occurring in infants.

struma (stroo′mah) enlargement of the thyroid gland. **Hashimoto's s., s. lymphomato′sa,** a progressive disease of the thyroid gland with degeneration of its epithelial elements and replacement by lymphoid and fibrous tissue. **s. malig′na,** carcinoma of the thyroid gland. **s. ova′rii,** an ovarian tumor containing iodine. **Riedel's s.,** a chronic, proliferating, fibrosing, inflammatory process involving usually one but sometimes both lobes of the thyroid gland, as well as the trachea and other adjacent structures.

strumectomy (stroo-mek′to-me) thyroidectomy.

strumitis (stroo-mi′tis) thyroiditis.

strumoderma (stroo″mo-der′mah) scrofuloderma.

strumous (stroo′mus) scrofulous.

strychnine (strik′nīn) an alkaloid from seeds of *Strychnos nux-vomica;* used as a central nervous stimulant.

strychninomania (strik″nin-o-ma′ne-ah) psychosis caused by strychnine.

strychnism (strik′nizm) poisoning by strychnine.

S.T.S. serologic test for syphilis.

stump (stump) distal end of a limb left after amputation.

stupe (stoōp) a hot, wet cloth or sponge, charged with a medication for external application.

stupefacient (stu″pē-fa′shent) 1. inducing stupor. 2. an agent that induces stupor.

stupefactive (-fak′tiv) producing narcosis or stupor.

stupor (stu′por) partial or nearly complete unconsciousness; a state of lethargy and immobility with diminished responsiveness to stimulation.

stuttering (stut′er-ing) a speech problem characterized chiefly by repetition of parts of words and whole words, prolongation of sounds, interjection of sounds or words, and unduly prolonged pauses.

sty (sti), pl. *sties,* hordeolum. **meibomian s.,** inflammation of a meibomian gland. **zeisian s.,** inflammation of a zeisian gland.

styl(o)- (sti′lo) word element [L., Gr.], *stake; pole; styloid process of the temporal bone.*

styloid (sti′loid) long and pointed, like a pen or stylus.

styloiditis (sti″loi-di′tis) inflammation of tissues around the styloid process.

stylomastoid (sti″lo-mas′toid) pertaining to styloid and mastoid processes of the temporal bone.

stylomaxillary (-mak′si-ler″e) pertaining to the styloid process of the temporal bone and the maxilla.

stylus (sti′lus) 1. a stilet. 2. a pencil or stick, as of caustic.

stype (stīp) a tampon or pledget of cotton.

stypsis (stip′sis) 1. astringency; astringent action. 2. use of styptics.

styptic (stip′tik) 1. arresting hemorrhage by means of an astringent quality. 2. a markedly astringent remedy.

Stypven (stip′ven) trademark for a preparation of Russell's viper venom; used as a hemostatic agent.

styramate (stir′ah-māt) a compound used as a skeletal muscle relaxant.

styrol (sti′rol) a liquid hydrocarbon from storax, or synthesized from benzene and ethylene.

styrone (sti′rōn) cinnamic alcohol, $C_9H_{10}O$.

Suavitil (swav′ĭ-til) trademark for a preparation of benactyzine.

sub (sub) [L.] preposition, *under;* used also as a prefix, *under; less than.*

subabdominal (sub″ab-dom′ĭ-nal) below the abdomen.

subacetate (sub-as′ĕ-tāt) a basic acetate.

subacid (-as′id) somewhat acid.

subacromial (sub″ah-kro′me-al) below the acromion.

subacute (-ah-kūt′) somewhat acute; between acute and chronic.

subalimentation (-al-ĭ-men-ta′shun) insufficient nourishment.

subaponeurotic (-ap-o-nu-rot′ik) below an aponeurosis.

subarachnoid (-ah-rak′noid) below the arachnoid.

subarachnoiditis (-ah-rak″noid-i′tis) inflammation on the lower surface of the arachnoid.

subareolar (-ah-re′o-lar) beneath the areola of the nipple.

subastragalar (-as-trag′ah-lar) below the astragalus.

subastringent (-ah-strin′jent) moderately astringent.

subaural (sub-aw′ral) below the ear.

subaurale (sub″aw-ra′le) an anthropometric landmark, the lowest point on the inferior border of the ear lobule when the subject is looking straight ahead.

subcapsular (sub-kap′su-lar) below a capsule, especially the capsule of the cerebrum.

subcarbonate (-kar′bon-āt) a basic carbonate.

subcartilaginous (-kar″tĭ-laj′ĭ-nus) 1. below a cartilage. 2. partly cartilaginous.

subchronic (-kron′ik) between chronic and subacute.

subclavian (-kla′ve-an) below the clavicle.

subclavicular (sub″klah-vik′u-lar) subclavian.

subclinical (sub-klin′ĭ-kal) without clinical manifestations.

subconjunctival (sub″kon-jungk-ti′val) beneath the conjunctiva.

subconscious (sub-kon′shus) imperfectly or partially conscious, yet capable of being made conscious by an effort of memory or by association of ideas.

subconsciousness (-kon′shus-nes) 1. partial unconsciousness. 2. the area of mental activity below the level of conscious perception.

subcoracoid (-kor′ah-koid) situated under the coracoid process.

subcortex (-kor′teks) the brain substance underlying the cortex. adj., **subcor′tical.**

subcostal (-kos′tal) below a rib or ribs.

subcostalgia (sub″kos-tal′je-ah) pain over the subcostal nerve.

subcostalis (sub″kos-ta′lis), pl. *subcosta′les* [L.] subcostal.

subcranial (sub-kra′ne-al) below the cranium.

subcrepitant (-krep′ĭ-tant) somewhat crepitant in nature.

subculture (-kul′tūr) culture of bacteria derived from another culture.

subcutaneous (sub″ku-ta′ne-us) beneath the layers of the skin.

subcuticular (sub″ku-tik′u-lar) below the cuticle.

subdelirium (sub″dĕ-lir′e-um) mild delirium.

subdiaphragmatic (sub-di″ah-frag-mat′ik) below the diaphragm.

subdural (sub-du′ral) below the dura.

subencephalon (sub″en-sef′ah-lon) the pons, oblongata, crura and corpora quadrigemina.

subendocardial (-en-do-kar′de-al) below the endocardium.

subendothelial (-en-do-the′le-al) below the endothelium.

subepidermal (-ep-ĭ-der′mal) below the epidermis.

subepithelial (-ep-ĭ-the′le-al) below the epithelium.

subfamily (sub-fam′ĭ-le) a taxonomic order sometimes established, subordinate to a family and superior to a tribe.

subfascial (-fash′al) below a fascia.

subfebrile (-feb′ril) somewhat febrile.

subfertility (sub″fer-til′ĭ-te) a state of less than normal fertility.

subfrontal (sub-frun′tal) below a frontal lobe or convolution.

subglenoid (-gle′noid) below the glenoid fossa.

subglossal (-glos′al) below the tongue.

subgrondation (sub″gron-da′shun) depression of one fragment of bone beneath another.

subhepatic (-hĕ-pat′ik) below the liver.

subhyoid (sub-hi′oid) below the hyoid bone.

subiculum (su-bik′u-lum) an underlying or supporting structure.

subiliac (sub-il′e-ak) below the ilium.

subilium (-il′e-um) the lowest portion of the ilium.

subinfection (sub″in-fek′shun) a mild infection.

subinvolution (-vo-lu′shun) incomplete involution.

subiodide (sub-i′o-dīd) that iodide of any series containing the least iodine.

subjacent (-ja′sent) located below.

subject (sub′jekt) 1. person or animal subjected to treatment or experiment. 2. a body for dissection.

subjective (sub-jek′tiv) perceived only by the individual involved, and not perceptible to the senses of another person.

subjugal (-ju′gal) below the malar bone.

sublatio retinae (-la′she-o ret′ĭ-ne) detachment of the retina of the eye.

sublesional (-le′zhun-al) performed or situated beneath a lesion.

sublethal (-le′thal) not sufficient to cause death.

sublimate (sub′lĭ-māt) a substance obtained by sublimation.

sublimation (sub″lĭ-ma′shun) 1. the con-

version of a solid directly into the gaseous state. 2. a mental mechanism operating outside of conscious awareness by which consciously unacceptable instinctual drives are expressed in personally and socially acceptable channels.

subliminal (sub-lim′ĭ-nal) below the threshold of sensation or conscious awareness.

sublingual (-ling′gwal) beneath the tongue.

sublinguitis (sub″ling-gwi′tis) inflammation of the sublingual gland.

sublumbar (sub-lum′bar) below the lumbar region.

subluxation (sub″luk-sa′shun) incomplete or partial dislocation.

submammary (sub-mam′ar-e) below the mammary gland.

submaxilla (sub″mak-sil′ah) the mandible.

submaxillaritis (sub″mak-sĭ-lar-i′tis) inflammation of the submaxillary gland.

submaxillary (sub-mak′sĭ-ler″e) below the maxilla.

submental (-men′tal) beneath the chin.

submetacentric (-met″ah-sen′trik) having the centromere almost, but not quite, at the metacentric position.

submicron (-mi′kron) a small particle invisible with the microscope, but visible with the ultramicroscope.

submicroscopic (-mi″kro-skop′ik) too small to be visible with the microscope.

submorphous (-mor′fus) neither amorphous nor perfectly crystalline.

submucosa (sub″mu-ko′sah) areolar tissue situated beneath a mucous membrane.

submucous (sub-mu′kus) below mucous membrane.

subnarcotic (sub″nar-kot′ik) moderately narcotic.

subnasale (sub″na-sa′le) an anthropometric landmark, the point at which the nasal septum merges, in the midsagittal plane, with the upper lip.

subnatant (sub-na′tant) 1. situated below or at the bottom of something. 2. the liquid lying beneath a layer of precipitated insoluble material.

subneural (-nu′ral) beneath a nerve or the neural axis.

subnormal (-nor′mal) below or less than normal.

subnormality (sub″nor-mal′ĭ-te) a state less than normal or that usually encountered, as *mental subnormality*, generally considered characterized by an intelligence quotient under 69.

subnucleus (sub-nu′kle-us) a partial or secondary nucleus.

suboccipital (sub″ok-sip′ĭ-tal) below the occiput.

suboperculum (-o-per′ku-lum) portion of occipital gyrus overlying the insula.

suborbital (sub-or′bĭ-tal) beneath the orbit.

suborder (-or′der) a taxonomic category sometimes established, subordinate to an order and superior to a family.

suboxide (-ok′sīd) that oxide in any series which contains the least oxygen.

subpapular (-pap′u-lar) indistinctly papular.

subpatellar (sub″pah-tel′ar) below the patella.

subpericardial (sub″per-ĭ-kar′de-al) beneath the pericardium.

subperiosteal (sub″per-e-os′te-al) beneath the periosteum.

subperitoneal (sub″per-ĭ-to-ne′al) beneath the peritoneum.

subpharyngeal (sub″fah-rin′je-al) beneath the pharynx.

subphrenic (sub-fren′ik) beneath the diaphragm.

subphylum (-fi′lum) a taxonomic category sometimes established, subordinate to a phylum and superior to a class.

subplacenta (sub″plah-sen′tah) the decidua parietalis.

subpleural (sub-ploor′al) beneath the pleura.

subpontine (-pon′tin) beneath the pons.

subpreputial (sub″pre-pu′shal) beneath the prepuce.

subpubic (sub-pu′bik) beneath the pubic bone.

subpulmonary (-pul′mo-nar″e) beneath the lung.

subretinal (-ret′ĭ-nal) beneath the retina.

subsalt (sub′sawlt) a basic salt.

subscapular (sub-skap′u-lar) below the scapula.

subscription (-skrip′shun) the third chief part of a drug prescription, comprising directions to be followed by the pharmacist in its preparation.

subserous (-se′rus) beneath a serous membrane.

subspinale (sub″spi-na′le) a cephalometric landmark, being the deepest midline point on the premaxillary between the anterior nasal spine and the prosthion.

substage (sub′stāj) part of the microscope underneath the stage.

substance (sub′stans) material constituting an organ or body. **agglutinable s.**, a substance in red blood corpuscles and bacteria, with which the agglutinin unites to produce specific agglutination. **agglutinating s.**, agglutinin. *α*-**s.**, **alpha s.**, reticular substance. **antidiuretic s.**, antidiuretic hormone. **autacoid s.**, autacoid. *β*-**s.**, **beta s.**, Heinz-Ehrlich bodies. **black s.**, substantia nigra. **cement s.**, the intercellular substance of certain tissues, as endothelium. **chromophil s.**, Nissl bodies. **colloid s.**, the jelly-like substance formed in colloid degeneration. **cytotoxin s.**, cytolysin. **depressor s.**, a substance that tends to decrease activity or blood pressure. **dotted s.**, a granular material which makes up a large part of the central nervous system of invertebrates. **gray s.**, nerve tissue composed of nerve cell bodies, unmyelinated nerve fibers and supporting tissue. **ground s.**, the basic homogeneous material of a tissue or organ, in which the specific components occur. **hemolytic s.**, the material in a serum which destroys the red blood cells of a serum added to it. **interfibrillar s. of Flemming**, hyaloplasm (1). **interspongioplastic s.**, cytochylema. **interstitial s.**, ground substance. **medullary s.**, 1. the white matter of the central nervous system, consisting of axons and their myelin sheaths. 2. the soft, marrow-like substance of

such structures as bone marrow, kidney, adrenal gland, etc. **Nissl s.**, chromatin-like material occurring in granules in the cytoplasm of nerve cells, consisting chiefly of ribonucleic acid and staining blue with certain basic dyes. **no-threshold s's**, those substances in the blood which are excreted into the urine in proportion to their absolute amount in the blood. **prelipoid s.**, degenerated nerve tissue which has not yet been converted into fat. **pressor s.**, a substance that raises blood pressure. **reaction s.**, a substance formed in the body of an animal on immunization with cellular products from an animal of another species. **reticular s.** the netlike mass of threads seen in red blood corpuscles after vital staining. **Rolando's gelatinous s.**, substantia gelatinosa. **Rollett's secondary s.**, the transparent material lying in narrow zones on each side of Krause's disks. **sarcous s.**, the porous material of a sarcous element. **sensibilizing s., sensitizing s.**, amboceptor. **Soemmerring's gray s.**, substantia nigra. **threshold s's**, those substances in the blood, such as sodium chloride, sugar, etc., which are excreted into the urine only when they exceed a certain (threshold) value. **thromboplastic s.**, zymoplastic s. **tigroid s.**, Nissl bodies. **transmitter s.**, a chemical substance (mediator) which induces activity in an excitable tissue. **white s.**, tissue consisting mostly of myelinated nerve fibers and constituting the conducting portion of the brain and spinal cord. **white s. of Schwann**, myelin (1). **zymoplastic s.**, a substance in the tissues which hastens the coagulation of the blood.

substantia (sub-stan′she-ah), pl. *substan′tiae* [L.] substance; used in anatomic nomenclature in naming various components of various tissues and structures of the body. **s. al′ba**, white substance. **s. ferrugin′ea**, pigmented nerve cell substance of the locus caeruleus. **s. gelatino′sa**, substance sheathing posterior horn of spinal cord and lining the central canal. **s. gris′ea**, gray substance. **s. ni′gra**, dark spot in the section of crus cerebri. **s. pro′pria**, lamina propria.

substernal (-ster′nal) below the sternum.

substrate (sub′strāt) the compound whose chemical transformation is catalyzed by an enzyme.

substructure (sub′struk-tūr) the underlying or supporting portion of an organ or appliance; in dentistry, that portion of an implant denture which is embedded in the tissues of the jaw.

subsylvian (sub-sil′ve-an) below the fissure of Sylvius.

subtarsal (-tar′sal) below the tarsus.

subtelocentric (-tel″o-sen′trik) having the centromere almost, but not quite, at the telocentric position.

subthalamic (sub″thah-lam′ik) below the thalamus.

subthalamus (sub-thal′ah-mus) a portion of the hypothalamus situated between the thalamus and the tegmentum of the mesencephalon.

subtle (sut′l) 1. very fine, as a subtle powder. 2. very acute, as a subtle pain.

subtribe (sub′trīb) a taxonomic category sometimes established, subordinate to a tribe and superior to a genus.

subtrochanteric (sub″tro-kan-ter′ik) below the trochanter.

subtympanic (sub″tim-pan′ik) somewhat tympanic in quality.

subungual (sub-ung′gwal) beneath a nail.

suburethral (sub″u-re′thral) beneath the urethra.

subvaginal (sub-vaj′ĭ-nal) under a sheath, or below the vagina.

subvertebral (-ver′tĕ-bral) on the ventral side of the vertebrae.

subvirile (-vir′il) having deficient virility.

subvitaminosis (-vi″tah-mĭ-no′sis) hypovitaminosis.

subvitrinal (-vit′rĭ-nal) beneath the vitreous.

subvolution (sub″vo-lu′shun) the operation of turning over a flap to prevent adhesions.

subzonal (sub-zo′nal) below the zona pellucida.

Sucaryl (soo′kah-ril) trademark for a noncaloric sweetening agent.

succagogue (suk′ah-gog) 1. inducing glandular secretion. 2. an agent which induces glandular secretion.

succinylcholine (suk″sĭ-nil-ko′lēn) a compound used as a skeletal muscle relaxant.

succinylsulfathiazole (-sul″fah-thi′ah-zōl) an antibacterial agent used in infections of the intestinal tract.

succorrhea (suk″o-re′ah) excessive flow of a natural secretion.

succus (suk′us), pl. *suc′ci* [L.] any fluid derived from living tissue; juice. **s. enter′-icus**, intestinal juice. **s. gas′tricus**, gastric juice.

succussion (sŭ-kush′un) a splashing sound elicited by shaking, indicative of fluid and air in a body cavity.

Sucostrin (su-kos′trin) trademark for a preparation of succinylcholine.

sucrase (soo′krās) invertin.

sucroclastic (soo″kro-klas′tik) splitting up sugar.

sucrose (soo′krōs) a sugar obtained from sugar cane, sugar beet or other sources; used as a food and sweetening agent.

suction (suk′shun) the withdrawal or uptake of fluid by creation of a partial vacuum. **post-tussive s.**, a sucking sound heard over a lung cavity just after a cough.

suctorian (suk-to′re-an) a protozoan of the subphylum Ciliophora, characterized by the presence of cilia only during the young developmental stages, the mature organisms having specialized tentacles which serve as locomotor and food-acquiring mechanisms.

Sudafed (soo′dah-fed) trademark for preparations of pseudoephedrine hydrochloride.

sudamen (su-da′men), pl. *sudam′ina* [L.] a whitish vesicle caused by retention of sweat in the stratum corneum.

Sudan (su-dan′) a substance used as a stain. **S. III,** a red stain used for tubercle bacilli.

sudanophilia (su-dan″o-fil′e-ah) a condition in which the leukocytes contain particles staining readily with Sudan red.

sudanophilous (su″dan-of′ĭ-lus) staining easily with Sudan.

sudarium (su-da′re-um) a sweat bath.

sudation (su-da′shun) 1. the process of sweating. 2. excessive sweating.

sudatoria (su″dah-to′re-ah) hyperhidrosis.

sudatorium (-to′re-um), pl. *sudato′ria* [L.] a hot-air bath or sweat bath.

sudogram (su′do-gram) a graph representing the sweating response of different areas of the body after injection of a dye which is excreted by the sudoriparous glands.

sudokeratosis (su″do-ker″ah-to′sis) keratosis of the sweat ducts.

sudomotor (-mo′tor) exerting an influence on the sweat glands.

sudor (su′dor) sweat; perspiration. **s. an′-glicus**, miliary fever. **s. cruen′tus**, the excretion of red sweat.

sudoral (su′dor-al) characterized by profuse sweating.

sudoresis (su″do-re′sis) profuse sweating.

sudorific (su″dŏ-rif′ik) an agent causing sweating.

sudoriparous (-rip′ah-rus) secreting or producing sweat.

suet (su′et) the hard internal fat of the abdomen of a food animal. **mutton s., prepared s.,** the internal fat of the abdomen of sheep, *Ovis aries;* used in formulating ointment bases.

suffocation (suf′ŏ-ka′shun) stoppage of respiration, or asphyxia due to such stoppage.

suffusion (sŭ-fu′zhun) the process of overspreading, or diffusion.

sugar (shoog′ar) a simple carbohydrate distributed universally in plants and animal tissues, containing carbon and hydrogen usually in the ratio of 1 to 2. **beet s.,** saccharose from root of beet. **cane s.,** sucrose. **diabetic s.,** glucose found in the urine in diabetes. **fruit s.,** levulose. **grape s.,** dextrose. **invert s.,** a natural mixture of dextrose and levulose. **liver s.,** dextrose from the liver. **malt s.,** maltose. **milk s.,** lactose. **muscle s.,** inositol. **starch s.,** dextrin.

suggestibility (sug-jes″tĭ-bil′ĭ-te) inclination to act on suggestions of others.

suggestible (sug-jes′tĭ-bl) inclined to act on the suggestion of another.

suggestion (sug-jes′chun) impartation of an idea to a subject from without. **hypnotic s.,** one imparted to a person in the hypnotic state. **posthypnotic s.,** implantation in the mind of a subject during hypnosis of a suggestion to be acted upon after recovery from the hypnotic state.

suggillation (sug″jĭ-la′shun) an ecchymosis.

suicide (soo′ĭ-sīd) the taking of one's own life. **psychic s.,** the termination of one's own life without use of any physical agent.

Sulamyd (sul′am-id) trademark for a preparation of sulfacetamide.

sulcate (sul′kāt) furrowed, or marked with sulci.

sulcation (sul-ka′shun) the formation of sulci; the state of being marked by sulci.

sulcus (sul'kus), pl. *sul'ci* [L.] a groove or furrow; used in anatomic nomenclature to designate a linear depression, as one separating the gyri of the brain or one on the surface of another organ. **s. centra'lis**, rolandic fissure. **sul'ci cu'tis**, fine depressions of the skin between the ridges of the skin. **gingival s.**, the groove between the surface of the tooth and the epithelium lining the free gingiva. **Harrison's s.**, Harrison's groove. **Jacobson's s.**, a groove in the middle ear containing branches of the tympanic plexus. **scleral s.**, a slight groove on the outer surface of the eyeball, at the junction of the sclera and cornea. **triradiate s.**, orbital fissure.

sulfacetamide (sul"fah-set'ah-mīd) an antibacterial agent used principally in infections of the urinary tract. **sodium s.**, an antibacterial compound used topically in ointment or solution.

sulfadiazine (-di'ah-zēn) a rapidly absorbed and readily excreted antibacterial agent. **sodium s.**, an antibacterial compound used intravenously in 5 per cent solution.

sulfadimetine (-di'mē-tēn) sulfisomidine.

sulfadimidine (-di'mī-dēn) sulfamethazine.

sulfadimethoxine (-di"meth-ok'sēn) a rapidly absorbed and slowly excreted antibacterial compound used in urinary tract and other infections.

sulfaethidole (-eth'ĭ-dōl) a compound used as an antibacterial agent.

sulfafurazole (-fu'rah-zōl) sulfisoxazole.

sulfaguanidine (-gwahn'ĭ-dēn) one of the sulfonamides used especially in intestinal tract infections.

sulfamerazine (-mer'ah-zēn) a readily absorbed antibacterial substance usually used in combination with sulfamethazine and sulfadiazine

sulfamethazine (-meth'ah-zēn) a readily acetylated antibacterial substance usually used in combination with sulfadiazine and sulfamerazine.

sulfamethizole (-meth'ĭ-zōl) an antibacterial compound used mainly in urinary tract infections.

sulfamethoxazole (-meth-ok'sah-zōl) an antibacterial agent used in both systemic and urinary tract infections.

sulfamethoxypyridazine (-meth-ok"se-pi-rid'ah-zēn) an antibacterial agent used in urinary tract and other infections.

sulfamethyldiazine (-meth"il-di'ah-zēn) sulfamerazine.

sulfamethylthiadiazole (-thi"ah-di'ah-zōl) sulfamethizole.

Sulfamezathine (sul"fah-mez'ah-thēn) trademark for a preparation of sulfamethazine.

Sulfamylon (-mi'lon) trademark for preparations of mafenide.

sulfanemia (-ne'me-ah) anemia resulting from use of sulfonamides.

sulfanilamide (-nil'ah-mīd) a potent antibacterial compound, the first of the sulfonamides discovered.

sulfanilate (sul-fan'ĭ-lāt) a salt of sulfanilic acid.

sulfapyridine (sul"fah-pir'ĭ-dēn) a sulfonamide synthesized in Great Britain, effective against pneumococci and staphylococci.

sulfarsphenamine (sulf"ars-fen'ah-min) an arsenic-containing compound formerly used in treatment of syphilis.

sulfasuxidine (sul"fah-suk'sĭ-dēn) trademark for preparations of succinylsulfathiazole.

sulfatase (sul'fah-tās) an enzyme which catalyzes the hydrolysis of sulfate esters.

sulfate (sul'fāt) a salt of sulfuric acid. **cupric s.**, a copper-containing compound used as a fungicide and an emetic. **ferrous s.**, an iron-containing compound used in treatment of iron deficiency anemia.

Sulfathalidine (sul"fah-thal'ĭ-dēn) trademark for phthalylsulfathiazole.

sulfathiazole (-thi'ah-zōl) a sulfonamide synthesized in the United States in 1939.

sulfhemoglobin (sulf"he-mo-glo'bin) Sulfmethemoglobin.

sulfhemoglobinemia (-glo"bin-e'me-ah) sulfmethemoglobin in the blood.

sulfhydryl (sulf-hi'dril) the univalent radical, −SH.

sulfide (sul'fīd) a binary compound of divalent sulfur, as one in which it is combined with two atoms of a monovalent metal, or with two monovalent organic radicals.

sulfinpyrazone (sul"fin-pi'rah-zōn) a compound used in gout to promote excretion of uric acid.

sulfisomidine (sul"fī-som'ĭ-dēn) a compound closely related to sulfamethazine, used in urinary tract infections.

sulfisoxazole (-sok"sah-zōl) an antibacterial compound used orally, topically and parenterally.

sulfite (sul'fīt) a salt of sulfurous acid.

sulfmethemoglobin (sulf"met-he"mo-glo'bin) a compound of hemoglobin and hydrogen sulfide.

sulfobromophthalein (sul"fo-bro"mo-thal'e-in) a sulfur- and bromine-containing compound used as the disodium salt in liver function tests.

sulfonamide (sul-fon'ah-mīd) generic name for an antibacterial substance derived from para-aminobenzene-sulfonamide (sulfanilamide).

sulfonamiduria (sul"fon-am"ĭ-du're-ah) the presence of a sulfonamide in the urine.

sulfone (sul'fōn) an organic compound of the type R_2SO_2 or R.SOOR, produced by oxidation of a sulfide.

sulfonethylmethane (sul"fōn-eth"il-meth'ān) colorless crystalline substance; hypnotic somnifacient.

sulfonmethane (-meth'ān) a compound with moderate hypnotic properties.

Sulfonsol (sul-fon'sol) trademark for oral trisulfapyrimidines suspension.

sulfoxide (-fok'sid) 1. the divalent radical, =SO. 2. an organic compound of the type R_2SO or R.SO.R, intermediate between a sulfide and a sulfone, and produced by oxidation of a mercaptan. **alkyl s.**, one in which the organic radicals are alkyl groups. **dimethyl s.**, one in which the organic radicals are methyl groups.

sulfoxone (sul-fok'sōn) a compound derived from dapsone. **sodium s.**, an antibacterial agent used in treatment of leprosy.

sulfur (sul'fer) chemical element (*see table*), at. no. 16, symbol S. **s. dioxide,** colorless, noninflammable gas, used as an antioxidant and pharmaceutic aid. **s. lo'tum,** washed sulfur. **precipitated s.,** a fine, pale yellow powder; used in an ointment as a scabicide. **s. sublima'tum, sublimed s.,** fine yellow crystalline powder; fungicide, parasiticide and keratolytic agent. **washed s.,** fine yellow crystalline powder, without odor or taste; used like sublimed sulfur.

sulfurated (sul'fu-rāt"ed)   combined with sulfur.

sulfuret (sul'fu-ret) sulfide.

sulph- for words beginning thus, see those beginning *sulf-*.

Sul-spansion (sul-span'shun) trademark for a suspension of sulfaethidole.

sunburn (sun'bern) injury to the skin, with erythema and vesiculobullous changes, caused by exposure to ultraviolet rays of the sun.

sunstroke (sun'strōk) a condition caused by excessive exposure to the sun, marked by high skin temperature, convulsions and coma.

super- (su'per) word element [L.], *above; excessive.*

superalimentation (su"per-al"ĭ-men-ta'shun) excessive feeding.

superalkalinity (-al"kah-lin'ĭ-te) excessive alkalinity.

superaurale (-aw-ra'le) an anthropometric landmark, the highest point on the superior border of the helix of the ear.

supercilia (-sil'e-ah) (pl., L.) the hairs on the arching protrusion over either eye.

supercilium (-sil'e-um) (sing., L.) eyebrow; the transverse elevation at the junction of the forehead and upper eyelid. adj., **supercil'iary.**

superclass (su'per-klas) a taxonomic category sometimes established, subordinate to a phylum and superior to a class.

super-ego (su"per-e'go) a part of the psyche derived from both the id and the ego, which acts, largely unconsciously, as a monitor over the ego.

superexcitation (-ek"si-ta'shun) excessive excitation.

superfamily (-fam'ĭ-le) a taxonomic category sometimes established, subordinate to an order and superior to a family.

superfatted (-fat'ed) containing more fat than can be combined with the quantity of alkali present.

superfecundation (-fe"kun-da'shun) fertilization of two ova, liberated at the same time, by sperm of different fathers.

superfemale (-fe'māl) a female organism whose cells contain more than the ordinary number of sex-determining (X) chromosomes.

superfetation (-fe-ta'shun) fertilization of an ovum when there is already a developing embryo in the uterus.

superficial (su"per-fish'al) situated on or near the surface.

superficialis (-fish"e-a'lis) superficial.

superficies (-fish'e-ēz) an outer surface.

superimpregnation (-im"preg-na'shun) successive fertilization of two ova.

superinduce (-in-dūs') to bring on in addition to an already existing condition.

superinfection (-in-fek'shun) sudden growth of a type of bacteria different from the original offender in a wound or lesion under treatment.

superinvolution (-in"vo-lu'shun) excessive involution.

superjacent (-ja'sent) located above.

superlactation (-lak-ta'shun) oversecretion of milk.

superlethal (-le'thal) more than sufficient to cause death.

supermaxilla (-mak-sil'ah) the maxilla.

supermedial (-me'de-al) situated above the middle.

supermicroscope (-mi'kro-skōp) electron microscope.

supermotility (-mo-til'ĭ-te) excess of motility.

supernatant (-na'tant) 1. situated above or at the top of something. 2. the liquid lying above a layer of precipitated insoluble material.

supernumerary (-nu'mer-ār"e) in excess of the regular number.

supernutrition (-nu-trish'un) excessive nutrition.

superphosphate (-fos'fāt) an acid phosphate.

super-regeneration (-re-jen"e-ra'shun) the development of superfluous tissue, organs or parts as a result of regeneration.

supersalt (su'per-sawlt) a salt with excess of acid.

supersaturate (su"per-sat'ū-rāt) to add more of an ingredient than can be held in solution permanently.

superscription (-skrip'shun) something written above; the first of the four chief parts of a drug prescription, the ℞, or prescription sign ("Take thou").

supersecretion (-se-kre'shun) excess of any secretory function.

supersoft (su'per-soft) extremely soft; applied to roentgen rays of extremely long wavelength and low penetrating power.

supersonic (su"per-son'ik) having a speed greater than that of sound (faster than about one fifth mile a second, or 720 miles an hour in air.

supersphenoid (-sfe'noid) above the sphenoid bone.

superstructure (-struk'tūr) the overlying or visible portion of an appliance.

supertension (-ten'shun) extreme tension.

supervirulent (-vir'u-lent) unusually virulent.

supinate (su'pĭ-nāt) to place in or assume a supine position.

supination (su"pĭ-na'shun) the act of assuming the supine position; placing or lying on the back.

supine (su'pīn) lying with the face upward, or on the dorsal surface.

suppository (sŭ-poz'ĭ-to″re) a cone-shaped mass of solid medicated substance for introduction into the rectum, urethra or vagina. **glycerin s.**, one made up of a mixture of glycerin and sodium stearate; used as a rectal evacuant.

suppressant (sŭ-pres'sant) an agent that stops secretion, excretion or normal discharge.

suppression (sŭ-presh'un) 1. sudden stoppage of a secretion, excretion or normal discharge. 2. the voluntary expulsion of ego-threatening ideas and impulses from the consciousness.

suppurant (sup'u-rant) 1. causing suppuration. 2. an agent causing suppuration.

suppuration (sup″u-ra'shun) formation or discharge of pus. adj., **sup'purative.**

supra- (su'prah) word element [L], *above.*

supra-acromial (su″prah-ah-kro'me-al) above the acromion.

supra-auricular (-aw-rik'u-lar) above an auricle.

suprabulge (su'prah-bulj) the surfaces of a tooth occlusal to the height of contour, or sloping occlusally.

supracerebellar (su″prah-ser″ĕ-bel'ar) on the upper surface of the cerebellum.

suprachoroid (-ko'roid) on the outer surface of the choroid.

suprachoroidea (-ko-roi'de-ah) the outermost layer of the choroid.

supraclavicular (-klah-vik'u-lar) above the clavicle.

supraclusion (-kloo'zhun) projection of a tooth beyond the normal occlusal plane.

supracommissure (-kom'ĭ-shūr) a cerebral commissure in front of the stalk of the pineal body.

supracondylar (-kon'dĭ-lar) above a condyle.

supracostal (-kos'tal) above or outside the ribs.

supracotyloid (-kot'ĭ-loid) above the acetabulum.

supracranial (-kra'ne-al) on the upper surface of the cranium.

supradiaphragmatic (-di″ah-frag-mat'ik) above the diaphragm.

supra-epicondylar (-ep″ĭ-kon'dĭ-lar) above the epicondyle.

suprahyoid (-hi'oid) above the hyoid bone.

supraliminal (-lim'ĭ-nal) above the threshold of sensation.

supralumbar (-lum'bar) above the loin.

supramalleolar (-mah-le'o-lar) above a malleolus.

supramaxilla (-mak-sil'ah) maxilla.

supramaxillary (-mak'sĭ-ler″e) pertaining to the upper jaw.

supramentale (-men-ta'le) a cephalometric landmark, being the most posterior midline point in the concavity between the infradentale and pogonion.

supranormal (-nor'mal) greater than normal; present in or occurring in excess of normal amounts or values.

supra-occlusion (-o-kloo'zhun) supraclusion.

supraorbital (-or'bĭ-tal) above the orbit.

suprapelvic (-pel'vik) above the pelvis.

suprapontine (su″prah-pon'tīn) above or in upper part of the pons.

suprapubic (-pu'bik) above the pubes.

suprarenal (-re'nal) above a kidney; adrenal.

suprarenalism (-re'nal-izm) adrenalism.

Suprarenin (-ren'in) trademark for a preparation of epinephrine bitartrate.

suprascapular (-skap'u-lar) above the scapula.

suprascleral (-skle'ral) on the outer surface of the sclera.

suprasellar (-sel'ar) above the sella turcica.

suprasonic (-son'ik) pertaining to vibrations of frequency greater than that of sound waves.

supraspinal (-spi'nal) above the spine.

suprasternal (-ster'nal) above the sternum.

supratrochlear (-trok'le-ar) above the trochlea.

supravaginal (-vaj'ĭ-nal) outside or above a sheath; specifically, above the vagina.

supraversion (-ver'zhun) abnormal elongation of a tooth from its socket.

sura (su'rah) [L.] calf of the leg. adj., **su'ral.**

suramin (soor'ah-min) a nonmetallic compound first used in therapy of protozoal infections in Germany. **sodium s.**, a compound effective in trypanosomal and filarial infections.

surdimutitas (ser'dĭ-mu'tĭ-tas) deaf-mutism.

surditas (ser'dĭ-tas) deafness.

Surfacaine (ser'fah-kān) trademark for preparations of cyclomethycaine.

surface (ser'fas) the outer part or external aspect of a solid body. **anterior s.**, that surface which is toward the front of the body in man, or toward the head in quadrupeds. **articular s.**, that surface of a bone or cartilage which forms a joint with another. **dorsal s.**, that surface which is toward the back of the body. **extensor s.**, the aspect of a joint of a limb on the side toward which the movement of extension is directed. **flexor s.**, the aspect of a joint of a limb on the side toward which the movement of flexion is directed. **inferior s.**, that surface which is lower. **lateral s.**, a surface nearer to or directed toward the side of the body. **medial s.**, a surface nearer to or directed toward the midline of the body. **posterior s.**, that surface which is toward the back of the body in man or directed toward the tail in quadrupeds. **superior s.**, that surface which is upper or higher. **ventral s.**, the anterior surface in man, and the lower surface, nearest the abdominal aspect, in quadrupeds.

surfactant (ser-fak'tant) 1. active on the surface. 2. a surface-active agent.

surgeon (ser'jun) a practitioner of surgery.

surgery (ser'jer-e) 1. that branch of medicine which treats disease by manual and operative procedures. 2. a place for the performance of surgical operations. adj., **sur'gical. antiseptic s.**, **aseptic s.**, surgery according to antiseptic or aseptic methods. **dental s.**, that branch of dentistry which deals with the surgical and adjunctive treatment of diseases, injuries and defects of the teeth. **major s.**, important surgical procedures, which are hazardous and incapacitate the patient. **minor s.**, surgical procedures of lesser importance, not involving incapacitation of the patient, as application of bandages, splints or dressings, catheterization, etc. **operative s.**, that concerned with procedures performed upon the human body with instruments, involving incision, excision, transection, etc., of various organs or parts. **oral s.**, that branch of medicine which deals with diagnosis and surgical and adjunctive treatment of diseases, injuries and defects of the mouth, jaws and associated structures. **orthopedic s.**, surgery dealing with the correction of deformities of the musculoskeletal system. **plastic s.**, surgery concerned with restoration of function and esthetic repair of parts damaged by trauma or disease, or with the correction of unsightly disfiguration. **veterinary s.**, the surgery of domestic animals.

Surital (sur'ĭ-tal) trademark for preparations of thiamylal.

surrogate (sur'o-gāt) a substitute; a thing or person that takes the place of something or someone else, as a drug used in place of another, or a person who takes the place of another in someone's affective existence.

sursumduction (sur″sum-duk'shun) sursumversion.

sursumvergence (-ver'jens) sursumversion.

sursumversion (-ver'zhun) the turning upward of a part, especially of the eyes.

susceptibility (sŭ-sep″tĭ-bil'ĭ-te) lack of resistance of a body to the effects of a deleterious or other agent, such as a pathogenic microorganism.

susceptible (sŭ-sep'tĭ-bl) capable of being affected; liable to contract a disease.

suscitate (sus'ĭ-tāt) to arouse to greater activity.

suscitation (sus″ĭ-ta'shun) arousal to greater activity.

suspension (sus-pen'shun) a preparation of finely divided, undissolved substance dispersed in a liquid vehicle. **colloid s.**, one in which the suspended particles are very small. **trisulfapyrimidines oral s.**, a preparation for oral administration containing sulfadiazine, sulfamerazine and sulfamethazine.

suspensoid (-pen'soid) a colloid system resembling a suspension, but in which the particles are so small they do not settle out on standing, but are kept in motion by brownian movement.

suspensory (-pen'sor-e) 1. serving to hold up a part. 2. a bandage or sling for supporting the testes.

suspirious (-pi're-us) breathing heavily.

sustentacular (sus″ten-tak'u-lar) supporting; sustaining.

sustentaculum (-tak'u-lum), pl. *sustentac'uli* [L.] a support.

susurrus (sū-sur'us) [L.] murmur.

sutura (su-tu'rah), pl. *sutu'rae* [L.] suture; used in anatomic nomenclature to designate a type of joint in which the apposed bony surfaces are united by fibrous tissue, permitting no movement; found only between bones of the skull. **s. denta'ta**, interlocking of bones by sawlike processes. **s. harmo'nia**, simple apposition of bones. **s. limbo'sa**, an inter-

locking by beveled surfaces. **s. no'tha**, a type of suture formed by apposition of the roughened surfaces of the two participating bones. **s. pla'na**, a type of suture in which there is simple apposition of the contiguous surfaces, with no interlocking of the edges of the participating bones. **s. serra'ta**, sutura dentata. **s. squamo'sa**, the overlapping of edges of bones. **s. ve'ra**, a true suture, in which no movement of the participating bones can occur.

suturation (su″tu-ra'shun) process or act of suturing.

suture (su'cher) 1. the line of union of adjoining bones of the skull. 2. a stitch or series of stitches made to secure apposition of the edges of a surgical or accidental wound; used also as a verb to indicate application of such stitches. 3. material used in closing a wound with stitches. adj., **su'tural. absorbable s.**, material for use in approximating the edges of disrupted tissues that is absorbed by tissue fluids and ultimately disappears. **apposition s.**, a superficial suture used for exact approximation of the cutaneous edges of a wound. **approximation s.**, a deep suture for securing apposition of the deep tissue of a wound. **basilar s.**, the line of union between the basilar process of the occipital bone and the sphenoid. **buried s.**, one placed deep in the tissues and concealed by the skin. **catgut s.**, material for approximating wound edges, prepared from submucous connective tissue of the small intestine of healthy sheep. **coaptation s.**, apposition suture. **cobblers' s.**, one made with suture material threaded through a needle at each end. **continuous s.**, one in which the stitches are made with one unbroken thread. **coronal s.**, the line of union between the frontal bone and the parietal bones. **Czerny s., Czerny-Lembert s.**, a stitch used in intestinal surgery. **dry s.**, suturation of edges of wound through adhesive plaster. **everting s.**, a method by which the approximated edges of a wound are everted. **false s.**, a line of junction between apposed surfaces without fibrous union of the bones. **Gély's s.**, a continuous stitch for wounds of the intestine, made with a thread having a needle at each end. **glover's s.**, a continuous suture in which the needle is, after each stitch, passed through the loop of the preceding stitch. **Halsted's s.**, a stitch used in suturing intestinal wounds. **harelip s.**, a twisted suture for harelip. **hemostatic s's**, sutures to control oozing of blood from raw areas. **interrupted s.**, a form in which each stitch is made with a separate piece of suture material, threaded on a different needle. **intradermic s.**, a stitch applied parallel with the edges of the wound, but below the surface of the skin. **inverting s.**, a method by which the approximated edges of a wound are inverted. **Jobert's s.**, a stitch for transverse intestinal wounds. **lambdoid s.**, line of union between the upper borders of occipital and parietal bones. **Lembert's s.**, a stitch for intestinal wounds. **lock-stitch s.**, a continuous hemostatic suture used in intestinal surgery.

loop s., interrupted suture. **mattress s.,** a continuous suture applied back and forth through the wound. **nonabsorbable s.,** material for use in approximating the edges of disrupted tissues that persists in the body and cannot be absorbed in the tissue fluids. **noose s.,** interrupted suture. **pin s.,** one in which the suture material is passed around pins inserted in the tissues at the side of the wound. **purse-string s.,** a type of inverting suture in which a continuous running suture is placed about an opening and then drawn tight. **relaxation s.,** a secondary line of stitches to relieve tension on edges of a wound. **retention s.,** a reinforcing suture for abdominal wounds, utilizing exceptionally strong material and including a large amount of tissue in each stitch. **sagittal s.,** the line of union of the parietal bones, dividing the skull anteroposteriorly into two symmetrical halves. **subcuticular s.,** a method of skin closure involving placement of stitches in the subcuticular tissues parallel with the line of the wound. **superficial s.,** one placed through the skin only or not including any deep tissue. **tension s.,** relaxation suture. **twisted s.,** harelip suture. **uninterrupted s.,** continuous suture.

Suvren (suv'ren) trademark for a preparation of captodiamine.

suxamethonium (suk"sah-mē-tho'ne-um) succinylcholine.

swab (swahb) a small pledget of cotton or gauze wrapped around the end of a slender wooden stick or wire for applying medications or obtaining specimens of secretions, etc., from body surfaces or orifices.

swage (swāj) 1. to shape metal by hammering or by adapting it to a die. 2. a tool or form for shaping metal by pressure.

sweat (swet) the excretion of the sudoriparous glands; perspiration.

sweeny (swe'ne) atrophy of the muscles in the shoulder of a horse.

swelling (swel'ing) abnormal enlargement or increase in volume, associated with accumulation in the tissue of a protein-containing exudate. **cloudy s.,** enlargement of cells and presence of granules in their cytoplasm, occurring in certain tissues in relatively mild infections and various other conditions. **white s.,** that produced by tuberculous arthritis.

sycephalus (si-sef'ah-lus) syncephalus.

sycoma (si-ko'mah) a condyloma.

sycosiform (si-ko'si-form) resembling sycosis.

sycosis (si-ko'sis) pustular inflammation of hair follicles, especially of the beard. **s. bar'bae,** sycosis of the beard. **lupoid s.,** a chronic, scarring form of deep sycosis barbae.

Sycotrol (si'ko-trol) trademark for a preparation of pipethanate hydrochloride.

syllepsiology (si-lep"se-ol'o-je) the department of medicine dealing with conception and pregnancy.

syllepsis (si-lep'sis) pregnancy.

symbiology (sim"bi-ol'o-je) the scientific study of symbiosis and symbiotic organisms.

symbiont (sim'bi-ont, sim'be-ont) one of the organisms or species associated biologically with an organism of another species.

symbiosis (sim"bi-o'sis) the biological association of two individuals or populations of different species, classified as mutualism, commensalism, parasitism or predation, depending on the advantage or disadvantage derived from the relationship. adj., **symbiot'ic.**

Symbiotes (-o'tez) a genus of Microtatobiotes (order Rickettsiales, family Rickettsiaceae, tribe Wolbachieae).

symblepharon (sim-blef'ah-ron) adhesion of the eyelids.

symblepharopterygium (-blef"ah-ro-tē-rij'e-um) symblepharon and pterygium.

symbolism (sim'bo-lizm) a mental state in which every occurrence is conceived of as a symbol of the patient's own thoughts.

symbolophobia (sim"bo-lo-fo'be-ah) a morbid fear that one's acts may contain some symbolic meaning.

symmelus (sim'ē-lus) a fetal monster with fused legs.

symmetry (sim'ē-tre) correspondence in size, form and arrangement of parts on opposite sides of a plane, line or point. **bilateral s.,** the state of an irregularly shaped body (such as the human body or that of higher animals) which can be divided into equivalent halves by one special cut. **radial s.,** the state of a round body in which a top and a bottom surface are distinguishable, which can be cut into equivalent halves by a plane from top to bottom through the center. **spherical s.,** the state of a completely round body which can be cut into two equivalent halves.

sympathectomize (sim"pah-thek'to-mīz) to deprive of sympathetic innervation.

sympathectomy (-thek'to-me) excision or interruption of a sympathetic nerve. **chemical s.,** the interruption of the transmission of impulses through a sympathetic nerve by chemicals. **periarterial s.,** surgical removal of the sheath of an artery containing the sympathetic nerve fibers.

sympathetic (-thet'ik) 1. pertaining to or caused by sympathy. 2. pertaining to the sympathetic nervous system.

sympatheticomimetic (-thet"ĭ-ko-mi-met'ik) sympathomimetic.

sympatheticoparalytic (-par"ah-lit'ik) caused by paralysis of the sympathetic nervous system.

sympatheticotonia (-to'ne-ah) sympathicotonia. adj., **sympatheticoton'ic.**

sympathicoblast (sim-path'ĭ-ko-blast") an embryonic cell which develops into a sympathetic nerve cell.

sympathicoblastoma (sim-path"ĭ-ko-blasto'mah) a tumor containing sympathicoblasts.

sympathicolytic (-lit'ik) sympatholytic.

sympathicomimetic (-mi-met'ik) sympathomimetic.

sympathiconeuritis (-nu-ri'tis) inflammation of the sympathetic nerves.

sympathicotonia (-to'ne-ah) a stimulated condition of the sympathetic nervous system, marked by vascular spasm and heightened blood pressure. adj., **sympathicoton'ic.**

sympathicotripsy (sim-path"ĭ-ko-trip'se) crushing of a ganglion or plexus of the sympathetic nervous system.

sympathicotropic (-trop'ik) having affinity for or exerting its principal effect on the sympathetic nervous system.

sympathicus (sim-path'ĭ-kus) the sympathetic nervous system.

sympathin (sim'pah-thin) a mediating substance formed at the peripheral ends of sympathetic nerves. **s. E.,** the excitatory form, which causes vasoconstriction. **s. I.,** the inhibitory form, which causes vasodilatation.

sympathism (sim'pah-thizm) suggestibility.

sympathoblast (sim-path'o-blast) sympathicoblast.

sympathoblastoma (sim"path-tho"blast-to'-mah) sympathicoblastoma.

sympathogonium (sim"pah-tho-go'ne-um), pl. *sympathogo'nia* [Gr.] an embryonic cell which develops into a sympathetic cell.

sympathogonioma (-go"ne-o'mah) a tumor composed of sympathogonia.

sympatholytic (-lit'ik) blocking transmission of impulses from the postganglionic fibers to effector organs or tissues, inhibiting smooth muscle contraction and glandular secretion; antisympathomimetic.

sympathoma (sim"pah-tho'mah) sympathicoblastoma.

sympathomimetic (sim"pah-tho-mi-met'ik) producing effects resembling those of impulses transmitted by the postganglionic fibers of the sympathetic nervous system.

sympathy (sim'pah-the) the emotional understanding of another person's feelings.

symphalangism (sim-fal'an-jizm) ankylosis of the proximal phalangeal joints.

symphyseal (-fiz'e-al) pertaining to a symphysis.

symphysial (-fiz'e-al) symphyseal.

symphysiectomy (-fiz"e-ek'to-me) resection of the symphysis pubis.

symphysion (-fiz'e-on) the middle point of the outer border of the alveolar process of the mandible.

symphysiorrhaphy (-fiz"e-or'ah-fe) suture of a divided symphysis.

symphysiotomy (-fiz"e-ot'o-me) division of the symphysis pubis to facilitate delivery.

symphysis (sim'fĭ-sis), pl. *sym'physes* [Gr.] a union; a type of joint in which the apposed bony surfaces are firmly united by a plate of fibrocartilage. **pubic s.,** the line of union of the bodies of the pubic bones in the median plane.

sympodia (sim-po'de-ah) fusion of the lower extremities.

symptom (simp'tom) an organic or physiologic manifestation of disease of which the patient is usually aware and frequently complains of. adj., **symptomat'ic. abstinence s's,** symptoms caused by sudden withdrawal of a customary stimulant, such as opium. **Anton's s.,** refusal of a patient to recognize his own blindness. **cardinal s's,** temperature, pulse,

respiration. **dissociation s.,** anesthesia to pain and to heat and cold, without impairment of tactile sensibility. **halo s.,** the appearance of colored rings around lights, occurring in incipient glaucoma. **objective s.,** one perceptible to others than the patient, as pallor, rapid pulse or respiration, restlessness, and the like. **signal s.,** a peculiar sensation or movement indicative of an impending epileptic attack. **subjective s.,** one perceptible only to the patient, as pain, pruritus, vertigo, and the like.

symptomatology (simp"to-mah-tol'o-je) the branch of medicine dealing with symptoms.

symptomatolytic (-to-lit'ik) causing the disappearance of symptoms.

symptosis (simp-to'sis) gradual wasting of the body or of an organ.

sympus (sim'pus) a fetal monster with feet and legs fused.

Synalar (sin'ah-lar) trademark for a preparation of fluocinolone acetonide.

synalgia (si-nal'je-ah) pain experienced in one place, but caused by stimuli originating in another. adj., **synal'gic.**

synanastomosis (sin"ah-nas"to-mo'sis) the anastomosis of several vessels.

Synangium (sin-an'je-um) a genus of Schizomycetes (order Myxobacterales, family Polyangiaceae).

synanthema (sin"an-the'mah) a local or grouped eruption.

synapse (sin'aps) the functional junction between two neurons, a region of protoplasmic contiguity, but not continuity. **axodendritic s.,** one between the axon of one neuron and dendrites of another. **axodendrosomatic s.,** one between the axon of one neuron and dendrites and body of another. **axosomatic s.,** one between the axon of one neuron and body of another.

synapsis (sĭ-nap'sis) the pairing off and union of homologous chromosomes from male and female pronuclei at start of mitosis.

synaptic (sĭ-nap'tik) pertaining to a synapse or to a synapsis.

synaptology (sin"ap-tol'o-je) the study of the synaptic correlations of the nervous system.

synarthrodia (sin"ar-thro'de-ah) synarthrosis. adj., **synarthro'dial.**

synarthrophysis (-thro-fi'sis) progressive ankylosis of joints.

synarthrosis (-thro'sis), pl. *synarthro'ses* [Gr.] a form of joint in which the bony elements are united by continuous intervening fibrous tissue.

syncanthus (sin-kan'thus) adhesion of the eyeball to the orbital structures.

syncephalus (-sef'ah-lus) a twin fetal monster with heads fused into one, there being a single face, with four ears.

synchilia (-ki'le-ah) congenital adhesion of the lips.

synchiria (-ki're-ah) reference of sensation to the opposite side on application of a stimulus.

synchondrectomy (sin"kon-drek'to-me) surgical excision of a synchondrosis.

synchondrosis (-dro'sis), pl. *synchondro'ses* [Gr.] a type of cartilaginous joint in which the cartilage is usually converted into bone before adult life.

synchondrotomy (sin″kon-drot′o-me) division of a synchondrosis.

synchronism (sin′kro-nizm) occurrence at the same time.

synchysis (sin′kĭ-sis) a softening or fluid condition of the vitreous body of the eye. **s. scintil′lans,** abnormal softness of the vitreous, with floating particles of cholesterol or other material.

synclitism (sin′klĭ-tizm) position of fetal head when the planes are parallel with those of the maternal pelvis.

synclonus (sin′klo-nus) muscular tremor or successive clonic contraction of various muscles together.

syncope (sin′ko-pe) 1. a sudden loss of strength. 2. suspension of consciousness due to cerebral anemia; a faint. adj., **syn′copal. digital s.,** a sudden, temporary loss of strength in the fingers.

Syncurine (sin′ku-rēn) trademark for a preparation of decamethonium bromide.

syncytiolysin (sin-sit″e-ol′ĭ-sin) an antibody which destroys syncytium.

syncytioma (sin-sit″e-o-mah) a tumor in which the uterine wall is infiltrated with large syncytial cells. **s. malig′num,** chorioadenoma.

syncytium (sin-sish′e-um) 1. a large cell with many nuclei. 2. the outermost fetal layer of the placenta, composed of epithelial cells. adj., **syncyt′ial.**

syndactylia (sin″dak-til′e-ah) syndactyly.

syndactyly (sin-dak′ti-le) persistence of webbing between adjacent digits of the hand or foot, so that they are more or less completely fused together. **quadruple s.,** webbing of the digits on all four extremities.

syndectomy (sin-dek′to-me) excision of a circular strip of conjunctiva in treatment of pannus.

syndesis (sin′dĕ-sis) artificial ankylosis.

syndesm(o)- (sin-des′mo) word element [Gr.], *connective tissue; ligament.*

syndesmectomy (sin″des-mek′to-me) excision of a ligament.

syndesmectopia (-mek-to′pe-ah) unusual situation of a ligament.

syndesmitis (-mi′tis) 1. inflammation of a ligament. 2. conjunctivitis.

syndesmology (sin″des-mol′o-je) scientific study or description of ligaments and other structures associated with joints.

syndesmoma (-mo′mah) a tumor of connective tissue.

syndesmoplasty (sin-des′mo-plas″te) plastic repair of a ligament.

syndesmosis (sin″des-mo′sis), pl. *syndesmo′-ses* [Gr.] a joint in which the bones are united by fibrous connective tissue forming an interosseous membrane or ligament.

syndesmotomy (-mot′o-me) incision of a ligament.

syndrome (sin′drōm) a combination of symptoms resulting from a single cause or so commonly occurring together as to constitute a distinct clinical entity. adj., **syndrom′ic.**

acute organic brain s., severe mental symptoms arising in a person previously psychologically normal. **Adams-Stokes s.,** sudden attacks of unconsciousness, with or without convulsions, accompanying heart block. **Adie's s.,** difference in size of the two pupils, the larger one being myotonic and often reacting abnormally to continued stimulation by direct light. **adiposogenital s.,** adiposogenital dystrophy; Frölich's syndrome. **adrenogenital s.,** hyperfunction of the adrenal cortex, causing pseudohermaphroditism and virilism in the female, usually evident at birth, and precocious sexual development in the male, usually not evident until age three to four. **Albright's s.,** asymmetric disease of the bones (osteitis fibrosa cystica), melanotic pigmentation of the skin and sexual precocity in the female. **Aldrich's syndrome,** chronic eczema, chronic suppurative otitis media, anemia and thrombocytic purpura, transmitted as a sex-linked recessive by an unaffected female to the male. **amyostatic s.,** a complex of symptoms in which involuntary muscular movements are prominent. **Ascher's s.,** blepharochalasis, adenoma of the thyroid gland and redundancy of the mucous membrane and submucous tissue of the upper lip. **Avelli's s.,** ipsilateral paralysis of the larynx and soft palate with contralateral loss of pain and temperature sense, in a lesion involving the nucleus ambiguus or vagus and spinal accessory nerve. **Banti's s.,** congestive splenomegaly. **Bassen-Kornzweig s.,** progressive ataxic neuropathy associated with atypical retinitis pigmentosa with involvement of the macula and presence in the blood of erythrocytes having pseudopodia or irregular length and number, giving them a crenated appearance (acanthocytes). **Benedikt's s.,** ipsilateral oculomotor paralysis with coarse tremor of the contralateral extremities, due to intramedullary lesion of the midbrain. **Bloch-Sulzberger s.,** incontinentia pigmenti. **Bonnevie-Ullrich s.,** a condition characterized by pterygium colli, lymphangiectatic edema of the hands and feet, ocular hypertelorism, short stature and other developmental anomalies. **Bouillaud's s.,** acute joint disorder, endocarditis and pericarditis. **Bouveret's s.,** idiopathic atrial paroxysmal tachycardia. **brain s.,** mental disorder associated with organic impairment of the brain, classified as *acute brain syndrome* if the disorder is reversible, *chronic brain syndrome* if it is not. **Brock's s.,** middle lobe syndrome. **Brown-Séquard s.,** a condition due to unilateral compression or section of the spinal cord as a result of neoplasm, inflammation or trauma, with motor paralysis and loss of touch, proprioception and vibratory sense on the same side and with pain and loss of temperature sense on the opposite side. **Burnett's s.,** milk-alkali syndrome. **Caffey's s.,** infantile cortical hyperostosis. **carpal tunnel s.,** pain and paresthesias in the fingers and hand, or extending to the elbow, due to compression of the median nerve at the wrist.

Cestan's s., **Cestan-Chenais s.**, anesthesia affecting the face and trunk, paralysis of the lateral conjugate gaze and contralateral hemiplegia, due to a lesion of the pyramidal tracts at the pons. **Charcot's s.**, amyotrophic lateral sclerosis. **chromosomal s.**, a complex of symptoms (congenital malformations or biochemical disorders) presumed to be causally related to an identifiable chromosomal aberration. **Clarke-Hadfield s.**, pancreatic infantilism. **Claude's s.**, ipsilateral paralysis of eye muscles, contralateral hemianesthesia and sometimes hemiataxia, in the paramedian mesencephalic lesion originating in the midbrain. **Conn's s.**, aldosteronism. **Costen's s.**, temporomandibular syndrome. **Crigler-Najjar s.**, congenital familial nonhemolytic jaundice in an infant, with excessive amounts of unconjugated bilirubin in the blood and kernicterus. **crush s.**, moderate to severe shock, myoglobinuria and lower nephron nephrosis subsequent to traumatic crushing of soft tissues. **Cruveilhier-Baumgarten s.**, splenomegaly, portal hypertension and patent umbilical vein. **cubital tunnel s.**, pain along the ulnar aspect of the hand and forearm and disability of the hand, due to compression of the ulnar nerve at the elbow. **Cushing's s.**, a condition usually occurring in females, due to excess adrenal cortical hormone and characterized by weakness and obesity of the face, neck and trunk. **defibrination s.**, incoagulability of the blood as a result of massive release of thromboplastic material and consumption of fibrinogen or destruction of formed fibrin; frequent after shock or in various obstetric complications. **Down's s.**, mongoloid features, disordered skeletal growth and anomalies of the eyes and heart, with moderate to severe mental retardation; usually associated with trisomy of chromosome 21. **Dubin-Johnson s.**, chronic idiopathic jaundice characterized by exacerbations and remissions, and presence of a brown pigment in the hepatic cells. **dumping s.**, a complex of symptoms, sometimes including diarrhea, occurring after ingestion of food by patients who have had partial gastrectomy. **effort s.**, neurocirculatory asthenia. **Ehlers-Danlos s.**, a tetrad of symptoms consisting of overextensibility of joints, hyperelasticity of the skin, fragility of the skin and pseudotumors following trauma. **Eisenmenger's s.**, displacement of the aorta to the right, defect of the septum, right ventricular hypertrophy and enlargement of the infundibulum, pulmonary artery and pulmonary vein. **Ellis-van Creveld s.**, chondroectodermal dysplasia. **Faber's s.**, Hayem-Faber syndrome. **Fabry's s.**, a genetically transmitted disorder characterized by remittent attacks of fever, lightning pains and burning dysesthesias of the extremities, proteinuria and hematuria, and cutaneous lesions. **Fanconi's s.**, a condition characterized by amino-acidura, renal glycosuria, hypophosphatemia and hyperphosphaturia. **Felty's s.**, rheumatoid arthritis with hepatosplenomegaly and leukopenia. **Frölich's s.**, adiposogenital dystrophy.

Gardner's s., multiple polyps of the colon and rectum, with multiple osteomas of the facial bones and other abnormal growths. **general adaptation s.**, the total of all nonspecific reactions of the body to prolonged systemic stress. **Gradenigo's s.**, ipsilateral paralysis of the abducens nerve and severe pain in the area supplied by the ophthalmic branch of the trigeminal nerve, in inflammation of the inner ear, mastoid sinus, or both. **Guillain-Barré s.**, infectious polyneuritis. **Hallervorden-Spatz s.**, a fatal, familial condition of unknown origin, characterized by neurologic symptoms and intellectual impairment. **Hamman-Rich s.**, diffuse interstitial pulmonary fibrosis. **Hand-Schüller-Christian s.**, a type of cholesterol lipoidosis, with defects in membranous bones, exophthalmos and diabetes insipidus. **Hayem-Faber s.**, severe hypochromic microcytic and sometimes hypoplastic anemia with achlorhydria or achylia. **Horner's s.**, miosis, apparent enophthalmos, narrowing of the palpebral fissure, hyperemia of the cheek, and absence of facial sweating, due to absence of sympathetic innervation. **Hurler's s.**, a genetically determined disorder marked by cloudy corneas, hepatosplenomegaly, mental deficiency, skeletal changes and dwarfed stature. **hyaline membrane s.**, idiopathic respiratory distress of newborn. **jugular foramen s.**, paralysis of the glossopharyngeal, vagus and spinal accessory nerves due to trauma or a lesion in the region of the jugular foramen. **Kartagener's s.**, chronic sinusitis, bronchiectasis and situs inversus. **Klinefelter's s.**, a condition associated with chromosomal abnormality in the male, with small testes, fibrosis and hyalinization of the seminiferous tubules and increase in urinary gonadotropins. **Klippel-Feil s.**, shortness of the neck with a low hairline, the number of cervical vertebrae being reduced, or several hemivertebrae being fused into one mass. **Kocher's s.**, leukopenia due to granulocytopenia with relative and absolute lymphocytosis and moderate eosinophilia, sometimes accompanying thyrotoxicosis. **Launois's s.**, gigantism due to overactivity of the pituitary gland. **Laurence-Moon-Biedl s.**, polydactyly, obesity, mental retardation, retinitis pigmentosa and hypogenitalism. **Leriche's s.**, fatigue in the hips, thighs or calves after exertion, pallor of the legs on elevation, and absence of pulsation in the arteries of the lower extremities, due to obstruction of the terminal aorta. **Libman-Sacks s.**, nonbacterial verrucous endocarditis. **Lichtheim's s.**, anemia occurring with degeneration of the spinal cord, producing various motor and sensory disturbances. **Lightwood's s.**, renal tubular acidosis. **Lowe's s.**, oculocerebrorenal syndrome. **Lutembacher's s.**, mitral stenosis of rheumatic origin associated with an atrial septal defect. **McArdle's s.**, myopathy due to inability of skeletal muscles to utilize muscle glycogen properly. **Maffucci's s.**, dyschondroplasia with multiple hemangiomas at the ends of bones. **malabsorption s.**, celiac disease.

Marchiafava-Micheli s., nocturnal paroxysmal hemoglobinuria. **Marfan's s.**, abnormal length of the extremities, especially of fingers and toes, with subluxation of the lens and other deformities. **Marie's s.**, a complex of symptoms due to excessive secretion of the anterior pituitary, with acromegaly a prominent feature. **middle lobe s.**, atelectasis of the middle lobe of the right lung, with chronic pneumonitis, due to compression of the bronchus by tuberculotic hilar lymph nodes. **Mikulicz's s.**, chronic lymphocytic infiltration and enlargement of the lacrimal and salivary glands, occurring in association with sarcoidosis, malignant lymphoma or collagen disease. **milk-alkali s.**, hypercalcemia without hypercalciuria or hypophosphatemia and with only mild alkalosis and other symptoms attributed to ingestion of milk and absorbable alkali for long periods. **Milkman's s.**, a generalized bone disease marked by multiple transparent stripes of absorption in the long and flat bones. **Morel-Moore s.**, **Morgagni's s.**, frontal internal hyperostosis. **Munchausen s.**, habitual seeking of hospital treatment for an apparent acute illness, the patient giving a plausible and dramatic history, all of which is false. **nephrotic s.**, a condition marked by massive edema, heavy proteinuria, hypoalbuminemia and unusual susceptibility to intercurrent infections. **oculocerebrorenal s.**, vitamin D-refractory rickets associated with glaucoma, mental retardation and faulty reabsorption of certain elements in the tubules of the kidney. **orofacial-digital s.**, a condition characterized by hypertrophy of the frenula, oligophrenia, trembling and anomalies of the hands. **Pancoast's s.**, 1. roentgenographic shadow at the apex of the lung, neuritic pain in the arm, atrophy of the muscles of the arm and hand, and Horner's syndrome, observed in tumor near the apex of the lung. 2. osteolysis in the posterior part of one or more ribs and sometimes involving also the corresponding vertebra. **Parinaud's s.**, paralysis of conjugate upward movement of the eye without paralysis of convergence. **Parinaud's oculoglandular s.**, unilateral conjunctivitis followed by chronic enlargement of the parotid gland and anterior cervical lymph nodes. **Peutz-Jeghers s.**, gastrointestinal polyposis with excessive melanin pigmentation of the skin and mucous membranes. **pickwickian s.**, exogenous obesity, somnolence, hypoventilation and erythrocytosis. **Pierre Robin s.**, micrognathia occurring in association with cleft palate and glossoptosis. **Plummer-Vinson s.**, difficulty in swallowing, with atrophy of buccal, glossopharyngeal and esophageal mucosa, deficiency of iron in plasma and often anemia. **postcommissurotomy s.**, fever, chest pain, pneumonitis and cardiomegaly occurring frequently after commissurotomy. **postgastrectomy s.**, dumping syndrome. **postirradiation s.**, signs and symptoms due to exposure to x-rays, gamma rays and fast and slow neutrons, its severity depending on the amount of radiation re-

ceived. **postpericardiectomy s.**, fever, chest pain and signs of pleural or pericardial inflammation after opening of the pericardium. **Putnam-Dana s.**, Lichtheim's syndrome. **respiratory distress s.**, a condition of the newborn characterized by acute difficulty in breathing, occurring most frequently in premature infants, infants of diabetic mothers or infants delivered by cesarean section. **Riley-Day s.**, familial dysautonomia. **rubella s.**, a complex of congenital abnormalities due to rubella in the mother during early pregnancy, including cataract, deafness, heart lesions, microcephaly and mental retardation. **scalenus anticus s.**, symptoms due to compression of the brachial plexus and subclavian artery by the scalenus anticus muscle. **Schaumann's s.**, a systemic condition involving lymph nodes, eyes, salivary glands, skin, lungs, liver and spleen. **Sézary reticulosis s.**, an exfoliative erythroderma associated with alopecia, edema, hyperkeratosis and changes in nails and pigmentation of the skin. **Sheehan's s.**, hypopituitarism occurring in a woman after severe hemorrhage or shock at delivery, with failure of lactation, loss of body hair, and amenorrhea. **shoulder-hand s.**, a disorder of the upper extremity characterized by pain and stiffness in the shoulder, with puffy swelling and pain in the ipsilateral hand, sometimes occurring after myocardial infarction, but also produced by other causes. **Siemon's s.**, congenital ectodermal defect. **Sjögren's s.**, keratoconjunctivitis sicca with pharyngitis sicca, enlargement of parotid glands and chronic polyarthritis. **Stein-Leventhal s.**, secondary amenorrhea and absence of ovulation associated with bilateral polycystic ovaries, but normal excretion of follicle-stimulating hormone and 17-ketosteroids. **Stevens-Johnson s.**, a systemic disease complex with fever and malaise, the clinical picture being dominated by lesions of the skin and mucous membranes. **Stewart-Morel s.**, frontal internal hyperostosis. **Stewart-Treves s.**, lymphangiosarcoma occurring in an edematous arm after radical removal of a breast cancer. **stiffman s.**, progressive fluctuating muscular rigidity and spasm. **Sturge-Kalischer-Weber s.**, nevoid amentia. **Sturge-Weber s.**, vascular nevi along the course of the superior and middle branches of the trigeminal nerve, glaucoma on the same side, and nevi of the pia. **subclavian steal s.**, deficiency of cerebral circulation as a result of drainage of blood from the brain to the upper extremity when the ipsilateral subclavian artery is obstructed proximal to the origin of the vertebral artery. **Taussig-Bing s.**, a combination of overriding large pulmonary artery, transposed aorta and ventricular septal defect. **temporomandibular joint s.**, tinnitus, vertigo, discomfort in the ears and other symptoms due to faulty articulation of the temporomandibular joint. **testicular feminization s.**, an extreme form of male pseudohermaphroditism, with external genitalia and secondary sex characters typical of the female, but with presence of testes and absence of uterus and uterine tubes. **transfusion s.,** a condition sometimes found in single-ovum, monochorial twins, due to unequal mutual circulation in the placenta, one twin being larger and edematous, the other small and dehydrated. **Treacher-Collins s.,** mandibulofacial dysostosis. **Turner's s.,** sexual infantilism, webbed neck and cubitus valgus in the female, due to a chromosomal abnormality. **van der Hoeve's s.,** a genetically determined condition characterized by blue scleras, deafness and abnormal brittleness of bones. **Vernet's s.,** jugular foramen syndrome. **Villaret's s.,** unilateral paralysis of the glossopharyngeal, vagus, spinal accessory and hypoglossal nerves due to a lesion in the space posterior to the parotid gland. **Waardenburg's s.,** congenital deafness with anomalies of the eyelids, eyebrows or nose root, with anomalous pigmentation of the iris and scalp hair. **Waterhouse-Friderichsen s.,** massive adrenal hemorrhage with profound shock and usually sudden death, often occurring with a severe infection or an overdose of anticoagulants. **Weber-Christian s.,** recurring febrile episodes, with nonsuppurative nodules developing in subcutaneous tissue. **Werner's s.,** premature age changes in an adult, with early graying and loss of hair, hyperkeratinization and scleroderma-like changes in the skin of the lower extremities, followed by chronic ulceration. **Wernicke's s.,** a condition due to acute thiamine deficiency, usually in alcoholics, with symptoms referable to the central nervous system. **Willebrand's s.,** a hemorrhagic disorder characterized by prolonged bleeding time, and normal clotting time and platelet count. **Wolff-Parkinson-White s.,** a defect in functioning of the heart in paroxysmal tachycardia, the electrocardiogram showing a short P-R interval and widened QRS complex. **Zollinger-Ellison s.,** intractable, sometimes fulminating, atypical peptic ulcers associated with extreme gastric hyperacidity and nonbeta cell, noninsulin-secreting islet cell tumors of the pancreas.

Syndrox (sin'droks) trademark for preparations of methamphetamine.

synechia (sĭ-nek'e-ah), pl. *synech'iae* [Gr.] adhesion, as of the iris to the cornea or lens. **annular s., circular s.,** adhesion of the whole rim of the iris to the lens. **anterior s.,** adhesion of the iris to the cornea. **s. pericar'dii,** concretio cordis. **posterior s.,** adhesion of the iris to the capsule of the lens. **total s.,** adhesion of the whole surface of the iris to the lens. **s. vul'vae,** a congenital or acquired condition in which the labia minora are sealed in the midline, with only a small opening below the clitoris through which urination and menstruation may occur.

synechotomy (sin"ĕ-kot'o-me) incision of a synechia.

synecology (sin"e-kol'o-je) the study of the environment of organisms in the mass.

synencephalocele (sin"en-sef'ah-lo-sēl") en-

cephalocele with adhesions to adjoining parts.

synencephalus (sin"en-sef'ah-lus) a fetal monster with two bodies and one head.

syneresis (sĭ-ner'ĕ-sis) a drawing together of the particles of the dispersed phase of a gel, with separation of some of the disperse medium and shrinkage of the gel.

synergism (sin'er-jizm) the joint action of agents so that their combined effect is greater than the algebraic sum of their individual parts. adj., **synergist'ic.**

synergist (sin'er-jist) a muscle or agent which acts with another.

synergy (sin'er-je) correlated action or cooperation. adj., **synerget'ic, syner'gic.**

synesthesia (sin"es-the'ze-ah) sensation experienced in association with stimuli producing another sensation.

synesthesialgia (-the"ze-al'je-ah) a painful synesthesia.

syngamy (sing'gah-me) a method of reproduction in protozoa in which two individuals (gametes) unite permanently and their nuclei fuse.

syngenesis (sin-jen'ĕ-sis) 1. the origin of an individual from a germ derived from both parents and not from either one alone. 2. the state of having descended from a common ancestor.

synizesis (sin"ĭ-ze'sis) contraction of the pupil of the eye.

synkaryon (sin-kar'e-on) a nucleus formed by fusion of two pronuclei.

Synkayvite (sin'ka-vīt) trademark for preparations of menadiol sodium diphosphate.

synkinesis (sin"ki-ne'sis) involuntary contraction of a muscle occurring synchronously with contraction of another.

synneurosis (sin"nu-ro'sis) syndesmosis.

synonychia (sin"o-nik'e-ah) fusion of the nails of two or more digits in syndactyly.

synophthalmus (sin"of-thal'mus) cyclops.

Synophylate (sin"o-fi'lāt) trademark for preparations of theophylline sodium glycinate.

synorchism (sin'or-kizm) congenital fusion of the testes into one mass.

synosteology (sin"os-te-ol'o-je) the study of joints and articulations.

synosteotomy (sin"os-te-ot'o-me) dissection of the joints.

synostosis (-to'sis), pl. *synosto'ses* [Gr.] normal or abnormal connection of two bones by osseous material.

synotia (sĭ-no'she-ah) developmental anomaly with fusion of the ears, or location near the midventral line in the upper part of the neck.

synotus (sĭ-no'tus) a fetal monster exhibiting synotia.

synovectomy (sin"o-vek'to-me) excision of a synovial membrane.

synovia (sĭ-no've-ah) the transparent, viscid fluid secreted by synovial membrane and found in joint cavities, bursae and tendon sheaths. adj., **syno'vial.**

synovialis (sĭ-no"ve-a'lis) the synovial membrane.

synovialoma (-ah-lo'mah) a tumor of synovial membrane origin.

synovianalysis (-ah-nal'ĭ-sis) laboratory examination of synovia in diagnosis of joint disease.

synovioma (sĭ-no″ve-o′mah) synovialoma.

synovitis (sin″o-vi′tis) inflammation of a synovial membrane, usually painful, particularly on motion, and characterized by fluctuating swelling, due to effusion in a synovial sac. **dry s.**, synovitis with little effusion. **purulent s.**, synovitis with effusion of pus in a synovial sac. **serous s.**, synovitis with copious nonpurulent effusion. **s. sic′ca**, dry synovitis. **simple s.**, synovitis with clear or but slightly turbid effusion. **tendinous s.**, inflammation of a tendon sheath.

synovium (sĭ-no′ve-um) a synovial membrane.

synthermal (sin-ther′mal) of the same temperature.

synthesis (sin′thĕ-sis) creation of a compound by union of elements composing it, done artificially or as a result of natural processes. adj., **synthet′ic. distributive s.**, in psychobiology, guided integration of a patient's total self and reactions.

synthetase (sin′thĕ-tās) an enzyme that catalyzes reactions necessary to the synthesis of a substance in the body.

Synthroid (sin′throid) trademark for a preparation of sodium levothyroxine.

Syntocinon (sin-to′sĭ-non) trademark for a solution of synthetic oxytocin.

syntonic (-ton′ik) pertaining to a stable, integrated personality.

Syntropan (sin′tro-pan) trademark for a preparation of amprotropine phosphate.

syntrophoblast (sin-trof′o-blast) the thick peripheral layer of the trophoblast, in which nuclei lie embedded in a common cytoplasmic mass.

syntropic (-trop′ik) turned in the same direction.

syntropy (sin′tro-pe) the state of felicitous and mutually satisfactory relationship.

synulotic (sin″u-lot′ik) 1. producing cicatrization. 2. an agent promoting cicatrization.

synxenic (sin-zen′ik) associated with a known number of microbic species.

syphilid (sif′ĭ-lid) a skin affection of syphilitic origin.

syphilis (sif′ĭ-lis) a venereal disease caused by *Treponema pallidum*, leading to many structural and cutaneous lesions. adj., **syphilit′ic. congenital s.**, syphilis existing at birth. **latent s.**, syphilis in the stage following the primary and secondary stages, when no signs or symptoms are present. **primary s.**, syphilis in its first stage. **secondary s.**, syphilis in the second of its three stages. **tertiary s.**, the stage characterized by peculiar skin affections.

syphiloderm (sif′ĭ-lo-derm″) a syphilitic skin disease.

syphilogenesis (sif″ĭ-lo-jen′ĕ-sis) the development of syphilis.

syphilography (sif″ĭ-log′rah-fe) a treatise on syphilis.

syphiloid (sif′ĭ-loid) 1. resembling syphilis. 2. a disease like syphilis.

syphilologist (sif″ĭ-lol′o-jist) a specialist in syphilology.

syphilology (sif″ĭ-lol′o-je) sum of knowledge about syphilis, its pathology and treatment.

syphiloma (sif″ĭ-lo′mah) a tumor of syphilitic origin.

syphilopathy (sif″ĭ-lop′ah-the) any syphilitic manifestation.

syphilophobia (sif″ĭ-lo-fo′be-ah) morbid fear of syphilis. adj., **syphilopho′bic.**

syphilophyma (-fi′mah) a syphilitic growth or excrescence.

syring(o)- (si-ring′go) word element [Gr.], *tube*; *fistula*.

syringe (sir′inj) instrument for introducing fluids into the body or a body cavity. **chip s.**, a small, fine-nozzled syringe for blowing away cuttings while excavating a tooth cavity. **dental s.**, a small syringe with a curved tip for use in dental work. **hypodermic s.**, one for introduction of liquids through a hollow needle into subcutaneous tissues. **Luer's s., Luer-Lok s.**, a glass syringe for intravenous and hypodermic use.

syringectomy (sir″in-jek′to-me) excision of a fistula.

syringitis (sir″in-ji′tis) inflammation of the eustachian tube.

syringoadenoma (si-ring″go-ad″ē-no′mah) adenoma of a sweat gland.

syringobulbia (-bul′be-ah) presence of fluid-filled cavities in the medulla oblongata and pons varolii.

syringocarcinoma (-kar″sĭ-no′mah) cancer of a sweat gland.

syringocele (si-ring′go-sēl) a cavity-containing herniation of the spinal cord through the bony defect in spina bifida.

syringocoele (sĭ-ring′go-sēl) the central canal of the spinal cord.

syringocystadenoma (si-ring″go-sist″ad-ē-no′mah) adenoma of a sweat gland.

syringocystoma (-sis-to′mah) cystic tumor of a sweat gland.

syringoma (sir″ing-go′mah) tumor of a sweat gland.

syringomeningocele (sĭ-ring″go-mĕ-ning′go-sēl) meningocele resembling syringomyelocele.

syringomyelia (-mi-e′le-ah) presence of fluid filled cavities in the substance of the spinal cord.

syringomyelitis (-mi″ĕ-li′tis) inflammation of spinal cord with formation of cavities.

syringomyelocele (-mi′ĕ-lo-sēl″) protrusion of the spinal cord, with central canal filled with fluid.

syringotomy (sir″ing-got′o-me) incision of a fistula.

syrosingopine (si″ro-sing′go-pēn) a white or slightly yellowish crystalline powder used as an antihypertensive.

syrup (sir′up) a concentrated solution of a sugar, such as sucrose, in water or other aqueous liquid; combined with other ingredients, such a solution is used as a flavored vehicle for medications. **acacia s.**, acacia with sodium benzoate, sucrose, vanilla tincture and distilled water. **simple s.**, one compounded with purified water and sucrose.

systaltic (sis-tal'tik) alternately contracting and dilating.

system (sis'tem) 1. a set or series of interconnected or interdependent parts or entities (objects, organs or organisms) that act together in a common purpose or produce results impossible by action of one alone. 2. an organized set of principles or ideas. adj., **systemat'ic, system'ic. alimentary s.**, the organs concerned with conversion of foodstuffs and absorption of nutritive elements in the body. **biological s.**, one composed of living material, ranging from a collection of separate molecules to an assemblage of separate organisms. **cardiovascular s.**, the heart and blood vessels, by which blood is pumped and circulated through the body. **centrencephalic s.**, the neurons in the central core of the brain stem from the thalamus down to the medulla oblongata, connecting the two hemispheres of the brain. **chromaffin s.**, cells of the body that characteristically stain strongly with chromium salts, considered collectively. **circulatory s.**, channels through which nutrient fluids of the body flow; often restricted to the vessels conveying blood. **digestive s.**, organs concerned with ingestion and digestion of food. **dosimetric s.**, a plan of exact or determinate dosage. **ecological s.**, ecosystem. **endocrine s.**, the glands which pour their secretions directly into the blood stream, including the pituitary, parathyroid, thyroid and adrenal glands; secretions of other organs, including the pancreas, testes and ovaries, also enter the blood directly. **genitourinary s.**, urogenital system. **Golgi s.**, Golgi complex. **haversian s.**, a haversian canal and its concentrically arranged lamellae, constituting the basic unit of structure in compact bone (osteon). **hematopoietic s.**, the tissues concerned in the production of blood. **heterogeneous s.**, a system or structure made up of mechanically separable parts, as an emulsion. **homogeneous s.**, a system or structure made up of parts which cannot be mechanically separated, as a solution. **limbic s.**, a system of brain structures common to the brains of all mammals, comprising the phylogenetically old cortex (archipallium and mesopallium) and its primarily related nuclei. **lymphatic s.**, the lymphatic vessels and lymphatic or lymphoid tissue, considered collectively. **masticatory s.**, all bony and soft structures of the face and mouth involved in mastication, and the vessels and nerves supplying them. **metric s.**, a system of weights and measures based on the meter and having all units based on some power of 10. **muscular s.**, the muscles of the body considered collectively; generally restricted to the voluntary, skeletal muscles. **nervous s.**, the chief organ system by which adjustment and reactions of an organism to internal and environmental conditions are correlated, comprising the central and the peripheral nervous systems. **nervous s., autonomic**, the portion of the nervous system concerned with regulation of activity of cardiac muscle, smooth muscle and glands. **nervous s., central**, the brain and spinal cord. **nervous s., parasympathetic**, part of the autonomic nervous system, the preganglionic fibers of which leave the central nervous system with cranial nerves III, VII, IX and X and the first three sacral nerves; postganglionic fibers are distributed to the heart, smooth muscle and glands of the head and neck, and thoracic, abdominal and pelvic viscera. **nervous s., peripheral**, all elements of the nervous system (nerves and ganglia) outside the brain and spinal cord. **nervous s., sympathetic**, part of the autonomic nervous system, the preganglionic fibers of which arise from cell bodies in the thoracic and first three lumbar segments of the spinal cord; postganglionic fibers are distributed to the heart, smooth muscle and glands of the entire body. **portal s.**, an arrangement by which blood collected from one set of capillaries passes through a large vessel or vessels and another set of capillaries before returning to the systemic circulation, as in the pituitary gland and liver. **respiratory s.**, the tubular and cavernous organs that allow atmospheric air to reach the membranes across which gases are exchanged with the blood. **reticuloendothelial s.**, highly phagocytic cells widely scattered throughout the body, identified by marked affinity for nontoxic colloidal dyes and inert particulate matter. **skeletal s.**, the bony framework which provides support for the body and associated elements that make possible movement and locomotion. **stomatognathic s.**, structures of the mouth and jaws, considered collectively, as they subserve the functions of mastication, deglutition, respiration and speech. **urogenital s.**, the organs concerned with production and excretion of urine, together with the organs of reproduction. **vascular s.**, the vessels of the body, especially the blood vessels. **vasomotor s.**, the part of the nervous system that controls the caliber of the blood vessels.

systema (sis-te'mah) system.

systole (sis'to-le) the contraction, or period of contraction, of the heart, especially of the ventricles. adj., **systol'ic. aborted s.**, a systole not appreciable through the pulse because of mitral regurgitation. **arterial s.**, the rhythmic contraction of an artery. **atrial s., auricular s.**, contraction of atria by which blood is forced into the ventricles; it precedes the true or ventricular systole. **catalectic s.**, an aborted or imperfect systole. **ventricular s.**, contraction of ventricles, forcing blood into aorta and pulmonary artery.

systremma (sis-trem'ah) a cramp in the muscles of the calf of the leg.

Sytobex (si'to-beks) trademark for a parenteral preparation of crystalline vitamin B_{12}.

syzygy (siz'ĭ-je) the intimate association (linkage) of separate structures (as organs or organisms) without loss of individual identity.

T

T. temperature; tension (of the eyeball); therm (thermal); time.

T — diminished intraocular tension.

T+ increased intraocular tension.

T.A. toxin-antitoxin.

Ta chemical symbol, *tantalum.*

T.A.B. a vaccine prepared from killed typhoid, paratyphoid A and paratyphoid B bacilli.

tabacism (tab′ah sizm) tabacosis.

tabacosis (tab″ah-ko′sis) poisoning by tobacco, chiefly by inhaling tobacco dust.

Tabanus (tah-ba′nus) a genus of flies of worldwide distribution; commonly known as horseflies, they serve as vectors of various species of Trypanosoma.

tabardillo (tah″bar-dēl′yo) an infectious disease of Mexico, resembling typhoid fever.

tabefaction (tab″e-fak′shun) wasting of the body; emaciation.

tabes (ta′bēz) 1. a wasting disorder. 2. tabes dorsalis. adj., **tabet′ic. cerebral t.,** general paresis. **cervical t.,** tabes dorsalis in which the upper extremities are first affected. **t. dorsa′lis,** a slowly progressive nervous disorder, resulting from degeneration of the dorsal columns of the spinal cord and sensory nerve trunks, with various trophic disturbances, especially of bones and joints. **hereditary t.,** Friedreich's ataxia. **marantic t.,** tabes dorsalis marked by great emaciation. **t. mesenter′ica, t. mesara′ica,** tuberculosis of mesenteric glands in children.

tabescent (tah-bes′ent) growing emaciated; wasting away.

tabetiform (tah-bet′ĭ-form) resembling tabes.

tablature (tab′lah-chūr) separation of the chief cranial bones into inner and outer tables, separated by a diploe.

table (ta′bl) a flat-surface structure. **inner t.,** the inner compact layer of the bones covering the brain. **operating t.,** a specially designed piece of furniture on which a patient is placed to undergo operation. **outer t.,** the outer compact layer of the bones covering the brain. **vitreous t.,** inner table. **water t.,** the upper surface of the impervious strata on which the ground water lies deep to the earth's surface.

tablet (tab′let) a solid dosage form containing a medicinal substance with or without a suitable diluent. **buccal t.,** a slowly dissolving tablet intended to be held in the mucosal pocket between cheek and jaw. **coated t.,** one covered with a thin film of another substance to improve its palatability or delay absorption. **enteric-coated t.,** one coated with material that delays release of the medication until after it leaves the stomach. **nitroglycerin t.,** a preparation of glyceryl trinitrate in tablet form; used as a vasodilator in angina pectoris. **sublingual t.,** a rapidly dissolving tablet intended to be inserted beneath the tongue. **trisulfapyrimidines t's,** tablets containing sulfadiazine, sulfamerazine and sulfamethazine.

taboparesis (ta″bo-par′ē-sis) tabes with general paralysis.

tabophobia (-fo′be-ah) a morbid fear of tabes.

tabular (tab′u-lar) resembling a table.

Tacaryl (tak′ah-ril) trademark for preparations of methdilazine.

Tace (tās) trademark for preparations of chlorotrianisene.

tache (tahsh) [Fr.] spot or blemish; applied to various blemishes on the skin, as *tache blanche* ("white spot"), *tache bleuâtre* ("blue spot") and *tache noir* ("black spot"), or to the slight enlargement of the fibril of a motor nerve on a muscle (*tache motrice*). adj., **tachet′ic.**

tachogram (tak′o-gram) the graphic record produced by tachography.

tachography (tah-kog′rah-fe) the recording of the movement and speed of the blood current.

tachy- (tak′e) word element [Gr.], *rapid; speed.*

tachycardia (tak″e-kar′de-ah) abnormally rapid heart rate. adj., **tachycar′diac. atrial t.,** a heart rate of 140–220 due to impulses arising in an irritable ectopic focus in the atrium. **ectopic t.,** rapid heart action in response to impulses arising outside the sino-atrial node. **essential t.,** a paroxysmal form resulting from functional disorder of the cardiac nerves. **orthostatic t.,** tachycardia occurring on arising from a reclining position. **paroxysmal t.,** rapid heart action that starts and stops abruptly. **ventricular t.,** a rapid, regular heart rate due to stimuli arising in an ectopic focus or ring in the ventricular conduction system.

tachygenesis (-jen′ē-sis) acceleration and compression of ancestral stages in embryonic development.

tachylalia (-la′le-ah) rapidity of speech.

tachymeter (tah-kim′ē-ter) instrument for measuring rapidity of motion.

tachyphagia (tak″e-fa′je-ah) rapid eating.

tachyphasia (-fa′ze-ah) rapid speech.

tachyphrasia (-fra′ze-ah) extreme volubility of speech.

tachyphrenia (-fre′ne-ah) mental hyperactivity.

tachyphylaxis (-fi-lak′sis) 1. reduction of reaction to a substance by repeated injection of small quantities of it. 2. reduction of response to a stimulus by repetitive slight stimuli. adj., **tachyphylac′tic.**

tachypnea (tak″ip-ne′ah) very rapid respiration.

tachypragia (tak″e-pra′je-ah) rapidity of action.

tachypsychia (-si′ke-ah) rapidity of psychic processes.

tachyrhythmia (-rith′me-ah) tachycardia.

tachysterol (tak-is′tĕ-rol) a compound produced by irradiation of ergosterol.

tachysystole (tak″e-sis′to-le) abnormally rapid systole.

Tacosal (tak′o-sal) trademark for a preparation of diphenylhydantoin.

tactile (tak'til) pertaining to touch.

tactometer (tak-tom'ĕ-ter) instrument for measuring tactile sensibility.

tactus (tak'tus) [L.] touch. adj., **tac'tual. t. erudi'tus,** delicacy of touch acquired by practice.

Taenia (te'ne-ah) a genus of tapeworms. **T. echinococ'cus,** Echinococcus granulosus. **T. sagina'ta,** a species 12–25 feet long, found in the adult form in the human intestine and in the larval state in muscles and other tissues of the ox. **T. so'lium,** the pork tapeworm, a common parasite of man where raw or poorly cooked pork is part of the normal diet; adult worms are usually 6–10 feet long and composed of 800–900 proglottids.

taenia (te'ne-ah) tenia.

taeniacide (te'ne-ah-sīd'') teniacide.

taeniafuge (te'ne-ah-fūj'') teniafuge.

Taeniarhynchus (te''ne-ah-ring'kus) a genus of tapeworms.

Tagathen (tag'ah-then) trademark for a preparation of chlorothen citrate.

Taka-diastase (tah'kah-di'as-tās) trademark for an amylolytic enzyme produced by action of a fungus on wheat bran.

talbutal (tal'bu-tal) a short- to intermediate-acting barbiturate.

talc (talk) a native hydrous magnesium silicate, sometimes with a small amount of aluminum silicate; used in pharmaceutical preparations.

talcosis (tal-ko'sis) a condition due to inhalation or implantation in the body of talc.

talcum (tal'kum) talc.

talipes (tal'ĭ-pēz) congenital deformity of the foot, which is twisted out of shape or position (clubfoot); the foot may be in dorsiflexion (talipes calca'neus) or plantar flexion (talipes equi'nus), abducted, everted (talipes val'gus), abducted, inverted (talipes va'rus) or various combinations of these (talipes calcaneoval'gus, talipes calcaneova'rus, talipes equinoval'gus or talipes equinova'rus).

talipomanus (tal''ĭ-pom'ah-nus) clubhand.

talocalcanean (ta''lo-kal-ka'ne-an) pertaining to talus and calcaneus.

talocrural (-kroo'ral) pertaining to talus and the leg bones.

talonid (tal'o-nid) the posterior part of a lower molar tooth.

talus (ta'lus) a bone of the ankle.

tambour (tam'boor) a drum-shaped appliance used in transmitting movements in a recording instrument.

tampon (tam'pon) a pack or plug made of cotton, sponge or other material, variously used in surgery.

tamponade (tam''po-nād') 1. the exertion of pressure or compression on a part, occurring as the result of a pathologic process or used as a means of arresting hemorrhage. 2. an instrument used in checking internal hemorrhage. **balloon t.,** a device with a triple-lumen tube and two inflatable balloons, the third lumen providing for aspiration of blood clots, designed for esophagogastric tamponade. **cardiac t., heart t.,** compression of the heart due to collection of blood in the pericardium. **esophagogastric t.,** the exertion of pressure against bleeding esophageal varices by means of an inflatable device, with one sausage-shaped balloon in the esophagus and a globular one in the stomach.

Tandearil (tan-de'ah-ril) trademark for a preparation of oxyphenbutazone.

tank (tank) a large artificial receptacle for the storage of fluid substances. **Hubbard t.,** a tank in which exercises may be performed under water.

tannate (tan'āt) a salt of tannic acid.

tannin (tan'in) tannic acid.

tantalum (tan'tah-lum) chemical element (see table), at. no. 73, symbol Ta; a noncorrosive and malleable metal used in surgery to repair defects in the skull or other tissues.

tantrum (tan'trum) a violent display of temper.

tap (tap) 1. a quick, light blow. 2. to drain off fluid by paracentesis.

Tapazole (tap'ah-zol) trademark for a preparation of methimazole.

tape (tāp) a long, narrow strip of fabric or other flexible material. **adhesive t.,** a strip of fabric or other material evenly coated on one side with a pressure-sensitive adhesive material.

tapeinocephalic (tah-pi''no-sĕ-fal'ik) characterized by tapeinocephaly; having a vertical index below 72.

tapeinocephaly (-sef'ah-le) flattening or depression of the skull.

tapetum (tah-pe'tum), pl. tape'ta [L.] a covering structure or layer of cells. **t. lu'cidum,** the iridescent epithelium of the choroid of animals which gives their eyes the property of shining in the dark.

tapeworm (tāp'werm) a parasitic intestinal cestode worm. **armed t.,** Taenia solium. **beef t.,** Taenia saginata. **broad fish t.,** Dibothriocephalus latus. **dog t.,** Dipylidium caninum. **hydatid t.,** Echinococcus granulosus. **pork t.,** Taenia solium. **unarmed t.,** Taenia saginata.

taphophilia (taf''o-fil'e-ah) morbid interest in graves and cemeteries.

taphophobia (-fo'be-ah) morbid fear of being buried alive.

tapotement (tah-pōt-maw') [Fr.] a tapping manipulation in massage.

tar (tar) a dark, viscid substance obtained from wood of different trees or from bituminous coal. **coal t.,** a by-product obtained in destructive distillation of bituminous coal; used in ointment or solution in treatment of eczema. **juniper t.,** volatile oil obtained from wood of Juniperus oxycedrus. **pine t.,** a product of destructive distillation of the wood of Pinus palustris or other species of pine; used as a local irritant and antibacterial agent.

Taraxacum (tah-rak'sah-kum) a genus of composite-flowered plants.

taraxacum (tah-rak'sah-kum) dried rhizome and root of a species of Taraxacum.

tare (tār) 1. the weight of the vessel in which a substance is weighed. 2. to weigh a vessel which is to contain a substance in order to allow for it when the vessel and substance are weighed together.

target (tar'get) that part of the x-ray tube on which the electrons impinge and from which the x-rays are sent out.

tars(o)- (tar'so) word element [Gr.], *edge of eyelid; tarsus of the foot.*

tarsalgia (tar-sal'je-ah) pain in a tarsus.

tarsalia (tar-sa'le-ah) the bones of the tarsus.

tarsalis (tar-sa'lis) [L.] tarsal.

tarsectomy (tar-sek'to-me) 1. excision of one or more bones of the tarsus. 2. excision of the cartilage of the eyelid.

tarsitis (tar-si'tis) inflammation of the cartilaginous portion of the eyelid.

tarsoclasis (tar-sok'lah-sis) surgical fracturing of the tarsus of the foot.

tarsomalacia (tar″so-mah-la'she-ah) softening of the tarsal cartilage.

tarsometatarsal (-met″ah-tar'sal) pertaining to tarsus metatarsus.

tarsophyma (-fi'mah) any tumor of the tarsus.

tarsoplasty (tar'so-plas″te) plastic repair of the tarsal cartilage of an eyelid.

tarsoptosis (tar″sop-to'sis) falling of the tarsus; flatfoot.

tarsorrhaphy (tar-sor'ah-fe) suture of the tarsal cartilage of an eyelid.

tarsotomy (tar-sot'o-me) incision of the tarsal cartilage of an eyelid.

tarsus (tar'sus) 1. the seven bones—talus, calcaneus, navicular, medial, intermediate and lateral cuneiform, and cuboid—composing the articulation between the foot and leg; the ankle. 2. the cartilaginous plate forming the framework of either (upper or lower) eyelid. adj., **tar'sal.**

tartar (tar'tar) 1. the recrystallized sediment of wine casks; crude potassium bitartrate. 2. dental calculus. **t. emetic,** antimony potassium tartrate.

tartrate (tar'trāt) a salt of tartaric acid.

tattooing (tah-too'ing) a process of applying permanent coloring to skin or cornea, to cover leukomatous spots.

taurine (taw'rēn) a crystallized acid, aminoethyl-sulfonic acid, from the bile.

taurocholate (taw″ro-ko'lāt) a salt of taurocholic acid.

taurocholemia (-ko-le'me-ah) taurocholic acid in the blood.

tautomer (taw'to-mer) a chemical compound exhibiting, or capable of exhibiting, tautomerism.

tautomeral (taw-tom'er-al) tautomeric.

tautomeric (taw″to-mer'ik) 1. sending axons to the white substance in the same side of the spinal cord; said of nerve cells. 2. exhibiting tautomerism.

tautomerism (taw-tom'er-izm) the dynamic equilibrium between two spontaneously interconvertible isomers.

taxis (tak'sis) 1. an orientation movement of a motile organism in response to a stimulus; it may be either toward (positive) or away from (negative) the source of the stimulus. 2. exertion of force in manual replacement of a displaced organ or part. **coughing t.,** manipu-

lation to reduce hernia while the patient coughs.

taxon (tak'son), pl. *tax'a* [Gr.] a particular category into which living organisms are classified on the basis of certain common features, as species, genus, family, order or class.

taxonomy (tak-son'o-me) the orderly classification of organisms into appropriate categories (taxa), with application of suitable and correct names. adj., **taxonom'ic.**

Tb chemical symbol, *terbium.*

tb tuberculosis; tubercle bacillus.

TBP bithionol.

Tc chemical symbol, *technetium.*

TCID tissue culture infective dose; that amount of a pathogenic agent that will produce pathologic change when inoculated on tissue cultures.

TCID$_{50}$ median tissue culture infective dose; that amount of a pathogenic agent that will produce pathologic change in 50 per cent of cell cultures inoculated.

Te chemical symbol, *tellurium.*

TEA tetraethylammonium.

tea (te) an aqueous beverage prepared by infusion of herbs or other substance. **pectoral t.,** an aqueous infusion of expectorant and demulcent herbs and aromatics.

TEAB tetraethylammonium bromide.

TEAC tetraethylammonium chloride.

tease (tēz) to pull apart gently with fine needles to permit microscopic examination of ultimate structure.

teat (tēt) the nipple of the mammary gland.

technetium (tek-ne'she-um) chemical element *(see table),* at. no. 43, symbol Te.

technic (tek'nik) technique.

technician (tek-nish'an) a person skilled in the performance of technical procedures.

technique (tek-nēk') the method of procedure and details of a mechanical process or surgical operation.

tectonic (tek-ton'ik) pertaining to plastic surgery.

tectorial (tek to're-al) of the nature of a roof or covering.

tectorium (tek-to're-um) the membrane of Corti.

tectum (tek'tum) a rooflike structure. **t. of midbrain,** the dorsal portion of the midbrain.

teething (tēth'ing) eruption of the teeth through the gingivae.

tegmen (teg'men), pl. *teg'mina* [L.] a covering structure or roof.

tegmentum (teg-men'tum), pl. *tegmen'ta* [L.] a covering; used in anatomic nomenclature to designate various structures. adj., **tegmen'tal.**

tegument (teg'u-ment) the integument or skin. adj., **tegumen'tal, tegumen'tary.**

teichopsia (ti-kop'se-ah) scintillating scotoma.

T-1824 Evans blue.

teinodynia (ti″no-din'e-ah) pain in the tendons.

tela (te'lah), pl. *te'lae* [L.] a weblike structure or tissue; used in naming various anatomic structures. **t. conjuncti'va,** connective tissue. **t. elas'tica,** elastic tissue. **t. subcuta'nea,**

the subcutaneous connective tissue or supeficial fascia.

telalgia (tel-al'je-ah) referred pain.

telangiectasia (tel-an"je-ek-ta'ze-ah) the presence of small red focal lesions, usually in skin or mucous membrane, caused by dilation of capillaries, arterioles or venules.

telangiectasis (-ek'tah-sis), pl. *telangiec'tases* [Gr.] the small red focal lesion of telangiectasia. **spider t.,** a focal network of dilated arterioles, radiating about a central core.

telangiitis (-i'tis) inflammation of capillaries.

telangioma (-o'mah) hemangioma.

telangiosis (-o'sis) any disease of the capillaries.

tele- (tel'e) word element [Gr.], *far away; operating at a distance; an end.*

telecardiography (tel"ĕ-kar"de-og'rah-fe) recording of changes in electric potential of the heart, the impulses being transmitted by telephone wires to the receiving apparatus located some distance from the subject.

telecardiophone (-kar'de-o-fōn") an apparatus for making heart sounds audible at a distance from the patient.

teleceptor (-sep'tor) a receptor which receives stimuli from a distance. adj., **telecep'tive.**

telecinesia (-si-ne'ze-ah) telekinesis.

telecurietherapy (-ku"re-ther'ah-pe) treatment with radium placed at a distance from the body.

telediastolic (-di"as-tol'ik) pertaining to the last phase of diastole.

telefluoroscopy (-floo"or-os'ko-pe) television transmission of images visualized by fluoroscopy for observation and study at a distant location.

telekinesis (-ki-ne'sis) movement of an object produced without contact.

telemetry (tĕ-lem'ĕ-tre) the making of measurements at a distance from the subject, the measurable evidence of phenomena under investigation being transmitted by radio signals.

telencephalon (tel"en-sef'ah-lon) the larger portion of the forebrain, comprising chiefly the cerebral hemispheres, but including also the area adjacent to the anterior part of the third ventricle and the anterior part of the hypothalamus. adj., **telencephal'ic.**

teleneurite (tel"e-nu'rīt) telodendron.

teleneuron (-nu'ron) a neuron at which the impulse ceases.

teleological (te"le-o-loj'ĭ-kal) serving an ultimate purpose in development.

teleology (te"le-ol'o-je) the doctrine of final causes or of adaptation to a definite purpose.

teleomitosis (tel"e-o-mi-to'sis) completed mitosis.

teleonomic (-nom'ik) pertaining to or having evolutionary survival value.

teleonomy (tel"e-on'o-me) the doctrine that existence of a structure or function in an organism implies that it has had evolutionary survival value.

teleorganic (tel"e-or-gan'ik) necessary to life.

Telepaque (tel'e-pāk) trademark for a preparation of iopanoic acid.

telepathy (tĕ-lep'ah-the) the communication of thought through extrasensory perception.

teleradiography (tel"e-ra"de-og'rah-fe) radiography with the radiation source 6–7 feet from the subject.

telergy (tel'er-je) automatism.

teleroentgenography (tel"e-rent"gen-og'rah-fe) roentgenography with the source of roentgen (x) rays 6–7 feet from the subject.

telesthesia (tel"es-the'ze-ah) 1. perception at a distance. 2. extrasensory perception.

telesystolic (tel"e-sis-tol'ik) pertaining to the end of systole.

teletherapy (-ther'ah-pe) treatment with ionizing radiation whose source is located at a distance from the body.

telethermometer (-ther-mom'ĕ-ter) a device for registering temperature at a distance from the body being studied.

telluric (tĕ-lu'rik) 1. pertaining to tellurium. 2. pertaining to or originating from the earth.

tellurium (tĕ-lu're-um) chemical element (*see table*), at. no. 52, symbol Te.

telo- (tel'o) word element [Gr.], *end.*

teloblast (tel'o-blast) a segmentation sphere at the end of a germinal band.

telocentric (tel"o-sen'trik) having the centromere at one end of the replicating chromosome.

telodendrion (-den'dre-on), pl. *teloden'dria* [Gr.] telodendron.

telodendron (-den'dron) one of the fine terminal branches of an axon.

telogen (tel'o-jen) the quiescent or resting phase of the hair cycle, following catagen, the hair having become a club hair and not growing further.

telognosis (tel"og-no'sis) diagnosis based on facsimiles of roentgenograms transmitted by radio or telephonic communication to a clinical or diagnostic center.

telolecithal (tel"o-les'ĭ-thal) having a yolk concentrated at one of the poles.

telolemma (-lem'ah) the covering of a motor end-plate.

telomere (tel'o-mēr) an extremity of a chromosome, which has specific properties, one of which is failure to fuse with other fragments of chromosomes.

telophase (tel'o-fāz) the last stage of division of the nucleus of a cell in either meiosis or mitosis.

TEM triethylene melamine.

Temaril (tem'ah-ril) trademark for preparations of trimeprazine tartrate.

temperament (tem'per-ah-ment) the peculiar physical character and mental cast of an individual. **lymphatic t.,** that characterized by a fair but not ruddy complexion, light hair, and a general softness or laxity of the tissues. **melancholic t.,** that characterized by a predominance of *black bile* (supposedly secreted by the spleen), rendering the disposition melancholy and morose. **nervous t.,** that characterized by predominance of the nervous element and by great activity or susceptibility of the brain. **phlegmatic t.,** lymphatic temperament. **sanguine t., sanguineous t.,** that characterized by a fair and ruddy complexion, full, muscular development, large, full veins and an active pulse.

temperature (tem'per-ah-chūr) an expression of heat or coldness in terms of a specific scale. **absolute t.,** that reckoned from absolute zero (−273.15°C. or −459.67°F.). **critical t.,** that below which a gas may be converted to a liquid by pressure. **normal t.,** that usually registered by a healthy person (98.6°F. or 37° C.).

temple (tem'pl) lateral region of the head above the zygoma.

tempolabile (tem"po-la'bil) subject to change with time.

temporal (tem'po-ral) pertaining to the temple.

temporomandibular (tem"po-ro-man-dib'u-lar) pertaining to temporal bone and mandible.

temporomaxillary (-mak"sĭ-lar"e) pertaining to temporal bone and maxilla.

temporo-occipital (-ok-sip'ĭ-tal) pertaining to temporal and occipital bones.

temporospatial (-spa'shal) pertaining to both time and space.

temporosphenoid (-sfe'noid) pertaining to temporal and sphenoid bones.

tempostabile (tem"po-sta'bil) not subject to change with time.

Tempra (tem'prah) trademark for preparations of acetaminophen.

tenaculum (tĕ-nak'u-lum) a surgical instrument for grasping and holding parts.

tenalgia (ten-al'je-ah) pain in a tendon.

tenderness (ten'der-nes) a state of unusual sensitivity to touch or pressure. **rebound t.,** a state in which pain is felt on the release of pressure over a part.

tendinitis (ten"dĭ-ni'tis) tenonitis.

tendinoplasty (ten'dĭ-no-plas"te) tenoplasty.

tendinosuture (ten"dĭ-no-su'chūr) tenorrhaphy.

tendinous (ten'dĭ-nus) pertaining to, or made up of, tendons.

tendo (ten'do), pl. *ten'dines* [L.] tendon; used in anatomic nomenclature. **t. Achil'lis, t. calca'neus,** Achilles tendon.

tendolysis (ten-dol'ĭ-sis) the freeing of a tendon from adhesions.

tendon (ten'don) a fibrous cord of connective tissue continuous with the fibers of a muscle and attaching the muscle to bone or cartilage. **Achilles t., calcaneal t.,** the powerful tendon at the back of the heel, attaching the triceps surae muscle to the calcaneus.

tendovaginal (ten"do-vaj'ĭ-nal) pertaining to a tendon and its sheath.

tenectomy (tĕ-nek'to-me) excision of a tendon.

tenesmus (tĕ-nez'mus) ineffectual and painful straining at stool or in urinating.

tenia (te'ne-ah), pl. *te'niae* [L.] 1. a flat band or strip of soft tissue; used in anatomic nomenclature to designate various structures. 2. an individual of the genus Taenia. **te'niae co'li,** the three thickened bands (*te'nia li'bera, te'nia mesocol'ica* and *te'nia omenta'lis*) formed by longitudinal fibers in the muscular tunic of the large intestine, extending from the root of the vermiform appendix to the rectum.

teniacide (te'ne-ah-sīd") a medicine for destroying tapeworms.

teniafuge (te'ne-ah-fūj") a medicine for expelling tapeworms.

teniasis (te-ni'ah-sis) presence of tapeworms in the body.

teno- (te'no) word element [Gr.], *tendon.*

tenodesis (ten-od'e-sis) suture of the end of a tendon to a bone.

tenodynia (ten"o-din'e-ah) pain in a tendon.

tenomyoplasty (-mi'o-plas"te) plastic repair of a tendon and muscle.

tenomyotomy (-mi-ot'o-me) excision of tendon and muscle.

tenonectomy (-nek'to-me) excision of part of a tendon.

tenonitis (-ni'tis) 1. inflammation of a tendon. 2. inflammation of Tenon's capsule.

tenontitis (ten"on-ti'tis) inflammation of a tendon.

tenonto- (ten-on'to) word element [Gr.], *tendon.*

tenontodynia (ten"on-to-din'e-ah) pain in the tendons.

tenontography (ten"on-tog'rah-fe) the written description of tendons.

tenontology (-tol'o-je) sum of what is known about the tendons.

tenontothecitis (ten-on"to-the-si'tis) tenosynovitis.

tenophyte (ten'o-fīt) an osseous growth in a tendon.

tenoplasty (ten'o-plas"te) plastic repair of a tendon.

tenoreceptor (ten"o-re-scp'tor) a nerve receptor in a tendon.

tenorrhaphy (ten-or'ah-fe) suture of a tendon.

tenositis (ten"o-si'tis) tenontitis.

tenostosis (ten"os-to'sis) conversion of a tendon into bone.

tenosuspension (ten"o-sus-pen'shun) suspension of head of humerus to acromion process by a strip of tendon.

tenosuture (-su'chūr) tenorrhaphy.

tenosynovectomy (-sin"o-vek'to-me) excision of a tendon sheath.

tenosynovitis (-sin"o-vi'tis) inflammation of a tendon and its sheath.

tenotomy (ten-ot'o-me) transection of a tendon. **graduated t.,** partial transection of a tendon.

tenovaginitis (ten"o-vaj"ĭ-ni'tis) tenosynovitis.

Tensilon (ten'sĭ-lon) trademark for a solution of edrophonium chloride.

tension (ten'shun) the quality of being stretched or strained, or under pressure. **gaseous t.,** the elasticity of a gas, or its tendency to expand. **intraocular t.,** intraocular pressure. **premenstrual t.,** a complex of symptoms, including emotional instability and irritability, sometimes occurring in the 10 days before menstruation. **surface t.,** tension or resistance which acts to preserve the integrity of a surface. **tissue t.,** a state of equilibrium between tissues and cells which prevents overaction of any part.

tensometer (ten-som'ĕ-ter) an apparatus by which the tensile strength of materials can be determined.

CELSIUS : FAHRENHEIT $°F = (°C \times {}^9/_5) + 32$				FAHRENHEIT : CELSIUS $°C = (°F - 32) \times {}^5/_9$					
C°	F°	C°	F°	F°	C°	F°	C°	F°	C°
−50	−58.0	49	120.2	−50	−46.7	99	37.2	157	69.4
−40	−40.0	50	122.0	−40	−40.0	100	37.7	158	70.0
−35	−31.0	51	123.8	−35	−37.2	101	38.3	159	70.5
−30	−22.0	52	125.6	−30	−34.4	102	38.8	160	71.1
−25	−13.0	53	127.4	−25	−31.7	103	39.4	161	71.6
−20	−4.0	54	129.2	−20	−28.9	104	40.0	162	72.2
−15	−5.0	55	131.0	−15	−26.6	105	40.5	163	72.7
−10	14.0	56	132.8	−10	−23.3	106	41.1	164	73.3
−5	23.0	57	134.6	−5	−20.6	107	41.6	165	73.8
0	32.0	58	136.4	0	−17.7	108	42.2	166	74.4
+1	33.8	59	138.2	+1	−17.2	109	42.7	167	75.0
2	35.6	60	140.0	5	−15.0	110	43.3	168	75.5
3	37.4	61	141.8	10	−12.2	111	43.8	169	76.1
4	39.2	62	143.6	15	−9.4	112	44.4	170	76.6
5	41.0	63	145.4	20	−6.6	113	45.0	171	77.2
6	42.8	64	147.2	25	−3.8	114	45.5	172	77.7
7	44.6	65	149.0	30	−1.1	115	46.1	173	78.3
8	46.4	66	150.8	31	−0.5	116	46.6	174	78.8
9	48.2	67	152.6	32	0	117	47.2	175	79.4
10	50.0	68	154.4	33	+0.5	118	47.7	176	80.0
11	51.8	69	156.2	34	1.1	119	48.3	177	80.5
12	53.6	70	158.0	35	1.6	120	48.8	178	81.1
13	55.4	71	159.8	36	2.2	121	49.4	179	81.6
14	57.2	72	161.6	37	2.7	122	50.0	180	82.2
15	59.0	73	163.4	38	3.3	123	50.5	181	82.7
16	60.8	74	165.2	39	3.8	124	51.1	182	83.3
17	62.6	75	167.0	40	4.4	125	51.6	183	83.8
18	64.4	76	168.8	41	5.0	126	52.2	184	84.4
19	66.2	77	170.6	42	5.5	127	52.7	185	85.0
20	68.0	78	172.4	43	6.1	128	53.3	186	85.5
21	69.8	79	174.2	44	6.6	129	53.8	187	86.1
22	71.6	80	176.0	45	7.2	130	54.4	188	86.6
23	73.4	81	177.8	46	7.7	131	55.0	189	87.2
24	75.2	82	179.6	47	8.3	132	55.5	190	87.7
25	77.0	83	181.4	48	8.8	133	56.1	191	88.3
26	78.8	84	183.2	49	9.4	134	56.6	192	88.8
27	80.6	85	185.0	50	10.0	135	57.2	193	89.4
28	82.4	86	186.8	55	12.7	136	57.7	194	90.0
29	84.2	87	188.6	60	15.5	137	58.3	195	90.5
30	86.0	88	190.4	65	18.3	138	58.8	196	91.1
31	87.8	89	192.2	70	21.1	139	59.4	197	91.6
32	89.6	90	194.0	75	23.8	140	60.0	198	92.2
33	91.4	91	195.8	80	26.6	141	60.5	199	92.7
34	93.2	92	197.6	85	29.4	142	61.1	200	93.3
35	95.0	93	199.4	86	30.0	143	61.6	201	93.8
36	96.8	94	201.2	87	30.5	144	62.2	202	94.4
37	98.6	95	203.0	88	31.0	145	62.7	203	95.0
38	100.4	96	204.8	89	31.6	146	63.3	204	95.5
39	102.2	97	206.6	90	32.2	147	63.8	205	96.1
40	104.0	98	208.4	91	32.7	148	64.4	206	96.6
41	105.8	99	210.2	92	33.3	149	65.0	207	97.2
42	107.6	100	212.0	93	33.8	150	65.5	208	97.7
43	109.4	101	213.8	94	34.4	151	66.1	209	98.3
44	111.2	102	215.6	95	35.0	152	66.6	210	98.8
45	113.0	103	217.4	96	35.5	153	67.2	211	99.4
46	114.8	104	219.2	97	36.1	154	67.7	212	100.0
47	116.6	105	221.0	98	36.6	155	68.3	213	100.5
48	118.4	106	222.8	98.6	37.0	156	68.8	214	101.1

tent (tent) 1. conical, expansible plug for dilating an orifice. 2. a portable shelter to be placed over a patient in bed, to limit dissemination of gases or vapors administered for therapeutic purposes. **oxygen t.**, a portable shelter used in administration of oxygen. **sponge t.**, a conical plug made of compressed sponge. **steam t.**, a portable shelter erected over a bed, into which steam or medicated vapor is passed.

tentacle (ten'tah-kl) a slender, whiplike organ for receiving stimuli or for motion.

tentigo (ten-ti'go) morbid lasciviousness.

tentorium (ten-to're-um), pl. *tento'ria* [L.] a covering structure or roof. adj., **tento'rial.**

tephrosis (tef-ro'sis) incineration or cremation.

tera- (ter'ah) word element [Gr.], *monstrosity*; used in naming units of measurement to designate an amount 10^{12} (a trillion, or million million) times the size of the unit to which it is joined, as teracurie; symbol T.

teracurie (ter"ah-ku're) a unit of radioactivity, being one trillion (10^{12}) curies.

teras (ter'as), pl. *ter'ata* [L., Gr.] a fetal monster. adj., **terat'ic.**

teratism (ter'ah-tizm) a fetal monster.

terato- (ter'ah-to) word element [Gr.], *monster; monstrosity*.

teratoblastoma (ter"ah-to-blas-to'mah) teratoma.

teratocarcinoma (-kar"si-no'mah) teratoma.

teratogen (ter'ah-to-jen) an agent or influence that causes physical defects in the developing embryo. adj., **teratogen'ic.**

teratogenesis (ter"ah-to-jen'ě-sis) the production of deformity in the developing embryo, or of a fetal monster. adj., **teratogenet'ic.**

teratogenous (ter"ah-toj'ě-nus) developed from fetal remains.

teratogeny (-toj'ě-ne) teratogenesis.

teratoid (ter'ah-toid) like a monster.

teratology (ter"ah-tol'o-je) the branch of embryology which deals with abnormal development and congenital malformations.

teratoma (-to'mah) a compound tumor; a growth containing cellular elements derived from more than one primary germ layer. **cystic t.**, a small neoplasm, lined by skin and filled with typical cheesy secretion, derived from the mainly ectodermal proliferation of totipotential cells.

teratophobia (ter"ah-to-fo'be-ah) morbid fear of giving birth to a teratism.

teratosis (ter"ah-to'sis) the condition of a monster.

terbium (ter'be-um) chemical element (see table), at. no. 65, symbol Tb.

terchloride (ter-klo'rīd) trichloride.

terebene (ter'ě-bēn) a mixture of hydrocarbons from turpentine oil; antiseptic and stimulant expectorant.

terebinth (ter'ě-binth) turpentine.

terebration (ter"ě-bra'shun) the process of boring.

teres (te'rēz) [L.] round.

Terfonyl (ter'fo-nil) trademark for prepara-

tions of sulfamethazine, sulfadiazine and sulfamerazine (trisulfapyrimidines).

ter in die (ter in de'a) [L.] three times a day.

term (term) 1. a limit or boundary. 2. a definite period, especially the period of gestation, or pregnancy.

terminal (ter'mĭ-nal) 1. pertaining to an end. 2. a termination, end or extremity, especially a nerve ending.

terminatio (ter"mi-na'she-o), pl. *termina-tio'nes* [L.] an ending; used in anatomic nomenclature to designate free nerve endings (*termina'tiones nervo'rum li'berae*).

terminology (-nol'o-je) nomenclature; a system of scientific or technical terms; the science which deals with the investigation, arrangement and construction of terms.

terminus (ter'mĭ-nus), pl. *ter'mini* [L.] 1. a term; expression. 2. an ending.

ternary (ter'nah-re) 1. third in a series or in order. 2. made up of three elements or radicals.

teroxide (ter-ok'sīd) trioxide.

terpene (ter'pēn) any hydrocarbon of the formula $C_{10}H_{16}$.

terpin (ter'pin) a product obtained by the action of nitric acid on oil of turpentine and alcohol. **t. hydrate**, a bitter, colorless, crystalline compound used as an expectorant.

Terramycin (ter'ah-mi"sin) trademark for preparations of oxytetracycline.

terror (ter'or) an attack of extreme fear or dread. **day t., daytime t.**, pavor diurnus. **night t., nighttime t.**, pavor nocturnus.

tertian (ter'shan) recurring every three days (every second day).

tertiary (ter'she-a"re) third in order.

tertigravida (ter"she-grav'ĭ-dah) a woman pregnant for the third time; gravida III.

tertipara (ter-tip'ah-rah) a woman who has had three pregnancies which resulted in viable offspring; para III.

Tessalon (tes'sah-lon) trademark for a preparation of benzonatate.

tessellated (tes'ě-lāt"ed) checkered; marked by little squares.

test (test) a procedure designed to demonstrate the existence or nonexistence of a certain quality or condition. **agglutination t.**, one whose results depend on agglutination of bacteria or other cells; used in diagnosing certain infections, diseases and rheumatoid arthritis. **Allen-Doisey t.**, one for detection of estrogenic activity. **Almen t's**, tests for detection of albumin, blood or dextrose in solutions, such as urine. **alpha t.**, a set of intelligence tests first used in 1917-1918 for evaluation of U.S. army recruits who were literate. **angiotensin-infusion t.**, one for determining the role of renal artery stenosis in the genesis of a patient's hypertension. **aptitude t.**, one designed to measure the capacity for developing general or specific skills. **Aschheim-Zondek t.**, one for pregnancy, based on the effects on ovaries of immature female mice produced by injection of the patient's urine. **association t.**, one based on associative reaction, usually by mentioning words to a patient and noting what other words the patient will give as the ones called up in his mind. **autohemolysis t.**, determination of spontaneous hemolysis in a blood specimen maintained under certain conditions, to detect the presence of certain hemolytic states. **Babcock's t.**, one for determination of the fat content of milk. **Benedict's t.**, a qualitative or quantitative test for the determination of sugar (glucose or dextrose) content of solutions. **bentonite t.**, a flocculation test for rheumatoid arthritis in which sensitized bentonite particles are used. **beta t.**, a set of intelligence tests first used in 1917-1918 for evaluation of U.S. army recruits who were unable to read. **Binet-Simon t's**, tests for the determination of mental capacity, the results being expressed numerically as the intelligence quotient. **biologic t's**, tests involving the use of living organisms to determine the effects of the test material. **blanche t.**, blanching of the tissues just lingual to the maxillary medial incisors after a tug on the upper lip indicates persistence of attachment of a heavy fibrous frenum which may interfere with normal developmental closure of the spacing between the teeth. **Bourdon's t.**, one based on the accuracy and time required for a subject to strike out certain letters, numbers or words as required. **breeding t's**, the rearing of successive generations of organisms as a means of genetic research. **Calmette t.**, ophthalmic reaction. **caloric t.**, Barany's sign. **Casoni's t.**, an intracutaneous test for hydatid disease. **Chautard's t.**, one for acetone in the urine. **Chediak t.**, a clotting and flocculation test for syphilis. **chromatin t.**, determination of genetic sex of an individual by examination of body cells for the presence of sex chromatin. **cis-trans t.**, a test in microbial genetics to determine whether two mutations that have the phenotypic effect, in a haploid cell or a cell with single phage infection, are located in the same gene or in different genes; the test depends on the independent behavior of two alleles of a gene in a diploid cell or in a cell infected with two phages carrying different alleles. **Clark t.**, profuse bleeding from the cervical canal when a probe is withdrawn from the uterus, indicative of carcinoma of the fundus. **coin t.**, a silver coin held flat on the anterior chest wall is struck with the edge of another silver coin; a clear, bell-like sound heard by stethoscope on the posterior chest wall indicates air in the pleural space. **Coombs t.**, one for detection of globulin antibodies on the surface of erythrocytes. **Dick t.**, one for determination of susceptibility to scarlet fever. **Donnath-Landsteiner t.**, one performed on the blood in the diagnosis of paroxysmal cold hemoglobinuria. **double-blind t.**, a study of the effects of a specific agent in which neither the administrator nor the recipient, at the time of administration, knows whether the active or an inert substance is being used. **euglobulin lysis t.**, one which measures blood fibrinolytic activity by determining the time required to dissolve an incubated clot composed of precipitated plasma euglobulin and exoge-

nous thrombin. **flocculation t.**, one whose results depend on the degree of flocculent precipitation produced. **Frei t.**, intracutaneous injection of antigen derived from infected chick embryos, used in the diagnosis of lymphogranuloma venereum. **Friedman t.**, one for pregnancy, based on the effects on ovaries of a mature, nonpregnant female rabbit, produced by injection of the patient's urine. **glucose tolerance t.**, a test of the body's ability to utilize carbohydrates by measuring the blood sugar level at stated intervals after ingestion or intravenous injection of a large quantity of glucose. **guaiac t.**, one for determination of blood in a stain. **Guenzburg t.**, one for free hydrochloric acid in the stomach contents. **Haagensen t.**, observation of the contour of the breasts when the patient leans forward as a means of detecting malignant changes in the mammae. **Ham t.**, one for congenital or acquired hemolytic anemia. **Heaf t.**, an intracutaneous test for sensitivity to the tubercle bacillus, a drop of solution of P.P.D. being forced to penetrate the outer layer of the skin by the pressure of six needle points. **Heller t.**, one for detection of albumin in the urine. **Hinton's t's**, serologic tests performed for the diagnosis of syphilis. **histidine loading t.**, one for determining folic acid deficiency. **Holmgren t.**, one for detection of imperfect perception of color, based on matching various strands of yarn. **Huhner t.**, determination of the number and condition of spermatozoa in mucus aspirated from the cervical canal within two hours after intercourse. **human erythrocyte agglutination t.**, one for rheumatoid arthritis, depending on agglutination by the patient's serum of human Rh-positive cells sensitized with incomplete anti-Rh antibody. **inkblot t.**, Rorschach test. **intracutaneous t.**, one which involves introduction of an antigen between the layers of the skin and evaluation of the reaction elicited by it. **Kahn t.**, a serologic test performed for the diagnosis of syphilis. **Kline t.**, a serologic test performed for the diagnosis of syphilis. **Koh t.**, one for the detection of emotional disorders in children. **Kolmer t.**, a complement-fixation technique used in the diagnosis of syphilis or other infections. **Kuhlmann t's**, tests for the determination of intelligence in infants. **Kurzrok-Miller t.**, an in-vitro test of compatibility of cervical mucus and spermatozoa. **Kveim t.**, an intracutaneous test for the diagnosis of sarcoidosis. **Lange colloidal gold t.**, one formerly used for the determination of the albumin-globulin ratio in the spinal fluid. **latex-fixation t.**, a serologic test for rheumatoid arthritis. **Leffmann-Beam t.**, a modification of the Babcock test used for determination of fat in human breast milk. **lysis time t.**, one for measuring blood fibrinolytic activity. **Mantoux t.**, an intracutaneous test for sensitivity to the tubercle bacillus, solutions of gradually increasing concentration of P.P.D. being used until a reaction occurs. **Master "2-step" exercise t.**, a test of coronary circulation, electrocardiograms being recorded while and after the subject repeatedly ascends and descends two steps, each 9 inches high. **Moloney t.**, one for detection of delayed hypersensitivity to diphtheria toxoid. **multiple-puncture t.**, an intracutaneous test in which the material used (e.g. tuberculin) is introduced into the skin by pressure of several needles or pointed tines or prongs. **neutralization t.**, one for the bacterial neutralization power of a substance by testing its action on the pathogenic properties of the organism concerned. **Nickerson-Kveim t.**, Kveim test. **nonverbal t.**, a mental test in which language is not used. **osmotic resistance t.**, one for determining the liberation of platelet factor 3. **Pandy t.**, one for globulin in cerebrospinal fluid. **Pap t.**, **Papanicolaou t.**, examination by special techniques of cells exfoliated from the uterine cervix, as a means of early detection of cervical carcinoma. **partial thromboplastin time t.**, a one-stage clotting test to detect deficiencies of the components of the intrinsic thromboplastin system. **patch t.**, a test for hypersensitivity, performed by observing the reaction to application to the skin of filter paper or gauze saturated with the substance in question. **paternity t.**, one to determine the blood groups of mother, child and alleged father for the purpose of excluding the possibility of paternity. **performance t.**, an intelligence test in which pieces of blocks, pictures, etc., are fitted together. **phlorizin t.**, a test of kidney function based on injection of phlorizin and sodium carbonate. **Pinter-Patterson t's**, a group of performance tests in which a form board is used. **plasmacrit t.**, a rapid screening test for syphilis, using plasma from microhematocrit tubes. **prothrombin consumption t.**, a test to measure the formation of intrinsic thromboplastin by determining the residual serum prothrombin after blood coagulation is complete. **Quick hippuric acid excretion t.**, measurement of hippuric acid in urine after ingestion of a standard dose of benzoic acid; formerly used as a test of liver function. **Quick one-stage prothrombin time t.**, a method of determining the integrity of the prothrombin complex of the blood, used in controlling anticoagulant therapy. **Quick tourniquet t.**, estimation of capillary fragility by counting the number of petechiae appearing in a limited area on the flexor surface of the forearm after obstruction to the circulation by a blood pressure cuff applied to the upper arm. **Rinne t.**, a test of hearing made with tuning forks of 256, 512 and 1024 cycle frequency, comparing the duration of perception by bone and by air conduction. **Roberts t.**, one for detection of albumin in urine. **Rorschach t.**, one for disclosing personality traits and conflicts by the patient's response to 10 cards bearing symmetrical ink blots in various colors and shading. **Rosenbach t.**, detection of cold hemolysins by hemoglobinuric response to immersion of the hands or feet in ice water. **Rose-Waaler t.**, a sheep cell agglutination test. **Rubin t.**, one for patency of

the uterine tubes, made by transuterine inflation with carbon dioxide gas. **Rubner t.**, one for detection of lactose in the urine. **Sachs-Georgi t.**, **Sachs-Witebsky t.**, serologic tests for the diagnosis of syphilis. **Schick t.**, one for determination of susceptibility to diphtheria. **Schiller t.**, one for early carcinoma, performed by painting the uterine cervix with a solution of iodine and potassium iodide, diseased areas being revealed by a failure to take the stain. **Schilling t.**, one for the diagnosis of primary pernicious anemia. **Schwabach t.**, a test of hearing made with tuning forks of 256, 512, 1024 and 2048 cycle frequency, the duration of perception of the patient by bone conduction being compared with that of the examiner. **serologic t.**, one involving examination of blood serum. **sheep cell agglutination t.**, a test for rheumatoid arthritis depending on agglutination by the patient's serum of sheep red blood cells sensitized with rabbit gamma globulin. **sickling t.**, one for demonstratingon of abnormal hemoglobin and the sickling phenomenon in erythrocytes. **single-blind t.**, a study of the effects of a specific agent in which the administrator, but not the recipient, knows whether the active or an inert substance is being used. **Snider match t.**, a screening test of pulmonary ventilation, based on the patient's ability to extinguish the flame of an ordinary book match under specified conditions. **Strauss t.**, one for the presence of lactic acid in stomach contents. **Terman t.**, a verbal test of general mental ability. **Thorn t.**, one for adrenal cortical function, based on a decrease of eosinophilic leukocytes in the blood after injection of adrenocorticotropic hormone. **thromboplastin generation t.**, one for delineation of defects in formation of intrinsic thromboplastin and hence deficiencies of the factors involved. **tine tuberculin t. (Rosenthal)**, a multiple-puncture test in which a steel disk bearing four 2-mm. long tines or prongs coated with dip-dried old tuberculin is pressed firmly against the skin, usually over the belly of a muscle on the forearm. **tolerance t.**, 1. an exercise test to determine the efficiency of the circulation 2. a test to determine the body's ability to metabolize a substance or to endure administration of a drug. **tourniquet t.**, one involving application of a tourniquet to an extremity, as in determination of capillary fragility or status of the collateral circulation. **T.P.A.** (*Treponema pallidum* agglutination) **t.**, **T.P.C.F.** (*Treponema pallidum* complement fixation) **t.**, **T.P.I.** (*Treponema pallidum* immobilization) **t.**, **T.P.I.A.** (*Treponema pallidum* immune-adherence) **t.**, tests related directly to the causative organism, used in the diagnosis of syphilis. **tuberculin t.**, a test for the existence of tuberculosis, consisting in the injection subcutaneously of 5 mg. of tuberculin. **two-stage prothrombin t.**, a method of quantitating prothrombin after tissue thromboplastin and excess factor V have converted it to thrombin. **Uffelmann t.**, one for the presence of lactic acid in stomach contents. **van den Bergh t.**, one for determination of the level of bilirubin in the blood serum. **Waaler-Rose t.**, sheep cell agglutination test. **Wassermann t.**, one used for the diagnosis of syphilis. **Watson-Schwartz t.**, one used in the diagnosis of acute porphyria. **Weber t.**, a hearing test made by placing a vibrating tuning fork at some point on the midline of the head and noting whether it is perceived in the midline or referred to either ear. **Widal t.**, one for the diagnosis of typhoid and paratyphoid fevers, based on agglutination of typhoid bacilli by the patient's serum.

test meal (test′ mēl) a portion of food or foods given for the purpose of determining the functioning of the alimentary or digestive tract. **Boas' t. m.**, a tablespoonful of oatmeal in a quart of water, boiled down to a pint. **Dock's t. m.**, Ewald's test meal, with one shredded wheat biscuit substituted for the rolls or bread. **Ewald's t. m.**, 2 rolls or slices of dry bread and 9 to 12 ounces of water. **Fischer's t. m.**, Ewald's test meal, with addition of ¼ pound of finely chopped, lean hamburger steak, broiled and slightly seasoned. **Klemperer's t. m.**, one consisting of 70 gm. of bread and 500 cc. of milk. **Leube-Riegel t. m.**, 12 ounces of soup, 4 ounces of minced steak, 2 ounces of white bread, 6 ounces of water. **motor t. m.**, food or drink whose progress through the stomach, pylorus and the intestinal tract is observed roentgenoscopically. **Schmidt-Strassburger t. m.**, a meal for testing gastric motility.

test type (test tīp) printed letters of varying size, used in the testing of visual acuity.

testectomy (tes-tek′to-me) removal of a testis; castration.

testibrachium (tes″tī-bra′ke-um) superior peduncle of cerebellum.

testicle (tes′tī-kĕl) testis.

testiculoma (tes-tik″u-lo′mah) a tumor containing testicular tissue.

testis (tes′tis), pl. *tes′tes* [L.] the structure in the male in which the spermatozoa develop; the male gonad corresponding with the ovary in the female. adj., **testic′ular. Cooper's irritable t.**, a testis affected with neuralgia. **ectopic t.**, one in an abnormal location. **retained t.**, **undescended t.**, one that has not completed its descent into the scrotum, but is still within the abdomen or the inguinal canal.

testitis (tes-ti′tis) orchitis.

testoid (tes′toid) 1. resembling a testis. 2. a rudimentary testis.

testosterone (tes-tos′tĕ-rōn) a secretion of the testes in the male that functions in the induction and maintenance of male secondary sex characters; a pharmaceutical compound is prepared synthetically or isolated from bull testes. **ethinyl t.**, pregneninolone. **methyl t.**, methyltestosterone. **t. propionate**, creamy white crystalline powder, used as replacement therapy in the male and in treatment of certain conditions in the female.

Testryl (tes′tril) trademark for a suspension of pure crystalline testosterone.

tetaniform (tě-tan′ĭ-form) resembling tetanus.

tetanism (tet′ah-nizm) persistent muscular hypertonicity.

tetanization (tet″ah-ni-za′shun) the induction of tetanic convulsions or symptoms.

tetanize (tet′ah-nīz) to induce tetanic convulsions or symptoms in the organism or in a muscle.

tetanode (tet′ah-nōd) the unexcited stage of tetany.

tetanoid (tet′ah-noid) resembling tetanus.

tetanolysin (tet″ah-nol′ĭ-sin) a hemotoxin produced by *Clostridium tetani.*

tetanophilic (tet″ah-no-fil′ik) having affinity for tetanus toxin.

tetanospasmin (-spaz′min) the neurotoxic component of the tetanus toxin, of primary importance in the pathogenesis of tetanus.

tetanus (tet′ah-nus) 1. a highly fatal disease caused by *Clostridium tetani*, and characterized by convulsive contractions of the voluntary muscles. 2. sustained contraction of a muscle, without intervening periods of relaxation. adj., **tetan′ic. idiopathic t.**, a form occurring without known cause. **infantile t.**, **t. neonato′rum**, a form due to infection at the umbilicus. **puerperal t.**, a form occurring in childbed. **traumatic t.**, tetanus following injury.

tetany (tet′ah-ne) a syndrome manifested by sharp flexion of the wrist and ankle joints (carpopedal spasm), muscle twitchings, cramps and convulsions, sometimes with attacks of stridor; due to abnormal calcium metabolism and occurring in parathyroid hypofunction, vitamin D deficiency, alkalosis, and as a result of ingestion of alkaline salts. **duration t.**, a continuous tetanic contraction in response to a strong continuous current, occurring especially in degenerated muscles. **gastric t.**, a severe form due to disease of the stomach, attended by difficult respiration and painful tonic spasms of the extremities. **hyperventilation t.**, tetany produced by forced inspiration and expiration continued for a considerable time. **latent t.**, tetany elicited by the application of electrical and mechanical stimulation. **parathyroid t.**, **parathyroprival t.**, tetany due to removal or hypofunctioning of the parathyroids. **thyroprival t.**, a form due to removal of hypofunctioning of the thyroid gland.

tetarcone (tet′ar-kōn) tetartocone.

tetartanopia (tet″ar-tah-no′pe-ah) 1. quadrantanopia. 2. a type of defective color vision.

tetartanopsia (-nop′se-ah) tetartanopia.

tetartocone (tet-ar′to-kōn) the posterior internal cusp of a lower bicuspid tooth.

tetra- (tě′trah) word element [Gr.], *four.*

tetrabasic (tě″trah-ba′sik) having four replaceable hydrogen atoms.

tetrabrachius (-bra′ke-us) a fetal monster having four arms.

tetracaine (tě′trah-kān) a white or light yellow, waxy solid, used as a local anesthetic; applied topically to the conjunctiva in 0.5 per cent ointment. **t. hydrochloride**, a fine white crystalline powder, used as a local anesthetic;

in solution intraspinally or topically to the conjunctiva or in the nose and throat.

tetrachloride (tĕ″trah-klo′rīd) a compound of a radical with four atoms of chlorine.

tetrachloroethylene (-klōr″o-eth′ĭ-lēn) a clear, colorless liquid; anthelmintic.

tetracrotic (-krot′ik) having four sphygmographic waves or elevations to one beat of the pulse.

tetracycline (-si′klēn) a chemical compound containing four benzene rings, originally derived from soil microorganisms and found to be highly effective against rickettsiae, several gram-positive bacteria and certain viruses; several closely related compounds are elaborated by different species of Streptomyces or produced semisynthetically. **t. hydrochloride,** an antiamebic, antibacterial, antirickettsial compound.

Tetracyn (tĕ′trah-sin) trademark for preparations of tetracycline.

tetrad (tĕ′trad) 1. an element with a valence of four. 2. a group of four similar bodies or units.

tetradactyly (tĕ″trah-dak′tĭ-le) the presence of four digits on the hand or foot.

tetraethylammonium (-eth″il-ah-mo′ne-um) the radical ($C_2H_5)_4N$, used as a ganglionic blocking agent in various compounds (tetraethylammonium bromide, tetraethylammonium chloride).

tetraethylthiuram disulfide (-thi′u-ram di-sul′fīd) a white or slightly yellow powder; used in treatment of alcoholism.

tetragenous (tĕ-traj′ĕ-nus) splitting into groups of four.

tetragonum (tĕ″trah-go′num) [L.] a four-sided figure. **t. lumba′le,** the quadrangle bounded by the four lumbar muscles.

tetrahydrozoline (-hi-dro′zo-lēn) a sympathomimetic agent used topically as a nasal decongestant.

tetraiodophthalein (-i″o-do-thal′e-in) iodothalein.

tetraiodothyronine (-thi′ro-nēn) thyroxine.

tetralogy (tĕ-tral′o-je) a group or series of four. **t. of Fallot,** a complex of congenital heart defects commonly found in adults: pulmonic stenosis, interventricular septal defect, hypertrophy of right ventricle, and dextroposition of the aorta.

tetrameric (tĕ″trah-mer′ik) having four parts.

tetramethylenediamine (-meth″ĭ-lēn-di-am′-ēn) a bacterial decomposition product of proteins, arising from the decarboxylation of ornithine.

tetranopsia (-nop′se-ah) obliteration of one quadrant of the field of vision.

tetraodontoxin (-o″don-tok′sin) a toxin derived from fishes of the suborder Tetraodontoidea.

tetraparesis (-par′ĕ-sis) muscular weakness affecting all four extremities.

tetraplegia (-ple′je-ah) paralysis of all four extremities.

tetraploid (tĕ′trah-ploid) 1. characterized by tetraploidy. 2. an individual or cell having four sets of chromosomes.

tetraploidy (tĕ′trah-ploi″de) the state of having four sets of chromosomes (4n).

tetrapus (tĕ′trah-pus) fetal monster with four feet.

tetrasaccharide (tĕ″trah-sak′ah-rīd) a sugar, each molecule of which yields four molecules of monosaccharide on hydrolysis.

tetrascelus (tĕ-tras′ĕ-lus) a fetal monster with four legs.

tetrasomy (tĕ′trah-so″me) the presence of two extra chromosomes of one type in an otherwise diploid cell (2n + 2).

tetraster (tĕ-tras′ter) a figure in mitosis produced by quadruple division of the nucleus.

Tetrastoma (tĕ″trah-sto′mah) a genus of trematodes found in urine.

tetratomic (-tom′ik) 1. containing four atoms in the molecule. 2. containing four replaceable hydrogen atoms. 3. containing four hydroxyl groups.

tetravalent (-va′lent) having a valence of four.

tetroxide (tĕ-trok′sīd) a binary compound containing four oxygen atoms in the molecule.

tetter (tet′er) a vesicular skin disease.

textiform (teks′tĭ-form) formed like a network.

textoblastic (teks″to-blas′tik) forming adult tissue; regenerative.

textoma (teks-to′mah) a tumor composed of completely differentiated tissue cells.

textural (teks′chūr-al) pertaining to the constitution of tissues.

TGT thromboplastin generation test.

Th chemical symbol, *thorium.*

thalamencephalon (thal″ah-men-sef′ah-lon) that part of the diencephalon including the thalami, metathalamus and epithalamus.

thalamocoele (thal′ah-mo-sēl″) the third ventricle.

thalamocortical (thal″ah-mo-kor′tĭ-kal) pertaining to thalamus and cerebral cortex.

thalamolenticular (-len-tik′u-lar) pertaining to thalamus and lenticular nucleus.

thalamus (thal′ah-mus), pl. *thal′ami* [L.] either of the two large masses of gray matter situated one on each side of the third ventricle. adj., **thalam′ic.**

thalassemia (thal″ah-se′me-ah) a genetically determined defect of hemoglobin synthesis, associated with hepatosplenomegaly, mongoloid features and changes in bones, occurring chiefly in children of Mediterranean stock.

thalassophobia (thah-las″o-fo′be-ah) morbid dread of the sea.

thalassoposia (-po′ze-ah) the drinking of sea water.

thalassotherapy (-ther′ah-pe) treatment of disease by sea bathing, sea voyages or sea air.

thalidomide (thah-lid′o-mīd) a sedative and hypnotic compound whose use during early pregnancy was frequently followed by the birth of infants showing serious developmental deformities, notably dysmelia.

thallium (thal′e-um) chemical element (*see table*), at. no. 81, symbol Tl.

thanato- (than′ah-to) word element [Gr.], *death.*

thanatobiologic (than″ah-to-bi″o-loj′ik) pertaining to life and death.

thanatognomonic (than″ah-tog″no-mon′ik) indicating the approach of death.

thanatoid (than′ah-toid) resembling death.

thanatomania (than″ah-to-ma′ne-ah) suicidal mania.

thanatophobia (-fo′be-ah) unfounded apprehension of imminent death.

thassophobia (thas″so-fo′be-ah) morbid dread of sitting idle.

thebaine (the-ba′in) a crystalline, poisonous and anodyne alkaloid from opium, having properties similar to those of strychnine.

thebaism (the′bah-izm) opium poisoning.

theca (the′kah), pl. *the′cae* [L.] a case or sheath. adj., **the′cal. t. cor′dis,** pericardium. **t. follic′uli,** the capsule of a graafian follicle. **t. vertebra′lis,** the membranes or meninges of the spinal cord.

thecodont (the′ko-dont) having the teeth inserted in sockets.

thecoma (the-ko′mah) a tumor of the ovary containing cells of the theca folliculi.

thecostegnosis (the″ko-steg-no′sis) contraction of a tendon sheath.

Theileria (thi-le′re-ah) a genus of minute protozoan parasites.

theileriasis (thi″lē-ri′ah-sis) infection with Theileria.

theine (the′in) the alkaloid of tea, isomeric with caffeine.

thelalgia (the-lal′je-ah) pain in the nipples.

thelarche (the-lar′ke) beginning of development of the breast at puberty.

theleplasty (the′le-plas″te) plastic reconstruction of the nipples.

thelerethism (thel-er′ĕ-thizm) erection of the nipple.

thelitis (the-li′tis) inflammation of a nipple.

thelium (the′le-um) a papilla.

thelorrhagia (the″lo-ra′je-ah) hemorrhage from the nipple.

thelyblast (thel′ĭ-blast) the feminonucleus.

thelygenic (thel″ĭ-jen′ik) producing only female offspring.

thelyplasty (thel′ĭ-plas″te) theleplasty.

thenad (the′nad) toward the thenar eminence or toward the palm.

thenar (the′nar) fleshy part of the hand at the base of the thumb. adj., **the′nal.**

thenyldiamine (then″il-di′ah-mēn) a compound used as an antihistaminic.

Thenylene (then′i-lēn) trademark for a preparation of methapyrilene hydrochloride.

thenylpyramine (then″il-pir′ah-mēn) methapyrilene.

theobromine (the″o-bro′min) an alkaloid prepared from dried ripe seed of *Theobroma cacao*; used as a diuretic and smooth muscle relaxant; available as *theobromine calcium salicylate, theobromine sodium acetate* and *theobromine sodium salicylate.*

Theoglycinate (-gli′sī-nāt) trademark for a preparation of theophylline sodium glycinate.

theomania (-ma′ne-ah) religious insanity; especially mental disorder in which the patient believes himself inspired by or possessed of divinity.

theophylline (the″o-fil′in) an alkaloid derived from tea or produced synthetically; used as a smooth muscle relaxant and diuretic; available as *theophylline ethanolamine, theophylline methylglucamine, theophylline sodium acetate* and *theophylline sodium glycinate.* **t. cholinate,** oxtriphylline. **t. ethylenediamine,** aminophylline.

theory (the′o-re) a proposition advanced in explanation of an occurrence or condition. **Adler's t.,** neuroses develop as compensation for some feeling of inferiority. **cell t.,** all organic matter consists of cells, and cell activity is the essential process of life. **clonal-selection t. of immunity,** the theory that immunologic specificity is preformed during embryonic life and is mediated through cell clones. **Cohnheim's t.,** true tumors are due to faulty development in the embryo. **Ehrlich's side-chain (lateral-chain) t.** (of immunity and cytolysis), the protoplasm of body cells contains highly complex organic molecules consisting of a tolerably stable central group to which are attached less stable lateral (side) chains of atoms or atomic groups (*receptors*) which carry on the ordinary chemical transformations in the protoplasm, the stable center of the molecule remaining unaffected. The lateral chains contain a group of atoms (*haptophore group*) capable of uniting with similar (haptophore) groups in toxins, bacteria, and other foreign cells. As the lateral chains are seized upon by the foreign cells, the stable central group is stimulated to produce new lateral chains (*intermediary bodies*), designated, according to their nature, *uniceptors* or *amboceptors.* The *uniceptors,* represented by the antitoxins, produce their effect by seizing the toxin by means of its haptophore group. The *amboceptors,* represented by the cytolysins and bacteriolysins, have two affinities, one for the invading foreign cells, and one for a body called the *complement, end-body* or *addiment,* which exists normally in the body juices. The complement, when united with the foreign cells by the amboceptor, is capable of causing their solution by means of a *zymotoxic group.* **germ t.,** 1. all organisms are developed from a cell. 2. infectious diseases are of microbic origin. **Hering's t.,** color perception depends on a visual substance in the retina which is variously modified by anabolism for black, green and blue, and by catabolism for white, red and yellow. **neuron t.,** the nervous system consists of innumerable neurons in contiguity, but not in continuity. **preformation t.,** the theory that the individuals of successive generations are contained, completely formed, within the reproductive cell of one of the parents. **quantum t.,** radiation and absorption of energy occur in quantities (quanta) which vary in size with the frequency of the radiation. **undulatory t., wave t.,** light, electricity and heat are propagated by undulations in an ether which pervades all space. **Young-Helmholtz t.,** color vision depends on three sets of retinal receptors, corresponding to the colors red, green and violet.

Thephorin (thef'o-rin) trademark for preparations of phenindamine tartrate.

therapeutic (ther"ah-pu'tik) pertaining to or effective in the treatment of disease.

therapeutics (-pu'tiks) 1. the science and art of healing. 2. a scientific account of the treatment of disease.

therapeutist (-pu'tist) therapist.

therapist (ther'ah-pist) a person skilled in the treatment of disease or other disorder. **physical t.**, a person skilled in the techniques of physical therapy and qualified to administer treatments prescribed by a physician. **speech t.**, a person specially trained and qualified to assist patients in overcoming speech and language disorders.

therapy (ther'ah-pe) treatment designated to eliminate disease or other bodily disorder or derangement. **anticoagulant t.**, the use of drugs to suppress coagulability of the blood and prevent formation of thrombi without incurring the risk of hemorrhage. **collapse t.**, collapse and immobilization of the lung in treatment of pulmonary disease. **electroconvulsive t.**, **electroshock t.**, the induction of convulsions by the passage of an electric current through the brain, as in the treatment of affective disorders. **fever t.**, induction of high body temperature by bacterial or physical means in the treatment of various morbid conditions, such as general or physical means in the treatment of various morbid conditions, such as general paresis. **immunosuppressive t.**, treatment with agents that depress the formation of antibody, used in patients with autoimmune disease or receiving organ grafts. **insulin shock t.**, induction of hypoglycemic coma by the administration of insulin in the treatment of affective disorders. **milieu t.**, in psychiatry, treatment by modification of the life circumstances or immediate environment of the patient. **nonspecific t.**, treatment of disease by agents which produce a general effect on cellular activity. **occupational t.**, use during the convalescent period of some type of work or occupation to promote recovery. **physical t.**, use of physical agents and methods in rehabilitation and restoration of normal bodily function after illness or injury; it includes massage and manipulation, therapeutic exercises, hydrotherapy and various forms of energy (electrotherapy, actinotherapy and ultrasound). **replacement t.**, substitution therapy. **serum t.**, serotherapy. **shock t.**, the suspension of cerebral function by various means (insulin, electric current or other agent) in the treatment of affective disorders. **specific t.**, measures which are effective against the organism causing the disease. **speech t.**, the use of special techniques for correction of speech and language disorders. **substitution t.**, administration of glandular substance or of hormones to compensate for deficiency of an endocrine secretion in the body. **vaccine t.**, injection of killed cultures of an organism to produce immunity to or modify the course of a disease.

therm (therm) a unit of heat: (1) the small calorie; (2) British thermal unit.

therm(o)- (ther'mo) word element [Gr.], *heat*.

thermal (ther'mal) pertaining to heat.

thermalgesia (ther"mal-je'ze-ah) painful sensation produced by heat.

thermalgia (ther-mal'je-ah) causalgia.

thermanalgesia (therm"an-al-je'ze-ah) absence of sensibility to heat.

thermanesthesia (-es-the'ze-ah) inability to recognize heat and cold.

thermatology (ther"mah-tol'o-je) the study of heat as a therapeutic agent.

thermelometer (ther"mel-om'ĕ-ter) an electric thermometer for measuring small temperature changes.

thermesthesia (therm"es-the'ze-ah) perception of heat or cold.

thermesthesiometer (-the"ze-om'ĕ-ter) an instrument for measuring sensibility to heat.

thermhyperesthesia (therm"hi-per-es-the'ze-ah) increased sensibility to high temperatures.

thermhypesthesia (-pes-the'ze-ah) decreased sensibility to high temperatures.

thermic (ther'mik) pertaining to heat.

thermistor (ther-mis'tor) a special type of resistance thermometer that measures extremely small changes in temperature.

Thermoactinomyces (ther"mo-ak"ti-no-mi'-sēz) a genus of Schizomycetes (order Actinomycetales, family Streptomycetaceae).

thermobiosis (-bi-o'sis) ability to live in high temperature. adj., **thermobiot'ic**.

thermocautery (-kaw'ter-e) cauterization by a heated wire or point.

thermochemistry (-kem'is-tre) the aspect of physical chemistry dealing with temperature changes that accompany chemical reactions.

thermocoagulation (-ko-ag"u-la'shun) coagulation of tissue with high-frequency currents.

thermocouple (ther'mo-kup"el) a pair of dissimilar electrical conductors so joined that they may be used for measuring temperature differences

thermodiffusion (ther"mo-dĭ-fu'zhun) diffusion by heat.

thermoduric (-du'rik) able to endure high temperatures.

thermodynamics (-di-nam'iks) the branch of science dealing with heat and energy, their interconversion, and problems related thereto.

thermoexcitory (-ek-si'tor-e) stimulating production of bodily heat.

thermogenesis (-jen'ĕ-sis) the production of heat in organisms. adj., **thermogenet'ic**, **thermogen'ic**.

thermogenics (-jen'iks) the science of heat production.

thermogram (ther'mo-gram) the film produced by thermography.

thermograph (ther'mo-graf) an instrument for registering heat variations.

thermography (ther-mog'rah-fe) a technique of photographically portraying surface temperature of a body, sometimes used as a means of diagnosing underlying conditions.

thermohyperalgesia (ther″mo-hi″per-al-je′ze-ah) extreme thermalgesia.

thermohyperesthesia (-es-the′ze-ah) extreme sensitiveness to heat.

thermoinactivation (ther″mo-in-ak″tĭ-va′-shun) destruction of the power to act by exposure to high temperature.

thermoinhibitory (-in-hib′ĭ-tor″e) retarding generation of bodily heat.

thermolabile (-la′bil) easily affected by heat.

thermology (ther-mol′o-je) the science of heat.

thermoluminescence (ther″mo-lu″mĭ-nes′ens) the production of light by a substance when its temperature is increased.

thermolysis (ther-mol′ĭ-sis) 1. dissociation by means of heat. 2. dissipation of bodily heat by radiation, etc. adj., **thermolyt′ic.**

thermomassage (ther″mo-mah-sahzh′) massage with heat.

thermomastography (-mas-tog′rah-fe) use of thermography for the detection of lesions of the breast.

thermometer (ther-mom′ĕ-ter) an instrument for determining temperatures, in principle making use of a substance with a physical property that varies with temperature and is susceptible of measurement on some defined scale. **Celsius t.,** one on which the melting point of ice is 0 and the boiling point of water is 100 degrees. For equivalents of Celsius and Fahrenheit temperatures, *see table* (p. 610). **clinical t.,** one used to determine the temperature of the human body. **Fahrenheit t.,** one on which the melting point of ice (freezing point of water) is 32 and the boiling point of water is 212 degrees. **fever t.,** clinical thermometer. **mercurial t.,** one in which the expansible material is mercury. **metallic t.,** one in which the expansible material is some metal other than mercury. **oral t.,** a clinical thermometer whose mercury-containing bulb is placed under the tongue. **Réaumur's t.,** one on which the freezing point of water is 0 and the boiling point is 80 degrees. **recording t.,** a temperature-sensitive instrument by which the temperature to which it is exposed is continuously recorded. **rectal t.,** a clinical thermometer which is inserted in the rectum for determining body temperature. **resistance t.,** one which uses the electric resistance of metals for determining temperature. **self-registering t.,** recording thermometer. **veterinary t.,** one designed for determining body temperature of animals.

thermometry (ther-mom′ĕ-tre) measurement of temperature.

thermophile (ther′mo-fīl) an organism that grows best at temperatures of 55–65°C. adj., **thermophil′ic.**

thermophobia (ther″mo-fo′be-ah) morbid dread or intolerance of heat.

thermophore (ther′mo-fōr) an apparatus for applying therapeutic heat.

thermopile (ther′mo-pīl) a number of thermocouples in series, used to increase sensitivity to change in temperature or for direct conversion of heat into electric energy.

thermoplacentography (ther″mo-plas″en-tog′rah-fe) use of thermography for determination of the site of placental attachment.

thermoplegia (-ple′je-ah) heatstroke or sunstroke.

thermopolypnea (-pol″ip-ne′ah) quickened breathing due to great heat.

thermoreceptor (-re-sep′tor) a nerve ending sensitive to stimulation by heat.

thermoresistance (-re-zis′tans) the quality of being neither easily nor greatly affected by heat. adj., **thermoresis′tant.**

thermostabile (-sta′bel) not affected by heat.

thermostasis (-sta′sis) maintenance of temperature, as in warm-blooded animals.

thermostat (ther′mo-stat) a device interposed in a heating system by which temperature is automatically maintained between certain levels.

thermosteresis (ther″mo-stĕ-re′sis) deprivation of heat.

thermosystaltic (-sis-tal′tik) contracting under the stimulus of heat.

thermotaxis (-tak′sis) 1. normal adjustment of bodily temperature. 2. movement of a freely motile organism in response to the stimulation of a temperature gradient. adj., **thermotac′tic, thermotax′ic.**

thermotherapy (-ther′ah-pe) therapeutic use of heat.

thermotics (ther-mot′iks) the science of heat.

thermotolerant (ther″mo-tol′er-ant) capable of enduring heat.

thermotonometer (-to-nom′ĕ-ter) instrument for measuring amount of muscular contraction produced by heat.

thermotoxin (-tok′sin) a toxic substance formed in the body by heat.

thermotropism (ther-mot′ro-pizm) a growth curvature occurring in response to a temperature gradient. adj., **thermotrop′ic.**

Theruhistin (ther″u-his′tin) trademark for preparations of isothipendyl.

thesaurismosis (the-saw″riz-mo′sis) a metabolic disorder in which some substance accumulates in certain cells in abnormal amounts.

thesaurosis (the″saw-ro′sis) a condition due to the storing up in the body of unusual amounts of normal or foreign substance.

thi(o)- (thi′o) word element [Gr.], *sulfur.*

thiabendazole (thi″ah-ben′dah-zol) a broad-spectrum anthelmintic found useful in ancylostomiasis and strongyloidiasis.

thiamazole (thi-am′ah-zōl) methimazole.

thiamine (thi′ah-min) a component of the B complex group of vitamins, found in various foodstuffs and present in the free state in blood plasma and cerebrospinal fluid. **t. hydrochloride, t. mononitrate,** preparations used therapeutically as a vitamin supplement. **phosphorylated t., t. pyrophosphate,** the active form of thiamine, serving as a cofactor in certain reactions in carbohydrate metabolism.

thiamylal (thi-am′ĭ-lal) an ultrashort-acting barbiturate. **sodium t.,** a compound used intravenously as a general anesthetic.

thiemia (thi-e′me-ah) sulfur in the blood.

thigh (thi) the portion of the leg above the knee.

thigmesthesia (thig″mes-the′ze-ah) tactile sensibility.

thigmocyte (thig′mo-sīt) a blood platelet.

thigmotaxis (thig″mo-tak′sis) movement of a freely motile organism in response to the stimulation of touch. adj., **thigmotac′tic, thigmotax′ic.**

thigmotropism (thig-mot′ro-pizm) a growth curvature occurring in response to the stimulation of touch. adj., **thigmotrop′ic.**

thimerosal (thi-mer′o-sal) a mercury-containing compound used as a local antibacterial agent.

thimethaphan (thi-meth′ah-fan) trimethaphan.

thinking (thingk′ing) the formulation of images or concepts in one's mind. **dereistic t.,** thinking in which the imagination is given free play.

Thiobacillus (thi″o-bah-sil′us) a genus of Schizomycetes (order Pseudomonadales, suborder Pseudomonadineae, family Thiobacteriaceae).

Thiobacteriaceae (-bak-te″re-a′se-e) a family of Schizomycetes (order Pseudomonadales, suborder Rhodobacteriineae) which oxidize sulfur compounds.

Thiobacterium (bak-te′re-um) a genus of Schizomycetes (order Pseudomonadales, suborder Pseudomonadineae, family Thiobacteriaceae) found in fresh or salt water or in the soil.

thiobarbiturate (-bar-bit′u-rāt) a compound due to condensation of malonic acid and thiourea, differing from barbiturates by the presence of a sulfur atom.

Thiocapsa (-kap′sah) a genus of Schizomycetes (order Pseudomonadales, suborder Rhodobacteriineae, family Thiorhodaceae).

thiocyanate (-si′ah-nāt) a salt analogous in composition to a cyanate, but containing sulfur instead of oxygen.

Thiocystis (-sis′tis) a genus of Schizomycetes (order Pseudomonadales, suborder Rhodobacteriineae, family Thiorhodaceae).

Thiodictyon (-dik′te-on) a genus of Schizomycetes (order Pseudomonadales, suborder Rhodobacteriineae, family Thiorhodaceae).

thiodiphenylamine (-di-fen″il-am′ēn) phenothiazine.

Thiomerin (-mer′in) trademark for a preparations of mercaptomerin sodium.

thiomersalate (-mer′sah-lāt) thimerosal.

thionine (thi′o-nin) a purple dye used as a nuclear stain.

Thiopedia (thi″o-pe′de-ah) a genus of Schizomycetes (order Pseudomonadales, suborder Rhodobacteriineae, family Thiorhodaceae).

thiopental (-pen′tal) an ultrashort-acting barbiturate. **sodium t.,** the sodium salt of thiopental, injected intravenously or rectally as an anesthetic.

thiopentone (-pen′tōn) thiopental.

thiopexy (thi′o-pek″se) the fixation of sulfur. adj., **thiopec′tic.**

thiophil (thi′o-fil) an organism which grows successfully in the presence of sulfur or requires sulfur for its growth. adj., **thiophil′ic.**

Thioploca (thi″o-plo′kah) a genus of Schizomycetes (order Beggiatoales, family Beggiatoaceae).

Thiopolycoccus (-pol″e-kok′us) a genus of Schizomycetes (order Pseudomonadales, suborder Rhodobacteriineae, family Thiorhodaceae).

thiopropazate (-pro′pah-zāt) a phenothiazine compound used as a tranquilizer.

Thiorhodaceae (-ro-da′se-e) a family of Schizomycetes (order Pseudomonadales, suborder Rhodobacteriineae) occurring in environments containing sulfides.

thioridazine (-rid′ah-zēn) a phenothiazine compound used as a tranquilizer.

Thiosarcina (-sar-si′nah) a genus of Schizomycetes (order Pseudomonadales, suborder Rhodobacteriineae, family Thiorhodaceae).

Thiospira (-spi′rah) a genus of Schizomycetes (order Pseudomonadales, suborder Pseudomonadineae, family Thiobacteriaceae).

Thiospirillopsis (-spi″ril-lop′sis) a genus of Schizomycetes (order Beggiatoales, family Beggiatoaceae).

Thiospirillum (-spi-ril′lum) a genus of Schizomycetes (order Pseudomonadales, suborder Rhodobacteriineae, family Thiorhodaceae).

thio-tepa (-te′pah) a compound used as a neoplastic suppressant.

Thiothece (-the′se) a genus of Schizomycetes (order Pseudomonadales, suborder Rhodobacteriineae, family Thiorhodaceae).

Thiothrix (thi′o-thriks) a genus of Schizomycetes (order Beggiatoales, family Beggiatoaceae).

thiouracil (thi″o-u′rah-sil) a derivative of thiourea, used in treatment of hyperthyroidism.

thiourea (-u′re-ah) urea with its oxygen replaced by sulfur, $CS(NH_2)_2$.

Thiovulum (thi-o′vu-lum) a genus of Schizomycetes (order Pseudomonadales, suborder Pseudomonadineae, family Thiobacteriaceae).

Thixokon (thik′so-kon) trademark for a preparation of acetrizoate sodium.

thixotropism (thik-sot′ro-pizm) thixotropy.

thixotropy (thik-sot′ro-pe) the property of certain gels of becoming fluid when shaken and then becoming solid again. adj., **thixotrop′ic.**

thlipsencephalus (thlip″sen-sef′ah-lus) fetal monster with a defective skull.

thonzylamine (thon-zil′ah-min) a compound used as an antihistaminic.

thoracalgia (thor″rah-kal′je-ah) pain in the chest.

thoracectomy (-sek′to-me) thoracotomy with resection of part of a rib.

thoracentesis (-sen-te′sis) puncture of the chest wall with aspiration.

thoracic (tho-ras′ik) pertaining to the chest.

thoracoacromial (tho″rah-ko-ah-kro′me-al) pertaining to chest and acromion.

thoracobronchotomy (-brong-kot′o-me) incision into the bronchus through the thoracic wall.

thoracocautery (tho″rah-ko-kaw′ter-e) division of pulmonary adhesions by cautery.

thoracoceloschisis (-se-los′ki-sis) fissure of thorax and abdomen.

thoracocentesis (-sen-te′sis) thoracentesis.

thoracocyllosis (-si-lo′sis) deformity of the thorax.

thoracocyrtosis (-sir-to′sis) abnormal curvature of the thorax.

thoracodelphus (-del′fus) a fetal monster with duplication of body parts below the thorax.

thoracodidymus (-did′i-mus) thoracopagus.

thoracodynia (-din′e-ah) pain in the thorax.

thoracogastroschisis (-gas-tros′ki-sis) developmental anomaly resulting from faulty closure of the body wall along the midventral line, involving both thorax and abdomen.

thoracograph (tho-rak′o-graf) an apparatus for recording the chest movements.

thoracolumbar (tho″rah-ko-lum′bar) pertaining to thoracic and lumbar vertebrae.

thoracolysis (tho″rah-kol′ĭ-sis) pneumonolysis. **t. praecordi′aca,** cardiolysis.

thoracomelus (-kom′ĕ-lus) a fetal monster with a limb of a twin fetus attached to the thorax.

thoracometer (-kom′ĕ-ter) stethometer.

thoracomyodynia (tho″rah-ko-mi″o-din′e-ah) pain in the muscles of the chest.

thoracopagus (tho″rah-kop′ah-gus) conjoined twins united at the thorax.

thoracopathy (-kop′ah-the) any disease of the thoracic organs.

thoracoplasty (tho″rah-ko-plas″te) surgical alteration of the shape of the thoracic cage by removal of ribs, allowing the chest wall and underlying lung to move inward.

thoracopneumoplasty (tho″rah-ko-nu′mo-plas″te) plastic surgery of chest and lung.

thoracoschisis (tho″rah-kos′ki-sis) fissure of chest wall.

thoracoscopy (-kos′ko-pe) endoscopic examination of the chest.

thoracostenosis (tho″rah-ko-stĕ-no′sis) abnormal contraction of the thorax.

thoracostomy (tho″rah-kos′to-me) incision of the chest wall, with maintenance of the opening.

thoracotomy (-kot′o-me) incision of the chest wall.

thorax (tho′raks) the part of the body between neck and abdomen, enclosed by the backbone, ribs and sternum.

Thorazine (thor′ah-zēn) trademark for preparations of chlorpromazine hydrochloride.

thorium (tho′re-um) chemical element (see table), at. no. 90, symbol Th.

thoron (tho′ron) a radioactive isotope of radon.

Thorotrast (tho′ro-trast) a proprietary contrast medium for use in roentgenography.

thoroughpin (thur′o-pin) distention of the synovial sheaths at the upper portion and back of the hock joint of a horse.

threadworm (thred′werm) any nematode worm, as *Enterobius vermicularis.*

thremmatology (threm″ah-tol′o-je) science of the laws of heredity and variation.

threonine (thre′o-nin) a naturally occurring amino acid, one of those essential for human metabolism.

threpsology (threp-sol′o-je) the scientific study of nutrition.

threshold (thresh′old) the level which must be exceeded for an effect to be produced, as the degree of intensity of a stimulus which must be surpassed for a sensation to be produced, or the concentration that must be present in the blood before certain substances are excreted by the kidney (*renal threshold*).

thrill (thril) tremor perceived in auscultation or palpation. **diastolic t.,** one felt over the precordium during diastole in advanced aortic insufficiency. **hydatid t.,** one felt on percussing over a hydatid cyst. **presystolic t.,** one occasionally felt just before the systole over the apex of the heart. **purring t.,** a thrill of a quality suggesting the purring of a cat. **systolic t.,** one felt over the precordium during systole in aortic stenosis, pulmonary stenosis and aneurysm of the ascending aorta.

thrix (thriks) hair. **t. annula′ta,** a condition in which the hair appears to be constricted with annular rings.

-thrix (thriks) word element [Gr.], *hair.*

throat (thrōt) 1. pharynx. 2. fauces. 3. anterior aspect of the neck.

thromb(o)- (throm′bo) word element [Gr.], *clot; thrombus.*

thrombase (throm′bās) thrombin.

thrombasthenia (throm″bas-the′ne-ah) a functional disorder of the blood platelets. **Glanzmann's t.,** a qualitative disorder of blood platelets, marked by ease of bruising and bleeding from mucous membranes.

thrombectomy (throm-bek′to-me) surgical removal of a clot from a blood vessel. **medical t.,** enzymatic dissolution of a blood clot in situ.

thrombin (throm′bin) an enzyme resulting from activation of prothrombin, which catalyzes the conversion of fibrinogen to fibrin; a preparation from prothrombin of bovine origin is used as a clotting agent.

thromboangiitis (throm″bo-an″je-i′tis) intravascular clot formation, with inflammation of the vessel wall. **t. oblit′erans,** thromboangiitis with contraction of the vessel about the clot, leading to diminution of blood flow distal to the site.

thromboarteritis (-ar″ter-i′tis) thrombosis with arteritis.

thromboclasis (throm-bok′lah-sis) the dissolution of a thrombus. adj., **thromboclas′tic.**

thrombocystis (throm″bo-sis′tis) the sac sometimes formed around a clot or thrombus.

thrombocyte (throm′bo-sīt) a blood platelet.

thrombocythemia (throm″bo-si-the′me-ah) a fixed increase in the number of circulating blood platelets. **essential t., hemorrhagic t.,** a clinical syndrome with repeated spontaneous hemorrhages, either external or into the tissues, and greatly increased number of circulating platelets.

thrombocytin (-si′tin) serotonin.

thrombocytocrit (-si′to-krit) an instrument for counting thrombocytes.

thrombocytolysin (throm"bo-si-tol'ĭ-sin) factor VIII.

thrombocytolysis (-si-tol'ĭ-sis) destruction of thrombocytes.

thrombocytopathy (-si-top'ah-the) any qualitative disorder of the blood platelets.

thrombocytopenia (-si"to-pe'ne-ah) decrease in number of platelets in circulating blood.

thrombocytopoiesis (-poi-e'sis) the production of thrombocytes. adj., **thrombocytopoiet'ic.**

thrombocytosis (throm"bo-si-to'sis) increase in number of platelets in circulating blood.

thromboelastogram (-e-las'to-gram) the graphic record of the values determined by thromboelastography.

thromboelastograph (-e-las'to-graf) an apparatus used in study of the rigidity of blood or plasma during coagulation.

thromboelastography (-e"las-tog'rah-fe) determination of the rigidity of the blood or plasma during coagulation by use of the thromboelastograph.

thromboembolism (-em'bo-lizm) obstruction of a blood vessel with a thrombus which has broken loose from its site of formation.

thromboendarterectomy (-end"ar-ter-ek'to-me) excision of an obstructing thrombus together with a portion of the inner lining of the obstructed artery.

thromboendarteritis (-end"ar-ter-i'tis) inflammation of the innermost coat of an artery, with thrombus formation.

thrombogen (throm'bo-jen) prothrombin.

thrombogenesis (throm"bo-jen'ē-sis) clot formation. adj., **thrombogen'ic.**

thromboid (throm'boid) like a thrombus.

thrombokinase (throm"bo-ki'nās) thromboplastin.

thrombokinesis (-ki-ne'sis) the clotting of blood.

thrombolymphangitis (-lim"fan-ji'tis) inflammation of a lymph vessel due to a thrombus.

thrombolysis (throm-bol'ĭ-sis) dissolution of a thrombus. adj., **thrombolyt'ic.**

thrombon (throm'bon) the circulating thrombocytes and their precursors.

thrombopathy (throm-bop'ah-the) thrombocytopathy.

thrombopenia (throm"bo-pe'ne-ah) thrombocytopenia.

thrombophilia (-fil'e-ah) a tendency to the occurrence of thrombosis.

thrombophlebitis (-fle-bi'tis) the development of venous thrombi in the presence of inflammatory changes in the vessel wall. **t. mi'grans,** a recurrent condition involving different vessels simultaneously or at intervals.

thromboplastic (-plas'tik) causing clot formation in the blood.

thromboplastid (-plas'tid) thrombocyte.

thromboplastin (-plas'tin) a factor essential to production of thrombin and proper hemostasis.

thromboplastinogen (-plas-tin'o-jen) factor VIII.

thrombopoiesis (-poi-e'sis) thrombocytopoiesis. adj., **thrombopoiet'ic.**

thrombosed (throm'bōsd) affected with thrombosis.

thrombosin (throm-bo'sin) thrombin.

thrombosinusitis (throm"bo-si"nu-si'tis) thrombosis and inflammation of a dural sinus.

thrombosis (throm-bo'sis) formation of thrombi within the lumen of the heart or blood vessels. adj., **thrombot'ic. propagating t.,** progressive clot formation upon an occlusive thrombus, producing an elongated mass sometimes extending into other blood vessels.

thrombosthenin (throm"bo-sthe'nin) a substance liberated by blood platelets that is important for clot retraction and firmness of the clot.

thrombostasis (throm-bos'tah-sis) stasis of blood in a part with formation of thrombus.

thrombus (throm'bus) a solid mass formed in the living heart or vessels from constituents of the blood. **mural t.,** one that is attached at only one side to the vessel wall and does not obstruct blood flow. **occluding t.,** one that occupies the entire lumen of a vessel and obstructs blood flow. **parietal t.,** mural thrombus.

thrush (thrush) infection of the oral mucous membrane by *Candida albicans*, characterized by superficial, confluent white patches on a red, moist, inflammatory surface.

thrypsis (thrip'sis) a comminuted fracture.

thulium (thoo'le-um) chemical element *(see table)*, at. no. 69, symbol Tm.

thumb (thum) the radial or first digit of the hand.

thym(o)- (thi'mo) word element [Gr.], *thymus gland; mind, soul or emotions.*

thymectomy (thi-mek'to-me) excision of the thymus.

thymelcosis (thi"mel-ko'sis) ulceration of the thymus.

thymergasia (thi"mer-ga'ze-ah) an affective or reaction-type psychosis, such as manic-depressive psychosis. adj., **thymergas'ic, thymergas'tic.**

-thymia (thi'me-ah) word element [Gr.], *condition of mind.* adj., **-thy'mic.**

thymicolymphatic (thi"mĭ-ko-lim-fat'ik) pertaining to the thymus and the lymphatic nodes.

thymidine (thi'mĭ-dēn) a compound isolated from the liver.

thymine (thi'min) a pyrimidine base obtained from nucleinic acid; used in treatment of pernicious anemia and sprue.

thymitis (thi-mi'tis) inflammation of the thymus.

thymocyte (thi'mo-sīt) a lymphocyte derived from the thymus.

thymogenic (thi'mo-jen'ik) of affective or hysterical origin.

thymol (thi'mol) a colorless or white crystalline compound; used as an anthelmintic, antibacterial and antifungal agent. **t. iodide,** mixture of iodine derivatives of thymol, containing not less than 43 per cent of iodine; mild antiseptic.

thymolysis (thi-mol'ĭ-sis) destruction of thymus tissue. adj., **thymolyt'ic.**

thymoma (thi-mo'mah) a tumor of the thymus.

thymopathy (thi-mop'ah-the) any disease of the thymus. adj., **thymopath'ic.**

thymopsyche (thi"mo-si'ke) the affective processes of the mind.

thymotoxin (thi"mo-tok'sin) an element that exerts a deleterious effect on the thymus gland.

thymus (thi'mus) a two-lobed ductless gland in the cavity of the chest, just above the heart. adj., **thy'mic.**

thymusectomy (thi"mus-ek'to-me) excision of the thymus.

thyr(o)- (thi'ro) word element [Gr.], *thyroid.*

thyroadenitis (thi"ro-ad"ĕ-ni'tis) inflammation of the thyroid.

thyroaplasia (-ah-pla'ze-ah) defective development of the thyroid.

thyroarytenoid (-ar"i-te'noid) pertaining to thyroid and arytenoid cartilages.

thyrocalcitonin (-kal'si-to"nin) a hormone derived from the thyroid gland which has hypocalcemic and hypophosphatemic actions, and is of physiologic significance in maintenance of calcium homeostasis in animals.

thyrocardiac (-kar'de-ak) pertaining to the thyroid and heart.

thyrocarditis (-kar-di'tis) heart disorder occurring with hyperthyroidism.

thyrocele (thi'ro-sēl) goiter.

thyrochondrotomy (thi"ro-kon-drot'o-me) surgical incision of the thyroid cartilage.

thyrocricotomy (-kri-kot'o-me) incision of the cricothyroid membrane.

thyrodesmic (-dez'mik) thyrotropic.

thyroepiglottic (-ep"i-glot'ik) pertaining to thyroid and epiglottis.

thyrogenic (-jen'ik) originating in the thyroid.

thyroglobulin (-glob'u-lin) an iodized glycoprotein characteristically present in the colloid of the thyroid follicles.

thyroglossal (-glos'al) pertaining to thyroid and tongue.

thyrohyal (-hi'al) pertaining to the thyroid cartilage and the hyoid bone.

thyrohyoid (-hi'oid) pertaining to thyroid gland or cartilage and hyoid bone.

thyroid (thi'roid) 1. resembling a shield. 2. the thyroid gland. 3. a pharmaceutical preparation of cleaned, dried, powdered thyroid gland, obtained from domesticated animals used for food by man.

thyroidectomize (thi"roi-dek'to-mīz) to deprive of the thyroid by excision.

thyroidectomy (-dek'to-me) excision of the thyroid. **medical t.**, diminution of thyroid function by the use of drugs.

thyroidism (thi'roid-izm) a morbid condition resulting from disorder of functioning of the thyroid gland or excessive use of thyroid.

thyroiditis (thi"roi-di'tis) inflammation of the thyroid. **chronic t.**, **chronic fibrous t.**, Riedel's struma. **chronic lymphadenoid t.**, **chronic lymphocytic t.**, **Hashimoto's t.**, struma lymphomatosa.

thyroidotomy (-dot'o-me) incision of the thyroid.

thyroiodine (thi"ro-i'o-dīn) an iodine-containing substance from the thyroid gland.

thyrolysin (thi-rol'ĭ-sin) a substance destructive to thyroid tissue. adj., **thyrolyt'ic.**

thyromimetic (thi"ro-mi-met'ik) producing effects similar to those of thyroid hormones or the thyroid gland.

thyroparathyroidectomy (-par"ah-thi"roi-dek'-to-me) excision of thyroid and parathyroids.

thyropenia (-pe'ne-ah) diminished thyroid action.

thyrophyma (-fi'mah) tumor of the thyroid.

thyroprival (-pri'val) due to decreased function or removal of the thyroid.

thyroptosis (thi"rop-to'sis) downward displacement of a goitrous thyroid.

thyrosis (thi-ro'sis) any disease based on disordered thyroid action.

thyrotomy (thi-rot'o-me) 1. surgical division of the thyroid cartilage. 2. the operation of cutting the thyroid gland.

thyrotoxic (thi"ro-tok'sik) marked by toxic activity of the thyroid.

thyrotoxicosis (-tok"sĭ-ko'sis) the condition due to excessive thyroid action.

thyrotoxin (-tok'sin) a cytotoxin specific for thyroid tissue.

thyrotrophic (-trof'ik) thyrotropic.

thyrotrophin (-trōf'in) thyrotropin.

thyrotropic (-trop'ik) 1. stimulating the thyroid gland. 2. pertaining to thyrotropism.

thyrotropin (-trop'in) a hormone secreted by the anterior pituitary which stimulates the thyroid gland.

thyrotropism (thi-rot'ro-pizm) predominance of the thyroid in the endocrine constitution.

thyroxine (thi-rok'sin) the hormone of the thyroid gland, 3,5,3',5'-tetraiodothyronine.

Ti chemical symbol, *titanium.*

tibia (tib'e-ah) the larger bone of the leg below the knee. adj., **tib'ial.**

tibialis (tib"e-a'lis) [L.] tibial.

tibiofemoral (tib"e-o-fem'o-ral) pertaining to tibia and femur.

tibiofibular (-fib'u-lar) pertaining to tibia and fibula.

tibiotarsal (-tar'sal) pertaining to tibia and tarsus.

tic (tik) an involuntary, spasmodic contraction of muscle fibers. **t. douloureux** (doo-loo-roo'), neuralgia of the trigeminal nerve.

tick (tik) an arthropod of the order Acarina (suborder Ixodides), characterized by relatively large size, a leathery integument and other typical body structures. **Gulf coast t.**, *Amblyomma maculatum.* **hard-bodied t.**, an individual of the family Ixodidae, which has a scutum in all stages of development. **Lone Star t.**, *Amblyomma americanum.* **soft-bodied t.**, an individual of the family Argasidae, which does not have a scutum in any stage of development.

t.i.d. [L.] *ter in di'e* (three times a day).

Tigan (ti'gan) trademark for preparations of trimethobenzamide hydrochloride.

tigrolysis (ti-grol'ĭ-sis) chromatolysis (2).

tilmus (til'mus) involuntary picking at the bed clothes.

timbre (tim'ber, tam'ber) musical quality of a tone or sound.

time (tīm) a measure of duration. **bleeding t.,** the duration of bleeding after puncture of the ear lobe. **circulation t.,** the time required for blood to flow between two given points. **clotting t., coagulation t.,** the time it takes a drop of blood to coagulate. **decalcification t.,** the interval required for clot formation when calcium ion is added to platelet-rich plasma; a measure of hemostatic function of the blood. **inertia t.,** the time required to overcome the inertia of a muscle after reception of a stimulus from a nerve. **persistence t.,** the time following contraction of the ventricle until the occurrence of relaxation. **reaction t.,** the time elapsing between the application of a stimulus and the resulting reaction.

timopathy (tim-op'ah-the) a state characterized by abnormal dread or apprehension.

Timovan (tim'o-van) trademark for a preparation of prothipendyl hydrochloride.

tin (tin) chemical element (*see table*), at. no. 50, symbol Sn.

tinct. tincture.

tinctorial (tingk-to're-al) pertaining to dyeing or staining.

tincture (tingk'chūr) an alcoholic or hydroalcoholic solution prepared from an animal or vegetable drug or a chemical substance. **belladonna t.,** a preparation of belladonna leaf in a menstruum of alcohol and water. **benzoin t., compound,** a mixture of powdered benzoin and aloe, storax and tolu balsam, with alcohol as the menstruum. **camphorated opium t.,** paregoric. **cardamom t., compound,** a preparation of powdered cardamom seed, cinnamon, caraway and cochineal, in a menstruum of glycerin and diluted alcohol. **digitalis t.,** finely powdered digitalis in a menstruum of alcohol and water. **green soap t.,** a mixture of green soap, lavender oil and alcohol. **iodine t.,** a mixture of iodine and sodium iodide in a menstruum of alcohol and water. **lemon t.,** a flavoring agent prepared by maceration of outer yellow rind of fresh ripe fruit of *Citrus limon* in alcohol. **nitromersol t.,** nitromersol, sodium hydroxide and alcohol in hydroalcoholic solution. **opium t.,** an alcoholic solution of opium, each 100 ml. of which yields 0.95–1.05 gm. of anhydrous morphine. **sweet orange peel t.,** a flavoring agent prepared by maceration of the outer rind of natural colored fresh ripe fruit of *Citrus sinensis* in alcohol. **thimerosal t.,** thimerosal, monoethanolamine, acetone, ethylenediamine solution, with alcohol and water; used as an antibacterial. **tolu balsam t.,** tolu balsam macerated in alcohol as the menstruum. **vanilla t.,** one prepared with small pieces of vanilla and coarse granules of sucrose in diluted alcohol.

Tindal (tin'dal) trademark for a preparation of acetophenazine dimaleate.

tinea (tin'e-ah) a skin disease caused by infection of fungi. (Trichophyton or Microsporum). **t. bar'bae,** infection of the bearded parts of the face and neck caused by Trichophyton. **t. cap'itis,** fungus infection of the scalp. **t. circina'ta,** a variety forming reddish circles on the trunk or limbs. **t. cru'ris,** fungus infection of the inside of the thighs. **t. favo'sa,** favus. **t. ke'rion,** a highly inflammatory and suppurative fungal infection, mainly of the scalp or the bearded area of the face and neck. **t. pe'dis,** a chronic, superficial fungal infection of the skin of the foot. **t. profun'da,** a deep, pustular form of tinea circinata. **t. syco'sis,** tinea barbae. **t. versico'lor,** a fungal infection of the skin, usually of the upper part of the trunk and the neck, with a macular eruption and brownish-red, scaling patches.

tingible (tin'ji-bel) stainable.

tinnitus (ti-ni'tus) a noise in the ears, which may at times be heard by others than the patient. **t. au'rium,** a subjective sensation of noises in the ears.

tintometer (tin-tom'ĕ-ter) an instrument for determining the relative proportion of coloring matter in a liquid, as in blood.

tintometry (-tom'ĕ-tre) the use of the tintometer.

tirefond (tēr-faw') [Fr.] an instrument like a corkscrew for raising depressed portions of bone.

tissue (tish'u) a group or layer of similarly specialized cells which together perform certain special functions. **adenoid t.,** connective tissue with meshes which lodge lymphoid cells. **adipose t.,** connective tissue made of fat cells in meshwork of areolar tissue. **areolar t.,** connective tissue made up largely of interlacing fibers. **bony t.,** bone. **cancellous t.,** the spongy tissue of bone. **cartilaginous t.,** cartilage. **chordal t.,** the tissue of the notochord. **chromaffin t.,** tissue which stains yellow or brown with chromium salts, typical of the adrenal medulla and ganglia of the sympathetic nervous system. **cicatricial t.,** tissue derived directly from granulation tissue. **compact t.,** the hard, external portion of a bone. **connective t.,** the stromatous or nonparenchymatous tissues of the body; that which binds together and is the ground substance of the various parts and organs of the body. **elastic t.,** connective tissue made up of yellow elastic fibers. **endothelial t.,** peculiar connective tissue lining serous and lymphoid spaces. **epithelial t.,** a general name for tissues not derived from the mesoblast. **erectile t.,** spongy tissue that expands and becomes hard when filled with blood. **extracellular t.,** the total of tissues and body fluids outside the cells. **fatty t.,** adipose tissue. **fibrous t.,** the common connective tissue of the body, composed of yellow or white parallel fibers. **gelatinous t.,** mucous tissue. **glandular t.,** a specialized form of epithelial tissue. **granulation t.,** material formed in repair of wounds of soft tissue, consisting of connective tissue cells and ingrowing young vessels. **indifferent t.,** undifferentiated embryonic tissue. **interstitial t.,** connective tissue between the cellular elements of a structure. **lymphadenoid t.,** the tissue constituting the lymph nodes, spleen, bone marrow, tonsils and lymphatic vessels. **lymphoid t.,** adenoid tissue. **mesenchymal t., mucous t.,**

the embryonic connective tissue. **muscular t.**, muscle. **myeloid t.**, red bone marrow. **nervous t.**, the specialized tissue forming the elements of the nervous system. **osseous t.**, the specialized tissue forming the bones. **podophyllous t.**, the tissue on the inner surface of the hoof of an animal. **reticular t.**, **retiform t.**, adenoid tissue. **scar t.**, cicatricial tissue. **sclerous t's**, the cartilaginous, fibrous and osseous tissue. **skeletal t.**, the bony, ligamentous fibrous and cartilaginous tissue forming the skeleton and its attachments. **splenic t.**, the spleen pulp. **subcutaneous t.**, the layer of loose connective tissue directly under the skin.

titanium (ti-ta′ne-um) chemical element (*see table*), at. no. 22, symbol Ti. **t. dioxide**, a white powder used in ointment or lotion to protect the skin from the rays of the sun.

titer (ti′ter) the quantity of a substance required to react with or to correspond to a given amount of another substance.

titration (ti-tra′shun) analysis by means of comparison with solutions of standard strength.

titrimetry (ti-trim′ĕ-tre) analysis by titration.

Tl chemical symbol, *thallium.*

TLC tender loving care; thin layer chromatography; total lung capacity.

T_m tubular maximum (in renal excretion).

Tm chemical symbol, *thulium.*

TNT trinitrotoluene.

tobacco (to-bak′o) the prepared leaves of *Nicotiana tabacum,* an annual plant widely cultivated in the United States, the source of various alkaloids, the principal one being nicotine.

Toclase (to′klās) trademark for preparations of carbetapentane citrate.

toco- (to′ko) word element [Gr.], *childbirth; labor.* See also words beginning *toko-.*

tocology (to-kol′o-je) science of reproduction and art of obstetrics.

tocomania (to″ko-ma′ne-ah) puerperal mania.

tocometer (to-kom′ĕ-ter) tokodynamometer.

tocopherol (to-kof′er-ol) a compound originally isolated from wheat germ oil, having antisterility properties. **alpha t.**, a biologically active compound separated from wheat germ oil or produced synthetically.

tocophobia (to″ko-fo′be-ah) abnormal dread of childbirth.

toe (to) a digit of the foot. **hammer t.**, deformity of a toe due to flexion contracture of the proximal interphalangeal joint and extension of the metatarsophalangeal joint. **Morton's t.**, a painful condition of the third and fourth toes due to thickening of the branch of the sensory nerve supplying them. **pigeon t.**, permanent toeing-in position of the feet. **webbed t's**, tocs abnormally joined by strands of tissue at their base.

Tofranil (to-fra′nil) trademark for preparations of imipramine hydrochloride.

toilet (toi′let) the cleansing and dressing of a wound.

toko- (to′ko) word element [Gr.], *childbirth; labor.* See also words beginning *toco-.*

tokodynagraph (to″ko-di′nah-graf) a tracing obtained by the tokodynamometer.

tokodynamometer (-di″nah-mom′ĕ-ter) an instrument for measuring and recording the expulsive force of uterine contractions.

tolazoline (tol-az′o-lēn) a compound used as a sympatholytic agent and a vasodilator.

tolbutamide (tol-bu′tah-mīd) a hypoglycemic agent effective when given orally.

tolerance (tol′er-ans) the ability to endure without effect or injury. **drug t.**, decrease of susceptibility to the effects of a drug due to its continued administration. **immunologic t.**, absence of reactivity to a substance normally expected to excite an immunologic response.

tolonium (to-lo′ne-um) a compound used to reduce bleeding tendency in certain hemorrhagic conditions associated with excess of heparinoid substances in the blood.

Tolserol (tol′ser-ol) trademark for preparations of mephenesin.

toluene (tol′u-ēn) the hydrocarbon C_7H_8.

toluidine (tol-u′ĭ-din) a compound made by reducing nitrotoluene.

tomatin (to-ma′tin) an antibiotic compound isolated from leaves and roots of common tomato plants.

-tome (-tōm) word element [Gr.], *an instrument for cutting; a segment.*

tomentum (to-men′tum) network of minute blood vessels of the pia and cortex cerebri.

tomo- (to′mo) word element [Gr.], *a section; a cutting.*

tomogram (to′mo-gram) a radiograph produced by tomography.

tomography (to-mog′rah-fe) a method of body-section roentgenography with the x-ray tube moved in only one direction, usually an arc. adj., **tomograph′ic.**

tomomania (to″mo-ma′ne-ah) 1. a craze for performing needless surgical operations. 2. hysterical desire to undergo surgery.

-tomy (to′me) word element [Gr.], *incision; cutting.*

tone (tōn) 1. normal degree of vigor and tension. 2. a particular quality of sound or voice.

tongue (tung) the movable muscular organ on the floor of the mouth. **bifid t.**, a tongue with a lengthwise cleft. **black t.**, blackening and elongation of the papillae of the tongue. **blue t.**, a disease of cattle and sheep in South Africa, characterized by necrotic ulceration of the tongue. **geographic t.**, tongue with denuded patches, surrounded by thickened epithelium. **hairy t.**, one with papillae elongated and hairlike. **raspberry t.**, diffusely reddened and swollen, uncoated tongue seen several days after onset of scarlet fever. **Sandwith's bald t.**, an unusually smooth tongue seen in pellagra. **strawberry t.**, coated tongue with enlarged red fungiform papillae, seen early in scarlet fever. **trombone t.**, involuntary movement of the tongue, consisting of vigorous alternating protrusion and retraction.

tongue-tie (tung′ti) ankyloglossia.

tonic (ton′ik) 1. producing and restoring

normal tone. 2. characterized by continuous tension. 3. an agent which tends to restore normal tone. **cardiac t.**, an agent that strengthens the heart's action. **general t.**, an agent that braces up the whole system. **hematic t.**, an agent that improves the quality of the blood. **intestinal t.**, an agent that gives tone to the intestinal tract. **nervine t.**, an agent that improves the tone of the nervous system. **stomachic t.**, an agent that aids digestive functions. **vascular t.**, an agent that improves the tone of blood vessels.

tonicity (to-nis'ĭ-te) the state of tone or tension.

tono- (to'no) word element [Gr.], *tone; tension.*

tonoclonic (ton″o-klon'ik) both tonic and clonic.

tonofibril (ton″o-fi″bril) one of the fine fibrils in epithelial cells.

tonogram (to'no-gram) the record produced by tonography.

tonograph (to'no-graf) a recording tonometer.

tonography (to-nog'rah-fe) recording of changes in intraocular pressure due to sustained pressure on the eyeball.

tonometer (to-nom'ĕ-ter) an instrument for measuring tension or pressure, especially for measuring intraocular pressure.

tonometry (to-nom'ĕ-tre) measurement of tension or pressure.

tonoplast (ton'o-plast) the limiting membrane of an intracellular vacuole, the vacuole membrane.

tonoscope (ton'o-skōp) an instrument for examining the head or cranium by means of sound.

tonsil (ton'sil) a small, rounded mass of tissue, especially of lymphoid tissue; generally used alone to designate the palatine tonsil. adj., **ton′sillar. t. of cerebellum**, a rounded mass of tissue on the inferior surface of the cerebellum. **faucial t.**, palatine tonsil. **lingual t.**, a mass of lymphoid tissue at the base of the tongue. **Luschka's t.**, pharyngeal tonsil. **palatine t.**, a small mass of lymphoid tissue between the pillars of the fauces on either side of the pharynx. **pharyngeal t.**, diffuse lymphoid tissue in the roof and posterior wall of the pharynx.

tonsilla (ton-sil'ah), pl. *tonsil'lae* [L.] tonsil.

tonsillectomy (ton″sĭ-lek'to-me) excision of a tonsil.

tonsillitis (-li'tis) inflammation of a tonsil. **follicular t.**, tonsillitis especially affecting the follicles. **pustular t.**, a variety characterized by formation of pustules. **suppurative t.**, quinsy.

tonsilloadenoidectomy (-lo-ad″ĕ-noi-dek'to-me) excision of lymphoid tissue from the throat and nasopharynx (tonsils and adenoids).

tonsillolith (ton-sil'o-lith) a calculus in a tonsil.

tonsillotomy (ton″sĭ-lot'o-me) incision of a tonsil.

tonus (to'nus) tone, or tonicity; the normal state of slight contraction of all skeletal muscles, maintained as long as innervation to the muscle is intact.

tooth (tooth), pl. *teeth*, one of the small, bone-like structures of the jaws for the biting and mastication of food. **accessional teeth**, the permanent molars, so called because they have no deciduous predecessors in the dental arch. **artificial t.**, one made of porcelain or other synthetic compound in imitation of a natural tooth. **auditory teeth**, toothlike projections in the cochlea. **azzle t.**, molar tooth. **bicuspid t.**, one of the premolar teeth. **canine t., cuspid t.**, the third tooth on either side from the midline in each jaw. **deciduous teeth**, the 20 teeth of the first dentition in man which are supplanted by the 32 teeth of the second dentition. **eye teeth**, the upper cuspid teeth of the first dentition. **Hutchinson teeth**, notched, narrow-edged teeth, indicative of congenital syphilis. **impacted t.**, one so placed in the jaw that it is unable to erupt or to attain its normal position in occlusion. **incisor teeth**, the four anterior teeth in each jaw. **milk teeth**, deciduous teeth. **molar teeth**, the three posterior teeth on either side in each jaw. **natal teeth**, true deciduous teeth that have erupted through the gingiva before birth. **peg t.**, a tooth whose sides converge or taper together incisally. **permanent teeth**, the 32 teeth of the second dentition. **postpermanent t.**, one that erupts after the permanent teeth have been extracted. **predeciduous t.**, a horrified epithelial structure, without roots, occurring on the gingiva over the crest of the ridge of the alveolar process. **premolar teeth**, the two teeth on either side in each jaw, anterior to the molar teeth. **primary teeth**, deciduous teeth. **stomach teeth**, the lower cuspid teeth of the first dentition. **successional teeth**, those of the permanent teeth that have deciduous predecessors in the dental arch. **temporary teeth**, deciduous teeth. **wisdom teeth**, the last molar tooth on either side in each jaw.

top(o)- (top'o) word element [Gr.], *particular place or area.*

topagnosia (top″ag-no'ze-ah) 1. loss of touch localization. 2. loss of ability to recognize familiar surroundings.

topectomy (to-pek'to-me) excision of a limited area of brain tissue.

topesthesia (top″es-the'ze-ah) ability to recognize the location of a tactile stimulus.

tophaceous (to-fa'shus) gritty or sandy.

tophus (to'fus) 1. a deposit of urates in the tissues about the joints in gout. 2. dental calculus. **t. syphilit'icus**, a syphilitic node.

topical (top'ĭ-kal) pertaining to a particular spot.

Topitracin (top″ĭ-tra'sin) trademark for a preparation of bacitracin.

topoalgia (to″po-al'je-ah) fixed or localized pain.

topoanesthesia (-an″es-the'ze-ah) inability to recognize the location of a tactile stimulus.

topographic (top″o-graf'ik) describing special regions.

topography (to-pog'rah-fe) a special description of a part or region.

toponarcosis (top″o-nar-ko'sis) local anesthesia.

toponeurosis (top"o-nu-ro'sis) neurosis of a limited region.

torcular Herophili (tor'ku-lar he-rof'ĭ-le) a depression in the occipital bone at the confluence of a number of venous sinuses.

torpor (tor'por) [L.] sluggishness adj., **tor'pid.**
t. ret'inae, sluggish response of retina to the stimulus of light.

torsion (tor'shun) act of twisting; state of being twisted. adj., **tor'sive.**

torsiversion (tor"sĭ-ver'zhun) turning of a tooth on its long axis out of normal position.

torso (tor'so) the body, exclusive of the head and limbs.

torticollis (tor"tĭ-kol'is) wryneck; a contracted state of cervical muscles, with torsion of the neck.

tortipelvis (-pel'vis) dystonia musculorum deformans.

Torula (tor'u-lah) Cryptococcus. **T. histo-lyt'ica,** Cryptococcus neoformans.

toruloid (tor'u-loid) knotted or beaded, like a yeast cell.

torulosis (tor"u-lo'sis) cryptococcosis.

torulus (tor'u-lus) [L.] a small elevation. **t. tac'tilis,** a tactile elevation in the skin of the palms and soles.

torus (to'rus), pl. *to'ri* [L.] a swelling or bulging projection.

totipotentiality (to"tĭ-po-ten"she-al'ĭ-te) the ability to differentiate along any line or into any type of cell. adj., **totip'otent.**

touch (tuch) 1. the sense by which contact of an object with the skin is recognized. 2. palpation with the finger.

tourniquet (toor'nĭ-ket) an instrument for the compression of blood vessels. **provisional t.,** one loosely applied, to be tightened when occasion may require.

toxalbumin (tok"sal-bu'min) a poisonous albumin of bacterial or other origin.

toxalbumose (tok-sal'bu-mōs) a poisonous albumose.

Toxascaris (tok-sas'kah-ris) a genus of nematode parasites. **T. leoni'na,** a species found in lions and tigers, as well as other animals.

toxemia (tok-se'me-ah) presence in the blood of toxic products formed in the body cells or by bacteria. **t. of pregnancy,** a pathologic condition occurring in pregnant women, including hyperemesis gravidarum, pre-eclampsia and eclampsia.

toxenzyme (tok-sen'zim) any poisonous enzyme.

toxic (tok'sik) poisonous; pertaining to poisoning.

toxic(o)- (tok'sĭ-ko) word element [Gr.], *poison; poisonous.*

toxicant (tok'sĭ-kant) 1. poisonous. 2. a poison.

toxicide (tok'sĭ-sīd) an agent which overcomes toxins or poisons.

toxicity (tok-sis'ĭ-te) the quality of exerting deleterious effects on an organism or tissue.

Toxicodendron (tok"sĭ-ko-den'dron) a genus name given plants sometimes classified as belonging to the genus Rhus, including poison ivy, etc.

toxicoderma (-der'mah) a skin disease due to a poison.

toxicogenic (tok"sĭ-ko-jen'ik) giving origin to poisons.

toxicohemia (-he'me-ah) toxemia.

toxicoid (tok'sĭ-koid) resembling a poison.

toxicologist (tok"sĭ-kol'o-jist) a specialist in toxicology.

toxicology (-kol'o-je) the science or study of poisons.

toxicomania (tok"sĭ-ko-ma'ne-ah) intense desire for poisons or intoxicants.

toxicomucin (-mu'sin) a poisonous substance derived from tubercle bacillus.

toxicopathy (tok"sĭ-kop'ah-the) a morbid condition caused by a poison. adj., **toxicopath'ic.**

toxicopexy (tok'sĭ-ko-pek"se) the fixation or neutralization of a poison. adj., **toxicopec'tic, toxicopex'ic.**

toxicophidia (tok"sĭ-ko-fid'e-ah) venomous serpents collectively.

toxicophobia (-fo'be-ah) morbid dread of poisons.

toxicophylaxin (-fi-lak'sin) a phylaxin which destroys the poisons produced by microorganisms.

toxicosis (tok"sĭ-ko'sis) a diseased condition due to poisoning.

toxiferous (tok-sif'er-us) conveying or producing a poison.

toxigenic (tok"sĭ-jen'ik) caused by or producing toxins.

toxigenicity (-jĕ-nis'ĭ-te) the property of producing toxins.

toxi-infection (tok"se-in-fek'shun) toxinfection.

toxin (tok'sin) a poison, especially a protein or conjugated protein substance produced by some higher plants, certain animals and pathogenic bacteria, that is highly poisonous for other living organisms. **animal t.,** zootoxin. **bacterial t's,** toxins produced by bacteria, including exotoxins, endotoxins and toxic enzymes. **Birkhaug's t.,** toxic filtrate of a streptococcus isolated from a patient with endocarditis and rheumatic fever; used in a skin test for rheumatic fever. **botulinus t.,** one of five type-specific, immunologically differentiable exotoxins (types A to E) produced by Clostridium botulinum. **dermonecrotic t.,** an exotoxin produced by certain bacteria that causes extensive local necrosis on intradermal inoculation. **Dick t.,** erythrogenic toxin. **diphtheria t.,** a preparation of toxic products of growth of Corynebacterium diphtheriae, used to indicate dermal reactivity, or in inactivated form as a control in such a test. **dysentery t.,** one produced by organisms of various species of Shigella. **erythrogenic t.,** a bacterial toxin that produces an erythematous reaction when injected intradermally. **extracellular t.,** exotoxin. **fatigue t.,** kenotoxin. **intracellular t.,** endotoxin. **plant t.,** phytotoxin. **scarlatinal t.,** erythrogenic toxin. **soluble t.,** exotoxin. **tetanus t.,** the exotoxin of Clostridium tetani, consisting of tetanolysin and tetanospasmin.

toxin-antitoxin (tok"sin-an'tĭ-tok"sin) a nearly neutral mixture of diphtheria toxin with its antitoxin.

toxinfection (tok″sin-fek′shun) infection by toxins or other poisonous agents.

toxipathic (tok″sĭ-path′ik) pertaining to or caused by the pathogenic action of toxins, of whatever origin.

toxipathy (tok-sip′ah-the) a disease due to poisoning.

toxisterol (tok-sis′ter-ol) a poisonous isomer of ergosterol.

toxitherapy (tok″sĭ-ther′ah-pe) therapeutic use of toxins.

Toxocara (tok″so-ka′rah) a genus of nematode parasites found in various animals and sometimes in man. **T. ca′nis,** a species common in man. **T. ca′tis,** a species common in cats.

toxocariasis (-ka-ri′ah-sis) infection by worms of the genus Toxocara.

toxoid (tok′soid) a toxin treated by heat or chemical agent to destroy its deleterious properties without destroying its ability to stimulate antibody production. **alum-precipitated t.,** a toxoid of diphtheria or tetanus precipitated with alum. **diphtheria t.,** a sterile preparation of formaldehyde-treated products of the growth of *Corynebacterium diphtheriae,* used as an active immunizing agent. **tetanus t.,** a sterile preparation of formaldehyde-treated products of the growth of *Clostridium tetani,* used as an active immunizing agent.

toxopeptone (tok″so-pep′ton) a poisonous peptone.

toxopexic (-pek′sik) toxicopexic.

toxophilic (-fil′ik) having affinity for toxins.

toxophore (tok′so-fōr) the group of atoms in a toxin molecule which produces the toxic effect.

toxophorous (tok-sof′o-rus) bearing poison; producing the toxic effect.

toxophylaxin (tok″so-fi-lak′sin) toxicophylaxin.

Toxoplasma (-plaz′mah) a genus of sporozoan parasites in man, other mammals and some birds; it includes one species, *T. gondii,* which is frequently transmitted from an infected mother to an infant in utero or at birth.

toxoplasmin (-plaz′min) an antigen that is injected intracutaneously as a test for toxoplasmosis.

toxoplasmosis (-plaz-mo′sis) infection with Toxoplasma.

Toxothrix (tok′so-thriks) a genus of Schizomycetes (order Chlamydobacteriales, family Chlamydobacteriaceae).

T.P.R. temperature, pulse, respiration.

trabecula (trah-bek′u-lah), pl. *trabec′ulae* [L.] a small beam or supporting structure; used in anatomic nomenclature to designate various fibromuscular bands or cords providing support in various organs, as heart, penis and spleen. adj., **trabec′ular.**

trabeculate (trah-bek′u-lăt) marked with cross bars or trabeculae.

trabs (trabz) [L.] beam. **t. cer′ebri,** corpus callosum.

tracer (trās′er) a means by which something may be followed, as (a) a mechanical device by which the outline or movements of an object can be graphically recorded, or (b) a material by which the progress of a compound through the body may be observed. **radioactive t.,** a radioactive isotope replacing a stable chemical element in a compound introduced into the body, enabling its metabolism, distribution and elimination to be followed.

trachea (tra′ke-ah) the passage from the larynx to the bronchi. adj., **tra′cheal.**

tracheaectasy (tra″ke-ah-ek′tah-se) dilatation of the trachea.

trachealgia (-al′je-ah) pain in the trachea.

tracheitis (-i′tis) inflammation of the trachea.

trachel(o)- (tra′ke-lo) word element [Gr.], neck; *necklike structure,* especially cervix uteri.

trachelagra (tra″ke-lag′rah) gout in the neck.

trachelectomy (-lek′to-me) excision of cervix uteri.

trachelematoma (-lem″ah-to′mah) a hematoma on the sternocleidomastoid muscle.

trachelismus (-liz′mus) spasm of the neck muscles.

trachelitis (-li′tis) cervicitis.

trachelocystitis (-lo-sis-ti′tis) inflammation of neck of bladder.

trachelodynia (-din′e-ah) pain in the neck.

trachelomyitis (-mi-i′tis) inflammation of muscles of neck.

trachelopexy (tra′ke-lo-pek″se) fixation of the cervix uteri.

tracheloplasty (tra′ke-lo-plas″te) plastic repair of the cervix uteri.

trachelorrhaphy (tra″ke-lor′ah-fe) suture of the cervix uteri.

trachelotomy (-lot′o-me) incision of the cervix uteri.

tracheo- (tra′ke-o) word element [Gr.], *trachea.*

tracheo-aerocele (tra″ke-o-a′er-o-sēl″) tracheal hernia containing air.

tracheobronchial (-brong′ke-al) pertaining to trachea and bronchi.

tracheobronchiomegaly (-brong″ke-o-meg′ah-le) abnormal dilatation of the trachea and bronchi.

tracheobronchoscopy (-brong-kos′ko-pe) inspection of the interior of the trachea and bronchus.

tracheocele (tra′ke-o-sēl″) 1. hernial protrusion of tracheal mucous membrane. 2. goiter.

tracheo-esophageal (tra″ke-o-e-sof′ah-je-al) pertaining to trachea and esophagus.

tracheofissure (-fish′ūr) incision of the trachea.

tracheolaryngotomy (-lar″ing-got′o-me) incision of larynx and trachea.

tracheomalacia (-mah-la′she-ah) softening of the tracheal cartilages.

tracheopathy (tra″ke-op′ah-the) disease of the trachea.

tracheopharyngeal (tra″ke-o-fah-rin′je-al) pertaining to trachea and pharynx.

tracheophony (tra″ke-of′o-ne) sound heard in auscultation over the trachea.

tracheoplasty (tra′ke-o-plas″te) plastic repair of the trachea.

tracheopyosis (tra″ke-o-pi-o′sis) purulent tracheitis.

tracheorrhagia (tra″ke-o-ra′je-ah) hemorrhage from the trachea.

tracheorrhaphy (tra″ke-or′ah-fe) suture of the trachea.

tracheoschisis (-os′ki-sis) fissure of the trachea.

tracheoscopy (-os′ko-pe) inspection of interior of the trachea.

tracheostenosis (tra″ke-o-stĕ-no′sis) constriction of the trachea.

tracheostomize (tra″ke-os′to-mīz) to perform tracheostomy.

tracheostomy (-os′to-me) creation of an opening into the trachea through the neck, with insertion of an indwelling tube to facilitate passage of air or evacuation of secretions.

tracheotome (tra′ke-o-tōm″) instrument for incising the trachea.

tracheotomy (tra″ke-ot′o-me) incision of the trachea for exploration, removal of a foreign body or for obtaining a biopsy specimen or removing a local lesion. **inferior t.**, performed below, and **superior t.**, above, the isthmus of the thyroid.

trachitis (trah-ki′tis) tracheitis.

trachoma (trah-ko′mah) contagious granular conjunctivitis.

trachychromatic (tra″ke-kro-mat′ik) having deeply staining chromatin.

trachyphonia (-fo′ne-ah) roughness of the voice.

tracing (trās′ing) a graphic record produced by copying another, or scribed by an instrument capable of making a visual record of movements.

tract (trakt) a longitudinal assemblage of tissues or organs, especially a bundle of nerve fibers having a common origin, function and termination, or a number of anatomic structures arranged in series and serving a common function. **alimentary t.**, digestive tract. **biliary t.**, the liver and gallbladder, and their various ducts. **digestive t.**, the passage from the mouth to the anus. **gastrointestinal t.**, the stomach and intestines; the portion of the digestive tract from the cardia to the anus. **intestinal t.**, the small and large intestines in continuity. **pyramidal t's**, collections of nerve fibers arising in the brain and passing down through the cord to motor cells in the anterior horns. **respiratory t.**, the organs which allow entrance of air into the lungs and exchange of gases with the blood, from air passages in the nose to the pulmonary alveoli. **urinary t.**, the organs concerned with the elaboration and excretion of urine: kidneys, ureters, bladder and urethra. **uveal t.**, the vascular tunic of the eye, comprising the choroid, ciliary body and iris.

traction (trak′shun) the act of drawing or pulling. **axis t.**, traction along an axis, as of the pelvis in obstetrics. **elastic t.**, traction by an elastic force or by means of an elastic appliance. **skeletal t.**, traction on a body part maintained by apparatus affixed through a bone. **skin t.**, traction on a body part maintained by apparatus affixed by dressings to the body surface.

tractotomy (trak-tot′o-me) transection of a nerve tract in the central nervous system.

tractus (trak′tus), pl. *trac′tus* [L.] tract; used in anatomic nomenclature to designate certain collections of nerve fibers in the central nervous system.

tragacanth (trag′ah-kanth) dried gummy exudation from *Astragalus gummifer* or other species of Astragalus; used as a suspending agent for drugs.

tragomaschalia (trag″o-mas-kal′e-ah) odorous perspiration from the axilla.

tragophonia (-fo′ne-ah) egophony.

tragopodia (-po′de-ah) knock-knee.

tragus (tra′gus), pl. *tra′gi* [L.] a cartilaginous projection anterior to the external opening of the ear; used also in the plural to designate hairs growing on the pinna of the external ear, especially on the anterior cartilaginous projection. adj., **tra′gal.**

trait (trāt) 1. a facial line. 2. a distinguishing quality or feature.

Tral (tral) trademark for preparations of hexocyclium methylsulfate.

trance (trans) profound or abnormal sleep.

Trancopal (tran′ko-pal) trademark for a preparation of chlormezanone.

tranquilizer (tran″kwī-lī′zer) an agent that calms or quiets an anxious or disturbed patient without affecting clarity of consciousness. **major t.**, a drug that is useful in the treatment of psychotic symptoms. **minor t.**, one that is useful in the treatment of milder symptoms of anxiety, tension or psychoneuroses.

trans- (trans) word element [L.], *through; across; beyond;* in names of chemical compounds it indicates certain atoms or radicals on opposite sides of the molecule.

transabdominal (trans″ab-dom′ĭ-nal) across the abdominal wall or through the abdominal cavity.

transacetylation (trans-as″ĕ-til-a′shun) a chemical reaction involving the transfer of the acetyl radical.

transacylase (-as′ĭ-lās) an enzyme that catalyzes transacylation.

transacylation (-as″ĭ-la′shun) a chemical reaction involving the transfer of the acyl radical between acetic and higher carboxylic acids.

transamidase (-am′ĭ-dās) an enzyme which catalyzes the transfer of an amide group from one molecule to another.

transaminase (-am′ĭ-nās) an enzyme which catalyzes the transfer of an amino group from one molecule to another. **glutamic-oxalacetic t.**, an enzyme normally present in serum and various tissues; it is released into serum as a result of tissue injury and present in increased concentration in myocardial infarction or acute damage to liver cells. **glutamic-pyruvic t.**, an enzyme normally present in the body, observed in higher concentration in the serum of patients with acute damage to liver cells.

transamination (trans″am-ĭ-na′shun) the reversible exchange of amino groups between different amino acids.

transanimation (trans-an″ĭ-ma′shun) resuscitation of an asphyxiated person by mouth-to-mouth breathing.

transaortic (trans″a-or′tik) performed through the aorta.

transatrial (trans-a′tre-al) performed through the atrium.

transaudient (-aw′de-ent) penetrable by sound waves.

transcalent (-ka′lent) penetrable by heat rays.

transcervical (-ser′vĭ-kal) performed through the cervical opening of the uterus.

transduction (-duk′shun) the transfer of a genetic fragment from one cell to another.

transduodenal (trans″du-o-de′nal) across or through the duodenum.

transection (tran-sek′shun) a section made across a long axis.

transepidermal (trans″ep-ĭ-der′mal) occurring through or across the epidermis.

transfaunation (trans″faw-na′shun) the transfer of animal parasites from one host organism to another.

transferase (trans′fer-ās) an enzyme that catalyzes the transfer, from one molecule to another, of a chemical group that does not exist in free state during the transfer.

transference (trans-fer′ens) 1. the passage of a symptom or affection from one part to another. 2. in psychiatry, the shifting of an affect from one person to another or from one idea to another; especially the transfer by the patient to the analyst of magnetic tones, of either affection or hostility, based on unconscious identification.

transferrin (-fer′rin) a serum globulin that binds and transports iron.

transfix (trans-fiks′) to pierce through or impale.

transfixion (-fik′shun) a piercing through.

transforation (trans″fo-ra′shun) perforation of the fetal skull.

transformer (trans-for′mer) an induction apparatus for changing electrical energy at one voltage and current to electrical energy at another voltage and current, through the medium of magnetic energy, without mechanical motion. **closed-core t.**, one having a continuous core of magnetic material (usually iron) without any air gap. **step-down t.**, one for lowering the voltage of the original current. **step-up t.**, one for raising the voltage of the original current.

transfusion (-fu′zhun) introduction into the body circulation of blood or other fluid. **arterial t.**, introduction of blood or other fluid into an artery. **direct t.**, transfer of blood directly from the donor to the recipient. **exchange t.**, successive withdrawal of small amounts of blood and transfusion of donor blood, until a large proportion of original volume has been replaced. **fetomaternal t.**, passage of blood of the fetus across the placenta into the circulation of the maternal organism. **intraperitoneal t.**, infusion of blood into the peritoneal cavity, as sometimes done in infants before birth. **intrauterine t.**, transfusion of blood into the peritoneal cavity of an unborn infant to prevent erythroblastosis fetalis at birth. **immediate t.** direct transfusion. **indirect t.**, introduction of blood which has been stored in a suitable container after withdrawal from the donor. **mediate t.**, indirect transfusion. **placental t.**, return to an infant after birth, through the intact umbilical cord, of the blood contained in the placenta. **replacement t.**, **substitution t.**, exchange transfusion. **venous t.**, introduction of blood or other fluid into a vein.

transiliac (trans-il′e-ak) across the two ilia.

transillumination (trans″ĭ-lu″mĭ-na′shun) the passage of strong light through a body structure, to permit inspection by an observer on the opposite side.

translateral (trans-lat′er-al) from side to side; in roentgenography, referring to the view obtained with the patient supine and the radiation directed horizontally.

translocation (trans″lo-ka′shun) the attachment of a fragment of one chromosome to a nonhomologous chromosome. **reciprocal t.**, the mutual exchange of fragments between two broken chromosomes, one part of one uniting with part of the other.

translucent (trans-lu′sent) slightly penetrable by light rays.

transmigration (trans″mi-gra′shun) 1. diapedesis. 2. change of place from one side of the body to the other.

transmission (trans-mish′un) the transfer, as of a disease, from one person to another.

transmutation (trans″mu-ta′shun) 1. evolutionary change to one species into another. 2. the change of one chemical element into another.

transorbital (trans-or′bĭ-tal) performed through the bony socket of the eye.

transovarial (trans″o-va′re-al) through the ovary; referring to transmission from the maternal organism through the ovum to individuals of the next generation.

transpalatal (trans-pal′ah-tal) performed through the roof of the mouth, or palate.

transpeptidase (-pep′tĭ-dās) an enzyme which catalyzes the transfer of a peptide group from one molecule to another.

transphosphorylase (-fos′fōr-ĭ-lās) an enzyme which catalyzes the transfer of a phosphate group from one molecule to another.

transpirable (trans-pi′rah-bel) permitting passage of perspiration.

transpiration (trans″pi-ra′shun) discharge of air, vapor or sweat through the skin.

transplacental (trans″plah-sen′tal) through the placenta.

transplant 1. (trans′plant) a portion of tissue used in grafting or transplanting. 2. (transplant′) to transfer tissue from one part to another.

transplantation (trans″plan-ta′shun) insertion or application in or on the body of tissue from another individual or another site in the same individual.

transport (trans′port) movement of materials in biological systems, particularly into and out of cells and across epithelial layers. **active t.**, movement of materials in biological systems resulting directly from expenditure of metabolic energy.

transposition (trans″po-zish′un) displacement to the opposite side; in genetics, the nonreciprocal insertion of material deleted from one chromosome into another, nonhomologous chromosome.

transsegmental (trans″seg-men′tal) extending across segments.

transseptal (trans-sep′tal) extending or performed through or across a septum.

trans-sexualism (-seks′u-al-izm″) conscious desire of a person for an anatomic change of sex.

transsphenoidal (trans″sfe-noi′dal) performed through the sphenoid bone.

transtemporal (trans-tem′po-ral) across the temporal lobe.

transthalamic (trans″thah-lam′ik) across the thalamus.

transthoracic (trans″tho-ras′ik) through the thoracic cavity or across the chest wall.

transthoracotomy (trans″tho-rah-kot′o-me) cutting across the thorax.

transtracheal (trans-tra′ke-al) performed through the wall of the trachea.

transtympanic (trans″tim-pan′ik) across the tympanic membrane or the cavity of the middle ear.

transudate (tran′su-dāt) a substance which has passed through a membrane.

transudation (tran″su-da′shun) passage of serum or other body fluid through a membrane or tissue surface.

transureteroureterostomy (trans″u-re″ter-o-u-re″ter-os′to-me) anastomosis of the distal end of the proximal portion of one ureter to the ureter of the opposite side.

transurethral (trans″u-re′thral) through the urethra.

transvaginal (trans-vaj′ĭ-nal) through the vagina.

transvector (-vek′tor) an organism that conveys or transmits a poison derived from another source.

transventricular (trans″ven-trik′u-lar) performed through a ventricle.

transversalis (trans″ver-sa′lis) [L.] transverse.

transverse (trans-vers′) extending from side to side; situated at right angles to the long axis.

transversectomy (trans″ver-sek′to-me) excision of a transverse process of a vertebra.

transversus (trans-ver′sus) [L.] transverse.

transvestism (-ves′tizm) the wearing of clothes appropriate to the opposite sex.

transvestite (-ves′tīt) a person who wears clothing appropriate to the opposite sex.

tranylcypromine (tran″il-si′pro-mēn) a compound used as an inhibitor of monoamine oxidase and as an antidepressant.

trapezium (trah-pe′ze-um) an irregular, four-sided figure.

Trasentine (tras′en-tin) trademark for preparations of adiphenine.

trauma (traw′mah) a wound or injury, especially damage produced by external force. **psychic t.**, injury to the subconscious mind by emotional shock, which may produce a lasting effect.

traumat(o)- (traw′mah-to) word element [Gr.], trauma.

traumatic (traw-mat′ik) pertaining to external force which damages the organism.

traumatism (traw′mah-tizm) morbid state resulting from infliction of an injury or wound by external force.

traumatology (traw″mah-tol′o-je) the science of wounds resulting from external force or violence.

traumatopnea (-top-ne′ah) passage of air through a wound in the chest wall.

tray (tra) a flat-surfaced utensil for the conveyance of various objects or material. **impression t.**, a contoured container to hold the material for making an impression of the teeth and associated structures.

treatment (trēt′ment) management and care of a patient or the combating of the existing disorder. **active t.**, treatment directed immediately to counteracting a disease. **causal t.**, treatment directed against the cause of a disease. **conservative t.**, 1. treatment designed to conserve the vital powers until clear indications develop. 2. conservative surgery. **empiric t.**, treatment by means which experience has proved to be beneficial. **envelope t.**, treatment of burns by covering with air-tight envelope of oiled silk, with openings for entrance and escape of fluid. **expectant t.**, treatment directed toward relief of untoward symptoms, leaving cure of the disease to natural forces. **Kenny t.**, treatment of poliomyelitis by wrapping patient in woolen cloths wrung out of hot water and re-educating muscles by passive exercise after pain has subsided. **light t.**, phototherapy. **organ t.**, organotherapy. **palliative t.**, treatment which is designed to relieve pain and distress, but which does not attempt a cure. **preventive t.**, **prophylactic t.**, that in which the aim is to prevent the occurrence of the disease. **rational t.**, that which is based upon a knowledge of disease and the action of the remedies given. **Sippy t.**, free administration of alkali to neutralize acid of gastric juice; used in gastric ulcer. **specific t.**, treatment particularly adapted to the special disease being treated. **supporting t.**, that which is mainly directed to sustaining the strength of the patient. **symptomatic t.**, expectant treatment.

tree (tre) 1. a perennial of the plant kingdom having a main stem or trunk and numerous branches. 2. an anatomic structure with branches resembling a tree. **bronchial t.**, the bronchi and their branching structures.

trehalose (tre-ha′lōs) sugar from manna or ergot.

Trematoda (trem″ah-to′dah) a class of animals (phylum Platyhelminthes) characterized by a noncellular layer covering the body, and including the flukes.

trematode (trem′ah-tōd) an individual of the class Trematoda.

trembles (trem′belz) milk sickness.

tremophobia (trem″o-fo′be-ah, tre″mo-fo′be-ah) morbid fear of trembling.

tremor (trem′or, tre′mor) involuntary movement due to alternating contractions of opposing muscles, occurring physiologically or pathologically. **coarse t.**, that involving large groups of muscle fibers contracting slowly. **fibrillary t.**, rapidly alternating contraction of small bundles of muscle fibers. **fine t.**, one in which the vibrations are rapid. **flapping t.**, asterixis. **forced t.**, movements persisting after voluntary motion, due to intermittent irritation of the nerve centers. **intention t.**, that occurring when the patient attempts voluntary movement. **volitional t.**, trembling of entire body during voluntary effort; seen in multiple sclerosis.

tremulous (trem′u-lus) trembling or quivering.

trepan (trē-pan′) trephine.

trepanation (trep″ah-na′shun) trephination.

trephination (tref″ĭ-na′shun) use of the trephine for creating an opening in the skull or in the sclera.

trephine (trē-fīn′, trē-fēn′) 1. a crown saw for removing a circular disk or button of tissue, chiefly from the skull. 2. to create an opening with the trephine.

trepidation (trep″ĭ-da′shun) 1. a trembling or oscillatory movement. 2. nervous anxiety and fear. adj., **trep′idant.**

Treponema (trep″o-ne′mah) a genus of Schizomycetes (order Spirochaetales, family Treponemataceae), some of them pathogenic and parasitic for man and other animals, and including *T. pallidum*, the cause of syphilis, and *T. pertenue*, the cause of yaws in man.

treponema (-ne′mah) an organism of the genus Treponema.

Treponemataceae (-ne″mah-ta′se-e) a family of Schizomycetes (order Spirochaetales) which commonly occur as parasites in vertebrates, some of them causing disease.

treponematosis (-to′sis) infection with organisms of the genus Treponema.

treponemicidal (trep″o-ne″mĭ-si′dal) destroying treponemas.

trepopnea (tre″pop-ne′ah) more comfortable respiration with the patient turned in a definite recumbent position.

treppe (trep′ĕ) [Ger.] the gradual increase in muscular contraction following rapidly repeated stimulation.

tresis (tre′sis) perforation.

tri- (tri) word element [Gr., L.], *three.*

triacetate (tri-as′ē-tāt) an acetate which contains three molecules of the acetic acid radical.

triacetin (-as′ē-tin) glyceryl triacetate; used as an antimycotic agent.

triacetyloleandomycin (-as″ē-til-o″le-an″do-mi′sin) a white, odorless, crystalline powder, used as an antibiotic.

triad (tri′ad) 1. an element with a valence of three. 2. a group of three similar bodies, or a complex composed of three items or units. **adrenomedullary t.**, three symptoms produced by activation of the adrenal medulla:

tachycardia, vasoconstriction and sweating. **Beck's t.**, rising venous pressure, falling arterial pressure and small, quiet heart, characteristic of cardiac compression. **Dieulafoy's t.**, skin sensitiveness, muscular contractions, and tenderness over McBurney's point, indicative of appendicitis. **Saint's t.**, hiatus hernia, colonic diverticula and cholelithiasis.

triakaidekaphobia (tri″ah-ki″dek-ah-fo′be-ah) abnormal dread of the number thirteen.

triamcinolone (tri″am-sin′o-lōn) a prednisolone compound used as an anti-inflammatory steroid.

triangle (tri′ang-gel) a three-cornered object, figure or area, as such an area on the surface of the body capable of fairly precise definition. **carotid t., inferior,** between median line of neck in front, the sternomastoid, and anterior belly of omohyoid. **carotid t., superior,** between anterior belly of omohyoid in front, posterior belly of digastric above, and sternomastoid behind. **cephalic t.**, on anteroposterior plane of skull, between lines from occiput to forehead and to chin, and from chin to forehead. **Codman's t.**, a triangular area visible roentgenographically where the periosteum, elevated by a bone tumor, rejoins the cortex of normal bone. **digastric t.**, the submaxillary triangle. **t. of elbow,** in front, the supinator longus on the outside and pronator teres inside the base toward the humerus. **t. of election,** superior carotid triangle. **facial t.**, its angles—basion, and alveolar and nasal points. **Farabeuf's t.**, a triangle in the upper part of the neck bound by the internal jugular vein, the facial nerve and the hypoglossal nerve. **femoral t.**, inguinal triangle. **frontal t.**, bounded by maximum frontal diameter and lines to the glabella. **Hesselbach's t.**, triangular space bounded by Poupart's ligament, rectus muscle and epigastric artery. **iliofemoral t.**, formed by Nélaton's line, another line through the superior iliac spine, and a third from this to the greater trochanter. **infraclavicular t.**, formed by the clavicle above, upper border of pectoralis major on inside, anterior border of deltoid on outside. **inguinal t.**, triangular area bounded by inner edge of sartorius, Poupart's ligament and outer edge of adductor longus. **Langenbeck's t.**, a triangle whose apex is the anterior superior iliac spine, its base the anatomic neck of the femur, and its external side the external base of the greater trochanter. **Lesser's t.**, formed by the hypoglossal nerve above, and the two bellies of the digastricus on the two sides. **lumbocostoabdominal t.**, lies between the obliquus externus, the serratus posticus inferior, the erector spinae and the obliquus internus. **Macewen's t.**, triangular space between lower posterior edge of root of zygoma and superior posterior edge of external auditory canal. **t. of necessity,** inferior carotid triangle. **t. of neck, anterior,** the two carotid and the submaxillary triangles together. **t. of neck, posterior,** the occipital and subclavian triangles together. **occipital t.** has the sternomastoid in front, the trapezius behind, and omohyoid below. **occipital t., inferior,** the bimastoid line as its base and inion its apex. **Pawlik's t.,** an area on the anterior vaginal wall corresponding to the trigone of the bladder. **Petit's t.,** space bounded by crest of ilium and latissimus dorsi and external oblique muscle of the abdomen. **Scarpa's t.,** inguinal triangle. **subclavian t.,** triangular area bounded by clavicle, sternocleidomastoid and omohyoid. **submaxillary t.,** lower jaw bone above, posterior belly of digastric and the stylohyoid below, and median line of neck in front. **suboccipital t.** lies between the rectus capitis posterior major and superior and inferior oblique muscles. **suprameatal t.,** Macewen's triangle.

triangularis (tri-ang″gu-la′ris) [L.] triangular.

Triatoma (tri″ah-to′mah) a genus of arthropods (order Hemiptera), numerous species of which, including *T. protracta* and *T. sanguisuga,* are naturally infected by trypanosomes.

triatomic (-tom′ik) 1. containing three atoms in the molecule. 2. containing three replaceable hydrogen atoms. 3. containing three hydroxyl groups.

tribe (trīb) a taxonomic category subordinate to a family (or subfamily) and superior to a genus (or subtribe).

triboluminescence (tri″bo-lu″mī-nes′ens) the production of light by a substance when it is rubbed to a fine powder.

tribrachius (tri-bra′ke-us) a fetal monster with three arms.

tribromoethanol (-bro″mo-eth′ah-nol) white crystalline powder, administered by rectum to produce general anesthesia.

Triburon (trib′u-ron) trademark for preparations of triclobisonium chloride.

tricephalus (tri-sef′ah-lus) a fetal monster with three heads.

trich(o)- word element [Gr.], *hair.*

trichangiectasis (trik″an-je-ek′tah-sis) dilatation of the capillaries.

trichiasis (trĭ-ki′ah-sis) 1. misplacement of the eyelashes so that they impinge on the cornea and bulbar conjunctiva. 2. appearance of hairlike filaments in the urine.

trichina (trĭ-ki′nah), pl. *trichi′nae* [Gr.] an individual organism of the genus Trichinella.

Trichinella (trik″i-nel′ah) a genus of nematode parasites. **T. spira′lis,** a species found in the striated muscle of various animals, a common cause of infection in man as a result of ingestion of poorly cooked pork.

trichinosis (-no′sis) infestation with Trichinella.

trichinous (trik′i-nus) affected with Trichinella.

trichion (trik′e-on) an anthropometric landmark, the point at which the midsagittal plane of the head intersects the hairline.

trichloride (tri-klo′rīd) a binary compound containing three chlorine atoms in the molecule.

trichlormethiazide (-klor″mĕ-thi′ah-zīd) a compound used as a diuretic and hypotensive and in the treatment of edema.

trichloroethylene (tri″klo-ro-eth′ĭ-lēn) a clear, mobile liquid used as an inhalation analgesic and anesthetic for short operative procedures.

trichlorophenol (-fe′nol) a disinfectant and external antiseptic.

trichlorthiazide (tri″klor-thi′ah-zīd) a compound used as a diuretic and hypotensive and in the treatment of edema.

trichoanesthesia (trik″o-an″es-the′ze-ah) loss of hair sensibility.

trichobacteria (-bak-te′re-ah) bacteria having flagella.

trichobezoar (-be′zōr) a bezoar composed of hair.

trichocardia (-kar′de-ah) hairy heart.

trichocephaliasis (-sef″ah-li′ah-sis) trichuriasis.

Trichocephalus (-sef′ah-lus) Trichuris.

trichoclasia (-kla′se-ah) brittleness of the hair.

trichocryptosis (-krip-to′sis) disease of the hair follicles.

trichodynia (-din′e-ah) painful sensation when the hair is touched.

trichoepithelioma (-ep″ĭ-the″le-o′mah) a skin tumor originating in the follicles of the lanugo hairs.

trichoesthesia (-es-the′ze-ah) sensibility of the hair to touch.

trichogenous (trī-koj′ĕ-nus) stimulating the growth of hair.

trichoglossia (trik″o-glos′e-ah) hairy tongue.

trichoid (trik′oid) resembling hair.

trichology (trī-kol′o-je) sum of knowledge about the hair.

trichome (tri′kōm) a filamentous or hairlike structure.

Trichomonas (trī-kom′o-nas) a genus of parasitic protozoa. **T. hom′inis,** a species found in the human mouth and intestines. **T. te′nax,** a species found in the mouth. **T. vagina′lis,** a species occurring in the vaginal secretions.

trichomoniasis (trik″o-mo-ni′ah-sis) infection by organisms of the genus Trichomonas.

trichomycosis (-mi-ko′sis) any disease of the hair caused by fungi. **t. favo′sa,** favus.

trichonocardiasis (-no-kar-di′ah-sis) a disease of pubic and axillary hair caused by *Nocardia tenuis.*

trichonodosis (-no-do′sis) a condition characterized by apparent or actual knotting of the hair.

trichopathy (trī-kop′ah-the) disease of the hair.

trichophobia (trik″o-fo′be-ah) morbid dread of hair.

trichophytic (-fit′ik) pertaining to Trichophyton.

trichophytid (trī-kof′ĭ-tid) a generalized eruption due to allergy to Trichophyton.

trichophytin (trī-kof′ĭ-tin) a filtrate from cultures of the Trichophyton; used in testing for trichophyton infection.

trichophytobezoar (trik″o-fi″to-be′zōr) a bezoar composed of animal hair and vegetable fiber.

Trichophyton (trī-kof′ĭ-ton) a genus of fungi which may cause various infections of the skin and its appendages.

trichophytosis (trik"o-fi-to'sis) infection with fungi of the genus Trichophyton. **t. bar'bae,** tinea sycosis. **t. cap'itis,** tinea capitis. **t. cor'-poris,** tinea corporis. **t. cru'ris,** tinea cruris. **t. un'guium,** fungal infection of the nails due to species of Trichophyton.

trichoptilosis (-tī-lo'sis) splitting of hairs at the end

trichorrhexis (-rek'sis) breaking of the hair. **t. nodo'sa,** a condition marked by fracture and splitting of the cortex of a hair into strands, giving the appearance of white nodes at which the hair is easily broken.

trichorrhexomania (-rek"so-ma'ne-ah) the morbid habit of breaking off one's hair by pinching it with the fingernails.

trichoschisis (trī-kos'kĭ-sis) trichoptilosis.

trichoscopy (trī-kos'ko-pe) examination of the hair.

trichosiderin (trik"o-sid'er-in) an iron-containing brown pigment found in normal human red hair.

trichosis (trī-ko'sis) any disease of the hair.

Trichosporon (trī-kos'po-ron) a genus of fungi which may infect the hair.

trichosporosis (trik"o-spo-ro'sis) infection with Trichosporon.

trichostasis spinulosa (trī-kos'tah-sis spin"u-lo'sah) formation of horny plugs containing bundles of hairs in the hair follicles of the scalp.

trichostrongyliasis (trik"o-stron"jī-li'ah-sis) infection by nematodes of the genus Trichostrongylus.

trichostrongylosis (-stron"jī-lo'sis) trichostrongyliasis.

Trichostrongylus (-stron'jī-lus) a genus of nematode parasites infecting animals and man.

trichotillomania (-til"o-ma'ne-ah) neurotic plucking of the hair.

trichotomous (trī-kot'o-mus) divided into three parts.

trichroism (tri'kro-izm) condition or quality exhibiting three different colors in three different aspects. adj., **trichro'ic.**

trichromatopsia (tri"kro-mah-top'se-ah) normal color vision for all three primary colors.

trichromic (tri-kro'mik) 1. pertaining to or exhibiting three colors. 2. able to distinguish only three of the seven colors of the spectrum.

trichuriasis (trik"u-ri'ah-sis) morbid condition caused by presence of Trichuris.

Trichuris (trik-u'ris) a genus of nematodes parasitic in the intestinal tract, including *T. trichiura,* found in man, and numerous other species found in various other mammals.

tricipital (tri-sip'ī-tal) 1. three-headed. 2. relating to the triceps.

triclobisonium (tri"klo-bi-so'ne-um) a compound used as an antimicrobial agent for skin and wound infections and as an antitrichomonal agent.

Tricofuron (tri"ko-fu'ron) trademark for preparations of furazolidone.

Tricoloid (tri'ko-loid) trademark for preparations of tricyclamol.

tricornute (tri-kor'nūt) having three cornua or processes.

tricrotism (tri'krot-izm) quality of having three sphygmographic waves or elevations to one beat of the pulse. adj., **tricrot'ic.**

tricuspid (tri-kus'pid) having three points or cusps.

tricyclamol (-si'klah-mol) a compound used in parasympathetic blockade.

tridactylism (-dak'tī-lizm) presence of only three digits on the hand or foot.

tridentate (-den'tāt) having three prongs.

tridermic (-der'mik) derived from the ectoderm, endoderm and mesoderm.

tridihexethyl (tri"di-heks-eth'il) a compound used in parasympathetic blockade.

Tridione (tri-di'ōn) trademark for preparations of trimethadione.

triethylamine (-eth"il-am'in) a ptomaine from putrefying fish.

triethylenemelamine (-eth"ī-lēn-mel'ah-mēn) a highly poisonous, white, crystalline powder used as an antineoplastic agent.

triethylenethiophosphoramide (-thi"o-fos-for'ah-mīd) thio-tepa.

trifid (tri'fid) split into three parts.

trifluoperazine (tri"floo-o-per'ah-zēn) a phenothiazine compound used as a tranquilizer.

triflupromazine (-pro'mah-zēn) a phenothiazine compound used as a tranquilizer.

trifluromethylthiazide (tri-flur"o-meth"il-thi'ah-zīd) flumethiazide.

trifurcation (tri"fer-ka'shun) division or the site of separation into three branches.

trigeminy (tri-jem'ī-ne) the condition of occurring in threes, especially the occurrence of three pulse beats in rapid succession.

triglyceride (-glis'er-īd) a compound consisting of three molecules of fatty acid esterified to glycerol; a neutral fat that is the usual storage form of lipids in animals.

trigocephalus (tri"go-sef'ah-lus) a fetal monster with forepart of the head triangular.

trigonal (tri'go-nal) 1. triangular. 2. pertaining to a trigone.

trigone (tri'gōn) a triangle. **t. of bladder,** vesical trigone. **Müller's t.,** a part of the tuber cinereum which folds over the optic chiasm. **olfactory t.,** triangular area of gray matter between the roots of the olfactory tract. **vesical t.,** a triangular region of the wall of the urinary bladder, the three angles corresponding with the orifices of the ureters and urethra, and an area in which the muscular fibers are closely adherent to the mucosa.

trigonectomy (tri"gon-ek'to-me) excision of the trigone of the bladder.

trigonid (tri-gon'id) the first three cusps of a lower molar tooth.

trigonitis (tri"go-ni'tis) inflammation of the trigone of the bladder.

trigonocephaly (tri"go-no-sef'ah-le) triangular shape of the head due to sharp forward angulation at the midline of the frontal bone. adj., **trigonocephal'ic.**

trigonum (tri-go'num), pl. *trigo'na* [L.] trigone, or triangle; used in anatomic nomenclature to designate various regions or structures.

trihexinol (-hek'sī-nol) a compound used in

parasympathetic blockade and in treatment of diarrhea.

trihexyphenidyl (tri-hek″se-fen′ĭ-dil) a compound used in parasympathetic blockade.

trihybrid (-hi′brid) a hybrid offspring of parents differing in three mendelian characters.

triiodothyronine (tri″i-o″do-thi′ro-nēn) a compound found in the thyroid gland, produced by conjugation of monoiodotyrosine and diiodotyrosine.

trilabe (tri′lāb) a three-pronged lithotrite.

Trilafon (tri′lah-fon) trademark for preparations of perphenazine.

Trilene (tri′lēn) trademark for a preparation of trichloroethylene.

trilobate (tri-lo′bāt) having three lobes.

trilocular (-lok′u-lar) having three loculi or cells.

trilogy (tril′o-je) a group or series of three. **t. of Fallot,** a term sometimes applied to concurrent pulmonic stenosis, atrial septal defect and right ventricular hypertrophy.

trimanual (tri-man′u-al) accomplished by use of three hands.

trimensual (-men′su-al) occurring every three months.

trimeprazine (-mep′rah-zēn) a compound used as a tranquilizer.

trimester (-mes′ter) a period of three months.

trimethadione (tri″meth-ah-di′ōn) a white, crystalline compound used as an anticonvulsant.

trimethaphan (tri-meth′ah-fan) a compound used in ganglionic blockade and as a hypotensive agent.

trimethidinium (-meth″ĭ-din′e-um) a compound used in ganglionic blockade and as a hypotensive agent.

trimethobenzamide (-meth″o-ben′zah-mīd) a compound used as an antiemetic.

trimethylene (-meth′ĭ-lēn) cyclopropane.

Trimeton (tri′me-ton) trademark for preparations of pheniramine maleate.

trimorphous (tri-mor′fus) crystallizing in three different forms.

trinitrate (-ni′trāt) a nitrate which contains three radicals of nitric acid.

trinitrin (-ni′trin) glyceryl trinitrate.

trinitroglycerol (-ni″tro-glis′er-ol) glyceryl trinitrate.

trinitrophenol (-fe′nol) pale yellow prisms or scales; germicide, antiseptic, and stimulant of epithelial growth.

trinitrotoluene (-tol′u-ēn) a highly explosive substance derived from toluene, sometimes a cause of poisoning in those working with it.

triocephalus (tri″o-sef′ah-lus) fetal monster with no organs of sight, hearing or smell.

triolism (tri′o-lizm) sexual interests or practices involving three persons of both sexes.

triorchidism (tri-or′kĭ-dizm) the presence of three testes.

triose (tri′ōs) a sugar containing three molecules of carbon.

trioxide (tri-ok′sīd) a binary compound containing three oxygen atoms in the molecule.

tripara (trip′ah-rah) tertipara.

triparanol (tri-par′ah-nol) a compound used to depress the synthesis of cholesterol.

tripelennamine (tri″pĕ-len′ah-min) a compound used as an antihistaminic.

tripeptide (tri-pep′tīd) a peptide formed from three amino acids.

triphalangism (-fal′an-jizm) three phalanges in a digit normally having only two.

triphasic (-fa′zik) having three phases.

triplegia (-ple′je-ah) paralysis of three extremities.

triplet (trip′let) 1. one of three offspring produced at one birth. 2. a combination of three objects or entities acting together, as three lenses or three nucleotides.

triplex (tri′pleks) triple or threefold.

triploid (trip′loid) having triple the haploid number of chromosomes (3n).

triploidy (trip′loi-de) the state of having three sets of chromosomes (3n).

triplokoria (trip″lo-ko′re-ah) the presence of three pupils in an eye.

triplopia (trī-plo′pe-ah) defective vision, objects being seen as threefold.

tripoding (tri′pod-ing) the use of three points of support, as adopted by paralyzed patients when changing from a sitting or standing position.

tripoli (trip′o-le) a mild abrasive and polishing agent used on the teeth.

triprolidine (tri-pro′lĭ-dēn) a compound used as an antihistaminic.

-tripsy (trip′se) word element [Gr.], *crushing*; used to designate a surgical procedure in which a structure is intentionally crushed.

tripus (tri′pus) a fetal monster with three feet.

trisaccharide (tri-sak′ah-rīd) a sugar each molecule of which yields three molecules of monosaccharides on hydrolysis.

trismoid (triz′moid) 1. resembling trismus. 2. a condition resembling tetanus neonatorum.

trismus (triz′mus) tetanic spasm of the jaw muscles. **t. nascen′tium, t. neonato′rum,** tetanus neonatorum.

trisomy (tri′so-me) existence in a cell of three instead of the normal diploid pair of a particular chromosome. adj., **triso′mic.**

trisplanchnic (tri-splangk′nik) pertaining to the three great visceral cavities.

tristichia (-stik′e-ah) the presence of three rows of eyelashes.

tristimania (tris″tĭ-ma′ne-ah) melancholia.

trisulcate (tri-sul′kāt) having three furrows.

trisulfate (-sul′fāt) a binary compound containing three sulfate (SO_4) groups in the molecule.

trisulfide (-sul′fīd) a binary compound containing three sulfur atoms in the molecule.

tritanopia (tri″tah-no′pe-ah) defective color vision, characterized by perception of only red and green and lacking blue and yellow.

tritiate (trit′e-āt) to treat with tritium.

tritium (trit′e-um, trish′e-um) the mass three isotope of hydrogen.

tritocone (tri′to-kōn) the distobuccal cusp of an upper bicuspid tooth.

tritoconid (tri″to-ko′nid) the distobuccal cusp of a lower bicuspid tooth.

triturable (trich′er-ah-bel) susceptible of being triturated.

triturate (trich′e-rāt) 1. to reduce to powder by

rubbing.   2. a substance powdered fine by rubbing.

trituration (trich″ĕ-ra′shun) 1. reduction to powder by friction or grinding. 2. a finely powdered substance.

triturator (-ra′tor) an apparatus in which substances can be continuously rubbed.

trivalent (tri-va′lent) having a valence of three.

trixenic (-zen′ik) associated with only three species of microorganisms, whose names are known.

trocar (tro′kar) sharp-pointed instrument used with a cannula for tapping. **Duchenne's t.,** a trocar for obtaining specimens of deep-seated tissues.

trochanter (tro-kan′ter) a broad, flat process on the femur, at the upper end of its lateral surface (*greater trochanter*), or a short conical process on the posterior border of the base of its neck (*lesser trochanter*). adj., **trochanter′ic, trochante′rian.**

troche (tro′ke) a medicinal preparation for solution in the mouth, consisting of an active ingredient incorporated in a mass made of sugar and mucilage or fruit base.

trochlea (trok′le ah), pl. *troch′leae* [L.] a pulley-shaped part or structure; used in anatomic nomenclature to designate various bony or fibrous structures through or over which tendons pass or with which other structures articulate. adj., **troch′lear.**

trochocardia (tro″ko-kar′de-ah) displacement of the heart due to rotation on its axis.

trochocephalia (-sē-fa′le-ah) abnormal or premature union of frontal and parietal bones.

trochoid (tro′koid) pivot-like, or pulley-shaped.

trochoides (tro-koi′dēz) a pivot joint.

trolnitrate (trol-ni′trāt) a compound used as a vasodilator.

Trombicula (trom-bik′u-lah) a widely distributed genus of mites, including several frequently encountered species, among them *T. akamushi, T. alfreddugesi, T. autumnalis* and *T. batatas.*

trombiculiasis (trom-bik″u-li′ah-sis) infestation with mites of the genus Trombicula.

Trombiculidae (trom-bik′u-li″de) a family of mites cosmopolitan in distribution, which infest vertebrates.

Tromexan (tro-mek′san) trademark for a preparation of ethyl biscoumacetate.

Tronothane (tron′o-thān) trademark for preparations of pramoxine.

troph(o)- (trof′o) word element [Gr.], *food; nourishment.*

trophectoderm (trof-ek′to-derm) the earliest trophoblast.

trophedema (trof″ē-de′mah) a chronic disease with permanent edema of the feet or legs.

trophema (tro-fe′mah) the nourishing blood of the uterine mucosa.

trophesy (trof′e-se) defective nutrition due to disorder of the trophic nerves.

trophic (trof′ik) pertaining to nutrition.

-trophic (trof′ik) word element [Gr.], *nourishing; stimulating.*

trophoblast (trof′o-blast) the peripheral cells of the blastocyst, which become the placenta

and the membranes that nourish and protect the developing organism.

trophoblastoma (trof″o-blas-to′mah) choriocarcinoma.

trophodermatoneurosis (-der″mah-to-nu-ro′sis) erythredema polyneuropathy.

trophology (tro-fol′o-je) the science of nutrition of the body.

trophoneurosis (trof″o-nu-ro′sis) 1. any functional nervous disease due to a trophic disorder. 2. trophesy. adj., **trophoneurot′ic.**

trophonosis (trof″o-no′sis) any disease due to nutritional causes.

trophonucleus (-nu′kle-us) macronucleus.

trophopathy (tro-fop′ah-the) any derangement of nutrition.

trophoplast (trof′o-plast) a granular protoplasmic body.

trophospongium (trof″o-spun′je-um) a network in the cytoplasm of certain cells which is instrumental in nutritive circulation.

trophotaxis (-tak′sis) taxis in relation to food supply.

trophotherapy (-ther′ah-pe) treatment of disease by dietary measures.

trophotropism (tro-fot′ro-pizm) tropism in relation to food supply.

trophozoite (trof″o-zo′īt) the active, motile feeding stage of a sporozoan parasite.

tropia (tro′pe-ah) heterotropia; deviation of the visual axis of one eye when the other eye is fixing.

-tropic (trop′ik) word element [Gr.], *turning toward.*

tropine (tro′pēn) a crystalline base from atropine.

tropism (tro′pizm) a growth response in a nonmotile organism elicited by an external stimulus, and either toward (*positive tropism*) or away from (*negative tropism*) the stimulus; used as a word element combined with a stem indicating nature of the stimulus (e.g. phototropism) or material or entity for which an organism (or substance) shows a special affinity (e.g. neurotropism).

tropopause (trop′o-pawz) a layer of the earth's atmosphere separating troposphere and stratosphere.

troposphere (trop′o-sfēr) the part of the atmosphere closest to the earth, in which most of the weather phenomena occur; it extends to an altitude of 30,000–40,000 feet near the equator and is less at the poles.

troxidone (trok′si-dōn) trimethadione.

T.R.U. turbidity reducing unit.

truncate (trung′kāt) to deprive of limbs or branches.

truncus (trung′kus), pl. *trun′ci* [L.] trunk; used in anatomic nomenclature. **t. arterio′sus,** an artery connected with the fetal heart, developing into the aortic and pulmonary arches. **t. brachiocephal′icus,** a vessel arising from the arch of the aorta and giving origin to the right common carotid and right subclavian arteries. **t. celi′acus,** celiac trunk. **t. pulmona′lis,** pulmonary trunk.

trunk (trungk) the main part, as the part of the body to which the head and limbs are attached, or a larger structure (e.g. vessel or nerve) from which smaller divisions or branches arise, or which is created by their union. adj., **trun'cal. celiac t.**, a vessel arising from the abdominal aorta and giving origin to the left gastric, common hepatic and splenic arteries. **pulmonary t.**, a vessel arising from the conus arteriosus of the right ventricle and bifurcating into the right and left pulmonary arteries.

truss (trus) device for retaining a reduced hernia in its place.

try-in (tri'in) a preliminary insertion of a dental prosthetic appliance to determine its fit and suitability.

trypaflavine (trip"ah-fla'vin) acriflavine hydrochloride.

trypanocidal (tri-pan"o-si'dal) destructive to trypanosomes.

trypanolysis (tri"pan-ol'ĭ-sis) the destruction of trypanosomes. adj., **trypanolyt'ic.**

Trypanoplasma (tri"pan-o-plaz'mah) a genus of protozoan parasites.

Trypanosoma (-so'mah) a genus of parasitic protozoa found in the blood of animals and men, including hundreds of species, all of which are parasitic in the blood and lymph of vertebrates and invertebrates. **T. cru'zi,** a species which causes Chagas' disease. **T. gambien'se,** found in man in cases of sleeping sickness and tropical cachexia. **T. rhodesien'se,** cause of African trypanosomiasis.

trypanosome (tri-pan'o-sōm) an individual of the genus Trypanosoma. adj., **trypanoso'mal, trypanoso'mic.**

trypanosomiasis (tri-pan"o-so-mi'ah-sis) infection with trypanosomes, marked by fever, anemia, erythema, etc. **African t.**, a fatal disease caused by *Trypanosoma rhodesiense,* and involving the central nervous system, the patient becoming lethargic and somnolent. **American t., Brazilian t., South American t.**, Chagas' disease.

trypanosomicide (-so'mĭ-sīd) an agent destructive to trypanosomes.

trypanosomid (-so'mid) a skin eruption occurring in trypanosomiasis.

tryparsamide (trip-ar'sah-mīd) white crystalline powder used in treatment of trypanosomiasis.

trypesis (tri-pe'sis) trephination.

trypsin (trip'sin) an enzyme that catalyzes the hydrolysis of practically all types of proteins, produced in the intestine by activation of trypsinogen. adj., **tryp'tic. crystallized t.**, a proteolytic enzyme crystallized from an extract of the pancreas of the ox.

trypsinize (trip'sĭ-nīz) to subject to the action of trypsin.

trypsinogen (trip-sin'o-jen) the inactive precursor of trypsin, the form in which it is secreted by the pancreas.

tryptophan (trip'to-fān) a naturally occurring amino acid, one of those essential for human metabolism.

tryptophanase (trip'to-fan"ās) an enzyme that catalyzes the cleavage of tryptophan into indole, pyruvic acid and ammonia.

T.S. test solution.

tsetse (tset'se) an African fly which is a vector of trypanosomes.

T.S.H. thyroid-stimulating hormone.

T.U. tuberculin unit.

Tuamine (too'ah-min) trademark for preparations of tuaminoheptane.

tuaminoheptane (tu-am"ĭ-no-hep'tān) a compound used as a sympathomimetic agent in congestion of the nasal mucosa.

tuba (tu'bah), pl. *tu'bae* [L.] tube.

Tubadil (too'bah-dil) trademark for a preparation of tubocurarine.

Tubarine (too'bah-rin) trademark for a preparation of tubocurarine.

tube (tūb) a hollow cylindrical organ or instrument. adj., **tu'bal. auditory t.**, the narrow channel connecting the middle ear and nasopharynx. **Chaoul t.**, a tube used in roentgen-ray therapy. **collecting t's**, the uriniferous tubules of the kidney. **Coolidge t.**, an x-ray tube with cathode consisting of tungsten spiral enclosed in a molybdenum tube. **Debove's t.**, a large tube for gastric lavage. **drainage t.**, tube used in surgery to facilitate escape of fluids. **Durham's t.**, a jointed tracheotomy tube. **eustachian t.**, canal from nasopharynx to tympanum. **fallopian t.**, uterine tube. **feeding t.**, a tube for introducing food into the stomach. **fermentation t.**, a bent tube, one portion of which is upright and closed at the end, for demonstrating the production of gas by bacteria or other material under study. **Geissler's t.**, an x-ray tube containing a highly rarefied gas. **intubation t.**, tracheostomy tube. **Jutte t.**, a form of duodenal tube for irrigation, aspiration and feeding. **Kimpton-Brown t.**, a tube for performing indirect transfusion of blood. **Lyster's t's**, tubes of calcium hypochlorite for sterilizing drinking water. **Miller-Abbott t.**, a double-channel intestinal tube for diagnosing and treating obstructive lesions of the small intestine. **nephrostomy t.**, one inserted through the abdominal wall into the pelvis of the kidney for direct drainage of the urine. **neural t.**, the epithelial tube produced by folding of the neural plate in the early embryo. **otopharyngeal t.**, eustachian tube. **Ryle's t.**, a thin rubber tube for giving a test meal. **safety t.**, the upper, open portion of the eustachian tube, by which air pressures on each side of the tympanum are equalized. **Schachowa's t.**, the spiral part of a uriniferous tubule. **Sengstaken-Blakemore t.**, an instrument used for tamponade of bleeding esophageal varices. **stomach t.**, one which is passed through the esophagus to the stomach, for introduction of nutrients or gastric lavage. **test t.**, a tube of thin glass, closed at one end; used in chemical tests and other laboratory procedures. **thoracostomy t.**, one inserted through an opening in the chest wall for application of suction to the pleural cavity to facilitate re-expansion of the lung in spontaneous pneumothorax. **tracheostomy t.**, a curved tube that is inserted into the trachea through the opening made in the neck at tracheostomy. **uterine t.**, a slender tube extending laterally from the uterus toward the ovary on the same side, conveying ova to the cavity of the uterus and permitting passage of spermatozoa in the opposite direction. **vacuum t.**, a tube of glass from which gaseous contents have been evacuated. **Wangensteen t.**, a suction apparatus connected with a duodenal tube for aspirating gas and fluid from the stomach and intestine.

tuber (tu'ber) a swelling or protuberance. **t. cine'reum**, an area of the under surface of the forebrain to which the stalk of the hypophysis is attached.

tubercle (tu'ber-kel) 1. a small, rounded nodule produced by the bacillus of tuberculosis. 2. a nodule or small eminence, especially one on a bone, for attachment of a tendon. adj., **tuber'cular**. **anatomic t.**, dissection tubercle. **caseous t.**, a tuberculous nodule which has undergone caseous degeneration. **darwinian t.**, an eminence sometimes seen on the edge of the helix of the ear. **dissection t.**, warty growth often occurring on the hand in persons performing dissection. **Farre's t's**, nodules on the surface of a carcinomatous liver. **fibrous t.**, tubercle of bacillary origin which contains connective-tissue elements. **genial t's**, two small eminences on either side of the midline, on the inner surface of the mandible. **Ghon's t.**, the primary lesion of tuberculosis in children. **Lisfranc t.**, an eminence on the first rib, for attachment of the scalenus anticus. **Lower's t.**, one in the right atrium, between the openings of the venae cavae. **lymphoid t.**, a lesion of tuberculosis consisting of lymphoid cells. **miliary t.**, a minute tubercle sometimes found in great numbers in various parts and organs in true bacillary tuberculosis. **scalene t.**, Lisfranc's tubercle **supraglenoid t.**, one on the scapula for attachment of the long head of the biceps. **zygomatic t.**, a small eminence on the zygoma, at the junction of its anterior root.

tuberculated (tu-ber'ku-lāt''ed) covered with tubercles.

tuberculid (tu-ber'ku-lid) a skin lesion representing a hypersensitivity reaction in a person with active tuberculosis. **papulonecrotic t.**, a condition characterized by crops of deep-seated papules or nodules, with central necrosis or ulceration.

tuberculigenous (tu-ber''ku-lij'ĕ-nus) causing tuberculosis.

tuberculin (tu-ber'ku-lin) a protein or protein derivative from cultures of tubercle bacilli (*Mycobacterium tuberculosis*), used in intradermal tests for sensitivity to the microorganism. **old t.**, a sterile solution of concentrated, soluble products of the growth of the tubercle bacillus, adjusted to standard potency by addition of glycerin and isotonic sodium chloride solution, final glycerin content being about 50 per cent. **t. P.P.D., purified protein derivative of t.**, a sterile, soluble, partially purified product of the growth of the tubercle bacillus in a special liquid medium free from protein.

tuberculitis (tu-ber''ku-li'tis) inflammation of a tubercle.

tuberculocele (tu-ber'ku-lo-sēl'') tuberculous disease of a testis.

tuberculocide (tu-ber'ku-lo-sīd'') an agent destructive to tubercle bacilli.

tuberculofibroid (tu-ber''ku-lo-fi'broid) characterized by tubercle that has undergone fibroid degeneration.

tuberculoid (tu-ber'ku-loid) resembling tuberculosis.

tuberculoma (tu-ber''ku-lo'mah) a tumor-like mass resulting from enlargement of a caseous tubercle.

tuberculomania (tu-ber''ku-lo-ma'ne-ah) a morbid belief that one is affected with tuberculosis.

tuberculophobia (-fo'be-ah) a morbid fear of tuberculosis.

tuberculosilicosis (-sil''ĭ-ko'sis) silicosis with tuberculosis.

tuberculosis (tu-ber''ku-lo'sis) an infectious disease caused by *Mycobacterium tuberculosis*, and characterized by formation of tubercles in the tissues. adj., **tuberculot'ic, tuber'culous. avian t.**, a form of tuberculosis affecting various birds. **bovine t.**, an infection of cattle due to *Mycobacterium bovis*. **disseminated t.**, acute miliary tuberculosis. **hematogenous t.**, infection carried through the blood stream to other organs from the primary site of infection. **t. indurati'va**, chronic tuberculosis of the skin, characterized by indurated nodules. **t. lupo'sa**, lupus vulgaris. **miliary t., acute**, an acute form in which minute tubercles are formed in a number of organs, due to dissemination of the bacilli through the body by the blood stream.

tuberculum (tu-ber'ku-lum), pl. *tuber'cula* [L.] a nodule or small eminence; used in anatomical nomenclature to designate principally a small eminence on a bone. **t. acus'ticum**, collection of nerve cells behind the accessory auditory nucleus. **t. arthrit'icum**, a gouty concretion in a joint. **t. doloro'sum**, a painful nodule or tubercle.

tuberosis (tu''ber-o'sis) a condition characterized by the presence of nodules. **t. cu'tis prurigino'sa**, prurigo nodularis.

tuberositas (tu''bĕ-ros'ĭ-tas), pl. *tuberosita'tes* [L.] tuberosity; used in anatomic nomenclature to designate elevations on bones to which muscles are attached.

tuberosity (-ros'ĭ-te) an elevation or protuberance.

tubo- (tu'bo) word element [L.], *tube*.

tubocurarine (tu''bo-ku-rah'rēn) an alkaloid from the bark and stems of *Chondrodendron tomentosum*, used as a skeletal muscle relaxant.

tuboligamentous (-lig''ah-men'tus) pertaining to uterine tube and broad ligament.

tubo-ovarian (-o-va're-an) pertaining to uterine tube and ovary.

tuboperitoneal (-per''ĭ-to-ne'al) pertaining to the uterine tube and the peritoneum.

tuborrhea (-re'ah) discharge from the eustachian tube.

tubo-uterine (-u'ter-in) pertaining to uterine tube and uterus.

tubule (tu'būl) a small tube. adj., **tu'bular.
collecting t's,** the terminal channels of the nephrons which open on the summits of the renal pyramids in the renal papillae. **dentinal t's,** the tubular structures of the teeth. **Ferrein's t.,** the cortical portion of a uriniferous tubule. **galactophorous t's, lactiferous t's,** small channels for the passage of milk from the secreting cells in the mammary gland. **mesonephric t's,** the tubules comprising the mesonephros, or temporary kidney, of amniotes. **metanephric t's,** the tubules comprising the permanent kidney of amniotes. **renal t's,** the minute canals made up of basement membrane and lined with epithelium, composing the substance of the kidney and secreting, collecting and conducting the urine. **segmental t's,** the tubules of the mesonephros. **seminiferous t's,** the tubules of the testis. **uriniferous t's,** renal tubules; channels for the passage of urine.

tubulorrhexis (tu″bu-lo-rek'sis) rupture of the tubules of the kidney.

tubulus (tu'bu-lus), pl. *tu'buli* [L.] tubule; a minute canal found in various structures or organs of the body.

tuft (tuft) a small clump, cluster or coil, especially a tassel-like cluster of capillaries. **malpighian t.,** renal glomerulus.

tularemia (tu″lah-re'me-ah) a disease of rabbits and other rodents, resembling plague, caused by *Pasteurella tularensis,* and transmissible to man.

tumefacient (tu″mě-fa'shent) producing tumefaction

tumefaction (-fak'shun) a swelling; puffiness.

tumescence (tu-mes'ens) congestion and swelling, especially of sexual organs.

tumor (tu'mor) a swelling or enlargement, especially one due to pathologic overgrowth of tissue. **Abrikossoff's t.,** a granular cell myoblastoma. **t. al'bus,** white swelling. **benign t.,** one not likely to recur after removal. **Brenner t.,** a benign fibroepithelioma of the ovary. **carotid body t.,** a firm, round mass at the bifurcation of the common carotid artery. **compound t.,** a teratoma. **cystic t.,** one containing cavities. **desmoid t.,** a neoplastic proliferation of fibrous tissue, midway between a benign fibroma and a malignant fibrosarcoma. **erectile t.,** one composed of erectile tissue. **Ewing's t.,** a malignant tumor of bone, arising in medullary tissue and more often in cylindrical bones. **false t.,** structural enlargement due to extravasation, exudation, echinococcus or retained sebaceous matter. **fibroid t.,** a fibroma. **fibroplastic t.,** a variety of spindle cell sarcoma. **follicular t.,** a dilated sebaceous follicle. **glomus t.,** glomangioma. **granulosa t., granulosa cell t.,** an ovarian tumor originating in the cells of the membrana granulosa. **heterologous t.,** one made up of tissue differing from that in which it grows. **homologous t.,** one made up of tissue resembling that in which it grows. **hylic t.,** hyloma. **infiltrating t.,** one which extends into surrounding tissue. **Krompecher's t.,** rodent ulcer. **Krukenberg's t.,** fibrosar-

coma of ovary which has undergone myxomatous degeneration. **Leydig cell t.,** a tumor of the Leydig cells of the testis. **malignant t.,** one which is likely to continue growing and eventually to cause death. **mixed t.,** one containing different types of cells derived from the same primary germ layer. **mucous t., muscular t.,** myoma. **organoid t.,** one composed of complex tissues, resembling an organ. **papillary t.,** papilloma. **pearl t.,** cholesteatoma. **phantom t.,** abdominal or other swelling not due to structural change, but, usually, to a neurosis. **sand t.,** psammoma. **sebaceous t.,** tumor of a sebaceous gland. **simple t.,** one containing a single type of cells. **teratogenous t., teratoid t.,** teratoma. **theca cell t.,** a fibroid tumor of the ovary containing yellow areas of fatty material. **true t.,** any tumor produced by proliferation of cells. **turban t's,** pink or maroon, grapelike, pedunculated tumors, occurring usually on the scalp, but sometimes on the trunk and extremities. **Wilms's t.,** embryonal carcinosarcoma of the kidney.

tumoricidal (tu″mor-ĭ-si'dal) destructive to cancer cells.

tumorigenesis (-jen'ĕ-sis) the production of tumors. adj., **tumorigen'ic.**

tumultus (tu-mul'tus) excessive organic action.

Tunga (tun'gah) a genus of fleas native to tropical and subtropical parts of South America. **T. pen'etrans,** the chigoe flea, which attacks man, dogs, pigs and other animals, as well as poultry.

tungsten (tung'sten) chemical element (*see table*), at. no. 74, symbol W.

tunic (tu'nik) a covering or coat. **Bichat's t.,** the intima of blood vessels.

tunica (tu'ni-kah), pl. *tu'nicae* [L.] a covering or coat; used in anatomic nomenclature to designate a membranous covering of an organ or a distinct layer of the wall of a hollow structure, as a blood vessel. **t. adna'ta oc'uli,** portion of conjunctiva in contact with the eyeball. **t. adventi'tia,** tunica extima. **t. albugin'ea,** 1. the sclera. 2. the fibrous coat of the testis or ovary. **t. ex'tima,** the outermost coat of blood vessels. **t. in'tima,** the innermost coat of blood vessels. **t. me'dia,** the middle coat of blood vessels. **t. muco'sa,** the mucous membrane lining of various tubular structures. **t. muscula'ris,** the muscular coat or layer surrounding the tela submucosa. **t. pro'pria,** the proper coat or layer of a part. **t. ruyschia'na,** lamina choriocapillaris. **t. sero'sa,** the membrane lining the external walls of the body cavities. **t. vagina'lis,** a serosa-lined sac immediately adjacent to the testis and epididymis. **t. vasculo'sa,** a vascular coat, or a layer well supplied with blood vessels.

tunicin (tu'nĭ-sin) substance resembling cellulose, from the tissues of certain low forms of animal life.

tunnel (tun'el) a circumscribed opening through a solid body, or a linear enclosed channel beneath a surface. **carpal t.,** the osseofibrous passage for the median nerve and the flexor tendons. **Corti's t.**, canal of Corti. **flexor t.**, carpal tunnel.

turbidimeter (ter″bī-dim′ĕ-ter) an apparatus for measuring turbidity of a solution.

turbidimetry (-dim′ĕ-tre) the measurement of the turbidity of a liquid.

turbidity (ter-bid′ĭ-te) cloudiness.

turbinal (ter′bī-nal) turbinate.

turbinate (ter′bī-nāt) 1. shaped like a top. 2. concha nasalis ossea.

turbinectomy (ter′bī-nek′to-me) excision of a nasal concha (turbinate).

turbinotomy (-not′o-me) incision of a turbinate.

turgescence (ter-jes′ens) distention or swelling of a part.

turgescent (ter-jes′ent) becoming swollen.

turgor (ter′gor) condition of being turgid; normal, or other fulness.

turnsickness (tern′sik-nes) staggers.

turpentine (ter′pen-tīn) concrete oleoresin from *Pinus palustris* and other species of Pinus; local irritant, sometimes used in ointments. **Canada t.**, liquid oleoresin from a fir tree, *Abies balsamea*, of Canada and Maine.

turricephaly (tur″ĭ-sef′ah-le) acrocephaly.

tussis (tus′is) [L.] cough. adj., **tus′sal, tus′sive. t. convulsi′va**, pertussis.

tutamen (tu-ta′men), pl. *tutam′ina* [L.] a protective covering or structure. **tutam′ina cer′ebri**, the hair, scalp, skull and meninges. **tutam′ina oc′uli**, the protecting appendages of the eye, as lids, lashes, etc.

Tween (twēn) trademark for a sorbitan polyoxyalkalene derivative; used as an emulsifier and detergent. **Tween 80**, trademark for polysorbate 80.

twin (twin) one of two offspring produced at one birth. **allantoido-angiopagous t's**, twins united by the umbilical vessels only. **binovular t's**, dizygotic twins. **conjoined t's**, monozygotic twins whose bodies are joined. **dizygotic t's**, twins developed from two separate ova fertilized at the same time. **enzygotic t's**, monozygotic twins. **equal t's**, two fetuses of similar development produced at the same gestation. **fraternal t's**, **heterologous t's**, dizygotic twins. **identical t's, monozygotic t's**, two individuals developed from one fertilized ovum. **omphalo-angiopagous t's**, allantoido-angiopagous twins. **similar t's**, monozygotic twins. **unequal t's**, two products of the same gestation period, one of which is imperfectly developed and shows disorganization that may be mild to severe. **uniovular t's**, monozygotic twins.

twinning (twin′ing) 1. the production of symmetrical structures or parts by division. 2. the simultaneous intrauterine production of two or more embryos.

twitch (twich) a brief, contractile response of a skeletal muscle elicited by a single maximal volley of impulses in the neurons supplying it.

twitching (twich′ing) the occurrence of a single contraction or a series of contractions of a muscle. **Trousseau's t.**, repetitive brief contraction involving muscles of the face.

tychastics (ti-kas′tiks) the study of industrial accidents.

Tylenol (ti′lĕ-nol) trademark for preparations of acetaminophen.

tylion (til′e-on) point on anterior edge of the optic groove in the median line.

tyloma (ti-lo′ma) a callus or callosity.

tylosis (ti-lo′sis) formation of callosities.

tympanectomy (tim″pah-nek′to-me) excision of the tympanic membrane.

tympanic (tim-pan′ik) 1. pertaining to the tympanum. 2. pertaining to or characterized by tympany.

tympanism (tim′pah-nizm) tympanites.

tympanites (tim″pah-ni′tēz) drumlike distention of the abdomen. adj. **tympanit′ic.**

tympanitis (-ni′tis) otitis media.

tympanoacryloplasty (tim″pah-no-ah-kril′o-plas″te) surgical obliteration of the mastoid cavity by instillation of an acrylic compound.

tympanohyal (-hi′al) part of the embryonic hyoid arch becoming fused with the styloid process.

tympanomastoiditis (-mas″toi-di′tis) inflammation of tympanum and mastoid cells.

tympanoplasty (tim′pah-no-plas″te) surgical reconstruction of the tympanic membrane and establishment of ossicular continuity from the tympanic membrane to the oval window.

tympanosclerosis (tim″pah-no-sklĕ-ro′sis) a condition characterized by the presence of masses of hard, dense connective tissue around the auditory ossicles in the tympanic cavity.

tympanotomy (tim″pah-not′o-me) myringotomy.

tympanous (tim′pah-nus) distended with gas.

tympanum (tim′pah-num) the part of the cavity of the middle ear, in the temporal bone, just medial to the tympanic membrane. adj., **tym′panal, tympan′ic.**

tympany (tim′pah-ne) a musical note elicited by percussion, of somewhat higher pitch than resonance. adj., **tympan′ic.**

type (tīp) 1. the general or prevailing character, as of an individual or a particular case of disease. 2. a block bearing a raised letter, or the impression of such a letter registered on a flat surface. **asthenic t.**, a type of physical constitution, with long limbs, small trunk, flat chest and weak muscles. **athletic t.**, a type of physical constitution, with broad shoulders, deep chest, flat abdomen, thick neck and good muscular development. **blood t's**, categories into which blood can be classified on the basis of M–N, P, Rh–Hr, etc., agglutinogens. **pyknic t.**, a type of physical constitution marked by rounded body, large chest, thick shoulders, broad head and short neck. **sympatheticotonic t.**, a type of physical constitution characterized by sympathicotonia. **vagotonic t.**, a physical type characteristic of deficient adrenal activity: there are slow pulse, low blood pressure, localized sweating, high sugar tolerance, and oculocardiac reflex.

typembryo (ti-pem′bre-o) an embryo in that

stage of development at which the characteristics of the type to which it belongs may be seen.

typhl(o)- (tif'lo) word element [Gr.], (1) *cecum;* (2) *blindness.*

typhlectasis (tif-lek'tah-sis) distention of the cecum.

typhlitis (tif-li'tis) inflammation of the cecum.

typhlocolitis (tif''lo-ko-li'tis) colitis in the region of the cecum.

typhlodicliditis (-dik''li-di'tis) inflammation of the ileocecal valve.

typhlohepatitis (-hep''ah-ti'tis) infectious enterohepatitis of turkeys.

typhlolexia (-lek'se-ah) word blindness.

typhlosis (tif-lo'sis) blindness.

typhlotomy (tif-lot'o-me) incision of the cecum.

typhoid (ti'foid) 1. resembling typhus. 2. typhoid fever.

typhoidal (ti-foi'dal) resembling typhoid fever.

typhomania (ti''fo-ma'ne-ah) the delirium accompanying typhus or typhoid fever.

typhopneumonia (-nu-mo'ne-ah) pneumonia with typhoid fever.

typhosepsis (-sep'sis) septic poisoning occurring in typhus.

typhotoxin (-tok'sin) a deadly ptomaine from cultures of typhoid bacillus.

typhus (ti'fus) an acute infectious disease caused by Rickettsia species and characterized by petechial eruption, high temperature and great prostration. adj., **ty'phous. endemic t.,** murine typhus. **epidemic t.,** the classic form, due to *Rickettsia prowazekii* and transmitted from man to man by body lice. **murine t.,** an infectious disease due to *Rickettsia typhi* and transmitted from rat to man by the rat flea and rat louse. **petechial t.,** epidemic typhus. **t. recur'rens,** relapsing fever. **scrub t.,** a self-limited, febrile disease due to *Rickettsia tsutsugamushi* and transmitted by chiggers; characterized by sudden onset of fever with a primary skin lesion and development of rash about the fifth day. **t. sid'erans,** a malignant

and quickly fatal form of typhus. **tropical t.,** scrub typhus.

typing (tip'ing) determination of the type of something. **t. of blood,** determining the character of the blood on the basis of the M–N, P, Rh–Hr, etc., agglutinogens.

tyramine (ti'rah-mēn) a decarboxylation product of tyrosine with a similar but weaker action like that of epinephrine and norepinephrine.

tyrocidin (ti''ro-si'din) a basic cyclic polypeptide present in tyrothricin.

tyrogenous (ti-roj'ĕ-nus) originating in cheese.

tyroid (ti'roid) of cheesy consistency.

tyroma (ti-ro'mah) a caseous mass.

tyromatosis (ti''ro-mah-to'sis) caseous degeneration.

tyrosiluria (-ti''ro-si-lu're-ah) presence in the urine of metabolites of tyrosine.

tyrosine (ti'ro-sēn) a naturally occurring amino acid produced in the body in the metabolism of phenylalanine to melanin, epinephrine and thyroxine.

tyrosinosis (ti''ro-si-no'sis) a condition characterized by a faulty metabolism of tyrosine in which an intermediate product, para-hydroxyphenyl pyruvic acid, appears in the urine and gives it an abnormal reducing power.

tyrosinuria (ti''ro-si-nu're-ah) presence of tyrosine in the urine.

tyrosis (ti-ro'sis) caseous degeneration.

tyrothricin (ti''ro-thri'sin) a substance produced by growth of a soil bacillus, *Bacillus brevis,* consisting principally of gramicidin and tyrocidin; used topically as an antibiotic.

tyrotoxin (-tok'sin) a toxin developed in cheese and milk by action of bacilli.

tyrotoxism (-tok'sizm) poisoning from a toxin present in milk or cheese.

tysonitis (ti''son-i'tis) inflammation of Tyson's glands.

Tyvid (ti'vid) trademark for a preparation of isoniazid.

Tyzine (ti'zēn) trademark for preparations of tetrahydrozoline hydrochloride.

tzetze (set'se) tsetse.

U

U chemical symbol, *uranium.*

U. unit.

uberous (u'ber-us) prolific.

uberty (u'ber-te) fertility.

udder (ud'er) the large mammary gland of various animals, provided with more than one nipple, as in cows.

ulalgia (u-lal'je-ah) pain in the gums.

ulatrophia (u''lah-tro'fe-ah) shrinkage of the gums.

ulcer (ul'ser) a local defect, or excavation of the surface of an organ, produced by sloughing of necrotic inflammatory tissue.

Curling's u., an ulcer of the duodenum seen after severe burns of the body. **Cushing's u.,** peptic ulcer associated with manifest or occult lesions of the central nervous system. **decubitus u.,** a lesion produced by breakdown of tissue due to localized pressure and lack of proper preventive measures in a patient at prolonged bed rest. **dental u.,** a lesion on the oral mucosa due to trauma inflicted by the teeth. **duodenal u.,** one on the mucous membrane of the duodenum. **gastric u.,** one on the inner wall of the stomach. **Hunner's u.,** one involving all layers of the bladder wall, occurring in chronic interstitial cystitis. **indolent u.**, one with indurated, elevated edge and nongranulating base, usually occurring on the leg. **marginal u.**, an ulcer along the site of a gastrojejunostomy. **penetrating u.**, an ulcerative lesion which involves also the wall or substance of an adjacent organ. **peptic u.**, one on the mucous membrane of stomach or duodenum. **phagedenic u.**, a necrotizing lesion in which tissue destruction is prominent. **rodent u.**, carcinomatous or epitheliomatous ulcer. **serpiginous u.**, one healing in one place and spreading in another. **stercoraceous u.**, ulcer of the colon caused by irritation from masses of feces. **trophic u.**, one due to imperfect nutrition of the part. **tropical u.**, 1. a chronic, sloughing ulcer usually on the lower extremities, occurring in tropical regions. 2. cutaneous leishmaniasis. **tuberculous u.**, one due to the tubercle bacillus. **varicose u.**, an ulcer due to varicose veins. **venereal u.**, chancre.

ulcerate (ul′sĕ-rāt) to produce an ulcer.

ulceration (ul″sĕ-ra′shun) formation of an ulcer.

ulcerative (ul′ser-ah-tiv) characterized by ulcer formation.

ulcerogangrenous (ul″ser-o-gang′grē-nus) characterized by both ulceration and gangrene.

ulcerogenic (-jen′ik) causing ulceration; leading to the production of ulcers.

ulcerous (ul′ser-us) of the nature of an ulcer.

ulcus (ul′kus), pl. *ul′cera* [L.] ulcer. **u. cancro′sum**, rodent ulcer. **u. hypostat′icum**, an ulcer due to hypostatic congestion. **u. mol′le cu′tis**, chancroid. **u. ser′pens**, serpiginous ulcer. **u. ventric′uli**, ulceration of the stomach. **u. vul′vae acu′tum**, a rapidly growing nonvenereal ulcer of the vulva.

ulectomy (u-lek′to-me) excision of scar tissue.

ulemorrhagia (u″lem-o-ra′je-ah) bleeding from the gums.

ulerythema (u″ler-i-the′mah) an erythematous disease with formation of cicatrices. **u. ophryog′enes**, keratosis pilaris affecting follicles of eyebrow hairs.

uletic (u-let′ik) pertaining to the gums.

uliginous (u-lij′i-nus) muddy or slimy.

ulitis (u-li′tis) inflammation of the gums.

ulna (ul′nah), pl. *ul′nae* [L.] one of the two bones between the elbow and the wrist. adj., **ul′nar.**

ulnad (ul′nad) toward the ulna.

ulnaris (ul-na′ris) [L.] ulnar.

ulnocarpal (ul″no-kar′pal) pertaining to ulna and carpus.

ulnoradial (-ra′de-al) pertaining to ulna and radius.

ulocace (u-lok′ah-se) ulceration of the gums.

ulocarcinoma (u″lo-kar″si-no′mah) carcinoma of the gums.

uloglossitis (-glos-si′tis) inflammation of gums and tongue.

uloid (u′loid) resembling a scar, but not due to any lesion of the skin.

uloncus (u-long′kus) swelling of the gums.

ulorrhagia (u″lo-ra′je-ah) free hemorrhage from the gums.

ulorrhea (-re′ah) bleeding from the gums.

ulosis (u-lo′sis) cicatrization. adj., **ulot′ic.**

ulotomy (u-lot′o-me) 1. incision of scar tissue. 2. incision of the gums.

ulotrichous (u-lot′ri-kus) having woolly hair.

Ultandren (ul-tan′dren) trademark for a preparation of fluoxymesterone.

ultimum (ul′ti-mum) [L.] ultimate.

ultra- (ul′trah) word element [L.], *beyond; excess.*

ultrabrachycephalic (ul″trah-brak″e-sē-fal′ik) having a cephalic index of more than 90.

ultracentrifugation (-sen-trif″u-ga′shun) subjection of material to centrifugal force 200,000 to 400,000 times the force of gravity.

ultrafiltration (-fil-tra′shun) filtration through a filter capable of removing very minute (ultramicroscopic) particles.

ultraligation (-li-ga′shun) ligation of a vessel beyond the point of origin of a branch.

ultramicropipet (-mi″kro-pi-pet′) a pipet designed to handle extremely small quantities of liquid (0.002–0.005 ml.).

ultramicroscope (-mi″kro-skōp) a special darkfield microscope for examination of particles of colloidal size.

ultramicroscopic (-mi″kro-skop′ik) 1. pertaining to the ultramicroscope. 2. too small to be seen with the ordinary light microscope.

ultramicroscopy (-mi-kros′ko-pe) use of an ultramicroscope.

Ultran (ul′tran) trademark for preparations of phenaglycodol.

ultrasonic (-son′ik) beyond the audible range; relating to sound waves having a frequency of more than 20,000 cycles per second.

ultrasonics (-son′iks) the science dealing with mechanical radiant energy of a frequency greater than 20,000 cycles per second.

ultrasonometry (-so-nom′ē-tre) measurement of certain physical properties of biologic fluids by means of ultrasound.

ultrasound (ul′trah-sownd) mechanical radiant energy of a frequency greater than 20,000 cycles per second.

ultrastructure (ul′trah-struk″chūr) the structural arrangement of the smallest particles composing a substance.

ultraviolet (ul″trah-vi′o-let) beyond the violet portion of the visible spectrum.

ultravirus (-vi′rus) an extremely small pathogenic agent.

umb. umbilicus.

umbilectomy (um″bi-lek′to-me) omphalectomy.

umbilical (um-bil′i-kal) pertaining to the umbilicus.

umbilicated (um-bil′i-kāt″ed) marked by depressed spots resembling the umbilicus.

umbilication (um-bil″i-ka′shun) a depression resembling the umbilicus.

umbilicus (um-bil′i-kus, um″bi-li′kus) the (usually) depressed scar marking the site of entry of the umbilical cord in the fetus.

umbo (um′bo), pl. *umbo′nes* [L.] a small protuberance at the center of a rounded surface.

unciform (un'sĭ-form) hooked or shaped like a hook.

Uncinaria (un"sĭ-na're-ah) a name formerly given a genus of hookworms.

uncinariasis (un"sĭ-nah-ri'ah-sis) ancylostomiasis.

uncinate (un'sĭ-nāt) unciform.

uncipressure (un'sĭ-presh"ur) pressure with a hook to stop hemorrhage.

unconscious (un-kon'shus) 1. not aware of surrounding environment; not responding to sensory stimulation. 2. the area or activity of the mind in which primitive or unacceptable ideas and impulses are concealed from awareness by the psychic censor. **collective u.**, the portion of the unconscious which is theoretically common to mankind.

unco-ossified (un"ko-os'ĭ-fĭd) not united into one bone.

unction (ungk'shun) 1. an ointment. 2. application of an ointment.

unctuous (ungk'chu-us) greasy or oily.

uncus (ung'kus) the medial protrusion of the anterior part of the para-hippocampal gyrus.

undifferentiation (un"dif-er-en"she-a'shun) lack of normal differentiation.

undine (un'dēn) a small glass flask for irrigating the eye.

undulation (un"du-la'shun) a wavelike motion in any medium.

ung. [L.] *unguen'tum* (ointment).

ungual (ung'gwal) pertaining to the nails.

unguent (ung'gwent) an ointment.

unguentum (ung-gwen'tum), pl. *unguen'ta* [L.] ointment.

unguiculate (ung-gwik'u-lāt) having claws; clawlike.

unguinal (ung'gwĭ-nal) pertaining to a nail.

unguis (ung'gwis), pl. *un'gues* [L.] the horny cutaneous plate on the dorsal surface of the distal end of finger or toe; a fingernail or toenail.

ungula (ung'gu-lah) an instrument for extracting a dead fetus.

ungulate (ung'gu-lāt) an animal with a horny covering on the distal end of certain digits (hoof), adapting it for unguligrade locomotion.

unguligrade (ung'gu-lĭ-grād") walking or running on the tips of one or two digits of each limb; characteristic of certain quadrupeds known as ungulates.

uni- word element [L.], *one.*

uniaxial (u"ne-ak'se-al) having only one axis.

unicellular (-sel'u-lar) made up of a single cell.

uniceptor (u'ni-sep"tor) a ceptor with a single combining group.

unicornous (u"nĭ-kor'nus) having only one cornu.

unidirectional (-di-rek'shun-al) flowing in only one direction.

uniglandular (-glan'du-lar) affecting only one gland.

unigravida (-grav'ĭ-dah) a woman pregnant for the first time; gravida I.

unilateral (-lat'er-al) affecting only one side.

unilocular (-lok'u-lar) having only one loculus or compartment.

uninucleated (u"nĭ-nu'kle-āt"ed) having a single nucleus.

uniocular (-ok'u-lar) pertaining to only one eye.

union (ūn'yun) the growing together of tissues separated by injury, as of the ends of a fractured bone, or of the edges of an incision. **immediate u.**, healing by first intention.

uniovular (u"ne-ov'u-lar) arising from one ovum.

unipara (u-nip'ah-rah) a woman who has had one pregnancy which resulted in a viable infant; para I.

uniparous (u-nip'ah-rus) having had only one pregnancy which resulted in a viable infant.

unipolar (u"nĭ-po'lar) having a single pole.

unipotent (u-nip'o-tent) unipotential.

unipotential (u"nĭ-po-ten'shal) having only one power, as giving rise to cells of one order only.

unit (u'nit) 1. a single thing; one segment of a whole that is made up of identical or similar segments. 2. a specifically defined amount of anything subject to measurement, as of activity, dimension, velocity, volume, or the like. **Allen-Doisy u.**, rat unit. **Ångström u.**, the unit of wavelength, being one ten-thousandth of a micron. **British thermal u.**, a unit of heat, being the amount necessary to raise the temperature of one pound of water from 39 to 40°F., generally considered the equivalent of 252 calories; abbreviated B.T.U. **u. of capacity**, farad. **cat u.**, that amount of a drug per kilogram of cat which is just sufficient to kill when slowly and continuously injected into the vein. **C.G.S. u.**, any unit in the centimeter-gram-second system. **Clauberg u.**, a unit of measurement of progestin activity. **Collip u.**, a unit of dosage of parathyroid extract. **coronary care u.**, a specially designed and equipped hospital area containing a small number of private rooms, with all facilities necessary for constant observation and possible emergency treatment of patients who have had myocardial infarction. **craw u.**, the amount of *Veratrum viride* that will cause cardiac arrest in the test animal, *Daphnia magna*, a fresh-water crustacean. **u. of current**, ampere. **u. of electricity**, ampere, coulomb, farad, ohm, volt, watt. **u. of electromotive force**, volt. **electrostatic u's**, that system of unit which is based on the fundamental definition of a unit charge as one which will repel a similar charge with a force of one dyne when the two charges are 1 cm. apart. **enzyme u.**, that amount of an enzyme that will, under defined conditions, transform 1 micromole of substrate per minute, or 1 microequivalent of a substrate in which more than one bond is attached. **u. of force**, dyne. **Hanson u.**, a unit of measurement of parathyroid activity. **u. of heat**, calorie, therm. **intensive care u.**, an area of a hospital provided with unusual equipment and facilities for observation and treatment of a small number of patients requiring special and possibly emergency attention, as after surgery. **International u.**, a unit established by the International Conference for the Unification of Formulas. **Lf u.**, the amount of diphtheria toxin or toxoid that gives the most rapid flocculation with one standard unit of antitoxin when mixed and incubated in vitro. **light u.**, foot candle. **motor u.**, the unit of motor activity formed by a motor nerve cell and its many innervated muscle fibers. **mouse u.**, the least amount of estrus-producing hormone which will cause a characteristic degeneration of the vaginal epithelium in a spayed mouse. **Oxford u.**, a unit of penicillin dosage, being that amount which, dissolved in 50 cc. of meat extract broth, just inhibits completely a test strain of *Staphylococcus aureus.* **u. of quantity,** coulomb. **rat u.**, the highest dilution of an estrus-producing hormone which, in three injections at four-hour intervals during the first day, will produce cornification and desquamation of the vaginal epithelium in a mature spayed rat. **u. of resistance,** ohm. **Somogyi u.**, that amount of amylase which will destroy 1.5 mg. of starch in 8 minutes at 37°C. **Svedberg u.**, a unit expressing the velocity of movement of a sedimenting molecule per unit of gravitational field, being 1×10^{-13} cm. per second per dyne per gram. **Thayer-Doisy u.**, a unit of vitamin K activity, equivalent to that of 1 microgram of pure vitamin K_1. **toxic u., toxin u.**, the smallest dose of a toxin which will kill a guinea pig weighing about 250 gm. in three to four days. **tuberculin u.**, 0.00002 mg. of purified protein derivative in 0.1 ml. of tuberculin solution, corresponding in potency to a 1:10,000 solution of old tuberculin. **U.S.P. u.**, one used in the United States Pharmacopeia in expressing potency of drugs and other preparations.

unitary (u″nĭ-ter″e) pertaining to a single object or individual.

Unitensen (u″nĭ-ten′sen) trademark for preparations of cryptenamine.

uniterminal (-ter″mi-nal) monoterminal.

univalent (-va′lent) having a valence of one

unof. unofficial.

unofficial (un″ŏ-fish′al) not authorized by an established dispensatory or formulary.

unphysiologic (un″fiz-e-o-loj′ik) not in harmony with the laws of physiology.

unsaturated (un-sat′u-rāt″ed) 1. not having all affinities of its elements satisfied. 2. not holding all of a solute which can be held in solution by the solvent.

unsex (un-seks′) to deprive of the gonads, making reproduction impossible.

urachus (u′rah-kus) a canal in the fetus extending from the bladder to the umbilicus, the lumen usually being obliterated after birth. adj., **u′rachal.**

uracil (u′rah-sil) a ureide dihydroxypyrimidin obtained from nucleinic acid.

uracrasia (u″rah-kra′ze-ah) disordered state of urine.

uracratia (-kra′she-ah) inability to retain urine.

uragogue (u′rah-gog) an agent which increases urinary secretion.

uraniscolalia (u″rah-nis″ko-la′le-ah) speech defect characteristic of cleft palate.

uranisconitis (u″rah-nis″ko-ni′tis) inflammation of the palate.

uraniscus (u″rah-nis′kus) the palate.

uranium (u-ra′ne-um) chemical element *(see table),* at. no. 92, symbol U.

uranophobia (u″rah-no-fo′be-ah) morbid fear of heaven.

uranoplasty (u-ran′o-plas″te) plastic repair of the palate.

uranorrhaphy (u″rah-nor′ah-fe) suture of the palate.

uranoschisis (-nos′kĭ-sis) cleft palate.

uranostaphyloschisis (u″rah-no-staf″ĭ-los′kĭ-sis) fissure of the soft and hard palates.

urarthritis (u″rar-thri′tis) gouty arthritis.

urate (u′rāt) a salt of uric acid.

uratemia (u″rah-te′me-ah) urates in the blood.

uratic (u-rat′ik) pertaining to urates or to gout.

uratolysis (u″rah-tol′ĭ-sis) the splitting up of urates. adj., **uratolyt′ic.**

uratoma (-to′mah) a concretion made up of urates; tophus.

uratosis (-to′sis) the deposit of urates in the tissues.

uraturia (-tu′re-ah) urates in the urine.

urceiform (er-se′ĭ-form) pitcher-shaped.

ur-defense (er″de-fens′) a belief essential to the psychological integrity of the individual.

urea (u-re′ah) a crystallizable compound, the chief end-product of amino acid metabolism in the body, a pharmaceutical preparation of which is sometimes used to promote diuresis. adj., **ure′al.**

ureagenetic (u-re″ah-jĕ-net′ik) forming urea.

ureameter (u″re-am′ĕ-ter) an apparatus for measuring urea in urine.

ureametry (-am′ĕ-tre) measurement of urea in urine.

ureapoiesis (u-re″ah-poi-e′sis) formation of urea. adj., **ureapoiet′ic.**

urease (u-re-ās) an enzyme which catalyzes the decomposition of urea to ammonia and carbon dioxide.

ureochysis (u-rek′ĭ-sis) an effusion of urine into cellular tissue.

Urecholine (u″re-ko′lin) trademark for preparations of bethanechol.

uredema (u″rĕ-de′mah) swelling from extravasated urine.

uredo (u-re′do) urticaria.

ureide (u′re-id) a compound of urea and an acid or aldehyde formed by the elimination of water.

urelcosis (u″rel-ko′sis) ulceration in the urinary tract.

uremia (u-re′me-ah) accumulation in the blood of substances ordinarily eliminated in the urine; specifically a toxic condition seen in nephritis and urinary suppression, marked by nausea, vomiting, vertigo, convulsions and coma. adj., **ure′mic.**

uremigenic (u-re″mĭ-jen′ik) caused by uremia.

ureolysis (u″re-ol′ĭ-sis) the disintegration or decomposition of urea into carbon dioxide and ammonia. adj., **ureolyt′ic.**

ureometer (-om′ĕ-ter) ureameter.

ureometry (-om′ĕ-tre) ureametry.

ureopoiesis (u-re″o-poi-e′sis) ureapoiesis.

ureosecretory (-se-kre′tor-e) pertaining to secretion of urea.

ureotelic (-tel′ik) having urea as the chief excretory product of nitrogen metabolism.

uresis (u-re′sis) secretion and excretion of urine.

-uresis (u-re′sis) word element [Gr.], *urinary excretion of.* adj., **-uret′ic.**

ureter (u-re′ter) the tubular organ through which urine passes from kidney to bladder. **ectopic u.,** a ureter which opens elsewhere than in the bladder wall.

ureter(o)- (u-re′ter-o) word element [Gr.], *ureter.*

ureteralgia (u-re″ter-al′je-ah) pain in the ureter.

ureterectasis (-ek′tah-sis) distention of the ureter.

ureterectomy (-ek′to-me) excision of a ureter.

ureteritis (-i′tis) inflammation of a ureter.

ureterocele (u-re′ter-o-sēl″) intravesical ballooning of the lower end of the ureter.

ureterocelectomy (u-re″ter-o-se-lek′to-me) excision of a ureterocele.

ureterocolostomy (-ko-los′to-me) anastomosis of a ureter to the colon.

ureterocutaneostomy (-ku-ta″ne-os′to-me) surgical creation of an opening of the ureter on the body surface (skin).

ureterocystoneostomy (-sis″to-ne-os′to-me) implantation of a ureter at a different site on the bladder wall.

ureterocystoscope (-sis′to-skōp) a cystoscope with a catheter for insertion into the ureter.

ureterocystostomy (-sis-tos′to-me) ureterocystoneostomy.

ureterodialysis (-di-al′ĭ-sis) rupture of a ureter.

ureteroduodenal (-du″o-de′nal) pertaining to or communicating with a ureter and the duodenum.

ureteroenterostomy (-en″ter-os′to-me) anastomosis of one or both ureters to the wall of the intestine.

ureterography (u-re″ter-og′rah-fe) roentgenography of the ureter, after injection of a contrast medium.

ureteroheminephrectomy (u-re″ter-o-hem″ĭ-nĕ-frek′to-me) excision of the diseased portion of a reduplicated kidney and its ureter.

ureteroileostomy (-il″e-os′to-me) anastomosis of the ureters to an isolated loop of the ileum, drained through a stoma on the abdominal wall.

ureterolith (u-re′ter-o-lith″) a calculus in the ureter.

ureterolithiasis (u-re″ter-o-lĭ-thi′ah-sis) formation of calculus in the ureter.

ureterolithotomy (-lĭ-thot′o-me) incision of ureter for removal of calculus; excision of a ureteral calculus.

ureterolysis (u-re″ter-ol′ĭ-sis) 1. rupture of the ureter. 2. paralysis of the ureter. 3. the operation of freeing the ureter from adhesions.

ureteromeatotomy (u-re″ter-o-me″ah-tot′o-me) incision of the opening of the ureter in the bladder wall.

ureteroneocystostomy (u-re″ter-o-ne″o-sis-tos′to-me) ureterocystoneostomy.

ureteroneopyelostomy (-pi″ē-los′to-me) ureteropyeloneostomy.

ureteronephrectomy (u-re″ter-o-nĕ-frek′to-me) excision of a kidney and ureter.

ureteropathy (u-re″ter-op′ah-the) any disease of the ureter.

ureteropelvioplasty (u-re″ter-o-pel′ve-o-plas″-te) ureteropyeloplasty.

ureteroplasty (u-re′ter-o-plas″te) plastic repair of a ureter.

ureteropyelitis (u-re″ter-o-pi″ē-li′tis) inflammation of ureter and kidney pelvis.

ureteropyelography (-pi-ē-log′rah-fe) roentgenography of the ureter and pelvis of the kidney.

ureteropyeloneostomy (-pi″ē-lo-ne-os′to-me) surgical creation of a new communication between a ureter and the kidney pelvis.

ureteropyelonephritis (-pi″ē-lo-nĕ-fri′tis) inflammation of ureter, renal pelvis and kidney.

ureteropyeloplasty (-pi″ē-lo-plas″te) plastic repair of ureter and renal pelvis.

ureteropyelostomy (-pi″ē-los′to-me) ureteropyeloneostomy.

ureteropyosis (-pi-o′sis) suppurative inflammation of ureter.

ureterorectal (-rek′tal) pertaining to or communicating with a ureter and the rectum.

ureterorrhagia (-ra′je-ah) discharge of blood from ureter.

ureterorrhaphy (u-re″ter-or′ah-fe) suture of the ureter.

ureterosigmoidostomy (u-re″ter-o-sig″moid-os′to-me) anastomosis of a ureter to the sigmoid colon.

ureterostomy (u-re″ter-os′to-me) creation of a new outlet for a ureter. **cutaneous u.,** implantation of a ureter to the body surface.

ureterotomy (-ot′o-me) incision of a ureter.

ureteroureterostomy (u-re″ter-o-u-re″ter-os′to-me) surgical anastomosis of two previously remote portions of a ureter, or of one ureter and the other.

ureterovaginal (-vaj′ĭ-nal) pertaining to ureter and vagina.

ureterovesical (-ves′ĭ-kal) pertaining to ureter and bladder.

urethan (u′rĕ-than) a compound formed by esterification of carbamic acid; a colorless crystalline or granular compound used as an antineoplastic agent.

urethane (u′rĕ-thān) urethan.

urethr(o)- (u-re′thro) word element [Gr.] *urethra.*

urethra (u-re′thrah) the passage through which urine is discharged from the bladder. adj., **ure′thral.**

urethralgia (u″re-thral′je-ah) pain in a urethra.

urethratresia (u-re″thrah-tre′ze-ah) imperforation of the urethra.

urethrectomy (u″re-threk′to-me) excision of the urethra.

urethremphraxis (-threm-frak′sis) obstruction of urethra.

645   urinophilous

urethrism (u-re'thrizm) chronic spasm of the urethra.

urethritis (u″re-thri'tis) inflammation of the urethra. **u. cys'tica,** inflammation of the urethra with formation of multiple submucosal cysts. **gonorrheal u.,** gonorrheal infection of the urethra. **gouty u.,** urethritis due to gout. **nonspecific u.,** simple urethritis. **u. petrif'icans,** urethritis with formation of calcareous matter in the urethral wall. **simple u.,** inflammation not due to a specific infection. **specific u.,** inflammation due to infection with *Neisseria gonorrhoeae.* **u. vene'rea,** gonorrhea.

urethrocele (u-re'thro-sēl) prolapse of female urethra through meatus urinarius.

urethrocystitis (u-re″thro-sis-ti'tis) inflammation of urethra and bladder.

urethrocystogram (-sis'to-gram) a radiogram of urethra and bladder.

urethrocystography (-sis-tog'rah-fe) radiography of urethra and bladder.

urethrodynia (-din'e-ah) urethralgia.

urethrography (u″re-throg'rah-fe) radiography of the urethra.

urethrometry (-throm'ĕ-tre) 1. determination of the resistance of various segments of the urethra to retrograde flow of fluid. 2. measurement of the urethra.

urethropenile (u-re″thro-pe'nīl) pertaining to urethra and penis.

urethroperineal (-per″ĭ-ne'al) pertaining to urethra and perineum.

urethroperineoscrotal (-per″ĭ-ne″o-skro'tal) pertaining to urethra, perineum and scrotum.

urethropexy (u-re'thro-pek″se) surgical correction of stress incontinence in the female by fixation of the urethra to the symphysis pubis and fascia of the rectus abdominis muscle.

urethrophraxis (u-re″thro-frak'sis) obstruction of the urethra.

urethrophyma (-fi'mah) a tumor in the urethra.

urethroplasty (u-re'thro-plas″te) plastic repair of the urethra.

urethrorectal (u-re″thro-rek'tal) pertaining to urethra and rectum.

urethrorrhagia (-ra'je-ah) flow of blood from the urethra.

urethrorrhaphy (u″re-thror'ah-fe) suture of a urethral fistula.

urethrorrhea (u-re″thro-re'ah) abnormal discharge from the urethra.

urethroscope (u-re'thro-skōp) instrument for viewing interior of the urethra.

urethroscopy (u″re-thros'ko-pe) visual inspection of the urethra.

urethroscrotal (u-re″thro-skro'tal) pertaining to or communicating with the urethra and scrotum.

urethrospasm (u-re'thro-spazm) spasm of the urethral muscular tissue.

urethrostaxis (u-re″thro-stak'sis) oozing of blood from the urethra.

urethrostenosis (-stĕ-no'sis) constriction of the urethra.

urethrostomy (u″re-thros'to-me) creation of a new opening in the urethra of the male to facilitate catheter drainage of the bladder.

urethrotome (u-re'thro-tōm) instrument for cutting a urethral stricture.

urethrotomy (u″re-throt'o-me) incision of the urethra.

urethrotrigonitis (u-re″thro-tri″go-ni'tis) inflammation of the urethra and trigone of the bladder.

urethrovaginal (-vaj'ĭ-nal) pertaining to urethra and vagina.

uretic (u ret'ik) promoting the secretion of urine.

urhidrosis (ur″hĭ-dro'sis) secretion of sweat containing increased amounts of urea and other nitrogenous waste products.

-uria (u're-ah) word element [Gr.], *condition of the urine.* adj., **-u'ric.**

uricacidemia (u″rik-as″ĭ-de'me-ah) uric acid in the blood.

uricaciduria (-as″ĭ-du're-ah) excess of uric acid in the urine.

uricase (u'rĭ-kās) an enzyme which catalyzes the first step in the decomposition of uric acid.

uricemia (u″rĭ-se'me-ah) uricacidemia.

uricocholia (-ko-ko'le-ah) uric acid in the bile.

uricolysis (u″rĭ-kol'ĭ-sis) the splitting up of uric acid. adj., **uricolyt'ic.**

uricometer (-kom'ĕ-ter) instrument for measuring uric acid in urine.

uricopoiesis (u″rĭ-ko-poi-e'sis) the formation of uric acid. adj., **uricopoiet'ic.**

uricosuria (u″rĭ-ko-su're-ah) excretion of uric acid in the urine. adj., **uricosu'ric.**

uricotelic (-tel'ik) having uric acid as the chief excretory product of nitrogen metabolism.

uricoxidase (u″rĭ-kok'sĭ-dās) an enzyme which oxidizes uric acid.

uriesthesis (u″re-es-the'sis) normal impulse to pass the urine.

urin(o)- (u'rĭ-no) word element [Gr., L.], *urine.*

urina (u-ri'nah) [L.] urine.

urinal (u'rĭ-nal) a receptacle for urine.

urinalysis (u″rĭ-nal'ĭ-sis) analysis of the urine.

urinate (u'rĭ-nāt) to void urine.

urination (u″rĭ-na'shun) the discharge of urine from the bladder.

urine (u'rin) the fluid secreted by the kidneys, stored in the bladder, and discharged through the urethra. adj., **u'rinary. residual u.,** urine remaining in the bladder after urination.

urinemia (u″rĭ-ne'me-ah) uremia.

uriniferous (-nif'er-us) transporting or conveying urine.

uriniparous (-nip'ah-rus) secreting urine.

urinogenital (-no-jen'ĭ-tal) urogenital.

urinogenous (u″rĭ-noj'ĕ-nus) of urinary origin.

urinology (-nol'o-je) urology.

urinoma (u″rĭ-no'mah) a cyst containing urine.

urinometer (u″rĭ-nom'ĕ-ter) instrument for determining specific gravity of urine.

urinometry (-nom'ĕ-tre) determination of specific gravity of urine.

urinophilous (-nof'ĭ-lus) having an affinity for urine, as microorganisms which grow best in urine or invade the urinary meatus of bathers in infested waters.

urinoscopy (u″rĭ-nos′ko-pe) uroscopy.

urinous (u′rĭ-nus) containing or resembling urine.

uriposia (u″rĭ-po′ze-ah) the drinking of urine.

urisolvent (-sol′vent) dissolving uric acid.

Uritone (u′rĭ-tōn) trademark for preparations of methenamine.

uro- (u′ro) word element [Gr.], *urine* (urinary tract, urination).

uroanthelone (u″ro-an′the-lōn) urogastrone.

urobilin (-bi′lin) a brownish pigment formed by oxidation of urobilinogen.

urobilinicterus (-bi″lin-ik′ter-us) brownish coloration of the skin from deposit of urobilin.

urobilinogen (-bi-lin′o-jen) a colorless compound formed in the intestines by reduction of bilirubin.

urocele (u′ro-sēl) distention of scrotum with extravasated urine.

urochesia (u″ro-ke′ze-ah) discharge of urine through the rectum.

urochrome (u′ro-krōm) a breakdown product of hemoglobin related to the bile pigments, found in the urine and responsible for its yellow color.

uroclepsia (u″ro-klep′se-ah) the involuntary escape of urine.

urocrisia (-kriz′e-ah) diagnosis by examining the urine.

urocrisis (-kri′sis) a crisis marked by copious discharge of urine.

urocriterion (-kri-te′re-on) an indication of disease observed in examination of urine.

urocyanogen (-si-an′o-jen) a blue pigment of urine, especially of cholera patients.

urocyanosis (-si″ah-no′sis) blueness of the urine.

urocyst (u′ro-sist) the urinary bladder.

urocystitis (u″ro-sis-ti′tis) inflammation of the urinary bladder.

urodialysis (-di-al′ĭ-sis) partial suppression of the urine.

urodynia (-din′e-ah) pain accompanying urination.

uro-edema (-ē-de′mah) edema from infiltration of urine.

uroenterone (-en′ter-ōn) urogastrone.

uroerythrin (-er′ĭ-thrin) a reddish pigment of urine.

urofuscohematin (-fus″ko-hem′ah-tin) a red-brown pigment of urine in certain diseases.

urogastrone (-gas′trōn) a principle derived from urine of man and other mammals which inhibits gastric secretion.

urogenital (-jen′ĭ-tal) pertaining to urinary apparatus and genitalia.

urogenous (u-roj′ĕ-nus) producing urine.

uroglaucin (u″ro-glaw′sin) a blue pigment from urine.

urogram (u′ro-gram) a film obtained by urography.

urography (u-rog′rah-fe) radiography of any part of the urinary tract. **ascending u.**, **cystoscopic u.**, retrograde urography. **descending u.**, **excretion u.**, **excretory u.**, **intravenous u.**, urography after intravenous injection of an opaque medium which is rapidly excreted in the urine. **retrograde u.**, urography after injection of contrast medium into the bladder through the urethra.

urogravimeter (u″ro-grah-vim′ē-ter) urinometer.

urohematin (-hem′ah-tin) the pigmentary substance of the urine.

urohematoporphyrin (-hem″ah-to-por′fĭ-rin) hematoporphyrin found in the urine.

urokinase (-ki′nās) a principle derived from urine of man and other mammals which acts enzymatically to split plasminogen and activates the fibrinolytic system.

urolith (u′ro-lith) a calculus in the urine or the urinary tract.

urolithiasis (u″ro-lĭ-thi′ah-sis) formation of urinary calculi.

urolithology (-lĭ-thol′o-je) sum of knowledge about urinary calculi.

urologist (u-rol′o-jist) a specialist in urology.

urology (u-rol′o-je) the branch of medicine dealing with the urinary system in the female and genitourinary tract in the male. adj., **urolog′ic.**

urolutein (u″ro-lu′te-in) a yellow pigment of the urine.

uromancy (u′ro-man″se) uroscopy.

uromelanin (u″ro-mel′ah-nin) a black pigment from urine.

uromelus (u-rom′ĕ-lus) a fetal monster with fused limbs.

urometer (u-rom′ĕ-ter) urinometer.

uroncus (u-rong′kus) a swelling caused by retention or extravasation of urine.

uronephrosis (u″ro-nĕ-fro′sis) distention of renal pelvis and tubules with urine.

uropathogen (-path′o-jen) an agent that causes disease of the urinary tract.

uropathy (u-rop′ah-the) any disease in the urinary tract. **obstructive u.**, any disease of the urinary tract caused by obstruction.

uropenia (u″ro-pe′ne-ah) deficiency of urinary secretion.

uropepsin (-pep′sin) a pepsin-like enzyme occurring in urine.

urophanic (-fan′ik) appearing in the urine.

uroplania (-pla′ne-ah) the secretion of urine from abnormal sites.

uropoiesis (-poi-e′sis) the formation of urine. adj., **uropoiet′ic.**

uroporphyrin (-por′fĭ-rin) a porphyrin occurring in urine.

uroporphyrinogen (-por″fĭ-rin′o-jen) a reduced, colorless compound readily giving rise to uroporphyrin by oxidation.

uropsammus (-sam′us) urinary gravel.

uropyonephrosis (-pi″o-nĕ-fro′sis) distention of renal pelvis and tubules with urine and pus.

uropyoureter (-u-re′ter) collection of urine and pus in the ureter.

urorrhagia (u″ro-ra′je-ah) excessive secretion of urine.

urorrhea (-re′ah) involuntary flow of urine.

urorrhodin (-ro′din) a rosy pigment from urine.

urorrhodinogen (-ro-din′o-jen) a chromogen

of the urine which is decomposed into uror-rhodin.

urorubin (u″ro-roo′bin) a red pigment from urine.

urorubrohematin (-roo″bro-hem′ah-tin) a red pigment occasionally found in urine.

urosaccharometry (-sak″ah-rom′ĕ-tre) estimation of sugar in the urine.

urosacin (-sa′sin) urorrhodin.

uroscheocele (u-ros′ke-o-sēl″) urocele.

uroschesis (u-ros′kĕ-sis) retention or suppression of the urine.

urosemiology (u″ro-se″me-ol′o-je) diagnostic study of the urine.

urosepsin (-sep′sin) a septic poison from urine in the tissues.

urosepsis (-sep′sis) septic poisoning from retained and absorbed urinary substances.

urosis (u-ro′sis) any disease of the urinary organs.

urotoxia (u″ro-tok′se-ah) 1. urosepsis. 2. a poisonous state of the urine. adj., **urotox′ic.**

Urotropin (u-rot′ro-pin) trademark for a preparation of methenamine.

uroureter (u″ro-u-re′ter) distention of the ureter with urine.

uroxanthin (-zan′thin) a yellow pigment of the urine.

Urtica (er-ti′kah) genus of plants; the true nettles.

urticaria (er″tĭ-ka′re-ah) a vascular reaction of the skin marked by transient appearance of slightly elevated patches which are redder or paler than the surrounding skin and often attended by severe itching; it may result from various causes (e.g. allergens, exercise, excitement). adj., **urtica′rial. u. bullo′sa, bullous u.,** a variety occurring mostly in children, with sudden outbreak of vesicles or bullae. **u. facti′tia, factitious u.,** a condition in which the lesions are produced by rubbing, pinching or scratching, instead of appearing spontaneously. **giant u., u. gigan′tea,** angioneurotic edema. **u. hemorrhag′ica,** purpura urticans. **u. medicamento′sa,** that due to use of a drug. **papular u., u. papulo′sa,** an allergic reaction to the bite of various insects, with appearance of lesions that evolve into inflammatory, increasingly hard, red or brownish, persistent papules. **u. photogen′ica,** that resulting from exposure to electromagnetic radiation of the range of visible light. **u. pigmento′sa,** a highly distinctive dermatosis developing usually in the first year of life, with only one or two or widespread yellowish to reddish-brown macules of varying shape, the lesions usually undergoing spontaneous involution. **solar u.,** that resulting from exposure to certain bands of the solar spectrum of electromagnetic radiation.

urtication (-ka′shun) 1. flogging of a part with nettles. 2. burning sensation, as of the sting of nettles.

USAEC United States Atomic Energy Commission.

USAN United States Adopted Name, a nonproprietary designation for any compound used as a drug, established by negotiation between its manufacturer and a council sponsored jointly by the American Medical Association, American Pharmaceutical Association and United States Pharmacopeial Convention, Inc.

U.S.M.H. United States Marine Hospital.

U.S.P. United States Pharmacopeia, a publication of the United States Pharmacopoeial Convention, first assembled in 1820, revised at regular intervals, to provide authoritative standards for substances and their preparations which are used in the science of medicine.

U.S.P.H.S. United States Public Health Service.

ustulation (us″tu-la′shun) the drying of a substance by heat.

ustus (us′tus) [L.] burnt.

U.S.V.B. United States Veterans Bureau.

uter(o)- word element [L.], *uterus.*

uteralgia (u″ter-al′je-ah) pain in the uterus.

uterectomy (-ek′to-me) hysterectomy.

uterine (u′ter-in, u′ter-īn) pertaining to the uterus.

uteritis (u″ter-i′tis) inflammation of the uterus.

uteroabdominal (u″ter-o-ab-dom′ĭ-nal) pertaining to uterus and abdomen.

uterocervical (-ser′vĭ-kal) pertaining to uterus and cervix uteri.

uterofixation (-fik-sa′shun) hysteropexy.

uterogenic (-jen′ik) formed in the uterus.

uterogestation (-jes-ta′shun) uterine gestation.

uterography (u″ter-og′rah-fe) x-ray examination of the uterus.

uterolith (u′ter-o-lith″) a uterine calculus.

uteromania (u″ter-o-ma′ne-ah) nymphomania.

uterometer (u″ter-om′ĕ-ter) an instrument for measuring the uterus.

utero-ovarian (u″ter-o-o-va′re-an) pertaining to uterus and ovary.

uteropexy (u′ter-o-pek″se) hysteropexy.

uteroplacental (u″ter-o-plah-sen′tal) pertaining to placenta and uterus.

uteroplasty (u′ter-o-plas″te) plastic repair of the uterus.

uterorectal (u″ter-o-rek′tal) pertaining to the uterus and rectum, or communicating with the uterine cavity and rectum.

uterosacral (-sa′kral) pertaining to uterus and sacrum.

uterosalpingography (-sal″ping-gog′rah-fe) roentgenography of uterus and oviducts.

uterosclerosis (-sklĕ-ro′sis) sclerosis of the uterus.

uteroscope (u′ter-o-skōp″) an instrument for viewing the interior of the uterus.

uterotome (u′ter-o-tōm″) hysterotome.

uterotomy (u″ter-ot′o-me) hysterotomy.

uterotonic (u″ter-o-ton′ik) increasing the tone of uterine muscle.

uterotropic (-trop′ik) having special affinity for or exerting its principal influence on the uterus.

uterotubal (-tu′bal) pertaining to uterus and oviducts.

uterovaginal (u″ter-o-vaj′ĭ-nal) pertaining to uterus and vagina.

uterovesical (-ves′ĭ-kal) pertaining to uterus and bladder.

uterus (u′ter-us) the hollow organ in the female mammal in which the young develops during gestation. **u. bicor′nis,** one with two cornua. **u. cordifor′mis,** a heart-shaped uterus. **u. du′plex,** a double uterus. **gravid u.,** one containing a developing fetus. **u. mas-culi′nus,** prostatic utricle. **u. unicor′nis,** one with a single cornu.

utricle (u′trĭ-kel) the larger of the two divisions of the membranous labyrinth of the internal ear. **prostatic u., urethral u.,** a small blind pouch in the substance of the prostate.

utricular (u-trik′u-lar) 1. bladder-like. 2. pertaining to the utricle.

utriculitis (u-trik″u-li′tis) inflammation of the prostatic utricle.

utriculosaccular (u-trik″u-lo-sak′u-lar) pertaining to utricle and saccule of the labyrinth.

utriculus (u-trik′u-lus) utricle. **u. hom′inis, u. masculi′nus, u. prostat′icus,** prostatic utricle.

uve(o)- word element, *uvea.*

uvea (u′ve-ah) the iris, ciliary body and choroid together. adj., **u′veal.**

uveitis (u″ve-i′tis) inflammation of the uvea. adj., **uveit′ic. heterochromic u.,** uveitis in which the diseased eye differs in color from the normal one. **sympathetic u.,** uveitis following the same affection in the other eye.

uveoparotitis (u″ve-o-par″o-ti′tis) uveoparotid fever.

uveoplasty (u′ve-o-plas″te) plastic repair of the uvea.

uveoscleritis (u″ve-o-skle-ri′tis) inflammation of uvea and sclera.

uviform (u′vĭ-form) shaped like a grape.

uviofast (u′ve-o-fast″) uvioresistant.

uviometer (u″ve-om′ĕ-ter) an instrument for measuring ultraviolet emanation.

uvioresistant (u″ve-o-re-zis′tant) resistant to ultraviolet rays.

uviosensitive (-sen′sĭ-tiv) sensitive to ultraviolet rays.

uvula (u′vu-lah), pl. *u′vulae* [L.] a pendent, fleshy mass, as the dependent triangular portion of the soft palate (*u′vula palati′na* or *palatine uvula*) above the root of the tongue. adj. **u′vular. u. of bladder,** a rounded elevation at the neck of the bladder, formed by convergence of muscle fibers terminating in the urethra. **u. cerebel′li,** a lobule which is the posterior limit of the fourth ventricle.

uvulectomy (u″vu-lek′to-me) excision of the uvula.

uvulitis (-li′tis) inflammation of the uvula.

uvuloptosis (-lop-to′sis) a relaxed, pendulous state of the uvula.

uvulotomy (-lot′o-me) incision of the uvula.

V

V chemical symbol, *vanadium.*

V. velocity; vision; visual acuity; volume; volt.

V.A. Veterans Administration.

vaccigenous (vak-sij′ĕ-nus) producing vaccine.

vaccinal (vak′sĭ-nal) pertaining to vaccinia or to inoculation of vaccinia virus.

vaccinate (vak′sĭ-nāt) to introduce vaccine into.

vaccination (vak″sĭ-na′shun) the introduction of vaccine into the body, as by injection or scarification.

vaccine (vak′sēn) a suspension of attenuated or killed microorganisms (viruses, bacteria or rickettsiae), administered for prevention, amelioration or treatment of infectious diseases. **autogenous v.,** a bacterial vaccine prepared from cultures of material derived from a lesion of the patient to be treated. **BCG v.,** a preparation for prophylactic inoculation of young infants against tuberculosis, consisting of living cultures of bovine tubercle bacilli that have been grown on glycerinated ox bile so that their virulence is greatly reduced. **cholera v.,** a preparation of killed cholera vibrios, used in immunization against cholera. **influenza virus v., polyvalent,** a preparation of inactivated or killed viruses causing different types of influenza, used to produce immunity. **measles virus v.,** a preparation from the causative virus grown in monkey kidney or chick embryo tissue, and inactivated or attenuated; used to produce immunity to the naturally occurring disease. **mixed v.,** polyvalent vaccine. **mumps v.,** a sterile suspension of mumps virus, inactivated and used to produce active immunity against mumps (epidemic parotitis). **pertussis v.,** a preparation derived from the organisms causing whooping cough, used to immunize against the disease. **plague v.,** a preparation of killed plague bacilli, used as an active immunizing agent. **poliomyelitis v., poliovirus v.,** a vaccine used to immunize against poliomyelitis, prepared from attenuated or killed viruses of the three types ordinarily causing the paralytic infection. **polyvalent v.,** one prepared from more than one strain or species of microorganisms. **rabies v.,** a preparation of rabies virus that has been treated with a virucidal agent, used to prevent development of rabies in an exposed person. **Sabin oral polio v.,** an orally administered vaccine consisting of live, attenuated polioviruses of the three types, grown in monkey kidney tissue culture. **Salk v.,** a preparation of killed polioviruses of the three types, grown in monkey kidney tissue culture, given intramuscularly to immunize against the disease. **smallpox v.**, a preparation of vaccinia virus, grown by various methods, used to produce immunity to smallpox. **tuberculosis v.**, BCG vaccine. **typhoid and paratyphoid v.**, a preparation of killed typhoid and paratyphoid A and B bacilli.

vaccinia (vak-sin'e-ah) a virus disease of cows usually manifest only by mild eruption of the skin on the udder and teats; communicated to man, usually after smallpox vaccination, it has a morbilliform eruption. **v. gangreno'sa,** progressive vaccinia. **generalized v.**, a condition of widespread vaccinal lesions resulting from sensitivity response to smallpox vaccination and delayed production of neutralizing antibodies. **progressive v.**, vaccinia in which the patient fails to produce antibodies, with spreading necrosis at the site of the inoculation, metastatic necrotic lesions throughout the body, and eventually death.

vacciniform (vak-sin'ĭ-form) resembling vaccinia.

vacciniola (vak"sĭ-ne-o'lah) secondary eruption of vesicles after vaccination.

vaccinoid (vak'sĭ-noid) spurious or modified vaccinia.

vaccinotherapy (vak"sĭ-no-ther'ah-pe) treatment with bacterial vaccines.

vacuolation (vak"u-o-la'shun) the formation of vacuoles.

vacuole (vak'u-ōl) a space or cavity in the protoplasm of a cell. **contractile v.**, a small cavity found in many protozoa that regularly fills with water from the surrounding protoplasm and empties it to the environment. **food v's,** small cavities in the protoplasm of protozoa and other simple animals into which food is taken and in which it is digested.

vacuolization (vak"u-o-li-za'shun) vacuolation.

vacuome (vak'u-ōm) the system of vacuoles in a cell which stain with neutral red.

vagal (va'gal) pertaining to the vagus.

vagina (vah-ji'nah) 1. the canal in the female, from the vulva to the cervix of the uterus, that receives the penis of the male in sexual congress. 2. any sheath or sheathlike structure; used in anatomic nomenclature to designate many enveloping tissues.

vaginal (vaj'ĭ-nal) pertaining to the vagina, the tunica vaginalis or any sheath.

vaginalectomy (vaj"ĭ-nal-ek'to-me) excision of the tunica vaginalis testis.

vaginalitis (-i'tis) inflammation of the tunica vaginalis testis.

vaginate (vaj'ĭ-nāt) enclosed in a sheath.

vaginismus (vaj"ĭ-niz'mus) painful spasm of the vagina.

vaginitis (-ni'tis) 1. inflammation of the vagina. 2. inflammation of a sheath. **v. adhae'siva,** senile vaginitis. **contagious granular v.**, vaginitis verrucosa. **diphtheritic v.**, diphtheritic inflammation of the vagina. **emphysematous v.**, a variety marked by the formation of gas in the meshes of the connective tissue. **glandular v.**, a form affecting only the vaginal glands. **granular**

v., the most common variety, in which the papillae are enlarged and infiltrated with small cells. **senile v.**, vaginitis occurring in old age and marked by the formation of raw patches, which often adhere to apposed surfaces, causing obliteration of the vaginal canal. **v. tes'tis,** perididymitis. **v. verruco'sa,** an infectious inflammation of the vagina in cows, prevalent in European countries.

vagino-abdominal (vaj"ĭ-no-ab-dom'ĭ-nal) pertaining to vagina and abdomen.

vaginocele (vaj'ĭ-no-sēl") colpocele.

vaginocutaneous (vaj"ĭ-no-ku-ta'ne-us) pertaining to the vagina and skin, or communicating with the vagina and the cutaneous surface of the body.

vaginodynia (-din'e-ah) pain in the vagina.

vaginofixation (-fik-sa'shun) colpopexy.

vaginogenic (-jen'ik) originating in the vagina.

vaginogram (vah-ji'no-gram) a roentgenogram of the vagina.

vaginography (vaj"ĭ-nog'rah-fe) roentgenography of the vagina.

vaginolabial (vaj"ĭ-no-la'be-al) pertaining to vagina and labia.

vaginometer (vaj"ĭ-nom'ĕ-ter) an instrument for measuring the vagina.

vaginomycosis (vaj"ĭ-no-mi-ko'sis) fungus disease of the vagina.

vaginopathy (vaj"ĭ-nop'ah-the) any disease of the vagina.

vaginoperineal (vaj"ĭ-no-per"ĭ-ne'al) pertaining to vagina and perineum.

vaginoperineorrhaphy (-per"ĭ-ne-or'ah-fe) suture of the vagina and perineum.

vaginoperineotomy (-per"ĭ-ne-ot'o-me) incision of the vagina and perineum.

vaginoperitoneal (-per"ĭ-to-ne'al) pertaining to vagina and peritoneum.

vaginopexy (vah-ji'no-pek"se) colpopexy.

vaginoplasty (vah-ji'no-plas"te) colpoplasty.

vaginoscopy (vaj"ĭ-nos'ko-pe) colposcopy.

vaginotomy (-not'o-me) colpotomy.

vaginovesical (vaj"ĭ-no-ves'ĭ-kal) pertaining to vagina and bladder.

vagitis (vah-ji'tis) inflammation of the vagus.

vagitus (vah-ji'tus) the cry of an infant. **v. uteri'nus,** the cry of an infant in the uterus.

vagolysis (va-gol'ĭ-sis) destruction of esophageal branches of the vagus for cardiospasm.

vagolytic (va"go-lit'ik) having an effect resembling that produced by interruption of impulses transmitted by the vagus nerve; parasympatholytic.

vagomimetic (-mi-met'ik) having an effect resembling that produced by stimulation of the vagus nerve.

vagosympathetic (-sim"pah-thet'ik) the vagus and cervical sympathetic together.

vagotomy (va-got'o-me) surgical transection of the fibers of the vagus nerve. **medical v.**, interruption of transmission of impulses by fibers of the vagus nerve by the use of drugs.

vagotonia (va"go-to'ne-ah) irritability of the vagus nerve, characterized by vasomotor instability, sweating, disordered peristalsis and muscle spasms. adj., **vagoton'ic.**

vagotonin (va-got'o-nin) a preparation of hormone from the pancreas which increases vagal tone, slows the heart and increases the store of glycogen in the liver.

vagotropic (va"go-trop'ik) having an effect on the vagus nerve.

vagotropism (va-got'ro-pizm) affinity of a drug for the vagus nerve.

vagovagal (va"go-va'gal) arising as a result of afferent and efferent impulses mediated through the vagus nerve.

valence (va'lens) 1. the power of an atom to combine with other atoms, the combining power of the hydrogen atom being considered unity, and the valence of atoms of other elements being the number of hydrogen atoms they combine with. 2. an expression of the number of reactive sites on the surface of the molecules by which homologous antigens and antibody specifically combine.

valethamate (val-eth'ah-māt) a compound used in parasympathetic blockade.

valgus (val'gus) [L.] bent; commonly used to designate angulation away from the midline of the body.

valine (va'lēn) a naturally occurring amino acid, one of those essential for human metabolism.

vallate (val'āt) surrounded with an elevation; cupped.

vallecula (vah-lek'u-lah), pl. *vallec'ulae* [L.] a depression or hollow. **v. cerebel'li,** a longitudinal fissure of the cerebellum. **v. syl'vii,** a depression made by the fissure of Sylvius at base of the brain. **v. un'guis,** the depression at the root of a nail.

Vallestril (val-les'tril) trademark for a preparation of methallenestril.

Valmid (val'mid) trademark for a preparation of ethinamate.

value (val'u) an expression of worth or efficiency, or of other measurable attribute. **liminal v., threshold v.,** that intensity of a stimulus which produces a just noticeable impression.

valva (val'vah), pl. *val'vae* [L.] a valve.

valve (valv) a membranous fold in a canal or passage that prevents backward flow of material passing through it. **aortic v.,** that guarding the entrance to the aorta from the left ventricle. **Bauhin's v.,** ileocecal valve. **Béraud's v.,** a fold at the beginning of the nasolacrimal duct. **bicuspid v.,** mitral valve. **cardiac v's,** valves that control the flow of blood through and from the heart. **coronary v.,** a valve at entrance of coronary sinus into right atrium. **Hasner's v.,** membranous fold at nasal orifice of the nasolacrimal duct. **Heister's v.,** a spiral fold in the mucous membrane lining the proximal part of the cystic duct. **Houston's v.,** the middle one of three transverse folds of mucous membrane in the rectum. **ileocecal v., ileocolic v.,** that guarding the opening between the ileum and cecum. **Kerckring's v's,** permanent transverse folds projecting into the lumen of the small intestine, involving both mucosa and submucosa. **mitral v.,** that guarding the opening between the left atrium and left ventricle. **pulmonary v.,** that at the entrance of the pulmonary trunk from the right ventricle. **pyloric v.,** a prominent fold of mucous membrane at the junction of the stomach and duodenum. **semilunar v's,** valves made up of semilunar segments or cusps *(val'vulae semiluna'res)*, guarding the entrances into the aorta and pulmonary trunk from the cardiac ventricles. **thebesian v.,** a fold of endocardium at the opening of the coronary sinus in the right atrium of the heart. **tricuspid v.,** that guarding the opening between the right atrium and right ventricle. **v. of Varolius,** ileocecal valve. **v. of Vieussens,** white layer connecting superior peduncles of cerebellum and roofing the fourth ventricle.

valvotomy (val-vot'o-me) incision of a valve; splitting of the commissures of a valve for dilation of the opening. **mitral v.,** splitting of the commissures of the valve between the left atrium and ventricle, with extension of the opening.

valvula (val'vu-lah), pl. *vul'vulae* [L.] a small valve. adj., **val'vular. val'vulae conniven'tes,** transverse mucous folds in small intestine.

valvulectomy (val"vu-lek'to-me) excision of a valve.

valvulitis (-li'tis) inflammation of a valve, especially of a valve of the heart.

valvuloplasty (val'vu-lo-plas"te) plastic repair on a valve, especially a valve of the heart.

valvulotome (val'vu-lo-tōm") an instrument for cutting a valve.

valvulotomy (val"vu-lot'o-me) valvotomy.

vanadium (vah-na'de-um) chemical element *(see table),* at. no. 23, symbol V.

vanadiumism (vah-na'de-um-izm") poisoning by vanadium.

Vancocin (van'ko-sin) trademark for a preparation of vancomycin.

vancomycin (van"ko-mi'sin) an antibacterial compound produced by a species of soil bacilli (Streptomyces).

vanilla (vah-nil'ah) cured, full-grown, unripe fruit of species of Vanilla; used as a flavoring agent.

vanillal (vah-nil'lal) ethyl vanillin.

vanillin (vah-nil'in) an aromatic, crystallizable principle used as a flavoring agent. **ethyl v.,** fine white or slightly yellowish crystals, with a taste and odor similar to those of vanilla; used as a flavoring agent.

vanillism (vah-nil'izm) dermatitis and pruritus from handling vanilla.

Vanogel (van'o-jel) trademark for an aqueous suspension of aluminum hydroxide gel.

vapor (va'por) a gas, especially of a compound which at ordinary temperatures is a liquid or solid.

vaporization (va"por-i-za'shun) dispersal of a liquid in the form of a gas.

vapotherapy (va"po-ther'ah-pe) treatment by vapor or spray.

varicella (var"ĭ-sel'ah) chickenpox.

variciform (vah-ris'ĭ-form) having the form of a varix.

varicoblepharon (var"ĭ-ko-blef'ah-ron) a varicose tumor of the eyelid.

varicocele (var'ĭ-ko-sēl") a cystic accumulation of blood in the spermatic cord.

varicocelectomy (var"ĭ-ko-se-lek'to-me) excision of a varicocele.

varicography (var"ĭ-kog'rah-fe) x-ray visualization of varicose veins.

varicomphalos (-kom'fah-los) a varicose tumor of the umbilicus.

varicophlebitis (var"ĭ-ko-fle-bi'tis) infection in varicose veins.

varicosity (var"ĭ-kos'ĭ-te) 1. a varix. 2. quality of being enlarged and tortuous.

varicotomy (-kot'o-me) excision of a varix or of a varicose vein.

varicula (vah-rik'u-lah) a varix of the conjunctiva.

Varidase (var'ĭ-dās) trademark for preparations of streptokinase and streptodornase.

variola (vah-ri'o-lah) smallpox. adj., **vari'olate. v. hemorrha'gica,** hemorrhagic smallpox. **v. ma'jor,** malignant smallpox. **v. milia'ris,** smallpox with an eruption of small vesicles. **v. mi'nor,** a mild form of smallpox having a low fatality rate.

variolation (var"re-o-la'shun) application or ingestion of crusts of dried variola pustules to produce immunity to natural infection by the virus of smallpox.

varioloid (va're-o-loid") infection by virus of smallpox producing no or slight symptoms in a previously vaccinated person who is capable of transmitting infection that may be fatal to a susceptible person.

variolous (vah-ri'o-lus) pertaining to smallpox.

variolovaccinia (vah-ri"o-lo-vak-sin'e-ah) a disease in the heifer caused by inoculation with smallpox virus.

varix (văr'iks), pl. **var'ices** [L] an enlarged, tortuous vein. adj., **var'icose. aneurysmal v.,** a varix due to direct communication with an adjacent artery as a result of a wound. **arterial v.,** an enlarged, tortuous artery. **v. lymphat'icus,** an enlarged and tortuous lymphatic vessel.

varolian (vah-ro'le-an) pertaining to the pons varolii.

varus (va'rus) [L.] bent; commonly used to indicate angulation toward the midline of the body.

vas (vas), pl. **va'sa** [L.] a vessel. adj., **va'sal. v. aber'rans,** 1. a blind tube sometimes connected with the epididymis or vas deferens. 2. any anomalous or unusual vessel. **va'sa afferen'tia,** vessels that convey fluid to a structure or part. **va'sa bre'via,** the small branches of the splenic artery going to the stomach. **v. def'erens,** ductus deferens. **va'sa efferen'tia,** vessels that convey fluid away from a structure or part. **v. lymphat'icum,** a vessel that conveys lymph. **va'sa pre'via,** appearance of the vessel of the umbilical cord ahead of the presenting part of the fetus at the onset of the uterus. **va'sa**

rec'ta, straight tubes formed by the seminiferous tubules. **va'sa vaso'rum,** vessels conveying blood to and from the outer and middle coats of the larger blood vessels. **va'sa vortico'sa,** vorticose veins.

vas(o)- (vas'o) word element [L.], *blood vessel; vas (ductus) deferens.*

vascular (vas'ku-lar) pertaining to or full of vessels.

vascularity (vas"ku-lar'ĭ-te) condition of being vascular.

vascularization (vas"ku-lar-i-za'shun) the process of becoming vascular.

vascularize (vas'ku-lar-īz) to supply with vessels.

vasculature (vas'ku-lah-chūr) 1. the vascular system of the body, or any part of it. 2. the supply of vessels to a specific region.

vasculitis (vas"ku-li'tis) inflammation of a vessel.

vasectomy (vah-sek'to-me) excision of the vas (ductus) deferens.

vasifactive (vas"ĭ-fak'tiv) producing new vessels.

vasiform (vas'ĭ-form) resembling a vas or vessel.

vasitis (vas-i'tis) inflammation of the vas (ductus) deferens.

vasoconstriction (vas"o-kon-strik'shun) decrease in the caliber of blood vessels. adj., **vasoconstric'tive.**

vasoconstrictor (-kon-strik'tor) 1. causing constriction of the blood vessels. 2. something that acts to decrease the caliber of blood vessels.

vasocorona (-kŏ-ro'nah) the assemblage of arteries passing radially into the spinal cord from its periphery.

vasodentin (-den'tin) dentin provided with blood vessels.

vasodepression (-de-presh'un) vasomotor depression or collapse.

vasodepressor (-de-pres'sor) 1. having a depressing effect on the circulation. 2. an agent that causes vasomotor depression.

Vasodilan (di'lan) trademark for preparations of isoxsuprine hydrochloride.

vasodilatation (-dil"ah-ta'shun) dilatation of blood vessels.

vasodilation (-di-la'shun) increase in the caliber of blood vessels.

vasodilator (-di-la'tor) 1. causing dilatation of blood vessels. 2. a nerve or agent which causes dilatation of blood vessels.

vaso-epididymostomy (-ep"ĭ-did'ĭ-mos'to-me) anastomosis of the vas (ductus) deferens and the epididymis.

vasoganglion (-gang'gle-on) a vascular ganglion or rete.

vasography (vas-og"rah-fe) radiography of the blood vessels.

vasohypertonic (vas"o-hi"per-ton'ik) increasing the tone of blood vessels.

vasohypotonic (-hi"po-ton'ik) decreasing the tone of blood vessels.

vasoinert (-in-ert') having no effect on the caliber of blood vessels.

vaso-inhibitor (-in-hib'ĭ-tor) 1. inhibiting the

vasomotor nerves. 2. an agent which inhibits vasomotor nerves. adj., **vaso-inhib'itory.**

vasoligation (vas"o-li-ga'shun) ligation of the vas (ductus) deferens.

vasomotion (-mo'shun) the change in caliber of blood vessels.

vasomotor (-mo'tor) having an effect on the caliber of blood vessels.

vasomotorium (-mo-to're-um) the vasomotor system of the body.

vasoneuropathy (-nu-rop'ah-the) a condition caused by combined vascular and neurologic defect, resulting from simultaneous action or interaction of the vascular and the nervous systems.

vasoneurosis (-nu-ro'sis) angioneurosis.

vaso-orchidostomy (-or"ki-dos'to-me) anastomosis of the epididymis to the severed end of the vas (ductus) deferens.

vasoparesis (-par'e-sis) paralysis of vasomotor nerves.

vasopressin (-pres'in) a water-soluble principle from the posterior lobe of the pituitary gland which increases blood pressure and influences the reabsorption of water by the kidney tubules.

vasopressor (-pres'or) an agent that stimulates contraction of the muscular tissue of capillaries and arteries.

vasopuncture (-pungk'chŭr) puncture of the vas (ductus) deferens.

vasoreflex (-re'fleks) a reflex of blood vessels.

vasorelaxation (-re"lak-sa'shun) decrease of vascular pressure.

vasoresection (-re-sek'shun) resection of the vas (ductus) deferens.

vasorrhaphy (vas-or'ah-fe) suture of the vas (ductus) deferens.

vasosection (vas"o-sek'shun) the severing of a vessel or vessels, especially of the ductus deferentes (vasa deferentia).

vasosensory (-sen'sor-e) supplying sensory filaments to the vessels.

vasospasm (vas'o-spazm) spasm of a vessel. adj., **vasospas'tic.**

vasospasmolytic (vas"o-spaz"mo-lit'ik) arresting spasm of the vessels.

vasostimulant (-stim'u-lant) stimulating vasomotor action.

vasothrombin (-throm'bin) a fibrin factor formed from the endothelial cells of the vessels, which takes part in the formation of thrombin.

vasotomy (vah-sot'o-me) incision of the vas (ductus) deferens.

vasotonic (vas"o-ton'ik) regulating the tone of a vessel.

vasotrophic (-trof'ik) affecting nutrition through alteration of the caliber of the blood vessels.

vasotropic (-trop'ik) exerting an influence on the blood vessels, causing either constriction or dilatation.

vasovasostomy (-vah-sos'to-me) restoration of the continuity of the divided vas (ductus) deferens.

vasovesiculectomy (-ve-sik"u-lek'to-me) excision of vas (ductus) deferens and seminal vesicle.

vasovesiculitis (vas"o-ve-sik"u-li'tis) inflammation of vas (ductus) deferens and seminal vesicle.

Vasoxyl (vas-ok'sil) trademark for preparations of methoxamine hydrochloride.

vastus (vas'tus) [L.] great.

V.C. acuity of color vision.

V-cillin (ve-sil'in) trademark for preparations of penicillin V.

V.D. venereal disease.

V.D.G. veneral disease – gonorrhea.

V.D.H. valvular disease of the heart.

VDM vasodepressor material.

V.D.R.L. Venereal Disease Research Laboratory.

V.D.S. venereal disease – syphilis.

vection (vek'shun) the mechanical transmission of disease germs from an infected person to a well person.

vectis (vek'tis) a curved lever for making traction on the fetal head in labor.

vector (vek'tor) a carrier, as (1) an arthropod that carries a protozoan parasite from a biological reservoir or an infected organism to another organism (animal or human), or (2) a vector quantity. adj., **vecto'rial.**

vectorcardiogram (vek"tor-kar'de-o-gram") the record, usually a photograph, of the loop formed on the oscilloscope in vectorcardiography.

vectorcardiography (-kar"de-og'rah-fe) the registration, by formation of a loop on an oscilloscope, of the direction and magnitude of the moment-to-moment electromotive forces of the heart during one complete cycle.

vegan (vej'an) a vegetarian who excludes from his diet all protein of animal origin.

veganism (vej'ah-nizm) strict adherence to a vegetable diet, with exclusion of all protein of animal origin.

vegetal (vej'e-tal) common to plants.

vegetarian (vej"e-ta're-an) one who eats only foods of vegetable origin.

vegetarianism (-ta're-ah-nizm") the restriction of man's food to substances of vegetable origin.

vegetation (-ta'shun) a plantlike neoplasm or growth.

vegetative (-ta"tiv) concerned with growth and nutrition.

vegeto-animal (vej"e-to-an'i-mal) common to plants and animals.

vehicle (ve'i-kl) a transporting agent, especially the component of a medication (prescription) serving as a solvent or to increase the bulk or decrease the concentration of the mixture.

veil (val) 1. a covering structure. 2. a caul or piece of amniotic sac occasionally covering the face of a newborn child. 3. slight huskiness of the voice.

Veillonella (va"yon-el'ah) a genus of Schizomycetes (order Eubacteriales, family Neisseriaceae) found as nonpathogenic parasites in the mouth, intestines and urogenital and respiratory tracts of man and other animals.

vein (van) a vessel in which blood flows toward the heart, in the systemic circulation carrying blood that has given up most of its oxygen. For names of veins of the body, *see the table*. **afferent v's,** veins that carry blood to an organ. **allantoic v's,** paired vessels that accompany the allantois, growing out from the primitive hindgut and entering the body stalk of the early embryo. **aqueous v's,** microscopic, blood vessel-like pathways on the surface of the eye, containing aqueous humor or diluted blood. **cardinal v's,** various (anterior, common and posterior) paired vessels in the early embryo. **central v.,** one occupying the axis of an organ. **emissary v.,** one passing through a foramen of the skull and draining blood from a cerebral sinus into a vessel outside the skull. **hypophyseoportal v's,** a system of venules connecting capillaries in the hypothalamus with sinusoidal capillaries in the anterior lobe of the hypophysis. **postcardinal v's,** paired vessels in the early embryo that return blood from regions caudal to the heart. **precardinal v's,** paired vessels that drain blood from the head region of the embryo. **pulp v's,** vessels draining the venous sinuses of the spleen. **subcardinal v's, supracardinal v's,** paired vessels in the embryo that successively replace and supplement the postcardinal veins. **sublobular v's,** tributaries of the hepatic veins that receive the central veins of hepatic lobules. **trabecular v's,** vessels coursing in splenic trabeculae, formed by tributary pulp veins. **umbilical v.,** a vessel contained in the umbilical cord that conveys blood from placenta to fetus. **varicose v.,** a permanently distended and tortuous vein, especially one in the leg. **vesalian v.,** an emissary vein connecting the cavernous sinus with the pterygoid venous plexus. **vitelline v's,** early veins of the developing embryo, communicating with the yolk sac.

Velacycline (vel″ah-si′klen) trademark for preparations of rolitetracycline.

velamen (ve-la′men), pl. *velam′ina* [L.] a membrane, meninx or tegument.

Velban (vel′ban) trademark for a preparation of vinblastine sulfate.

vellication (vel″ĭ-ka′shun)· a twitching of a muscle.

vellus (vel′us) the coat of fine hairs of the prepuberal years, which appear after the lanugo hairs are cast off.

velopharyngeal (vel″o-fah-rin′je-al) pertaining to the velum palatinum and pharynx.

velum (ve′lum), pl. *ve′la* [L.] a covering structure or veil. adj., **ve′lar. v. interpos′itum,** membranous roof of the third ventricle. **medullary v.,** one of the two portions *(superior medullary velum* and *inferior medullary velum)* of the white matter of the hindbrain that form the roof of the fourth ventricle. **v. palati′num,** the dependent portion of the soft palate, including the uvula and the palatoglossal and palatopharyngeal arches.

VEM vasoexcitor material.

vena (ve′nah), pl. *ve′nae* [L.] vein. **v. ca′va, inferior,** vein returning blood to the heart from the lower part of the body (see table of veins). **v. ca′va, superior,** vein returning blood to the heart from the upper part of the

body *(see table of veins).* **ve′nae comitan′tes,** veins accompanying arteries.

venacavography (ve″nah-ka-vog′rah-fe) radiography of a vena cava; usually denoting that of the inferior vena cava.

venectasia (ve″nek-ta′ze-ah) phlebectasia.

venectomy (ve-nek′to-me) phlebectomy.

venenation (ven″ĕ-na′shun) poisoning; a poisoned condition.

venenific (-nif′ik) forming poison.

venenosa (-no′sah) venomous snakes collectively.

venenous (ven′ĕ-nus) poisonous or toxic.

venereal (vĕ-ne′re-al) propagated by sexual intercourse.

venereologist (vĕ-ne″re-ol′o-jist) a specialist in venereology.

venereology (-ol′o-je) the study and treatment of venereal diseases.

venereophobia (-o-fo′be-ah) morbid fear of contracting venereal disease.

venerupin (ven″ĕ-roo′pin) a toxic principle derived from certain Japanese mollusks.

venery (ven′er-e) coitus.

venesection (ven″ĕ-sek′shun) the opening of a vein for letting blood.

veniplex (ven′ĭ-pleks) a venous plexus.

venipuncture (ven″ĭ-pungk′chur) surgical puncture of a vein.

venisuture (-su′chur) phleborrhaphy.

venoclysis (ve-nok′lĭ-sis) injection of medicinal or nutrient fluid into a vein.

venogram (ve′no-gram) phlebogram.

venography (ve-nog′rah-fe) phlebography.

venom (ven′om) poison, especially a toxic substance normally secreted by a serpent, insect or other animal. **Russell's viper v.,** the venom of the Russell viper, which acts in vitro as an intrinsic thromboplastin and is useful in defining deficiencies of blood coagulation factor X

venomization (ven″om-i-za′shun) treatment of a substance with snake venom.

venomotor (ve″no-mo′tor) controlling dilation or contraction of the veins.

veno-occlusive (ve″no-ŏ-kloo′siv) pertaining to or characterized by obstruction of the veins.

venosclerosis (-sklĕ-ro′sis) sclerosis of veins.

venosity (ve-nos′ĭ-te) 1. the characteristic quality of venous blood. 2. excess of venous blood in a part.

venostasis (ve″no-sta′sis) checking of return flow of blood by compressing veins in the four extremities.

venostat (ve′no-stat) an instrument for performing venostasis.

venotomy (ve-not′o-me) phlebotomy.

venous (ve′nus) pertaining to the veins.

venovenostomy (ve″no-ve-nos′to-me) phlebophlebostomy.

vent (vent) an opening or outlet, such as an opening that discharges pus, or the anus.

venter (ven′ter), pl. *ven′tres* [L.] the belly or any belly-like part; the anterior or inferior surface of the body.

ventilation (ven″tĭ-la′shun) 1. the process of supplying with fresh air. 2. free discussion, as of one's problems or grievances.

TABLE OF VEINS

COMMON NAME	NA TERM	REGION	RECEIVES BLOOD FROM	DRAINS INTO
accompanying v. of hypoglossal nerve	v. comitans nervi hypoglossi	accompanies hypoglossal nerve	formed by union of deep v. of tongue and sublingual v.	facial, lingual or internal jugular v.
anastomotic v., inferior	v. anastomotica inferior	interconnects superficial middle cerebral v. and superior sagittal sinus		
anastomotic v., superior	v. anastomotica superior	interconnects superficial middle cerebral v. and transverse sinus		
angular v.	v. angularis	between eye and root of nose	formed by union of supratrochlear v. and supraorbital v.	continues as facial v. behind facial artery
antebrachial v., median	v. mediana antebrachii	forearm between cephalic v. and basilic v.	a palmar venous plexus	cephalic v. and/or basilic v., or median cubital v.
appendicular v.	v. appendicularis	accompanies appendicular artery		joins anterior and posterior cecal vv. to form ileocolic v.
v. of aqueduct of vestibule	v. aqueductus vestibuli	passes through aqueduct of vestibule	internal ear	superior petrosal sinus
arcuate vv. of kidney	vv. arcuatae renis	a series of complete arches across the bases of the renal pyramids, formed by union of interlobular vv. and straight vv. (venules) of kidney		interlobar vv.
auditory vv., internal. See labyrinthine vv.				
auricular vv., anterior	vv. auriculares anteriores	anterior part of auricle of external ear		superficial temporal v.
auricular v., posterior	v. auricularis posterior	passes down behind auricle	a plexus on side of head	joins retromandibular v. to form external jugular v.
axillary v.	v. axillaris	the upper limb	formed at lower	at lateral border of first rib be-

				comes subclavian v.
azygos v.	v. azygos	intercepting trunk for right intercostal vv. as well as connecting branch between superior and inferior venae cavae; it ascends in front of and on right side of vertebrae	ascending lumbar v.	superior vena cava
azygos v., left. *See* hemiazygos v.				
azygos v., lesser superior. *See* hemiazygos v., accessory				
basal v.	v. basalis	passes from anterior perforated substance backward and around cerebral peduncle	anterior perforated substance	internal cerebral v.
basilic v.	v. basilica	forearm, superficially	ulnar side of dorsal rete of hand	joins brachial vv. to form axillary v.
basilic v., median	v. mediana basilica	sometimes present as medial branch of a bifurcation of median antebrachial v.		basilic v.
basivertebral vv.	vv. basivertebrales	venous sinuses in cancellous tissue of bodies of vertebrae, which communicate with external and internal vertebral plexuses		
brachial vv.	vv. brachiales	accompany brachial artery	border of teres major muscle by junction of basilic v. and brachial v.	join basilic v. to form axillary v.
brachiocephalic vv.	vv. brachiocephalicae (dextra et sinistra)	thorax	head, neck and upper limbs; formed at root of neck by union of ipsilateral internal jugular and subclavian vv.	unite to form superior vena cava

TABLE OF VEINS (Continued)

COMMON NAME	NA TERM	REGION	RECEIVES BLOOD FROM	DRAINS INTO
bronchial vv.	vv. bronchiales		larger subdivisions of bronchi	azygos v. on left; hemiazygos or superior intercostal v. on right
v. of bulb of penis	v. bulbi penis		bulb of penis	internal pudendal v.
v. of bulb of vestibule	v. bulbi vestibuli		bulb of vestibule of vagina	internal pudendal v.
cardiac vv., anterior	vv. cordis anteriores		anterior wall of right ventricle	right atrium of heart, or lesser cardiac v.
cardiac v., great	v. cordis magna		anterior surface of ventricles	coronary sinus
cardiac v., middle	v. cordis media		diaphragmatic surface of ventricles	coronary sinus
cardiac v., small	v. cordis parva		right atrium and ventricle	coronary sinus
"cardiac vv., smallest"	vv. cordis minimae	numerous small veins arising in myocardium, draining independently into cavities of heart and most readily seen in the atria		
carotid v., external. See retromandibular v.				
cavernous vv. of penis	vv. cavernosae penis		corpora cavernosa	deep vv. and dorsal v. of penis
central vv. of liver	vv. centrales	in middle of hepatic lobules	liver substance	hepatic v.
central v. of retina	v. centralis retinae	eyeball	retinal vv.	superior ophthalmic v.
central v. of suprarenal gland	v. centralis glandulae suprarenalis	the large single vein into which the various veins within the substance of the gland empty, and which continues at the hilus as the suprarenal v.		

cephalic v.	v. cephalica	winds anteriorly to pass along anterior border of brachioradialis muscle; above elbow, ascends along lateral border of biceps muscle	axillary v.
cephalic v., accessory	v. cephalica accessoria	forearm	joins cephalic v. just above elbow
cephalic v., median	v. mediana cephalica	sometimes present as lateral tributary of a bifurcation of median antebrachial v.	cephalic v.
cerebellar vv., inferior	vv. cerebelli inferiores	inferior surface of cerebellum	transverse, sigmoid and inferior petrosal sinuses, or occipital sinus
cerebellar vv., superior	vv. cerebelli superiores	upper surface of cerebellum	straight sinus and great cerebral v., or transverse and superior petrosal sinuses
cerebral v., anterior	v. cerebri anterior	accompanies anterior cerebral artery	basal v.
cerebral v., great	v. cerebri magna	curves around splenium of corpus callosum	straight sinus
cerebral vv., inferior	vv. cerebri inferiores	veins that ramify on inferior surface of brain, those on inferior surface of frontal lobe draining into inferior sagittal sinus and cavernous sinus, those on temporal lobe into superior petrosal sinus and transverse sinus, and those on occipital lobe into straight sinus	
cerebral vv., internal (2)	vv. cerebri internae	pass backward from interventricular foramen through tela choroidea	unite at splenium of corpus callosum to form great cerebral v.
cerebral v., middle, deep	v. cerebri media profunda	accompanies middle cerebral artery in floor of lateral sulcus	basal v.

TABLE OF VEINS (Continued)

COMMON NAME	NA TERM	REGION	RECEIVES BLOOD FROM	DRAINS INTO
cerebral v., middle, superficial	v. cerebri media superficialis	follows lateral cerebral fissure	lateral surface of cerebrum	cavernous sinus
cerebral vv., superior	vv. cerebri superiores	about 12 veins draining superolateral and medial surfaces of cerebrum toward longitudinal fissure		superior sagittal sinus
cervical v., deep	v. cervicalis profunda	accompanies deep cervical artery down neck	a plexus in suboccipital triangle	vertebral v. or brachiocephalic v.
cervical vv., transverse	vv. transversae colli	accompany transverse artery of neck		subclavian v.
choroid v.	v. choroidea	runs whole length of choroid plexus	choroid plexus, hippocampus, fornix, corpus callosum	joins thalamostriate v. to form internal cerebral v.
ciliary vv.	vv. ciliares	anterior vessels follow anterior ciliary arteries; posterior follow posterior ciliary arteries	arise in eyeball by branches from ciliary muscle; anterior ciliary vv. also receive branches from sinus venosus, sclerae, episcleral vv. and tunica conjunctiva of eyeball	superior ophthalmic v.; posterior ciliary vv. empty also into inferior ophthalmic v.
circumflex femoral vv., lateral	vv. circumflexae femoris laterales	accompany lateral circumflex femoral artery		femoral v. or profunda femoris v.
circumflex femoral vv., medial	vv. circumflexae femoris mediales	accompany medial circumflex femoral artery		femoral v. or profunda femoris v.
circumflex iliac v., deep	v. circumflexa ilium profunda	a common trunk formed by veins accompanying deep circumflex iliac artery	accompanying deep	external iliac v.

circumflex iliac v., superficial	v. circumflexa illium superficialis	accompanies superficial circumflex iliac artery		great saphenous v.
v. of cochlear canaliculus	v. canaliculi cochleae		cochlea	superior bulb of internal jugular v.
colic v., left	v. colica sinistra	accompanies left colic artery		inferior mesenteric v.
colic v., middle	v. coiica media	accompanies middle colic artery		superior mesenteric v.
colic v., right	v. colica dextra	accompanies right colic artery		superior mesenteric v.
conjunctival vv. coronary vv. See entries under cardiac vv.	vv. conjunctivales		conjunctiva	superior ophthalmic v.
cubital v., median	v. mediana cubiti	a large connecting tributary passing obliquely upward across cubital fossa	cephalic v., below elbow	basilic v.
cutaneous v.	v. cutanea	one of the small veins that begin in papillae of skin, from subpapillary plexuses, and open into the subcutaneous veins		
cystic v.	v. cystica	within substance of liver	gallbladder	right branch of portal v.
deep vv. of clitoris	vv. profundae clitoridis		clitoris	vesical venous plexus
deep vv. of penis	vv. profundae penis	accompany deep artery of penis	penis	dorsal v. of penis
digital vv., palmar	vv. digitales palmares	accompany proper and common palmar digital arteries		superior palmar venous arch
digital vv., plantar	vv. digitales plantares	plantar surfaces of toes		unite at clefts to form plantar metatarsal vv.
digital vv. of foot, dorsal	vv. digitales dorsales pedis	dorsal surfaces of toes		unite at clefts to form dorsal metatarsal vv.
diploic v., frontal	v. diploica frontalis		frontal bone	supraorbital v. or superior sagittal sinus

TABLE OF VEINS (Continued)

COMMON NAME	NA TERM	REGION	RECEIVES BLOOD FROM	DRAINS INTO
diploic v., occipital	v. diploica occipitalis		occipital bone	occipital v. or transverse sinus
diploic v., temporal, anterior	v. diploica temporalis anterior		lateral portion of frontal bone, anterior part of parietal bone	sphenoparietal sinus or a deep temporal v.
diploic v., temporal, posterior	v. diploica temporalis posterior		parietal bone	transverse sinus
dorsal v. of clitoris	v. dorsalis clitoridis	accompanies dorsal artery of clitoris		vesical plexus
dorsal vv. of clitoris, superficial	vv. dorsales clitoridis superficiales		clitoris, subcutaneously	external pudendal v.
dorsal v. of penis	v. dorsalis penis	a single median vein lying subfascially in penis between the dorsal arteries; it begins in small veins around corona glandis, is joined by deep veins of penis as it passes proximally, and passes between arcuate pubic and transverse perineal ligaments, where it divides into a left and a right vein to join prostatic plexus		
dorsal vv. of penis, superficial	vv. dorsales penis superficiales		penis, subcutaneously	external pudendal v.
dorsal vv. of tongue	vv. dorsales linguae	veins that unite with a small vein accompanying lingual artery and join main lingual trunk		
emissary v., condylar	v. emissaria condylaris	a small vein running through condylar canal of skull, connecting sigmoid sinus with vertebral v. or internal jugular v.		
emissary v., mastoid	v. emissaria mastoidea	a small vein passing through mastoid foramen of skull, connecting sigmoid sinus with occipital v. or posterior auricular v.		

emmissary v., occipital	v. emissaria occipitalis	an occasional small vein running through a minute foramen in occipital protuberance of skull, connecting confluence of sinuses with occipital v.	
emissary v., parietal	v. emissaria parietalis	a small vein passing through parietal foramen of skull, connecting superior sagittal sinus with superficial temporal vv.	
epigastric v., inferior	v. epigastrica inferior	accompanies inferior epigastric artery	external iliac v.
epigastric v., superficial	v. epigastrica superficialis	accompanies superficial epigastric artery	great saphenous v. or femoral v.
epigastric vv., superior	vv. epigastricae superiores	accompany superior epigastric artery	internal thoracic v.
episcleral vv.	vv. episclerales	around cornea	vorticose vv. and ciliary vv.
esophageal vv.	vv. esophageae	esophagus	hemiazygos v. and azygos v., or left brachiocephalic v.
ethmoidal vv.	vv. ethmoidales	accompany anterior and posterior ethmoidal arteries and emerge from ethmoidal foramina	superior ophthalmic v.
facial v.	v. facialis	a vein beginning at medial angle of eye as angular v., descending behind facial artery, and usually ending in internal jugular v.; formerly called anterior facial v.; this vessel sometimes joins retromandibular v. to form a common trunk previously known as common facial vein	
facial v., common. *See* facial v.			
facial v., deep	v. faciei profunda	pterygoid plexus	facial v.
facial v., posterior. *See* retromandibular v.			
facial v., transverse	v. transversa faciei	passes backward with transverse facial artery just below zygomatic arch	retromandibular v.

COMMON NAME	NA TERM	REGION	RECEIVES BLOOD FROM	DRAINS INTO
femoral v.	v. femoralis	follows course of femoral artery in proximal two thirds of thigh	continuation of popliteal vv.	at inguinal ligament becomes external iliac v.
femoral v., deep. *See* profunda femoris v.				
fibular vv. *See* peroneal vv.	vv. fibulares (official alternative for vv. peroneae)			
gastric v., left	v. gastrica sinistra	accompanies left gastric artery		portal v.
gastric v., right	v. gastrica dextra	accompanies right gastric artery		portal v.
gastric vv., short	vv. gastricae breves		left portion of greater curvature of stomach	splenic v.
gastroepiploic v., left	v. gastroepiploica sinistra	accompanies left gastroepiploic artery		splenic v.
gastroepiploid v., right	v. gastroepiploica dextra	accompanies right gastroepiploic artery		superior mesenteric v.
genicular vv.	vv. genus	accompany genicular arteries		popliteal v.
gluteal vv., inferior	vv. gluteae inferiores	accompany inferior gluteal artery; unite into a single vessel after passing through greater sciatic foramen	subcutaneous tissue of back of thigh, muscles of buttock	internal iliac v.
gluteal vv., superior	vv. gluteae superiores	accompany superior gluteal artery and pass through greater sciatic foramen	muscles of buttock	internal iliac v.
hemiazygos v.	v. hemiazygos	an intercepting trunk for lower	ascending lumbar	azygos v.

				v.
hemiazygos v., accessory	v. hemiazygos accessoria	left posterior intercostal vv.; ascends on left side of vertebrae to eighth thoracic vertebra, where it may receive accessory tributary, and crosses vertebral column	the descending intercepting trunk for upper left posterior intercostal vv.; it lies on left side and at eighth thoracic vertebra joins hemiazygos v. or crosses to right side to join azygos v. directly; above, it may communicate with left superior intercostal v.	
hemorrhoidal vv. *See* entries under rectal vv.				
hepatic vv.	vv. hepaticae	central vv. of liver	2 or 3 large veins in an upper group and 6 to 20 small veins in a lower group, forming successively larger vessels	inferior vena cava on posterior aspect of liver
hypogastric v. *See* iliac v., internal				
ileal vv.	vv. ilei	walls of ileum		superior mesenteric v.
ileocolic v.	v. ileocolica		accompanies ileocolic artery	superior mesenteric v.
iliac v., common	v. iliaca communis	arises at sacroiliac joint by union of external and internal iliac vv.	ascends to right side of fifth lumbar vertebra	unites with fellow of opposite side to form inferior vena cava
iliac v., external	v. iliaca externa	continuation of femoral v.	extends from inguinal ligament to sacroiliac joint	joins internal iliac v. to form common iliac v.
iliac v., internal	v. iliaca interna	formed by union of parietal branches	extends from greater sciatic notch to brim of pelvis	joins external iliac v. to form common iliac v.
iliolumbar v.	v. iliolumbalis		accompanies iliolumbar artery	internal iliac v. and/or common iliac v.

COMMON NAME	NA TERM	REGION	RECEIVES BLOOD FROM	DRAINS INTO
innominate vv. *See* brachiocephalic vv.				
intercapital vv.	vv. intercapitales	veins at clefts of fingers which pass between heads of metacarpal bones and establish communication between dorsal and palmar venous systems of hand		
intercostal vv., anterior (12 pairs)	vv. intercostales anteriores	accompany anterior thoracic arteries		internal thoracic vv.
intercostal v., highest	v. intercostalis suprema	first posterior intercostal vein of either side, which passes over apex of lung		brachiocephalic, vertebral or superior intercostal v.
intercostal vv., posterior, IV and XI	vv. intercostales posteriores (IV et XI)	accompany posterior intercostal arteries IV and XI		azygos v. on right; hemiazygos or accessory hemiazygos v. on left
intercostal v., superior, left	v. intercostalis superior sinistra	crosses arch of aorta	formed by union of second, third and sometimes fourth posterior intercostal vv.	left brachiocephalic v.
intercostal v., superior, right	v. intercostalis superior dextra		formed by union of second, third and sometimes fourth posterior intercostal vv.	azygos v.
interlobar vv. of kidney	vv. interlobares renis	pass down between renal pyramids	venous arcades of kidney	unite to form renal v.
interlobular vv. of kidney	vv. interlobulares renis		capillary network of renal cortex	venous arcades of kidney
interlobular vv. of liver	vv. interlobulares hepatis	arise between hepatic lobules	liver	portal v.

interosseous vv. of foot, dorsal.
See metatarsal vv., dorsal

				veins of the region
intervertebral v.	v. intervertebralis	vertebral column	vertebral venous plexuses	
jejunal vv.	vv. jejunales		walls of jejunum	superior mesenteric v.
jugular v., anterior	v. jugularis anterior	arises under chin and passes down neck		external jugular or subclavian v., or jugular venous arch
jugular v., external	v. jugularis externa	begins in parotid gland, passes down neck	formed by union of retromandibular v. and posterior auricular v.	subclavian, internal jugular, or brachiocephalic v.
jugular v., internal	v. jugularis interna	from jugular fossa, descends in neck with internal carotid artery and then with common carotid artery	begins as superior bulb, draining much of head and neck	joins subclavian v. to form brachiocephalic v.
labial vv., anterior	vv. labiales anteriores		anterior aspect of labia in female	external pudendal v.
labial vv., inferior	vv. labiales inferiores		region of lower lip	facial v.
labial vv., posterior	vv. labiales posteriores		labia in female	vesical venous plexus
labial v., superior	v. labialis superior		region of upper lip	facial v.
labyrinthine vv.	vv. labyrinthi	pass through internal acoustic meatus	cochlea	inferior petrosal sinus or transverse sinus
lacrimal v.	v. lacrimalis		lacrimal gland	superior ophthalmic v.
laryngeal v., inferior	v. laryngea inferior		larynx	inferior thyroid v.
laryngeal v., superior	v. laryngea superior		larynx	superior thyroid v.

COMMON NAME	NA TERM	REGION	RECEIVES BLOOD FROM	DRAINS INTO
lingual v.	v. lingualis	a deep vein, following distribution of lingual artery		internal jugular v.
lingual v., deep. *See* deep v. of tongue				
lingual vv., dorsal. *See* dorsal vv. of tongue				
lumbar vv., I and II	vv. lumbales (I et II)	accompany first and second lumbar arteries		ascending lumbar v.
lumbar vv., III and IV	vv. lumbales (III et IV)	accompany third and fourth lumbar arteries		usually, inferior vena cava
lumbar v., ascending	v. lumbalis ascendens	an ascending intercepting vein for lumbar vv. of either side; it begins in lateral sacral region and ascends to first lumbar vertebra, where by union with subcostal v. it becomes on right side the azygos v. and on left the hemiazygos v.		
maxillary vv.	vv. maxillares	usually form a single short trunk with pterygoid plexus		joins superficial temporal v. in parotid gland to form retromandibular v.
mediastinal vv.	v. mediastinales		anterior mediastinum	brachiocephalic v., azygos v. or superior vena cava
meningeal vv.	vv. meningeae	accompany meningeal arteries	dura mater (also communicate with lateral lacunae)	regional sinuses and veins
meningeal vv., middle	vv. meningeae mediae	accompany middle meningeal artery		pterygoid venous plexus
mesenteric v., inferior	v. mesenterica inferior	follows distribution of inferior mesenteric artery		splenic v.

mesenteric v., superior	v. mesenterica superior	follows distribution of superior mesenteric artery		joins splenic v. to form portal v.
metacarpal vv., dorsal	vv. metacarpeae dorsales	veins arising from union of dorsal veins of adjacent fingers and passing proximally to join in forming	dorsal venous network of hand	deep palmar venous arch
metacarpal vv., palmar	vv. metacarpeae palmares	accompany palmar metacarpal arteries		
metatarsal vv., dorsal	vv. metatarseae dorsales		arise from dorsal digital vv. of toes at clefts of toes	dorsal venous arch
metatarsal vv., plantar	vv. metatarseae plantares	deep veins of foot	arise from plantar digital veins at clefts of toes	plantar venous arch
musculophrenic vv.	vv. musculophrenicae	accompany musculophrenic artery	parts of diaphragm and wall of thorax and abdomen	internal thoracic vv.
nasal vv., external	vv. nasales externae	small ascending branches from nose	supraorbital v.	angular v., facial v.
nasofrontal v.	v. nasofrontalis			superior ophthalmic v.
oblique v. of left atrium	v. obliqua atrii sinistri	left atrium of heart		coronary sinus
obturator vv.	vv. obturatoriae	enter pelvis though obturator canal	hip joint and regional muscles	internal iliac and/or inferior epigastric v.
occipital v.	v. occipitalis	scalp; follows distribution of occipital artery		opens deep to trapezius muscle into suboccipital venous plexus, or accompanies occipital artery to end in internal jugular v.
ophthalmic v., inferior	v. ophthalmica inferior	a vein formed by confluence of muscular and ciliary tributaries, and running backward either to join superior ophthalmic vein or to open directly into cavernous sinus; it sends a communicating branch through inferior orbital fissure to join pterygoid venous plexus		

TABLE OF VEINS (Continued)

COMMON NAME	NA TERM	REGION	RECEIVES BLOOD FROM	DRAINS INTO
ophthalmic v., superior	v. ophthalmica superior	a vein beginning at medial angle of eye, where it communicates with frontal, supraorbital and angular vv.; it follows distribution of ophthalmic artery, and may be joined by inferior ophthalmic v. at superior orbital fissure before opening into cavernous sinus		
ovarian v., left	v. ovarica sinistra		pampiniform plexus of broad ligament on left	left renal v.
ovarian v., right	v. ovarica dextra		pampiniform plexus of broad ligament on right	inferior vena cava
palatine v., external	v. palatina externa		tonsils and soft palate	facial v.
palpebral vv.	vv. palpebrales	small branches from eyelids		superior ophthalmic v.
palpebral vv., inferior	vv. palpebrales inferiores		lower eyelid	facial v.
palpebral vv., superior	vv. palpebrales superiores		upper eyelid	angular v.
pancreatic vv.	vv. pancreaticae		pancreas	superior ophthalmic v.
pancreaticoduodenal vv.	vv. pancreaticoduodenales	4 veins that drain blood from pancreas and duodenum, closely following pancreaticoduodenal arteries, a superior and an inferior vein originating from an anterior and a posterior venous arcade; anterior superior v. joins right gastroepiploic v., and posterior superior v. joins portal v.; anterior and posterior inferior vv. join, sometimes as one trunk, uppermost jejunal v. or superior mesenteric v.		splenic v., superior mesenteric v.
paraumbilical vv.	vv. paraumbilicales	veins that communicate with portal v. above and descend to anterior abdominal wall to anastomose		

668

		with superior and inferior epigastric and superior vesical vv. in region of umbilicus, they form a significant part of collateral circulation of portal v. in event of hepatic obstruction	
parotid vv.	vv. parotideae		superficial temporal v.
perforating vv.	vv. perforantes	accompany perforating arteries of thigh	profunda femoris v.
pericardiac vv.	vv. pericardiaceae	pericardium	brachiocephalic, inferior thyroid and azygos vv., superior vena cava
pericardiacophrenic vv.	vv. pericardiacophrenicae	pericardium and diaphragm	left brachiocephalic v.
peroneal vv.	vv. peroneae	accompany peroneal artery	posterior tibial v.
pharyngeal vv.	vv. pharyngeae	pharyngeal plexus	internal jugular v.
phrenic vv., inferior	vv. phrenicae inferiores	accompany inferior phrenic arteries	on right, enters inferior vena cava; on left, enters left suprarenal or renal v., or inferior vena cava
phrenic vv., superior. See pericardiacophrenic vv.			
popliteal v.	v. poplitea	follows popliteal artery	formed by union of anterior and posterior tibial vv.	at adductor hiatus becomes femoral v.
portal v.	v. portae	a short, thick trunk formed by union of superior mesenteric and splenic vv. behind neck of pancreas; it ascends to right end of porta hepatis, where it divides into successively smaller branches, following branches of hepatic artery, until it forms a capillary-like system of sinusoids that permeates entire substance of liver	

TABLE OF VEINS (*Continued*)

COMMON NAME	NA TERM	REGION	RECEIVES BLOOD FROM	DRAINS INTO
posterior v. of left ventricle	v. posterior ventriculi sinistri cordis		posterior surface of left ventricle	coronary sinus
prepyloric v.	v. prepylorica	accompanies prepyloric artery, passing upward over anterior surface of junction between pylorus and duodenum		right gastric v.
profunda femoris v.	v. profunda femoris	accompanies profunda femoris artery		femoral v.
profunda linguae v.	v. profunda linguae		deep part of tongue	joins sublingual v. to form accompanying v. of hypoglossal nerve
v. of pterygoid canal	v. canalis pterygoidei	passes through pterygoid canal		pterygoid plexus
pudendal vv., external	vv. pudendae externae	follow distribution of external pudendal artery		great saphenous v.
pudendal v., internal	v. pudenda interna	follows course of internal pudendal artery		internal iliac v.
pulmonary v., inferior, left	v. pulmonalis inferior sinistra		lower lobe of left lung (from superior apical branch and common basal v.)	left atrium of heart
pulmonary v., inferior, right	v. pulmonalis inferior dextra		lower lobe of right lung (from apical branch and common, superior and inferior basal vv.)	left atrium of heart
pulmonary v., superior, left	v. pulmonalis		upper lobe of left	left atrium of heart

	superior sinistra		lung (from apicoposterior, anterior and lingular branches)	left atrium of heart
pulmonary v., superior, right	v. pulmonalis superior dextra		upper and middle lobes of right lung (from apical, anterior and posterior branches and middle lobar branch)	left atrium of heart
pyloric v. *See* gastric v., right				
radial vv.	vv. radiales	accompany radial artery		brachial vv.
ranine v. *See* profunda linguae v.				
rectal vv., inferior	vv. rectales inferiores		rectal plexus	internal pudendal v.
rectal vv., middle	vv. rectales mediae		rectal plexus	internal iliac and superior rectal vv.
rectal v., superior	v. rectalis superior	establishes connection between portal and systemic systems	upper part of rectal plexus	inferior mesenteric v.
renal vv.	vv. renales	short, thick trunks, one from either kidney, the one on the left being longer than that on the right	kidneys	inferior vena cava
retromandibular v.	v. retromandibularis	a vein formed in upper part of parotid gland behind neck of mandible by union of maxillary and superficial temporal vv.; it passes downward through the gland, communicates with facial v. and, emerging from the gland, joins with posterior auricular v. to form external jugular v.		
sacral vv., lateral	vv. sacrales laterales	follow lateral sacral arteries		help form lateral sacral plexus, empty into internal iliac v. or superior gluteal vv.

COMMON NAME	NA TERM	REGION	RECEIVES BLOOD FROM	DRAINS INTO
sacral v., middle	v. sacralis mediana	follows middle sacral artery		common iliac v.
saphenous v., accessory	v. saphena accessoria		medial and posterior superficial parts of thigh	great saphenous v.
saphenous v., great	v. saphena magna	extends from dorsum of foot to just below inguinal ligament		femoral v.
saphenous v., long. *See* saphenous v., great				
saphenous v., short. *See* saphenous v., small				
saphenous v., small	v. saphena parva	back of ankle and leg		popliteal v.
scrotal vv., anterior	vv. scrotales anteriores		anterior aspect of scrotum	external pudendal v.
scrotal vv., posterior	vv. scrotales posteriores	scrotum		vesical venous plexus
v. of septum pellucidum	v. septi pellucidi	septum pellucidum		thalamostriate v.
sigmoid vv.	vv. sigmoideae		sigmoid colon	inferior mesenteric v.
spinal vv.	vv. spinales	anastomosing networks of small veins that drain blood from spinal cord and its pia mater into internal vertebral venous plexuses		
spiral v. of modiolus	v. spiralis modioli	modiolus		labyrinthine vv.
splenic v.	v. lienalis	passes from left to right of neck of pancreas	formed by union of several branches at hilus of spleen	joins superior mesenteric v. to form portal v.
stellate vv. of kidney	venulae stellatae renis		superficial parts of renal cortex	interlobular vv. of kidney

sternocleidomastoid v.	v. sterno-cleidomastoidea	follows course of sternocleidomastoid artery		internal jugular v.
striate v.	v. striata		anterior perforated substance of brain	basal v.
stylomastoid v.	v. stylomastoidea	follows stylomastoid artery		retromandibular v.
subclavian v.	v. subclavia	follows subclavian artery	continues axillary v. as main venous channel of upper limb	joins internal jugular v. to form brachiocephalic v.
subcostal v.	v. subcostalis	accompanies subcostal artery		joins ascending lumbar v. to form azygos v. on right, hemiazygos v. on left
subcutaneous vv. of abdomen	vv. subcutaneae abdominis	superficial layers of abdominal wall		
sublingual v.	v. sublingualis	follows sublingual artery		lingual v.
submental v.	v. submentalis	follows submental artery		facial v.
supraorbital v.	v. supraorbitalis	passes down forehead lateral to supratrochlear v.		joins supratrochlear vv. to form angular v.
suprarenal v., left	v. suprarenalis sinistra		left suprarenal gland	left renal v.
suprarenal v., right	v. suprarenalis dextra		right suprarenal gland	inferior vena cava
suprascapular v.	v. suprascapularis	accompanies suprascapular artery (sometimes as 2 veins that unite)		usually into external jugular v., occasionally into subclavian v.
supratrochlear vv. (2)	vv. supra-trochleares		venous plexuses high up on forehead	join supraorbital v. to form angular v.

673

TABLE OF VEINS (Continued)

COMMON NAME	NA TERM	REGION	RECEIVES BLOOD FROM	DRAINS INTO
temporal vv., deep	vv. temporales profundae		deep portions of temporal muscle	pterygoid plexus
temporal v., middle	v. temporalis media	descends deep to fascia to zygoma	arises in substance of temporal muscle	superficial temporal v.
temporal vv., superficial	vv. temporales superficiales	veins that drain lateral part of scalp in frontal and parietal regions, the tributaries forming a single superficial temporal v. in front of ear, just above zygoma; this descending vein receives middle temporal and transverse facial vv. and, entering parotid gland, unites with maxillary v. deep to neck of mandible to form retromandibular v.		
testicular v., left	v. testicularis sinistra		left pampiniform plexus	left renal v.
testicular v., right	v. testicularis dextra		right pampiniform plexus	inferior vena cava
thalamostriate v.	v. thalamostriata		corpus striatum and thalamus	joins choroid v. to form internal cerebral v.
thoracic vv., internal	vv. thoracicae internae	2 veins formed by junction of the veins accompanying internal thoracic artery of either side; each continues along the artery to open into brachiocephalic v.		
thoracic v., lateral	v. thoracica lateralis	accompanies lateral thoracic artery		axillary v.
thoracoacromial v.	v. thoracoacromialis	follows thoracoacromial artery		subclavian v.
thoracoepigastric vv.	vv. thoracoepigastricae	long, longitudinal, superficial veins in anterolateral subcutaneous tissue of trunk		superiorly into lateral thoracic v.; inferiorly into femoral v.

674

thymic vv.	vv. thymicae		thymus
thyroid v., inferior	v. thyroidea inferior	either of 2 veins, left and right, that drain thyroid plexus into left and right brachiocephalic vv.; occasionally they may unite into a common trunk to empty, usually, into left brachiocephalic v.	left brachiocephalic v.
thyroid vv., middle	vv. thyroideae mediae		thyroid gland
thyroid v., superior	v. thyroidea superior	arises from side of upper part of thyroid gland	thyroid gland
tibial vv., anterior	vv. tibiales anteriores	accompany anterior tibial artery	internal jugular v.
tibial vv., posterior	vv. tibiales posteriores	accompany posterior tibial artery	internal jugular v., occasionally in common with facial v.
tracheal vv.	vv. tracheales		join posterior tibial vv. to form popliteal v.
tympanic vv.	vv. tympanicae	small veins from tympanic cavity that pass through petrotympanic fissure and open into the plexus around temporomandibular joint	join anterior tibial vv. to form popliteal v.
ulnar vv.	vv. ulnares	accompany ulnar artery	brachiocephalic v.
umbilical v.	v. umbilicalis	in the early embryo, either of the paired veins that carry blood from chorion to sinus venosus and heart; they later fuse and a single vessel persisting in umbilical cord carries all the blood from placenta to ductus venosus of fetus	retromandibular v.
uterine vv.	vv. uterinae		join radial vv. at elbow to form brachial vv.
vena cava, inferior	vena cava inferior	the venous trunk for the lower limbs and for pelvic and abdominal viscera; it begins at level of fifth lumbar vertebra by union of common iliac vv. and ascends on right of aorta	trachea
		uterine plexus	internal iliac vv.
			right atrium of heart

COMMON NAME	NA TERM	REGION	RECEIVES BLOOD FROM	DRAINS INTO
vena cava, superior	vena cava superior	the venous trunk draining blood from head, neck, upper limbs and thorax; it begins by union of 2 brachio-cephalic vv. and passes directly downward		right atrium of heart
vertebral v.	v. vertebralis	passes with vertebral artery through foramina transversaria of upper 6 cervical vertebrae	suboccipital venous plexus	brachiocephalic v.
vertebral v., accessory	v. vertebralis accessoria	descends with vertebral vein and emerges through foramen transversarium of seventh cervical vertebra	a plexus formed around vertebral artery by vertebral v.	brachiocephalic v.
vertebral v., anterior	v. vertebralis anterior		venous plexus around transverse processes of upper cervical vertebrae	vertebral v.
vesical vv.	vv. vesicales		vesical plexus	internal iliac v.
vestibular vv.	vv. vestibulares		vestibule of labyrinth	labyrinthine vv.
vorticose vv. (4)	vv. vorticosae	eyeball	choroid	superior and inferior ophthalmic vv.

ventr(o)- (ven'tro) word element [L.], *belly; abdomen; ventral aspect.*

ventrad (ven'trad) toward a belly, venter or ventral aspect.

ventral (ven'tral) 1. pertaining to the abdomen or to any venter. 2. directed toward or situated on the belly surface; opposite of dorsal.

ventralis (ven-tra'lis) ventral.

ventricle (ven'trĭ-kel) a small cavity or chamber, as in the brain or heart. adj., **ventric'ular. v. of Arantius,** lower end of fourth ventricle. **fifth v.,** narrow space between layers of septum lucidum. **fourth v.,** a median cavity in the hindbrain, containing cerebrospinal fluid. **v. of larynx,** space between the true and false vocal cords. **lateral v's,** cavities in the forebrain, one in each cerebral hemisphere, containing cerebrospinal fluid. **left v.,** the lower chamber of the left side of the heart, which pumps oxygenated blood out through the aorta to all the tissues of the body. **Morgagni's v.,** ventricle of the larynx. **v. of myelon,** the central canal of spinal cord. **pineal v.,** the cavity beneath or within the pineal body. **right v.,** the lower chamber of the right side of the heart, which pumps venous blood through the pulmonary trunk and arteries to the capillaries of the lung. **third v.,** a median cavity in the forebrain, containing cerebrospinal fluid. **Verga's v.,** occasional space between the callosum and fornix.

ventricornu (ven″trĭ-kor'nu) the ventral horn of gray matter in the spinal cord. adj., **ventricor'nual.**

ventriculitis (ven-trik″u-li'tis) inflammation of the cerebral ventricles.

ventriculoatriostomy (ven-trik″u-lo-a″tre-os'to-me) surgical creation of a passage permitting drainage of cerebrospinal fluid from a cerebral ventricle to the right atrium for relief of hydrocephalus.

ventriculocisternostomy (-sis″ter-nos'to-me) introduction of a catheter for drainage of cerebral spinal fluid from a lateral ventricle of the brain into the cisterna magna or cervical subarachnoid space.

ventriculocordectomy (-kor-dek'to-me) punch resection of the vocal cords.

ventriculogram (ven-trik'u-lo-gram″) a radiograph of the cerebral ventricles.

ventriculography (ven-trik″u-log'rah-fe) radiography of the cerebral ventricles after introduction of air.

ventriculomastoidostomy (ven-trik″u-lo-mas″toi-dos'to-me) surgical provision for drainage of cerebrospinal fluid from the lateral ventricle into the mastoid antrum, in treatment of hydrocephalus.

ventriculometry (ven-trik″u-lom'ĕ-tre) measurement of intracranial pressure.

ventriculomyotomy (ven-trik″u-lo-mi-ot'o-me) incision of the obstructing muscular band in subaortic stenosis.

ventriculonector (ven-trik″u-lo-nek'tor) the atrioventricular bundle.

ventriculopuncture (-pungk'chūr) puncture of a lateral ventricle of the brain.

ventriculoscopy (ven-trik″u-los'ko-pe) endoscopic examination of cerebral ventricles.

ventriculoseptopexy (ven-trik″u-lo-sep'to-pek″se) surgical correction of a defect in the interventricular septum.

ventriculoseptoplasty (-sep'to-plas″te) plastic repair of the interventricular septum of the heart.

ventriculostomy (ven-trik″u-los'to-me) creation of a communication with a cerebral ventricle for drainage of cerebrospinal fluid in hydrocephalus.

ventriculosubarachnoid (ven-trik″u-lo-sub″ah-rak'noid) pertaining to cerebral ventricles and subarachnoid space.

ventriculotomy (ven-trik″u-lot'o-me) incision of a ventricle for repair of cardiac defects.

ventriculovenostomy (ven-trik″u-lo-ve-nos'to-me) creation of a communication from a cerebral ventricle to the internal jugular vein, in hydrocephalus.

ventriculus (ven-trik'u-lus), pl. *ventric'uli* [L.] 1. a ventricle. 2. the stomach.

ventricumbent (ven″trĭ-kum'bent) prone; lying on the belly.

ventriduct (ven'trĭ-dukt) to bring or carry ventrad.

ventriflexion (ven″trĭ-flek'shun) flexion toward the ventral aspect.

ventrimeson (ven″trĭ-mes'on) the median line on the ventral surface.

ventripyramid (-pir'ah-mid) the ventral pyramid of the oblongata.

ventrofixation (ven″tro-fik-sa'shun) fixation of a viscus to the abdominal wall.

ventrohysteropexy (-his'ter-o-pek″se) ventrofixation of the uterus.

ventroscopy (ven-tros'ko-pe) illumination of the abdominal cavity for purposes of examination.

ventrose (ven'trōs) having a belly.

ventrosuspension (ven″tro-sus-pen'shun) suspension from the abdominal wall, as in fixation of the uterus.

ventrotomy (ven-trot'o-me) celiotomy.

venula (ven'u-lah), pl. *ven'ulae* [L.] one of the small vessels receiving blood from capillary plexuses and joining to form veins.

venule (ven'ūl) a small vein. adj., **ven'ular.**

Veralba (ver-al'bah) trademark for preparations of protoveratrines A and B.

veratrine (ver'ah-trĭn) a mixture of alkaloids from *Veratrum viride.*

Veratrum (ver-a'trum) a genus of plants common in North America (*V. viride*) and Europe (*V. album*), which are the source of alkaloids used widely in treatment of hypertensive disorders.

verbigeration (ver-bij″er-a'shun) abnormal repetition of meaningless words and phrases.

verbomania (ver″bo-ma'ne-ah) abnormal talkativeness.

verdigris (ver'dĭ-grēs, ver'dĭ-gris) a mixture of basic copper acetates.

verge (verj) a circumference or ring. **anal v.,** the opening of the anus on the surface of the body.

vergeture (ver'jĕ-chur) a stripe or stria, especially on the skin.

Veriloid (ver′ĭ-loid) trademark for a preparation of alkavervir.

vermicide (ver′mĭ-sīd) an agent that destroys worms.

vermicular (ver-mik′u-lar) wormlike.

vermiculation (ver-mik″u-la′shun) peristaltic motion; peristalsis.

vermiculous (ver-mik′u-lus) 1. wormlike 2. infested with worms.

vermiform (ver′mĭ-form) worm-shaped.

vermifugal (ver-mif′u-gal) expelling intestinal worms.

vermifuge (ver′mĭ-fūj) an agent that expels worms.

vermilionectomy (ver-mil″yon-ek′to-me) excision of the vermilion border of the lip.

vermin (ver′min) an external animal parasite. adj., **ver′minous.**

vermination (ver″mĭ-na′shun) infestation with vermin.

verminosis (ver″mĭ-no′sis) infestation with worms.

vermis (ver′mis) [L.] a worm, or wormlike structure. **v. cerebel′li,** the median part of the cerebellum, between the two hemispheres.

vernix (ver′niks) [L.] varnish. **v. caseo′sa,** unctuous substance covering the skin of the fetus.

verruca (vĕ-ru′kah) 1. a lesion of the skin of viral origin, commonly small, round and raised, with a rough, dry surface; a wart. 2. a wartlike growth on any surface, as on the endocardium. adj., **ver′rucose, verru′cous. v. acumina′ta,** condyloma acuminatum. **v. necrogen′ica,** a nodular lesion occurring on the hands of persons performing autopsies. **v. perua′na, v. peruvia′na,** verruga peruana. **v. pla′na,** one that is only slightly elevated, sometimes occurring in great numbers, most frequently in children (*verru′ca pla′na juveni′lis*). **v. planta′ris,** a viral epidermal tumor on the sole of the foot.

verruciform (vĕ-roo′sĭ-form) resembling a wart.

verruga (vĕ-roo′gah) wart. **v. perua′na,** a hemangioma-like tumor or nodule occurring in Carrion's disease.

version (ver′zhun) the act of turning; especially the manual turning of the fetus in delivery. **bipolar v.,** turning effected by acting upon both poles of the fetus. **Braxton Hicks v.,** a combined external and internal method of changing the position of the fetus in utero. **cephalic v.,** turning of fetus so that the head presents. **combined v.,** external and internal versions together. **external v.,** turning effected by outside manipulation. **internal v.,** turning effected by the hand or fingers inserted through the dilated cervix. **pelvic v.,** version by manipulation of the breech. **podalic v.,** conversion of a more unfavorable presentation into a footling presentation. **spontaneous v.,** one which occurs without aid from any extraneous force.

vertebro(o)- (ver′tĕ-bro) word element [L.], *vertebra; spine.*

vertebra (ver′tĕ-brah), pl., *ver′tebrae* [L.] one of the segments of the spine (vertebral

column, or backbone). adj., **ver′tebral. basilar v.,** the lowest lumbar vertebra. **cervical vertebrae,** the seven vertebrae closest to the skull, constituting the skeleton of the neck. **coccygeal vertebrae,** the three to five segments of the vertebral column most distant from the skull, which fuse to form the coccyx. **cranial v.,** one of the segments which become fused to form the bones of the skull and face. **v. denta′ta,** the second cervical vertebra, or axis. **dorsal vertebrae,** thoracic vertebrae. **false vertebrae,** those vertebrae which normally fuse with adjoining segments: the sacral and coccygeal vertebrae. **lumbar vertebrae,** the five segments of the vertebral column between the twelfth thoracic vertebra and the sacrum. **v. mag′num,** the sacrum. **odontoid v.,** the second cervical vertebra, or axis. **v. pla′na,** a condition of spondylitis in which the body of the vertebra is reduced to a sclerotic disk. **sacral vertebrae,** the segments (usually five) below the lumbar vertebrae, which normally fuse to form the sacrum. **sternal v.,** sternebra. **thoracic vertebrae,** the 12 segments of the vertebral column between the cervical and the lumbar vertebrae, giving attachment to the ribs and forming part of the posterior wall of the thorax. **true vertebrae,** those segments of the vertebral column that normally remain unfused throughout life: the cervical, thoracic and lumbar vertebrae.

vertebrarium (ver″tĕ-bra′re-um) the vertebral column.

vertebrate (ver′tĕ-brāt) 1. having a spinal column (vertebrae). 2. an animal with a vertebral column.

vertebrectomy (ver″tĕ-brek′to-me) excision of a vertebra.

vertebrochondral (ver″tĕ-bro-kon′dral) pertaining to a vertebra and a costal cartilage.

vertebrocostal (-kos′tal) pertaining to a vertebra and a rib.

vertebrosternal (-ster′nal) pertaining to a vertebra and the sternum.

vertex (ver′teks) the summit or top, especially the crown of the head.

verticalis (ver″tĭ-ka′lis) [L.] vertical.

verticillate (ver-tis′ĭ-lāt) arranged in whorls.

vertigo (ver′tĭ-go) dizziness; a sensation of rotation or movement of one's self (*subjective vertigo*) or of one's surroundings (*objective vertigo*) in any plane. adj., **vertig′inous. auditory v., aural v.,** a type of vertigo due to disorder of the inner ear. **central v.,** that due to disorder of the central nervous system. **cerebral v.,** due to some brain disease. **encephalic v.,** a sensation of movement of tissues within the skull. **epileptic v.,** attends or follows an epileptic attack. **essential v.,** without discoverable cause. **gastric v.,** associated with disease of the stomach. **hysterical v.,** associated with hysteria. **labyrinthine v.,** a form associated with disease of the labyrinth of the ear. **lithemic v.,** associated with gout and lithemia. **objective v.,** a sensation of movement of stationary objects in one's environment in relation to one's self. **ocular v.,** caused by eye diseases. **organic v.,** caused by lesion of brain or cord. **peripheral v.**, due to noncentral irritation. **positional v.**, that occurring when the head is placed in a certain position, due to disorder of the utricle (aural vertigo) or a lesion in the central nervous system, usually the brainstem (central vertigo). **special-sense v.**, aural or ocular vertigo. **subjective v.**, a sensation of movement by the patient in relation to objects in his environment. **toxemic v.**, due to some poison in the blood.

vertigraphy (ver-tig′rah-fe) body-section roentgenography.

verumontanitis (ver″u-mon″tah-ni′tis) inflammation of the verumontanum.

verumontanum (-mon-ta′num) a rounded projection on the floor of the prostatic portion of the urethra.

ves. [L.] *vesi′ca* (the bladder).

vesalianum (vĕ-sa″le-a′num) a sesamoid bone in the tendon of origin of the gastrocnemius muscle, or in the angle between the cuboid and fifth metatarsal.

vesic. [L.] *vesic′ula* (a vesicle); [L.] *vesica-to′rium* (a blister).

vesic(o)- (ves′ĭ-ko) word element [L.], *blister; bladder.*

vesica (vĕ-si′kah), pl. *vesi′cae* [L.] bladder. adj., **ves′ical. v. fel′leae**, gallbladder. **v. uri-na′ria**, urinary bladder.

vesicant (ves′ĭ-kant) 1. producing blisters. 2. an agent that produces blisters.

vesication (ves″ĭ-ka′shun) the production of blisters or the state of being blistered.

vesicle (ves′ĭ-kel) 1. a small, saclike cavity. 2. a circumscribed, elevated, fluid-containing lesion of the skin, 5 mm. or less in diameter. **air v.**, a saccule in lung tissue into which the air is drawn in breathing. **allantoic v.**, internal hollow portion of allantois. **auditory v.**, an ovoid sac formed by closure of the auditory pit in the early embryo, from which percipient parts of the ear develop. **Baer's v.**, graafian follicle. **blastodermic v.**, blastocyst. **brain v's, primary**, three expanded regions separated by two zones of relative constriction at the cephalic end of the closed neural tube in the early embryo. **cerebral v.**, embryonic expansion of neural canal whence the brain is formed. **chorionic v.**, the developing ovum at the time of its invasion of the endometrium of the uterus. **compound v.**, one which has more than one chamber. **ear v.**, auditory vesicle. **encephalic v's**, brain vesicles. **germinal v.**, the fluid-filled nucleus of an oocyte toward the end of prophase of its meiotic division. **graafian v.**, graafian follicle. **lens v.**, the primordium of the lens in the developing eye of the early embryo, formed by invagination of the lens placode. **olfactory v.**, part of cerebral vesicle whence the olfactory bulb and tract are formed. **optic v.**, a swelling on either side of the anterior of the three primary brain vesicles in the early embryo, from which the percipient parts of the eye develop. **otic v.**, auditory vesicle. **pituitary v.**, Rathke's pouch. **Purkinje's v.**, germinal vesicle. **seminal v's**, paired lobulated

structures in close apposition to the bladder in the male, opening into the deferent duct. **umbilical v.**, portion of yolk sac outside the body of the embryo.

vesicocele (ves′ĭ-ko-sēl″) hernia of bladder.

vesicocervical (ves″ĭ-ko-ser′vĭ-kal) pertaining to bladder and cervix uteri.

vesicoclysis (ves″ĭ-kok′lĭ-sis) introduction of fluid into the bladder.

vesicocolonic (ves″ĭ-ko-ko-lon′ik) pertaining to or communicating with the urinary bladder and the colon.

vesicoenteric (-en-ter′ik) vesicointestinal.

vesicointestinal (-in-tes′tĭ-nal) pertaining to or communicating with the urinary bladder and intestine.

vesicoperineal (-per″ĭ-ne′al) pertaining to or communicating with the urinary bladder and the perineum.

vesicoprostatic (-pros-tat′ik) pertaining to bladder and prostate.

vesicopubic (-pu′bik) pertaining to bladder and pubes.

vesicosigmoidostomy (-sig″moi-dos′to-me) creation of a permanent communication between the urinary bladder and the sigmoid flexure.

vesicospinal (-spi′nal) pertaining to bladder and spine.

vesicotomy (ves″ĭ-kot′o-me) incision of the bladder.

vesico-uterine (ves″ĭ-ko-u′ter-ĭn) pertaining to bladder and uterus.

vesicovaginal (-vaj′ĭ-nal) pertaining to bladder and vagina.

vesicula (vĕ-sik′u-lah), pl. *vesic′ulae* [L.] vesicle. adj., **vesic′ular.**

vesiculation (vĕ-sik″u-la′shun) formation of vesicles.

vesiculectomy (-lek′to-me) excision of a vesicle, especially the seminal vesicle.

vesiculiform (vĕ-sik′u-lĭ-form″) shaped like a vesicle.

vesiculitis (vĕ-sik″u-li′tis) inflammation of a seminal vesicle.

vesiculocavernous (vĕ-sik″u-lo-kav′er-nus) both vesicular and cavernous.

vesiculogram (vĕ-sik′u-lo-gram″) a roentgenogram of the seminal vesicles.

vesiculography (vĕ-sik″u-log′rah-fe) radiography of the seminal vesicles.

vesiculopapular (vĕ-sik″u-lo-pap′u-lar) marked by vesicles and papules.

vesiculopustular (-pus′tu-lar) marked by vesicles and pustules.

vesiculotomy (vĕ-sik″u-lot′o-me) incision into a vesicle, especially the seminal vesicles.

vesiculotympanic (vĕ-sik″u-lo-tim-pan′ik) both vesicular and tympanic.

Vesprin (ves′prin) trademark for preparations of trifluromazine.

vessel (ves′sel) 1. a channel for carrying a fluid, such as blood or lymph. 2. a receptacle used in laboratory work, of glass, porcelain or other material. **absorbent v's**, the lacteals and other lymphatic vessels. **blood v.**, one of the vessels conveying the blood. **collateral v's**, channels other than the principal ones supplying or draining an area which serve in the event of obstruction of the main vessels. **hemorrhoidal v's,** varicose veins of the rectum. **lymph v's,** channels conveying lymph. **nutrient v's,** vessels supplying nutritive elements to special tissues, as arteries entering the substance of bone or the walls of large blood vessels.

vestibule (ves'tĭ-būl) a space or cavity at the entrance to another structure. adj., **vestib'ular. v. of aorta,** small space at root of aorta. **v. of ear,** cavity at entrance to cochlea in the internal ear. **v. of mouth,** the portion of the oral cavity bounded on the one side by teeth and gingivae, or residual alveolar ridges, and on the other by the lips (*labial vestibule*) and cheeks (*buccal vestibule*). **v. of nose,** the anterior part of the nasal cavity. **v. of pharynx,** the fauces. **v. of vagina,** the space between the labia minora into which the urethra and vagina open.

vestibuloplasty (ves-tib'u-lo-plas"te) surgical modification of gingiva-mucous membrane relations in the vestibule of the mouth.

vestibulotomy (ves-tib"u-lot'o-me) incision into the vestibule of the ear.

vestibulo-urethral (ves-tib"u-lo-u-re'thral) pertaining to vestibule of vulva and urethra.

vestibulum (ves-tib'u-lum), pl. *vestib'ula* [L.] vestibule.

vestige (ves'tij) the remnant of a structure that functioned in a previous stage of species or individual development. adj., **vestig'ial.**

vestigium (ves-tij'e-um), pl. *vestig'ia* [L.] vestige.

veterinarian (vet"er-ĭ-na're-an) one who treats diseases and injuries in animals.

veterinary (vet'er-ĭ-ner"e) pertaining to animals.

V.F. visual field; vocal fremitus.

via (vi'ah), pl. *vi'ae* [L.] way; channel. **pri'mae vi'ae,** the alimentary canal. **secun'dae vi'ae,** the lacteals and blood vessels.

viability (vi"ah-bil'ĭ-te) the state or quality of being viable.

viable (vi'ah-bl) able to maintain an independent existence; able to live after birth.

Viadril (vi'ah-dril) trademark for a preparation of hydroxydione sodium.

vial (vi'al) a small bottle.

vibesate (vi'bĕ-sāt) a modified polyvinyl plastic applied topically as a spray to form an occlusive dressing for surgical wounds and other surface lesions.

vibex (vi'beks), pl. *vib'ices* [L.] a linear ecchymosis or streak of effused blood.

vibratile (vi'brah-tĭl) swaying or moving to and fro.

vibrator (vi'bra-tor) an apparatus used in vibratory treatment.

vibratory (vi'brah-tor"e) having a vibrating or to-and-fro movement.

Vibrio (vib're-o) a genus of Schizomycetes (order Pseudomonadales, suborder Pseudomonadineae, family Spirillaceae).

vibrio (vib're-o) an organism of the genus Vibrio, or other spiral motile organism. **cholera v.,** the causative agent of cholera.

vibriocidal (vib"re-o-si'dal) destructive to organisms of the genus Vibrio.

vibrissa (vi-bris'ah), pl. *vibris'sae* [L.] one of the hairs growing in the vestibule of the nose in man or about the nose (muzzle) of an animal.

vibrocardiogram (vi"bro-kar'de-o-gram") the record produced by vibrocardiography.

vibrocardiography (-kar"de-og'rah-fe) graphic recording of vibrations of the chest wall of relatively high frequency that are produced by action of the heart.

vibrotherapeutics (-ther"-ah-pu'tiks) the therapeutic use of vibrating appliances.

viburnum (vi-ber'num) a preparation of the bark of various species of Viburnum, shrubs or bushes native to the United States. **v. op'ulus,** dried bark of *Viburnum opulus*; used in treatment of functional uterine disorders. **v. prunifo'lium,** dried bark of root or stem of *Viburnum prunifolium* or *Viburnum rufidulum*; formerly used as a uterine sedative.

Vicia (vish'e-ah) a genus of herbs, including the vetch and broad bean. **V. fa'ba (V. fa'va),** a species whose beans or pollen may cause poisoning.

videognosis (vid"e-og-no'sis) diagnosis in a clinical center based on facsimiles of roentgenograms transmitted by television techniques.

vigilambulism (vij"il-am'bu-lizm) a state resembling somnambulism, but not occurring in sleep; double or multiple personality.

vigor (vig'or) strength or force; a combination of attributes of living organisms expressed in rapid growth, high fertility and fecundity, large size and long life. **hybrid v.,** that shown by certain hybrids which exceeds that of either parent.

villiferous (vil-lif'er-us) provided with villi.

villikinin (vil"ĭ-ki'nin) a hormone which activates the intestinal villi.

villitis (vĭ-li'tis) inflammation of the villous tissue of the coronet and plantar substance of the horse's foot.

villoma (vĭ-lo'mah) a villous tumor, especially of the rectum.

villose (vil'ōs) shaggy with soft hairs.

villositis (vil"o-si'tis) a bacterial disease with alterations in the villosities of the placenta.

villosity (vĭ-los'ĭ-te) 1. condition of being covered with villi. 2. a villus.

villus (vil'us), pl. *vil'li* [L.] a small vascular process or protrusion, as from the free surface of a membrane. **chorionic villi,** threadlike projections originally occurring uniformly over the external surface of the chorion. **intestinal villi,** multitudinous threadlike projections covering the surface of the mucous membrane lining the small intestine. **synovial villi,** slender projections from the surface of the synovial membrane into the cavity of a joint.

villusectomy (vil"ŭ-sek'to-me) synovectomy.

Vinactane (vin-ak'tān) trademark for a preparation of viomycin.

vinbarbital (vin-bar'bĭ-tal) a short- to intermediate-acting barbiturate. **sodium v.**, a compound used as a central nervous system depressant.

vinblastine (vin-blas′tēn) an alkaloid derived from *Vinca rosa*, used as an antineoplastic agent.

vinculum (ving′ku-lum), pl. *vin′cula* [L.] a band or bandlike structure. **vin′cula ten′dinum**, filaments which connect the phalanges with the flexor tendons.

vinegar (vin′ĕ-gar) 1. a weak and impure dilution of acetic acid. 2. a medicinal preparation of dilute acetic acid.

Vinethene (vin′ĕ-thēn) trademark for vinyl ether.

vinyl (vi′nil) the univalent group, CH_2CH, from vinyl alcohol.

viocid (vi′o-sid) methylrosaniline.

Viocin (vi′o-sin) trademark for a preparation of viomycin sulfate.

Vioform (vi′o-form) trademark for preparations of iodochlorhydroxyquin.

violet (vi′o-let) 1. the reddish-blue color produced by the shortest rays of the visible spectrum. 2. a dye which produces a reddish-blue color. **crystal v., gentian v., methyl v.**, methylrosaniline chloride.

viomycin (vi″o-mi′sin) an antibiotic substance produced by a species of Streptomyces and used in treatment of tuberculosis.

viosterol (vi-os′ter-ol) calciferol.

viral (vi′ral) pertaining to or caused by a virus.

Virales (vi-ra′lēz) an order of Microtatobiotes.

viremia (vi-re′me-ah) the presence of viruses in the blood.

viridin (vir′ĭ-din) an alkaloid of *Veratrum viride*.

virile (vir′il) characterized by virility.

virilescence (vir″i-les′ens) development of male qualities in women of advanced age.

virilism (vir′ĭ-lizm) the presence of male characteristics in women. **prosopopilary v.**, virilism with presence of hair on the face.

virility (vĭ-ril′ĭ-te) strength and sexual potency in the male.

virilization (vir″ĭ-li-za′shun) induction or development of male secondary sex characters, especially appearance of such changes in the female.

virogenetic (vi″ro-jĕ-net′ik) having a viral origin.

virology (vi-rol′o-je) the study of viruses and virus diseases.

virose (vi′rōs) having poisonous qualities.

virosis (vi-ro′sis), pl. *viro′ses*, a disease caused by a virus.

virucidal (vi″rŭ-si′dal) capable of neutralizing or destroying a virus.

virucide (vi′rŭ-sīd) an agent which neutralizes or destroys a virus.

virulence (vir′u-lens) competence of a noxious agent to produce its effect. adj., **vir′ulent.**

viruliferous (vir″u-lif′er-us) conveying a virus or infectious agent.

viruria (vi-roo′re-ah) the presence of viruses in the urine.

virus (vi′rus) a minute infectious agent which, with certain exceptions, is not resolved by the light microscope, lacks independent metab-

olism and is able to replicate only within a living host cell; the individual particle, or elementary body, consists of DNA or RNA, but not both, contained within a protein coat, which may be multilayered. **animal v's**, viruses that produce disease only in animals. **arbor v's** (*ar*thropod-*borne*), a group of viruses, including the causative agents of yellow fever, viral encephalitides and certain febrile infections such as dengue, which are transmitted to man by various mosquitoes and ticks. **attenuated v.**, one whose pathogenicity has been reduced by serial animal passage or other means. **bacterial v.**, one that is capable of producing transmissible lysis of bacteria. **CELO** (*c*hicken-*e*mbryo *l*ethal *o*rphan) **v.**, an orphan virus which is lethal for chicken embryos and induces tumors in newborn and weanling hamsters. **Coxsackie v.**, one of a heterogeneous group of enteroviruses producing in man a disease resembling poliomyelitis, but without paralysis. **ECHO** (*e*nteric *c*ytopathogenic *h*uman *o*rphan) **v.**, an orphan virus isolated from intestines of man, sometimes found in association with aseptic meningitis. **encephalomyocarditis v.**, an arbor virus which causes mild aseptic meningitis and a nonparalytic poliomyelitis-like disease. **enteric v.**, enterovirus. **v. fixé**, rabies virus of maximum virulence obtained by passage through a series of 25 to 40 rabbits. **herpes v.**, herpesvirus. **latent v., masked v.**, one which ordinarily occurs in a noninfective state and is demonstrable by indirect methods which activate it. **orphan v.**, one isolated in tissue culture, but not found specifically associated with any disease. **plant v.**, one pathogenic for plants. **street v.**, virus obtained from a natural case of rabies. **vaccine v.**, the virus of cowpox, used in inoculating against smallpox.

vis (vis), pl. *vi′res* [L.] force, energy. **v. a fron′te**, force exerted from the front, obstructing or retarding. **v. a lat′ere**, force exerted from the side, tending to support. **v. a ter′go**, force exerted from the back, pushing or propelling. **v. formati′va**, energy manifesting itself in formation of new tissue. **v. medica′trix natu′rae**, the power of recovery inherent in an organism.

viscerad (vis′er ad) toward the viscera.

visceralgia (vis″er-al′je-ah) pain in the viscera.

visceralism (vis′er-al-izm″) the opinion that the viscera are the main seats of disease.

viscero-inhibitory (vis″er-o-in-hib′ĭ-tor″e) arresting the activity of the viscera.

visceromegaly (-meg′ah-le) abnormal enlargement of the viscera.

visceromotor (-mo′tor) conveying motor stimuli to the viscera.

visceroparietal (-pah-ri′ĕ-tal) pertaining to the viscera and the abdominal wall.

visceroperitoneal (-per″ĭ-to-ne′al) pertaining to the viscera and peritoneum.

visceropleural (-ploo′ral) pertaining to the viscera and the pleura.

visceroptosis (vis″er-op-to′sis) splanchnoptosis.

viscerosensory (vis″er-o-sen′sor-e) pertaining to sensation in the viscera.

visceroskeletal (-skel′ĕ-tal) pertaining to the visceral skeleton.

viscerosomatic (-so-mat′ik) pertaining to the viscera and the body.

viscerotonia (-to′ne-ah) a group of traits characterized by general relaxation, and love of comfort, sociability and conviviality; considered typical of an endomorph.

viscerotropic (-trop′ik) having a special affinity for the abdominal viscera.

viscid (vis′id) having a glutinous consistency.

viscidity (vĭ-sid′ĭ-te) the property of being glutinous.

viscosimeter (vis″ko-sim′ĕ-ter) an apparatus used in measuring viscosity of a substance.

viscosity (vis-kos′ĭ-te) a physical property of a substance that is dependent on the friction of its component molecules as they slide by one another.

viscous (vis′kus) sticky or gummy.

viscus (vis′kus), pl. *vis′cera* [L.] any large interior organ in any of the four great body cavities, especially those in the abdomen.

vision (vizh′un) faculty of seeing; sight. adj., **vis′ual. achromatic v.,** vision characterized by lack of color vision. **binocular v.,** that resulting from simultaneous stimulation of the receptors of both eyes; termed *single binocular vision* when the resulting images are properly fused into one. **central v.,** that produced by stimulation of receptors in the macula lutea. **chromatic v.,** chromatopsia. **color v.,** perception of the different colors making up the spectrum of visible light. **daylight v.,** visual perception in the daylight or under conditions of bright illumination. **dichromatic v.,** that in which color perception is restricted to a pair of primaries, either blue and yellow or red and green. **direct v.,** central vision. **double v.,** diplopia. **finger v.,** alleged ability to recognize, as a result of stimuli received through the skin of the fingertips, qualities (such as color) ordinarily recognized by sight. **half v.,** hemianopia. **indirect v.,** peripheral vision. **monocular v.,** vision with one eye. **multiple v.,** polyopia. **night v.,** visual perception in the darkness of night or under conditions of reduced illumination. **oscillating v.,** oscillopsia. **peripheral v.,** that produced by stimulation of receptors in the retina outside the macula lutea. **solid v., stereoscopic v.,** visual perception of depth (relative distance) as well as height and width of objects. **tunnel v.,** a condition of great reduction in the visual field, as though the subject were looking through a long tunnel.

visualization (vizh″u-al-i-za′shun) the act of viewing or of achieving a complete visual impression of an object.

visuo-auditory (vizh″u-o-aw′dĭ-tor″e) pertaining to sight and hearing.

visuometer (vizh″u-om′ĕ-ter) an instrument for measuring range of vision.

visuopsychic (vizh″u-o-si′kik) pertaining to both visual and psychic processes.

visuosensory (-sen′so-re) pertaining to perception of visual impressions.

vital (vi′tal) pertaining to life; necessary to life.

vitalism (vi′tah-lizm) the theory that bodily functions are produced by a distinct principle called vital force. adj., **vitalis′tic.**

vitalist (vi′tah-list) a believer in vitalism.

vitallium (vi-tal′e-um) a cobalt-chromium alloy used for cast dentures and surgical appliances.

vitamer (vi′tah-mer) a substance or compound which has vitamin activity.

vitamin (vi′tah-min) a factor necessary for normal growth or functioning of the body; an organic substance occurring in small amounts in fresh native foods, such as plants and the flesh of animals. As a result of the effect produced by their absence in the diet, various vitamins have acquired such names as antixerophthalmic factor (A), antineuritic factor (B₁), anti-black tongue factor (nicotinic acid), antiacrodynia factor (pyridoxine), antirachitic factor (D), antisterility factor (E), antihemorrhagic factor (K), etc. Other factors, which have been found essential to the growth of microorganisms or lower animals, bear such names as citrovorum factor (essential to growth of *Leuconostoc citrovorum*) or tenebrio factor (essential to growth of the meal worm, *Tenebrio molitor*), **antihemorrhagic v.,** a substance that counteracts a hemorrhagic tendency. **antineuritic v.,** thiamine. **antipellagra v.,** nicotinic acid. **antiscorbutic v.,** ascorbic acid. **permeability v.,** a substance necessary to ensure integrity of the capillary walls.

v. A, a high-molecular weight alcohol, $C_{20}H_{29}OH$, essential for regeneration of rhodopsin when bleached by light in the visual cycle, and for integrity of epithelial cells and for new cell growth, and an aid in maintaining resistance to infections and delaying senility. Vitamin A is formed in the body from various precursors, such as the yellow pigments of vegetables and fruits.

v. A₁, the form of vitamin A found in mammals and salt-water fish.

v. A₂, an isomeric form of vitamin A found in fresh-water fish.

v. B, a name originally applied to a water-soluble substance later found to consist of various constituents essential to proper functioning of the body, including biotin, choline, folic acid, inositol, nicotinic acid, nicotinic acid amide, para-aminobenzoic acid, pantothenic acid, pyridoxine, riboflavin and thiamine, known collectively as vitamin B complex.

v. B₁, thiamine.

v. B₂, riboflavin.

v. B₃, nicotinamide.

v. B₆, pyridoxine.

v. B₁₂, a water-soluble, hematopoietic vitamin.

v. C, ascorbic acid.

v. D, a chemical compound derived from sterol, capable of enhancing absorption of calcium, regulating blood calcium, and promoting conversion of inorganic phosphorus to organic compounds in bone.

v. D₂, calciferol.

v. D₃, a highly active antirachitic compound, 7-dehydrocholesterol, produced by ultraviolet irradiation of cholesterol.

v. E, one of a group of chemically related substances originally isolated from wheat germ oil, and later produced synthetically, which were found to influence the reproductive ability in animals, leading to the name "antisterility vitamin."

v. F, a term formerly applied to various unsaturated fatty acids (linoleic acid, linolenic acid, arachidonic acid) essential to the storage of fat in the body.

v. G, riboflavin.

v. H, biotin.

v. K, a factor originally identified in green leaves, which is essential for synthesis of prothrombin and the normal clotting of blood.

v. K₁, phytonadione.

v. K₃, menadione.

v. M, folic acid.

v. P, citrin.

vitaminogenic (vi-tam″ĭ-no-jen′ik) caused by or due to a vitamin.

vitaminoid (vi-tam′ĭ-noid) resembling a vitamin.

vitaminology (vi″tah-min-ol′o-je) the study of vitamins.

vitellin (vi-tel′in) the phosphoprotein found in egg yolk.

vitellolutein (vi″tel-o-lu′te-in) yellow pigment obtainable from egg yolk.

vitellorubin (-roo′bin) reddish pigment obtainable from egg yolk.

vitellus (vi-tel′us) the yolk of egg. adj., **vitel′line.**

vitiligo (vit″ĭ-li′go) a condition due to failure of melanin formation in the skin, producing sharply demarcated, milky-white patches with hyperpigmented borders.

vitiligoidea (vit″ĭ-li-goi′de-ah) xanthoma.

vitodynamic (vi″to-di-nam′ik) pertaining to vital force.

vitreocapsulitis (vit″re-o-kap″su-li′tis) inflammation of membrane which enfolds the vitreous body.

vitreodentin (-den′tin) a dense and glasslike form of dentin.

Vitreoscilla (vit″re-os-sil′lah) a genus of Schizomycetes (order Beggiatoales, family Vitreoscillaceae).

Vitreoscillaceae (-sil-la′se-e) a family of Schizomycetes (order Beggiatoales) found in decaying organic matter.

vitreous (vit′re-us) 1. glasslike or hyaline. 2. vitreous body.

vitriol (vit′re-ol) any crystalline sulfate. **blue v.,** copper sulfate. **green v.,** ferrous sulfate. **white v.,** zinc sulfate.

vitropression (vit″ro-presh′un) exertion of pressure on the skin with a slip of glass, forcing blood from the area.

vitrum (vit′rum) [L.] glass.

vivi- (viv′e) word element [L.], *alive; life.*

vividialysis (viv″ĭ-di-al′ĭ-sis) dialysis through a living membrane.

vividiffusion (-dĭ-fu′zhun) circulation of the blood through a closed apparatus in which it is passed through a membrane for removal of substances ordinarily removed by the kidneys.

vivification (-fi-ka′shun) conversion of lifeless into living protein matter by assimilation.

viviparous (vi-vip′ah-rus) giving birth to living young which have derived nutrition directly from the maternal organism through a special organ, the placenta, which is an outgrowth of the embryo.

viviperception (viv″ĭ-per-sep′shun) the study of the vital processes of a living organism.

vivisection (-sek′shun) surgical procedures performed upon a living animal for purpose of physiologic or pathologic investigation.

vivisectionist (-sek′shun-ist) one who practices or defends vivisection.

V.M. voltmeter.

vocal (vo′kal) pertaining to the voice.

voice (vois) sound produced by vibrations of the vocal cords.

void (void) to cast out as waste matter, especially the urine.

vol. volume.

vola (vo′lah) a concave or hollow surface. **v. ma′nus,** the palm. **v. pe′dis,** the sole.

volar (vo′lar) pertaining to sole or palm.

volaris (vo-la′ris) palmar.

volatile (vol′ah-til) evaporating rapidly.

volatilization (vol″ah-til-ĭ-za′shun) conversion into a vapor.

volley (vol′e) a number of impulses of energy, as nerve impulses, transmitted in rapid succession.

volsella (vol-sel′ah) vulsella.

volt (vōlt) the unit of electromotive force; 1 ampere of current against 1 ohm of resistance. **electron v.,** the energy acquired by an electron when accelerated by a potential of 1 volt, being equivalent to 3.82 × 10⁻²⁰ calories, or 1.6 × 10⁻¹² ergs.

voltage (vōl′tij) electromotive force measured in volts.

voltaic (vōl-ta′ik) pertaining to Volta, an Italian physicist.

voltaism (vōl′tah-izm) galvanism.

voltmeter (vōlt′me-ter) instrument for measuring electromotive force in volts.

volume (vol′ūm) the measure of the quantity of a substance. **blood v.,** the total quantity of blood in the body. **circulation v.,** the amount of blood pumped through the lungs and out to all the organs of the body. **expiratory reserve v.,** the maximal amount of gas that can be expired from the end-expiratory level. **inspiratory reserve v.,** the maximal amount of gas that can be inspired from the end-inspiratory position. **minute v.,** the total flow of blood through the heart per minute, or the total volume of air breathed per minute. **packed-cell v.,** the volume of the blood corpuscles in a centrifuged sample of blood. **residual v.,** the amount of gas remaining in the lung at the end of a maximal expiration. **stroke v.**, the quantity of blood ejected from a ventricle at each beat of the heart. **tidal v.**, the amount of gas passing into and out of the lungs in each repiratory cycle.

volumetric (vol″u-met′rik) pertaining to or accompanied by measurement in volumes.

volumometer (vol″u-mom′ĕ-ter) an instrument for measuring volume or changes in volume.

volute (vo-lūt′) rolled up.

volvulosis (vol″vu-lo′sis) infestation with *Onchocerca volvulus*, producing cutaneous or subcutaneous fibrous tumors.

volvulus (vol′vu-lus) [L.] torsion of a loop of intestine, causing obstruction with or without strangulation.

vomer (vo′mer) a bone forming part of the nasal septum. adj., **vo′merine.**

vomica (vom′ĭ-kah) 1. abnormal cavity in an organ, especially in the lung, 2. profuse and sudden expectoration of pus or putrescent matter.

vomit (vom′it) 1. matter expelled from the stomach by the mouth. 2. to eject stomach contents through the mouth. **bilious v.**, vomit stained with bile. **black v.**, darkened blood cast up from the stomach in yellow fever. **coffee-ground v.**, dark granular material ejected from the stomach, produced by mixture of blood with the gastric contents, in malignant disease of the stomach.

vomiting (vom′it-ing) forcible ejection of contents of stomach through the mouth. **cyclic v.**, recurring attacks of vomiting. **dry v.**, attempts at vomiting, with the ejection of nothing but gas. **pernicious v.**, vomiting in pregnancy so severe as to threaten life. **v. of pregnancy**, vomiting occurring in the morning during the early months of pregnancy. **projectile v.**, vomiting with the material ejected with great force. **stercoraceous v.**, vomiting of fecal matter.

vomitory (vom′i-to″re) an emetic.

vomiturition (vom″ĭ-tu-rish′un) repeated ineffectual attempts to vomit; retching.

vomitus (vom′ĭ-tus) 1. vomiting. 2. matter

vomited. **v. matuti′nus**, the morning vomiting of chronic gastric catarrh.

vortex (vor′teks), pl. *vor′tices* [L.] a pattern of curving lines radiating from a common center.

vox (voks) [L.] voice. **v. choler′ica**, the peculiar suppressed voice of true cholera.

voyeurism (voi′yer-izm) a form of sexual aberration in which gratification is derived from looking at sexual objects or acts.

V.R. vocal resonance.

V.S. vibration seconds; volumetric solution.

vuerometer (vu″er-om′ĕ-ter) instrument for measuring distance between the eyes.

vulgaris (vul-ga′ris) [L.] ordinary; common.

vulnerary (vul′ner-er″e) an agent which promotes the healing of wounds.

vulnus (vul′nus), pl. *vul′nera* [L.] wound.

vulsella (vul-sel′ah) a forceps with clawlike hooks at the end of each blade.

vulva (vul′vah) the external genital organs of the female, including the labia majora and minora, clitoris and vestibule of the vagina. adj., **vul′var. v. cer′ebri**, an opening into the third ventricle of the brain, below the anterior crus of the fornix. **v. clau′sa, v. coni′vens**, a vulva with labia majora plump and closed. **fused v.**, synechia vulvae. **v. hi′ans**, a vulva with labia majora flaccid and gaping.

vulvectomy (vul-vek′to-me) excision of the vulva.

vulvismus (vul-viz′mus) vaginismus.

vulvitis (vul-vi′tis) inflammation of the vulva.

vulvocrural (vul″vo-kroo′ral) pertaining to vulva and thigh.

vulvopathy (vul-vop′ah-the) any disease of the vulva.

vulvorectal (vul″vo-rek′tal) pertaining to or communicating with the vulva and rectum.

vulvo-uterine (-u′ter-in) pertaining to vulva and uterus.

vulvovaginal (-vaj′ĭ-nal) pertaining to vulva and vagina.

vulvovaginitis (-vaj″ĭ-ni′tis) inflammation of the vulva and vagina.

vv. venae (L. pl.); veins.

v./v. volume (of solute) per volume (of solvent).

W

W chemical symbol, *tungsten (wolfram).*

W. watt; Wehnelt *(a unit of roentgen tube hardness);* weight; work.

waist (wāst) the portion of the body between the thorax and the hips.

wall (wawl) a structure bounding or limiting a space or a definitive mass of material. **cell w.**, a structure outside of and protecting the cell membrane, present in all plant cells and in many bacteria and other types of cells. **nail w.**, a fold of skin overlapping the sides and proximal end of a fingernail or toenail. **parietal w.**, somatopleure. **splanchnic w.**,

splanchnopleure. **vessel w.**, the multiple layers bounding a channel conveying blood or lymph.

ward (wōrd) a large room in a hospital, with beds for the accommodation of many patients. **isolation w.**, a special room or section of a hospital for the care of patients with infectious or communicable diseases. **probationary w.**, a ward for temporary detention of patients suspected of having a contagious disease. **psychopathic w.**, a ward in a general hospital for care of patients with mental disease.

warfarin (wōr'fer-in) a compound used as an anticoagulant. **potassium w., sodium w.,** an anticoagulant compound.

wart (wort) a small, round, usually elevated lesion on the skin, with rough, dry surface, caused by a virus; such growth may also occur on mucous membrane, near the mucocutaneous junction. **anatomic w.,** verruca necrogenica. **fig w.,** condyloma acuminatum. **fugitive w.,** one which disappears spontaneously. **moist w.,** condyloma acuminatum. **mosaic w.,** an irregularly shaped lesion on the sole of the foot, with a granular surface, formed by an aggregation of contiguous plantar warts. **necrogenic w.,** verruca necrogenica. **Peruvian w.,** verruga peruana. **plantar w.,** a wart occurring on the sole of the foot. **pointed w.,** condyloma acuminatum. **postmortem w., presector's w.,** verruca necrogenica. **soot w.,** chimneysweeps' cancer. **telangiectatic w.,** angiokeratoma. **tuberculous w.,** verruca necrogenica. **venereal w.,** condyloma acuminatum.

wash (wosh) a solution used for cleansing or bathing a part, as an eye or the mouth.

Wassermann-fast (wos'er-man-fast") showing a positive Wassermann reaction despite antisyphilitic treatment.

water (wot'er) 1. clear, colorless, odorless, tasteless liquid, H_2O. 2. an aqueous solution of a medicinal substance. 3. (plural) liquor amnii. **ammonia w.,** diluted ammonia solution. **ammonia w., stronger,** a practically saturated solution of ammonia in water. **aromatic w's,** a clear, saturated aqueous solution of a volatile oil or other aromatic or volatile substance. **chlorine w.,** a saturated solution of chlorine in water. **cinnamon w.,** a clear, saturated solution of cinnamon oil in purified water. **egg w.,** water containing fertilizin exuded from ripe eggs of sea urchins and other aquatic animals by which spermatozoa are agglutinated. **ground w.,** water lying deep to the surface of the earth, maintained at its level by a layer of impervious material. **w. for injection,** water that has been purified by distillation and contains no added substance. **w. for injection, bacteriostatic,** sterile water for injection to which one or more suitable bacteriostatic agents have been added. **w. for injection, sterile,** water for injection that has been sterilized. **lime w.,** calcium hydroxide solution. **orange flower w.,** a saturated solution of odoriferous principles of fresh flowers of *Citrus aurantium,* separated from excess volatile oil. **peppermint w.,** a clear, saturated solution of peppermint oil in purified water. **purified w.,** water obtained by either distillation or ion-exchange treatment. **rose w., stronger,** a saturated solution of odoriferous principles of fresh flowers of *Rosa centifolia,* separated from excess volatile oil.

water-borne (wot'er-born") spread or transmitted by water.

watt (wot) amount of pressure developed by 1 volt of potential with 1 ampere of current.

wattage (wot'ij) the output or consumption of an electric device expressed in watts.

wattmeter (wot'me-ter) an instrument for measuring wattage.

wave (wāv) a gradual increase and subsidence, as a progressing disturbance in the surface of a liquid, the rhythmic variation occurring in the transmission of electromagnetic energy, or the sensation of nausea. **alpha w's,** waves in the electroencephalogram having a frequency of 8 to 13 per second. **beta w's,** waves in the electroencephalogram having a frequency of 18 to 30 per second. **brain w's,** changes in electric potential of different areas of the brain. **delta w's,** waves in the electroencephalogram having a frequency of $1/2$ to 3 per second. **electrical w's,** electromagnetic radiation of wavelength between 10^6 and 10^{11} cm. and frequency of 10^4 to 10^{-1} cps. **electromagnetic w's,** electromagnetic radiation. **light w's,** a form of radiant energy causing the individual particles of the medium to vibrate perpendicularly to the direction of advance of the waves, particularly those of the wavelengths which stimulate the sensation of sight. **P w.,** a deflection in the normal electrocardiogram produced by the wave of excitation passing over the atria **radio w's,** electromagnetic radiation of wavelength between 10^{-1} and 10^6 cm. and frequency of about 10^{11} to 10^4 cps. **sound w's,** a form of radiant energy causing the individual particles of the medium to vibrate in the direction of advance of the waves, particularly those of the wavelengths which stimulate the sensation of hearing. **T w.,** the final deflection of the normal electrocardiogram, recording the potential variations associated with repolarization of the heart. **ultrashort w's,** waves of electric energy of less than 15 meters wavelength.

wavelength (wāv'length) the distance between identical phases in the advance of waves of radiant energy.

wax (waks) a plastic solid of plant or animal origin or produced synthetically. adj., **wax'y. ear w.,** cerumen. **grave w.,** adipocere. **white w.,** bleached, purified wax from the honeycomb of the bee, *Apis mellifera.* **yellow w.,** purified wax from the honeycomb of the bee, *Apis mellifera.*

waxing (wak'sing) the shaping of a wax pattern or the wax base of a trial denture into the contours desired.

W.B.C. white blood cell; white blood (cell) count.

wean (wēn) to discontinue the breast feeding of an infant, with substitution of other feeding habits.

weanling (wēn'ling) an animal newly changed from breast feeding to other forms of nourishment.

webbed (webd) connected by a membrane or strand of tissue.

weight (wāt) heaviness; downward pressure due to gravity. (See *Table of Weights and Measures,* pp. 687-694.) **atomic w.,** weight of an atom of a chemical element, compared with the weight of an atom of hydrogen taken as 1. **equivalent w.**, the weight in grams of a substance that is equivalent in a chemical reaction to 1.008 gm. of hydrogen. **molecular w.**, the weight of a molecule of a chemical compound as compared with the weight of an atom of hydrogen.

weightlessness (wāt'les-nes) absence of downward pressure due to gravity, experienced by bodies in outer space or in certain high-speed flying maneuvers.

well (wel) a container for fluid, of greater depth than cross-sectional area. **atrial w.**, a device used in open-heart surgery, being attached to the atrium to permit blood to rise within it while the surgeon explores and repairs a defect inside the heart.

wen (wen) a sebaceous cyst.

wet-nurse (wet'ners) a woman who suckles other infants than her own.

wet-scald (wet'skawld) eczema in sheep.

wheal (hwēl) a localized area of edema on the body surface, often attended with severe itching and usually evanescent.

wheeze (hwēz) a whistling respiratory sound.

whipworm (hwip'werm) *Trichuris trichiura*.

whistle (hwis'l) 1. a shrill musical breath sound. 2. an instrument for making a shrill whistling sound. **Galton's w.**, a whistle used in hearing tests.

whitlow (hwit'lo) felon.

W.H.O. World Health Organization.

whoop (hōōp) a sonorous and convulsive inspiration.

whooping cough (hōōp'ing kof) an infectious disease characterized by coryza, bronchitis and violent spasmodic cough.

whorl (hwerl) a spiral arrangement.

Willia (wil'e-ah) a genus of fungi, some of which are parasitic in man.

williasis (wil-li'ah-sis) the presence of Willia in the body.

Wilpo (wil'po) trademark for a preparation of phenyl tertiary butylamine hydrochloride.

window (win'do) a circumscribed opening in a plane surface. **aortic w.**, a transparent area below the aortic arch in the left anterior oblique radiograph of the heart and great vessels. **oval w.**, an opening in the inner wall of the middle ear, in which the base of the stapes fits. **round w.**, an opening in the inner wall of the middle ear covered by the mucous membrane lining the chamber.

windpipe (wind'pīp) the trachea.

Winstrol (win'strol) trademark for a preparation of stanozolol.

wire (wīr) a slender, elongated structure of steel or other metal. **Kirschner w.**, steel wire for applying skeletal traction in cases of fracture.

W.M.A. World Medical Association.

Wolbachia (wol-bak'e-ah) a genus of Microtatobiotes (order Rickettsiales, family Rickettsiaceae, tribe Wolbachieae).

Wolbachieae (wol"bah-ki'e-e) a tribe of Microtatobiotes (order Rickettsiales, family Rickettsiaceae).

wolfram (wool'fram) tungsten (symbol W).

womb (wōōm) uterus.

worm (werm) a small, slender, elongated, softbodied animal, often found as a parasite in man and other animals. **eye w.**, an individual of the species *Loa loa*. **flat w.**, platyhelminthes. **guinea w.**, an individual of the species *Dracunculus medinensis*. **macaco w.**, larva of a South American worm, which burrows under the skin. **medina w.**, an individual of the species *Dracunculus medinensis*. **spiny-headed w.**, **thorny-headed w.**, an individual of the phylum Acanthocephala.

wound (wōōnd) any interruption of the continuity of an external or internal surface caused by violence. **contused w.**, one made by a blunt object. **incised w.**, one caused by a cutting instrument. **lacerated w.**, one in which the tissues are torn. **open w.**, one having a free outward opening. **penetrating w.**, one reaching an important cavity of the body. **puncture w.**, one made by a pointed instrument, with a very small external opening in the skin.

W.P. working point.

W.R. Wassermann reaction.

wreath (rēth) an encircling structure, resembling a circlet of flowers or leaves such as may be worn about the head. **hippocratic w.**, the sparse peripheral rim of scalp hair which is the ultimate stage of male pattern alopecia.

wrist (rist) the region of the joint between the forearm and hand; the carpus. **drop w.**, wristdrop. **tennis w.**, tenovaginitis of the tendons of the wrist in tennis players.

wristdrop (rist'drop) paralysis of the extensor muscles of the hand and fingers, mainly due to metallic poisoning.

writing (rīt'ing) the recording of a visible impression, such as the inscription of letters and words on paper. **automatic w.**, 1. a dissociative phenomenon in which a person writes while his attention is distracted. 2. that which follows the suggestions made to a patient while he is in a hypnotic trance. **mirror w.**, the writing of letters and words in reversed form, as if seen in a mirror.

wryneck (ri'nek) torticollis.

wt. weight.

Wuchereria (voo"ker-e're-ah) a genus of nematode parasites of the superfamily Filarioidea. **W. bancrof'ti**, a species widely distributed in tropical and subtropical countries, producing important pathologic changes in the lymphatic system in human hosts.

Wuchepriasis (voo"ker-i'ah-sis) infestation with worms of the genus Wuchereria.

w./v. weight (of solute) per volume (of solvent).

Wyamine (wi'ah-min) trademark for preparations of mephentermine.

Wycillin (wi-sil'lin) trademark for a preparation of penicillin G procaine.

Wydase (wi'dās) trademark for preparations of hyaluronidase for injection.

Measures of Mass

Avoirdupois Weight

GRAINS	DRAMS	OUNCES	POUNDS	METRIC EQUIVALENTS, GRAMS
1	0.0366	0.0023	0.00014	0.0647989
27.34	1	0.0625	0.0039	1.772
437.5	16	1	0.0625	28.350
7000	256	16	1	453.5924277

Apothecaries' Weight

GRAINS	SCRUPLES (ϑ)	DRAMS ($\mathfrak{Z}$)	OUNCES ($\mathfrak{Z}$)	POUNDS(lb.)	METRIC EQUIVALENTS, GRAMS
1	0.05	0.0167	0.0021	0.00017	0.0647989
20	1	0.333	0.042	0.0035	1.296
60	3	1	0.125	0.0104	3.888
480	24	8	1	0.0833	31.103
5760	288	96	12	1	373.24177

Troy Weight

GRAINS	PENNYWEIGHTS	OUNCES	POUNDS	METRIC EQUIVALENTS, GRAMS
1	0.042	0.002	0.00017	0.0647989
24	1	0.05	0.0042	1.555
480	20	1	0.083	31.103
5760	240	12	1	373.24177

MEASURES OF MASS

METRIC WEIGHT

MICROGRAM	MILLIGRAM	CENTIGRAM	DECIGRAM	GRAM	DECAGRAM	HECTOGRAM	KILOGRAM	EQUIVALENTS	
								AVOIRDUPOIS	APOTHECARIES'
1	...	...	...	...	...	...	...		0.000015 grains
10^3	1	...	...	...	...	...	...		0.015432 grains
10^4	10	1	...	...	...	...	...		0.154323 grains
10^5	10^2	10	1	...	...	...	...		1.543235 grains
10^6	10^3	10^2	10	1	...	...	...		15.432356 grains
10^7	10^4	10^3	10^2	10	1	...	...	5.6438 dr.	7.7162 scr.
10^8	10^5	10^4	10^3	10^2	10	1	...	3.527 oz.	3.215 oz.
10^9	10^6	10^5	10^4	10^3	10^2	10	1	2.2046 lb.	2.6792 lb.
10^{12}	10^9	10^8	10^7	10^6	10^5	10^4	10^3	2204.6223 lb.	2679.2285 lb.

Measures of Capacity

Apothecaries' (Wine) Measure

MINIMS	FLUID DRAMS	FLUID OUNCES	GILLS	PINTS	QUARTS	GALLONS	CUBIC INCHES	MILLI-LITERS	CUBIC CENTIMETERS
								EQUIVALENTS	
1	0.0166	0.002	0.0005	0.00013	...	...	0.00376	0.06161	0.06161
60	1	0.125	0.0312	0.0078	0.0039	...	0.22558	3.6966	3.6967
480	8	1	0.25	0.0625	0.0312	0.0078	1.80468	29.5729	29.5737
1920	32	4	1	0.25	0.125	0.0312	7.21875	118.2915	118.2948
7680	128	16	4	1	0.5	0.125	28.875	473.167	473.179
15360	256	32	8	2	1	0.25	57.75	946.333	946.358
61440	1024	128	32	8	4	1	231	3785.332	3785.434

Tables of Weights and Measures—*Continued*

Measures of Capacity

Metric Measure

MICROLITER	MILLILITER	CENTILITER	DECILITER	LITER	DEKALITER	HECTOLITER	KILOLITER	MYRIALITER	EQUIVALENTS (APOTHECARIES' FLUID)
1	...	...	...	...	...	...	...	...	0.01623108 min.
10^3	1	...	...	...	...	...	...	...	16.23 min.
10^4	10	1	...	...	...	...	...	...	2.7 fl. dr.
10^5	10^2	10	1	...	...	...	...	...	3.38 fl. oz.
10^6	10^3	10^2	10	1	...	...	...	...	2.11 pts.
10^7	10^4	10^3	10^2	10	1	...	...	...	2.64 gal.
10^8	10^5	10^4	10^3	10^2	10	1	...	...	26.418 gal.
10^9	10^6	10^5	10^4	10^3	10^2	10	1	...	264.18 gal.
10^{10}	10^7	10^6	10^5	10^4	10^3	10^2	10	1	2641.8 gal.

1 liter = 2.113363738 pints (Apothecaries').

MICRON	MILLI-METER	CENTI-METER	DECI-METER	METER	DEKA-METER	HECTO-METER	KILO-METER	MYRIA-METER	MEGA-METER	EQUIVALENTS
1	0.001	10^{-4}	...	...	...	...	...	...	...	0.000039 inch
10^3	1	10^{-1}	...	...	...	...	...	...	...	0.03937 inch
10^4	10	1	...	...	...	...	...	...	...	0.3937 inch
10^5	10^2	10	1	...	...	...	...	...	...	3.937 inch
10^6	10^3	10^2	10	1	...	...	...	...	...	39.37 inch
10^7	10^4	10^3	10^2	10	1	...	...	...	...	10.9361 yards
10^8	10^5	10^4	10^3	10^2	10	1	...	...	...	109.3612 yards
10^9	10^6	10^5	10^4	10^3	10^2	10	1	...	...	1093.6121 yards
10^{10}	10^7	10^6	10^5	10^4	10^3	10^2	10	1	...	6.2137 miles
10^{11}	10^8	10^7	10^6	10^5	10^4	10^3	10^2	10	1	62.1370 miles

CONVERSION TABLES

AVOIRDUPOIS—METRIC WEIGHT		APOTHECARIES'—METRIC LIQUID MEASURE	
Ounces	Grams	Minims	Milliliters
1/16	1.772	1	0.06
1/8	3.544	2	0.12
1/4	7.088	3	0.19
1/2	14.175	4	0.25
1	28.350	5	0.31
2	56.699	10	0.62
3	85.049	15	0.92
4	113.398	20	1.23
5	141.748	25	1.54
6	170.097	30	1.85
7	198.447	35	2.16
8	226.796	40	2.46
9	255.146	45	2.77
10	283.495	50	3.08
11	311.845	55	3.39
12	340.194	60 (1 fl.dr.)	3.70
13	368.544		
14	396.893	Fluid drams	
15	425.243	1	3.70
16 (1 lb.)	453.59	2	7.39
		3	11.09
Pounds		4	14.79
		5	18.48
1 (16 oz.)	453.59	6	22.18
2	907.18	7	25.88
3	1360.78 (1.36 kg.)	8 (1 fl.oz.)	29.57
4	1814.37 (1.81 ")		
5	2267.96 (2.27 ")	Fluid ounces	
6	2721.55 (2.72 ")	1	29.57
7	3175.15 (3.18 ")	2	59.15
8	3628.74 (3.63 ")	3	88.72
9	4082.33 (4.08 ")	4	118.29
10	4535.92 (4.54 ")	5	147.87
		6	177.44
		7	207.01
		8	236.58
		9	266.16
		10	295.73
		11	325.30
		12	354.88
		13	384.45

METRIC—AVOIRDUPOIS WEIGHT		14	414.02
		15	443.59
GRAMS	OUNCES	16 (1 pt.)	473.17
0.001 (1 mg.)	0.000035274	32 (1 qt.)	946.33
1	0.035274	128 (1 gal.)	3785.32
1000 (1 kg.)	35.274 (2.2046 lb.)		

METRIC—APOTHECARIES' LIQUID MEASURE

MILLILITERS	MINIMS	MILLILITERS	FLUID DRAMS	MILLILITERS	FLUID OUNCES
1	16.231	5	1.35	30	1.01
2	32.5	10	2.71	40	1.35
3	48.7	15	4.06	50	1.69
4	64.9	20	5.4	500	16.91
5	81.1	25	6.76	1000 (1 L.)	33.815
		30	7.1		

CONVERSION TABLES

APOTHECARIES'—METRIC WEIGHT		METRIC—APOTHECARIES' WEIGHT	
Grains	Grams	Milligrams	Grains
1/150	0.0004	1	0.015432
1/120	0.0005	2	0.030864
1/100	0.0006	3	0.046296
1/80	0.0008	4	0.061728
1/64	0.001	5	0.077160
1/50	0.0013	6	0.092592
1/48	0.0014	7	0.108024
1/30	0.0022	8	0.123456
1/25	0.0026	9	0.138888
1/16	0 004	10	0.154320
1/12	0.005	15	0.231480
1/10	0.006	20	0.308640
1/9	0.007	25	0.385800
1/8	0.008	30	0.462960
1/7	0.009	35	0.540120
1/6	0.01	40	0.617280
1/5	0.013	45	0.694440
1/4	0.016	50	0.771600
1/3	0.02	100	1.543240
1/2	0.032		
1	0.065	Grams	
1 1/2	0.097 (0.1)	0.1	1.5432
2	0.12	0.2	3.0864
3	0.20	0.3	4.6296
4	0.24	0.4	6.1728
5	0.30	0.5	7.7160
6	0.40	0.6	9.2592
7	0.45	0.7	10.8024
8	0.50	0.8	12.3456
9	0.60	0.9	13.8888
10	0.65	1.0	15.4320
15	1.00	1.5	23.1480
20 (1ᴈ)	1.30	2.0	30.8640
30	2.00	2.5	38.5800
Scruples		3.0	46.2960
1	1.296 (1.3)	3.5	54.0120
2	2.592 (2.6)	4.0	61.728
3 (1ᴣ)	3.888 (3.9)	4.5	69.444
Drams		5.0	77.162
1	3.888	10.0	154.324
2	7.776		
3	11.664		Equivalents
4	15.552	10	2.572 drams
5	19.440	15	3.858 "
6	23.328	20	5.144 "
7	27.216	25	6.430 "
8 (1ᴣ)	31.103	30	7.716 "
Ounces		40	1.286 oz.
1	31.103	45	1.447 "
2	62.207	50	1.607 "
3	93.310	100	3.215 "
4	124.414	200	6.430 "
5	155.517	300	9.644 "
6	186.621	400	12.859 "
7	217.724	500	1.34 lb.
8	248.828	600	1.61 "
9	279.931	700	1.88 "
10	311.035	800	2.14 "
11	342.138	900	2.41 "
12 (1 lb.)	373.242	1000	2.68 "

METRIC DOSES WITH APPROXIMATE APOTHECARY EQUIVALENTS*

These *approximate* dose equivalents represent the quantities usually prescribed, under identical conditions, by physicians trained, respectively, in the metric or in the apothecary system of weights and measures. In labeling dosage forms in both the metric and the apothecary systems, if one is the approximate equivalent of the other, the approximate figure shall be enclosed in parentheses.

When prepared dosage forms such as tablets, capsules, pills, etc., are prescribed in the metric system, the pharmacist may dispense the corresponding *approximate* equivalent in the apothecary system, and vice versa, as indicated in the following table.

Caution—For the conversion of specific quantities in a prescription which requires compounding, or in converting a pharmaceutical formula from one system of weights or measures to the other, *exact* equivalents must be used.

LIQUID MEASURE		LIQUID MEASURE	
METRIC	APPROX. APOTHECARY EQUIVALENTS	METRIC	APPROX. APOTHECARY EQUIVALENTS
1000 ml.	1 quart	3 ml.	45 minims
750 ml.	1 1/2 pints	2 ml.	30 minims
500 ml.	1 pint	1 ml.	15 minims
250 ml.	8 fluid ounces	0.75 ml.	12 minims
200 ml.	7 fluid ounces	0.6 ml.	10 minims
100 ml.	3 1/2 fluid ounces	0.5 ml.	8 minims
50 ml.	1 3/4 fluid ounces	0.3 ml.	5 minims
30 ml.	1 fluid ounce	0.25 ml.	4 minims
15 ml.	4 fluid drams	0.2 ml.	3 minims
10 ml.	2 1/2 fluid drams	0.1 ml.	1 1/2 minims
8 ml.	2 fluid drams	0.06 ml.	1 minim
5 ml.	1 1/4 fluid drams	0.05 ml.	3/4 minim
4 ml.	1 fluid dram	0.03 ml.	1/2 minim

WEIGHT		WEIGHT	
METRIC	APPROX. APOTHECARY EQUIVALENTS	METRIC	APPROX. APOTHECARY EQUIVALENTS
30 Gm.	1 ounce	30 mg.	1/2 grain
15 Gm.	4 drams	25 mg.	3/8 grain
10 Gm.	2 1/2 drams	20 mg.	1/3 grain
7.5 Gm.	2 drams	15 mg.	1/4 grain
6 Gm.	90 grains	12 mg.	1/5 grain
5 Gm.	75 grains	10 mg.	1/6 grain
4 Gm.	60 grains (1 dram)	8 mg.	1/8 grain
3 Gm.	45 grains	6 mg.	1/10 grain
2 Gm.	30 grains (1/2 dram)	5 mg.	1/12 grain
1.5 Gm.	22 grains	4 mg.	1/15 grain
1 Gm.	15 grains	3 mg.	1/20 grain
0.75 Gm.	12 grains	2 mg.	1/30 grain
0.6 Gm.	10 grains	1.5 mg.	1/40 grain
0.5 Gm.	7 1/2 grains	1.2 mg.	1/50 grain
0.4 Gm.	6 grains	1 mg.	1/60 grain
0.3 Gm.	5 grains	0.8 mg.	1/80 grain
0.25 Gm.	4 grains	0.6 mg.	1/100 grain
0.2 Gm.	3 grains	0.5 mg.	1/120 grain
0.15 Gm.	2 1/2 grains	0.4 mg.	1/150 grain
0.12 Gm.	2 grains	0.3 mg.	1/200 grain
0.1 Gm.	1 1/2 grains	0.25 mg.	1/250 grain
75 mg.	1 1/4 grains	0.2 mg.	1/300 grain
60 mg.	1 grain	0.15 mg.	1/400 grain
50 mg.	3/4 grain	0.12 mg.	1/500 grain
40 mg.	2/3 grain	0.1 mg.	1/600 grain

Note—A milliliter (ml.) is the approximate equivalent of a cubic centimeter (cc.).

*Adopted by the latest Pharmacopeia, National Formulary, and New and Nonofficial Remedies, and approved by the Federal Food and Drug Administration.

X

X. symbol, *Kienböck's unit.*

xanth(o)- (zan'tho) word element [Gr.], *yellow.*

xanthate (zan'thāt) any salt of zanthic acid.

xanthein (zan'the-in) the soluble part of the yellow pigment of flowers.

xanthelasma (zan"thel-az'mah) xanthoma affecting the eyelids and characterized by soft yellow spots.

xanthelasmoidea (-az-moi'de-ah) disease of infants marked by formation of brownish wheals followed by pigmentation.

xanthematin (zan-them'ah-tin) a yellow substance derivable from hematin.

xanthemia (zan-the'me-ah) the presence of yellow coloring matter in the blood.

xanthic (zan'thik) 1. yellow. 2. pertaining to xanthine.

xanthine (zan'thēn) a compound, $C_5H_4N_4O_2$, found in most bodily tissues.

xanthinuria (zan"thin-u're-ah) excess of xanthine in the urine.

xanthochromatic (zan"tho-kro-mat'ik) yellow-colored.

xanthochromia (-kro'me-ah) yellowish discoloration of the skin or spinal fluid.

xanthochrous (zan-thok'ro-us) having a yellowish complexion.

xanthocreatinine (zan"tho-kre-at'ĭ-nēn) a poisonous yellow leukomaine, $C_5H_{10}N_4O$, from muscle tissue.

xanthocyanopsia (-si"ah-nop'se-ah) inability to perceive red or green tints, vision being limited to yellow and blue.

xanthoderma (-der'mah) yellowish discoloration of the skin.

xanthodontous (-don'tus) having yellowish teeth.

xanthoma (zan-tho'mah) a disease with formation of yellow neoplastic growths on the skin, composed of large numbers of fat-laden foam cells. **x. diabetico'rum,** skin disease associated with diabetes mellitus. **x. dissemina'tum,** xanthoma distributed throughout the body. **x. mul'tiplex,** xanthoma distributed over the whole body. **x. palpebra'rum,** xanthoma affecting the eyelids. **x. pla'num,** xanthoma in which the lesions appear as smooth plates. **x. tubero'sum,** xanthoma in which the lesions appear as nodules. **x. tubero'sum mul'tiplex,** rare disease with formation of nodules of lipoid material on the soles and palms, and extensor surfaces of the extremities.

xanthomatosis (zan"tho-mah-to'sis) an accumulation of excess lipids in the body. **x. bul'bi,** fatty degeneration of the cornea. **chronic idiopathic x.,** Hand-Schüller-Christian disease. **x. generalisa'ta os'sium,** lipid granulomatosis of bone.

Xanthomonas (zan"tho-mo'nas) a genus of Schizomycetes (order Pseudomonadales, suborder Pseudomonadineae, family Pseudomonadaceae).

xanthomyeloma (-mi"ĕ-lo'mah) xanthosarcoma.

xanthophane (zan'tho-fān) a yellow pigment from the retinal cones.

xanthophyll (zan'tho-fil) the yellow coloring matter of plants.

xanthoplasty (zan'tho-plas"te) xanthoderma.

xanthoprotein (zan"tho-pro'te-in) an orange pigment produced by heating proteins with nitric acid.

xanthopsia (zan-thop'se-ah) perversion of color vision in which objects are seen as yellow.

xanthopsin (zan-thop'sin) a compound produced by the action of light on rhodopsin.

xanthopsydracia (zan"tho-si-dra'she-ah) presence of small yellow pustules in the skin.

xanthopterin (zan-thop'ter-in) a yellow pigment from wasps, hornets and butterflies having hemopoietic activity in anemic animals.

xanthosarcoma (zan"tho-sar-ko'mah) giant cell sarcoma of tendon sheaths and aponeuroses containing xanthoma cells.

xanthosis (zan-tho'sis) yellowish discoloration. **x. cu'tis,** yellowish pigmentation of the skin, without involvement of the sclera, sometimes resulting from excessive consumption of carotene-rich foods.

Xe chemical symbol, *xenon.*

xenodiagnosis (zen"o-di"ag-no'sis) diagnosis of disease by finding causative microorganisms in laboratory-bred bugs permitted to feed on the patient.

xenogenesis (-jen'ĕ-sis) alternation of generation, or heterogenesis.

xenogenous (ze-noj'ĕ-nus) caused by a foreign body, or originating outside the organism.

xenomenia (zen"o-me'ne-ah) vicarious menstruation.

xenon (ze'non) chemical element *(see table),* at. no. 54, symbol Xe.

xenoparasite (zen"o-par'ah-sīt) an organism not usually parasitic on a particular species, but present because of a weakened condition of the individual host.

xenophobia (-fo'be-ah) morbid dread of strangers.

xenophonia (-fo'ne-ah) alteration in the quality of the voice.

xenophthalmia (zen"of-thal'me-ah) inflammation caused by a foreign body in the eye.

Xenopsylla (zen"op-sil'lah) a genus of fleas, including more than 30 species, many of which transmit disease-producing microorganisms. **X. cheo'pis,** a species that is a major vector for *Pasteurella pestis.*

xenorexia (zen"o-rek'se-ah) a perversion of appetite leading to the repeated swallowing of foreign bodies not ordinarily ingested. adj., **xenorec'tic.**

xer(o)- (ze'ro) word element [Gr.], *dry; dryness.*

xeransis (ze-ran'sis) loss of moisture. adj., **xeran'tic.**

xerasia (ze-ra'ze-ah) a disorder marked by brittleness and dryness of the hair.

xerocheilia (ze"ro-ki'le-ah) dryness of the lips.

xeroderma (ze"ro-der'mah) dryness of the skin. **x. of Kaposi, x. pigmento'sum,** a rare pigmentary and atrophic disease appearing in childhood, progressing to early development of senile changes in the skin, and ending in death.

xerography (ze-rog'rah-fe) an x-ray method of obtaining images of breast structures on selenium-coated metal plates.

xeroma (ze-ro'mah) abnormal dryness of the conjunctiva.

xeromenia (ze"ro-me'ne-ah) the appearance of constitutional symptoms at the menstrual period without any flow of blood.

xerophagia (-fa'je-ah) the eating of dry food.

xerophthalmia (ze"rof-thal'me-ah) abnormal dryness of the surface of the conjunctiva.

xeroradiography (ze"ro-ra"de-og'rah-fe) the making of radiographs by a dry, totally photoelectric process, using metal plates coated with a semiconductor.

xerosis (ze-ro'sis) abnormal dryness, as of the conjunctiva (xerophthalmia) or skin (xeroderma). adj., **xerot'ic.**

xerostomia (ze"ro-sto'me-ah) dryness of the mouth.

xerotocia (-to'se-ah) dry labor.

xerotripsis (-trip'sis) dry rubbing.

xiph(o)- (zif'o) word element [Gr.], *xiphoid process.*

xiphisternum (zif"i-ster'num) xiphoid process.

xiphocostal (zif"o-kos'tal) pertaining to xiphoid process and ribs.

xiphoid (zif'oid, zi'foid) sword-shaped.

xiphoiditis (zif"oi-di'tis) inflammation of the xiphoid process.

xiphopagus (zi-fop'ah-gus) symmetrical conjoined twins united in the region of the xiphoid process.

xylene (zi'lēn) dimethylbenzene, C_8H_{10}; used in medicine and as a solvent in microscopy.

xylenol (zi'lē-nol) any of a series of colorless crystalline substances resembling phenol.

Xylocaine (zi'lo-kān) trademark for preparations of lidocaine.

xylol (zi'lol) xylene.

xylometazoline (zi"lo-met"ah-zo'lēn) a compound used as a nasal decongestant.

xylose (zi'lōs) a sugar, $C_5H_{10}O_5$, from beechwood and jute.

xylosuria (zi"lo-su're-ah) the presence of xylose in the urine.

xysma (zis'mah) material resembling bits of membrane in stools of diarrhea.

xyster (zis'ter) a file-like instrument used in surgery.

Y

Y chemical symbol, *yttrium.*

yaw (yaw) the raspberry-like excrescence of yaws. **mother y.,** the original lesion in yaws.

yaws (yaws) a treponemal infection with a clinical picture similar to that of early syphilis, but without its serious late manifestations.

Yb chemical symbol, *ytterbium.*

yeast (yēst) a term applied to unicellular, nucleated microorganisms which reproduce by budding and to other organisms which exist usually or predominantly in similar form; some are used in production of various foodstuffs and beverages, and some are pathogenic for man. **brewer's y.,** yeast obtained as a by-product from the brewing of beer. **dried y.,** dried cells of any suitable strain of *Saccharomyces cerevisiae* or certain other fungi, used as a source of protein and of vitamins of the B complex.

yellow (yel'o) 1. the color produced by stimulation by light waves of wavelength of 571.5 to 578.5 millimicrons. 2. a dye or stain which produces a yellow color. **visual y.,** xanthopsin.

yoghurt (yo'gert) a cheeselike preparation from milk, used as a food.

yoke (yōk) a connecting structure; a depression or ridge connecting two structures.

yolk (yōk) the material of an egg or ovum which serves as food for the developing organism until it obtains nourishment in some other way.

ytterbium (i-ter'be-um) chemical element *(see table),* at. no. 70, symbol Yb.

yttrium (i'tre-um) chemical element *(see table),* at. no. 39, symbol Y.

Z

Z symbol, *atomic number.*

Zactane (zak'tān) trademark for a preparation of ethoheptazine citrate.

Zanchol (zan'kol) trademark for a preparation of florantyrone.

Zarontin (zah-ron'tin) trademark for a preparation of ethosuximide.

zea (ze'ah) the fresh styles and stigmas of *Zea mays,* Indian corn, or maize; formerly used as a diuretic.

zein (ze'in) a soft yellow protein from maize.

zeiosis (zi-o'sis) budding or blebbing activity, giving the appearance of boiling in slow motion. adj., **zeiot'ic.**

zeismus (ze-is'mus) skin disease, said to be due to excessive diet of maize.

zeoscope (ze'o-skōp) apparatus for determining the alcoholic strength of a liquid by means of its boiling point.

zeotropy (ze-ot'ro-pe) production of change in composition of a mixture of substances when it is boiled under a given pressure. adj., **zeotrop'ic.**

Zephiran (zef'ĭ-ran) trademark for preparations of benzalkonium.

zero (ze'ro) the point on a thermometer scale from which the degrees are numbered, the zero of the centigrade and Réaumur thermometers is the freezing point of water; on the Fahrenheit thermometer it is 32 degrees below the freezing point of water. **absolute z.,** the lowest possible temperature, designated as 0 on the Kelvin or Rankin scale, the equivalent of −273.15°C. or −459.67°F. **ground z.,** the ground area immediately below an exploding atomic or thermonuclear bomb. **physiologic z.,** the temperature at which a thermal stimulus ceases to cause a sensation.

zinc (zingk) chemical element (*see table*), at. no. 30, symbol Zn. **z. acetate,** a salt used as an astringent solution in ophthalmia, and an irrigation in gonorrhea. **z. carbonate,** a salt used as a dusting powder. **z. chloride,** a white or nearly white crystalline compound used in dentistry as an astringent or dentin desensitizer. **z. gelatin,** a mixture of zinc oxide, gelatin, glycerin and purified water, used topically as a protectant. **z. hydroxide,** a white powder, an ingredient of medicinal zinc peroxide. **z. oxide,** a fine, amorphous white or yellowish-white powder, used as an astringent and protectant. **z. peroxide,** a yellowish-white, odorless powder used in pharmaceuticals. **z. phenolsulfonate,** colorless prisms or crystals, or white granules or powder; antiseptic and astringent. **z. stearate,** a compound of zinc and stearic acid used as a tablet lubricant. **z. sulfate,** a compound used as an ophthalmic astringent. **z. undecylenate,** a fine white powder used topically in 20 per cent ointment as a fungistatic agent. **white z.,** zinc oxide.

zirconium (zir-ko'ne-um) chemical element (*see table*). at. no. 40, symbol Zr.

Zn chemical symbol, *zinc.*

zo(o)- word element [Gr.], *animal*

zoanthropy (zo-an'thro-pe) delusion that one has become a wild animal.

zoetic (zo-et'ik) pertaining to life.

zoetrope (zo'ĕ-trōp) stroboscope.

zona (zo'nah) pl. *zo'nae* [L.] 1. zone. 2. herpes zoster. **z. arcua'ta,** the tunnel formed by the combined arches of Corti. **z. cartilagin'ea,** limbus of spiral lamina. **z. cilia'ris,** ciliary processes taken together. **z. denticula'ta,** the inner zone of the lamina basilaris ductus cochlearis with the limbus of the osseous spiral lamina. **z. facia'lis,** herpes zoster of face. **z. fascicula'ta,** the intermediate layer of the adrenal cortex. **z. glomerulo'sa,** the outermost layer of the adrenal cortex. **z. hemorrhoida'lis,** that part of the anal canal extending from the anal valves to the anus and containing the rectal venous plexus. **z. incer'ta,** a mixture of gray and white substance between the nucleus subthalamicus and the dorsal layer of white substance of the hypothalamus. **z. ophthal'mica,** herpetic infection of the cornea. **z. orbicula'ris,** thick ring of capsular ligament around the acetabulum. **z. pectina'ta,** the outer part of the lamina basilaris ductus cochlearis running from the rods of Corti to the spiral ligament. **z. pellu'cida,** the transparent, noncellular secreted layer surrounding an ovum. **z. perfora'ta,** the inner portion of the lamina basilaris ductus cochlearis. **z. radia'ta,** a zona pellucida exhibiting conspicuous radial striations. **z. reticula'ris,** the innermost layer of the adrenal cortex. **z. stria'ta,** a zona pellucida exhibiting conspicuous striations. **z. tec'ta,** canal of Corti. **z. vasculo'sa,** a region in the supramastoid fossa containing many foramina for the passage of blood vessels.

zone (zōn) 1. a girdle or belt. 2. a restricted area. **biokinetic z.,** the range of temperatures within which the living cell carries on its life activities, lying approximately between 10 and 45°C. **comfort z.,** an environmental temperature between 13 and 21°C. (55-70°F.) with a humidity of 30 to 55 per cent. **epileptogenic z.,** a superficial area, stimulation of which provokes an epileptic seizure. **erogenous z's, erotogenic z's,** areas of the body whose stimulation produces erotic desire. **hypnogenic z., hypnogenous z.,** an area of the body, pressure on which will characteristically induce sleep. **Lissauer's z.,** the area of white substance at the tip of the posterior cornu of gray matter in the spinal cord. **root z.,** that part of the white substance of the spinal cord connected with the anterior and posterior nerve roots. **superficial z.,** the outermost of the four layers of cortical cells of the cerebrum. **transitional z.,** the posterior part of the lens sac during the stage of growth.

zonesthesia (zo"nes-the'ze-ah) a sensation of constriction, as by a girdle.

zonifugal (zo-nif'u-gal) passing outward from a zone or region.

zoning (zōn'ing) the occurrence of a stronger fixation of complement in a lesser amount of suspected serum.

zonipetal (zo-nip'ĕ-tal) passing toward a zone or region.

zonula (zōn'u-lah) pl. *zon'ulae* [L.] zonule.

zonule (zōn'ūl) a small encircling structure or zone. adj. **zon'ular. ciliary z., z. of Zinn,** a series of fibers connecting the ciliary body and lens of the eye.

zonulitis (zōn"u-li'tis) inflammation of the ciliary zonule.

zonulolysis (zon"u-lol'ĭ-sis) dissolution of the ciliary zonula by use of enzymes, to permit surgical removal of the lens.

zonulotomy (zon″u-lot′o-me) incision of the ciliary zonule.

zoo- word element [Gr.], *animal; an organism of the animal kingdom.*

zoobiology (zo″o-bi-ol′o-je) the biology of animals.

zoochemistry (-kem′is-tre) chemistry of animal tissues.

zoodermic (-der′mik) performed with the skin of an animal.

zoodetritus (-de-tri′tus) detritus produced by disintegration and decomposition of animal tissues and organisms.

zoodynamics (-di-nam′iks) animal physiology.

zoogenous (zo-oj′ĕ-nus) acquired from animals.

zoogeny (zo-oj′ĕ-ne) the production or generation of animals.

zoogeography (zo″o-je-og′rah-fe) the scientific study of the distribution of animals.

zooglea (-gle′ah) a colony of microbes embedded in a jelly-like matrix.

Zoogloea (-gle′ah) a genus of Schizomycetes (order Pseudomonadales, suborder Pseudomonadineae, family Pseudomonadaceae).

zoogony (zo-og′o-ne) the production of living young from within the body. adj., **zoog′onous.**

zoograft (zo′o-graft) a graft of tissue from an animal; a zooplastic graft.

zoography (zo-og′rah-fe) a treatise on animals.

zooid (zo′oid) resembling an animal.

zoology (zo-ol′o-je) a science of the form, nature and classification of animals.

zoonosis (zo″o-no′sis) a disease of animals that may secondarily be transmitted to man.

zoonosology (-no-sol′o-je) zoopathology.

zooparasite (-par′ah-sīt) an animal parasite.

zooparasitic (-par″ah-sit′ik) living as a parasite on an animal organism.

zoopathology (-pah-thol′o-je) the science of the diseases of animals.

zoophagous (zo-of′ah-gus) carnivorous.

zoopharmacy (zo″o-far′mah-se) veterinary pharmacy.

zoophilia (-fil′e-ah) abnormal fondness for animals.

zoophobia (-fo′be-ah) abnormal fear of animals.

zoophyte (zo′o-fīt) any plantlike animal.

zooplankton (zo″o-plangk′ton) minute animal organisms floating free in practically all natural waters.

zooplasty (zo′o-plas″te) transplantation of tissue from animal to man.

zoopsia (zo-op′se-ah) hallucination with vision of animals.

zoopsychology (zo″o-si-kol′o-je) animal psychology.

zooscopy (zo-os′ko-pe) 1. zoopsia. 2. observation of physiologic phenomena in animals.

zoosis (zo-o′sis) any disease due to animal agents.

zoosmosis (zo″os-mo′sis) passage of living protoplasm from blood vessels into the tissues.

zoospermia (zo″o-sper′me-ah) presence of live spermatozoa in ejaculated semen.

zoospore (zo′o-spōr) any spore moving by means of cilia.

zoosterol (zo-os′ter-ol) a sterol of animal origin.

zootechnics (zo″o-tek′niks) the breeding and handling of animals in domestication.

zootherapeutics (-ther″ah-pu′tiks) the treatment of diseases of animals.

zootomy (zo-ot′o-me) the dissection or anatomy of animals.

zootoxin (zo″o-tok′sin) a toxin produced by higher animals, especially snakes, scorpions and spiders, which is usually a mixture of hemotoxin and neurotoxin.

zoster (zos′ter) herpes zoster.

zosteriform (zos-ter′ĭ-form) resembling herpes zoster.

zoxazolamine (zok″sah-zol′ah-mēn) a compound used as a skeletal muscle relaxant and uricosuric agent.

Z-plasty (ze′plas-te) repair of a skin defect by the transposition of two triangular flaps.

Zr chemical symbol, *zirconium.*

zyg(o)- (zi′go) word element [Gr.], *yoked; joined; a junction.*

zygal (zi′gal) shaped like a yoke, or pertaining to a yoke-shaped structure.

zygapophysis (zi″gah-pof′ĭ-sis) the articular process of a vertebra.

zygion (zij′e-on) the most lateral point on the zygomatic arch.

zygocyte (zi′go-sīt) zygote.

zygodactyly (zi″go-dak′ti-le) union of digits by soft tissues (skin), without bony fusion of the phalanges involved.

zygoma (zi-go′mah) the process of the temporal bone that connects with the zygomatic bone. adj., **zygomat′ic.**

zygomaxillare (zi″go-mak′sī-lār″e) a craniometric point at the lower end of the zygomaticomaxillary suture.

zygon (zi′gon) the stem connecting the two branches of a zygal fissure.

zygoneure (zi′go-nūr) a nerve cell connecting other nerve cells.

zygosity (zi-gos′ĭ-te) the condition of conjugation; specifically, whether derived from one ovum or more than one (monozygotic or dizygotic), or whether having identical or unlike genes in respect to a certain character (homozygous or heterozygous).

zygote (zi′gōt) the cell produced by the union of two gametes; the fertilized ovum; by extension applied to the organism developing therefrom at any stage of its growth. adj., **zygot′ic.**

zym(o)- (zi′mo) word element [Gr.], *enzyme; fermentation.*

zymase (zi′mās) enzyme.

zymic (zi′mik) pertaining to enzymes or fermentation.

Zymobacterium (zi″mo-bak-te′re-um) a genus of Schizomycetes (order Eubacteriales, family Propionibacteriaceae), nonpathogenic, but occurring as parasites in the intestinal tract.

zymocyte (zi′mo-sīt) an organism which causes fermentation.

zymogen (zi′mo-jen) an inactive material that

may be converted into an enzyme by action of an acid, another enzyme or by other means; a proenzyme. adj., **zymogen'ic.**

zymogram (zi'mo-gram) a graphic representation of enzymatically active components of a material separated by electrophoresis.

zymoid (zi'moid) any poison from decaying tissue.

zymology (zi-mol'o-je) the sum of knowledge about fermentation. adj., **zymolog'ic.**

zymolysis (zi-mol'ĭ-sis) digestion by means of an enzyme. adj., **zymolyt'ic.**

zymome (zi'mōm) an enzyme.

zymometer (zi-mom'ĕ-ter) instrument for measuring degree of fermentation.

Zymomonas (zi"mo-mo'nas) a genus of Schizomycetes (order Pseudomonadales, suborder Pseudomonadineae, family Pseudomonadaceae) found in fermenting beverages.

Zymonema (-ne'mah) a genus of yeast fungus.

zymonematosis (-ne"mah-to'sis) infestation with Zymonema.

zymophore (zi'mo-fōr) the group of atoms in a molecule of an enzyme that is responsible for its effect. adj., **zymoph'orous.**

zymophyte (zi'mo-fīt) a bacterium causing fermentation.

zymoplastic (zi'mo-plas"tik) forming ferment.

zymoprotein (zi"mo-pro'te-in) a protein having catalytic powers.

zymosan (zi'mo-san) a mixture of lipids, polysaccharides, proteins and ash, derived from the cell walls or the entire cell of yeast.

zymoscope (zi'mo-skōp) an apparatus for determining the fermenting power of yeast.

zymose (zi'mōs) invertin.

zymosimeter (zi"mo-sim'ĕ-ter) zymometer.

zymosis (zi-mo'sis) 1. fermentation. 2. the development of any zymotic disease. 3. any infectious or contagious disease. adj., **zymot'ic. z. gas'trica,** the presence of an organic acid in the stomach.

zymosterol (zi-mos'ter-ol) a sterol occurring in fungi and molds.

zymurgy (zi'mer-je) the science of the industrial use of enzymes.